HANDBOOK OF
CLINICAL AUDIOLOGY

SECOND EDITION

HANDBOOK OF
CLINICAL
AUDIOLOGY

second edition

Edited by

Jack Katz, Ph.D.

Professor, Department of Communicative Disorders and Sciences
State University of New York
Buffalo, New York

Editorial Assistant: WILMA LAUFER GABBAY, M.S.

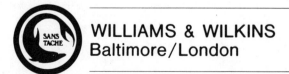

WILLIAMS & WILKINS
Baltimore/London

Made in the United States of America

Reprinted 1979
Reprinted 1981

Library of Congress Cataloging in Publication Data

Katz, Jack.
    Handbook of clinical audiology.

    Includes bibliographies and index.
    1. Hearing disorders. 2. Audiology. I. Title.[DNLM: 1. Hearing disorders.
WV270 H2371]
RF290.K38 1978   617.8′9   77-23902
ISBN 0-683-04550-4

Composed and printed at the
Waverly Press, Inc.
Mt. Royal and Guilford Aves.
Baltimore, Md. 21202, U.S.A.

Dedication

This book is dedicated to:

Robert W. West
Louis M. Di Carlo
Aubrey Epstein

because of their high ideals and capabilities, and their significant contributions to my own education and to the field.

J.K.

Preface

SINCE 1972, students, audiologists, and other professionals have used the *Handbook of Clinical Audiology*. Although the original edition was well received, the many new developments in the field make it desirable to have a second edition.

As in the first edition we have attempted, "to provide between one set of covers a summary of the current state of the science-art of clinical audiology." In order to maintain an up-to-date view of the field it has been necessary to revise and delete previous materials and add new information.

Audiology has grown in scope and depth in the past several years. The six-year period between the planning of the first and second editions led to a 16% increase in the number of chapters (from 41 to 49). Twenty-two chapters (45%) are completely new and the 27 chapters remaining from the first edition have been modified in varying degrees. About half of the 43 contributors to the new edition contributed to the previous one.

The second edition of the *Handbook* required even more help from more people than the first edition. I am indebted to Norma Hopkinson, Bill Hodgson, Derek Sanders and Tom White for their guidance. Wilma Gabbay meticulously proofread the entire manuscript in its various stages and gave invaluable suggestions. I am grateful to Ruby Richardson at The Williams & Wilkins Co. who has given me advice and support over the past several years. My wife, Irma, helped a great deal in various phases of the book and especially with compiling the massive index.

The following students, former students and secretaries aided me in getting out what seemed like a million manuscripts, letters and forms: Walter Appling, Carmel Basile, Regina Bryde, Sherry Gottlieb, Margaret Kovel, Steve Perlow, Kim Reinson, Linda Ronis, Peggy Ross and Andrea Segmond. To the above and any others whom I may have inadvertently omitted, my sincere thanks.

The acronym for the *Handbook of Clinical Audiology*, "HOCA," is quite interesting. In Turkish *hoca* (pronounced /hodʒə/) means a clergyman, a revered teacher or a schoolmaster. From some of the very nice comments that I have received on the first edition, it seems that the acronym is well suited. I hope that the second edition will be as valuable, or more so, than the first.

J. K.

List of Contributors

CHARLES V. ANDERSON, PH.D., Associate Professor, Departments of Otolaryngology and Speech Pathology and Audiology, University of Iowa, Iowa City, IA 52242 (Chapter 5).

JOAN M. BILLGER, M.A., Instructor and Coordinator of Pediatric Audiology, Department of Communication Disorders, Colorado State University, Fort Collins, CO 80523 (Chapter 34).

ROBERT J. BRISKEY, M.A., Advisor on Professional Affairs, Administrative Division, Beltone Electronics Corporation, 4201 West Victoria Street, Chicago, IL 60646 (Chapter 41).

MICHAEL BRUNT, PH.D., Associate Professor, Department of Speech Pathology and Audiology, Illinois State University, Normal, IL 61761 (Chapter 23).

WILLIAM F. CARVER, PH.D., Director, Division of Audiology, Department of Otolaryngology, Washington University School of Medicine, 517 South Euclid Avenue, St. Louis, MO 63110 (Chapters 15 and 39).

DONALD D. DIRKS, PH.D., Professor, Division of Head and Neck Surgery, Audiology Research, University of California at Los Angeles, 1000 Veteran Avenue, 32–34 Rehabilitation Center, Los Angeles, CA 90025 (Chapter 10).

TIMOTHY N. DOYLE, PH.D., Chief of Audiology, Veterans Administration Hospital, Minneapolis, MN 55417 and Assistant Professor, Department of Communication Disorders, University of Minnesota, Minneapolis, MN and Assistant Professor, Department of Otolaryngology, University of Minnesota, Minneapolis, MN (Chapter 4).

CAROL H. EHRLICH, PH.D., Director, Audiology and Speech Pathology Department, The Children's Hospital, 1056 East 19th Avenue, Denver, CO 80218 (Chapter 32).

ALAN S. FELDMAN, PH.D., Professor/Director, SUNY Upstate Medical Center/Communication Disorder Unit, 766 Irving Avenue, Syracuse, NY 13210 (Chapter 30).

IRWIN A. GINSBERG, M.D., Clinical Professor of Otolaryngology, School of Medicine, State University of New York at Buffalo; Chief, Section of Otology, Buffalo General Hospital; Chief of Otology, Buffalo Otological Group, 897 Delaware Avenue, Buffalo, New York 14209 (Chapter 2).

THEODORE J. GLATTKE, PH.D., Associate Professor, Department of Speech and Hearing Sciences, The University of Arizona, Tucson, AZ 85721 (Chapters 28 and 31).

CORNELIUS P. GOETZINGER, PH.D., Professor of Audiology and Director of Audio-ENG Clinic, Department of Otorhinolaryngology, Room 312, Sudler Hall, University of Kansas Medical Center College of Health Sciences and Hospital, Rainbow at 39th Streets, Kansas City, KS 66103 and Consultant Psychologist, Kansas School for Deaf, Olathe, KS (Chapters 13 and 37).

DAVID S. GREEN, PH.D., Director of Audiology, Communication Disorders Department, Southern Connecticut State College, 501 Crescent Street, New Haven, CT 06515 (Chapters 9 and 17).

ALISON M. GRIMES, M.A., Clinical Audiologist, San Francisco Hearing and Speech Center, San Francisco, CA 94115 (formerly: Research Assistant, Audiology Division, Department of Otolaryngology, University of Colorado Medical Center, 4200 East 9th Avenue, Denver, CO) (Chapter 29).

WILLIAM R. HODGSON, PH.D., Professor, Department of Speech and Hearing Sciences, University of Arizona, Tucson, AZ 85721 (Chapters 33 and 44).

JAMES E. HOFFMAN, M.D., Associate Professor, Head of Clinical Sciences, University of Minnesota (Duluth) School of Medicine, Duluth, MN 55812 (Chapter 4).

NORMA T. HOPKINSON, PH.D., Clinical Associate Professor, Department of Otolaryngology, University of Pittsburgh, School of Medicine and Eye and Ear Hospital, E321 Eye and Ear Hospital, 230 Lothrop Street, Pittsburgh, PA 15213 (Chapters 12 and 25).

* RICHARD L. HUGHES, PH.D., (formerly) Audiologist, Consultant in Audiology, Otologic Medical Group, Los Angeles Foundation of Otology, 2122 West 3rd Street, Los Angeles, CA 90057 (Chapter 18).

RAYMOND H. HULL, PH.D., Chairperson, Department of Communication Disorders, Director of Audiology, School of Special Education and Rehabilitation, University of Northern Colorado, Greeley, CO 80639 (Chapters 35 and 49).

E. W. JOHNSON, PH.D., Director, Clinical Audiology, Otologic Medical Group, Inc., 2122 West 3rd Street, Los Angeles, CA 90057 (Chapter 18).

ROGER N. KASTEN, PH.D., Professor of Audiology, Department of Logopedics, Wichita State University, Wichita, KS 67208 (Chapter 40).

JACK KATZ, PH.D., Professor, Department of Communicative Disorders and Sciences, State University of New York at

* Deceased.

Buffalo, 4226 Ridge Lea Road, Buffalo, NY 14226 (Chapters 1, 3 and 20).

VINCENT H. KNAUF, PH.D., Audiologist and Speech Pathologist, Ear, Nose and Throat Clinic, 129 West Sixth Street, Reno, NV 89503 (Chapter 45).

ALBERT W. KNOX, PH.D., Chief, Audiology and Speech Pathology Service, Veterans Administration Hospital, 4801 Linwood, Kansas City, MO 64128 and Professor of Audiology and Speech Pathology, Kansas University, Kansas City, MO (Chapter 26).

SAMUEL F. LYBARGER, B.S. (Physics), Acoustical Consultant, 101 Oakwood Road, McMurray, PA 15317 (Chapter 42).

FREDERICK N. MARTIN, PH.D., Professor, Department of Speech Communication, University of Texas, Austin, TX 78712 (Chapters 16 and 24).

WILLIAM MELNICK, PH.D., Associate Professor, Department of Otolaryngology, The Ohio State University, University Hospital Clinic, 456 Clinic Drive, Columbus, OH 43210 (Chapter 6).

JERRY L. NORTHERN, PH.D., Associate Professor, Otolaryngology/Pediatrics and Head, Audiology Division, University of Colorado Medical Center, 4200 East 9th Avenue, Denver, CO 80262 (Chapter 29).

MICHAEL RODEL, M.A.T., Instructor and Coordinator of Audiologic Rehabilitation, Department of Communication Disorders, Colorado State University, Fort Collins, CO 80523 (Chapter 47).

PHILIP E. ROSENBERG, PH.D., Professor of Audiology, Department of Otorhinology, Temple University, School of Medicine, 3400 North Broad Street, Philadelphia, PA 19140 and Professor of Speech and Audiology, Department of Speech, Temple University, Weiss Hall, Philadelphia, PA (Chapters 7 and 14).

MARK ROSS, PH.D., Professor, Department of Speech, University of Connecticut, Storrs, CT 06268 (Chapters 38 and 43).

JAY W. SANDERS, PH.D., Professor of Audiology, Division of Hearing and Speech Sciences, Vanderbilt University, Nashville, TN 37232 (Chapter 11)

DONALD G. SIMS, PH.D., Research Associate, Department of Audiology, National Technical Institute for the Deaf, 1 Lomb Drive, Rochester, NY 14623 (Chapter 46).

PAUL SKINNER, PH.D., Chairman, Department of Speech and Hearing Sciences, University of Arizona, Speech Building, Room 104, Tucson, AZ 85721 (Chapter 27).

WALTER J. SMOSKI, M.S., Instructor, Departments of Speech Pathology and Audiology, Illinois State University, Normal, IL 61761 (Chapter 36).

JAMES H. STEVENS, PH.D., Administrative Manager, Department of Otoneurologic Services, Bishop Clarkson Memorial Hospital, Dewey Avenue at 44th, P.O. Box 3328, Omaha, NB 68103 (Chapter 21).

J. CURTIS TANNAHILL, PH.D., Director, Eckelmann-Taylor Speech and Hearing Clinic, Department of Speech Pathology and Audiology, Illinois State University, Normal, IL 61761 (Chapter 36).

LEON WEISBERG, M.D., Assistant Professor of Neurology, Department of Psychiatry, Tulane University School of Medicine, 1430 Tulane Avenue, New Orleans, LA 70112 (Chapter 3).

THOMAS P. WHITE, M.A., Assistant Professor of Audiology, Department of Communicative Disorders and Sciences, State University of New York at Buffalo; Chief of Audiology, Buffalo Otological Group, 897 Delaware Avenue, Buffalo, New York 14209 (Chapter 2).

LAURA ANN WILBER, PH.D., Professor and Director of Hearing Clinics, Audiology Program, Department of Communication Disorders, Northwestern University, Frances Searle Building, 2299 Sheridan Road, Evanston, IL 60201 (Chapter 8).

JACK A. WILLEFORD, PH.D., Professor and Director, Division of Audiology, Department of Communication Disorders, Colorado State University, Center and Pitkin Streets, Fort Collins, CO 80523 (Chapters 22 and 34).

H. N. WRIGHT, PH.D., Associate Professor, Department of Otolaryngology and Communication Sciences, State University of New York, Upstate Medical Center, 750 East Adams, Syracuse, NY 13210 (Chapter 19).

VERNA V. YATER, PH.D., Program Specialist, Santa Barbara County Schools, 4400 Cathedral Oaks Road, Santa Barbara, CA 93110 (Chapter 48).

Contents

---

* Deceased.

SECTION 8

EVALUATION OF YOUNG CHILDREN AND THE ELDERLY

SECTION 9

INTRODUCTION TO THE MANAGEMENT OF THE HEARING IMPAIRED

SECTION 10

HEARING AIDS

SECTION 11

COMMUNICATION TRAINING

Nature of Problem

chapter 1

CLINICAL AUDIOLOGY

Jack Katz, Ph.D.

In the six years between the planning of the first and second editions of the *Handbook of Clinical Audiology,* many changes have taken place in this field and in the world around it. The variations in clinical audiology reflect both internal and external dynamics.

One of the external influences on the field has been a great social change. This includes the status of women, the acceptance of individual differences and an increased awareness of the need for accuracy in interpersonal communication. Vast political change has taken place, including the demand for accountability in government and the desire of citizens to make institutions more responsive to the constituents' needs. The economic change has been no less drastic causing people at every level to take stock and make adjustments.

In recent years the number of audiologists has increased, the sex distribution in the field has been altered, the variety of work settings has been increased and there is a greater average income (Fricke, 1972; Curlee, 1975). At the same time the methods used by audiologists have undergone modification. Some newer procedures have come to the fore gradually or sometimes precipitously in a relatively short space of time. Other methods have lessened in popularity. There is a trend toward more extensive testing, both in scope and in depth.

In the second edition of the *Handbook,* we have attempted to retain the vital and current features of the first edition, weed out the obsolete, update the references, and present the recent information and approaches. New information has been added to the appropriate chapters and in some cases entirely new chapters seemed warranted. While the main purpose of this book is to provide a picture of the current state of the science-art of clinical audiology, background information is also presented as well as thorough bibliographies in various areas of study. We have included published and unpublished research findings, a wealth of clinical insights and a touch of humor.

As in the first edition the contributors represent an outstanding group of audiologists and related professionals. These individuals are actively involved in the work which they discuss. This helps make the chapters more vital and applicable.

AUDIOLOGY A PROFESSION

In recent years clinical audiology has developed and grown as a profession. One measure of growth is the sheer numbers of individuals who are trained and working in the field.

Between 1969 (the year the first edition was being planned) and 1975 (the year the second edition was being planned) the number of American Speech and Hearing Association (ASHA) members with the Certificate of Clinical Competence in Audiology (CCC-A) more than doubled. In 1969 there were about 1500 certified audiologists compared to over 3000 CCC-A members in 1975. Judging from the enrolment figures in graduate training programs the number of students choosing audiology continues to increase.

At the same time new positions have been opening up in both traditional audiology settings and in new areas. Clinical audiology services are being added or expanded across the country in community and university clinics, elementary and secondary schools, hospitals, industry, hearing aid work and in private practices.

It is interesting, according to the records of ASHA, that one-third of all CCC audiologists work for a college or university; another one-third work in community clinics or hospitals, almost 15% in elementary and secondary schools and another 15% in other work settings.

A full one-half of CCC audiologists have direct clinical work as their major activity. The next largest group is involved primarily in college or university teaching (19%), followed by administration (10%) and clinical supervision (7%). Three percent are primarily in research and about 8% of audiologists work in various other types of activities. About 4% were not employed for any of various reasons.

Audiology has become quite specialized over the years. The breadth of this *Handbook* underscores the wide scope of audiologic activities. Some newer areas of audiology were unknown 5 to 10 years ago. Such terms as educational audiology, geriatric audiology, hearing aid audiology, neuro-audiology, and industrial audiology did not appear in the first edition of the *Handbook*. Electrophysiologic work, acoustic impedance, and services to the learning disabled child have shown marked increases in the past few years.

One of the important professional developments has been the growth of private practices in audiology. Well trained audiologists in increasing numbers are providing direct services to the public in either individual or group practice settings. Group practices involve two or more audiologists, or an audiologist might associate himself with other related professionals. By the middle of 1974 over 30% of all CCC-As had full or part-time private practices. Six percent of all audiologists were in full-time private practices.

Private practice is probably the most professional setting in which an audiologist can ply his skill. It offers (1) a high level of rapport between the patient and the clinician, (2) a maximum degree of freedom and job satisfaction, and (3) the potential for greater financial remuneration. The more audiologists who are involved in the private practice option, the stronger the footing and the taller the standing of our entire profession.

An interesting change has taken place in the last few years. Monetary gain was almost an unmentionable topic and the word *money* was rather taboo. This no doubt sprung up because speech pathologists and audiologists thought of themselves in the most altruistic terms without "contamination by material impulses." This followed the model of the social worker and nurse who for many years were overtrained, underpaid and underregarded (aside from being underutilized).

In the past, more so than presently, institutions and referral sources were willing to receive less than the full impact of the audiologist. From the point of view of service to the public and the economic advantage of getting the full value for every salary dollar, it behooves the parent institution to take full advantage of what the audiologist knows and can do.

Fortunately, audiology has matured to the point where gainful and rightful profit is clearly differentiated from unscrupulous preying on the misfortunes of others. Money is not a dirty word. Rather it is a strong motivation and without it no program can exist. While greed in our society has in some cases reached unconscionable limits, the audiologist must be adamant to receive appropriate compensation.

Hand in hand with the growth in stature of audiology has come an increasing responsibility and influence. In the past, the reputations of audiologists generally rose and fell with the institution of which they were a part. Institutions do have a profound influence on one's professional activities; however, now a fine clinician can often rise above a weak institution.

The greater independence of action and communication that audiologists have earned make them more in control of their own destiny. The audiologist plans, evaluates, reports, rehabilitates, counsels and consults, thereby quickly demonstrating what he can and cannot do. The weak audiologist, as a distinct professional entity, is able to float along only for a short while on the good reputation of his employer.

Social Influences

It is difficult to separate social influences from political and economic influences. Certainly, each aspect conditions the others. In recent years there has been a greater trend toward the study of social sciences and people-oriented vocations. This has influenced many bright people who are willing to serve others to enter audiology in increasing numbers. Thus, universities and colleges can be more selective in their choice of students. It would be folly to train all students who wish to enter the field since there must be a balance between supply and demand. Because of the need for reasonable limits we are in an enviable position to admit the most capable and best suited student to the study of audiology. This selection process will continue to have a beneficial effect on the practice of audiology.

Another influence on the field which we might term primarily social is the changing role and attitude of women in our society. No longer are the technical and scientific areas considered exclusively male oriented activities, nor nurturing and giving fields female oriented. Audiology is typically thought of as a technical-scientific field (but has important nurturing-giving aspects as well) and yet reflects a healthy balance between men and women. As of 1974, a full 50% of all CCC-As were women. This represents a distinctive change from a highly male represented field of 10 years ago.

Political, Legal and Economic Influences

There have been a considerable number of changes in the political, legal and economic sectors which have had an effect on the practice of audiology. For example, there are both legal and moral reasons why a patient or family has "the right to know." At one time, professionals (including audiologists) felt free to withhold information, reports or audiograms from the very people who sought out or paid for the services for themselves or family members. The information might then be sent to a professional person (frequently without interest or background). These professionals would be expected to digest the report and explain and counsel the patient appropriately. Needless to say, this was not a practical approach.

With all of its attendant difficulties and complications, it is the current feeling that the patient has the right to know what is wrong and to be given to understand to the best of his knowledge what was found and what needs to be done. Therefore, it is appropriate to permit a patient to have a current audiogram or to have the information explained to him. The audiologist is the person most qualified to do this, except in certain special or complex cases.

The growing influence of government into health and education has an increasing influence on audiology. By their funding regulations the federal and state governments could strengthen or weaken an entire profession. Medicare could strengthen the position of audiology by stating that a licensed audiologist (or one who holds CCC-A or equivalent) must evaluate the patient in order that the service be covered by insurance. It would also encourage an employer and worker who is less well trained to pursue a higher level of attainment.

If an agency indicates that a problem of hearing is determined solely by an unspecified physician, the functions of audiology (and no doubt otology) are undermined. This might encourage some general practitioners, dermatologists or gynecologists to think that they had the needed skills for evaluating hearing. I recall such a case when a general practitioner in the community wanted to use the audiometers and test chamber in a hospital to evaluate a patient with a suspected disorder. He did not even have the most meager of credentials in audiology and was of course denied permission.

In the interest of better patient care it is necessary to establish guidelines for the qualifications required for evaluating and rehabilitating hearing. In this regard many states have enacted legislation to define and license audiologists. In most cases this has served to protect the public by putting the evaluation of hearing in the hands of the audiologist (while not excluding the physician and surgeon who we hope will show reasonable restraint).

Because of the growing outside influence upon health and educational services, audiologists and speech pathologists have become more vocal in influencing legislation and regulations. Some of the current concerns involve licensure, national health insurance (Klar, 1975), and Professional Standards Review Organizations (PSROs). PSROs permit a peer review of services provided to the public. It seems reasonable that each health team member should be evaluated on the basis of his own performance by individuals in his own profession rather than to have to satisfy those who lack in depth and current knowledge of the field (American Speech and Hearing Association, 1975).

Related to PSROs is the entire question of *accountability*. There are many conflicting interests which influence audiology. Patients, the judicial system, referral sources and professional organizations are demanding high quality services. They also expect that new and valid procedures will be added as needed. At the same time the patient, insurance companies and others insist that the cost be held to a minimum and only costs related to the standard acceptable services can be charged. That is, no funds should be expended for fringe activities like research.

From these somewhat conflicting guidelines, the audiologist must establish a reasonably up-to-date program with costs that are not excessive. In order to account for his charges, the audiologist must decide on what basis a charge will be made (American Speech and Hearing Association, 1971). Is it the time spent by the audiologist that is the crucial commodity in establishing a fee or is it the test or service rendered (training the audiologist, buying the specific equipment, supplies used and time)? If most of the services require comparable equipment, supplies and personnel it is simplest to use time as the unit for charging fees.

Specialization in Audiology

One measure of development and sophistication in a field is the level of specialization. A number of years ago audiologists were content to limit their hearing evaluation procedures to air- and bone-conduction threshold tests. It is easy to see why the referral source would ask to see the audiogram without audiologic interpretation. With a little training many people were able to interpret "the audiogram" practically as well as the audiologist.

With increased knowledge and technical advances audiology has become highly specialized. It is safe to say that only the rarest of audiologists could read the *Handbook* from cover to cover with relaxed familiarity. Thus, we no longer hear from our physician colleagues that they know as much about audiology as the audiologist. Reading an audiogram provides only the grossest form of audiological analysis. The audiologist who spends his entire professional life studying cannot feel content that he ever knows enough about his area of specialization.

Clinical audiology can be divided (albeit not too neatly) into two main branches, diagnostic and rehabilitative audiology. The former deals primarily with evaluation, particularly site of lesion testing, and the latter with the management of the hearing impaired person. One can further subdivide the two branches into those audiologists dealing mostly with children and those who work with adults. Other subgroups cluster around the work setting (e.g., private practice or V.A. Hospitals).

There are already a number of offshoots from the two main branches of clinical audiology. Some of these areas have a recognized label (e.g., educational audiology) or in some cases they are unnamed but are evolving divisions of labor (e.g., electrophysiological measurement).

Educational audiology has come into existence along with the impetus to get the hearing impaired or any handicapped children integrated into the general school population. This effort at mainstreaming has required an educationally oriented breed of audiologist to help the child into the regular classroom. This includes screening programs, testing, hearing aid work, visual and auditory training, and counseling. As more schools realize the availability of such professionals they have been quick to make a place for them.

Unlike the audiologists of old, we now have more objective measurements which tap physiological function. This trend started rather meekly with raw data obtained from changes in skin resistance (EDA) and progressed to the present work with computer assisted bioelectrical potentials measured at the vertex of the skull (ERA) including brain stem evoked responses (BSER), or at the round window (ECoG). During the years between the first and second editions of the *Handbook,* acoustic impedance measurement became a rather standard test in most clinics. Its influence on the entire field is reflected in many chapters in the *Handbook.*

In the past several years there has been a growth of clinical interest in the patient with central auditory disturbances. This represents an extension of the site of lesion testing. Neuroaudiology refers to the study of the central auditory nervous system. The central auditory system is within the province of the neurologist and neurosurgeon. One reason for this term is to replace the current misnomer oto-neurology or neuro-otology when they are used to refer to audiologic procedures. The neuro-audiologist (or the audiologist using neuro-audiologic techniques) is able to contribute site of lesion information about the brain stem and brain. This aspect of audiology is growing rapidly as neurologists and other physicians realize the investigative potential of audiology deep into the skull, without potential danger to the patient.

Professionally trained audiologists have entered into the area of dispensing hearing aids. While audiologists have been involved with various aspects of hearing aid selection, modification and dispensing as long as the field of audiology existed, there has been a recent spurt of private and institutional dispensing. This is due to the advances and the increasingly technical nature of the work in ear mold acoustics, and measurement of hearing aid output, as well as the wide variety of options open in the selection of hearing instruments.

Geriatric audiology is also growing as a subspecialty. New positions in audiology clinics and geriatric centers have come about because of the increasing number of older people and their demand to live useful and active lives.

The audiologist has directed his attention to the learning disabled child and his hearing and perceptual difficulties. There is much in the evaluation and management of these children which requires the skills of the audiologist.

TERMS

Since this book has almost 50 chapters and nearly as many contributors, it was necessary to decide on some uniform terminology. Terms come into usage to accomodate new observations or to make distinctions. Certain terms may become popular if they serve a useful purpose and finally give way to other labels as knowledge continues. Not infrequently words which were used previously return, sometimes with the same meaning but oftentimes representing a new variation. Terms are by no means permanent but deserve careful consideration because they serve an important purpose in professional communication.

Typically one has a theoretical or practical rationale for deciding on a term, however, sometimes it is chosen because of familiarity or emotional reasons. Some decisions on terms used in the *Handbook* are mentioned below. A number of terms differ from the ones used in the earlier edition.

Signal

The term signal is used to designate the tone, noise or speech which is delivered to the listener. It is a signal whether it is heard or not; whether for the purpose of establishing threshold or for comparing two or more sounds. If a signal is sufficient to elicit a response (behavioral or physiologic) we could designate it also as a stimulus since it obviously stimulated the system to respond. However, it would not be appropriate to refer to a "stimulus" if the signal is below threshold. Because the term stimulus is used widely in the electrophysiology literature its use was not completely discontinued. Rather it was deemphasized here to encourage the generic term *signal*.

Sensitivity

Hirsh (1952) aptly points out that we have misused the term *acuity* when referring to a threshold measure. The visual acuity test requires that we distinguish one letter from the others. This is a visual discrimination, not a visual threshold task. Thus, a test to determine an individual's hearing threshold should be a measure of hearing sensitivity and not a measure of hearing acuity.

Unfortunately, the literature is rampant with the term hearing acuity. Sometimes it is used for sensitivity and sometimes for discrimination. Although it would be well to reestablish this word with its more proper meaning (auditory discrimination), it must be given time to go into disuse before it can be revived and used in a consistent manner. For this reason the word acuity is not used here at all as a reference to auditory function.

Sensory-neural

The term *sensory-neural* has almost completely supplanted the former terms *neural* and *perceptive* as the indication of a nonconductive hearing loss. Sensory-neural is also spelled *sensori-neural* or *sensorineural* (on rare occasions it is written *neurosensory*) in various publications. There are reasons for using any of these spellings, however, sensory-neural is used here to preserve the important reason for establishing the term. Nonconductive hearing losses are almost exclusively a result of sensory (cochlear) or neural (referring to retrocochlear) dysfunction. In rare instances they may also result from cerebral disorder. The term *sensory-neural* separates sensory from neural, just as the audiologist is trained to separate these two aspects of disorder central to the middle ear. In some clinics where in depth testing is not carried out there is a tendency to equate *sensorineural* with cochlear pathology. Equally depressed air- and bone-conduction thresholds might be due to end organ dysfunction or to a disorder somewhere in the retrocochlear system. By using the spelling *sensory-neural* we maintain before us the knowledge that the cause might be either cochlear or retrocochlear (or a combination of these two factors).

Hearing Level

In the previous edition the term hearing threshold level (HTL) was used throughout in referring to the number on the audiometer dial. HTL was used for the ISO-1964 standard (Davis and Kranz, 1964) to distinguish it from the ASA-1951 standard. There is presently some momentum to revert back to hearing level (HL) for the ANSI-1969 standard (ASHA Committee on Audiometric Evaluation, 1974). HL seems simpler and more widely applicable than HTL. Since the period of maximum confusion is over we are free to return to HL. However, since there is no agreement at this time we shall use HL and HTL interchangeably.

CANS

In the first edition of the *Handbook*, one of the contributors (Hodgson) suggested that we use CANS to represent *central auditory nervous system*. This acronym is easy to remember and has saved a great deal of space in this book.

Pseudohypacusis

We have given way primarily, but not exclusively, to *pseudohypacusis*. The term *nonorganic* which was used previously has not been completely abandoned in this book.

Audiometric Symbols

Recently a set of audiometric symbols was developed by the Committee on Audiometric Evaluation of the American Speech and Hearing Association (1974) and was approved by the Executive Board of ASHA. We shall follow this system in the *Handbook*. Tables 1.1 and 1.2 show the symbols for unmasked and masked signals.

Hearing Loss Classification

To maintain consistency throughout this volume it was necessary to adopt one classification system of hearing impairment. Several systems have been proposed for describing or predicting the hearing problems associated with various test results (Davis, 1948; Davis, 1965; Goodman, 1965). Davis (1965) and Goodman (1965) have proposed comparable systems for classifying the pure tone speech averages (for 500, 1000 and 2000 Hz). Although the hearing threshold ranges which they refer to differ by no more than 2 dB, they use different descriptive names for some of the classifications. Since Goodman's descriptions are more generally recognized by audiologists, his system has been adopted for the *Handbook*. This scale of hearing impairment is shown in Chapter 9 and elsewhere.

TABLE 1.1 *Recommended Symbols for Threshold Audiometry*

Unless otherwise specified, symbols are to indicate that test signals used were pure tones. The same symbols may be used for warble tones and narrow-band noise, if so noted on the audiogram.

MODALITY	EAR+		
	RIGHT	BOTH	LEFT
AIR CONDUCTION - EARPHONES			
UNMASKED	◯		✕
MASKED	△		☐
BONE CONDUCTION - MASTOID			
UNMASKED	‹		›
MASKED	⊏		⊐
BONE CONDUCTION - FOREHEAD			
UNMASKED		˅	
MASKED	˥		˩
AIR CONDUCTION - SOUND FIELD		S	

+ The fine vertical lines represent the vertical axis of an audiogram.

TABLE 1.2. *Recommended "No Response" Symbols for Threshold Audiometry*

MODALITY	EAR+		
	RIGHT	BOTH	LEFT
AIR CONDUCTION - EARPHONES			
UNMASKED	◯		✕
MASKED	△		☐
BONE CONDUCTION - MASTOID			
UNMASKED	‹		›
MASKED	⊏		⊐
BONE CONDUCTION - FOREHEAD			
UNMASKED		˅	
MASKED	˩		˥
AIR CONDUCTION - SOUND FIELD		S	

+ The fine vertical lines represent the vertical axis of an audiogram.

THE FIRST EDITION, THE SECOND EDITION

The proliferation of printed materials has been great. So much is being written in so many places that it is difficult to keep up with the literature or to find what you are looking for. The second edition of this book seems warranted in that it brings together current information about the state of the science-art of clinical audiology. It provides both recent and classical references as well as the landmark literature along the way.

Some of the information from the first edition

is reprinted here with only minor changes and updating while much of it has been completely rewritten by the same or other authors. Obsolete information has been omitted. Some chapters which have considerable merit were nevertheless deleted for a variety of reasons. Of particular value is the information contained in the following chapters from the first edition: Clinical Audiology; Temporal and Dichotic Factors in Central Auditory Testing; Acoustic Impedance at the Tympanic Membrane; Auditory Perception in Children with Learning Disabilities; and Industrial Noise and Hearing Conservation.

There were 32 contributors to the first edition and 43 in the second. There is an increase from 41 chapters to 49. Three-quarters of the original contributors have written on the same or new topics and almost an equal number of new contributors have offered their knowledge for the second edition.

The format of the second edition differs from the first. The sections follow a logical sequence from the nature of the problem (4 chapters) to efforts at hearing conservation (2 chapters). The following 6 sections concern the evaluation of auditory impairments (29 chapters). The final 3 sections are on the management of the hearing impaired including the use of amplification (14 chapters).

In the first section there are chapters which outline the broad range of disorders which affect hearing (otologic, neurologic and general medical). They provide useful terminology, basic information and case studies. The conservation of hearing includes the screening of children and industrial audiology.

The sections on diagnostic procedures begin with the basic evaluation methods as well as the case history and calibration. This is followed by sections dealing with differentiating cochlear, retrocochlear and central dysfunction. Chapters on brief tone audiometry, clinical use of central tests, monosyllabic tests and sentence tests of central function have been added.

The six chapters on physiological procedures include a new chapter on electrocochleography and two chapters on acoustic impedance measurement. Among the chapters on the evaluation of children and the elderly is a new chapter dealing with the older patient.

The section introducing management procedures and problems begins with an overview of aural rehabilitation, psychology of hearing impairment and classroom acoustics. There are six chapters in the section on hearing aids and finally five chapters dealing with communication training. Chapters on educational audiology and geriatric audiology have been added.

REFERENCES

American Speech and Hearing Association, Report on the state of the art of activities related to PSRO's, June 20, 1975.

American Speech and Hearing Association, Determining cost of speech and hearing services: A guide to developing cost analysis procedures, October, 1971.

ASHA Committee on Audiometric Evaluation, Guidelines for audiometric symbols. *ASHA*, 16, 260–264, 1974.

Curlee, R., Personal incomes in the speech and hearing profession. *ASHA*, 17, 21–30, 1975.

Davis, H., The articulation area and the social adequacy index for hearing. *Laryngoscope*, 58, 761–778, 1948.

Davis, H., Guide for the classification and evaluation of hearing handicap in relation to the international audiometric zero. *Trans. Am. Acad. Ophthalmol. Otolaryngol.* 69, 740–751, 1965.

Davis, H., and Kranz, F. W., The international standard reference zero for pure-tone audiometers and its relation to the evaluation of impairment of hearing. *J. Speech Hear. Res.*, 7, 7–16, 1964.

Fricke, J. E., Personal incomes in the speech and hearing profession. *ASHA*, 14, 10–16, 1972.

Goodman, A., Reference zero levels for pure tone audiometer. *ASHA*, 7, 262–263, 1965.

Hirsh, I. J., *The Measurement of Hearing*, p. 89. New York: McGraw-Hill Book Co., 1952.

Klar, R., National health insurance; the federal perspective. *ASHA*, 17, 388–391, 1975.

chapter 2

OTOLOGICAL CONSIDERATIONS IN AUDIOLOGY

Irwin A. Ginsberg, M.D. and Thomas P. White, M.A.

Without modern audiology, otology would never have made its dramatic gains over the past 25 years. This short space of time has seen an almost total change in the treatment of hearing loss. The concerns and sympathetic understanding of the otologist have been strengthened by a real ability to correct the problems of conductive hearing loss and he now can be of greater help with sensory-neural problems. The disciplines of audiology and otology are mutually dependent and the practice of either demands a good working knowledge of the other. There is real beauty in the inter-relationships of these clinical sciences which can only be appreciated after mutual understanding is gained. It is the purpose of this chapter to promote that understanding.

Otology and audiology are young pursuits and the level of sophistication that we take so casually for granted was not even suspected a scant few years ago. The audiometer is about 55 years old (Bunch, 1943). Recruitment was first reported by Fowler in 1936; Bekesy described automatic audiometry in 1947; the short increment sensitivity index (SISI) was devised by Jerger, Shedd and Harford in 1959; ANSI specifications for audiometers were adopted in 1969; marked advancements were made in the clinical application of electroacoustic impedance concepts in the 1960s and electrocochleography in the 1970s. In the 1940s many otologists dismissed bone-conduction measurements as unreliable and of no value. The Lempert fenestration operation was reported in 1938. Rosen reported the stapes mobilization renaissance in 1953. Tympanoplasty was first described by Wullstein in 1953. Ultrasound labyrinthectomy in Meniere's disease dates back to 1953 (Arslan, 1953). Translabyrinthine surgery in acoustic neurinomas was reported in 1961 (House, 1961). The first cochlear implants for sensory deafness were by Michelson in 1971. The refinements in otological treatment are inextricably associated with the refinements in diagnostic audiology. They progress together and must be constantly correlated.

There are two kinds of ear disorders presented to otologists. The first is the easy kind; obvious and apparent and consisting of such conditions as cerumen blocking the external auditory canal, acute otitis media, acute otitis externa, sensory-neural hearing loss of the aged, and others. The second kind represents the less obvious problems such as presented by a young adult with mixed deafness, the vertiginous patient, the young child with a hearing loss, and the hearing loss of the patient in litigation. It is in this less obvious group that the audiologist shines and where his importance to an otologic diagnosis is so quickly appreciated. It is no longer sufficient to know whether a loss is conductive or sensory-neural for we must know where the problem is in the conductive pathway and in the sensory-neural pathway. Precision in otologic treatment now must be matched by precision in localization by audiologic measurement and vice versa. Of course the audiologist has parallel responsibilities in the nonmedical management of hearing impairment. This information will be discussed in other chapters of the *Handbook*.

We shall consider the approach of the otologist to various ear disorders and simultaneously describe the role of the audiologist in the assessment of their effects. Abnormalities, for simplification, will be grouped into those affecting the external, the middle and the inner ear and those involving the central nervous system.

EXTERNAL EAR

Congenital Atresia

This rather serious problem is discovered early because of the high visibility of the deformity. Many times the atresia of the canal is associated with malformation of the auricle of the ear such as microtia, and multiple rudimentary auricular anlage presenting as auricular tags or accessory auricles. Whenever one sees these obvious external deformities he must immediately suspect associated deformities in the middle ear as well as in the inner ear. Because the embryology of the ear is complex, involving all three germ layers, and because all germ layers take part in such a synchronized manner, when one "gets out of step" the development of the others may also be affected. It is this interrelationship that results in the myriads of possible combinations of malformations. One may have a pure canal atresia with a normal auricle and with a normal middle and inner ear, or a canal atresia which is only a part of the problem and where some or all of the other portions of the ear are involved. It is in this latter type of case that audiometric studies are so important (Fig. 2.1). What is the

8

status of the inner ear? Do we have an intact cochlea and an intact neural mechanism? Is it merely a question of establishing some type of conducting mechanism and reconstructing the canal? In cases of partial atresia where a drum is present, impedance studies may be of great help. The audiologist can help determine whether any surgical attempts should be made. X-ray studies using polytomographic techniques also can be of help in providing the otosurgeon with valuable preoperative information. As a general rule complete, unilateral atresia with a normal opposite ear provides insufficient hearing handicap to warrant a surgical approach. The reconstruction of an ear with congenital atresia has some serious risks to the facial nerve, the inner ear and the frequent need for multiple surgical procedures. One may not wish to assume these risks with

only a fair chance for hearing improvement. Unilateral conductive loss rarely merits assumption of these risks.

Treacher Collins Syndrome

The interrelationships of deformities due to embryologic mishap at first seem strange but quickly make sense when the embryology is understood. Abnormalities of the mandible associated with hearing loss as in the Treacher Collins syndrome result because of the common first branchial arch origin of the mandible, malleus and incus. Pure tone audiometry and impedance studies are of course necessary in establishing a diagnosis.

Impacted Cerumen

A much more ordinary and less exciting "lesion" of the external ear is impacted cerumen. This condition is the worm in the otologic apple! Tremendous amounts of time are expended in the otologic office purging ear canals of this obstructing material. Because it is time-consuming and not particularly pleasant to remove, the tendency is to test around it and also to look around it. Incomplete visualization of the tympanic membrane because of accumulated cerumen is risky just as is audiometric testing of the same obstructed ear. Of course the ear need not be cerumen-free for testing, but there certainly must be an open canal and a visible tympanic membrane. The old idea that appreciable conductive losses cannot be caused by cerumen plugs is not true and losses of as much as 40 dB are possible, (Fig. 2.2, A and B). This brings up the interesting question of the audiologist and the otoscope. All audiologists should have an otoscope close at hand. Unless the patient has been checked by the otologist immediately before testing, the au-

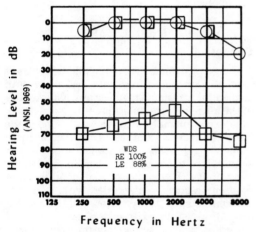

Fig. 2.1. Audiometric results of 14-year-old boy with congenital atresia, left ear.

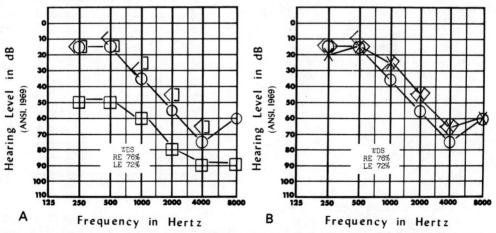

Fig. 2.2. (A) Hearing test results of patient showing effects of impacted cerumen, left ear. (B) Hearing test results of same patient as A, after removal of impacted cerumen.

diologist should perform the pretest otoscopy. If cerumen is present he should refer the patient for its removal. A clean external canal is even of greater importance in impedance measurement since the presence of cerumen will give misleading information regarding the status of the middle ear.

Otitis Externa

Otitis externa, usually a bacterial infection of the external canal skin and erroneously referred to as fungus ear infection, can cause a conductive hearing loss. Usually the canal skin is red and edematous and only a small amount of discharge is present in which case there is no resulting hearing loss. If the swelling of the canal is so marked that it obstructs the canal or if the discharge is so copious, a conductive element will result. Some varieties of otitis externa are associated only with dry, scaling canal skin with little discharge and little swelling. These obviously have no audiologic effect.

Foreign Body Obstruction

Obstruction of the external canal by foreign bodies can produce a conductive impairment especially in children. Small foreign bodies leave no audiologic consequences, thus a hearing loss discovered on routine school audiometry rarely is caused by this problem. The foreign object would have to be totally obstructive such as a bead or a pencil eraser. Foreign bodies should always be thought of in cases of unilateral conductive loss but their presence is soon discovered on otoscopy.

Osteoma, Hyperostosis, Exostosis

Growths of the bony external canal are not uncommon but rarely produce a hearing loss. They can occur as either osteomas which are discrete rounded excrescences of bone, or as a diffuse bony narrowing of the canal called hyperostosis. Osteomas usually occur medially in the bony canal rather close to the tympanic membrane. They usually are small whitish rounded masses which on cursory examination may be confused with the whitish pearly cholesteatoma which occurs in the attic of the ear. A closer look reveals that they are in fact lateral to Shrapnell's membrane. Ordinarily they are too small to cause any degree of canal obstruction and are best left untreated. Uncommonly they may become large and completely obstructing in which case they must be removed. Exostoses are covered with canal skin and are hard on palpation. They must not be confused with middle ear polyps which present in the external canal as soft, shiny, rounded masses covered with moist mucous membrane and which have a totally different significance

and effect on hearing as we shall see later. Hyperostosis, the diffuse narrowing of the bony canal wall, also must be completely obstructing to produce a change in the pure tone results.

Collapsed Canal

Audiologists and otologists are sometimes baffled by an air-bone gap with a flat air-conduction curve for which there is no apparent cause. The drum appears quite normal as does the canal, and tuning fork tests fail to confirm the presence of an air-bone gap. This proves to be due to an anatomical variation of the outermost part of the cartilaginous canal and tragus. The pressure of the ear phone produces a valve-like closing of the meatus, so complete as to produce a very significant conductive loss as shown in Figure 2.3. This must be looked for and, if suspected, a device should be placed in the canal to prevent collapse when the phones are applied.

MIDDLE EAR

Congenital

Congenital anomalies of the middle ear have been alluded to as a frequent concurrence with congenital atresia. Whenever any abnormality of the auricle or meatus is present, suspicion of middle ear anomaly should be high. One of the most common anomalies is that of a fused malleus and incus. Sometimes the incus is solidly fixed to the posterior bony annulus by a bony bridge. There may be a congenital stapes fixation frequently associated with a grossly deformed stapes. Many varieties of more minor congenital defects exist such as absence of the stapedius tendon, completely uncovered facial

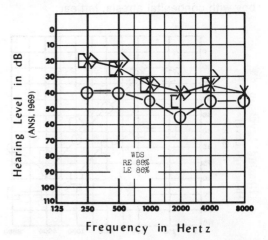

Fig. 2.3. Audiometric findings of individual showing influence of collapsed canal while under test (right ear).

nerves with deficiencies in the bony canal, aberrant courses of the facial nerve and partial bony plate formation in the region of the bony annulus. Hearing loss of course will depend on the degree of abnormality of ossicular transmission as well as on the presence or absence of associated inner ear deficiencies. Air-bone gaps of 60 dB are not infrequent in patients with a congenitally malformed middle ear. The audiologist helps to establish the indication for surgical reconstruction and with the help of tympanometry can predict the pathology. Quite often impedance measurements reveal a normal shallow tympanogram with absent reflexes (Fig. 2.4, *A* and *B*).

Acute Otitis Media

Acute otitis media is almost always associated with a conductive hearing loss, certainly in its exudative stage and during the recovery stage until the middle ear is again well ventilated. A certain number of these cases do not go on to complete resolution and a conductive loss may persist because of unresolved or unevacuated products of infection. Sterile fluid may persist with its effect on hearing. In any case where incomplete resolution is suspected the audiometric findings are all important in determining further course of treatment. Certainly it is extremely important for the otologist to know whether or not a conductive loss persists. If one does, treatment must be extended. Tympanometric studies may play an extremely important role as negative middle ear pressure or fluid may exist without a sig-

nificant hearing loss, as shown in Figure 2.5, *A* and *B*.

Chronic Otitis Media Tympanic Membrane Perforation

It is from these cases of acute otitis media that cases of chronic otitis media arise. Some infections are caused by particularly virulent organisms which early in the course of the infection can produce destruction of drum substance with a resulting perforation. Sometimes a perforation results because of long standing, low grade infection or as the sequela of an incompletely treated acute otitis media, not followed to complete resolution. In some cases, the now subacute rather than acute infection results in ossicular damage with frequent incus necrosis. The lenticular process and lower half of the long process of the incus most frequently are involved when the ossicular chain is damaged. Long standing infection leaves the ear with defects in the tympanic membrane, damage to the ossicular chain, or both. The effect on audiometric findings can be very protean indeed. Not only is the size of the perforation important in determining the degree of hearing loss but its location as well. The larger the perforation the more the loss of sound pressure which can be transmitted to the inner ear. However, if the perforation is small but located directly over the round window, the loss may be even greater than that due to a larger perforation located elsewhere. Size and location are therefore both important factors. In some cases surprisingly large perforations may be

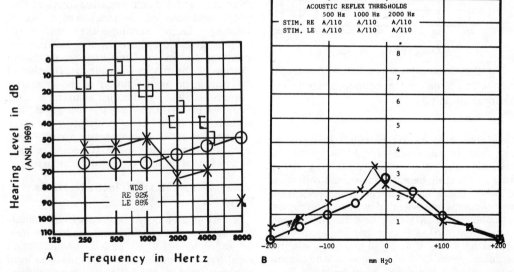

Fig. 2.4. (*A*) Audiogram of 11-year-old boy with surgically confirmed, bilateral, congenital stapes fixation. (*B*) Tympanogram of patient in *A*, with congenital stapes fixation.

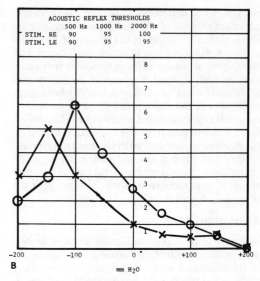

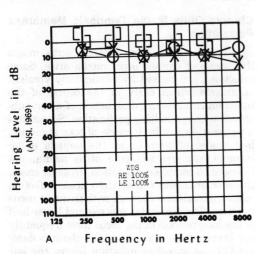

Fig. 2.5. (A) Audiometric results of girl, age 5, with bilateral acute otitis media. (B) Tympanometry curves of girl, age 5, with bilateral acute otitis media.

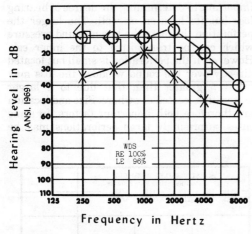

Fig. 2.6. Hearing test results of 50-year-old man with a large central tympanic membrane perforation, left ear.

associated with relatively small losses (Fig. 2.6). The round window could be getting a valuable amount of sound protection either from a protecting band of mucosa or a collection of thick mucus or discharge. The perforation may of course be associated with an interrupted ossicular chain in which case the advancing sound front strikes the mobile stapes directly producing a loss of 30 to 40 dB. Surprisingly, an intact drum in the presence of a discontinuous ossicular chain can be responsible for a 60-dB loss since its very presence prevents the sound wave from striking the stapes directly.

Myringostapediopexy, Tympanosclerosis

A perforation may be associated with an incus necrosis but the drum remnant may have attached itself to the stapes head producing a spontaneous "tympanoplasty" known as a myringostapediopexy. In this case, if the perforation is not very large and is not located directly over the round window, the hearing loss may be very slight or nonexistent. A perforation may be small or even healed and yet the conductive loss might be great because of masses of tympanosclerosis which have formed about the ossicular chain causing fixation. This tympanosclerosis can be considered a form of scarring. Large cartilage-like masses or plaques grow anywhere in the middle ear, involving the mucosa and ossicles, producing fixation of the malleus and incus, fixation of the stapes, or even fixation of the tympanic membrane. The tympanic membrane may therefore be intact and yet the loss great. The otologist could well be forewarned by the accurate assessment of a preoperative air-bone gap, low compliance and absent stapedial reflexes demonstrated on impedance measurements.

Malleus Head Fixation, Incus Necrosis, Polyp

A very small amount of disease in the middle ear may cause a considerable conductive loss, for example, cases of malleus head fixation resulting from otitis media. The malleus head becomes fixed to the attic wall markedly increasing impedance and producing a loss which might easily be mistaken for otosclerosis. Incus necrosis behind an intact drum is very common and may cause up to a 60-dB loss. In these cases compliance is very high. In some cases of chronic otitis media with perforation, the middle ear mucosa may become so thick and hypertrophied that polypoid changes occur and actual polyps may form. These may extend through the perforation and present as a mass in the external canal. Polyps, as opposed to bony exostoses, are soft, shiny and covered with mucosa. In cases of polypoid chronic otitis media there may be a severely damaged middle ear with damage to the ossicular chain and a conductive loss increased further by the very presence of the polyp. Merely removing the polyp and not correcting the underlying disease is rarely recommended. The surgery should be directed to the middle ear and sometimes the mastoid.

Serous Otitis Media

Serous or secretory otitis media, the most common cause of conductive loss in children, has certainly become more common in recent years. Although one might be tempted to believe that the increased incidence represents cases previously missed and that the figures indicate better diagnosis, this would probably be an incorrect conclusion. Politzer described the entity over 60 years ago and even developed and used vulcanite collar button tubes (Noyes, 1869). The condition was known to exist and, although some cases may have been missed because of the absence of modern diagnostic audiologic techniques, it seems apparent that fewer cases actually existed. The cause is probably variable ranging from infection to allergy and all that is known with any degree of certainty is that the middle ear is not ventilating, presumably because of faulty Eustachian tube function. Once the stage has been set and the middle ear is under negative pressure, a vicious cycle is established. The histology of the mucosa in the middle ear undergoes morphologic changes and the pavement type of epithelium becomes secretory and glandular in nature. The longer the ear is unventilated the greater these changes. The greater these changes the more adverse the effect on ventilation since the Eustachian tube is obstructed by even thicker and more viscid secretions. Diagnosis may be fairly simple with obvious fluid seen on otoscopic examination. In other cases, it might be difficult to recognize any abnormality of the tympanic membrane and yet a significant conductive hearing loss may be present (Fig. 2.7A and B). Audiologically, this problem manifests itself as a flat pure conductive hearing loss. The air-conduction curve initially will show a greater loss in the high frequencies and spread to the lows. Bone conduction responses may be depressed slightly in the high frequencies. Tympanometry is exceedingly helpful showing in advanced cases a relatively flat curve and in less severe cases merely a negative pressure with a diminished compliance.

In short term cases a conservative approach might be tried with Eustachian tube inflation and decongestant medication. In the case of long-standing serous otitis media this approach usually fails and the best approach is to perform myringotomy with the insertion of a ventilation tube which in a sense replaces the

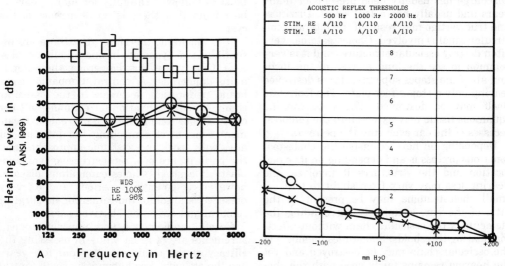

Fig. 2.7. (A) Audiometric findings of 7-year-old girl with bilateral serous otitis media. (B) Tympanograms of same patient as shown in A, with bilateral serous otitis media.

function of the inoperative Eustachian tube. After tubes have remained in place for a sufficient length of time, the mucosa may return to normal, with resumption of normal Eustachian tube function and the return of normal hearing. Audiometric and tympanometric follow-up, after the tubes have been extruded or been removed, will determine the success of the treatment. Some cases with serous otitis media may have other middle ear pathology as well and a conductive deficit will still be present even after complete control of the middle ear fluid. This may be due to incus necrosis, an underlying congenital anomaly, tympanosclerosis, or cholesteatoma to mention some of the possibilities. When audiometric and tympanometric follow-up are carried out the presence of this additional pathology can be diagnosed accurately. Appropriate corrective measures may then be taken.

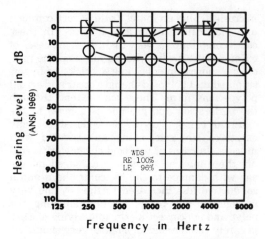

Fig. 2.8. Audiometric results of 34-year-old woman with large cholesteatoma, right ear.

Cholesteatoma

In some ears, associated with long periods of negative middle ear pressure and with recurring infection one will find cysts called cholesteatoma. These cysts are squamous-lined and usually begin in the attic of the ear, extending into the mastoid antrum, sometimes all the way to the mastoid tip. Cholesteatomas are filled with cast-off epithelial debris and slowly increase in size. They erode the bone with which they come in contact and can produce serious intracranial complications if they erode through the dura of the middle or posterior fossa of the skull, through the lateral sinus, or into the lateral semicircular canal. They may also produce a facial paralysis if the facial nerve is eroded in the middle ear or mastoid. Discharge has usually been present for many years and usually has a foul smell. Dizziness and true vertigo may result if the lateral semicircular canal is involved. Cholesteatomas very often destroy ossicular structures and it is very common to see the long process of the incus and all of the stapes superstructures destroyed leaving only a stapes foot plate. The foot plate itself may be destroyed. The wide ranging squamous tissue may extend into the remotest recesses of the ear even into the petrosa.

Depending on how extensive the cholesteatomatous process is and depending on its exact location and the structures it involves, the hearing loss may vary from slight to total. A small cholesteatoma may be present in the attic of the ear, completely surrounding the elements of the ossicular chain without affecting hearing thresholds. Sometimes members of the ossicular chain may be destroyed and yet the hearing remains fairly good with the cholesteatoma itself bridging the gap and helping in sound transmission (Fig. 2.8). Since the

cholesteatoma must be removed as a potentially fatal disease it may in situations like these, be necessary to lose hearing in order to eradicate it. It is usually necessary to enter both the mastoid and the middle ear at the time of surgery in order to properly expose and remove all of the cyst. In cases where the hearing was poor or becomes poor as a result of the surgery a secondary procedure may be planned at the time of the original removal and a reconstructive procedure performed at least one year later, as a secondary tympanoplasty. On rare occasion, when the cyst is small and easily removed, it might be possible to remove the cyst and during the same procedure reconstruct the drum and ossicular chain in a one stage mastoid-tympanoplasty. These ears must be followed carefully for many years to be certain that there is no recurrence of the cyst.

It is apparent, therefore, that there are essentially two types of chronic middle ear disease. One type is not dangerous, the other is quite dangerous. A central tympanic membrane perforation, a break in the ossicular chain, a malleus fixation for example will not cause serious complications if untreated. Treatment consists of controlling the infection, if any, with local and systemic approaches and the performance of a reconstructive tympanoplasty if desired. Cholesteatomatous disease, however, is potentially serious and its very presence is absolute indication for its surgical removal and not on an elective basis.

Careful audiometric and impedance measurements are of great value in assessing the efficacy of the treatment. A scant few years ago the otologist was happy if he could control the infection, stop the discharge and make the ear safe. As otosurgery has progressed the goals are ever higher and hearing improvement is more to be expected. A careful audiologic evaluation is important not only for determining the baseline hearing but also to suggest or support surgical intervention and the maximum amount of possible hearing improvement that can be expected. Recent developments in the application of impedance measurement may also help the surgeon anticipate the pathology he will find at surgery.

Trauma, Nonorganic Hearing Loss

Various degrees of damage to the conductive mechanism may result from mechanical trauma, although most damage to the drum or ossicular chain is due to the results of infection. A blow to the ear with the open palm (frequently in play) may easily produce a traumatic perforation, a hemotympanum (a collection of blood in the middle ear) or damage to the ossicular chain (Fig. 2.9A and B). Sensory-neural elements also may be damaged. Because of the frequent medicolegal implications of ear trauma, especially in cases of automobile accidents or industrial accidents, a very complete battery of audiometric tests is needed. Many times in these cases, the audiologist must be particularly astute. When litigation and possible enrichment exist together it is not uncommon for the patient to exaggerate the loss. In some cases there may be actual malingering. It is a truism which the audiologist is well advised to heed, that all litigated cases and all compensation cases are exaggerating or malingering until proven otherwise. When performing audiometric tests on these cases one is struck with the poor reliability of the responses and must be prepared to spend the requisite amount of time to establish true thresholds (frequently many decibels better than found on the first audiometric curve). Actual techniques in audiologic measurement may require modification in these cases. Tests for confirmation of nonorganic hearing loss are often in order such as Stenger (Newby, 1972) and Doerfler-Stewart (Doerfler and Stewart, 1946). Electroacoustic impedance measurements, especially the finding of the acoustic reflex, have been invaluable in substantiating the presence of hearing. This is not to say that all patients in these classifications are "out to cheat" but there are certainly a goodly number who try.

Otosclerosis

One of the most interesting of all ear diseases is that known as otosclerosis. It is this disease and the exciting surgical developments concerning it in 1952 which sparked the entire renaissance in the surgery of the ear. Valsalva was the first to report that ankylosis or fixation of the stapes could cause hearing impairment back in 1735.

In 1841, Toynbee and others observed, in a large number of postmortem examinations done on patients who were known to be hard-of-hearing during their lifetime, that ankylosis of the stapes was a common cause of hearing loss. Politzer in 1893 determined that this ankylosis was due to particular disease of the bone forming the otic capsule and not to chronic

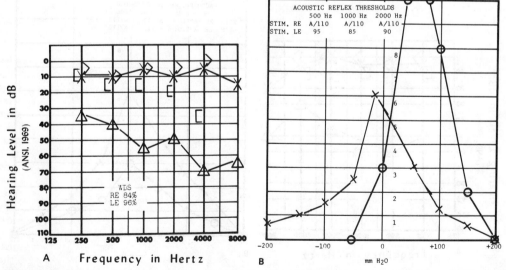

Fig. 2.9. (A) Hearing test results of 14-year-old girl with reported history of head trauma and subsequent surgically confirmed ossicular discontinuity (right ear). (B) Tympanograms of patient shown in A.

middle ear catarrh as previously thought. The cause still remains unknown but certain characteristics are consistent with its presence. A comprehensive computer analysis of 2405 surgically confirmed cases of otosclerosis has confirmed the previously known fact that it occurs twice as often in women as in men. Results also showed that tinnitus is present approximately 50% of the time and the average age of noticed impairment is 36 years (Ginsberg, Hoffman and White, 1975). The condition is also aggravated in a good number of cases by pregnancy. The hearing loss is insidious in onset, slowly progressive and in most cases largely conductive. Many cases, however, show mixed loss and some purely sensory-neural hearing loss.

The actual bone changes in otosclerosis consist of a simultaneous laying down of new bone with a concomitant resorption of the older bone producing a spongy type of bone. This abnormal bone may occur anywhere in the otic capsule and depending on where it occurs will determine whether the hearing loss is conductive, sensory-neural, mixed or not present at all. If none of the elements of hearing are involved one may have otosclerosis of the temporal bone and not be aware of it. This might account for negative family histories in some patients with otosclerosis. The main site of predilection for otosclerosis is that portion of the oval window just anterior to the foot plate causing the foot plate to fix in position wedging it posteriorly.

The drums are almost always normal except in those few cases especially in younger adults where the increased vascularity of the actively growing bone is reflected through the drum as a pink discoloration. This sign is known as the Schwartze sign and is very inconsistent. It has also been referred to as the "flamingo flush." Since the drum is almost always normal one must depend on the history and the audiometric findings, the latter of which have characteristic features. Audiometric results augmented by impedance measurements are of great help in establishing the diagnosis of otosclerosis. Knowledge of the size of the air-bone gap and the absence of acoustic reflexes with a normal tympanogram is indispensable as an indication for surgery (Fig. 2.10A and B). The classical example shows a conductive impairment with a greater loss in the low than in the high frequencies and follows the impedance formula for stiffness. The less typical case is a patient with a mixed loss and a greater or lesser degree of sensory-neural involvement. More recently we have recognized the fact that otosclerosis may cause a purely sensory-neural loss. In these cases the conduction mechanism is not involved but the sensory-neural elements are directly or indirectly affected. The diagnosis of sensory-neural loss due to otosclerosis can only be made after special x-ray studies of the temporal bone are done. This type of study is called polytomography and can delineate on the x-ray film small foci of otosclerosis.

It might be well to stress here the fact that all surgery for hearing improvement depends upon the ability of the audiologist to consistently identify the existence and the size of the

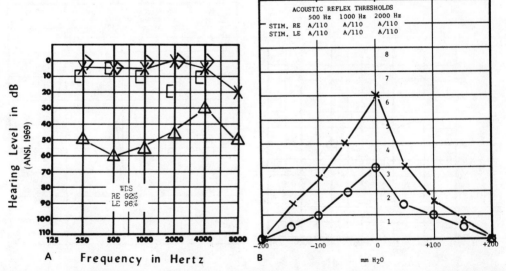

Fig. 2.10. (A) Results of audiometric studies performed on 46-year-old woman with surgically confirmed otosclerosis, right ear. (B) Tympanometric results of patient described in A.

air-bone gap. The preoperative bone conductive curve is the target for the otosurgeon and everything possible must be done in the testing suite to accurately determine it. In the more difficult case every aspect of bone conduction measurement must be carefully controlled in order to avoid false estimates of the remaining cochlear potential.

INNER EAR AND RETROCOCHLEAR SYSTEM

Not many years ago the otologist had to be content with an audiologic assessment telling only whether the loss was conductive, sensory-neural or mixed. As audiology evolved it became possible to determine where in the sensory-neural pathway the site of lesion was, and for that matter, where in the conductive pathway as well. Impedance measurements have recently added a whole new dimension to the location of the site of lesion. Cochlear, retro-cochlear and central lesions can be identified in an ever increasing percentage of cases. When dealing with conductive losses the otologist looks to the audiologist not only for the site of lesion but for the size of the air-bone gap. When dealing with sensory-neural hearing loss the otologist looks to the audiologist for the site of the pathology. Caring for a patient with a hearing loss is one thing. Missing a brain stem tumor is quite another. The audiologist and otologist, working as a team, can discover early cerebellopontine angle tumors such as acoustic neurinomas and by their cooperative efforts actually perform a lifesaving function. Careful, meticulous audiology reaps its largest rewards in these cases.

Cochlear problems are the most usual and are due to the greatest variety of pathologic entities. The following are common types.

Congenital Deafness

Hereditary hearing loss may be defined as those cases where the causative factors are present in the fertilized ovum. Congenital loss, on the other hand, means merely that the impairment was present at birth and includes both the hereditary cases as well as the acquired cases. Acquired cases have causative factors acting while the fetus was in utero but not contained in the germ cells.

Hereditary hearing loss may be transmitted as a dominant or recessive characteristic. It may be associated with other stigmata such as renal involvement, degenerative diseases of the nervous system, albinism, mental retardation, and metabolic abnormalities. There are many named syndromes to describe various combinations of abnormalities such as Alport's, Waardenburg's and Hurler's syndromes. The diag-

nosis of any particular entity can rarely be made from audiometric findings alone but is the result of the total clinical picture.

Some examples of congenital hearing loss acquired in utero are maternal rubella in the first and second trimesters of pregnancy, and the breakdown of red blood cells with resulting neonatal jaundice most often the result of erythroblastosis fetalis (Rh incompatibility). In addition sensory-neural hearing loss may be due to birth injury often associated with anoxia, drug ingestion by the mother such as Thalidomide and quinine, and in general cases associated with significant degrees of prematurity (possible because many premature infants have periods of hypoxia). The diagnosis of a hearing loss in the young infant is quite challenging. The otologist can do little more than observe gross reflexes. It falls to the audiologist to determine and quantify the hearing loss. Impedance measurement has helped greatly in assessing middle ear function and objectively predicting the presence and degree of hearing loss (Jerger et al., 1974).

There are of course, many types of cochlear disorders which are not congenital. The following are the more common types.

Meniere's Disease

Many patients who consult the otologist do not complain of a hearing loss but rather imbalance, dizziness or vertigo. What must be determined first is whether or not true vertigo (hallucination of movement) is present. Unless it is, the likelihood of a labyrinthine cause is remote. Symptoms of dizziness which can mean anything from weakness, "blacking out" to loss of consciousness are not otitic in origin. The otologist seeing a patient with this type of complaint usually finds normal ear drums. After a complete history has been taken to try to establish a pattern characteristic enough to identify, the patient is referred to the audiologist in the hopes that a characteristic audiometric picture will appear. The typical clinical picture of Meniere's disease includes episodic true rotatory vertigo, associated with tinnitus, frequently roaring in type, a "fullness" or a sense of pressure in the offending ear, nausea and vomiting. There is usually a definite hearing loss during and bracketing the actual period of vertigo. There may be marked intolerance to loud sounds. The attacks come in clusters and are usually followed by periods of complete freedom from them. There are variations however and hearing loss need not be reported. Conversely there may be periods of hearing impairment without associated vertigo. Because of the variability of the clinical picture the audiologist usually must provide the data before a diagnosis of Meniere's disease can be established. When a hearing loss is present it usually begins as a low frequency, sensory-neural loss which over a long period of time tends to flatten (Fig. 2.11). A small number of cases can present first as a high frequency loss and later show flattening as the low end is affected. In more than 80% of the cases the disease is unilateral and recruitment can be determined by the alternate binaural loudness balance test. Complete or even over-recruitment is the rule in this disease. Discrimination scores are usually fair and in keeping with the degree of sensory-neural loss. There is absence of tone decay and usually a high SISI score. The hearing thresholds will fluctuate from day to day and this fact may be noted both by the audiologist and the patient. Impedance studies may help to confirm these findings. Presence of recruitment is indicated by a positive stapedial reflex produced by stimulus levels in the affected ear at or nearly equal to those levels required to elicit the reflex in the unaffected ear (Metz, 1946). This occurs despite the reduced hearing levels. Bekesy audiometry will confirm the cochlear nature of the problem with absence of abnormal threshold shift in the continuous tracing.

Unless reasonably typical audiometric findings match a reasonably typical clinical picture the diagnosis is in doubt. Using the phrase "Meniere's syndrome" rather than "Meniere's disease" so as to indicate an atypical case is a dangerous practice. It tends to serve as a catchall "wastebasket" for incompletely understood cases. The diagnosis of Meniere's disease must be a definite one—indicating endolymphatic hydrops only, for Meniere's disease under the microscope almost always shows dilatation of

the endolymphatic spaces—the result of increased volume of endolymph. It is not a syndrome; it is a disease state.

Noise Induced Loss

More and more attention has been given to the adverse effects of noise on the human organism. As civilization has "progressed" the noise in man's environment has increased. The adverse effects of noise are widespread with respect to human physiology and produce changes in many biosystems other than the ear. It is however the ear which concerns us here.

Traumatic noise levels almost invariably affect the threshold at 4000 Hz. As the exposure continues the damage extends to either side of this area and what was once a slight dip at 4000 Hz becomes a wide notch involving lower and higher frequencies as well, and the loss for 4000 Hz increases. The pathologic process involves outer hair cell damage first as it progressively involves the other cells of the cochlea and later the inner hair cells. Finally, as reported by Siebenmann and Yoshii in 1908, the cochlear neurons may atrophy.

Industrial hearing loss resulting from noise exposure is usually equal bilaterally. Hearing impairment induced by the noise of gunfire may show different degrees of loss in each ear. A right handed rifleman shooting a shotgun exposes his left ear to more sound than his right because of the proximity of the breech to the left ear. Consequently a right handed rifleman shows a greater loss in the left ear and vice versa (Fig. 2.12A and B). This may be a good lead in attempting to determine the cause of a particular loss and may, for example, reveal that a case of industrial hearing loss was in fact due to many years of skeet and trap shooting. There is, of course, no therapy for this type of loss and prophylaxis is the only possible approach. This requires the cooperation of the employee as well as the employer and hearing conservation programs in industry must be supported vigorously by both groups.

Drug Induced Hearing Loss

There is a group of ototoxic drugs which has a predilection for causing cochlear and in some cases, vestibular damage. Drugs which are particularly toxic to the ear are certain antibiotics, salicylates and quinine. There are others as well but they are less commonly used and therefore of lesser importance in this discussion. Streptomycin, dihydrostreptomycin, kanamycin, neomycin, gentamicin, and viomycin are ototoxic and should therefore be utilized in the treatment of infection only when there is not a less toxic, or nontoxic drug

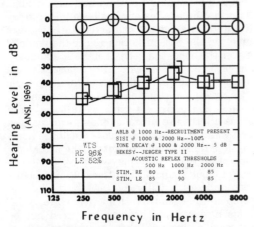

Fig. 2.11. Audiogram indicating findings obtained in a 47-year-old man with diagnosed Meniere's disease, left ear.

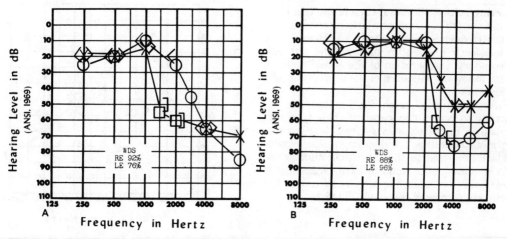

Fig. 2.12. (A) Audiometric findings of 44-year-old, right handed man, with significant history of noise exposure from rifle fire. (B) Audiometric findings of 46-year-old, left handed woman with significant history of noise exposure from rifle fire.

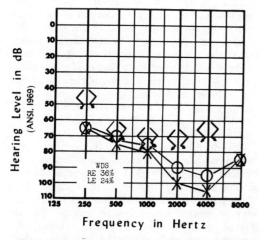

Fig. 2.13. Pure tone and speech discrimination results of 52-year-old man who had received large doses of neomycin, producing subsequent sensory-neural hearing loss.

available. Streptomycin is essentially vestibulo-toxic while dihydrostreptomycin usually is more toxic to the cochlea. Neither is exclusively so. Neomycin and kanamycin are essentially cochleo-toxic whereas gentamicin and viomycin seem to be more vestibulo-toxic. Ordinarily the losses due to streptomycin are not as severe as those due to kanamycin and neomycin which usually produce profound hearing loss as shown in Figure 2.13. The point to be stressed is that none of these ototoxic drugs should be used unless less toxic drugs are not suitable for treatment of the infection.

Virus Induced Hearing Loss

The inner ear may be affected both by specific and nonspecific viruses. The viruses of measles and mumps are well known offenders. The measles virus usually produces moderate to severe bilateral losses involving both the cochlear and vestibular systems. Mumps usually causes a total unilateral loss with no involvement of the vestibular organs. Uncommonly it may cause a high frequency loss only. Some mumps infections may be unsuspected and yet be the cause of sudden deafness. Determination of the mumps virus as the etiologic agent requires the performance of antibody studies, for the absence of the typical parotid swelling might result in the actual cause not being suspected. That group of viruses which for example, can be the cause of respiratory infections may also involve the cochlea producing a viral cochleitis. This too can be a cause of a sudden loss but fortunately some cases of this have been shown to have recovered very well, or at least to have regained some of the lost hearing.

Presbycusis

Presbycusis is that type of sensory-neural loss due to the degenerative changes of aging. Most persons if they live long enough will exhibit this type of hearing loss to some degree. The degenerative changes of aging involve a variety of locations and cell types in the inner ear with more or less specific effects on the pure tone thresholds. It is for this reason that presbycusis in some may cause profound difficulties while in others the deficit is small. When the changes involve the sensory or supporting cells of the basal turn of the cochlea a characteristic audiometric pattern of an abrupt high frequency loss is produced. Hearing for the speech frequencies may not be affected. Secondary degeneration of the actual neurons may follow degeneration of the supporting cells (Fig. 2.14).

Another type of presbycusis is that due primarily to neural degeneration. This type also causes a high frequency hearing loss but discrimination scores are disproportionately poor when compared to the pure tone audiogram. As a consequence amplification is usually of less help than when the sensory or supporting cells are primarily involved (Fig. 2.15).

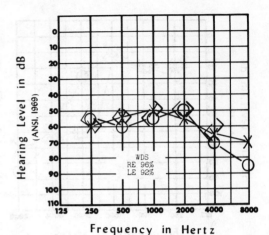

Fig. 2.16. Hearing test results of 76-year-old woman with loss due to strial atrophy.

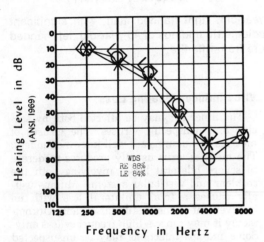

Fig. 2.14. Audiometric results of 82-year-old man showing typical results of sensory presbycusis.

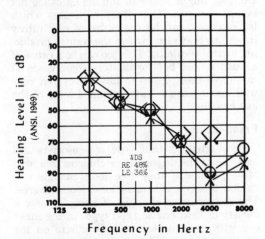

Fig. 2.15. Audiogram of 75-year-old woman indicating results consistent with neural presbycusis.

Atrophy of the stria vascularis usually results in a flat loss, essentially equal for all frequencies but with preservation of excellent speech discrimination. Because the stria is felt to be responsible for maintaining the DC potential of the scala media loss of its function may produce effects similar to those in a DC radio with spent batteries. The sounds are clear but the volume reduced. The patient with strial atrophy usually is an excellent candidate for amplification (Fig. 2.16).

A fourth type of presbycusis which results in a straight line descending audiometric configuration has been called cochlear conductive presbycusis. It appears that this type is due to altered physical responses in the cochlear duct since there are inadequate changes in the sensory or neural structures to account for the degree of loss. Generally the steeper the straight line audiometric pattern the poorer the discrimination and the less effectively the patient can wear a hearing aid (Fig. 2.17).

Patients with presbycusis may not manifest any of these degenerative changes in a pure form but rather a mixture of these various types. Their audiograms will therefore be summations of the effects of these various changes.

Meningitis

Bacterial meningitis despite the advent of antibiotic therapy is still a cause of severe sensory-neural hearing loss although less frequently than in the preantibiotic era. The infection may extend through the cochlear aqueduct or through the internal auditory meatus involving the spaces of the inner ear. Bacterial labyrinthitis results in fibrosis and destruction of the cochlear and vestibular elements. Most often a profound hearing loss is produced.

Retrocochlear Hearing Loss

It has been mentioned earlier that it is important for the otologist to learn the site of the lesion in sensory-neural hearing loss cases. When audiometric findings suggest a retrocochlear site the case must be thoroughly investigated in an attempt to discover or rule out the presence of an acoustic neurinoma. Acoustic neurinoma, although a benign tumor of the vestibular nerve, is nevertheless life-threatening. The skilled audiologist is crucial in discovering the presence of one of these tumors. In this respect a unilateral sensory-neural loss should be considered a potential acoustic neurinoma until proven otherwise. The audiologist should in this case have a high index of suspicion and should perform the complete battery of audiometric studies which are helpful in determining the site of the lesion (Fig. 2.18). This should include the traditional tests which have been used to distinguish cochlear from retrocochlear losses. These include tests for presence of recruitment, tone decay, detection of excessive sensitivity to small increases in sound intensity, and speech discrimination tests. These tests should be supplemented by automatic audiometry and newer advancements in impedance measurements utilizing the stapedial reflex response.

Electronystagmography is of great help in establishing retrocochlear disease. Characteristically, but not invariably, the caloric response on the affected side is severely depressed or absent in the ear with retrocochlear hearing loss. The study of retrocochlear pathology again points out the need for close cooperation between the otologist and the audiologist and a

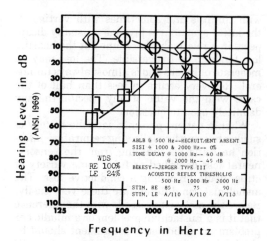

Fig. 2.18. Results of audiologic studies carried out on 44-year-old woman with surgically confirmed cerebellopontine angle tumor, left side.

mutual understanding of the two disciplines. Corroboration should be further provided by x-rays of the internal auditory meati, polytomography (a more sophisticated x-ray technique) and the even more reliable posterior fossa myelogram where radiopaque dye is used to outline the tumor.

Whenever the test battery indicates a retrocochlear site of lesion one must remember that processes other than acoustic neurinoma may be responsible for the test results. This includes viral neuritis, trauma, hemorrhage, or neurologic disorders such as multiple sclerosis. X-ray studies help to distinguish these from acoustic neurinoma.

Sudden Deafness

Sensory-neural hearing loss although usually having a gradual onset with slow progression may also have a sudden onset. Sudden hearing loss of known cause may be due to drugs, trauma, infection or disease. Those cases of sudden loss without apparent etiology have been explained by two hypotheses. The first is viral labyrinthitis producing changes in the inner ear similar to those caused by known viral invaders such as the virus of mumps. Further evidence of this as a likely cause is that of the frequent relationship to respiratory infection which often seems to precede the hearing loss. The second hypothesis is that of vascular occlusion causing abrupt interruption of blood supply. The fact that sudden loss occurs at any age tends to mitigate against this as a frequent factor.

Sudden hearing loss is usually associated

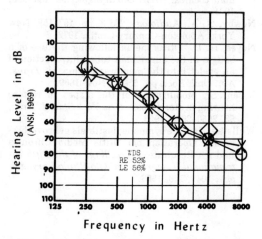

Fig. 2.17. Audiometric findings of 69-year-old man showing pure tone and speech discrimination patterns typical of cochlear conductive presbycusis.

with tinnitus and sometimes with vertigo. If the latter symptom is present it usually disappears in a relatively short time but the hearing loss tends to be irreversible. The loss may be moderate or severe and is almost always unilateral. Recovery occurs in less than half of the cases with the value of any specific therapy definitely open to question.

When a patient presents with the history of sudden hearing loss following respiratory infection he could be suffering from the sensory-neural loss described or from some variety of otitis media producing a conductive loss. The audiologist can differentiate these very easily. Before the otologist proceeds with the inference that it is a Eustachian problem or a middle ear problem an audiometric assessment should be obtained, sparing the patient from much treatment foredoomed to failure.

Nephritis and Hearing Loss

Alport (1927) reported an unusually high incidence of sensory-neural deafness in association with hereditary nephritis. The sensory-neural loss begins in childhood, affects all frequencies and may become quite severe. Many of these patients may die of the renal disease before the hearing loss becomes very great. The exact mechanism of this hearing loss is not known nor is the exact nature of the pathology in the cochlea.

CONCLUSION

A realization of the complexity of the ear and its neural pathways and an awareness of the many disorders which involve the auditory system make one very much aware of the diagnostic effort which must be made to define the pathology in any given case. The otologist may view only the drum head or the middle ear. Deeper portions are hidden from his view and may be examined only functionally by the audiologist. The diagnostic and rehabilitative work of the audiologist finds roots in the work of the otologist. It is the work of the otologist to treat conditions of the ear medically or surgically to the best of his ability. When hearing impairment remains, the audiologist is again called upon to ease the burden of hearing handicap by consideration of a hearing aid or other forms of aural rehabilitation.

REFERENCES

Alport, A., Hereditary familial congenital haemorrhagic nephritis. Br. Med. J., 1, 504–506, 1927.

American National Standards Institute, Specifications for audiometers. ANSI S3.6–1969. New York: American National Standards Institute, Inc., 1970.

Arslan, M., Treatment of Meniere's syndrome by direct application of ultrasound waves to the vestibular system. Proceedings of the Fifth International Congress in Otolaryng, pp. 629–635, 1953.

Bekesy, G. v., A new audiometer. Acta Otolaryngol., 35, 411–422, 1947.

Bunch, C. C., Clinical Audiometry, p. 171. St. Louis: C. V. Mosby, 1943.

Doerfler, L. G., and Stewart, K., Malingering and psychogenic deafness. J. Speech Disord, 11, 181–186, 1946.

Fowler, E. P., A method for the early detection of otosclerosis. Arch. Otolaryngol., 24, 731–741, 1936.

Ginsberg, I., Hoffman, S., and White, T., In depth computer analysis of aspects of otosclerosis (unpublished information), 1975.

House, W., Surgical exposure of the internal auditory canal and its contents through the middle, cranial fossa. Laryngoscope, 71, 1363–1385, 1961.

Jerger, J., Shedd, J., and Harford, E., On the detection of extremely small changes in sound intensity. Arch. Otolaryngol., 69, 200–211, 1959.

Jerger, J., Burney, P., Mauldin, L., and Crump, B., Predicting hearing loss from the acoustic reflex. J. Speech Hear. Disord. 39, 11–22, 1974.

Lempert, J., Improvement of hearing in cases of otosclerosis: A new one-stage surgical technic. Arch. Otolaryngol., 28, 42–97, 1938.

Metz, D., The acoustic impedance measures on normal and pathological ears. Acta Otolaryngol (Suppl), 63, 1–254, 1946.

Michelson, R. P., Electrical stimulation of the human cochlea. Arch. Otolaryngol., 93, 317–323, 1971.

Newby, H. A., Audiology, Ed 3, pp. 157–159. New York: Appleton-Century-Crofts, 1972.

Noyes, H. D., Otitis media following the use of a bougie in the eustachian tube—introduction of an eyelet into the membrana tympani. Trans. Am. Otol. Soc., pp. 55–61, Nov. 1869.

Rosen, S., Mobilization of the stapes to restore hearing in otosclerosis. New York State J. Med., 53, 2650–2653, 1953.

Wullstein, H., Die tympanoplastik als gehroverbessernde Operation bei Otitis Media Chronica und irh Resultate. Proceedings of the Fifth International Congress on Oto-Rhino-Laryngology, 1041, 108, 1953.

chapter 3

NEUROLOGIC CONSIDERATIONS IN AUDIOLOGY

Leon Weisberg, M.D., and Jack Katz, Ph.D.

Some audiologists may consider a chapter on neurologic aspects of audiology to be premature, while others might consider this *Handbook* to be incomplete without it. The authors feel that an exchange of information between neurology and audiology is long overdue.

For a number of years audiologists and neurologists have worked closely in arriving at accurate differential diagnoses. In one community hospital 70 to 80% of all neurology patients were referred for audiologic evaluations because the neurologists found the auditory battery to be important with a wide variety of cases. Neuro-audiology (Baker, 1973) has great potential value in several areas. Not only do these tests help the patient and the neurologist but they aid the audiologist professionally in broadening his service base and upgrading the care he provides to his current patients.

The present chapter will briefly review the auditory anatomy from cranial nerve VIII to the brain. We shall then review the symptoms of neurologic disease; the neurologic and other medical tests which are generally used for diagnosis; specific disorders which disrupt central auditory function; and finally some case studies which illustrate the input of audiologic information into the neurologic diagnosis. Definitions are provided in parenthesis in the text and additional terms are listed in the glossary.

This chapter will complement the otologic and general medical information from the preceding and following chapters. Together, they provide a rather broad view of the disorders which affect the auditory process. These chapters provide an introduction or guide for the audiologist in understanding the terminology and test procedures used by his medical colleagues. It is hoped that by studying these and other chapters in the *Handbook* that the medical specialist will understand more fully how the study of hearing and central auditory function can help his patients.

For many years the field of audiology has been inextricably associated with problems of the "ear" and the medical specialty of otology. While the ear is unquestionably a most vital aspect, the concept of audiology is much broader. The name *audiology* refers to the study of the auditory process and not just to the ear alone. Many patients who are seen for evaluation have intact ears but significant auditory difficulty in the form of central dysacusis. Many individuals have hearing loss as well as central auditory nervous system (CANS) dysfunction. Audiologists should be in a position to understand both peripheral and central problems but to be able to evaluate them independently.

Patients who have hearing problems will usually complain of having difficulty in communication or not hearing certain aspects of their environment. This is not the case with many CANS disorders. Patients with subtle CANS problems are frequently unaware of auditory dysfunction in everyday situations because the internal redundancy of the auditory mechanism compensates for the lost or distorted information. Although there may be no gross abnormalities on standard hearing test performance, by simply adding one or two more specialized central procedures important information can be derived about CANS. The central auditory system primarily refers to the brain stem and brain.

ANATOMY

Audiologic tests are primarily "where" oriented. Like the radiologist and pathologist who are studying a disordered system, the audiologist is aided by a knowledge of the anatomy, symptoms and other test findings. We shall begin this brief anatomical review at cranial nerve VIII.

The eighth cranial nerve is a special sensory nerve which is concerned with hearing and equilibrium. The cochlear and vestibular nerves originate in the inner ear and pass through the internal auditory canal in the temporal bone along with the facial nerve to enter the brain stem in the region of the cerebellopontine angle at the caudal aspect of the pons. The cochlear nerve enters the dorsolateral brain stem and synapses in either the ventral or dorsal cochlear nucleus. Some fibers which synapse in the ventral nucleus have secondary fibers which pass upward ipsilaterally in the lateral lemniscus. The other fibers pass through the ventral cochlear nucleus decussate and synapse either in the trapezoid body or the superior olive and then enter the lateral lemniscus. Fibers entering the dorsal cochlear nucleus either synapse there and decussate to pass upward in the contralateral lemniscus or may continue through the nucleus without synapse and course to the contralateral superior olive where they ascend in the tract of the lateral lemniscus. Therefore, some second order fibers ascend ipsilaterally and others contralaterally in the lateral lemnisci.

The inferior colliculus in the midbrain receives afferent fibers from the lateral lemnisci which synapse there and also fibers from the dorsal cochlear nucleus which pass through the colliculus on their way directly to the medial geniculate body of the thalamus. At this level fiber connections exist between the two inferior colliculi to interconnect both sides. Third order fibers arise from the neurons of the inferior colliculus and project ipsilaterally to the medial geniculate body via the brachium of the inferior colliculus. Auditory fibers synapse in the thalamus and give rise to the major cortical projection system (auditory radiations) located in the sublenticular portion of the posterior limb of the internal capsule. The midportion of the anterior and posterior transverse gyrus of Heschl is the primary auditory reception area (Brodmann's area 41). The secondary auditory association area (area 42) lies inferiorly but adjacent to area 41. The majority of the geniculotemporal fibers from the medial geniculate body to the temporal lobe project to area 41 and the minority project to area 42. In addition, area 22 which lies medially and directly in front of areas 41 and 42 receives fibers from these two regions and has fiber connections with the parietal, occipital and insular cortex (Doig, 1972).

The primary auditory reception area is located on the opercular surface of the superior temporal gyrus. The auditory cortices are interconnected by associational fibers passing through the anterior commissure and the corpus callosum. Electrical stimulation of the cortical area of the superior temporal gyrus rostral to the primary auditory region evokes the sensation of vertigo and this area may be the primary vestibular cortical area. Electrical stimulation of Brodmann's areas 41 and 42 elicits the sensation of whistle-like noises which are usually heard in the ear contralateral to the stimulation (Truex and Carpenter, 1976). In addition to the classical language centers of the brain (Broca's and Wernicke's areas) there are centers for musical reception and expression (Kimura, 1961). These are thought to be located in the nondominant hemisphere for language but the exact location in either the frontal or temporal lobe is not clear (Wertheim and Botez, 1961).

SYMPTOMS

Sensory-neural involvement of the auditory system may be *peripheral* (i.e., inner ear or auditory nerve) or *central* as the nerve passes through the brain stem, cerebellum, thalamus, and cortex. To determine the anatomical level of involvement requires a knowledge of the associated signs and symptoms that accompany the auditory dysfunction. Auditory symptoms include hearing loss or tinnitus or they can be more complex and include poor speech discrimination and sound localization, hyperacusis, auditory misperceptions and hallucinations (DeJong, 1967). It is important to know if the auditory dysfunction is associated with other symptoms. Vertigo is a hallucination of movement. The patient has a disturbed sense of his relation to space in which he feels that he is spinning about his stationary environment or that his surroundings are spinning about him in either the horizontal or vertical direction. These episodes may be intermittent or constant, modified by position, and may be associated with nausea and vomiting. Dizziness is a sensation of light-headedness, giddiness, or floating, but there is no sensation of movement. These latter sensations usually do not result from dysfunction of the vestibular system.

The presence of headache is an important neurologic symptom. Most headaches are due to tension, i.e. muscular contraction, or vascular changes in the extra- and intracranial blood vessels. Tension-type headaches consist of a band-like quality, worse in the evening, occurring in the occipital cervical region. Vascular headaches are throbbing in nature and worse in the morning. Headaches due to a brain tumor may be related to the presence of increased intracranial pressure or traction on pain sensitive structures. These may be associated with nausea, vomiting, as well as blurring and double vision. The headache is increased by a change in the patient's position and may even awaken the patient from sleep at night. Symptoms of brain stem and cerebellar dysfunction include double vision, facial pain or numbness, difficulty with swallowing, hoarseness, slurred speech, unsteadiness or clumsiness, weakness, sensory disturbance in the body and limbs.

NEUROLOGIC EXAMINATION

The purpose of the neurologic examination is to delineate the abnormalities and localize lesions in the central nervous system. It is important to examine the patient's gait and station. The patient with cerebellar disease has a broad base, unsteady reeling gait, and cannot walk unsupported. Tandem (walking a straight line) gait requires a level of coordination not possible for a patient with cerebellar disease. If the pyramidal motor system is involved, the patient's base is normal and he is not unsteady but will demonstrate frank weakness when asked to arise from the sitting position or walk on his heels or toes. In patients with sensory or proprioceptive abnormalities the Romberg test is positive. In this test the patient is asked to stand with his feet together, first with his eyes open and then with his eyes closed. If the patient has proprioceptive impairment, he is able to remain steady with his eyes open but falls when asked to close his eyes. Patients with cerebellar disease cannot maintain the position with either eyes open or closed. In hysteria or conversion symptoms the patient sways from his hips and not from his ankles. He sways with a wide arc as if he will fall but is always able to regain his balance quite gracefully although with much effort.

If the patient's gait is abnormal because of balance difficulties, other tests of cerebellar function should be performed. These involve the ability to do rapid alternating movements including moving the heel down the shin and touching the finger to the nose rapidly. If the gait is abnormal because of weakness, the problem should be localized to both lower extremities or present on one side only. The patient's muscle tone and reflexes should be checked. If the pyramidal or corticospinal tract is involved, the weakness should be unilateral, tone increased on the side involved, and the reflexes brisk on the involved side with the presence of a pathologic Babinski response. The Babinski response is the most important indication of a pyramidal motor tract lesion and is characterized by extension of the great toe when the lateral aspect of the foot is stroked with a pin. If the peripheral nerve is involved (neuropathy) both the lower extremities should be weak with sensation and reflexes absent, and the tone of the extremities should be decreased. In patients with peripheral nerve disease different modalities of sensation should be checked and these include the ability to appreciate a pin prick as sharp, to recognize touch with a wisp of cotton, discriminate temperature correctly, and recognize the movement of his limb. In patients with a peripheral neuropathy these modalities would be lost first in the feet, then in the hands and later spread to involve the proximal portions of these extremities.

Cranial nerve function should be checked. Olfaction may be lost in patients who have suffered basilar skull fractures. The patient's sense of smell is tested by his ability to identify common odors such as peppermint and tobacco. Optic nerve function is evaluated by a visual acuity test and the use of an ophthalmoscope to check for papilledema (evidence of increased intracranial pressure) or optic atrophy. In patients with double vision (diplopia), extraocular muscle function is evaluated by asking the patient to look in all directions of gaze. The eyes should be conjugate in all planes. If there is double vision and dysconjugate eye move-

ments, further evaluation of extraocular muscle function is necessary with the use of a red glass cover test. Also, eye movements are studied for evidence of nystagmus in both the horizontal and vertical directions.

In patients with facial numbness or pain, the corneal reactivity to a wisp of cotton is checked and facial sensitivity evaluated with the use of the pin. In addition, motor function of the jaw muscles should be tested. Facial weakness can best be evaluated by judging the symmetry of both sides of the face around the eyes, the nasolabial fold, and the mouth. A gross neurologic test of auditory function is done by checking the patient's ability to hear a watch tick, understand spoken and whispered speech, and the use of tuning fork (Weber and Rinne) tests. To evaluate the lower cranial nerves the neurologist checks for the gag reflex, movement of the palate, shoulder shrug, and weakness of the tongue muscles.

LABORATORY STUDIES

Skull Radiographs

Conventional radiographic examination includes posteroanterior, anteroposterior, and lateral views. These should be adequate to determine evidence of a midline calcified pineal body, the size of the sella turcica, abnormal calcification, fracture lines, radiodense or radiolucent areas of the skull. In a patient with symptoms referable to cranial nerve VIII, special views which best demonstrate the temporal bone are carried out. Transorbital, Stenvers views and tomographic sections through the temporal bone are necessary in patients who present with: cerebrospinal fluid otorrhea (which can be caused by a fracture extending from the superior wall of the external auditory canal to the floor of the middle cranial fossa); facial nerve palsy; hearing loss; vertigo; or tinnitus. Stenvers projection allows a comparison of the symmetry of the internal auditory canal on the two sides and will demonstrate enlargement first of the canal and then erosion of the petrous pyramids in patients with acoustic neurinoma (Crabtree and House, 1964). Enlargement, erosive change, and asymmetry of the foramina at the base of the skull through which the cranial nerves emerge can best be demonstrated with carefully sectioned tomograms done in the coronal, sagittal, and horizontal planes. Glomus jugulare tumors arise in the region of the jugulare ganglion and may extend into the middle ear cavity. The earliest radiographic changes occur in the petrous, mastoid, and occipital bone and the hypoglossal canal. In addition, there is bony destruction of the jugulare foramen. Linear skull fractures can usually be detected with conventional radiographs but fracture lines at the base of the skull also require tomograms and in some instances may not be detected despite clinical indications of the presence of such a fracture. Standard skull radiographs may give an early clue to the presence of meningiomas, osteomas, chordomas, and cholesteatomas in the temporal bone.

Echoencephalography

This involves the use of high frequency sound to evaluate a possible shift of midline intracranial structures caused by a space occupying lesion—subdural hematoma, brain abscess, intracranial tumor, or intracerebral hemorrhage. It is a valuable test and involves no risk or discomfort to the patient. It can accurately predict a shift of the midline third ventricle. This shift usually occurs in patients with a large unilateral hemispheric (supra- or subtentorial) mass lesion in association with increased intracranial pressure and herniation of intracranial structures. A shift is unlikely to occur in patients with an intrinsic brain stem tumor or a small acoustic neurinoma.

Brain Scan

This involves the intravenous injection of a gamma-emitting radio isotope to detect the presence of intracranial lesions. Normally, the isotope remains in the intravascular space, but, if a lesion is present, the isotope accumulates in the abnormal region and can be detected by the scan. In evaluating patients with a possible hemispheric lesion, the brain scan is an effective screening procedure to detect the presence of a meningioma, glioblastoma, metastatic lesion, brain abscess, cerebral infarction, or subdural hematoma. It is less effective in evaluating the organs of the posterior fossa (brain stem, cerebellopontine angle, and cerebellum) because such tumors are usually small and are missed due to the limited resolving capacity of the isotope scan. In order to detect a tumor it must have a critical volume. Small tumors including acoustic neurinomas confined to the internal auditory canal will be undetectable by this scan, but, when they expand to involve the posterior fossa, they can be detected. In addition, slow growing and relatively benign tumors (gliomas, pituitary adenomas) will also give negative results.

Electroencephalography

EEG monitors the electrical events which occur in the brain and are picked up on the scalp by a series of unipolar and bipolar electrodes. EEG reflects superficial activity but frequently cannot detect activity originating in the deeper midline structures. Lesions distort normal tissue and normal electrical activity to produce abnormal discharges—slow waves and spikes. Epileptic spikes are seen both in patients with documented neuropathologic lesions and in those in whom no lesion can be detected (idiopathic epilepsy). The origin of the electrical discharges is not known but probably is generated by the cerebral hemispheres and upper diencephalon. Lesions involving the posterior fossa are unlikely to affect the EEG. A positive or abnormal EEG is an indication for a more careful study, but a single negative study does not rule out CNS disease as 20% of patients with epilepsy can have a single normal EEG. In addition, 5 to 10% of normal people without any neurologic symptoms or disease have nonspecifically abnormal EEGs (Kiloh, McComas and Osselton, 1972).

Cerebrospinal Fluid (CSF) Examination

Lumbar puncture should be done on any patient suspected of having meningitis or subarachnoid hemorrhage. If the clinical situation raises the suspicion of an expanding intracranial lesion, a lumbar puncture should be done unless there is evidence of increased intracranial pressure as demonstrated by the presence of papilledema. In that case lumbar puncture should be avoided because it can cause a shift of intracranial structures leading to tonsillar or tentorial herniation with clinical worsening of the patient's condition. Complete examination includes pressure determination, appearance of the fluid and cells, protein and sugar content determination, serology, and gammaglobulin determination.

Normally CSF pressure is 60 to 100 mm of water; if above this, it is diagnostic of intracranial hypertension and reflects the presence of a mass lesion. The CSF should be clear and colorless; if it is cloudy, meningitis or encephalitis should be suspected. If it is bloody or xanthochromic, subarachnoid hemorrhage should be suspected. The fluid should be acellular; the presence of white cells reflects infection and the presence of red blood cells suggests intracranial hemorrhage. The normal protein content is 15 to 50 mg per 100 ml; if elevated, it is a nonspecific indication of CNS pathology. The CSF sugar content should be two-thirds of the blood sugar content and if it is lower this suggests the presence of bacterial or tuberculous infection. Gammaglobulin should be 12% of the total protein content and if it is elevated, it suggests the presence of multiple sclerosis.

Pneumoencephalography (PEG)

This is a radiologic study of the ventricular system and subarachnoid spaces (cisterns). PEG uses air as the contrast medium. Air is injected through a lumbar puncture to fill the

CSF pathways. Following this procedure it is possible for the patient to develop an aseptic meningitis or a severe headache which may last up to 2 weeks. In this procedure air enters and outlines the ventricles and cisterns. A mass lesion will produce asymmetry and distortion of these structures. Lesions in the posterior fossa and enlargement of the ventricular system (hydrencephalus) are best detected by this procedure. Supratentorial lateralized mass lesions can be detected by PEG, but are best studied by arteriography.

Arteriography

This involves the injection of radiopaque contrast material into the arterial system (via the brachial, femoral, or carotid artery) to visualize accurately the intracranial vessels. This method best demonstrates vascular malformations, aneurysms, stenosis, and occlusion of the intracranial vessels and supratentorial lateralized mass lesions. Tumors produce displacements, stretching, shifts of intracranial structures and distortions of vessels. Posterior fossa lesions are best studied by brachial arteriograms which outline the vertebral basilar system.

Computerized Axial Tomography (EMI Scan)

This is a new noninvasive radiologic technique which utilizes scintillation detectors and a computer to calculate small changes in radiodensity. It can detect the presence of pathologic conditions and define their composition—hemorrhagic, cystic, necrotic, or solid—in a manner not previously available. The exact limitations of this procedure have not yet been defined, but it may bring about extraordinary changes in our ability to diagnose the CNS lesions accurately.

DISEASES AFFECTING AUDITORY FUNCTION

Congenital

Progressive hearing impairment is found in patients with Charcot-Marie-Tooth syndrome, Freidrich ataxia, and hereditary sensory neuropathy. In addition to the sensory-neural hearing loss, these patients have difficulty with balance, walking, and have impaired sensation (temperature, pain, vibration, and position sense) in their lower extremities and later in their hands. In these conditions abnormalities exist in the spinal cord, cerebellum, peripheral and cranial nerves which account for these symptoms. Progressive sensory-neural hearing loss is associated with retinitis pigmentosa, polyneuropathy and ataxia which comprise the Refsum syndrome. It is inherited as an autoso-

mal recessive trait and is due to an abnormality in the metabolism of phytanic acid. Other neurologic syndromes characterized by optic atrophy, mental retardation, nerve or muscle disease, pyramidal tract involvement with spasticity have been associated with deafness and have a known inheritance pattern. These syndromes have been reviewed by Konigsmark (1969).

Infection

Acute and chronic meningitis can produce significant nerve VIII involvement to cause hearing loss and vestibular dysfunction. The pathogenesis is related to the production of the meningeal inflammatory exudate about the nerve at the base of the brain. In addition, the microorganisms have a toxic effect on the nerve and may produce a vasculitis involving nerve VIII. Hearing loss, optic nerve atrophy and extraocular nerve palsies are the most common sequelae of cranial nerve involvement in meningitis but are less common in fungal meningitis. In addition, antibiotics used to treat meningitis can have a deleterious effect on an already damaged nerve VIII. Chronic granulomatous meningitis can occur with sarcoid and syphilis of the central nervous system and lead to prominent nerve VIII dysfunction. Rubella, syphilis, toxoplasmosis, and cytomegalic inclusion body disease can cause hearing loss in the newborn as a sequela to maternal infection.

Trauma

Basilar skull fractures present with bleeding from the inner ear, ecchymotic areas over the mastoid region (Battle's sign) and around the orbits (racoon eyes), rhinorrhea, anosmia (absence of smell), visual loss due to optic nerve damage, double vision due to extraocular nerve palsy, otorrhea, and decreased hearing. Fractures of this type may be missed unless tomograms through the base of the skull are done to show a small area of fracture. Closed head trauma can produce a fracture in the temporal bone and petrous pyramids which may lead to damage of the facial and acoustic nerves. Transverse fractures through the temporal bone are commonly associated with permanent hearing loss due to contusion or transection of the auditory nerve and also these patients may present with peripheral total unilateral facial nerve paralysis (Haymaker, 1969).

Toxins

Many drugs used as antibiotics and diuretics can produce hearing loss but are thought to be toxic to the hair cells of the inner ear rather than toxic to the eighth nerve. Metallic toxins—lead, mercury, and arsenic—and organic compounds can produce damage to the optic and peripheral nerves but have not been clinically noted to cause dysfunction of the auditory or vestibular nerve.

Metabolic Conditions

In patients with myxedema (hypothyroidism) the auditory component of nerve VIII is the cranial nerve most frequently involved. The incidence of diminished hearing sensitivity is 15 to 30% and both conductive and sensoryneural losses have been noted (Sanders, 1962). Tinnitus and vertigo are common symptoms in myxedema even in the presence of normal hearing sensitivity. Myxedema is treated by thyroid replacement.

Synthetic oral contraceptives have been implicated in stroke syndromes in young women by altering the coagulation mechanism and producing thromboembolic phenomena. These hormones have not been definitely implicated in hearing loss, but such patients frequently complain of dizziness and vertigo. Infants and children suffering from kernicterus due to blood incompatibility hemolytic disease often develop neurologic dysfunction which may be manifested as an extrapyramidal syndrome with athetosis and chorea. One-half of these patients will also have hearing loss and auditory imperception. The pathology is found in nerve VIII, cochlear nuclei, and central auditory connections as well as in the basal ganglion and cerebellum (Dublin, 1951).

Demyelinating Disease

Multiple sclerosis is a disorder involving abnormalities in the myelin sheath and in the white matter of the nervous system, such that there are multiple areas of demyelination scattered throughout the brain. Clinically, these patients tend to have periods of exacerbations and remissions so that the neurologic findings may be constantly changing and it is very difficult to predict the future course of the disease. The most frequent sites of lesions are the optic nerve, brain stem, cerebellum, spinal cord, and pyramidal motor system. Patients may present with visual loss, double vision, instability of gait, tremor of the extremities, urinary symptoms, spastic extremities or weakness of their extremities.

When the brain stem is involved, hearing abnormalities and vertigo may be prominent symptoms. Decreased hearing occurs in 6 to 20% of patients, but the actual incidence of involvement of the auditory system in patients with multiple sclerosis as determined by audiometry may be even higher. Equilibratory symptoms ranging from giddiness to true vertigo occur in 12 to 75% of patients with multiple sclerosis. Lateral or rotatory nystagmus is a

common sign in patients who complain of vertigo. Although some patients with multiple sclerosis will have diffuse but extensive demyelination involving both temporal lobes, it is rare for them to present with bilateral deafness which would occur on a cortical basis (McAlpine, Lumsden and Acheson, 1968).

Vascular Disease

Vascular disease of the CNS involves abnormalities in both the anterior (internal carotid, midline anterior cerebral arteries) and posterior (vertebral-basilar arteries) circulation. Vascular accidents (stroke syndromes) are defined as the onset of episodes of focal neurologic deficit due to hemorrhage, thrombotic or embolic phenomena involving cerebral blood vessels. The sudden onset differentiates the stroke syndrome from the more gradual and progressive history seen in patients who harbor tumors. When the symptoms and signs of neurologic dysfunction last less than 24 hours, they are called transient ischemic attacks (TIA) and may be repetitive and forewarn of future stroke syndrome.

The most common vascular syndrome involves the middle cerebral artery which supplies the frontal, parietal, temporal and part of the occipital lobe. Clinically, patients with this syndrome have contralateral hemiparesis, hemisensory loss, and homonymous visual field disturbance. If the dominant hemisphere is involved the patient presents with aphasia. Dysarthria is another symptom which is frequently noted. In most cases there is no hearing loss which is clinically detectable, but in some cases pure tone audiometric thresholds have been elevated in the ear contralateral to the involved hemisphere (Karp, Belmont and Birch, 1969; Goldstein et al., 1956). Etiology of the vascular disease is frequently stenosis or occlusion of the internal carotid artery with extension of the thrombosis to the middle cerebral artery. In addition, the patient with heart disease—rheumatic, arteriosclerotic or hypertensive—frequently embolizes to the middle cerebral artery from the endocardium or from the valvular system.

The vertebral basilar arterial system supplies the brain stem. The basilar artery is formed by the union of the two vertebral arteries at the lower edge of the pons and terminates by dividing into two posterior cerebral arteries at the pontine midbrain junction. A lesion in one or more of the several branching vessels in this system will produce characteristic brain stem syndromes which may involve audiologic and vestibular dysfunction (Haymaker, 1969). The vessels most frequently involved include the posterior inferior cerebellar artery (PICA), anterior inferior cerebellar artery (AICA), superior cerebellar artery, internal auditory artery, and quadrigeminal artery. Etiology of these vascular syndromes includes thrombosis of vessels with subsequent infarction of the brain stem, enlargement of the vessel wall due to aneurysmal dilatation with subsequent compression of the brain stem and its emergent cranial nerves or sudden hemorrhage from a vascular malformation.

The specific vascular syndromes of the posterior circulation include the following.

a. Wallenberg Syndrome Due to Involvement of the PICA. The PICA arises from the vertebral artery and supplies the dorsolateral brain stem. Patients present with sudden onset of vertigo, nausea, vomiting, incoordination or a stumbling gait. Neurologic signs include nystagmus, ipsilateral facial anesthesia, Horner's syndrome, ipsilateral cerebellar signs and contralateral anesthesia of the body and limbs. No obvious hearing loss has been reported but prominent vertigo and nystagmus are believed to be due to vestibular nuclei involvement.

b. AICA Syndrome. The AICA arises from the basilar artery and extends laterally across the pons into the cerebellopontine angle. It is rostral to nerve VIII as it supplies the cerebellum and dorsolateral pons. Patients with the AICA syndrome have a stumbling gait, double vision, facial paralysis. Neurologic findings include ipsilateral facial anesthesia, cerebellar signs, Horner's syndrome, facial paralysis, paralysis of the lateral rectus muscle, and contralateral anesthesia of the body and limbs. Frequently this vessel is injured with subsequent thrombosis and infarction during the course of the removal of an acoustic neurinoma.

c. Lateral Pontine Branch of the Basilar Artery Syndrome. The branch supplies the lateral lemniscus, trapezoid body, and superior olive. Thrombosis with infarction can produce unilateral or bilateral deafness (Haymaker, 1969). Usually it is associated with ipsilateral facial anesthesia, cerebellar signs, facial paralysis, and contralateral sensory loss of the body and limbs.

d. Quadrigeminal Artery Syndrome. The quadrigeminal artery is derived from the superior cerebellar artery and supplies the lateral lemniscus, trapezoid body, and tegmentum of the midbrain. Patients present with ipsilateral or bilateral hearing loss, hyperacusis associated with paralysis of the upward gaze and ptosis (Haymaker, 1969).

e. Internal Acoustic Artery Syndrome. Occlusion of this vessel which supplies the inner ear may produce sudden unilateral deafness associated with tinnitus. If the branch supplying the vestibular system is also involved vertigo may be a prominent part of this syndrome.

Syndromes producing hearing loss and ver-

tigo may be caused by vascular malformations. Abnormal communications between the arterial and venous systems are referred to as A-V malformations. These abnormalities can originate in the posterior fossa, but most frequently occur in the cerebral hemispheres. Posterior fossa vascular malformations may compress the lateral pons to produce a cerebellopontine angle syndrome, distort and thrombose branches of the basilar artery, or rupture to produce a subarachnoid hemorrhage. In patients with a cerebellopontine angle syndrome a possible diagnostic clue to the presence of vascular malformation is the fact that the patient had an episode of sudden worsening in symptoms and signs rather than a gradually progressive course. Arteriography is necessary to make the correct diagnosis. A-V malformations occurring in the posterior fossa are infrequent and comprise less than 15% of all cerebral malformations (Pool, Pava and Greenfield, 1970).

Other vascular malformations include aneurysms which are due to congenital weakness in a localized portion of the medial segment of an intracranial vessel. This results in a dilatation or bulging of the vessel. Intracranial aneurysms most frequently occur at the branch points of arteries and the most likely locations are the anterior cerebral-anterior communicating junction, the trifurcation of the middle cerebral artery and the junction of the posterior communicating-internal carotid artery. Aneurysms may rupture to cause subarachnoid hemorrhage. Patients present with headaches, stiff neck, abnormalities of consciousness, seizures and focal neurologic signs. CSF examination shows increased intracranial pressure and bloody CSF. Arteriograms will demonstrate the presence of the aneurysm and its exact location. Treatment is usually surgical removal because of the threat that the aneurysm may bleed repeatedly. When an aneurysm ruptures it does so at arterial pressure and blood may be directed into the plane of the temporal bone and therefore patients with subarachnoid hemorrhage may present with profound vertigo and nystagmus in addition to the headache and stiff neck.

Tumors

Of the tumors that produce audiologic and neurologic dysfunction, the most frequent is the acoustic neurinoma which is associated with the cerebellopontine angle syndrome. These tumors arise from the Schwann cells covering the eighth nerve and usually arise first from the vestibular portion and originate within the internal acoustic canal. As the tumor grows it expands out of the canal and into the posterior fossa producing the cerebellopontine angle syndrome. Early signs and symptoms relate to nerve VIII dysfunction (Dix and Hallpike, 1958; Hitselberger and House, 1964). Vertigo associated with nausea and vomiting may be the first symptoms. Hearing loss may first be noted by the patient as an inability to understand spoken speech and conversation on the telephone (Johnson, 1966). In addition, there may be an intermittent or constant ringing (tinnitus) in the ipsilateral ear. In association with the vertigo, unsteadiness is an early and frequently annoying symptom to the patient. The patient may be so unsteady that he is constantly falling and walks with a staggering gait as if drunk. In addition, patients harboring a small acoustic neurinoma have headaches which are occipital or posterior cervical in location, more severe in the evening, often awaken the patient from sleep, and are aggravated by coughing, straining, or sneezing. The origin of these headaches is unclear but it may be related to the barrage of aberrant vestibular impulses which are also responsible for producing the unsteadiness. Later in the course when the tumor has expanded and reached large dimensions it may distort and block the ventricular system so that the intracranial pressure is elevated. At this stage the headaches are of a different character and intensity as they now become pulsatile, associated with nausea and vomiting, and blurred double vision, and examination of the optic discs demonstrates papilledema.

As the tumor expands out of the internal acoustic canal into the posterior fossa, other cranial nerves in the cerebellum become involved and the clinical symptoms become related to involvement of these structures. Numbness and paresthesias (tingling sensation or burning) may occur over the upper face in the distribution of the ophthalmic branch of the trigeminal nerve if the sensory branch becomes involved. Occasionally, patients will have intermittent or paroxysmal sudden bursts of pain which simulate trigeminal neuralgia but do not respond to conventional treatment with Tegretol or Dilantin and are associated with decreased corneal sensitivity suggesting that a lesion is compressing the trigeminal nerve. Weakness of the jaw muscles due to involvement of the motor division of the nerve is less common. Facial paralysis due to involvement of the motor division of the seventh nerve also occurs later when the tumor reaches large dimensions. The tumor compresses the cerebellum and in addition to the unsteadiness which occurred in the early stage the patient now has difficulty with coordination and difficulty in carrying out fine coordinated movements. On examination the patient falls constantly toward the side of the lesion, has difficulty in performing rapid alternating movements which include the heel-to-shin and finger-to-nose test and also has slurred dysarthric speech. As the tumor further enlarges, other cranial nerves become involved. The patient complains of double vision due to involvement of the extraocular muscles supplied by the abducens, trochlear, and oculomotor nerves. Most frequently involved is the abducens nerve and such patients have double vision which is prominent on far gaze because of their inability to diverge their eyes. Involvement of the other lower cranial nerves can produce dysphagia, hoarseness, weakness of the gag reflex, palate, and tongue. Further involvement of the motor and sensory tracts which traverse the brain stem occurs very rarely and later in the course, but when they are involved they produce weakness, spasticity, hyperreflexia, and pathologic Babinski signs.

Acoustic tumors are the most common cause of the cerebellopontine angle syndrome, but other lesions which can mimic this tumor include cholesteatomas, ependymomas (glioma which grows into ventricle), meningitis, medulloblastomas, carcinomatous deposits, chordomas, choroid plexus papillomas, vascular malformations and arachnoiditis (Hambley, Gorshenin and House, 1964). Neurinomas most frequently arise from nerve VIII but can arise from cranial nerves V, VII and IX as well. When the tumor arises from the fifth nerve — in the region of the gasserian ganglion — the earliest symptom is upper facial pain or paresthesias, corneal anesthesia, jaw weakness, and lateral rectus weakness. Hearing loss, vertigo, and unsteadiness occur less frequently and later than in patients with an acoustic neurinoma. In facial nerve neurinomas unilateral facial paralysis and paresthesias occur early in the course. In glossopharyngeal neurinomas evidence of vestibular and auditory dysfunction occur early but swallowing difficulty and hoarseness are also present early. These latter symptoms would occur late in the course of patients with an acoustic neurinoma. Despite these distinguishing features patients with neurinomas arising from the other three cranial nerves may present with early evidence of nerve VIII dysfunction and mimic the angle syndrome.

Almost all acoustic neurinomas occur unilaterally but occasionally there is evidence of bilateral acoustic nerve involvement. Bilateral tumors may occur in patients with neurofibromatosis (Von Recklinghausen syndrome) and are associated with cafe-au-lait spots, neurofibromas, or depigmented skin lesions (Pool, Pava and Greenfield, 1970).

Acoustic neurinomas which grow into the cerebellopontine angle to compress the brain stem represent an extra-axial (extrinsic) mass.

Glial tumors (gliomas) of the brain stem are intra-axial (intrinsic) and arise in the substance of the pons and medulla. These tumors present with evidence of unilateral or bilateral cranial nerve involvement, prominent cerebellar and pyramidal tract findings and only in the late stages with evidence of elevated intracranial pressure.

Intra-axial tumors when present in childhood and early adolescence frequently produce multiple cranial nerve involvement. Early symptoms include double vision due to abducens nerve palsy and facial paralysis due to nerve VII involvement. These symptoms are later accompanied by prominent gait disturbance, dysequilibrium and dysarthria due to cerebellar involvement and weakness, hyperreflexia and Babinski reflex due to pyramidal tract involvement. The course is progressive and more cranial nerves are involved as the tumor extends to the midbrain and the lower medullary level. Because these tumors grow within the substance of the brain stem, the symptoms and the signs would be expected to be bilateral but not infrequently the hearing loss begins unilaterally. The peripheral part of the auditory nerve is less commonly involved and therefore hearing loss is usually less severe but there have been cases of intra-axial brain stem tumors producing hearing loss without evidence of peripheral auditory nerve involvement (Dix and Hood, 1973; Parker, Decker and Richards, 1968; Katz, 1970). The presence of hearing loss makes differentiation with an extra-axial tumor more difficult. Because the vestibular nerve is not involved, the caloric response is normal. If the central connections of the auditory and vestibular systems are involved in the brain stem, pure tone threshold may be elevated bilaterally or unilaterally and vertical nystagmus may be present on neurologic examination.

Other extra-axial tumors which compress the brain stem and produce an angle syndrome include meningiomas, cholesteatomas as well as tumors arising from the cerebellum, fourth ventricle, sella region (pituitary adenoma) and suprasellar region (craniopharyngioma, pinealoma). Meningiomas arise from the venous sinus of the petrous tip of the temporal bone and can mimic an acoustic neurinoma. Cholesteatomas are of two types; they may be congenital epidermoid tumors or may be secondary to chronic middle ear and mastoid infection. Otoscopy will show a perforation of the eardrum and the CSF protein is normal compared to the elevated level in acoustic neurinomas and meningiomas. Patients with cerebellar tumors present with headache, nausea, vomiting, and have early papilledema and prominent cerebellar signs and only late in their course of develop-ment will there be evidence of brain stem compression. Tumors of the ventricular system (ependymomas, choroid plexus papilloma) also present with early signs of increased intracranial pressure due to obstructive hydrocephalus but occasionally may present as a unilateral cerebellopontine angle syndrome. Tumors of the sella and suprasellar region present with endocrine disturbance, bitemporal visual field defects, and headache. Rarely they may extend in a retrosellar direction to compress the upper brain stem and can cause usually unilateral but occasionally bilateral deafness. Intrinsic gliomas of the midbrain cause aqueductal obstruction in hydrocephalus with early and prominent signs of increased intracranial pressure. These patients are unable to look in an upward direction and have impaired pupillary reaction to light. Occasionally, the lateral lemnisci and inferior colliculi are involved and the patients have bilateral hearing loss and hyperacusis (Bray, Carter and Traveras, 1958).

Tumors involving the temporal lobe include meningiomas, metastases, gliomas, and oligodendrogliomas (slow growing glioma). The symptomatology of such tumors can be very diverse depending upon the predominant area of involvement. If the dominant hemisphere is involved, the patient may be aphasic and have difficulty with language function. The visual projection system passes through the temporal lobe and if involved, the patient may have a homonymous field defect (contralateral to the involved hemisphere). Seizures occur frequently when the temporal lobe is involved and may be of grand mal or psychomotor type. In psychomotor seizures the patient may first complain of a taste, smell, visual or auditory hallucination which is then followed by an impairment of consciousness; the EEG shows abnormal discharges arising from the temporal region. The auditory and vestibular system terminate in the superior temporal gyrus. Each ear projects bilaterally but tests of auditory recognition and localization usually are impaired in tumors of the temporal lobe on the side contralateral to the tumor. Tinnitus and vertigo can occur with temporal lobe tumors and occasionally auditory hallucinations both of a formed and unformed type may precede the psychomotor seizures.

CASE STUDIES

In this chapter we have attempted to show that there is a large area of mutual interest among neurologists and audiologists. Most of the auditory anatomy and a great many of the conditions which involve hearing and auditory function lie in the realm of the neurologist. In our experience neuro-audiology has played an important role in the differential diagnosis of patients with neurologic disorders.

Four cases will be presented in this section. They were chosen simply on the basis of locus of lesion. For this reason they do not show the wide range of disorders which were discussed previously. We have seen many patients with multiple sclerosis, vascular disorders of the brain and brain stem, infection, trauma and numerous other conditions.

The tests which were used by the audiologists in each case were sufficient to locate the lesion. However, it would be premature to endorse any one test or test battery over any other.

Tumor of Cranial Nerve VIII and Brain Stem

A 21-year-old man was referred by an otologist for a hearing evaluation in December 1971. He complained of both tinnitus and decreased hearing in the right ear for 4 months. By December he had also begun to have headaches. Figure 3.1, A and B, shows his pure tone air-conduction thresholds (bone-conduction thresholds were equivalent to air-conduction) and word discrimination scores (WDS) for the right and left ears. The initial test shows thresholds and WDS to be essentially normal bilaterally except perhaps for 250 Hz threshold and slightly lowered WDS in the right ear. We have frequently found low frequency sensory-neural hearing loss in the early stages of brain stem disorders. Hearing loss is first noted in the *ipsilateral* ear in these cases (Katz, 1970).

The patient was retested four times in February 1972 because of a sudden drop in hearing

(February 2) followed by threshold improvement and fluctuations (February 10, 15 and 17). A 55-dB sensory-neural notch was found in the right ear on February 2 but not afterward. During February the patient noted some difficulty hearing in his left ear but a cursory test on February 17 did not demonstrate any significant change from that found in December.

In February a physician summarized some of the mounting evidence: (1) positive tone decay, right ear; (2) marked reduction in discrimination, right ear; (3) slurred speech at times; (4) when marching in place the patient deviated slightly to the right side; (5) positive Romberg (tending to fall to the right); (6) slightly decreased sensation in the left ear canal. Corneal sensations and reflexes were normal bilaterally and the caloric test was unremarkable.

In March the patient complained of an aching in his left ear and sharp pains in the back of his right ear. In April a posterior fossa myelogram showed the presence of a probable cranial nerve VIII tumor on the right side. There was elevated spinal fluid protein (120 mg/100 ml) and some unsteadiness of gait. By early April hearing had decreased further especially in the low frequencies (Fig. 3.1). In addition, WDS was very poor, tone decay reached the limit of the audiometer and the short increment sensitivity index (SISI) was 0%. At the same time the speech reception threshold (SRT) in the left ear was 0 dB and WDS 90%. In May 1972 a SISI test was administered but no increments of 4 dB or smaller were detected at 500, 1000 or 2000 Hz in the

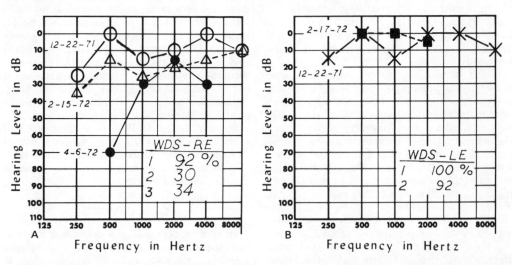

Fig. 3.1. Pure tone air conduction and WDS results for a patient with a right cerebellopontine angle tumor: (A) shows the information for the right ear from December, 1971 to April, 1972; (B) shows the results from December, 1971 to February, 1972. (Courtesy of Dr. Robert C. Meyer.)

right ear. They were easily identified in the left.

A right suboccipital craniectomy was performed in June 1972 to remove the tumor. It was located in the region of the internal acoustic meatus and extended medially. A partial removal of the tumor was necessary before the extent of the tumor could be visualized. Superiorly, it extended up to and possibly through the tentorium. The tumor was classified as a right cerebellopontine angle meningioma.

Because of the lengthy operation, it was decided to complete it in two stages. Two weeks later the patient was reoperated to remove the remainder of the tumor. However, respiratory complications arose and the patient expired. An autopsy showed the tumor to measure 3 × 3 × 3 cm, severely compressing the pons and the proximal portion of the medulla on the right side. It had extended into and enlarged the internal acoustic meatus. There was moderate vascularization with areas of vessel thrombosis. This might account for some of the fluctuations which had been found.

The staggered spondiac word (SSW) test of central auditory function was administered twice during the patient's illness (February 17 and April 6, 1972). The first time was when the patient's hearing was improving (speech averages: right ear = 22 dB, left ear = 2 dB, and WDSs were right ear = 30%, left ear = 92%). Figure 3.2 A shows the SSW-gram (for detailed

information about the test, see Chapter 23). This test suggested a lesion involving much of the right brain stem. The presence of severe tone decay on the right side indicates a retrocochlear disorder on the right (nerve VIII or brain stem). The poor discrimination indicates nerve VIII or low brain stem disorder but the moderate SSW score ipsilaterally indicates that the lesion also involves the middle or upper brain stem. Thus, there was evidence of upper and lower brain stem pathology and no evidence that it was not also a nerve VIII lesion, all on the right side (Katz, 1970; also see Chapter 20).

The second SSW test was given when hearing was more depressed in the right ear but WDS was essentially unchanged. The SSW-gram on the right side shows a greater nerve VIII or low brain stem effect than the previous SSW test. That is, the second test showed evidence of moderate as well as overcorrected scores in the right ear. The overcorrected portion in retrocochlear cases relates to nerve VIII or low brain stem locus, ipsilaterally. The moderate score indicates high brain stem dysfunction.

Tumor of the Cerebellum

A 48-year-old man was seen in April 1965 by an otologist because of "progressively increasing postural vertigo" over a period of 3 months with nausea and vomiting for the last month. The patient was referred for various medical studies (which were unremarkable) and an audiologic assessment.

Figure 3.3, A and B, shows the pure tone and WDS results for the right and left ears on two visits 1 year apart (January 1965 and January 1966). The initial test results in the left ear showed the patient to have normal hearing for the speech frequencies and a sensory-neural loss in the higher frequencies (bone-conduction and air-conduction thresholds were equivalent). There was a mild air-conduction loss in the right ear (speech average = 32 dB re ANSI-1969) and an air-bone gap of 12 dB for the same frequencies. WDSs were normal bilaterally and the Rush Hughes difference scores (see Chapter 21 for details about this test) were depressed (right ear = 30%, left ear = 28%). On the median plane lateralization test the patient had considerable difficulty locating the image in the left ear. The so called "final diagnosis" which was made at that time was focal brain stem encephalitis.

Due to the progression of symptoms the patient was seen again in December 1965. His dizziness was now termed "ataxia." For 3 to 4 months prior to the visit the patient had progressive headaches and visual loss. A neurologic examination revealed longstanding evi-

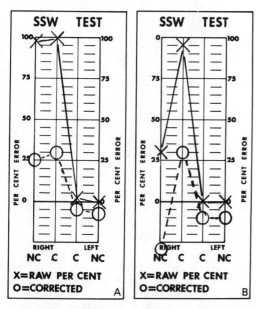

Fig. 3.2. R-SSW and C-SSW results for a patient with a right cerebellopontine angle tumor: (A) results for February 17, 1972; (B) results for April 6, 1972. (Courtesy of Dr. Robert C. Meyer.)

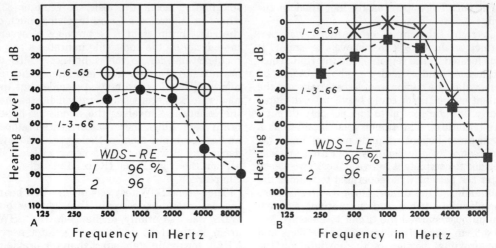

Fig. 3.3. Pure tone air conduction and WDS results for a patient with a tumor of the cerebellar vermis: (A) and (B) show information for the right and left ears, respectively. (Courtesy of Dr. C. P. Goetzinger.)

dence of papilledema, marked ataxia with sparing of the extremities, marked hypotonic and pendular reflexes.

On January 3, 1966, the patient was seen for an audiologic reevaluation. There was evidence of a small shift in threshold in the left ear, however, the high frequencies in the right ear were now similar to the loss in the left. The air-bone gap in the speech frequencies remained essentially unchanged (right ear = 10 dB) from the initial evaluation. WDS remained normal and essentially unchanged from the previous test, and lateralization continued to be markedly weakened in the left ear.

The SSW test was also administered to supplement the Rush Hughes difference test. Figure 3.4 shows the SSW-gram for this patient. Performance in the right ear was significantly depressed. Of considerable interest was the Order Effect low/high. In this case the patient made 20 errors on the second spondee and only 6 on the first spondee (although they were counterbalanced for left and right ears). We have noted the Order Effect low/high in a large percentage of cases with cerebellar lesions.

A brain scan was repeated at this time and it showed evidence of a lesion high in the cerebellar vermis. Surgery was performed and a nodular tumor was found in the vermis. The "final diagnosis" was papillary adenocarcinoma with metastasis to the vermis.

Cerebrovascular Accident Involving the Auditory Reception Center

A left-handed 41-year-old woman who complained about headaches was admitted to a hospital for examination on July 18, 1970. Although almost all of the tests were negative

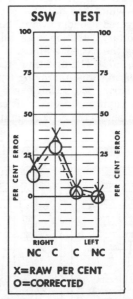

Fig. 3.4. R-SSW and C-SSW results for a patient with a cerebellar vermis tumor. The patient tended to make more errors on the second spondee, regardless of ear. This order effect was significant.

(e.g., brain scan and skull films), the lumbar puncture demonstrated some red blood cells. During this hospital stay she experienced a motor loss on the right side and aphasia.

She was transferred to a second hospital on July 21 because of more complete facilities. The standard physical examination was not remarkable. The neurologic examination showed "slight receptive aphasia and/or apraxia in that she follows directions poorly." The examination indicated flaccid paralysis and sensory deficit on the right side, as well as slightly increased reflexes as compared to the left side. Hoffmann and Babinski signs were not present at that time.

Bilateral carotid arteriograms were performed and a large aneurysm of the posterior communicating artery was noted at the junction with the carotid artery on the left side. An arteriogram was repeated because of the concern that a tumor was present but not visualized on the first arteriogram. No tumor was found but the impression was further enlargement of the aneurysm with slight upward displacement of the Sylvian vessels. A repeat of the brain scan now showed diffuse progression of radioactive uptake in the left hemisphere.

During the hospital stay the hemiparesis progressed and the patient developed a right homonymous hemianopsia. It was felt that surgery would be almost surely fatal and therefore she was treated conservatively and finally discharged. The diagnosis was "aneurysm, left posterior communicating artery; encephalomalacia secondary to intracranial hemorrhage from aneurysm."

Three years later the patient consulted another neurologist who was concerned about her general condition. On October 16, 1973, he admitted her to a hospital where speech, hearing, and other diagnostic services were available. By this time strong Hoffmann and positive Babinski signs were noted on the right side.

With regard to communication, the patient could point to pictures correctly but not to letters. When questions were composed of a number of words she was inconsistent in her responses. Her articulation contained distorted and substituted sounds. She was scheduled for aphasia therapy.

The patient's discharge summary noted, "Her major purpose in being in the hospital was for speech, occupational and physical therapy. These proceeded well and she was able to be discharged on November 21, 1973. Her speech has remarkably improved."

During the patient's stay she was tested twice using the SSW test. Figure 3.5 shows the patient's pure tone thresholds. Tone decay was negative and the SISI test was positive at 4K Hz. The second SSW test was much like the first except that the patient's WDS had stabilized at 90% in each ear. This test is shown in Figure 3.6. The *A curve* shown in this figure represents the adjusted SSW scores (the effects of response bias were compensated).

One unusual finding at this time was that the patient had extreme intolerance (hyperacusis) for signals in the left ear. The WDS and

SSW tests were administered at 30 dB to the left ear because she had severe pain above this level.

The severe SSW score in the right ear indicates an auditory reception problem in the left hemisphere. There were two reversals and a significant Ear (32/50) and Order (59/28) Effect. This combination suggested a disturbance in the shaded region shown in Figure 3.7. A neurologist's drawing of the affected region is also shown on the figure. The auditory recep-

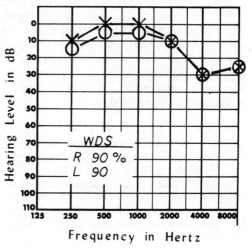

Fig. 3.5. Pure tone air conduction and WDS results for a patient with a left CVA involving the AR center.

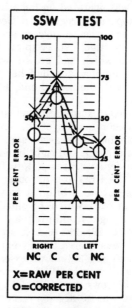

Fig. 3.6. R-SSW, C-SSW and A-SSW results for a patient with a left CVA involving the AR center. There were two reversals.

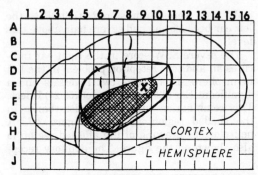

Fig. 3.7. The *shaded area* is the region implicated by the SSW test for a patient with a left CVA. The *unshaded area* was drawn by the neurologist as the region implicated by the neurologic examination and radiologic studies. The AR center which is included in both drawings is marked by X.

tion center is marked by an ×. The central auditory test was quite accurate in locating the brain dysfunction in the auditory reception center and the anterior temporal lobe.

It is quite possible that auditory tests would have revealed early evidence of this disorder. One advantage of audiologic tests beside their sensitivity is that CANS tests do not endanger the patient's health.

Nonauditory Reception Area Brain Tumor (Meningioma)

A 37-year-old woman with an 8-year history of seizures was operated on for a brain tumor (right frontoparietal region) on December 23, 1966. One year prior to surgery she developed "episodes of vertigo," suboccipital headaches, and dizziness which had grown progressively worse. In September she had her first grand mal seizure and, the second one, 1 week prior to surgery.

The neurologic examination revealed a slight decrease in coordination of the left arm and there was slightly decreased sensation on the right side of the face and right hand. A carotid arteriogram demonstrated a right frontoparietal tumor. The EEG and all other neurologic tests were negative. A brain survey was made using mercury-203 which revealed increased uptake in the right frontal region.

On December 29, 1966 (6 days after surgery) the patient was seen at the request of the audiologist. Figure 3.8 shows essentially normal hearing bilaterally. WDSs were normal.

Figure 3.9 shows the SSW test results. The C-SSW score was mildly depressed (indicating a nonauditory reception disorder), there was an Order Effect high/low, and a surprising 28 reversals. The Order Effect suggested that the

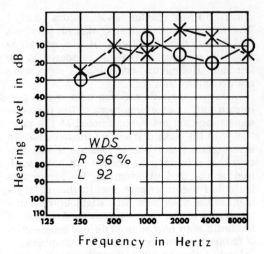

Fig. 3.8. Pure tone air conduction and WDS results for a patient with a right NAR tumor (removed).

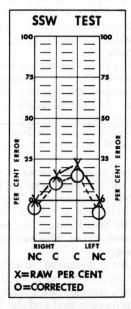

Fig. 3.9. R-SSW and C-SSW results for a patient with a right NAR tumor (removed). There were 28 maximum reversals.

disorder was in the anterior half of the brain and the reversals narrowed this down to an area along the fissure of Rolando shown by an × in Figure 3.10. The lesion drawn by the neurosurgeon is superimposed on it.

Summary

The four cases which were described are just a few of the hundreds of cases in our files which demonstrate that the brain and brain

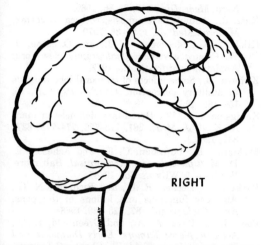

RIGHT

Fig. 3.10. Neurosurgeon's drawing of the tissue he removed in operating on this patient with a right NAR tumor. The region around the × was implicated by the large number of reversals on the SSW test.

stem are not outside the purview of the audiologist. A hearing-auditory assessment can provide surprisingly accurate indications of dysfunction in the CNS. Frequently, the audiologic manifestations have appeared before other signs so that early diagnosis was possible.

In order to provide this accurate, safe and relatively inexpensive service it will be necessary for both audiologists and neurologists to become familiar with neuro-audiology. The first step is for the audiologist to obtain training in the administration and interpretation of CANS tests. The next step is to incorporate central auditory tests into the routine or special test battery and the third step is to disseminate this information (the potentials and limitations of CANS tests) to the appropriate physicians.

GLOSSARY

Anosmia: loss of sense of smell usually due to impairment of the olfactory cranial nerve.

Battle's sign: discoloration (black and blue) due to ecchymosis behind the ear in the distribution of the posterior auricular artery occurring in skull fractures at the base of the skull.

dysphagia: difficulty in swallowing due to paralysis of lower cranial nerve function or direct muscular weakness.

fossa: compartment of brain: anterior—contains frontal lobe and parietal lobe; middle—contains temporal; posterior—contains brain stem and cerebellum.

glioma: an infiltrative and invasive tumor derived from the glial cells of low grade malignant quality. Glioblastoma is a highly malignant and rapidly progressive form of a glial tumor.

Horner's syndrome: the constellation of drooping of the eyelid (ptosis), small size of the pupil (miosis) and absent sweating (anhidrosis) on one side of the face.

hyperacusis: an abnormality of hearing characterized by a painful sensitivity to an intensity of sound not painful to normal individuals.

hyperreflexia: increase in reactivity of the deep tendon reflexes implying dysfunction of the pyramidal tract.

infarction: area of necrosis due to insufficient blood circulating or obstruction of blood flow by thrombosis or embolus to the blood vessel.

medulloblastoma: a malignant brain tumor which has a tendency to spread to the meninges.

meningioma: a well encapsulated benign brain tumor derived from the arachnoid villus.

neurinoma: tumor derived from Schwann cell origin and most likely involving the acoustic and vestibular nerve.

papilledema: elevation and blurring of optic disc margins and signifying increased intracranial pressure.

paroxysmal: sudden and episodic.

pyramidal tract: contains motor fibers which are involved in motor voluntary movement.

sarcoidosis: a multisystem disorder characterized pathologically by tuberculoid-like granuloma with predominant pulmonary involvement but not of infectious etiology.

subdural hematoma: a collection of blood and fluid in the subdural space acting as a space occupying lesion usually secondary to trauma.

tentorium: extension of dura that forms a partition between cerebral hemispheres and cerebellum.

vasculitis: inflammatory disease of blood vessels, i.e. systemic lupus erythematosus.

REFERENCES

Baker, R. H., The clinical neuroaudiologist (Letter to the Editor). *ASHA*, **15**, 683, 1973.

Bray, P. F., Carter, S., and Taveras, J. M., Brain stem tumors in children. *Neurology*, **8**, 1–7, 1958.

Crabtree, J. A., and House, W. F., X-ray diagnosis of acoustic neuromas. *Acta Otolaryngol.*, **80**, 695–697, 1964.

DeJong, R. N., *The Neurologic Examination.* New York: Harper & Row, 1967.

Dix, M. R., and Hallpike, C. S., The otoneurological diagnosis of tumors of the VIII nerve. *Proc. R. Soc. Med.*, **51**, 889–899, 1958.

Dix, M. R., and Hood, J. D., Symmetrical hearing loss in brain stem lesions. *Acta Otolaryngol.* **75**, 165–177, 1973.

Doig, J. A., Auditory and vestibular function and dysfunction. In Critchley, M. (Ed.), *Scientific Foundations of Neurology*. Philadelphia: F. A. Davis Co., 1972.

Dublin, W., Neurological lesions in erythroblastosis fetalis in relation to nuclear deafness. *Am. J. Clin. Pathol.*, **21**, 935–938, 1951.

Goldstein, R., Goodman, A. C., and King, R. B., Hearing and speech in infantile hemiplegia before and after hemispherectomy. *Neurology*, **6**, 869–875, 1956.

Hambley, W. M., Gorshenin, A. N., and House, W. F., The differential diagnosis of acoustic neuroma. *Arch. Otolaryngol.*, **80**, 708–719, 1964.

Haymaker, W., Localization of lesions involving the statoacoustic nerve. In *Bing's Local Diagnosis in Neurological Diseases*. St. Louis: C. V. Mosby Co., 1969.

Hitselberger, W. E., and House, W. F., Tumors of the cerebellopontine angle. *Arch. Otolaryngol.* **80**, 720–731, 1964.

Johnson, E. W., Confirmed retrocochlear lesions; Auditory results in 163 patients. *Arch. Otolaryngol.*, **84**, 247–254, 1966.

Karp, E., Belmont, I., and Birch, H. G., Unilateral hearing loss in hemiplegic patients. *J. Nerv. Ment. Dis.*, **148**, 83–86, 1969.

Katz, J., Audiologic diagnosis; cochlea to cortex. *Menorah Med. J.*, **1**, 25–38, 1970.

Kiloh, L. G., McComas, A. J., and Osselton, J. W., *Clinical electroencephalography*. New York: Appleton-Century-Crofts, 1972.

Kimura, D., Some effects of temporal lobe damage in auditory perception. *Can. J. Psychol.*, **15**, 156–165, 1961.

Konigsmark, B. W., Hereditary deafness in man. *N. Engl. J. Med.*, **281**, 713–720, 774–778, 827–832, 1969.

McAlpine, D., Lumsden, C. E., and Acheson, E. D., *Multiple Sclerosis: Reappraisal*. Baltimore: Williams & Wilkins Co., 1968.

Parker, W., Decker, R. L., and Richards, N. G., Auditory functions and lesions of the pons. *Arch. Otolaryngol.*, **87**, 228–240, 1968.

Pool, J. L., Pava, A. A., and Greenfield, E. C., *Acoustic Nerve Tumors: Early Diagnosis and Treatment*. Springfield, Ill.: Charles C Thomas, 1970.

Sanders, V., Neurologic manifestations of myxedema. *N. Engl. J. Med.*, **266**, 547–552, 1962.

Truex, R. C., and Carpenter, M. B., *Human Neuroanatomy*, Ed. 7. Baltimore: Williams & Wilkins Co., 1976.

Wertheim, N., and Botez, M. I., Receptive amusia; a clinical analysis. *Brain*, **84**, 19–30, 1961.

chapter 4

GENERAL MEDICAL CONSIDERATIONS IN AUDIOLOGY

Timothy N. Doyle, Ph.D., and
James E. Hoffman, M.D.

Hearing loss is known to occur in some systemic disease processes and is suspected in others. It is beyond the scope of this chapter to list the many genetic and congenital disorders associated with hearing loss as they may be readily found in standard texts (McKusick, 1968). Instead we have limited our discussion to the relatively more common disorders of hypothyroidism, diabetes mellitus and chronic renal disease.

For each disorder there will be a description of the anatomy and physiology of the involved organ, a resume of diagnostic tests, clinical features, management of the disease and selected literature dealing with audiologic aspects.

HYPOTHYROIDISM

Anatomy and Physiology

The thyroid gland is situated in the lower part of the neck at the level of the fifth, sixth and seventh cervical and first thoracic vertebrae. It is a bilobed organ with each lobe positioned laterally against the trachea, the isthmus being adapted to the second and third cartilaginous rings of the trachea. The vascular supply is the superior and inferior thyroid arteries and venous drainage is via the superior, middle, and inferior thyroid veins. Histologically, the thyroid gland is composed of secretory follicles. These follicles are the site of thyroid hormone synthesis and storage. The average weight of the adult human thyroid is 30 g.

The thyroid utilizes iodine in the synthesis of the biologically active hormones thyroxine (T_4) and triiodothyronine (T_3). The synthesis and release of these hormones is regulated by the pituitary thyroid stimulating hormone (TSH) and a hypothalamic thyrotropin releasing factor (TRF) (Fig. 4.1). The servomechanism for regulation of hormone release is basically a negative-feedback system where TSH release is inversely affected by the circulating level of T_3 and T_4. The circulating levels of thyroid hormone modulate the release of TSH from the anterior pituitary gland. When the thyroid hormone level falls, the inhibitory ef-

fect on the anterior pituitary is removed and TSH is released. This release of TSH again stimulates the thyroid gland to synthesize and to release T_3 and T_4 into the peripheral circulation. The hypothalamic releasing factor (TRF) effects the synthesis and release of TSH from the anterior pituitary gland, however, its complete role in the regulatory cycle is not completely understood. The complex integration of neurohormonal control of TSH synthesis and release can be reviewed in detail in other texts (Reichlin, 1971).

The metabolically active hormones affect cellular function by incompletely understood mechanisms. Data currently available suggest that specific sites in the cell nucleus are involved in the initiation of hormonal action (Oppenheimer, 1975). Since hearing loss is presently associated only with hypothyroidism, we will describe the signs and symptoms of this disorder.

Symptoms, Classification and Management

In the adult patient, symptoms of hypothyroidism are multisystem in origin and can include lethargy, cold intolerance, constipation, slowing of intellectual and motor function, and weight gain. Women frequently report menstrual disturbances. There may be loss of hair, dry skin, and hoarseness or change in voice. If untreated, the adult may develop mild hypothermia, puffiness of the face, enlargement of the tongue, nonpitting edema (myxedema), paresthesias and, on occasion, a psychosis referred to as "myxedema madness."

Severe hypothyroidism in infancy is called cretinism. The symptoms include somnolence, feeding problems and a hoarse cry. Abdominal protuberance, poor growth of hair and nails, and severe retardation of mental and physical development are characteristic features.

Although elaborate classifications of hypothyroidism are to be found, one can simplify the disorder by considering it to be either primary or secondary. The former places the failure of the system in the thyroid gland while secondary failure refers to defects in either the hypothalamus or pituitary. In secondary hypothyroidism the thyroid gland fails to produce T_3 and T_4 because of a TSH deficiency. Since T_3, T_4, and TSH assays are, in most instances, readily available, the diagnosis of hypothyroidism is easily confirmed and classified as either primary or secondary. Because of the existing variance in methodology for determining and reporting T_3, T_4 and TSH, we have not included any "normal" values.

The management of either primary or sec-

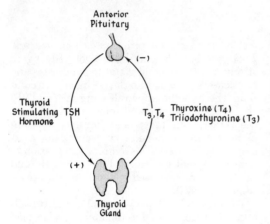

Fig. 4.1. Simplified feed-back loop process for thyroid function.

ondary hypothyroidism in the adult patient or infant involves the replacement of thyroid hormone. Although numerous preparations are available for replacement, including mixtures of T_3 and T_4, current data suggest the L-thyroxine (T_4) alone is the agent of choice for the treatment of hypothyroidism.

Review of Selected Literature

Hilger (1956), in a general discussion of the ear, nose and throat problems encountered with the hypothyroid patient, presented the first audiometrically documented cases of reversal of sensory-neural hearing loss. With hypothyroid patients presenting pure "inner ear," mixed, and otosclerotic hearing loss, administration of thyroid medication resulted in the improvement of bone-conduction sensitivity. Improvement of as much as 45 dB was seen at some frequencies, with typical improvement of 20 to 30 dB. Interestingly, in two patients with conductive hearing loss, the air-bone gaps remained constant.

Howarth and Lloyd (1956) discussed seven female patients with clinical hypothyroidism who ranged from 30 to 75 years of age. Pure tone air- and bone-conduction audiometry and some speech audiometry were obtained. These data were obtained prior to treatment. The three frequency (500, 1000 and 2000 Hz) averages were used to categorize degree of loss as well as improvement in hearing sensitivity after thyroid medication was administered. Five patients had sensory-neural hearing losses ranging from slight to very severe and two patients had severe mixed hearing losses. Pure tone improvement was more than 20 dB (three frequency average) for one patient with a sensory-neural hearing loss and one with a mixed hearing loss. Two of the patients with sensory-

neural hearing loss had slight improvement (5 to 10 dB). The three remaining patients had no improvement. In the patient with mixed hearing loss, threshold sensitivity improved bilaterally, but relative air-bone gaps were retained. Howarth and Lloyd (1956) concluded that, in hypothyroidism, any related hearing loss was sensory-neural.

Ritter and Lawrence (1960) discussed two patients with sensory-neural hearing loss documented by air- and bone-conduction audiometry. In one patient, the hearing loss and hypothyroidism were thought to be the result of ingestion of potassium thiocyanate (a thyroid depressive medication) for management of myocardial infarction. Thirty-three days after thiocyanate therapy was discontinued, audiometry revealed a substantial improvement in bone-conduction sensitivity (Fig. 4.2). The other hypothyroid patient was placed on thyroid supplement. Hearing improvement was determined by air- and bone-conduction audiometry about 3 months later and did not show the same magnitude of improvement demonstrated by the first patient. However, the three frequency average improved 12.5 dB for the right ear and 18 dB for the left ear. It is interesting that with these two patients the sensory-neural hearing loss was reversed in one case by eliminating a thyroid depressant medication. In the other case, the loss was reversed by introduction of a thyroid supplement medication.

DeVos (1963) discussed 32 hypothyroid patients who were evaluated audiometrically and otologically and were reported to be free of conductive hearing loss. Normal hearing was found in 15 of these patients. Two patients had severe hearing impairment and were diagnosed as having Pendred's syndrome. Ten of the patients had 20 to 30-dB losses; three were described as moderately severe due to additional loss at the high frequencies. There was one patient with unilateral loss and one with severe bilateral hearing loss with vertigo. All were treated medically for hypothyroidism. When thyroid and metabolic function had returned to normal and "a number" of cases were retested audiometrically, no hearing improvement was demonstrated. Unspecified tests for "fatigue" and "variation in limen differences" were administered pre- and post-treatment. The author reported that there was a lack of recruitment by these measures, and therefore, the results were suggestive of "neural" or "central" sensory-neural hearing loss.

Post (1964) discussed two groups of hypothyroid patients. The first group ($N = 7$) was primary hypothyroid patients who were evaluated by air- and bone-conduction audiometry

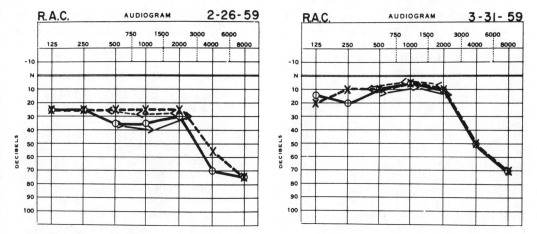

Fig. 4.2. Improvement in pure tone sensitivity following withdrawal of a thyroid depressant medication (potassium thiocyanate). (From F. N. Ritter and M. Lawrence: *Laryngoscope, 70,* 393–407, 1960. Reprinted with permission.)

and in some instances by speech audiometry. In this group, treated with thyroid supplement, only one patient demonstrated improved pure tone threshold sensitivity. For this patient the three frequency average improvement was less than 5 dB for the right ear and 15 dB for the left ear. It should be noted that there was threshold improvement at 8000 Hz of 35 dB for the left and 40 dB for the right ear. The second group of hypothyroid patients ($N = 35$) was hypothyroid as a result of thyroidectomy for carcinoma. In the course of treatment, these patients were hypothyroid (without thyroid supplement) for "generally" 6 weeks when audiometric data were obtained. Hearing loss was present for nine of the patients. These patients were retested 3 to 12 months after the thyroid supplement was reintroduced. In this group, improvement in hearing, compared to the hypothyroid state, was "minimal/mild" for three patients by audiometry and there was subjective improvement for one patient without improvement by audiometry. However, no audiometric data were reported. There were five patients who had "abnormal" audiograms while hypothyroid, but no improvement was noted in the loss when euthyroid (normal). The other 26 patients had "normal" audiograms while hypothyroid and reported no subjective change in hearing when euthyroid. It should be noted that of the 35 patients in this group, 31 were hypothyroid for 6 weeks or less and 4 were hypothyroid for 8 to 12 weeks. This duration of a hypothyroid state may not be sufficient to induce hearing loss.

Ritter (1967), in a major study of ear, nose and throat problems associated with hypothy-roidism, reported that in acquired hypothyroidism nasal discharge and obstruction, while not common, do occur. The nasal symptoms resulted from fluid accumulation (myxedema) in the submucosa as well as hypertrophy of the mucous glands. In the larynx, fluid accumulation in the submucosa of the vocal cords results in hoarseness and an easily fatigued "raspy" voice. Ritter attempted to determine the relationship between hypothyroidism and hearing loss using laboratory rats conditioned to respond to pure tone signals. Behavioral audiograms were obtained before and after radioiodine destruction of the thyroid gland. Results obtained from 166 rats suggested no causal relation between hearing loss and hypothyroidism. Of the 166 rats, 5 developed some degree of hearing loss. However, all 5 had middle ear disease when temporal bones were examined. The hearing loss in 4 of the rats was 30 dB, not inconsistent with a "pure" conductive loss and the analysis of the temporal bones revealed no significant changes. The single remaining rat had a hearing loss of 45 dB as well as some edematous swelling of inner ear tissues. Ritter reported that the experimental rats may have resisted any auditory effects of hypothyroidism in some unknown manner particular to the animal. For example, it was known that these rats were immune to dihydrostreptomycin ototoxicity.

Kohonen et al. (1971) used 19 hypothyroid guinea pigs. The hypothyroid state was artificially produced by the destruction of the thyroid gland with injections of radioiodine. Cochlear microphonic potentials were recorded and compared with the potentials of 17 control guinea pigs. Analysis of iodine uptake suggested that 6 to 8 months were required for maximum hypothyroidism to occur in these animals. Otitis media was observed in 10% of the experimental ears and these ears were excluded from the study. Results of cochlear microphonic measures obtained at 250 to 4000 Hz at sound pressure levels (SPLs) of 60 to 100 dB suggested lower microphonic potentials for the hypothyroid guinea pigs at all frequencies and all SPLs. The lower potentials were most obvious at 500 Hz and 1000 Hz. Analysis of 33 temporal bones for the hypothyroid group suggested that for 8 ears there was a slight to moderate loss of hair cells in the apical end of the cochlea. However, when cochlear microphonic recordings were compared, there was no significant difference between hypothyroid guinea pigs with or without hair cell loss.

The same experiments were repeated in 14 *hyper*thyroid guinea pigs. There were no significant differences in the cochlear microphonics or in the histologic results when compared to the control guinea pigs.

Summary

The incidence and severity of hearing loss with the hypothyroid patient have not been adequately described. Apparently, a reversible sensory-neural hearing loss can be expected in a small proportion of these patients. However, in our judgment, the paucity of data in the literature reviewed by the authors suggests that an adequate description of the auditory function of the hypothyroid patient might be obtained with more careful research from the audiologist and physician. Factors such as medical history, drug regimens, thyroid function assays, and duration and severity of the hypothyroidism must be coordinated with more complete audiologic evaluations.

DIABETES MELLITUS

Anatomy and Physiology

Diabetes mellitus is a disease process caused by a relative or absolute deficiency of the pancreatic hormone insulin. The pancreas is a bilobed gland with a convoluted surface which extends across the posterior abdominal wall from the region of the duodenum to the spleen. It is approximately 15 cm in length. The arterial supply to the pancreas is from the splenic artery and the pancreaticoduodenal arteries. Venous drainage is into the portal, splenic, and superior mesenteric veins. The pancreas, in addition to secreting enzymes necessary for digestive processes, synthesizes and secretes the hormone insulin. Insulin production occurs in specialized ductless tissue (islets of Langer-

hans). Although these islets comprise only about 1% of the gland's total weight, each gland has approximately 2 million islets.

Etiology, Symptoms and Management

As many factors can be involved in causing diabetes, it would be an oversimplification to say that all diabetics have the same basic cellular dysfunction. It is known that the disease is a familial disorder with a multifactorial pattern of inheritance and is clearly influenced by environmental factors such as diet, obesity, infections, medication and aging.

In the absence of insulin, glucose utilization is impaired and hyperglycemia (elevated blood glucose) develops. As impaired glucose utilization deprives the body of its primary source of energy, the metabolism of the other substrates, protein and fat, occurs. In acute diabetes mellitus the inability to utilize glucose for energy promotes the breakdown of fat stores (lipolysis) and causes an excess production of "ketones" by the liver. This excess production results in ketonemia (ketones in the blood) and ketonuria (ketones in the urine). Excessively high ketonemia can cause ketoacidosis which may result in coma and death.

In the chronic form of diabetes mellitus, weight loss, increased susceptibility to infections, loss of strength, polyuria (excessive urination), polydypsia (excessive water drinking), and polyphagia (excessive hunger) may be observed. Other symptoms develop over longer periods of time and appear to be the end result of microvascular complication. These symptoms are organ-specific complications that can involve the kidneys, myocardium, eyes and nervous system.

The mechanism by which elevated glucose levels are suspected to cause complications may be attributed to "alternative pathways of glucose metabolism" (Gabbay, 1973). Since glucose utilization in the body is primarily an insulin dependent process, the lack of insulin increases the flow of glucose into other metabolic pathways.

The pathway which has generated the most interest is the "polyol pathway." In this pathway glucose is first reduced to sorbitol (sugar alcohol) and is then oxidized to form fructose. Since the oxidation of sorbitol to fructose cannot be accelerated or increased (rate-limiting step), significant quantities of the osmotically active sorbitol accumulate intracellularly. The intracellular hypertonicity or disequilibrium that exists between the extracellular and intracellular fluids promotes an influx of water into the cell causing cell damage and dysfunction. This non-insulin dependent pathway has been found in most tissues in the body including the lens of the eye, major arteries, brain and peripheral nerves and is thought to play a prominent role in the development of diabetic complications.

In diabetes mellitus there is extreme variability in the clinical expression of the disease. The onset of angiopathy (disease of the blood vessels) is unpredictable, as is the onset of the neuropathy (disease of the nerves). In the case of diabetic neuropathy, exacerbations and remissions of the clinical symptoms are common.

In an otherwise healthy individual, a fasting blood glucose level in excess of 110 mg/100 ml or an abnormal glucose tolerance test confirms the diagnosis of diabetes. The delayed disappearance of glucose from the peripheral circulation constitutes an abnormal glucose tolerance test. The procedure and upper range of normal are seen in Figure 4.3.

The treatment of diabetes mellitus involves a controlled diet frequently in combination with either insulin or the use of medication that enhances the release of insulin from the pancreas. The therapeutic regimen is designed for the individual diabetic and, ideally, the goal is to maintain the blood sugar level within a normal range at all times. With the currently available agents, the "ideal" is infrequently accomplished.

Review of Selected Literature

Jorgensen and Buch (1961) discussed 69 diabetic patients ranging from 16 to 73 years of age. The duration of the diabetes ranged from 1 month to 33 years. Based on air-conduction audiometry, 39 patients were found to have hearing loss, 28 of which were felt to be the result of diabetes. Of these 28 patients, 20 were 53 years of age or younger. While there tended to be more hearing loss in the older patients, there was significant loss present for all age groups. There did not appear to be a "distinct" correlation between duration of the diabetes and degree of hearing loss. However, it was reported that hearing loss was twice as common in patients with severe retinopathy (disease of the retina) compared to those with no retinopathy. In addition, for patients under the age of 40, 7 of 14 had hearing loss and nephropathy, but in cases without nephropathy (disease of the kidney), only 6 of 30 had hearing loss. The authors concluded that when hearing loss occurs, the loss tends to be sensory-neural, slowly progressive and bilateral with more loss at the high frequencies. Tests for cranial nerve function, vestibular function, and cerebellar function were essentially negative.

In a later article, Jorgensen (1963) found that there were obvious histologic changes in the temporal bones of diabetics, namely thickening of the capillaries in the stria vascularis, but such changes are not specific to diabetes. These changes are also found in arteriosclerosis, although according to Jorgensen (1961) the effect of arteriosclerosis decreased the more peripheral the vascular system, while diabetic angiopathy had a "predilection" for only the stria vascularis in the inner ear.

Zelenka and Kozak (1965) discussed 17 diabetic patients ranging from 8 to 40 years of age. While none of the diabetic patients complained of hearing loss or vestibular symptoms, air- and bone-conduction audiometry suggested some slight sensory-neural loss for the group. For those patients who had been diagnosed as

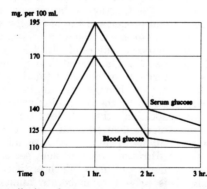
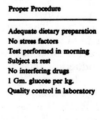

Fig. 4.3. Upper limits of normal glucose tolerance test. At least two glucose determinations must be elevated before a diagnosis of diabetes mellitus can be made. The glucose in plasma or serum is 15% higher than in whole blood. (From J. M. Moss, D. E. DeLawter, and C. R. Meloni: *Monograph:2 Diabetes*, 1974. Published by American Family Physician. Reprinted with permission.)

diabetic for less than 3 years, there was a "slight" hearing loss with a maximum 18 dB loss at 3000 Hz (reference unspecified). For those patients diagnosed as diabetic for more than 3 years, the maximum loss was approximately 35 dB at 3000 Hz (reference unspecified). In addition, data suggested some slight conductive losses. Vestibular testing suggested "minute but perceptible" deviations from normal. No descriptions of these deviations were presented. Based on these data and angiologic reports, the authors concluded that 75% of these diabetic patients had hearing loss and/or vestibular problems resulting from diabetic angiopathy.

Marshak and Anderson (1968) discussed 30 diabetic patients ranging from 11 to 43 years of age. The mean duration of the medically diagnosed diabetes was 11 years. All subjects reported a negative history of ototoxic medication, head trauma, noise exposure, familial hearing loss, or otologic disease and were otologically normal at the time of testing. For each patient air- and bone-conduction thresholds were obtained and fixed-frequency Bekesy thresholds (pulsed and continuous) were obtained from the better ear at 500, 2000 and 4000 Hz. No subject demonstrated poorer than 20 dB (ISO-1964) pure tone thresholds and air- and bone-conduction gaps did not exceed 5 dB. Results of the Bekesy tracings suggested "positive" (continuous poorer than pulsed by more than 5 dB) responses in 43% of the subjects at 4000 Hz. The possible interpretations of these results were: (1) the established angiopathy in diabetes resulted in pathologic response on Bekesy audiometry or (2) this group simply reflected a normal range of auditory function for Bekesy tracings. Marshak and Anderson (1968) favored the former interpretation, but noted that further investigation would be necessary to validate this interpretation.

Brunt (1969) obtained audiometric data from 40 diabetic subjects and 40 control subjects matched for age and sex. These subjects ranged from 16 to 61 years of age. The purpose of the study was to evaluate diabetics and controls on the following measures: air conduction (250 to 8000 Hz), bone conduction (500 to 4000 Hz), Owens tone decay, staggered spondaic word test, median plane localization, speech discrimination (W-22 and Rush Hughes recordings), speech reception threshold, fixed frequency Bekesy audiometry, and short increment sensitivity index (SISI). Blood sugar levels were monitored by blood analysis, samples being obtained before, during and after audiometry. Results suggested that for all measures except the Owens tone decay and the Rush Hughes discrimination test, there were no significant differences between the diabetic group and the matched controls. Brunt (1969) concluded that

while the diabetic may "exhibit somewhat less efficient auditory function," no generalized statement regarding hearing loss could be made. It is possible that retrocochlear pathology may result from the widespread angiopathy and/or neuropathy in the diabetic. Additional research utilizing distorted speech and measures of threshold fatigue should be used to clarify the effect of diabetes on the auditory system.

Summary

The lack of uniformity in the literature regarding diabetes mellitus and hearing loss underscores the variability in the disease process itself. As noted earlier, the clinical profile of diabetes is extremely varied. In addition, the manifestations of the disease at the individual level are equally difficult to predict. As an example, some relatively severe diabetics may not develop "diabetic" retinopathy for 25 years or more. Therefore, hearing loss directly related to diabetes may be difficult to isolate and describe.

CHRONIC RENAL DISEASE

Anatomy and Physiology

The kidneys are positioned on each side of the vertebral column extending in length from the twelfth thoracic vertebra to approximately the third lumbar vertebra. Each kidney weighs approximately 150 g in the adult male and 135 g in the adult female. They are surrounded by adipose tissue and are behind the peritoneal lining of the abdominal cavity, which separates the kidneys from the abdominal viscera. The vascular supply to the kidneys is the right and left renal arteries arising from the aorta. Venous return is via the right and left renal veins to the inferior vena cava.

The function of the kidneys is to excrete the end products of the body's metabolic processes and to control the concentrations of the constituents of body fluids. In this process, a plasma-like fluid is filtered through glomerular capillaries into the renal tubules. As this filtrate passes through the tubule, the volume is reduced by the removal of water and solutes. In addition, the tubules, through a secretory mechanism add solutes to the filtrate in the tubule. The net result of all these processes (filtration, reabsorption, secretion) is the formation of urine. Each of these intricate steps is subject to elaborate humoral and neural control mechanisms (homeostatic regulatory mechanisms).

Symptoms and Management

The normal kidney, through these mechanisms, protects the cells of the body from changes in electrolytes and water concentrations that would otherwise cause dysfunction. The kidneys are able to preserve the intra- and extracellular homeostasis until approximately 90% of normal functional capacity is destroyed. The abnormal water and electrolyte concentrations and end products of metabolic processes accumulate because the residual renal function is incapable of the adjustments necessary for normal cellular function. Specific symptoms develop as a consequence of renal dysfunction and will be mentioned individually.

1. Water and Sodium. With renal failure, the ability to excrete water may be impaired, resulting in water retention and, by dilution, a lowering of serum sodium levels. This can cause irritability and confusion, followed by lethargy and finally convulsions as the sodium levels fall from the normal range of 135 to 145 meq/L (a standard method of expressing the relationship of the weight of a dissolved substance to a given volume of fluid) to 100 meq/L. This state is referred to as water intoxication.

2. Potassium. In the terminal stages of renal failure, elevated serum potassium levels are common. Levels of 7 meq/L (normal 3.5 to 5.5 meq/L) may occur without producing clinical symptoms and cause death by cardiac arrest. Occasionally complaints of muscle weakness and paresthesias may precede death.

3. Magnesium. With the progression of renal failure, hypermagnesemia may develop with serum levels reaching 3.5 to 8.0 meq/L (normal 1.5 to 2.5 meq/L). This is due in part to medications such as antacids and cathartics which contain magnesium. In these instances, drowsiness and muscle weakness have been observed. Impaired nerve conduction occurs in hypermagnesemia, however, the role of hypermagnesemia in the neuropathy of chronic renal disease is unclear.

4. Acid-Base Disorders. A metabolic acidosis develops in renal failure with bicarbonate levels reaching less than 10 meq/L (normal 24 to 30 meq/L) in the preterminal patient. The acid produced in the body is only partially excreted by the failing kidneys, ultimately causing a fall in plasma bicarbonate levels. Another compensatory mechanism for the correction of the acidosis involves the respiratory system where deep, rapid breathing originally described by Kussmaul may develop.

Other compounds implicated in the production of clinical symptomatology are urea, uric acid, and the "uremic toxins" (guanidines, amines, and phenolic acids). The uremic toxins have, in animal models, caused vomiting, convulsions, and coma much like those observed in humans with renal failure.

Other findings in chronic renal disease include high blood pressure, which may occur in as many as 80% of those involved, anemia, edema, muscle weakness and peripheral neuropathy. The latter is characterized by numbness of the toes and feet with the painful sensation of burning hyperesthesia (abnormally increased sensitivity of the skin or of an organ of special sense). Nerve biopsies show the histologic appearance of demyelination and degeneration. The cause of the sensory and motor dysfunction remains speculative. However, correction of these symptoms can follow intensive hemodialysis or renal transplantation (Mitschke et al. 1975).

While both acute and chronic renal failure may require the same medical procedures (medication, hemodialysis, and/or transplantation), the relationship between renal disease and hearing loss has been established primarily with chronic renal disease.

Since the description of the relationship between renal disease and hearing loss by Alport (1927), there is clear evidence that the medical treatment of renal disease may involve the hearing mechanism. As the treatment for renal disease has become more efficient and the life expectancy for the renal disease patient has increased, hearing loss has become a significant side effect.

Review of Selected Literature

Beaney (1964) reported that of 262 chronic hemodialysis patients, 5 had some degree of vestibular disturbance and 1 had a hearing loss. At autopsy the patient with hearing loss was discovered to have had a cerebellopontine angle abscess. The 5 patients with vestibular defects reported a remission of symptoms with dialysis. Beaney discussed other ear, nose and throat problems with these patients which included epistaxis (nosebleed) and respiratory insufficiency.

Beaney also suggested that hemodialysis might explain the *low* order of apparent ototoxicity in his patients. As an example, while the half-life of streptomycin with normally functioning kidneys is 2.4 hours, in cases with severe renal failure the drug may not be cleared for 20 days. Thus, the partial clearing of the non-plasma bound streptomycin by hemodialysis might reduce ototoxic effects.

Ransome et al. (1966) discussed 20 patients with renal disease; 14 were treated with hemodialysis and Polybrene (hexadimethrine bromide). Five of the 14 developed severe sensory-neural hearing loss which was documented by pure tone audiometry. However, due to the illness of these patients, pretreatment audiometric data were not obtained. Further, while the configuration of the air-conduction losses would suggest a sensory-neural hearing loss, no other audiometric data were obtained. Ransome et al. concluded that the use of Polybrene was the significant factor in causing hearing loss in these patients. In addition, hearing loss became evident 3 to 8 months post-dialysis/ Polybrene treatment. Finally, after use of Polybrene was discontinued there were no additional cases of hearing loss resulting from dialysis for a period of more than 2 years.

Audiometric data were obtained on 71 of the 114 patients in renal failure discussed by Yassin et al. (1970). These cases included both chronic and acute renal failure. Of these 71 patients, 53 were reported to have moderate to very severe sensory-neural hearing loss. The degree of loss was determined by computing the American Medical Association percentage of hearing loss. Audiometry and recruitment test data were not presented and there was no discussion of pre-renal failure hearing function or other otologic history. The renal disease was treated "in most cases" by hemodialysis.

The authors reported that after hyponatremia (low blood sodium) was returned to normal levels, hearing improved in 80% of the acute renal cases and 52% of the chronic cases. Unfortunately, no audiometric data were presented nor was the degree of improvement discussed. In addition, it was stated that for 23 patients who reported tinnitus, normalization of hyponatremia resulted in improvement or "cure" of the tinnitus. There were no changes in hearing related to blood urea, serum potassium, blood hemoglobin, sex or age.

Bergstrom et al. (1973) discussed selected cases from a population of 224 patients with chronic renal disease. Audiometry included air- and bone-conduction, speech discrimination, high frequency (8 to 18 kHz) thresholds, and a retrocochlear battery. In addition, caloric and electronystagmography (ENG) data were obtained. Although pure tone data and speech results were reported in selected cases, there was no audiometric description of the population. Of the 224 cases, 80% were 40 years of age or younger, most had been managed by hemodialysis and transplantation, and 97 had hearing loss. There were 91 patients with sensory-neural or mixed hearing loss, and 6 patients with conductive hearing loss.

The authors also noted that while emphasis was placed on the patients with hearing loss, there were 127 patients who did not have hearing loss. In addition, of those patients who did present sensory-neural hearing loss, approximately 80% of the losses could be traced to etiologies other than renal failure.

Of the 290 patients with renal failure discussed by Oda et al. (1974), 43 demonstrated significant hearing loss "which could be directly attributable to the therapy of the kidney problem." The most common etiology of the hearing loss in these patients was ototoxicity, either diuretic or antibiotic. A most significant aspect of the study was the suggestion that hearing loss increased with the number of hemodialysis treatments and/or transplantations. Further, in the temporal bones from the 7 patients who received transplants, there were "blue stained concretions in the stria vascularis and/or vestibular receptors." The cause and effect of these concretions have not been explained. The authors did suggest possible factors such as electrolyte imbalance due to hemodialysis, drug ototoxicity, vascular injury or osmotic changes due to frequent hemodialysis. In addition, Quick, Fish and Brown, (1973) demonstrated that, for guinea pigs, cochlear pathology can be induced by injecting kidney (nephron) antibodies and, conversely, kidney pathology can be induced by injecting cochlear antibodies. Thus, the possibility exists that unknown immunologic factors with transplanted patients could account for the "concretions." The fact that there were cases who did not develop hearing loss due to hemodialysis or transplantation again underscores the complex nature of the hearing loss factor in the renal disease patient.

Johnson and Mathog (1974) reported audiometric and blood chemistry data on 61 renal patients who were undergoing hemodialysis. The study was concerned with description of hearing loss in the renal patients, fluctuating pure tone thresholds, and possible correlation of hearing change with factors such as blood urea nitrogen, calcium, creatine, glucose, potassium, sodium, blood pressure, and body weight. Blood samples, blood pressure, body weight and pure tone thresholds (250 to 8000 Hz) were assessed before and after dialysis treatment. Results suggested that the renal patient has a sensory-neural hearing loss above 2000 Hz when compared to normative data for sex and age. There was no trend toward better or poorer pure tone sensitivity when pre- and post-dialysis measures were compared. However, the authors did report that the variability of pure tone sensitivity was higher than expected and concluded that this variability was a function of hemodialysis.

In this study, there were no significant correlations between pure tone sensitivity and measures of blood chemistry, blood pressure, or body weight. Of importance, Johnson and Mathog felt that their subject population was not significantly contaminated by other etiologic factors such as drug ototoxicity, heredity, head trauma or noise exposure.

Summary

There is no question that a significant number of renal failure patients will develop hearing loss. However, when factors such as hemodialysis, drug therapy, transplantation and physiologic changes resulting from these treatments are considered, the effect of renal dysfunction on the auditory system has not been adequately documented.

CONCLUSIONS

It is apparent that much of the available data are conflicting and that the hearing disorders seen in hypothyroidism, diabetes mellitus and renal failure are highly variable. This variability is in part due to the individual differences in disease severity. Other factors also known to affect hearing such as ototoxic medications and underlying vascular disease which may not be clinically detectable make controlled studies difficult and existing data subject to cautious interpretation. Individuals with these disease processes frequently receive multiple drugs whose effect on hearing are currently unknown, but warrant further evaluation themselves. Other medical disorders, whose effect on hearing have not been studied, frequently become worse when hypothyroidism, diabetes mellitus or renal failure are superimposed. Thus, the complex relationships between hearing loss and any medical disorder will require careful research efforts of audiologists and physicians in the future.

REFERENCES

Alport, A. C., Hereditary familial congenital haemorrhagic nephritis. *Br. Med. J.*, 1, 504–506, 1927.

Beaney, G. P. E., Otolaryngeal problems arising during the management of severe renal failure. *J. Laryngol. Otol.*, 78, 507–515, 1964.

Bergstrom, L., Jenkins, P., Sando, I., and English, G. M., Hearing loss in renal disease; clinical and pathological studies. *Ann. Otol. Rhinol. Laryngol.*, 82, 555–576, 1973.

Brunt, M. A., Auditory sequelea of diabetes mellitus. Ph.D dissertation, University of Kansas, 1969.

Devos, J. A., Deafness in hypothyroidism. *J. Laryngol. Otol.*, 77, 390–414, 1963.

Gabbay, K. H., The sorbitol pathway and the complications of diabetes. *N. Engl. J. Med.*, 288, 831–836, 1963

Hilger, J. A., Otolaryngologic aspects of hypometabolism. *Ann. Otol. Rhinol. Laryngol.*, 65, 395–413, 1956.

Howarth, A. E., and Lloyd, H. E. D., Perceptive deafness in hypothyroidism. *Br. Med. J.*, 1, 431–433, 1956.

Johnson, D. W., and Mathog, R. H., Hearing function and chronic renal failure treated with chronic hemodialysis. Presented at the American Speech and Hearing Association Convention, Las Vegas, Nevada, 1974 (also see: Johnson, D. W., and Mathog, R. H., Hearing function and chronic renal failure, *Ann. Otol.*

Rhinol. Laryngol., 85, 43–49, 1976).

Jorgensen, M., The inner ear in diabetes mellitus. *Arch. Otolaryngol.*, 74, 373–381, 1961.

Jorgensen, M., and Buch, N., Studies on the inner ear function and cranial nerves in diabetes. *Acta Otolaryngol.*, 55, 350–364, 1961.

Jorgensen, M., Changes of aging in the inner ear, and the inner ear in diabetes mellitus: Histologic studies. *Acta Otolaryngol.* (Suppl.), 188, 125–128, 1963.

Kohonen, A., Jauhiainen, T., Liewendahl, K., Tarkkanen, J., and Kaimo, M., Deafness in experimental hypo- and hyperthyroidism. *Laryngoscope*, 81, 947–956, 1971.

McKusick, V. A., *Mendelian Inheritance in Man. Catalogues of Autosomal Dominant, Autosomal Recessive and X-linked Phenotypes.* Baltimore: The Johns Hopkins Press, 1968.

Marshak, G., and Anderson, C. V., Bekesy audiometry with juvenile-onset diabetics. *J. Audio. Res.*, 8, 323–330, 1968 (also see: Friedman, S. A., and Schulman, R. H., Hearing and diabetic neuropathy. *Arch. Intern. Med.*, 135, 573–576, 1975).

Mitschke, H., Schmidt, P., Kopsa, H. and Zazgornik, J., Reversible uremic deafness after successful renal transplantation. *N. Engl. J. Med.*, 292, 1062–1063, 1975.

Oda, M., Preciado, M. D., Quick, C. A., and Paparella, M. M., Labyrinthine pathology of chronic renal failure patients treated with hemodialysis and kidney transplantation. Presented at the Middle Section Meeting of the American Laryngological, Rhinological, and Otological Society, Kansas City, Mo., 1974.

Oppenheimer, J. H., Initiation of thyroid-hormone action. *N. Engl. J. Med.*, 292, 1063–1068, 1975.

Post, J. T., Hypothyroid deafness: A clinical study of sensori-neural deafness associated with hypothyroidism. *Laryngoscope*, 74, 221–232, 1964.

Quick, C. A., Fish, A., and Brown, C., The relationship between cochlea and kidney. *Laryngoscope*, 83, 1469–1482, 1973.

Ransome, J., Ballantyne, J. C., Shaldon, S., Bosher, S. K., and Hallpike, C. S., Perceptive deafness in subjects with renal failure treated with haemodialysis and Polybrene. *J. Laryngol. Otol.*, 80, 651–677, 1966.

Reichlin, S., Neuroendocrine-pituitary control. In Werner, S. C., and Ingbar, S. H. (Eds.), *The Thyroid*, ed. 3, p. 95. New York: Harper & Row, 1971.

Ritter, F. N., The effects of hypothyroidism upon the ear, nose, and throat. *Laryngoscope*, 77, 1427–1479, 1967.

Ritter, F. N., and Lawrence, M., Reversible hearing loss in human hypothyroidism and correlated changes in the chick inner ear. *Laryngoscope*, 70, 393–407, 1960.

Yassin, A., Badry, A., and Fatt-Hi, A., The relationship between electrolyte balance and cochlear disturbances in cases of renal failure. *J. Laryngol. Otol.*, 84, 429–435, 1970.

Zelenka, J., and Kozak, P., Disorder in blood supply of the inner ear as early symptom of diabetic angiopathy. *J. Laryngol. Otol.*, 79, 314–319, 1965.

chapter 5

HEARING SCREENING FOR CHILDREN

Charles V. Anderson, Ph.D.

The technique of screening has as its purpose the identification, as quickly and as economically as possible, of individuals in a large population who are in need of some special service. As audiologists, we are interested in finding those individuals who may have existing or potential hearing impairments. Our screening procedures are generally an integral part of hearing conservation programs which have as their goals the evaluation, treatment, rehabilitation and education of persons who have communication and/or health problems. Most often, these programs have the dual purpose of meeting both educational and health needs.

Hearing conservation programs for preschool and school age children are usually directed by an audiologist in a school or health agency with interest in the overall education, development and health of children. For over one-quarter century, many public and private schools have provided such services for school age children. Preschool children were often overlooked if they were not fortunate enough to fall under the care of a well baby clinic or nursery school which offered these services or could arrange for them. In recent years, with the development of Head Start and other comprehensive education and health programs for preschool children, hearing conservation programs have proliferated; in some instances, they have become mandatory for preschool as well as school age children. These developments have increased the demand for effective and efficient hearing screening procedures for children of all ages.

Hearing conservation programs which are truly comprehensive in their coverage and in the services they offer are laudable undertakings. Unfortunately, such excellence has at times been elusive, and many programs have fallen far short of providing adequate coverage, especially with regard to subsequent referral of individuals with hearing problems and providing follow-up and necessary services. Many hearing conservation programs have been active in surveying populations through hearing screening procedures and identifying hearing impairments, but they have not delivered the much needed treatment, rehabilitation and educational consultative services these individuals so desperately need. Screening procedures provide impressive incidence statistics, but these data, by themselves, are of little value to the children who need special services. Hearing screening without follow-up services is of less value than no screening at all since those involved in the program and the public whom they serve are deluded into thinking a hearing conservation program exists when indeed there is only a labeling service.

The purpose of this chapter is to present the major types of hearing screening procedures and techniques which are in use today and their application to populations of preschool children, age 3 years and above, and to children of school age. A discussion of hearing testing procedures with infants and younger children is presented in Chapter 33. The procedures discussed in the present chapter are designed to help answer the question: According to the criteria of this program, can this child be considered to have hearing within the normal limits of hearing? If the answer to this question is "yes" for a given child, he/she has passed the screening test, and no further attention need be given to the question of hearing at this time. If the answer is "no," he/she has failed the particular screening test. In this case, further testing must be done to determine if referral for more comprehensive evaluation and treatment is appropriate. The use of the evaluative terms "pass" and "fail" should be avoided, for obvious reasons, when discussing or communicating the test results to the child or parents.

Traditionally, hearing screening procedures have had, as their basis, air-conduction hearing sensitivity measures. Such procedures are considered fairly adequate for identifying children with peripheral hearing impairments serious enough to cause hearing communication problems. Certain inadequacies still exist, however, in their use for identifying children with medical problems. Melnick, Eagles and Levine (1964) provided the most dramatic illustration of this inadequacy when they reported that nearly one-half of the cases with active otologic pathology in their population were overlooked when the program recommended by the National Conference on Identification Audiometry (Darley, 1961) was applied. Until a feasible resolution of this dilemma is offered, we must make the most efficient use of the procedures which we have available while recognizing the limitations which may be inherent in their use.

The recent widespread acceptance of acoustic impedance and reflex testing provides additional measures which, if used judiciously, can improve our ability to identify health problems dramatically. A thorough discussion of such measures is given in Chapters 29 and 30. We are all anxiously awaiting meaningful guidelines for "pass-fail" criteria which will make impedance and reflex measures efficient and effective as routine aspects of identification programs.

HEARING SCREENING PROCEDURES

A number of specific techniques for screening the hearing of large populations have been described in the literature over the years. The major classifications of these techniques will be summarized below. Aspects of these procedures which have general application will not be discussed for each individual test or procedure but rather, will be presented in a later section. The procedure or technique chosen for any given group or hearing conservation program is typically some variation of one of these basic techniques. The modifications used are often dictated by the local situation.

Hearing screening procedures are administered in either individual or group settings with the groups numbering as large as 40 children for one administration of the test. The signals are most often individual pure tones or speech; however, noisemakers and environmental or animal sounds have been used on occasion with varying degrees of success.

Group Hearing Screening Procedures

The obvious advantage of group hearing screening procedures is that several children can be screened with each administration of the test procedure with the end result that more children can be seen in any given period of time. There are some disadvantages which must be taken into account when evaluating

the overall efficiency of group as opposed to individually administered techniques. These are the maintenance of equipment and its calibration, the necessity of insuring against cheating and the typically higher rate of false-positive identifications obtained with group screening.

Procedures Using Speech Signals

The fading numbers test was the first hearing screening procedure to be used on a large scale. With this technique, pairs and triplets of digits were recorded on a phonograph disc with each set of numbers presented at a level 3 dB less intense than the preceding set. These discs were played on a Western Electric 4-A or 4-B phonograph speech audiometer, the output of which could be directed to 40 different earphones. The children were given blanks on which they were to write the numbers heard each time they were alerted to listen. The answer sheets were designed in such a way that they could be scored easily to determine the lowest dB level at which each child was able to identify the digits correctly. A cut-off level, usually "the 9-dB level" (Newhart and Reger, 1956, p. 13), was chosen and any child who could hear at this level or lower was considered to have hearing within normal limits.

One obvious disadvantage with the fading numbers test was that the children had to be able to respond by writing the digits, a requirement which limited its use with younger or intellectually limited children. The major disadvantage, however, was first pointed out by Ciocco (1936) and has since been supported repeatedly. Many children with high frequency losses of hearing sensitivity above 1000 Hz were able to identify the digits correctly on the basis of the acoustic information contained in the lower frequencies and, therefore, their hearing losses were not identified with this procedure. For this reason, the procedure has fallen into disfavor and, hopefully, is no longer in use.

Several other procedures using speech signals have been developed since the fading numbers test in attempts to overcome some of its disadvantages. Watson and Tolan (1949) report the use of the Maico RS audiometer employing equipment similar to the Western Electric 4 series audiometers to play disc recordings of individual monosyllables which could be represented by pictures which the child identified. This fading word test used the same technique as the fading numbers test of reducing the level of each succeeding word by 3 dB. Watson and Tolan felt that having the child identify pictures representing monosyllabic words overcame both the problem of a written response and the failure to identify children with high frequency hearing losses. They indicated that consonant identification was necessary in order to recognize the words in their lists. This latter assumption may be in question.

In 1951, Bennett reported a procedure similar to the Maico RS test which used monosyllabic words as the auditory signals with pictures as the response mode. In the Bennett test, a closed response set of four phonetically similar words is presented for each trial. Bennett reported a rather strong positive relationship between his procedure and pure tone screening in identifying 6-year-old children with hearing losses.

As part of a much larger investigation of hearing for speech in children, Meyerson (1956) reported the use of spondaic words to screen the hearing of children. He used spondees which could be pictured and instructed the children to point to the picture of the word heard each time. In addition to the standard presentation of the words, he also had high-pass filtered presentations. It was Meyerson's impression that his verbal audiometric test was adequate for identifying children with losses of hearing sensitivity in the range of the speech frequencies.

In an attempt to find a more effective procedure for identifying preschool children with hearing impairments, a group in Minnesota developed a procedure called Verbal Auditory Screening for Children or VASC audiometry (Griffing, Simonton and Hedgecock, 1967). Twelve spondees which can be pictured are recorded on tape as speech signals. The first word is presented at a level of 51 dB (re normal speech reception threshold (SRT) of 22 dB sound pressure level (SPL)), and each succeeding word is attenuated 4 dB to the lowest level which is 15 dB (re normal SRT) where the last three words are presented. The test is administered to two children at a time while an observer records the responses of each child as he/she points to the pictures. It has been noted that children who have hearing impairments may be labeled as having hearing within normal limits when only the words are used. In an attempt to overcome this problem of false-negative identification on the basis of low frequency recognition of the words, a lion's roar and a bird's whistle have been added to the signals to be identified in the pictures. A survey of the control group data presently available in the literature leads one to evaluate the efficiency of this test as inadequate. Mencher and McCulloch (1970) reported that the VASC was inadequate in identifying hearing losses in kindergarten children. Of a group of 53 kindergarten children, they found that 31% of those passing the VASC failed to meet the pure tone

screening criteria for hearing within normal limits. Despite the fact that children with hearing impairments may not be identified with the VASC, it has gained popularity since volunteers can be trained to administer it. It is available commercially on cartridge tape and is currently being used in a number of hearing conservation programs for preschool children.

Procedures Using Pure Tone Signals

The pulse tone test described by Reger and Newby (1947) was one of the first group hearing screening tests to use pure tone signals. In this test, the listener records the number of bursts of tone heard with each alert to listen. In Reger and Newby's description, two descending series of presentations of tones are given in each ear for each frequency chosen for presentation. The lowest level at which the listener correctly identifies the number of pulses in one of the two series is considered to be an estimate of threshold for that frequency. The responses are recorded on answer sheets which can be checked after the test is administered. Depending upon the equipment which is available, this test can be automated and administered to as many as 40 listeners at a time.

With the Reger-Newby pulse tone screening procedure, it is necessary to test one ear at a time. Glorig (1965) reports a modification of this technique whereby some of the pulses in each group are presented to one ear, and others are presented to the opposite ear. In this way, it is possible to evaluate the response in both ears at the same time by scoring the number of pulses reported as heard at each level.

The Massachusetts test (Johnston, 1948) uses a single pure tone audiometer and 40 earphones and requires that the listener mark the answer sheet "yes" or "no" each time a tone is presented. Six presentations are made at each frequency, using three levels of signal. On a prearranged schedule, a certain number of responses are requested when no signal has been presented in order to control for guessing. The test is scored on the basis of the number of "no" responses; more than two incorrect "no" responses constitute a failure at that level.

In an attempt to make the Massachusetts test applicable to younger children who are unable to read or to otherwise respond in a "yes-no" situation, Johnston (1952) later offered a modification which has been called the Johnston group pure tone screening test. In this procedure, 10 children, each with an earphone, are seated in a semicircle and asked to close their eyes. They are to raise their hands when a tone is heard and the person administering the test or an assistant records any lack of response when a signal is presented. Johnston also suggests having a switch available to cut out certain earphones at times. In this way, the person administering the test can be reassured that the children are responding to the tones and not to other cues.

Individual Hearing Screening Procedures

One of the most popular hearing screening procedures over the years has been the individual pure tone sweep test which was originally discussed by Newhart (1938). This test may be used as the only hearing screening procedure or, as is often the case, as a second screening for those who have failed one of the previously discussed group procedures. In this test, preselected frequencies are presented at predetermined levels, and the child is asked to raise a hand, press a button or give a similar response each time a tone is heard. The series of frequencies is presented, first to one ear and then to the other, to each child individually. The lack of response to any one of the tones is often used as the criterion for failure of the screening test. Modifications of this basic procedure have been numerous and reflect local custom, supervisor preferences and examiner ingenuity.

Although many people feel that it is often difficult for preschool and lower elementary school age children to respond to pure tones, simple conditioning procedures and play audiometry techniques often make this a useful hearing screening procedure with youngsters as young as 3 years of age. Classroom teachers, technicians and volunteers can easily incorporate training in these techniques into the daily program of activities during the week or two preceding the actual testing. In addition, the tester can present an introduction to the equipment and test procedures in the classroom or play area. If the test procedure is introduced to the group as a whole with volunteers for demonstration, the test administrator can usually alleviate fears about what will occur and instruct in the procedures at the same time. It may also help to test the children in front of one another so the more reticent will gain confidence in seeing others do the task.

In view of the development of portable acoustic impedance and reflex measuring equipment, such tests need to be included in any discussion of individual hearing screening procedures. The use of tympanometry can be especially helpful in identifying medical problems which might otherwise go unnoticed through the use of behavioral techniques. In addition, the child who is difficult or impossible to test behaviorally may well be able to be screened for hearing through the use of tympanometry and acoustic reflexes.

CHOICE OF PROCEDURE

The choice of hearing screening procedure for any given program is obviously not a simple matter. Each advocate of the basic procedures reviewed here, as well as others reported elsewhere, feels that his/her procedure is the one of choice for the population of interest. Since no one procedure enjoys any clear-cut superiority for all ages or groups, people responsible for local hearing conservation programs must determine the most efficient and appropriate procedures for their population. They must give consideration to the following factors: (1) the goals of the program, (2) the ability of the children to accomplish the task required of them for any given procedure, (3) the testing environments which are available, (4) the equipment which is currently or potentially available and the maintenance of this equipment, and (5) the personnel who can carry out the program. All of these factors will be important in decisions which have to be made under each of the headings which follow.

Speech or Pure Tone Signal

The hearing screening procedures currently in use suggest whether or not the child has hearing within normal limits in relation to some reference group and lead to inferences about a range within which his/her hearing threshold levels fall. Signals have to be chosen to provide the most efficient estimate of hearing status. It is standard procedure in the measurement of hearing to sample at least the hearing threshold levels across a given range of frequencies. The frequencies represented in more complex auditory signals such as speech, noisemakers and animal sounds usually cover a broad range; however, we have to recognize that the detection or recognition of the presence of one of these signals may be dependent upon a very small portion of that range. Hearing screening procedures using these signals may not sample the hearing sensitivity adequately across the frequency range and, therefore, may result in a significant number of false-negative identifications.

It is common practice in hearing screening to use the simpler, more easily defined pure tone as the signal of choice. Speech, noisemakers and various animal and environmental sounds continue to be used when, for some reason, it appears that it is too difficult to get children to respond to pure tones. Despite the heavy criticism which has been leveled at screening procedures relying on signals other than pure tones, these procedures continue to emerge.

Group or Individual Procedures

When the time involved in administering one hearing screening test to each child in a program is considered, group procedures appear to be far more efficient than individual screening. This is especially true for children above the second or third grade in the typical school. Dahl (1949) indicated that, in her experience, up to three times as many children could be given group hearing screening tests in a day as could be administered individual tests. However, as many as 40% of the population may fail the first administration of the group hearing screening test and have to be retested. Upon retest, it may be found that only 5 to 12% of the population actually exhibit hearing impairments. This high rate of false-positive identification should be reduced considerably when using the individual screening methods. In order to evaluate the overall efficiency of the group versus the individual tests, one must assess the total time and personnel needed to arrive at the final identification figures for the population.

Other practical matters to be considered in comparing group and individual hearing screening procedures are the equipment, test environments and personnel needed for the administration of the tests. As with any hearing testing procedure, it is necessary that only durable, precisely calibrated equipment be used in screening testing. Neither this equipment nor its maintenance is inexpensive; however, the equipment for group testing is more expensive to purchase and to maintain per testing unit than that used for individual hearing screening. Furthermore, each active earphone that is added to a testing unit adds at least one more source of error and must be monitored for correct calibration.

A room that meets the dual requirements of being large enough to accommodate the size of group to be tested and quiet enough in which to do the testing may not exist, especially in many of our crowded schools. Obviously, the testing cannot be done if the signals cannot be detected or recognized because of masking from environmental noise. Difficulty in finding usable space may dictate that the hearing screening procedure which requires the least amount of space can be chosen for a program.

Many group hearing screening procedures have been simplified in administration and response so that they can be conducted for initial screening by an audiometric technician who has limited training. The interpretation of responses on the individual screening procedure may require greater skill and a higher level of training. Therefore, it may be more efficient to have a technician administer an initial screening procedure and leave the time of the skilled tester or clinical audiologist for retests and threshold examinations.

Probably the most common resolution of the vexing problem of whether to use group or individual hearing screening procedures is to use both, beginning with the initial group screening by a skilled technician followed by individual screening and threshold testing by an audiologist.

The combination of tympanometry, acoustic reflex, and behavioral procedures is growing in popularity. It should be noted that we still need research to help us resolve the question of which children should receive which screening procedure in order to avoid unproductive duplication of effort.

Criteria for Identification

It is assumed that the goal of hearing screening testing in preschool and school age children is to identify the children with actual or potential hearing impairments of significance as communication or health problems; the criteria for identification will have to be consistent with this goal. The signals used in behavioral testing which must be correctly detected or recognized in order for the child to demonstrate hearing within normal limits must be representative of the frequency range considered to be important for these purposes and must be at a level at which it is reasonable to expect their detection. The level of the signal must not be so high, nor the frequency range so restricted however, that the child with an existing or potential hearing problem is not identified. What criteria represent a happy medium between these extremes and are relevant for children's needs?

In 1961, the National Conference on Identification Audiometry (Darley, 1961, p. 31) recommended that pure tones can be used as the signals for hearing screening and that:

. . . *only four frequencies shall be considered in the criteria for referral: 1000, 2000, 4000, and 6000 cps. It is recommended that screening be done at the 10 dB level with reference to the present American Standard audiometric zero (ASA-1951) for the frequencies of 1000, 2000, and 6000 cps, and at the 20 dB level for the frequency of 4000 cps.* A child would be judged to have failed the screening test and to be a candidate for referral for the next step if he failed to hear . . .

any of the signals at these levels in either ear.

Anderson (1965) and Lloyd (1966) have pointed out that an easy and useful conversion of these levels to the ISO-1964 reference levels is made by using a level of 20 dB (ISO-1964) at all frequencies. Because of the close similarities between ISO-1964 and ANSI-1969 reference levels, this is also true for the new American standard.

The justification of the National Conference for recommending these frequencies was that children often failed to hear the frequencies below 1000 Hz simply on the basis of interference from noise in the testing environment and that threshold information at 8000 Hz was rarely used clinically. Their justification for the levels recommended was to insure the identification of the child with 25 dB (ISO-1964) hearing threshold levels. These reasons may be adequate in many situations. Many practitioners still prefer to include 500 Hz in the screening frequencies and referral criteria when feasible. A review of the data of Eagles, Wishik, and Doerfler (1967) and Roberts (1972) does not support the impression that children with middle ear disorders will be identified any more readily with the inclusion of 500 Hz. Assumptions such as the above which are based upon individual experiences in hearing screening often do not hold up when studied more rigorously. It is recommended here that, whenever possible, at least 500 Hz be added to the frequencies used for referral criteria.

Since many children have hearing threshold levels at 4000 and 6000 Hz of 30 dB (ANSI-1969) or greater and do not have a problem of medical significance, Newby (1964) recommends that priorities for medical referral be given to the children identified according to these criteria. The otologist or physician in the program can then determine, on the basis of these priorities, which children should be given individual medical examinations. He suggests that the highest priority be given to those children failing to meet the criteria for hearing within normal limits at 500, 1000 and 2000 Hz. Second highest priority should go to those demonstrating reduced hearing sensitivity at any one of these frequencies, and lowest priority to those with a loss of hearing sensitivity at only 4000 and/or 6000 Hz.

The ASHA Committee on Audiometric Evaluation (1975) recommends the use of the following priorities for an audiologic referral:

a. Binaural loss in both ears at all frequencies
b. Binaural loss at 1000 and 2000 Hz only
c. Binaural loss at 1000 or 2000 Hz only
d. Monaural loss at all frequencies
e. Monaural loss at 1000 and 2000 Hz
f. Binaural or monaural loss at 4000 Hz only.

Compatible but simpler referral guidelines are given at the end of this chapter.

It appears to be generally accepted today that one should use at least the frequencies 1000, 2000, and 4000 Hz at levels no higher than 25 dB (ANSI-1969) in the criteria for referral. House and Glorig (1957) once suggested the use of limited frequency audiometry in which only 4000 Hz or 2000 and 4000 Hz were used. This practice appears to be more appropriate for populations where one is inter-

ested in obtaining information in relation to noise-induced hearing loss than it is for preschool and school age children. A more precise procedure, especially for identifying hearing impairment of medical significance, might be to use 500 and 6000 Hz in addition to 1000, 2000, and 4000 Hz and perhaps to lower the dB level to 15 dB (ANSI-1969) for all frequencies as suggested by Glorig (1965). A higher incidence and referral rate will result from these more stringent criteria, and only close scrutiny of the results of the individual referral program will suggest if more children with medical problems but minimal hearing losses will be referred for medical examinations and possible early intervention.

With the addition of acoustic impedance measures to the hearing screening battery, it will undoubtedly be possible in the future to modify the criteria in such a way that the relatively high false-positive identification resulting from using low hearing levels and a large number of frequencies can be limited. Currently it is not possible to arrive at criteria based upon tympanometric measures which are commonly accepted. One of the more common sets of criteria for failure of impedance screening is that described by McCandless and Thomas (1974), i.e. -100 mm H_2O pressure and the absence of acoustic reflex. As we gain experience and report more research using acoustic impedance in hearing screening, clearer guidelines for pass-fail criteria will become evident.

Testing Environment

The noise level and distractions in the testing environment can be crucial in determining or undermining the effectiveness of any hearing screening program. For this reason, specific attention needs to be given to the testing environment when choosing a place to administer the tests. Observations of the environment need to be made during actual testing as well as prior to the selection of a location. Especially in busy, crowded schools, the hearing testing environment can change dramatically without notice, resulting in a high rate of misidentification. Although most standards for acceptable ambient noise levels in hearing testing rooms (e.g., ANSI, S3.1-1960) are written in order to avoid situations where the environmental noise will mask the signals being used in the test, examiners must also be alert for any distracting visual or acoustic signals in the environment which will take the attention of the children away from the listening task at hand.

Sites for the hearing screening and testing need to be selected so the children can be placed out of visual or auditory contact with other activities in the school. Room selection will depend upon the daily schedule in the building, the general environment, availability of electrical outlets and appropriate size for administering the test. The test site should be chosen to avoid any major noise sources such as boiler rooms, recess areas, physical education classes, shops or choral music and band rehearsal areas during periods of use. Rooms which often make good testing sites include auditorium stages with the curtains drawn, libraries, private offices, cafeterias, conference rooms, music rooms and church sanctuaries. The music rooms often offer several advantages; for instance, in some modern school buildings, the music rooms are sound-treated and are away from the major flow of traffic in the building. Hopefully, while you are testing in the room, students cannot be practicing, and you have eliminated one of the major sources of environmental noise. If you are having difficulty convincing the administrators and teachers of the necessity for quiet, it is often helpful to test their hearing in the setting. No more dramatic demonstration of the effect of noise on testing can be made.

In choosing the site for the testing, beware of the room which appears to be quiet because of the time of day or because noise sources within the room or in the vicinity are not currently in operation. Fluorescent lights, milk and water coolers, exhaust fans, adjacent rest rooms, elevators, stairways and hallways are all sources of noise which may be overlooked until they suddenly become operational during a testing session.

There are some sites in which it is simply impossible to conduct hearing screening and testing in a reasonable fashion. The options in these situations are (1) to transport the children to another site or (2) to bring an acceptable testing "environment" to the school. Many systems have resolved this problem by investing in a motor van or trailer in which the hearing screening and, especially, the threshold testing can be done. These transportable testing sites are obviously a major investment since they must be sound-treated, provided with cooling and heating systems, and most important, the hearing testing equipment must be installed in such a way that it is not damaged or otherwise altered in calibration while in transit.

Within recent years we have also seen the development of small portable hearing test booths which rarely match the specifications of a clinical testing booth but nevertheless reduce the ambient noise to a tolerable level for screening purposes. These small portable test booths are far less expensive than the mobile van in both initial investment and upkeep.

An acoustic environment which is too loud for behavioral testing may be acceptable for acoustic impedance measures. Thus, the procedure of choice may be influenced by the test environment.

A SUGGESTED PROGRAM

Although no single set of procedures will work for every group, there are some guidelines which can be applied generally in the decision making. The discussion which follows is intended to assist in making those decisions and carrying out the process of identifying children with hearing impairments and referring them for further services. A type of program which has been found useful is given in outline form at the end of this section.

First of all, the community or group to be served must be informed and shown the necessity for having an effective hearing conservation program for their preschool and school age children. Those individuals in the health and education professions must take an especially active role and understand the goals and activities, if the program is to work at all. The most logical person to direct such efforts is an audiologist who is well informed about the implications of hearing impairment, hearing testing procedures and equipment, and the importance of early educational and medical services for children with hearing impairments. One of the first steps in this program development may be to survey the population through hearing screening procedures so the extent of the problem can be pointed out. The program will become effective much sooner if demonstration referral and follow-up services are provided with this initial survey so that people can see the merit of these procedures.

For the initial survey of the population, it will undoubtedly be necessary to arrange to screen the hearing of all the children in the system. Once the program is established, however, it is probably advisable to follow the guidelines of the National Conference on Identification Audiometry (Darley, 1961) or ASHA Committee on Audiometric Evaluation (1975). Because of the higher incidence of medically treatable hearing problems in the younger age group, the National Conference recommended that all preschool, kindergarten and first grade children be screened annually. Children above the first grade level can probably be screened effectively once each 3 years. The Committee on Audiometric Evaluation recommends annual hearing screening of children in preschool through the first three grades with subsequent screening optional.

Certain preparations must be made before the actual screening of the pupils. The person who is planning the program will find it helpful to visit each setting in which testing is to be done. During this visit, the purposes and needs of the hearing screening will be explained to the administrators and teachers. Schedules can be checked to find the best days and times of day for the testing. If alterations in the schedule are necessary, they can also be worked out at this time. Especially if the hearing screening procedures are new to the group, the participants should be informed of the upcoming activities, how they will be carried out and what the results will mean. Prior knowledge of the program can reduce considerably the number of rumors and other signs of test anxiety on the day of the screening. If the teachers are to participate in training the children for response to the hearing screening, instructions and activities can be demonstrated in the classroom on the day of this visit as well. A room for administering the test must be selected and arrangements made for its use. Be sure to learn about all of the activities which are likely to take place on the day of the screening in the vicinity of any room to be used. A plan for getting the children to be screened to and from

the testing room should guarantee a constant flow of youngsters to be tested.

Class lists and reports which are necessary for the hearing screening should be obtained in advance. This is also a time when it can be determined if administrative rules require special parental permission for the administration of the hearing tests. A common practice is to have class lists, such as that shown in Figure 5.1, available ahead of time so the names can be placed on a composite record form. This allows for recording, in an efficient manner, the results of each test and the action to be taken for each child. In addition, each child brings a slip of paper to the test. This paper should contain name, grade, age, room, teacher and/or other pertinent information. The results of the hearing screening or test are also recorded on this slip and kept so this information can be transferred to the master lists. An example of this form is given in Figure 5.2.

Prior planning should have been done so that on the day of the hearing screening the procedures can begin as early in the day as possible. This means that all of the master lists and individual forms should have been

School _____ Grade _____

Teacher _____ Room _____

HEARING SCREENING RECORD

Name Last (Please Print) First	First Screening			Second Screening			Threshold	Notes
	Date	N	R	Date	N	RT	Date	
TOTALS								

N = Considered normal on all screening procedures
R = Rescreen (mark as P = pure-tone, T = Tympanometry, X = Reflex)
RT = Refer for threshold test

Fig. 5.1. Master list for each classroom. (The line across the form indicates that the form has been condensed to save space. Line represents a tear.)

prepared. Any training for participation in the hearing screening should have taken place prior to this time.

Upon arriving at the test site, the equipment should be arranged for the most efficient administration of the procedures. Adequate time should be allowed for the equipment to warm up. The technicians or audiologists should then do a routine check to determine if each earphone and audiometer is operating within acceptable limits. These checks will most often be done by listening tests, inadequate as they may be for calibration purposes. If equipment to measure environmental noise levels is not available for use, part of the listening test should include a determination that the signals can indeed be detected in this environment. This one check of the equipment, by the way, will not insure that the equipment will operate satisfactorily for the remainder of the day. Each earphone and audiometer should be spot-checked by listening throughout the day. Any piece of equipment thought to be out of calibration or otherwise malfunctioning, i.e., reporting an unaccountably high rate of failures, should be retired from use until proper functioning can be assured. For these reasons, it is always helpful to have stand-by equipment available which can be put into use.

After determining that the procedures are understood by all personnel and that provisions have been made for getting the children to and from the testing room, the screening testing is ready to begin. Each group or individual to be screened should be given clear, concise and meaningful instructions regarding the task to be completed. Be sure that each step of the procedure is covered in the instructions, but do not overinstruct to the point of confusion. Following the instructions for behavioral testing, either place the earphones over the ears of each listener, or ask the children to put on the earphones themselves. Assure yourself that each earphone is properly placed on each child. Two earphones should be used per child, even if only one is active and the earphones have to be reversed before the testing of the second ear. The presence of an earphone over the ear not under the test will assist in reducing, at least to a small degree, the effects of environmental noise upon the children's responses.

The behavioral test procedure is now ready to begin. It is recommended that only pure tones be used as signals and that the frequencies of 1000, 2000 and 4000 Hz be presented at levels of 20 dB (ANSI-1969). The order of presentation of frequencies and which ear is being tested first should be routinized so the test administrator will be able to monitor the procedure at any given time should it be interrupted. One useful procedure is to begin with a 1000 Hz tone at 45 dB (ANSI-1969) in the right ear, reduce the level to 20 dB and present a second 1000 Hz signal. All succeeding signals are presented at 20 dB (ANSI-1969) in the following order: 2000 and 4000 Hz to the right ear. If two active earphones are available, you can switch to the left earphone and present 4000, 2000 and 1000 Hz. If there are any responses about which you are uncertain, that

HEARING SCREENING RECORD

Name _____ Date _____
    Last   (Please Print)   First

School _____ Grade _____

Teacher _____ Age _____ Room _____

	250 Hz			500 Hz			1000 Hz			2000 Hz			4000 Hz			6000 Hz			Tympanometry
	I	II	X	I	II	X	I	II	X	I	II	X	I	II	X	I	II	X	
Right ear																			
Left ear																			

I = 1st screening at _____ dB HL, II = 2nd screening at _____ dB HL, X = Reflex

☐ Normal, ☐ Rescreen, ☐ Refer for threshold test

Fig. 5.2. Individual screening form.

frequency can be presented again as a double check. This order of presentation is chosen so that a signal readily recognizable for a vast majority of the children is presented first; it is followed by an orderly sequence of signals which also provides for the least manipulation of the typical pure tone audiometer.

Any children failing to respond to any one signal in either ear should be referred to a second tester for a rescreening, preferably on the same day. Anyone failing the second screening is then referred for a threshold determination, either that day or within the next 2 weeks.

As each child leaves the room for the last hearing screening or test for the day, he should be given a note for his parents. This note should contain a brief explanation of the purposes of the hearing screening procedures, a statement that the child had a hearing test on that day, and some indication as to our knowledge of the current hearing status — whether the child's hearing is considered to be within normal limits or whether responses to the hearing test warrant further evaluation and referral to determine if a hearing loss is present. For those who fail the hearing screening, impedance screening, or hearing threshold test, it should be clear to the parent that this is not a final determination of the child's hearing status. The name of a person whom they may contact for further explanation should be included. None of the notes should carry any reference to the terms "pass" or "fail." For examples of these forms see Figures 5.3 and 5.4.

Within 1 week after the final screening determination, a referral sheet (Fig. 5.5) should be sent home with those children for whom a medical (or hearing) evaluation referral is being made. This sheet should contain an explanation of the program as well as a clear statement as to the need for following through with the referral. Especially for medical refer-

Date _____

Dear Parent or Guardian:

As part of our overall hearing conservation program we are conducting the hearing screening testing for this year. We do this every year in order to identify those individuals who may have a hearing problem which needs attention.

We are pleased to inform you that your child was given a hearing screening test today and was found to have hearing within normal limits.

If you have any questions about the hearing tests or the hearing conservation program, please feel free to contact me at (give address and telephone number).

Sincerely yours,

Fig. 5.3. Notification to parents that hearing is within normal limits.

Date _____

Dear Parent or Guardian:

As part of our overall hearing conservation program, we are conducting the hearing screening testing for this year. We do this every year in order to identify those individuals who may have a hearing problem which needs attention.

Your child was given a hearing screening test today. Because we were uncertain about some of the responses to the sounds, we will be re-testing your child's hearing in the near future. We will inform you of the results of the next hearing test as soon as we have completed it.

If you have any questions about the hearing tests or the hearing conservation program, please feel free to contact me at (give address and telephone number).

Sincerely yours,

Fig. 5.4. Notification to parents that further hearing testing will be done.

rals, the bottom portion of the referral form should contain a place for the physician or other professional to indicate quickly the findings of the examination and the recommended follow-up procedures. This information portion of the form should then be returned to the program for follow-up data on the hearing screening procedures. Information should be obtained on those children for whom no form is returned to determine if the parents have followed the recommendation for referral and if not, why not. Perhaps a home visit by the

Name _____   Date _____

       Last   (Please Print)   First

School _____   Grade _____

Teacher _____   Age _____   Room _____

Dear Parent or Guardian:

    As part of our overall hearing conservation program we have recently completed the hearing screening testing for this year. We do this every year in order to identify those individuals who may have a hearing problem which needs attention.

    Your child was given a hearing test in school. From the results of these tests, which are reported below, it appears that a hearing problem may be present.

    Since many hearing problems can be corrected with prompt medical attention, we recommend that you take your child to your physician or ear specialist (otolaryngologist) for a medical evaluation.

    Please take this form with you when you go to the doctor. Have him complete the information on the bottom of this form and return it to us.

    If your child has already been seen or is currently under a physician's care for his hearing, please note this on this form and return it to us.

    If you have any questions about the hearing tests and what they mean or about our recommendations, please feel free to contact me.

Sincerely yours,

	Ear	250 Hz	500 Hz	1000 Hz	2000 Hz	4000 Hz	6000 Hz	Tympanometry	
dB HL	R							R	
	L								
Reflex	R							L	
	L								

Please return this portion of form to _____

Medical Report
Impressions and Recommendations

Right ear: _____

Left ear: _____
_____
_____

Physician: _____   Date: _____

Fig. 5.5. Medical referral form.

audiologist, nurse or home visitor is necessary to determine if assistance is needed in order to carry out the referral.

The results of the hearing screening, referral and follow-up information should become a part of the child's permanent record and should advance with progress through the school system or be forwarded if school systems are changed.

A summary of the results of the hearing screening testing for each school or group should be provided for the administrator's records and information. In addition, a summary of each year's hearing screening activities should be made an integral part of the records and reports for the overall hearing conservation program. These types of summaries and reports can be quite useful in evaluating the efficiency of the program as well as noting the accomplishments during the year.

Although it is difficult to state figures concerning incidence and testing time per child which can be applied to all programs, some generalizations can be made which can serve as guidelines. When using the behavioral procedures, signals and criteria suggested in this chapter, an incidence of referral on the basis of threshold determinations of between 5 and 10% of the population is within reasonable limits. If one is finding lower or higher incidence than this, an investigation should be made to determine if changes are needed in procedures, equipment, instructions, testing sites or personnel. Remember, however, that it is possible that the incidence of hearing impairment for one group may be higher or lower than an average and for legitimate reasons.

The time involved in testing varies from group to group and from one tester to the next. The length and variation in testing time will usually increase as the ages of the children decrease. This is especially true for children below the third grade. Generally speaking, when all is going well, with children in the third grade and above, one tester can screen the hearing of at least 300 children in one school day, using the Johnston group pure tone screening test. At least 150 students can be screened in a day by one examiner using the individual pure tone sweep test or impedance and reflex measurements. Air conduction thresholds can be obtained for both ears in from 8 to 12 min per child.

An outline for the hearing screening portion of a hearing conservation program follows:

I. Program development and community education
   A. Enlisting cooperation and assistance of professionals and citizens
   B. Education of the community to needs and services
   C. Selection of procedures
   D. Acquisition of equipment and arranging for maintenance and calibration
   E. Selection and training of personnel
   F. Development of forms and materials
   G. Visits to schools, test sites and individuals to whom referrals are to be made

II. Individuals to be screened for hearing each year
   A. All preschool, kindergarten and first grade children
   B. Grades 3, 6, 9, and 12
   C. All new children
   D. All children with known hearing impairments or ear disease
   E. All referrals from teachers and those children with complaints related to hearing

III. Basic procedures to be used
   A. For preschool, kindergarten, first and second grade children—individual pure tone sweep test using conditioning and play audiometry as necessary which is administered by an audiologist assisted by a technician
   B. For third grade children and above—Johnston group pure tone screening test with controls for cheating followed by a second screening for failures using individual pure tone sweep test, all administered by a technician
   C. Acoustic impedance and reflex measurements to supplement needs for identifying medical referrals not identified with pure tone screening. To be used at the discretion of the director. Incidence figures based upon acoustic impedance and reflex measurements are not now sufficiently documented to provide guidelines.
   D. Individual pure tone threshold determination administered by an audiologist or a technician under the supervision of an audiologist from which referrals are made by the audiologist

IV. Forms (Figs. 5.1 to 5.5)
   A. Brochure giving purpose and description of program
   B. Master lists of children by school, grade, room and teacher
   C. Individual forms for recording test information for each child
   D. Form for informing child or parent of test administration and test results
   E. Medical referral form to be returned with a report
   F. Final reports

V. Referral criteria
   A. For second screening or threshold determination—failure to respond to any one or more frequencies (1000, 2000 or 4000 Hz

frequencies, at 20 dB ANSI-1969), in either ear

B. Medical Referral

1. Priority one—failure to respond to either 1000 or 2000 Hz at 20 dB (ANSI-1969) or lower in either ear and any child whose thresholds have become poorer by 10 dB or more

2. Priority two—failure to respond to 4000 Hz at 20 dB (ANSI-1969) or lower in either ear

3. A report but not necessarily a referral is made for any child who (a) is presently under medical care for a hearing impairment or (b) has been evaluated medically as the result of a previous hearing screening and found not to have a medical problem nor have hearing threshold levels changed by more than 5 dB at any one frequency

4. Any child complaining of an earache or drainage from the ear

5. Any child failing the established impedance and reflex screening criteria

C. Hearing evaluation referral

1. Any child who is not presently being followed and has hearing threshold levels of 25 dB (ANSI-1969) or higher for either 1000 or 2000 Hz in the poorer ear

2. Any child failing hearing screening who gives no response, inconsistent responses or responses inconsistent with other communication behavior

3. Any child who appears to have more difficulty than peers understanding speech in relatively normal communication situations or complains of hearing problems

VI. On-going evaluation of program efficiency and service.

REFERENCES

American Speech and Hearing Association (ASHA) Committee on Audiometric Evaluation, Guidelines for Identification Audiometry. *ASHA*, 17, 94–99, 1975.

American Standard Criteria for Background Noise in Audiometer Rooms (ANSI S3.1-1960), New York: American National Standards Institute, Inc., 1960.

Anderson, C. V., The new international audiometric zero. *ISHA, J. Ind. Speech Hear. Assoc.*, 24, 1–9, 1965.

Bennett, S. M., A group test of hearing for six-year-old children. *Br. J. Educ. Psychol.*, 21, 45–52, 1951.

Ciocco, A., Consistency and significance of tests made with the 4-A audiometer. *Public Health Rep.*, 51, 1402–1406, 1936.

Dahl, L. A., *Public School Audiometry: Principles and Methods*. Danville, Ill.: The Interstate, 1949.

Darley, F. L. (Editor), Identification audiometry. *J. Speech Hear. Disord.*, Monograph Suppl. 9, 1961.

Eagles, E. L., Wishik, S. M., and Doerfler, L. G. *Hearing Sensitivity and Ear Disease in Children: A Prospective Study*. St. Louis: Laryngoscope (Monograph), 1967.

Glorig, A. (Editor), *Audiometry: Principles and Practices*. Baltimore: Williams & Wilkins Co., 1965.

Griffing, T. S., Simonton, D. M., and Hedgecock, L. D. Verbal auditory screening for preschool children. *Trans. Am. Acad. Ophthalmol. Otolaryngol.*, 71, 105–111, 1967.

House, H. P., and Glorig, A. A new concept of auditory screening. *Laryngoscope*, 67, 661–668, 1957.

Johnston, P. W., The Massachusetts hearing test. *J. Acoust. Soc. Am.*, 20, 697–703, 1948.

Johnston, P. W., An efficient group screening test. *J. Speech Hear. Disord.*, 17, 8–12, 1952.

Lloyd, L. L., Comments on "dilemmas in identification audiometry." *J. Speech Hear. Disord.*, 31, 161–165, 1966.

McCandless, G. A., and Thomas, G. K., Impedance audiometry as a screening procedure for middle ear disease. *Trans. Am. Acad. Ophthalmol. Otolaryngol.*, 78, 98–102, 1974.

Melnick, W., Eagles, E. L., and Levine, H. S. Evaluation of a recommended program of identification audiometry with school age children. *J. Speech Hear. Disord.*, 29, 3–13, 1964.

Mencher, G. T., and McCulloch, B. F., Auditory screening of kindergarten children using the VASC. *J. Speech Hear. Disord.*, 35, 241–247, 1970.

Meyerson, L., Hearing for speech in children: A verbal audiometric test. *Acta Otolaryngol. (Suppl.)*, 128, 1–165, 1956.

Newby, H. A., *Audiology*, Ed. 2. New York: Appleton-Century-Crofts, 1964.

Newhart, H. A new pure tone audiometer for school use. *Arch. Otolaryngol.*, 28, 777–779, 1938.

Newhart, H. and Reger, S. N., *Manual for a School Hearing Conservation Program. Second Revision*. Rochester, Minn.: American Academy of Ophthalmology and Otolaryngology, 1956.

Reger, S. N., and Newby, H. A., A group pure tone hearing test. *J. Speech Hear. Disord.*, 12, 61–66, 1947.

Roberts, J., Hearing sensitivity and related medical findings among children in the United States. *Trans. Am. Acad. Ophthalmol. Otolaryngol.*, 76, 355–359, 1972.

Watson, L., and Tolan, T., *Hearing Tests and Hearing Instruments*. Baltimore: Williams & Wilkins Co., 1949.

chapter 6

INDUSTRIAL HEARING CONSERVATION

William Melnick, Ph.D.

The word "conservation" is defined as "a careful preservation or protection of something; the planned management of a natural resource to prevent exploitation, destruction, or neglect." "Preservation" means "to keep safe from injury, harm, or destruction; to keep alive, intact, free from decay" (*Webster*, 1969). The conservation of hearing is a function of an audiologist. Conservation and rehabilitation — attempts to minimize the handicap of a hearing loss — form the foundation for the existence of the field of audiology. The fundamental purpose of industrial hearing conservation is not appreciably different from the aims of hearing conservation in general. There must be something unique about the industrial environment which permits us specifically to label these efforts "industrial hearing conservation." The most distinctive feature of hearing conservation in an industrial environment is that we have been able to identify a noxious agent which has a pervasive effect on the hearing of people working in this environment. That agent is noise. The National Safety Council has recognized the importance of hearing conservation in industry and has published a comprehensive reference (Olishifski and Harford, 1975) for use by the involved professional.

The link between the existence of noise in the environment and the production of hearing loss in people working in that environment is beyond question. There is no doubt that hazardous noise conditions produce destruction of auditory sensory cells, the hair cells (Lim and Melnick, 1971; see Fig. 6.1), in the cochlea, and that sufficient destruction of these elements will produce hearing loss (Sataloff and Michael, 1973). Many of the hazardous properties of noise have been defined. The physical characteristics of noise can be measured, and hearing loss produced by noise can be prevented, unlike many other conditions which produce sensory-neural hearing loss.

LEGAL BASIS

Legislation has been and is being written with a regulating effect on hearing conservation programs. This has stimulated the development of new conservation programs in industries which might otherwise have ignored the problem. Legal interpretations of compensation laws have made hearing losses resulting from exposure to industrial noise compensable. The economic realities of court decisions have made the problem of noise-induced hearing loss difficult to ignore.

Federal regulation of occupational noise exposure started with regulations issued under the authority of the Walsh-Healey Public Contracts Act in May, 1969. The Walsh-Healey Act stated that noise must be reasonably controlled to minimize fatigue and industrial accidents. This Act applied to all industries having government contracts of $10,000 or more. Passage of the 1970 Occupational Safety and Health Act set minimum standards for industrial hearing conservation programs and extended the applicability of acceptable noise exposure levels to all industries participating in interstate commerce.

A major reason for increased interest in industrial noise problems is the payment of compensation for occupationally caused loss of hearing. The intent of the original Workmen's Compensation Acts was to protect workers from loss of earnings and to cover medical costs arising from injuries occurring on-the-job. Landmark legal action has led to the inclusion of hearing loss as a compensable injury (Sataloff and Michael, 1973). In 1948, the New York Court of Appeals ruled that a person who developed a hearing loss as a result of his employment was entitled to compensation, even though there was no lost time and no loss of earnings. This departure from the original wage-loss concept of Workmen's Compensation resulted in an increased number of claims. In 1962, a court in Georgia ruled that an employee's hearing loss resulted from a cumulative effect of a succession of injuries caused by each daily noise insult on the ear. This court action resulted in a decision that hearing loss was compensable under the accidental injury provisions of the Workmen's Compensation law. Wisconsin had a Workmen's Compensation Act in force since 1931 which recognized a schedule of payments for loss of hearing. The first significant number of claims under this act were filed in 1951. Following several court cases, a bill was passed in Wisconsin establishing payment for occupational hearing loss in 1955.

The activities of federal and state legislatures and judicial systems have provided stimulus and motivation for development of industrial hearing conservation programs. The legal activities continue, with refinement and consideration of the present legislation specifying in more detail not only who will be covered by hearing conservation programs, but also the composition of these programs.

61

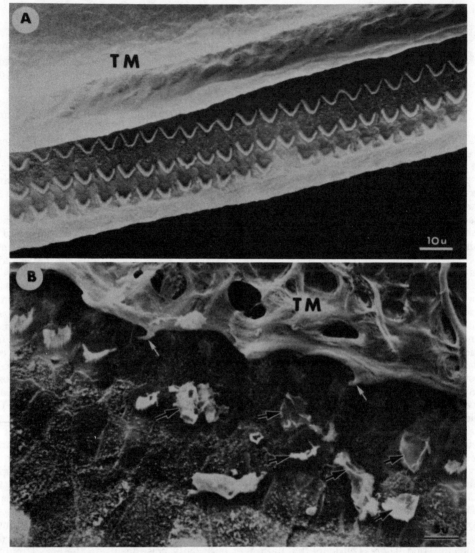

Fig. 6.1. (*A*) Scanning electron micrograph showing normal appearance of three rows of outer hair cells and tectorial membrane (TM). (*B*) Degenerating outer hair cells (arrows) resulting from a 6-hour exposure to a 1 to 2 kHz octave band of noise of 117 dB SPL. (From D. J. Lim and W. Melnick: *Archives of Otolaryngology*, **94**, 294–305, 1971. Reproduced with permission.)

EFFECTS OF NOISE ON HEARING

Noise has been reported to have many effects on people working in industry; such as, annoyance, decrease in working efficiency, physiologic changes in heart rate and blood pressure, and psychological distress. More direct auditory effects include the obvious interference with speech communication produced by the masking due to background noise, and the primary auditory effect, the capacity of noise to produce hearing loss. Industrial hearing con-servation programs are, for the most part, concerned only with the loss of hearing. Thus far, no conclusive evidence has been found that physiologic effects other than hearing loss can be produced at sound levels known to be hazardous to hearing. Even if it is found that other physiologic effects are produced at sound levels which result in hearing loss, it is probable that these secondary effects of noise would be eliminated incidentally by controlling the effect on hearing.

Effects of noise on hearing may be divided

generally into three categories: temporary threshold shift, permanent threshold shift, and acoustic trauma (Miller, 1971; Guignard, 1973). The term "acoustic trauma" is restricted to the effects of single exposures or relatively few exposures to very high levels of sound (e.g., an explosion). In the case of acoustic trauma, the sound levels reaching the structures in the inner ear exceed the physiologic limits of those structures, frequently producing complete breakdown and disruption of the organ of Corti. People who experience these very intense noise exposures may also have ruptured eardrums and damaged ossicles. Hearing loss from acoustic trauma is to a large degree permanent. The precipitating episode is usually very dramatic and pronounced in the memory of the person experiencing the event. The person involved has no difficulty in specifying the onset of the hearing problem.

Temporary threshold shift (TTS) is a short-term effect which may follow an exposure to noise. TTS refers to an elevation in the threshold of hearing which recovers gradually following the noise exposure. Since the noise produces a transient shift in the threshold, it has become known as temporary threshold shift, or even more specifically as noise-induced temporary threshold shift (NITTS).

Permanent threshold shifts (PTS) are those hearing changes which persist throughout the life of the affected person. When a threshold shift is permanent, there is no possibility for further recovery with the passage of time following exposure. Permanent threshold shifts which result from acoustic trauma or a single encounter to very destructive noise exist, but are relatively uncommon. More frequently, hearing loss produced by the effects of noise is a result of an accumulation of noise exposures which are repeated on a daily basis over a period of many years. This kind of hearing loss has become known as noise-induced permanent threshold shift (NIPTS). Thus, the loss in hearing sensitivity from chronic noise exposure is called noise-induced temporary threshold shift if the decrease in sensitivity eventually disappears, and it is called noise-induced permanent threshold shift if there is no recovery. An excellent, thorough treatment of temporary and permanent noise induced shift as well as consideration of the relationship of these two auditory phenomena has been published by Kryter (1970).

Temporary Threshold Shift (TTS)

Despite the large number of experiments in many laboratories throughout the world, the factors influencing TTS and the recovery from these shifts have not been completely defined.

A number of variables have been relatively uninvestigated. TTS can vary hearing sensitivity from an insignificant few decibels in a narrow frequency range to changes that render the ear temporarily deaf. After the termination of the noise, hearing sensitivity can return to the preexposure levels in a few minutes to several weeks.

Generalizations about TTS can be made from the experimental data (Miller, 1971). Low frequency noises are not as effective in producing TTS as high frequencies (Ward, 1973). Noises with energy concentrated in the frequency range of 2000 to 6000 Hz produce more TTS than noises with energy elsewhere in the frequency range. Sound levels must exceed a certain intensity before the average person will experience any TTS, even for exposures as long as 8 to 16 hours. If everything else is held constant, noise levels must exceed 60 to 80 dBA (60 to 80 dB on the A-scale of a sound level meter) to produce TTS. Above this intensity level, TTS will increase with an increase in intensity and with an increase in the duration of the noise (Miller, 1971). Recently, however, there is evidence that, at least for moderate intensity levels of noise, exposure durations that exceed 8 to 16 hours may not produce any further increase in the magnitude of the threshold shift (Mills et al., 1970; Mosko, Fletcher and Luz, 1970; Melnick, 1974; Melnick and Maves, 1974). For low level noises which produce very slight changes in threshold, most of the effect is observed in the frequency range of the noise or fatiguing sound. As the intensity of the noise increases, the frequency of maximum threshold shift occurs $\frac{1}{2}$ octave to an octave above the frequency region of greatest concentration of noise energy (Ward, 1963). Another observation is that a noise exposure with frequent interruptions will produce less TTS than a continuous noise exposure of equivalent sound energy (Ward, 1973).

People vary considerably in their susceptibility to NITTS (Ward, 1968). For classification purposes it would be convenient if individuals were grouped into two categories, those with ears particularly susceptible and those with ears minimally susceptible, if susceptibility to TTS were to be used as a predictor of susceptibility to permanent hearing losses from noise exposure. However, evidence from investigations of TTS indicates that the distribution of threshold shift shows a relatively good fit to a normal distribution, rather than a bimodal distribution of susceptibility (Burns, 1973).

TTS should be more than just of academic interest to those involved with industrial hearing conservation. There is usually an element of TTS which may accompany any permanent component of hearing loss following noise exposure. Hearing testing programs designed to provide evidence of the existence of permanent hearing loss must be wary of the possibility of a contaminating temporary component. This is especially true in obtaining valid preemployment audiograms or baseline audiograms in an industrial setting. The tester must be sure that the person tested is given ample opportunity for any TTS resulting from recent noise exposure to recover.

Information from systematic investigations of the relationship of noise exposure to NIPTS is difficult to obtain. Based on the assumption that the same processes involved in the growth and recovery of NITTS are also involved in the establishment of NIPTS, TTS data have been used to predict the hazardous effects of noise (Kryter et al., 1966; Burns, 1973).

Permanent Hearing Loss

NIPTS is found primarily among industrial workers who have been exposed repeatedly to high intensity noise for a relatively long period of employment. A common assumption is that the noise exposure component is the result of repeated NITTS. NIPTS is usually accompanied by NITTS. Apparently, with repeated exposure over a long work life the temporary component is reduced, while the magnitude of permanent hearing loss increases.

PTS found in the noise-exposed people usually results from combined effects of aging and chronic noise exposure. Gallo and Glorig (1964) studied the effects of age and duration of a continuous noise exposure as factors in developing PTS. In that investigation, several of the characteristics of NIPTS were described. Magnitude of PTS is related to the exposure levels and to the length of time a person worked in the noisy environment. A typical pattern of NIPTS showed that the maximum loss was in the range of 4000 to 6000 Hz, with smaller losses occurring at the frequencies above and below this range. Figure 6.2 illustrates the familiar air-conduction hearing loss pattern for noise-induced hearing loss (Maas, 1972). The growth of NIPTS at 4000 Hz is most rapid during the first 10 to 15 years of exposure, after which the loss seemed to slow down and plateau. As with NITTS, there were large individual differences in susceptibility to NIPTS.

Because of the many similarities in the effects of noise-produced TTS and PTS, there have been persistent attempts to demonstrate that the susceptibilities to TTS and PTS are related. If sensitivity to the temporary effects of noise could be demonstrated as an index of potential susceptibility to hearing loss, this predictor would be a major aid in industrial hearing conservation programs. Unfortunately, this relationship of TTS and PTS has

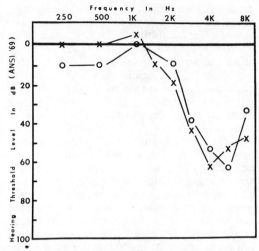

Fig. 6.2. Typical pure tone air-conduction threshold hearing levels for a patient exposed to high noise levels (Maas, 1972).

not been supported by any investigations thus far. A reliable test of susceptibility to PTS as a result of exposure to industrial noise has yet to be developed. The most that can be said about the relationship of TTS to PTS is that a noise which does not produce TTS will not produce permanent hearing loss. It is likely that a hearing loss produced by a specified exposure over a long period will not exceed the TTS produced by a short-term exposure to the same signal. Also, the audiometric pattern of TTS will resemble the pattern of the permanent hearing loss.

HAZARDOUS NOISE

The relation of noise exposure to hearing loss is not completely understood or well defined. From the data available from laboratory investigations of TTS and permanent hearing loss observed in industrial populations, four major factors emerge which contribute to the noise hazard (AAOO, 1973). These factors are:

1. The overall noise level.
2. The spectrum, or frequency content, of the noise.
3. Time distribution of noise exposure over an entire work day.
4. The total duration of noise exposure over an entire work day.

Review of these major factors makes it obvious that both the physical characteristics of the noise and the temporal patterns of the noise exposure are equally important. Noise exposure represents the product of the sound energy contained in the hazardous noise and the time this hazardous noise is experienced.

The type of industrial noise environment

must also be considered. The noise might be steady state, fluctuating, intermittent, or impulsive. Steady state noise can be described as continuous daily exposures in which the overall levels do not vary more than ± 5 dB (Guignard, 1973). Most frequently, noise encountered in industry is fluctuating; that is, the noise is continuous, but the levels rise and fall more than 5 dB during a particular exposure period. An intermittent noise is described as being discontinuous. During the work period, the noise level may fall to low or nonhazardous levels between periods of hazardous noise exposure. Impulsive noise can be described as one or more short, transient acoustical events which last less than 0.5 sec. A single impulse is usually heard as a discrete event occurring in otherwise quiet conditions or superimposed on a background of steady state ongoing noise.

The predicted effect of a particular noise on hearing has been based on the information developed in investigations of TTS and studies of industrially induced permanent hearing loss. A universal finding of all of these studies is a significant variation in susceptibility of people to NIPTS. In developing hazardous noise specifications, a decision must be made about the degree of hearing preservation that will be accomplished by these specifications. A criterion must be established which specifies the risk which is considered acceptable and serves as a basis for establishing predictive noise contours (Burns, 1973). In popular usage, the noise specifications or noise contours themselves have become known as the damage risk criteria, with the actual risk criteria being unknown or ignored by the users. Several specifications have been developed since the mid-1950s. Most of these noise specifications have made concessions in the amount of protection offered industrial employees from noise-induced TTS. Specifications usually are a compromise between an impractical aim of complete protection for all people exposed and the less stringent requirement of adequate protection for the speech frequencies, 500, 1000 and 2000 Hz.

The starting point, then, for the development of noise-risk specifications is the degree of deterioration of hearing which is regarded as acceptable. If all people reacted in the same way to noise, this would be an easy task. A limit could be established which would separate the damaging noise from the safe noise. However, the variability of normal hearing, the variability of change resulting from the aging process, and the variance in susceptibility to noise-induced change make this ideal difficult to accomplish.

For the most part, noise specifications assume that the noise experienced is a continuous, broad-band noise which is fairly flat throughout the audible spectrum without any prominent tonal components or narrow frequency bands. This noise is assumed to be continuous during the working day, for 5 days a week, over a period of years. Noise specifications usually take the form of acceptable sound pressure levels in octave bands covering the audible frequency range. If the noise is of a different character—discontinuous, impulsive or contains pure tones—the noise specifications are modified to include these noise variations. The present state of knowledge is not able to account for all of the relevant variables and, consequently, the specifications available today are less precise than desirable. Because specific sound pressure levels are stated in the specifications, the tendency is to attribute more precision to the predictions than is warranted.

Perhaps the most familiar and certainly the most detailed and elaborate noise specifications published thus far are the recommendations made by the National Research Council Committee on Hearing, Bioacoustics, and Biomechanics (CHABA), (Kryter et al., 1966). The criterion of acceptability underlying the CHABA proposal regards noise conditions as acceptable if, after 10 years or more of daily exposure, a hearing loss of not more than 10 dB at 1000 Hz and below, or 15 dB at 2000 Hz, or 20 dB at 3000 Hz and above, is produced. The CHABA specifications cover the frequencies between 100 and 7000 Hz and have been published in the form of noise curves or damage risk contours as shown in Figure 6.3. A distinct feature of these contours is that not only are maximum allowable sound pressures for bands of noise indicated, but also the duration to which a person might be exposed to any given level is specified. Another distinctive feature of the CHABA contours indicates that the contours for 8- and 4-hour exposures are almost exactly the same. This recommendation is questionable in view of the information coming from current studies using noise exposures longer than 8 hours (Mills et al., 1970; Melnick, 1974; Melnick and Maves, 1974). The CHABA specifications predict that continuous noises having tonal components are more hazardous, and that acceptable noise levels for these tones would have to be decreased by approximately 5 dB over that proposed for broad band noise for a comparable exposure time. At the time the CHABA recommendations were made, available data were insufficient for proposing specifications for impulsive noise, although the observation was made that repeated exposure to acoustic impulses exceeding peak levels of 140 dB could result in significant losses of hearing.

Many of the early hazardous noise specifications were stated in terms of octave band or

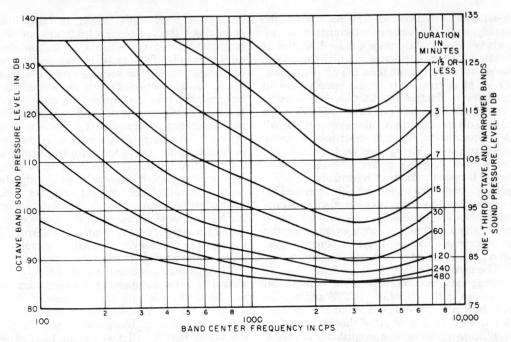

Fig. 6.3. Damage risk contours for octave and third octave bands of noise recommended by National Research Council Committee on Hearing, Bioacoustics, and Biomechanics (CHABA). (From K. D. Kryter et al.: *Journal of the Acoustical Society of America*, **39**, 451–464, 1966. Reproduced with permission.)

third octave band measurements. With accumulation of information about noise and its effects on hearing, the feeling arose that in many instances an octave band analysis was a needlessly complicated way to evaluate noise, and that it could be replaced by use of a single index of noise magnitude, the A-weighted sound level (Botsford, 1970). The A-weighting network in a sound level meter makes the meter less sensitive to low frequency sounds in much the same way that the ear is less sensitive to these same low frequency sounds (Fig. 6.2). The use of the dBA values as quantitative descriptions of noise exposures is likely to gain in acceptance. It has been incorporated in many of the federal and state regulations concerning noise exposure.

The American Conference of Governmental Industrial Hygienists developed recommendations for limits of permissible noise exposure (Botsford, 1970). These recommendations were incorporated in the Walsh-Healey Public Contracts Act and in subsequent federal regulations in the Occupational Safety and Health Act. These values are shown in Table 6.1, and incorporate the so-called "5-dB rule." This rule assumes that time-intensity trades will maintain equal noxiousness of noise exposures. If the intensity of the noise is increased 5 dB, then the permissible duration must be reduced by $\frac{1}{2}$. For instance, if the noise level were

TABLE 6.1. *Permissible Noise Exposures*[*]

Duration per Day (Hours)	Sound Level dBA Slow Response
8	90
6	92
4	95
3	97
2	100
1 1/2	102
1	105
1/2	110
1/4 or less	115

[*] Taken from Part 50-204 Safety and Health Standards for Federal Supply Contracts, *Federal Register*, May 20, 1969, with correction of July 15, 1969.

measured at 90 dBA, it would be permissible for a worker to be exposed to that noise for an entire 8 hours. If the noise level were measured at 95 dB, the maximum permissible duration would be reduced to 4 hours; at 100 dB, it would be reduced to 2 hours, and so on. These regulations specify 115 dBA to be the absolute maximum level to which anyone should be exposed, and levels beyond that should not be endured for any length of time. The federal regulations (Walsh-Healey, 1969) also adapted these dBA levels to approximately equivalent noise contours, so that noise data in the form of octave band sound pressure levels may be easily used in determining when noise exposure might be in excess of the proposed limits. These contours are shown in Figure 6.4.

The noise specifications just described are usually for a continuous steady state noise. This certainly is not the usual noise environment in industry. When the daily noise exposure is composed of two or more periods of noises at different levels, their combined effect should be considered. This kind of exposure is expressed as a noise exposure rating, which is defined as a ratio of the observed duration of the dangerous noise to that duration allowable under the specifications for regulatory limits. Noise exposure is considered acceptable for all values of exposure if the combined ratios do not exceed unity (one). The hazard to hearing increases as the noise exposure ratio becomes progressively greater than one. The hazardous noise rating may be calculated using the following equation:

$$\frac{C_1}{T_1} + \frac{C_2}{T_2} + \frac{C_n}{T_n} = \text{Noise rating}$$

C_n indicates the total time of exposure at a specified noise level, while T_n indicates the total time of an exposure permitted at that level (U.S. Department of Labor, 1974).

For impulsive noise, a recommendation has been made that the impact noise should not exceed 140 dB peak sound pressure level. With impulsive noises, there is usually a trade-off between intensities of the pulse and the number of pulses that can be experienced. A current recommendation is that with a 10-dB decrease in peak sound pressure level there would be a corresponding increase in the number of allowable pulses in a work day by a factor of 10. The base is assumed to be 100 pulses per day. If the peak level increases to 150 dB, then only 10 pulses per day would be permissible (U.S. Department of Labor, 1974).

HEARING CONSERVATION PROGRAM

Indication of the need for a hearing conservation program may be judged by simple observation of the environment. In the *Guide for the Conservation of Hearing in Noise*, prepared by the Subcommittee on Noise of the Committee on Conservation of Hearing of the American Academy of Ophthalmology and Otolaryngology (AAOO, 1973), the following three conditions are listed as indications of a need for such a program:

1. Difficulty in communicating by speech while in noise.

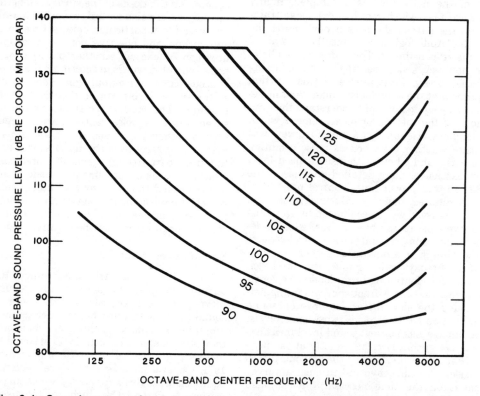

Fig. 6.4. Sound contours for determining equivalent A-weighted sound level. (Taken from Part 50–204, Safety and Health Standards for Federal Supply Contracts, *Federal Register*, May 20, 1969, with correction of July 15, 1969.)

2. Head noises or ringing in the ears after working in the noise for several hours.
3. A temporary loss of hearing that has the effect of muffling speech and changing the quality of other sounds after several hours of exposure to noise.

The *Guide* further points out that pain and annoyance are not reliable indicators of a potentially hazardous noise. Pain may be felt in the ear during exposure to noise over 120 dB, while noise-induced hearing loss may be produced at considerably lower levels.

An industrial hearing conservation program should involve three activities:

1. Assessment of noise exposure.
2. The control of the noise exposure.
3. The measurement of hearing.

NOISE SURVEY

As stated earlier, whether a noise is hazardous depends on the intensity of the noise, the spectrum of the noise, the duration and distribution of exposure during a typical work day, and the overall exposure during a work life. Each of these areas must be evaluated to determine the need for instituting noise control and hearing conservation programs. Detailed analysis of the noise field is a complex, highly technical task which requires extensive training on the part of the person performing the analysis. Audiologists are typically not trained for this responsibility. The industrial audiologist, however, should be capable of conducting a noise survey. Performance of this function requires that the audiologist understand noise-measuring equipment and understand the limitations of the method of measurement which he employs. Generally, a noise survey will indicate whether a hazardous noise condition does exist, and whether there is a need for a more extensive, more detailed analysis of the noise, so that proper noise control procedures can be initiated. In many industrial situations, the noise survey will be conducted by an industrial hygienist or safety engineer, while a detailed noise analysis and noise control require the services of an acoustical engineer.

Most of today's rules, guidelines, and specifications for identifying hazardous noise conditions state that the A-frequency weighting network and the slow meter response on sound level meters be used to measure noise levels. In a damage risk survey, sound level measurements are generally required only at the position that will be occupied by the person exposed to noise. The time involved in such a survey depends on the time necessary to establish typical temporal patterns of noise exposure. If the noise is continuous and does not change from day to day, then a fairly small sample is all that is required. If, however, there are unpredictable on-off times, intermittencies, and rather complex exposure patterns, then the noise survey may require many days or weeks in order to accomplish a meaningful description of the noise environment. If the noise is a simple continuous type then the measurements can be made simply by reading the sound level meter and recording the observation. A new sound measurement would not be necessary until there was some noticeable change in the noise source, or there was a change in the location of the worker. However, for the very complex noise exposure patterns which exist in many industries, the variation makes direct sound level measurements very difficult, and usually this kind of sound field requires the use of automatic sound recording equipment.

When a survey is conducted for purposes of noise control, the analysis requires the use of octave band or even narrower frequency band sound analyzers. These analyses are geared to pin-point and describe individual noise source contributions. Narrow band analyzers are used to isolate particular noise sources in high background noise levels. The measurement locations for a noise control survey will vary depending on the needs of the survey. Generally, the purpose of noise control surveys is to isolate and describe a particular noise source so that appropriate and effective noise control measures can be chosen. Another purpose for the noise control survey is to determine the amount of acoustical power output from a noise source, so that noise levels can be predicted in other locations. The method for recording the measurements in a noise control survey depends upon whether the person doing the measurement has control over the noise source and if the time patterns are generally predictable. However, if the measurement is made at many points around the noise source and is made in a special environment, such as an anechoic or reverberation chamber, the use of automatic recording equipment may be required.

Sound Level Meter

Surveying an industrial environment to determine whether the noise is hazardous requires the use of the sound level meter. The sound level meter consists of a microphone, an amplifier, attenuator circuit, and some sort of indicating meter. Characteristics of sound level meters are specified in ANSI standard S1.4-1971. General purpose sound level meters are equipped with three frequency weighting networks—A, B and C—which can be used to approximate frequency distribution of noise in the audible frequency range. These three frequency weighting networks were chosen because they approximate the ear response characteristics at different sound levels and because these circuits are easy to construct. The A-weighting network approximates the ear's response characteristics for low level sound below about 55-dB sound pressure level. The B-weighting network is intended to approximate the ear's response for levels between 55 and 85 dB, and the C-weighting network corresponds to the ear's response for levels above 85 dB (Sataloff and Michael, 1973). The frequency characteristics of these weighting networks are shown in Figure 6.5.

Sound level meters usually have two types of response characteristics built into the meter. These characteristics have been labeled "fast" and "slow" response. The fast response enables the meter to reach within 4 dB of its calibrated reading for 1000 Hz in 0.2 sec. It can be used to measure levels which do not change substantially in less than 0.2 sec. The slow response is intended to provide an averaging effect that will reduce the fluctuations of sound levels and make these noise levels easier to read. The slow setting will not provide accurate readings if the sound levels change in less than 0.5 sec. Neither the fast nor the slow response is adequate for measuring impulse or impact types of noise. Measurement of the acoustic properties of these noises requires special equipment or special circuits in the sound level meter.

Three basic types of microphones are used in noise measurements. These are the piezo electric, the dynamic, and the condenser microphones. Each has advantages and disadvantages, and all three may be used with sound level meters. Those making noise measure-ments should be aware of the limitations of the microphone on their meter. Particularly, they should be interested in the frequency response characteristics of the microphone, the intensity range that can be covered by the microphone, the effects of temperature and humidity on the properties of the microphone, and the directional characteristics.

Lack of understanding of the directional properties of microphones is a frequent source of error. A microphone calibrated with a randomly incident sound should usually be held at an angle with respect to the major noise source. This angle should be specified by the manufacturer. A free field microphone is calibrated to measure sounds emanating from a source perpendicular to the microphone diaphragm. A pressure type microphone that is designed for use in a coupler for calibrating audiometers can also be used to measure noise over most of the audible spectrum. The noise, however, should be measured at a grazing incidence to the diaphragm, and the proper microphone calibration curve should be used.

Vibration of the sound measuring equipment may cause erroneous sound level readings. Sound measuring equipment should, whenever possible, be mechanically isolated from any vibrating sources. Simply hand holding of the equipment or placement of it on a foam rubber pad is usually satisfactory.

Most general purpose sound measuring instruments have built-in calibration circuits for checking electrical gain. These sound level meters may also be used in connection with acoustical calibrators, which are either built-in or can be purchased as a separate accessory. The electrical and acoustical calibration should be made according to the manufacturer's in-

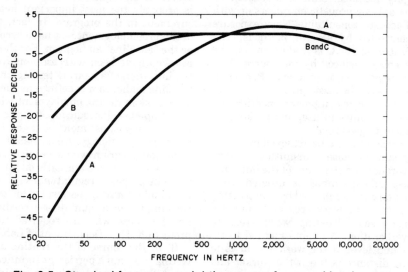

Fig. 6.5. Standard frequency weighting curves for sound level meters.

structions at the beginning and end of each day's measurements. If the equipment is battery-powered, a battery check should also be made at these times. These field calibration procedures are not of the highest accuracy, but will serve to warn of most common instrument failures. Periodically, (at least once a year), the sound measuring equipment should be sent back to the manufacturer or to an independent acoustic laboratory for complete calibration. How often a laboratory calibration is conducted depends upon the purpose of the measurements and how frequently and roughly the meter has been handled. It is a good rule of thumb that a complete calibration should be made if changes of greater than ± 2 dB are seen in the daily field calibrations (Sataloff and Michael, 1973).

The amount of noise exposure actually experienced by a given employee is difficult to measure with the usual sound level meter. During the course of a work day, the noise environment is likely to fluctuate because of changes in the noise source, or because of changes of the employee's position in the noise field. One attempted solution to this problem is the use of personal noise dosimeters. A noise dosimeter is a type of sound level meter which integrates the A-weighted sound pressure over a period of time and usually compares the measured exposure with a criterion sound exposure, for example with an 8-hour exposure to 90 dBA. The dosimeter is carried by the individual employee with the microphone mounted on the shoulder, on the chest, or at the ear. This device also could be used to monitor a particular area in the industrial environment.

NOISE CONTROL

The control of the noise environment requires highly technical skills and should be undertaken only by acoustic engineers or with the help of acoustic consultants. Noise exposure may be controlled by several methods. The most desirable method is reduction in the amount of noise produced by the source. This is not always possible or practical. Reduction of source noises can be accomplished by careful acoustic design of new equipment, modification of designs of machines in use, and by keeping the equipment in good repair.

Noise control may also be achieved by reducing the amount of noise transmitted through the air or through the structure of the building. If the noise source cannot be quieted, then noise reduction can be achieved by constructing barriers between the work area and the noise source, or by sound-treating work areas to reduce reverberation. A simple method to reduce the sound level at the worker's ear is to increase the distance between the worker and the noise sources. Placing noise generating equipment on vibration mounts can reduce transmission of noise through the structural properties of the building.

Noise exposure may also be reduced through administrative or procedural changes. Work schedules could be adjusted so that noise exposures would be interrupted regularly. Personnel who are routinely exposed to high levels of noise could be rotated to other areas and/or other jobs. Work schedules might be arranged so that a minimum number of people are in a particular work area during high noise conditions. Any procedure which will reduce the noise level or reduce the total exposure time will be effective for the purposes of hearing conservation.

MEASUREMENT OF HEARING

The main interest of an audiologist in industrial hearing conservation, because of his orientation, training, and experience, will be in the area of hearing measurement. Audiometric examinations are the only available way to detect an individual's susceptibility to noise. By comparing the results of periodic examinations, an estimate can be made of how the employee is being affected by the noisy working environment. People who are particularly sensitive to the stresses of noise can be identified, and corrective measures can be instituted before the hearing loss becomes permanent and handicapping.

An industrial hearing measurement program should involve preemployment testing and periodic follow-up tests. Preemployment tests should be made at the time the employee is hired. The preemployment audiogram establishes an employee's hearing status before he is exposed to noise in his job. This audiogram serves as a comparative baseline, and as such is probably the most important hearing measurement in the program. In fact, the results of the preemployment test have become known as the "baseline" audiogram. For those employees who have been with an employer prior to the initiation of a hearing testing program, the baseline audiogram is defined as the first audiogram taken during employment with the current employer. Periodic follow-up tests serve to monitor any subsequent changes in hearing, regardless of etiology. An optimal hearing conservation program would require that the follow-up test be made annually on all employees. Current proposed regulations suggest that annual audiograms be performed for those people working in noise equal to or exceeding 85 dBA, and for those who are required to wear ear protection (U.S. Department of Labor, 1974).

If, in the course of the routine audiometric testing program a persistent significant threshold shift is observed, then the employee should be retested more frequently. The frequency of retest may be at the discretion of the person responsible for the testing program, or it may in fact be regulated by legislation. Recently proposed federal legislation recommends that the employee be retested within 1 month if the hearing levels averaged for the frequencies 2000, 3000 and 4000 Hz show a shift of more than 10 dB relative to the baseline audiogram in either ear. If the shift of threshold hearing level persists, then employees should undergo further medical and audiologic evaluation in an effort to determine the etiology of the apparent hearing loss.

As mentioned earlier, one of the effects of working in a noise environment is a temporary change in threshold hearing levels. Those participating in a testing program in industry should be careful to minimize the influence of the temporary change on their audiograms. This reduction can be accomplished by allowing sufficient time for recovery of hearing sensitivity before testing the employee's hearing. Current guidelines (U.S. Department of Labor, 1974) suggest that audiometric tests be preceded by a period of at least 14 hours during which there is no exposure to sound levels of 80 dBA. This condition can be achieved either by insuring that the worker is away from the noise for that period of time, or by having the employee wear some type of effective hearing protection which would reduce his noise exposure to acceptable levels. Because of problems in scheduling tests around the work schedule of an employee, frequently the most feasible and practical method for achieving the noise rested condition is the use of hearing protection.

Audiometers

The cornerstone of an industrial hearing testing program is a pure tone air-conduction threshold test. At a minimum, threshold should be measured at the frequencies 500, 1000, 2000, 3000, 4000 and 6000 Hz in each ear. The testing may make use of either a manual audiometer or a self-recording "automatic" audiometer. Manual pure tone audiometers are manufactured in three basic types: wide range, limited range, or narrow range (ANSI S3.6-1969). For industrial testing purposes, the limited range pure tone air-conduction audiometer is appropriate. This audiometer is capable of handling the frequency and intensity requirements for the testing program. For "automatic" audiometry, the fixed frequency type of audiometer is preferable in the industrial setting. With this type of instrument, the test frequency is usually presented sequentially in periods of 30 sec for each test frequency. The test frequency and test ear are automatically selected

by the instrument. The intensity level is controlled by a switch manipulated by the person who is being tested, in a similar fashion to the Bekesy test procedure. For an automatic test to be valid, the test record should indicate at least six threshold crossings at each test frequency. The threshold is taken to be the average of the midpoints of the tracing.

There is no simple answer to the question of whether automatic audiometers are more suitable for industrial hearing testing than manual audiometers. With use of a manual audiometer, the tester has greater flexibility regarding the testing procedures and more control over the test situation than with the automatic variety. Some employees find that the task in manual pure tone audiometry is easier to understand and perform than the automatic test. Neither of these two audiometric techniques shows an advantage over the other in terms of the time required for the test. Experience shows, however, that young adults with normal hearing can be tested more quickly using the manual audiometer. The main advantage of the automatic audiometer is that it reduces the influence of one of the main sources of variation in measuring hearing threshold; that is, the technician himself. The testing technique is more standardized from situation to situation. Manual audiometry can become tedious, and technicians quickly may fall into bad habits. The self-recording audiometric technique, however, is not completely automatic. It still requires the attention of the audiometric technician. The technician can turn his attention to another task only when he is certain that the person being tested is responding properly. In larger industrial situations, self-recording audiometry will permit testing of several persons at the same time; the limiting factor would be the number of persons that a technician can visually monitor. Even though there are some automatic features to the self-recording audiometer, the industrial audiometric technician still should have the fundamental information and training regarding the testing of hearing as is needed for manual pure tone hearing tests (Rintelmann, 1973).

Test Method

A major source of variation in manual pure tone audiometry is the test technique. The people who perform these tests in industry vary widely in terms of their background, training, and experience with hearing testing. Consequently, there have been attempts to develop a standardized test procedure to minimize these individual tester differences. Because of the demand arising primarily out of the industrial hearing conservation program, efforts are being made to adopt a standard pure tone air conduction measuring technique as an American National Standard.

The proposed method involves a familiarization procedure. During the familiarization period, the listener is presented with a signal of sufficient intensity to evoke a clear response. This can be accomplished by turning the tone on continuously and starting from a completely attenuated signal, gradually increasing the sound pressure level until a response occurs. The tone is then switched off, and then again presented at the same level. If there is a second positive response, the tester proceeds to the threshold measurements. The first presentation of the tone for threshold measurement is 10 dB below the level at which the subject first responded during the familiarization process. Each succeeding presentation is determined by the preceding response. After each failure to respond to a signal, the level is increased 5 dB until the first response occurs. After this response, the intensity is again decreased 10 dB and another ascending series is begun. Threshold is taken to be the lowest level at which responses occurred in at least half of the ascending trials, with a minimum of three responses required at a single level.

Audiometer Calibration

The test equipment is another source of possible variation in hearing test results. If threshold measurements are to be reliable and valid indications of hearing status, the audiometer must be accurately calibrated. The person doing the testing should check the audiometer daily for malfunction: listening for distortion, intermittency, and extraneous noises, as well as checking grossly his own threshold. An additional more thorough check should be made at least once a month. This monthly check should consist of testing a person or persons having known stable audiometric patterns which do not exceed 25 dB hearing level at any frequency between 500 and 6000 Hz. A comparison can then be made with the subjects' known baseline audiograms. If the tester is suspicious of the performance, or if the monthly biologic check indicates that there may be some problem, the audiometer should be subjected to a more exhaustive laboratory calibration.

A detailed laboratory calibration of an audiometer should determine if the equipment meets the requirements stated in the American National Standard S3.6-1969, "Specifications for Audiometers." These specifications include tolerances for output sound pressure level, test frequency, harmonic distortion, attenuation linearity, tone presentation switching, and many other aspects of equipment performance. If the specifications are exceeded, the audiometer should be repaired and made to conform to the provisions of S3.6-1969. Proposed federal regulations (U.S. Department of Labor, 1974) for industrial hearing conservation programs recommend a complete laboratory calibration of audiometers at least every five years and a more frequent (annual) acoustic check of the audiometer's output sound pressure levels, attenuator linearity and frequency. Laboratory calibration of the audiometer should be carried out whenever results of the biological checks or the annual acoustic checks make the tester suspicious of the test equipment.

Test Environment

Reliable measures of hearing sensitivity require that the ambient background noise levels in the test environment be of a sufficiently low level so as not to interfere with the measurement of the pure tone threshold. Criteria for acceptable background noise levels to permit the measurement of normal hearing threshold under the old American Standards (see ANSI S3.1-1960) are not acceptable for measuring 0 dB HL *re* ANSI S3.6-1969. A rough approximation of more acceptable background noise levels can be calculated by subtracting the ANSI-1969 threshold hearing levels from the ASA-1951 levels and then reducing by those amounts the allowable background noise stated in the standard S3.1-1960 for the appropriate octave bands for each test frequency. These approximations are shown in Table 6.2. A new standard for allowable background noise levels for audiometry is in the process of preparation.

Frequently, testing in an industrial situation takes place in a quiet area in the plant or factory. Obtaining a quiet environment may dictate that a sound-isolating test room be constructed. If an industry is sufficiently large, and there are a number of employees involved in the hearing conservation program, the situation may warrant construction of a test facility on the premises. However, this is not always the case, and frequently hearing testing is accomplished using mobile test facilities.

Mobile test units are particularly useful when a number of different locations are to be surveyed. At the simplest level, the mobile facility could be an enclosure in the form of an audiometric room mounted on a trailer. On the other hand, the mobile unit may be more elaborate, containing several test rooms and including complete laboratory calibration facilities. In any case, whether the testing area is a quiet room in the industrial facility, a specially constructed sound-isolating test chamber built on the premises, or a mobile testing facility, the background noise levels should be sufficiently low to test air conduction threshold at the desired hearing level.

TABLE 6.2. *Estimated Allowable Background Noise Levels for Testing at Zero dB re ANSI-1969**

	Octave Band Center Frequency (Hz)				
	500	1000	2000	4000	8000
Permissible levels S3.1-1960 (based on ASA-1951)	40	40	47	52	62
Difference ASA-1951 minus ANSI-1969 (rounded off to nearest 5 dB)	15	10	10	10	10
Estimated allowable octave band levels for ANSI-1969 thresholds	25	30	37	42†	52‡

* These estimates are based on measurements made with earphones having attenuation characteristics of TDH-39 earphones with MX-41/AR cushions. A more general American National Standard is in the process of development.

† For test frequencies 3000 Hz; would be adequate for 4000 Hz.

‡ For test frequencies 6000 Hz; would be adequate for 8000 Hz.

Test Personnel

The accuracy of the audiometric measurements stems from the skill of the tester. It would be ideal if an audiologist were responsible for this service, but in fact under present conditions most hearing tests are conducted by an industrial nurse or by a technician who has a minimal background in audiometry. In an effort to reduce the variation attributable to the skill and training of the technician, training programs have been devised to establish minimal educational foundations and to introduce a standard air conduction test technique. In 1965, an Intersociety Committee—composed of the Industrial Medical Association, the American Industrial Hygiene Association, the American Association of Industrial Nurses, and the American Speech and Hearing Association—developed a 20-hour training course for the industrial audiometric technician (Maas, 1972, Appendix). In 1973, the responsibility for quality control of these training programs for industrial audiometric technicians was assumed by the Council for Accreditation in Occupational Hearing Conservation (CAOHC). These training courses should provide the prospective technician with a brief background in sound, the ear, and hearing. A major portion of the suggested training program is devoted to introducing a standard procedure for measurement of pure tone air-conduction thresholds, and practice in using this method. This includes the recognition of an adequate test environment, care and maintenance of test equipment, and accurate record keeping. Another area of concentration is the function and fitting of ear protectors. Successful completion of these training programs usually results in a certificate for the trainee. Test results produced by a certified audiometric technician are legally acceptable. Clinical audiologists have been extremely active in participating in these training programs and in the supervision of the work of these technicians in industrial hearing conservation programs.

EAR PROTECTION

The main goal of an industrial hearing conservation program is to prevent noise-induced hearing loss. This can be accomplished by reducing the noise exposure. The best method for this reduction is to prevent the noise generation at the source. When this is not possible, the next most desirable method is to reduce the opportunity for the employee to be exposed to noise through administrative controls. There will be many situations in which neither of these solutions to the noise problem are possible. Under these conditions, the method of choice would be to provide ear protectors.

An effective ear protector serves as a barrier between the noise and the inner ear, where the noise-induced damage occurs. Ear protectors usually take one of two forms: the ear muff, which is worn over the external ear and provides an acoustic seal against the head; or ear plugs, which seal the entrance to the external ear canal. The protection provided by an ear protector depends upon its design and on the physical characteristics of the person wearing the protector.

It is impossible to totally isolate the inner ear from noise by means of an ear protector. Sound energy can reach the inner ears of persons wearing ear protectors by three different paths:

1. By passing directly to the cochlea through vibration of the bones and tissues of the skull (bone conduction).
2. By vibration of the ear protector itself, which generates sound in the ear canal.
3. By passing through leaks in the ear protector, or around the protector because of poor fit.

The absolute limit of attenuation provided by an ear protector, of course, depends upon the sensitivity of the bone conduction pathway.

Ear Plugs

There are many kinds of protectors on the market. The insert type of protector, or ear plug, could be semipermanent, molded of soft rubber or soft plastic material that is sized. No single-sized molded ear plug has been found that would fit the large range of ear canal sizes and shapes. Most of the accepted molded ear plugs come in four or five different sizes.

Ear plugs may also be malleable, and made of materials such as cotton, paper, wax, glass wool, or some of the more recent plastic compounds. These plugs, which can be shaped by the wearer, are usually made of nonporous, easily formed materials, and they are capable of providing attenuation that compares favorably with the best of the semipermanent molded variety of ear plugs. The malleable ear plugs are usually designed for short term use and are frequently disposable.

Ear Muffs

Most of the muff protectors are similar in design. The protector ear cups are usually formed of a rigid, dense, imperforate material. These hard shells are fitted into soft, pliable seals, generally made of a smooth plastic envelope filled with a foam or some fluid material. The cup encloses a volume of air which is directly related to low frequency attenuation. The inside of the ear cup is partially filled with material that absorbs high frequency resonant noises.

Most protective devices available commercially will provide sufficient attenuation to offset the hazardous noise exposures typically found in industrial environments. The chief problem has been in developing motivation for employees to wear the ear protectors. Experience has shown that no one type satisfies all employees. It is therefore a good practice to stock more than one variety of ear protector.

There are advantages and disadvantages to the muff or insert types of ear protectors (Sataloff and Michael, 1973).

Advantages of ear plugs:

1. Small and easily carried.
2. Can be worn conveniently.
3. More comfortable to wear in hot environments.
4. Convenient to use when the head of the wearer must be in close, cramped quarters.
5. Cost is generally significantly less than ear muffs.

Disadvantages of insert-type protection:

1. The semi-permanent type and molded ear protectors require more time and effort to fit.
2. The amount of protection provided by an earplug is generally less and varies considerably among wearers.
3. Can become dirty and unsanitary through use.
4. Difficult to see at a distance, making it difficult to insure that employees are wearing them.

5. Cannot be worn by individuals with external and middle ear infections.

Advantages of muff-type protectors:

1. A single-size will fit most heads.
2. Can be easily seen, so the effectiveness of ear protector program can be easily monitored.
3. Usually more readily accepted by employee than ear plugs.
4. Generally more comfortable than plugs.
5. Not as easily misplaced or lost as ear plugs.

Disadvantages of ear muffs:

1. In general, more expensive than insert protectors.
2. Bulky and not as easily worn in cramped quarters.
3. Uncomfortably warm in hot environments.
4. Not as easily carried or stored as ear plugs.
5. Muff protection depends upon the spring force of the head band. Through usage, the force may be considerably weakened, and the protection significantly reduced.

Ultimately, the type of protection chosen will depend on the noise and environmental conditions in the industry. The chief function of an ear protector is to reduce the noise reaching the inner ear. The persons responsible for ear protector programs should be aware of the amount of attenuation provided by the various types of protectors they intend to use. The attenuation properties of the protectors are usually listed by the manufacturer. The person supervising the ear protector program should be aware that usually the specifications listed by the manufacturer are the average results obtained under relatively good laboratory conditions. It is a good rule of thumb to reduce these reported attenuation characteristics by 5 to 10 dB to get an estimate of actual performance in the field. Frequently, the manufacturer also provides an estimate of variation of effectiveness of the ear protector in terms of standard deviations. When this information is available, the effectiveness of the ear plug in the field can be better estimated by reducing the specified performance by one or two standard deviations. Examples of attenuation of various types of ear protectors are shown in Figure 6.6. Note the minimal protection provided by dry cotton. For some marginally hazardous noise conditions, even this minimal sound reduction by cotton would provide acceptable protection. The decision about the type of protection to use depends on the noise problem and the needs of the worker. Notice also that in Figure 6.6 the combination of the ear plugs and ear muffs does not provide additive protection afforded by either of these devices alone. Remember that the maximum amount of pro-

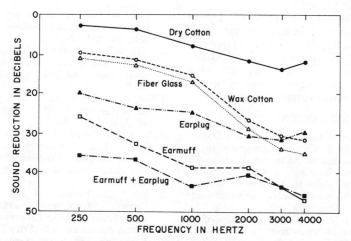

Fig. 6.6. Sound reduction properties of different types and combinations of ear protectors. (From W. Melnick: *Occupational Health Nursing*, **17**, 28–31, 1969. Reproduced with permission.)

tection is limited by the sensitivity of the transmission pathway through the skull.

RECORD KEEPING

Keeping accurate records is important in any clinical or hearing conservation program. Records assume a particular importance in an industrial situation, because of the potential for compensation and the implications for legal action. Federal and state legislation may in fact dictate the types of records to be maintained, the form in which these records will be kept, and the length of time the records will be stored.

The employer will need to keep accurate records of noise exposure measurements. These records should include the specifications on the location, date, and time the measurements were made, the noise levels obtained, and the name of the person making the measurement. The employer may also be required to keep the names of the employees and the daily noise dose experienced by each of these employees. Certainly there is a need for records specifying the type, model, and calibration of the noise measuring equipment.

The employer will probably be required to keep an accurate record of audiometric testing information for all employees. These records should include identification of the employee; the date of the audiogram; the employee's job location; the name of the tester; the tester's credentials (certification); the make, model, and serial number of the audiometer; and the date of the last calibration of test equipment.

Accurate records of all audiometric calibrations and checks must be kept. These records should specify the type of check, the date, and the measurements obtained.

The length of time these records need to be kept will vary from state to state and from regulation to regulation. Audiologists involved in industrial hearing conservation should be familiar with the requirements pertaining to the industries which are being served. Usually these records are required to be kept for a minimum of 5 years.

Initiating and maintaining an industrial hearing conservation program may involve a single professional or a group of people with relevant interests. Today there are relatively few audiologists employed full-time in industrial hearing conservation programs. More frequently, they are used in consulting roles. As a consultant, the audiologist comes in contact with industrial physicians, consulting otolaryngologists, safety engineers, industrial hygienists, industrial nurses, industrial relations and personnel managers, and officials of management and union. If an audiologist is to function effectively in such a program, he must be aware of his own skills and limitations, as well as the skills and potential services offered by each of the other members of the hearing conservation team. If an audiologist is to be a respected member of the team, he must understand the problems of business and industry as well as the problems of the employee who is liable to encounter hazardous noise environments. There must be a particular sensitivity to the need to maintain testing schedules which cause minimal interruption in the major mission of industry, that of production. An audiologist can help to supply hearing testing services, must be concerned with the provision of hearing protection devices, can serve as an educational source for audiometric technicians, and should be available as a consultant to employers and employees alike. The services offered by audiologists to industry will depend on the experience and training of the individual audiologist, as well as the need in the particular industry which he serves. Audiologists should promote interest in all forms of hearing conservation, and particularly now in the industrial hearing conservation program.

REFERENCES

American Academy of Ophthalmology and Otolaryngology, *Guide for Conservation of Hearing in Noise,* Revised edition. Rochester, Minn., 1973.

American National Standards Institute, "Criteria for Background Noise in Audiometer Rooms," ANSI S3.1-1960, American National Standards Institute, Inc., New York, 1960.

American National Standards Institute, "Specifications for General-Purpose Sound Level Meters," ANSI S1.4-1971, American National Standards Institute Inc., New York, 1971.

American National Standards Institute, "Specifications for Audiometers," ANSI S3.6-1969, American National Standards Institute, Inc., New York, 1969.

Botsford, J. H., Current trends in hearing damage risk criteria. *Sound Vibration,* 4, 16–19, 1970.

Burns, W., *Noise and Man,* Ed. 2, pp. 189–251. Philadelphia: J. B. Lippincott Co., 1973.

Gallo, R., and Glorig, A., Permanent threshold shift changes produced by noise exposure and aging. *Am. Ind. Hyg. Assoc. J.,* 25, 237–245, 1964.

Guignard, J. C., A basis for limiting noise exposure for hearing conservation, prepared for Environmental Protection Agency, EPA-550/9-73-001-A, pp. 4–21, 1973.

Kryter, K. D., *The Effects of Noise on Man.* New York: Academic Press, 1970.

Kryter, K. D., Ward, W. D., Miller, J. D., and Eldredge, D. H., Hazardous exposure to intermittent and steady-state noise. *J. Acoust. Soc. Am.* 39, 451–464, 1966.

Lim, D. J., and Melnick, W., Acoustic damage of the cochlea. *Arch. Otolaryngol.,* 94, 294–305, 1971.

Maas, R. B., Industrial noise and hearing conservation, in Katz, J. (Ed.), *Handbook of Clinical Audiology,* Ch. 41, pp. 772–818. Baltimore: Williams & Wilkins Co., 1972.

Melnick, W., Ear protectors. *Occup. Health Nurs.,* 17, 28–31, 1969.

Melnick, W., Human temporary threshold shift from 16-hour noise exposures. *Arch. Otolaryngol.,* 100, 180–189, 1974.

Melnick, W., and Maves, M., Asymptotic threshold shift (ATS) in man from 24-hour exposure to continuous noise. *Ann. Otol. Rhinol. Laryngol.,* 83, 820–829, 1974.

Miller, J. D., Effects of noise on people, prepared for Environmental Protection Agency, MTID 300.7, pp. 15–33, 1971.

Mills, J. H., Gengel, R. W., Watson, C. S., and Miller, J. D., Temporary changes of the auditory system due to exposure to noise for one or two days. *J. Acoust. Soc. Am.,* 48, 524–530, 1970.

Mosko, J. D., Fletcher, J. L., and Luz, G. A., Growth and recovery of temporary threshold shifts following extended exposure to high level continuous noise, U.S. Army Medical Research Laboratory, Ft. Knox, Kentucky, Report 911, 1970.

Olishifski, J. B., and Harford, E. R. (Editors), *Industrial Noise and Hearing Conservation.* Chicago: National Safety Council, 1975.

Rintelmann, W. F., Manual and automatic audiometry; a comparison. *Natl. Safety News,* pp. 95–102, October 1973.

Sataloff, J., and Michael, P. L. *Hearing Conservation, pp.* 70–83, 161–165, 315–316. Springfield, Ill., Charles C Thomas Co., 1973.

United States Department of Labor, Proposed Requirements and Procedures, Occupational Noise Exposure, *Federal Register,* 39, No. 207, October 24, 1974.

Walsh-Healey Public Contracts Act, *Federal Register,* 34, No. 96, May 1969.

Ward, W. D., Auditory fatigue and masking. In Jerger, J. (Ed.), *Modern Developments in Audiology,* Ed. 1, Ch. 7, pp. 240–286. New York: Academic Press, 1963.

Ward, W. D., Susceptibility to auditory fatigue, in Neff, W. D. (Ed.) *Contributions to Sensory Physiology,* Vol. 3, pp. 191–226. New York: Academic Press, 1968.

Ward, W. D., Adaptation and fatigue, in Jerger, J. (Ed.), *Modern Developments in Audiology,* Ed. 2, ch. 9, pp. 323–328. New York: Academic Press, 1973.

Webster's Seventh New Collegiate Dictionary, Springfield, Mass.: G. C. Merriam Co., 1969.

Williams-Steiger Occupational Safety and Health Act of 1970, PL 91-596, December 29, 1970.

chapter **7**

CASE HISTORY: THE FIRST TEST

Philip E. Rosenberg, Ph.D.

While it is not necessarily true that the best things in life are free, the case history in diagnostic audiology lends support to this thesis. The skilled, experienced diagnostician knows full well that the information gleaned from the patient prior to the examination may be of equal importance to the examination itself. Indeed, the case history is the first test. It is a test of both the clinician and the patient.

THE GIVEN INFORMATION

The primary purpose of the case history is to obtain information which will assist the audiologist in his job. This information may or may not be directly relevant to an existing hearing problem. The information obtained becomes a portion of the official record of the patient and is utilized in conjunction with examination findings in the decision-making processes concerning his welfare.

The wise audiologist is often able to predict with uncanny accuracy the specific results of the auditory examination from the case history data alone. While this procedure is certainly not recommended in lieu of the examination it is both reassuring and adds strength to the obtained results. The audiologist, however, must be wary not to permit the case history information to bias his test procedures. The given information may suggest to him new avenues of exploration and specific diagnostic procedures which might be relevant in the particular instance.

ACQUIRING THE INFORMATION

The Easy Conversational Approach

Some audiologists obtain specific case history information in a rather casual, friendly, conversational manner. The proponents of this method claim that the establishment of rapport is of great importance and that the utilization of the case history for this purpose is ideal. In this approach the primary purpose of the case history, obtaining information, is subverted in order to allay the patient's apprehensions, to relax him and to gain his trust and confidence. In this conversational method the interviewer rarely asks direct and specific questions. Rather, through skillful conversation he leads the patient through a recapitulation of his difficulty and those factors associated with it. The interviewer makes few notes during the interview and relies upon his memory to write out the specific information after the patient has left his office. Occasionally the examiner makes no notes whatever, relying instead on a tape recorder (sometimes hidden) which he may review later at his leisure. This interview technique is one favored by psychiatrists, clinical psychologists and our brethren in speech pathology. It is rarely well suited to the practice of audiology.

The Authoritarian Approach

The authoritarian approach of gathering case history information is best exemplified by the medical model. The physician asks simple, direct questions and actively writes down the patient's answers. No attempt is made at concealment or subterfuge. Questions are frequently highly specific and briefly stated. This method provides the maximum amount of information in the minimum amount of time. Little time is spent in the social amenities and still less in the conscious establishment of an interpersonal relationship between the examiner and the patient.

These two different approaches to the acquisition of case history information are in some opposition. The authoritarian approach tends to be more suitable for the audiologist, particularly in the diagnostic audiologic evaluation. In the first place, the establishment of rapport is not only not beneficial but is, in fact, frequently detrimental. The audiologist does not want the patient to be completely relaxed and at ease. Rather, an edge of apprehension and anxiety will often contribute to the reliability and validity of the total examination procedure. Second, the patient has not come to the audiologist for friendship and conviviality. He is there because he has a problem and the audiologist is the expert who can deal with his problem. The audiologist's authority becomes diluted by an overly friendly approach and the confidence of the patient in this authority may well be shaken. The authoritarian approach, while not overly friendly, should not be construed as an arrogant or rude interaction with the patient. Third, there need be no shame in asking direct and probing questions nor in writing down the patient's answers in his presence. The subterfuge of the tape recorder and the remembered answer is totally·unnecessary and may result in mistakes and misinterpretations. Fourth, the case history should be completed as rapidly as possible. As the audiologic examination has become more detailed and prolonged, the problems of physical and psychological fatigue have become very real ones. If an inordinate amount of time is consumed in obtaining information, the patient may become weary before the actual examination begins. It should take no longer than 10 min to obtain the most detailed and comprehensive case history.

SPECIFIC CASE HISTORY DATA

The Adult Case History

The clinical audiologist frequently has several different case history forms from which to choose. The simplest of these is the standard adult case history. The word "adult" when used in this manner refers less to the age of the patient than to the status of his language and the reason for the referral. The adult case history is used not only for "adults" but for children who have developed speech and language or who have symptoms of Meniere's disease, otosclerosis, or other problems which are most common in adulthood.

Identifying Information

Each case history must begin with certain basic information identifying the patient. This should include the patient's name and his case number, the date of the examination, the patient's address and telephone number. His birthdate and age, his marital status and his occupation also should be noted. If the patient is a child, his parents' names, his school and grade should be obtained. The source of the referral as well as the reason for the referral should be entered in this portion of the case history form.

Hearing Loss History

This section deals rather specifically with the patient's primary problem. He should be asked to describe in his own words the onset and progression of his hearing difficulty. This description should reflect his impressions of his disorder rather than those of other examiners. The patient should also be asked in some detail whether anyone in his family has a hearing impairment. Since a far greater number of hearing handicaps than previously suspected have some genetic basis, one should pursue this question diligently. One particular patient, when asked if anyone in the family had trouble hearing, responded, "No." Subsequent history revealed that his mother and two brothers were deaf. When asked to explain this seeming discrepancy he replied that his mother and two brothers truly did not have any *trouble* hearing since they were deaf. Needless to say, his idea of "trouble" and the clinician's were entirely different. One must guard against this type of misunderstanding. The patient should be questioned not only about his parents but his aunts, uncles and cousins as well.

The patient should be asked the cause of his hearing loss. While this will often be in error it will give the examiner some insight into what he may have been told previously and how he approaches his own defect. The patient should also be asked whether he notices any fluctuation in his hearing. This is a particularly interesting question in that its primary value is not necessarily in picking up truly fluctuating hearing losses but, rather, in giving the examiner information concerning the severity of the loss. Hearing fluctuation is reported not only by patients with endolymphatic hydrops and similar disorders, which are characterized by variability in hearing, but, more often, by people with hearing impairments of from 30 to 40 dB HL (ANSI-1969). The very slight hearing fluctuations which occur as a result of fatigue, weather and general state of the organism are negligible to people with normal hearing or very mild hearing impairments. Likewise, these minor changes are unnoticed by patients with more severe hearing losses. For those with 30 to 40 dB hearing levels, however, even a change of 2 or 3 dB in the course of a day is viewed as marked fluctuation. Patients often report that they can hear perfectly well in the morning but that as they get tired during the course of the day they cannot hear a thing. This report will most often suggest a mild to moderate hearing deficit.

The patient should also be asked whether he hears better in quiet or in noise. This question will assist the examiner in predicting the general type of the hearing loss in that those patients with conductive hearing impairments will claim better hearing in noise while those with sensory-neural hearing losses will hear better in quiet. The patient should be asked if he hears well over the phone and which ear he uses on the telephone. Telephone listening is often not impaired, surprisingly, until the loss exceeds 55 to 60 dB HL in the speech range. The patient should be questioned on his radio and television listening habits. If he responds that he can hear television but cannot understand it, one may anticipate difficulty in auditory discrimination. Typically, a patient will reply, "No, I have no trouble at all with hearing television." His wife will respond, "Neither does the entire neighborhood." Questions concerning hearing in groups as opposed to hearing while talking to a single individual are also helpful in this section. Similarly, hearing at a distance versus hearing close-up yields information of value. The patient should always be asked if he can determine from which direction sound comes. Good localization of sound means that the two ears are quite similar. Lack of the ability to localize sound direction suggests a difference between ears of more than 15 dB.

The history of the hearing loss would not be complete without a detailed statement about occupational and environmental noise. A brief job history must be obtained and it is the audiologist's responsibility to know which are high noise level jobs. For example, one does not usually think of a baker as being exposed to a substantial amount of noise. However, a bakery is among the noisiest of job environments. The patient's service record should also be reviewed. Exposure to gunfire, even in basic training, may often show up on later audiometric evaluation. Service in the artillery or combat infantry carries with it invariable audiologic stigmata. The patient should be asked if he hunts or uses guns in other hobbies such as skeet shooting and target practice and whether he uses ear protection. Habitual travel in extraordinarily noisy conveyances such as the Philadelphia Subway System should also be recorded. Indeed, few people in our modern civilization can escape the scourge of damaging noise.

Medical History

It is important to know which physicians have been consulted by the patient, what diagnoses were proposed and what treatment instituted. Many patients present a list of past medical consultation to the questioner. A history of previous drainage of the ears should also be elicited again with dates and treatment. Ear pain should be investigated as well.

The patient should be asked to describe his head noises in some detail. He should be questioned about tinnitus, its onset, severity, duration, frequency and whether it sounds like a ring, a whistle, seashell noise, surf, trainwhistle, rushing water or hiss. Is the noise present all the time, occasionally, or only at night? An attempt should be made to assess how well he is able to tolerate the intrusion of tinnitus in his life. Should the patient describe his tinnitus as "voices" he is probably in the wrong place. We did see one patient, however, who came to us in search of a hearing aid because the voices that spoke to him in his head were too soft.

The presence of dizziness or vertigo should be investigated. Its date of onset, severity and frequency should be noted. An entire constellation of terms may be subsumed under the heading of vertigo. Many patients describe unsteadiness, wooziness, lightheadedness, poor balance, and "nervousness" all of which may prove to be symptoms of vestibular disorder.

A history of allergy should be recorded. Include not only the obvious upper respiratory manifestations of allergy but such less common considerations as hives, eczema, and asthma. All types of allergic reactions could affect hearing. A history of headache should be elicited including severity, date of onset, frequency of occurrence, and location.

A patient's general health history may reveal important clues. Diseases such as meningitis, scarlet fever, mumps, measles, tuberculosis, syphilis, diabetes, multiple sclerosis and seizures are important to include. Also include any history of injury and in particular closed head injury, concussion, skull fracture or whiplash of the neck because they may be followed by an auditory impairment. Severe trauma, either physical or psychological, may well be associated with the hearing deficit. The investigator should also attempt to review the patient's usages of ototoxic drugs, including not only ototoxic antibiotics, but the consumption of aspirin and quinine.

Hearing Aid History

A comprehensive and detailed review of the patient's experience with amplification is mandatory. The patient should be questioned regarding the hearing aids he has worn in the past, how long he has worn them and how well he thinks they worked. Note the specific brand names and models. He should be questioned concerning the satisfaction he achieved from the hearing aid and whether he thinks it worked as well as expected. Frequently, of course, the patient's expectations are totally unrealistic and this is a good point to determine whether or not this is the case. His relationship to the hearing aid dealers could be probed and his satisfaction or dissatisfaction noted for future reference.

Miscellaneous Case History Data

The final portion of the case history is often less structured than the preceding part. It contains those items of information which the data gathered thus far suggest for further probing. The content of the personal meanderings of the patient may be written here. Notes concerning possible medical-legal action or compensation judgment should be entered. A review of special educational training as a child can be noted as well as childhood or adult experiences with lip reading, auditory training, speech correction or speech conservation. The patient's comments regarding previous examinations and his personal opinions of the examiners should also be recorded on this separate sheet. The audiologist's own observations should be jotted here regarding such things as physical appearance of the patient, his personal quirks, his personality and moods. One of the most revealing behaviors to consider is the patient's speech and language and his facility in communication. Possible stigmata of more general syndromes such as Waardenburg's, Marfan's and others may be recorded for future investigation and follow-up.

CONCLUSION

The first and possibly the most valuable single test is the case history. An enormous amount of information can be obtained by a skillful interviewer in a minimum amount of time. The information gleaned from the case history may well determine the specific test approach and influence the test conclusions.

The information should be acquired directly and specifically without subterfuge. The patient should be questioned concerning his hearing loss history, medical history and hearing aid history with a space left at the end for miscellaneous observations. A careful case history, skillfully obtained and well written, is the hallmark of a good clinical audiologist. It, as well as specific examination findings, reflects on the competence of the audiologist. The case history contains four qualities that make it rare indeed in this modern world: it is not fattening, it is not sinful, it is rewarding, and it is free.

chapter 8

CALIBRATION, PURE TONE, SPEECH AND NOISE SIGNALS

Laura Ann Wilber, Ph.D.

WHY CALIBRATE?

Some years ago when this chapter appeared in the first edition of this *Handbook,* we asked the question, "Why calibrate?" Although we had hoped the question was answered, it seems apparent that it must still be raised. While it is true that most audiologists pay lip service to the necessity of calibration procedures, it appears to be equally true that not all calibration procedures are carried out routinely or with the precision which one might wish. As our equipment budgets become tighter, however, we will be forced into paying more attention to the maintenance and checking of current equipment instead of simple replacement by newer and brighter machines. Studies by Martin (1968), by Thomas et al. (1969) and by Walton, Williams and Labiak (1971) all indicated the importance of routine calibration by illustrating problems which were found when audiometers were checked from various settings. In the Walton study, for example, 44% of the wide range audiometers checked had one or more intensity errors, 30% had one or more frequency errors, 6% had one or more purity errors, 3% one or more rise-fall errors. Eighty percent of those audiometers had one or more errors of some type or other. The authors do point out that these were not all major errors, however, it is far easier to check and fix equipment than patients or clinicians. Thus, audiometers should be kept in good calibration. The Walton data were perhaps less disturbing than the Thomas data since the latter indicated that 89% of the audiometers which they checked were out of calibration with regard to intensity.

Audiometers have been found which emitted no frequencies above 1500 Hz, but produced only low frequency tones. Other brand new audiometers have been found with differences of as much as 20 dB between air and bone conduction. One audiometer had no output below 25 dB. Thomas et al. reported an audiometer that would not attenuate below 50 dB. Any of those problems may be found with new audiometers and those which have been in use and initially were well calibrated. Regardless of whether the audiometer is new or has been used for some time, it must be the responsibility of the user to check its calibration or to provide for the regular calibration of the equipment by outside sources.

Checking calibration is necessary to be sure that an audiometer produces a pure tone at the specified level and frequency, that the signal is present only in the transducer to which it is directed, and that the signal is free from distortion or unwanted noise interference. When the audiologist has demonstrated his equipment to be "in calibration" he will be able to report his results with greater confidence. When the audiologist checks the calibration of his audiometer, (1) he can establish whether this new equipment is in line with national norms and standards and (2) he can establish a reference point for his own equipment to determine if it changes over time.

Therefore, it is the purpose of this chapter to show the audiologist who does not have an extensive electronic background how to check his equipment to meet the criteria of the national standards. It is not as easy to control the mood or behavior of the client or the clinician, as it is to control the performance of the test equipment.

PARAMETERS OF CALIBRATION

Much "how to calibrate" information is available in the manuals which accompany audiometers and pieces of equipment used in calibration. The first step, then, in learning how to calibrate should always be to read the appropriate manuals. A good source of general information on calibration procedures is the United States Government Printing Office which offers among others: *Basic Electronics, Introduction to Electronics, Systems of Electrical Units, Guide to Instrumentation Literature,* and *Theory and Use of Electronic Test Equipment.* The specific parameters which must be checked in an audiometer are outlined in standards provided by the American National Standards Institute (ANSI) and the International Electrotechnical Commision (IEC). As of this writing new standards are under consideration by each organization and they are being voted upon. It is hoped that, before this book goes to press, the ANSI standard will have been approved, however, if it is not, the specific applicable standard may be obtained by writing to the American National Standards Institute at 1430 Broadway, New York, New York 10018. The ANSI standard which is currently in the last stages of review will be referred to throughout this chapter as the proposed standard. It will behoove the reader to obtain a copy of the precise standard after it has been approved to make sure that one knows the exact parameters and limitations on those parameters which will be permitted.

To better understand the procedures for checking calibration, one must first understand the parameters to be checked. For pure tone and speech audiometers, these parameters are frequency, intensity and time (phase and signal duration). Table 8.1 shows equipment which can be used to check each of these. Although there are no rigid requirements, in this author's opinion, frequency and time should be checked when the audiometer is purchased and at yearly intervals thereafter; however, it is advisable to check the intensity output at least once a month. (Research facilities generally check calibration weekly and in some instances daily.) If the clinician notices anything unusual in the audiometer's performance, calibration should be checked immediately. It is always better to check the equipment first rather than assume that the problem lies in the client or clinician.

Upon discovering a fault in the frequency or time components of the audiometer, the clinician should contact the manufacturer or his representative for immediate repair and proper calibration of the machine. Unless the user of the audiometer is a qualified electronics technician, he should not attempt to take the machine apart to rectify the problem himself; a qualified manufacturer's representative is responsible for such major operations. When checking the intensity parameter, if there is a stable deviation, calibration corrections can be made simply by posting a note on the front of the audiometer for plus or minus corrections by frequency and transducer. Figure 8.1 shows an example of such a correction form. Unstable intensity variations may require further investigation by a qualified repair technician.

TABLE 8.1. *Equipment Useful for Checking Various Parameters of Audiometer Calibration*

Parameter	Suggested Equipment
Intensity	Oscilloscope
	Vacuum tube voltmeter
	Microphone
	Spectrometer
	Graphic level recorder
	Sound level meter
	Coupler
	Artificial Headbone
Frequency	Oscilloscope
	Electronic counter
	Frequency analyzer
	Distortion meter
Time	Oscilloscope
	Electronic counter
	Graphic level recorder

BASIC EQUIPMENT

A list of basic calibration equipment for checking intensity should include: (1) a vacuum tube voltmeter (VTVM), (2) a condenser microphone (Western Electric 640 AA or equivalent), (3) a 6-cc coupler (National Bureau of Standards (NBS) 9A), (4) a 500-g weight, (5) a cathode follower with preamplifier, (6) an artificial headbone (mastoid) and (7) an ohmmeter.

When purchasing any of the above equipment it is usually helpful if there is a manufacturer's representative nearby to aid in the use and maintenance of the calibration equipment. It is also wise to check with other audiologists or acousticians, such as physicists or electronic engineers who use similar types of equipment, to find the best specific brands available locally.

There are several name brand vacuum tube voltmeters which are adequate. Certain characteristics should be looked for in a voltmeter. For example: it should read in true root mean square (RMS), it is helpful if there is a mirror behind the meter needle to avoid parallax problems, it should be portable, and it should have a high input impedance.

The microphone, coupler, weight and cathode follower may be purchased collectively as an "artificial ear." It should be noted that there is a "true" artificial ear which is described in the IEC Publication 318 entitled: "An Artificial Ear of the Wide Band Type, for the Calibration of Earphones Used in Audiometry" (1970). However, the proposed ANSI standard relates to the NBS 9A coupler rather than the IEC artificial ear. When purchasing these items it is important to ascertain that the coupler truly conforms to the NBS 9A type and that the condenser microphone fits snugly into the coupler. (The specifications for the NBS 9A coupler may be found in the ANSI S3.6-1969 (ANSI-1970) Specifications for Audiometers standard and in the proposed ANSI Standards Document). Local audiologists or members of a university speech and hearing center should be able to give advice on specific brands. Other equipment such as an oscilloscope (preferably a storage type), a graphic level recorder, an electronic counter, a frequency analyzer, or a distortion meter will also prove invaluable in checking the acoustic parameters of the audiometer. In many instances the latter equipment can be shared by laboratories.

CHECKING THE CALIBRATION OF PURE TONE AUDIOMETERS

Basic Signal

The first thing one should do upon obtaining a new audiometer is to read its manual and follow its calibration instructions, if any are given. These instructions generally have been

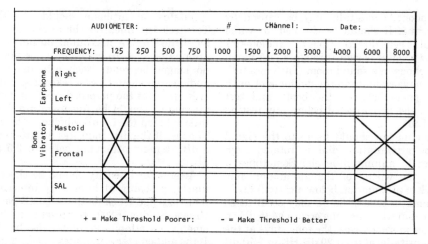

FREQUENCY:	125	250	500	750	1000	1500	2000	3000	4000	6000	8000
Earphone Right											
Earphone Left											
Bone Vibrator Mastoid											
Bone Vibrator Frontal											
SAL											

+ = Make Threshold Poorer: - = Make Threshold Better

Fig. 8.1. Correction sheet for audiometer.

designed as the most effective way to check the performance of the specific audiometer.

After the audiometer has been installed, plugged in, turned on and allowed to warm up for 10 to 15 min, the operator should listen to the signal at different dial settings through each transducer (earphone, loudspeaker and bone vibrator). Although few audiologists are equipped with "golden ears," with a little practice one can hear basic faults in audiometric equipment. Although a vague complaint to the audiometer repairman that it "sounds funny" is as futile as it would be to tell an automobile repairman the same thing, a specific description of the sound and circumstances can help determine the source of the trouble. The repairman may be able to focus in on the fault immediately without wasting his time and your money to do the "trouble shooting" himself.

A great deal of information on the source of the problem may be determined by just listening to the audiometer as well as inspecting it physically. Below are some difficulties which the clinician should check for periodically.

1. Check the earphone and vibrator cords for signs of wearing or cracking. One way to determine if the cord is defective is by listening to a tone through the transducer while twisting and jiggling the cords. A defective cord will usually produce static or will cause the tone to be intermittent. Sometimes tightening the earphone screws is all that is necessary. If this does not alleviate the problem, it is wise to replace the cord and/or the transducer.

2. Check the audiometer for loose dials or for dials that are out of alignment. If such faults exist the dial readings will not be meaningful. Defective dials should be repaired immediately, and the audiometer should be recalibrated to determine outputs at the new dial settings.

3. The audiologist should listen to see if mechanical clicks are audible through the earphone when the attenuator, frequency dial or interrupter switch are manipulated. The proposed standard suggests that a normal hearing listener listen with the earphones in place but disconnected and with a proper resistive load across the circuit while manipulating the interrupter switch, etc., to make sure that there are no audible signals which would clue the subject to the presence of the test signal. A mechanical click can best be detected by listening.

4. To determine if electronic clicks are audible it is wise to listen to the output at both a moderate, e.g., 50 dB hearing level (HL), and below the threshold of hearing. Electronic clicks will show up on an oscilloscope as an irregularity when the problem switch or dial is moved. The danger of an audible click whether it be mechanical or electronic is that the patient may respond to the click rather than to the stimulus tone. If the clicks are present the audiometer should be repaired immediately.

5. The clinician should listen for hum or static at high dial intensity levels both when a stimulus signal is present and when it is absent.

6. "Cross-talk" may occur between earphones; that is, the signal which is sent to one earphone may be heard in the contralateral earphone. Such a problem could greatly affect the measurements obtained on that audiometer, especially for cases with unilateral hearing loss. Cross-talk may be detected by sending a signal to one phone, disconnecting the earphone jack to this phone, inserting a resistive load in its place and listening for the signal in the opposite phone where it should not be. Cross-talk may also be detected as a change in voltage or oscilloscopic pattern of the test phone when the signal is presented to the opposite,

nontest phone. Cross-talk may be caused by faulty wiring. It should be checked for when the signal is sent directly from the audiometer as well as when it is sent through a jack panel to an earphone in a sound room. The cross-talk problem may originate in the audiometer or in the jack panel between the booth and test room. It must be corrected before any testing is carried out.

7. The clinician should listen to the signal while the attenutation dial is rotated from maximum to minimum levels. Sometimes a break in the wiring of the attenuator may cause lack of attenuation below a certain level. For instance, a tone of 20 dB may occur at 20 dB on the dial while no tone occurs at 15 dB on the dial (or in some cases, the tone stays at the same intensity level from 20 dB HL to −10 dB HL on the dial). This problem is readily perceived only by listening to the audiometer.

Aside from these gross problems which can be detected by listening, the precise accuracy of the dial output levels must be evaluated. Frequency, intensity, linearity of attenuation, and percentage of distortion should be measured.

The frequency output from the audiometer should be checked either using an electronic counter or an oscilloscope. By following the directions for either of those pieces of equipment, one can readily ascertain if the frequency dial settings are equivalent to the actual output for the audiometer. The proposed standard for audiometers allows a tolerance of ± 3% for frequency from a fixed frequency pure tone audiometer. That is, if the audiometer dial reads 500 Hz it must be between 485 and 515 Hz. At 1000 Hz it must be from 970 to 1030 Hz and so on. Frequency needs to be checked on initial receipt of the audiometer and at yearly intervals thereafter, however, by listening to the audiometer each day it is possible to assess whether the frequencies are reasonably accurate and if they are all being emitted.

If there is no electronic counter or oscilloscope available one may check certain octave frequencies (such as 1000 Hz) by beating the output of the audiometer against the signal from U.S. Government radio calibration stations. The electronics technician at your local radio station can help with this procedure. However, its usefulness is limited since it only enables one to ascertain if the output frequencies are identical or not. There is no room for the allowable frequency error.

Linearity of attenuation may be checked either electrically directly from the audiometer or acoustically from the audiometer through an earphone or bone vibrator. If measurements are made electrically the earphone should be in the line or a dummy load which electrically simulates the earphone, should be in the line. To check the linearity the audiometer should be turned to its maximum output and then attenuated in 5-dB steps until the output can no longer be read. Each attenuator on the audiometer should be checked separately. In order to meet the proposed ANSI standard the attenuator should be linear within 0.3 of the interval step (or 1.5 dB whichever is smaller). That is, if the dial indicates an attenuation of 5 dB, it must attenuate between 3.5 and 6.5 dB.

Attenuator linearity should be checked regularly, probably at bimonthly intervals. If a fixed-loss pad (such as the ± 20 dB pad on the Grason-Stadler E800) is present in the audiometer, its attenuation must also be checked. If the audiometer attenuates in 1- or 2-dB steps, these smaller attenuation steps should be checked if they are used in the typical, or special use of the equipment; however, calibration equipment accuracy itself precludes measurement of intervals of 0.5 dB or less. Linearity measurements may also help detect distortion in a transducer or in the audiometer itself. Distortion will appear as a lack of linear attenuation especially at high output levels. If the distortion is in the audiometer, appropriate repairs should be made. If it is in the transducer, the transducer should be replaced. It should be noted that almost all of today's small hearing aid type bone vibrators have harmonic distortion, especially at 250 Hz, which cannot be eliminated due to the size (and lack of mass) of these vibrators. The proposed standard considers this by allowing higher (6 to 12%) distortion for bone vibrators at 250 Hz. It is hoped that in the future as new vibrators are designed distortion at 250 Hz will no longer be a problem. The maximum permissible distortion is listed by transducer and hearing level output in the proposed standard. The audiometer user should check the ANSI standard for the precise figures, but in general for pure tone air-conduction calibration, the maximum permissible total harmonic distortion is 3%. More detailed "how to" check the output of transducers will be discussed in subsequent sections.

Earphone Calibration

Basically, there are two procedures for calibration of earphones. One is the "real ear" method and the other is the "artificial ear" or coupler method. With the original real ear method one simply tested the hearing of a group of normal hearing individuals, averaged the results and checked to see that the average hearing of this group was at zero on the dial for each frequency. Although this method is theoretically feasible when one has a large population to sample, it is not a recommended procedure. In order to do the procedure properly the sample should consist of at least 25 young (18 to 25 years of age) otologically normal hearing adults. The equipment used should allow the examiner to measure thresholds at least 10 to 20 dB below zero to account for those subjects who will have extremely sensitive hearing. Consequently, it is clear that although this precedure is possible, it is unwieldy, especially if it is to be followed weekly or even monthly. In addition, it is technically incorrect since the International Standards Organization (ISO) reference is not tied to normal hearing.

Another type of real ear earphone calibration procedure consists of comparing the output of a known earphone with that of an unknown earphone. If one has an audiometer and earphones which are in perfect calibration, one may compare the output from the known audiometer with the unknown by using a loudness balance procedure such as described by Stewart and Burgi (1970). Studies in our laboratory have suggested that, while this procedure is apparently a valid one, individual subjects may vary from one another from test to retest unless they are highly sophisticated. Even sophisticated subjects may vary as much as 10 dB from one test session to another in their estimate of equal loudness. However, in three trials, one right after the other at the same time, on the same day and under the same conditions there will be very little variability. Some individuals are able to repeat the estimate without varying as much as a single decibel. However, one sees that this technique, while feasible, is unwieldy. In addition, it presupposes that one has access to an earphone and audiometer system whose output is truly known. This is generally not so.

The most commonly used procedure today is that of the "artificial ear" or coupler. The "artificial ear" consists of a condenser microphone and a 6-cc coupler. The 6-cc coupler was originally chosen because it was thought that the enclosed volume was approximately the same as the volume under an earphone for a human ear (Corliss and Burkhard, 1953). However, since volume displacement is only one component of acoustic impedance it cannot be assumed that the coupler actually represents a human ear. Burkhard and Corliss (1954) pointed out that the impedance characteristics of a 6-cc coupler probably simulate the impedance of the human ear only over a small part of the audio range. Because the 6-cc coupler does not replicate the impedance of the human ear it cannot be considered a true artificial ear. In addition, to the problem of impedance characteristics, the present 6-cc coupler (NBS

9A) is known to have a natural resonance at 6000 Hz (Rudmose, 1964). This, of course, interferes with the measurement of the output of an audiometer earphone around that frequency. In addition, the size of the coupler and its shape with hard walls permits the possibility of standing waves at frequencies above 6000 Hz. Despite these difficulties the 6-cc coupler has been accepted as a standard device for measuring acoustic output from the audiometer through an earphone. It should be mentioned that there are two couplers, the IEC coupler mentioned earlier and the Zwislocki coupler (Zwislocki, 1970, 1971) which appear to more closely approximate the acoustic impedance of the human ear. However, the proposed standard for audiometers will still relate its threshold values to the NBS 9A coupler.

The procedure for using an artificial ear is a simple one. The earphone is placed on the coupler and a 500-g weight is then placed on top of the earphone. The output is read in voltage and then transformed to dB (or read directly in dB) *re* 20 μPa (20 micro Pascals will now replace 0.0002 dyne/sq cm). After initial placement of the earphone on the coupler, introduce a low frequency tone (125 or 250 Hz) and readjust the earphone on the coupler until the highest output intensity is read. This helps assure best placement on the coupler. This output may then be compared to the expected output per frequency. The intensity values which are used are given in ISO Recommendation R 389 (1964), ANSI S3.6-1969 (1970) and the proposed standard. These values were evolved through a "round robin" from various laboratories throughout the world (Weissler, 1968).

Previous audiometer standard threshold values were related to the Western Electric 705-A earphone. However, that earphone has not been commercially available for some years now. The proposed audiometer standard will give "standard reference equivalent threshold sound pressure level" for the TDH-39, TDH-49 and Telex-1470 earphones as measured using the NBS 9A coupler. Figure 8.2 shows an audiometer earphone calibration worksheet and contains the values which may be expected at each frequency with TDH-39 and TDH-49 earphones in MX-41/AR cushions on an NBS 9A coupler when no grid is used on the microphone.

A word of caution should be inserted here. The output measurements reported above are only valid when a supra-aural type earphone cushion (which touches the pinna) such as the MX-41/AR cushion is used. They are not valid when a circumaural earphone cushion (which encircles the pinna) is used. Benson et al. (1967) pointed out the lack of an approved

Audiometer: _____ # _____ Earphone: _____ Channel: _____ Place: _____

Calibrated by: _____ Date: _____ Equipment: _____

FREQUENCY:	125	250	500	750	1000	1500	2000	3000	4000	6000	8000
1. SPL *											
2. Audiometer Dial Reading											
3. Line 1 minus Line 2											
4. Equipment & Mike Correct.											
5. Line 3 minus Line 4											
6. ANSI -TDH-39 **	45.0	25.5	11.5	8.0	7.0	6.5	9.0	10.0	9.5	15.5	13.0
ANSI -TDH-49***	47.5	26.5	13.5	8.5	7.5	7.5	11.0	9.5	10.5	13.5	13.0
7. Line 5 minus Line 6											
8. CORRECTION'''											

Fig. 8.2. Calibration worksheet for audiometer earphones. (*) SPL = sound pressure level in dB *re* 20 μPa. (**) ANSI-TDH-39 proposed ANSI-69 threshold values for TDH-39 earphones in MX-41/AR cushions. (***) ANSI-TDH-49 proposed ANSI-69 threshold values for TDH-49 earphones in MX-41/AR cushions. (''') Correction — rounded to the nearest 5 dB: − = audiometer weak, make threshold better: + = audiometer strong, make threshold poorer.

reference threshold for circumaural earphones. It is hoped that the Zwislocki coupler will eliminate this problem, but as of this writing it has not yet been approved by the American National Standards Institute. It is possible in one's own clinic to obtain a reasonable estimate of the output differences between circumaural and supra-aural earphones by using the loudness balance procedure mentioned earlier. This procedure will allow one to know what difference, if any, should be used to compensate for the difference between the standard supra-aural and circumaural earphone cushion. Although it is possible to place the earphone receiver itself on the American Standards Association (ASA) Type I coupler, this in no way ensures that the sound pressure level (SPL) at the ear drum will be the same when the earphone is placed in a circumaural cushion. Readings can also be obtained with a flat-plate coupler between the earphone and microphone. The above procedures and outcome of measurements have been described by Shaw and Thiessen (1962), by Stein and Zerlin (1963) and by Tillman and Gish (1964). The authors indicate some of the differences which may be found between earphones in supra-aural and circumaural cushions. Until such time as these differences are taken into consideration and a standard calibration procedure is devised for circumaural cushions one must be aware that any audiometer using these earphone cushions does not conform to the present or proposed national standard.

When the output of the earphone has been established it can be compared to a standard to determine if it is in calibration or not. When corrections are less than 15 dB, a calibration correction card (shown earlier in Fig. 8.1) may be placed on an audiometer showing the discrepancy between the established norm and one's own audiometer. Such corrections must then be taken into consideration when an audiogram is plotted. If an audiometer is off by more than 15 dB at any frequency or by 10 dB at 3 or more frequencies, it is advisable to have the audiometer recalibrated by the manufacturer or manufacturer's representative. If the audiometer is new, it should be in calibration within 3 dB from 125 to 4000 Hz and within 5 dB at 6000 and 8000 Hz.

Bone Vibrator Calibration

Checking calibration of the bone vibrator presents a different problem than that of an earphone. While earphones can be checked easily by using a microphone as a pickup, bone vibrators cannot. The original technique for checking bone vibrator calibration was to use real ears (AMA, 1951). The real ear method for bone vibrator checking is somewhat different from that used for earphones. The method assumes that air- and bone-conduction thresholds are equivalent for humans; therefore, if 6 to 10 normal hearing subjects are tested for both air and bone conduction with an audiometer whose air-conduction system is in proper calibration, bone-conduction corrections for the audiometer can be determined by using the difference obtained between air- and bone-conduction thresholds. This procedure makes a few assumptions which are not always met. For example, it presupposes that one can obtain true thresholds for all the normal hearing subjects using the given audiometer. Since many audiometers do not go below 0 dB HL, it is difficult to determine true threshold. To avoid the above problem, Roach and Carhart (1956) suggested using individuals with pure sensory-neural losses for calibrating bone vibrators. Such a procedure eliminates ambient noise problems, and it increases the possibility that one will obtain true thresholds. A problem arises when trying to single out subjects with "pure" sensory-neural losses who have no conductive component and who have thresholds which do not extend beyond the bone-conduction limits of the audiometer.

In the real ear bone-conduction calibration procedure, acoustic radiations can also present a problem. The proposed standard for audiometers indicates that there should be no acoustic radiation at frequencies of 4000 Hz and below. The procedure for determining isolation is described in detail in the proposed standard. The sound radiated from the vibrator should be at least 10 dB below the bone-conduction threshold. Another basic problem with real ear bone vibrator calibration is the original supposition that air- and bone-conduction thresholds are equivalent. While this is certainly true for a large group of individuals, it cannot be expected to be true for any one small group. Studebaker (1967) hypothesized that one should expect that a certain percentage of "normal" individuals will have results in which the air- and bone-conduction thresholds deviate by as much as 25 dB by chance (according to normal distribution theory). Previous experimental studies by Wilber and Goodhill (1967) and Wilber (1972a) have shown that in real life groups of subjects can vary dramatically and that individuals with otologically normal ears and allegedly normal hearing may at a given time have thresholds in which air- and bone-conduction thresholds vary by as much as 15 dB.

The preferred procedure for calibrating bone vibrators involves the use of an artificial headbone or artificial mastoid. Artificial mastoids were proposed as early as 1939 by Hawley. However, it was not until Weiss (1960) developed his artificial mastoid that they became commercially available. The greatest problem in building an accurate artificial mastoid was in replicating the mechanical impedance of the human mastoid. Although there appears to be some disagreement as to what the human mastoid mechanical impedance is, a working agreement has been decided upon (IEC 373-1971, ANSI S3.13-1972). As of this writing no artificial mastoid (headbone) conforms to the IEC or ANSI standard. As of this writing a few bone vibrators do conform physically to the ANSI standard but threshold values for those vibrators have not yet been accepted. The proposed audiometer standard refers to ANSI S3.13-1972 for threshold values for bone conduction. The mastoid on which these bone values were obtained was the Weiss mastoid. Later comparisons by Lybarger (1966) and by Wilber (1972b) related values obtained on the Weiss mastoid to those on the B & K artificial mastoid. It is hoped that in the near future precise threshold standards will be established for vibrators which conform to the ANSI standard as measured on an artificial headbone that conforms to the ANSI and IEC standard. The values first reported by Lybarger (1966) on behalf of the Hearing Aid Industry Conference are essentially the same as those used in ANSI S3.13 and are the ones which should be used at the present time. The reader is strongly advised to check with the American National Standards Institute for a possible revision of the S3.13 standard or the acceptance of a new standard listing bone-conduction threshold values for the newer vibrators. Note that the values currently reported in ANSI S3.13 are for both mastoid and frontal bone placement. It is also extremely important to note that both sets of values were based on masked thresholds obtained with non-occluded ears. This presupposes that audiometric testing will be done using masking on the contralateral ear. Figure 8.3 shows a sample calibration worksheet for bone vibrators.

In both earphone and bone vibrator calibration it is important to check not only the overall intensity output but also the distortion through the transducer. Distortion may be measured directly with a distortion meter or a frequency analyzer. One may obtain a visual picture of the distorted wave by using an oscilloscope. The allowable distortion levels for both earphones and bone vibrators are reported in the proposed standard.

Along with the above physical measurement procedures the importance of just listening to the audiometer cannot be overly stressed. The

Audiometer: _____ Channel: _____ Vibrator: _____

Place: _____ Calibrated by: _____ Date: _____

Equipment Used: _____ + B & K Mastoid

FREQUENCY:	250	500	750	1000	1500	2000	3000	4000
Voltage Reading:								
1. dB re 1 dyne								
2. HAECOM B & K Mast. Correct. *							+1.0	+9.5
3. Line 1 minus/plus Line 2								
4. Audiometer Dial								
5. Line 3 minus Line 4								
6a. MASTOID Bone'	41.4	30.7	19.3	16.9	15.4	8.1	6.6	11.2
6b. FRONTAL Bone''	54.9	45.7	31.8	26.9	24.4	16.6	14.1	17.7
7. Line 5 minus Line 6								
8. CORRECTIONS **								

Fig. 8.3. Calibration sheet for bone vibrators. (*) Corrections specific to HAECOM B & K mastoid (B & K Model 4930 S.N. 331268). (') Threshold for *MASTOID* placement of RE B 70-A re ANSI S3.13-1972 norm incorporating Wilber B & K corrections (*Journal of the Acoustical Society of America*, 52, 1265, 1972). ('') Threshold for *FOREHEAD* placement of RE B 70-A re ANSI S3.13-1972 Norm incorporating Wilber B & K corrections (*Journal of the Acoustical Society of America* 52, 1265, 1972). (**) Corrections rounded to nearest 5 dB: + = strong, make threshold poorer, − = weak, make threshold better.

normal sophisticated ear should be able to perceive gross attenuation and distortion problems. The electronic procedures will serve to precisely describe the problems which the human ear approximates.

CALIBRATION OF SPEECH AUDIOMETERS

The speech audiometer or speech circuit of the diagnostic audiometer presents some of the same problems encountered with pure tone audiometers. For example, the linearity of attenuation should be checked. Since running speech itself fluctuates in intensity (and frequency and time) the preferred method is to introduce a pure tone (usually 1000 Hz) into the microphone, phonograph or tape input of the speech audiometer. The input impedance of the audiometer must be matched by the output of the signal-presenting instrument (such as a beat-frequency oscillator). The input intensity should be adjusted so that the volume unit meter on the face of the audiometer may be monitored at a suitable level, usually zero.

The output from the transducer is then measured. The attenuator linearity should be checked in the same way as described above for pure tone audiometers. In our clinics we use a separate pure tone oscillator whose output is fed into the speech audiometer input. If a pure tone oscillator is not available, one may use the 1000-Hz tone which precedes the test words on most commercially available speech material recordings. The proposed standard for speech audiometers suggests that the output for the 1000 Hz tone at 0 dB HL should be 12.5 dB above 1000 Hz reference standard sound pressure level for the appropriate earphone which would be 19.5 dB re 20 μPa using a TDH-39 earphone or 20 dB re 20 μPa using a TDH-49 earphone. If a bone vibrator is to be used as a transducer it must be calibrated separately. The 1000-Hz tone should be introduced into the audiometer as described above and in the proposed standard, and the output measured at an HL of 60 dB or above to preclude measurement of ambient room noise.

All subsequent speech testing must be carried out with the volume unit meter peaking at the same point as during the calibration check. If, for example, one prefers −3 on the volume unit meter rather than 0 then calibration of the 1000-Hz tone must be peaked at −3 or an appropriate correction made in reporting measurements.

The frequency response of the speech audiometer should be plus or minus 5 dB from 1000 Hz for the frequencies 200 through 4000 Hz and should not be greater than 10 dB different from the 1000-Hz signal for frequencies outside of the band. The procedures for this measurement for live voice and for recorded speech audiometers are given in the proposed standard for calibration of audiometers.

Harmonic distortion should be checked through the earphones after it has been ascertained that the pure tone being fed *into* the audiometer has no more than 1% harmonic distortion. The proposed standard requires that no output harmonic should exceed 3%. If the pure tone and speech audiometers are separate machines, the speech audiometer must also be checked for cross-talk and internal noise as described earlier.

Volume Unit Meter

Volume unit (VU) meters are indicators of intensity and are found on the face of most audiometers. The VU meter is calibrated relative to the input signal which it monitors and should not be interpreted as yielding any absolute value such as 0 dB *re* 20 μPa. On a speech audiometer the VU meter is used to monitor the speech signal or to aid the operator in adjusting the input calibration tone which precedes recorded speech material. The exact specifications for VU meters may be found in ANSI C 16.5-1954 (R 1961) and as VU meters relate to speech audiometers in the proposed standard.

In general, it is important that the VU meter be stable, that there is no undershoot or overshoot of the needle indicator relative to the actual signal and that any dB change is accurately represented on the meter. It is possible to either remove the VU meter from the audiometer or to remove the front panel along with the VU meter from its casing to accurately check its characteristics. However, if this is impractical, the audiologist may check the VU meter and its entire accompanying input system as described below.

A pure tone should be fed from an oscillator through an electronic switch to the input of the audiometer. The pure tone should be monitored by a voltmeter. By activating the electronic switch to produce a rapidly interrupted signal one can watch the VU meter to ascertain if there is any overshoot or undershoot relative to the signal in its steady state. One must also check the response time of the needle on the VU meter. Olsen (1975) suggests using a tape recording of a 270-, 300-, and 330-msec tone to ensure that the needle reaches its 99% state deflection in 300 msec ± 10%. To be certain of the nature of the input signal itself, it is recommended that an electronic switch with known characteristics be used. To check the relative accuracy of the VU meter's dB scale, one may insert a linear attenuator in the line between the oscillator and the audiometer input, or one may reduce the output from the oscillator by a known amount (as monitored by a voltmeter). The change in input should be accurately reflected by a corresponding change on the VU meter. When inserting an electronic switch or attenuator in the line it is, of course, important that all electrical impedances are properly matched.

LOUDSPEAKERS

If at all possible the calibration of loudspeakers should be checked initially in an anechoic chamber so that one can obtain precise frequency response characteristics of the loudspeaker. It is not possible to check the frequency characteristics of a loudspeaker in a standard test booth since standing waves will be set up in the room and will thus create a misleading interpretation of the output from the loudspeaker. Ideally a sweep-frequency oscillator and graphic level recorder are used to check the frequency response curve of the loudspeaker. The output from the oscillator is sent directly to the loudspeaker. A condenser microphone is placed 1 meter from the face of the loudspeaker, taking care to account for the angle of incidence of the signal from the speaker. The signal from the microphone is led through the necessary equipment (which will vary depending on brand) to the graphic level recorder. The total frequency response curve may be obtained quite rapidly and accurately. If, however, the above equipment is not available, the audiologist may introduce discrete tones into the loudspeaker and record the output through the condenser microphone from a spectrometer or voltmeter. In general, the loudspeaker should be relatively flat within its entire range. The necessary frequency response will depend upon the use. If the speakers are used with a speech audiometer for production of speech signals they should be flat (± 10 dB) within the range of 500 to 4000 Hz. If the speakers are to be used to measure pure tone thresholds in an anechoic chamber they should probably be within ± 3 dB from 125 to 8000 Hz. If it is not possible to measure the output of the loudspeaker in an anechoic chamber one may use narrow bands of noise to make this measurement. The microphone should be placed where the listener would be seated. Although this procedure is not as precise as using pure tones in an anechoic chamber, it will tell one the approximate frequency response curve in the test room. If the measurements are not made in an anechoic chamber a precise statement about the frequency response characteristics of the speaker cannot be stated. However, for audiometric testing purposes the narrow band noise method will allow one to ascertain the relative frequency response of the loudspeaker. It should be remembered that even within an anechoic chamber introduction of any object (such as a chair for the subject to sit on) can change the apparent response characteristics by as much as 5 to 10 dB.

Harmonic distortion measurements of the loudspeakers should also be carried out in an anechoic chamber as described above. In this instance a distortion meter or other device, as discussed in conjunction with earphone measurements, should be used. If an anechoic chamber is not available, it is theoretically possible to carry out the measurements in an open field free of reflecting surfaces. At the present time there is no standard for harmonic distortion of loudspeakers used in conjunction with speech audiometers. However, it seems reasonable to assume that the requirements for distortion should be as stringent as that mentioned above for other transducers.

The proposed standard for audiometers will describe some of the characteristics of sound field testing, such as the test room, frequency response, method for describing the intensity of the speech signal, and the location of the speakers. It does not give specific values for pure tones or warble tones in the sound field. It is well known that the classic study by Sivian and White (1933) demonstrated an average difference of approximately 6 dB between minimal audible pressure (MAP) and minimal audible field (MAF) thresholds for pure tone signals in the range of 200 through 6000 Hz. Their results demonstrated that thresholds are approximately 6 dB better in a free field situation than under earphones. So, one would infer that it should require less intensity to obtain thresholds for speech by free field than under earphones. More complete data are presented in studies by Stream and Dirks (1974) who discussed the effect of loudspeaker position on differences between earphone (minimal audible pressure) and sound field (minimal audible field) thresholds. This information can serve as a guide to the audiologist. Tillman, Johnson and Olsen (1966) compared thresholds with

TDH-39 earphones in MX-41/AR cushions to sound field. About 7.5 dB greater sensitivity was noted for the sound field. In order to conform to the proposed standard for earphones, the output from a loudspeaker should be 13 dB sound pressure level (SPL). This relationship should yield equivalent thresholds for sound field and earphone measurements of speech reception threshholds (SRTs) using spondee words.

Since pure tones should not be used to calibrate a loudspeaker except in an anechoic chamber, it is recommended that white noise or preferably speech spectrum noise be used for this calibration. Speech spectrum noise is white noise with equal energy from 250 to 1000 Hz and a 12 dB/octave fall-off from 1000 to 6000 Hz. In this procedure the noise is sent through the loudspeaker and is picked up by a condenser microphone placed where the center of the subject's head will be during test conditions. To conform to the procedure used by Tillman et al. (1966) the distance should be 6 feet from the loudspeaker face. The proposed standard for audiometers suggests in the appendix that the loudspeaker should be at least 1 meter from the listener. The output from the audiometer to the loudspeaker will be monitored to 0 on the VU meter. The signal from the loudspeaker through the condenser microphone is read on the linear scale of the spectrometer or sound level meter. The examiner must be careful to use a signal (approximately 80 dB HL) which is loud enough to avoid contamination of output measurements by ambient room noise. Even when white noise is used it is essential that no object be present between the loudspeaker and the microphone. If possible the examiner should be in another room to avoid any reflection or absorption from his presence. The attenuation of loudspeakers should be checked in the same way as that described earlier for earphones, except that speech spectrum noise rather than pure tones should be sent through the loudspeaker. The output should be measured in discrete steps. The amplifier hum or internal noise of the loudspeaker system should be checked. This is done by adjusting the attenuator dial to some setting (between 80 and 90 dB HL) and then measuring the output from the loudspeaker with no signal being presented. That is, everything is in normal position for testing except that there is no direct input signal to the speaker. The equipment noise should be at least 50 dB below the dial setting.

Figure 8.4 is a worksheet which may be used on a monthly basis to include most of the above calibration checks.

CALIBRATION OF ANCILLARY EQUIPMENT

Masking Generator

One of the major differences between the ANSI-1969 standard and the proposed standard is the greatly increased attention to the masking stimulus. The proposed standard defines white noise, spectrum level, weighted random noise, band level, narrow band noise and speech spectrum noise. The band widths for narrow bands are recommended and are those specified by Fletcher (1953). If narrow band noise is being used it will be necessary to have a frequency analyzer to determine if the band widths from the audiometer do conform to specification. Normally we have used the same transducer that we intend to use when delivering the masking source to make final calibration measurements. However, because the characteristics of various transducers are different it is sensible to first make an electronic check to verify that any possible variation from the band width is due to the transducer rather than to the audiometer itself.

The masking sound should be checked periodically through the earphones which are used to present that noise. The intensity of the masking signal may be checked in the same way as pure tones by presenting the noise through an earphone which is in place on an "artificial ear." The examiner should be careful to use a signal which is intense enough (80 to 90 dB HL) to avoid interference by extraneous room noise. If white noise (see Chapter 11, "Masking," for description) is the only masking signal on the audiometer, one need only check the output through the earphone with a linear setting (no filter). The overall output and attenuation characteristics should be checked in the same basic manner as described for pure tones.

If the output is measured through insert receivers, using a 2-cc coupler, the examiner should be aware that this output cannot be related directly to that obtained through a TDH-39 earphone measured via a 6-cc coupler. The 2-cc and 6-cc couplers are not equivalent in representing the SPL at the ear drum. Olsen, Jabaley and Pappas (1967) point out that since thresholds may vary as much as 20 dB between insert receivers and TDH-39 earphones extreme caution must be observed in considering the SPL values found for insert receivers. Part of the difference is due to the difficulty of obtaining a tight seal with insert receivers (both in the coupler and in the ear), and part of the difference may be due to individual ear canal volume difference ratios (between the volume under each type of receiver) which will affect the acoustic impedance at the ear drum.

If complex or narrow band noise is used rather than broad band (unfiltered) white noise, the characteristics of the noise should be checked by sending the noise through a wave analyzer and recording the intensity levels via a graphic level recorder. A rough approximation of the characteristics of the noise may be obtained by using a third octave filter. One should remember that more Hertz (cycles) are in the third octave centering around 8000 Hz than in the band centering around 1000 Hz, hence white noise will have less energy in the latter than in the former.

Figure 8.5 gives a worksheet which may be used in checking the calibration of the masking sound. In this procedure one uses an artificial ear in the manner described for checking the calibration of pure tones. The audiologist must be aware that when making measurements of noise, the characteristics of his measuring equipment are critical. Since noise is not a clean (i.e., uniform and unvarying) signal it is highly susceptible to errors of overshoot and undershoot on a VU meter and to damping on a graphic level recorder.

Tape Recorders and Phonographs

Tape recorders which are used in a clinic for reproducing speech signals should be checked at least once every 6 months. However, if the tape recorder is in regular use, weekly maintenance must be carried out, such as cleaning and demagnetizing the heads. The instruction manual should outline this procedure. (If it does not, any good tape recorder dealer can explain the procedure.) In addition, the frequency response and time characteristics of the tape recorder should be checked.

At the present time there are no standards for tape recorders used with speech audiometers per se, but there is a very comprehensive document dealing with tape recording and reproducing systems. This document (IEC-94, 1968) is entitled: "Magnetic Tape Recording and Reproducing Systems: Dimensions and Characteristics," and may be obtained through the American National Standards Institute. In addition, several ANSI and National Association of Broadcasters (NAB) documents deal with specific problem areas. ANSI S4.3-1972, for example, provides a method for determining flutter content of sound recorders.

The frequency response and time characteristics of the tape recorder may be checked by using a standard commercial tape recording of pure tones of various frequencies. By checking the exact frequency of the tone with an electronic counter, one learns whether the tape recorder is playing at the proper speed. By checking the output from the tape recorder one can also determine the flatness of the response

Audiometer: _____ # _____ Place: _____ Date: _____

TRANSDUCER	EARPHONES				BONE VIBRATOR				LOUDSPEAKER*			
CHANNEL	I		II			I	II			I		II
EAR	Rt.	Lft.	Rt.	Lft.						Rt.	Lft.	Rt.	Lft.
125	47.5												
250	26.5					41.4		15.0					
500	13.5					30.7		9.0					
750	8.5					19.3							
1000	7.5					16.9		3.0					
1500	7.5					15.4							
2000	11.0					8.1		-3.0					
3000	9.5					6.6							
4000	10.5					11.2		-4.0					
6000	13.5					X							
8000	13.0					X							
Speech	20.0					29.4		13.0					
White Noise	20.0							13.0					
Speech Spectrum	20.0							13.0					

FREQUENCY IN HZ

ANSI - '69 TDH - 49's

ANSI - '72 RE B 70-A

Expected Output

* warble tone

A

Fig. 8.4. Monthly calibration check summary

curve. If one does not have access to such a tape it is possible to make one by introducing pure tones from an audio oscillator into the machine, recording them, and playing them back. This enables the operator to check both the record and playback sections of the tape recorder. Of course, if both the record and playback are equally reduced (or increased) in speed the output will appear normal. The output from the oscillator should be monitored with a voltmeter to make certain that a constant intensity signal is used. Distortion of the pure tone from the tape recorder should also be checked. If none of the above is possible, one should at least check the speed of the tape recorder by marking a tape and then, after timing a segment as it goes across the tape recorder heads, measuring to see how many inches did pass over the heads per second.

Phonographs require weekly and daily maintenance such as cleaning the turntable and stylus. Their frequency response and time characteristics should also be checked. If it is not possible to procure a phonograph record of pure tones, one may check the turntable speed by using a time disc and stroboscopic light. One must be sure that the stylus on the phonograph is of the proper size for the recordings. It will be recalled that some speech materials have been recorded for a larger stylus than that normally found on phonographs. An improper match will create some distortion and greatly increase the wear of the phonograph record.

It must be remembered that the tape recorder or phonograph used to reproduce speech materials is an integral part of the audiometer system. Thus, it cannot be ignored when checking the calibration of test equipment.

NARROW BAND NOISE CALIBRATION

TRANSDUCER	EARPHONES					LOUDSPEAKER				
CHANNEL		I		II			I		II	
EAR (FREQUENCY IN HZ)	Expected Output	Rt.	Lft.	Rt.	Lft.	Expected Output	Rt.	Lft.	Rt.	Lft.
125	47.5									
250	26.5					15.0				
500	13.5					9.0				
750	8.5									
1000	7.5					3.0				
1500	7.5									
2000	11.0					-3.0				
3000	9.5									
4000	10.5					-4.0				
6000	13.5									
8000	13.0									

ATTENUATION

HL Attenuator Dial	I (1k-Rt. Phone)	II
110		
105		
100		
95		
90		
85		
80		
75		
70		
65		
60		
55		
50		
45		
40		
35		
30		
25		
20		
15		
10		
5		
0		

LISTENING CHECK:

Mechanical Click: Yes ___ No ___ (Where ______________)

Attenuation complete Ch. I Yes ___ No ___

" " Ch. II Yes ___ No ___

Earphones Cords: OK ___ Worn ___ Crackle ___ Need Replacing ___

Bone Vibrator Cord: OK ___ Worn ___ Crackle ___ Need Replacing ___

B

Examiner ______________________

Short Increment Sensitivity Index (SISI) Units

Although at the present time there is still no standard for SISI units, one should check the intensity increments to see if the dial readings (1 through 5 dB) are accurate. The intensity may be checked by sending the output directly from the SISI unit, or by sending the output through earphones and an artificial ear to a graphic level recorder. The signal is then displayed on recording paper. One should check the output at each frequency and at each increment setting. In order to properly administer the SISI test the increments must be exactly 1 dB (see Chapter 16). The above procedure will also enable the examiner to determine the time intervals between stimulus increment presentations. In using this procedure one must be certain of the damping characteristics of the graphic level recorder. If the SISI unit does not produce increments of precisely 1 dB at the point indicated on the dial, and if there is a variable potentiometer dial to control the output increments, one may mark the SISI dial to show the setting needed for the 1-dB increment. It is important for the examiner to listen to the unit to make sure there are no clicks or other distorting influences. If possible the output of the unit should be displayed on an oscilloscope. The scope may also be used to check increment size. For example, we noted that on one SISI unit an abnormally high percentage of patients obtained 100% scores at 2000 Hz. On checking

Masking Source: _____ Transducer: _____

Channel: _____ Date: _____ Examiner: _____

FREQUENCY:	125	250	500	750	1000	1500	2000	3000	4000	6000	8000
1. Total Intensity of noise											
2. Dial Setting											
3. Equals Line 1 minus Line 2 Equals Noise Intensity at 0 on Dial											
4. Bandwidth * (# of cycles)											
5. Line 3 Minus Line 4 Equals LPC **											
6. Critical Bandwidth ***	18.5	17.0	17.0	17.8	18.1	19.0	20.0	21.4	23.1	26.1	27.7
7. Line 5 + 6											
8. ANSI - 1969 Threshold	45.0	25.5	11.5	8.0	7.0	6.5	9.0	10.0	9.5	15.5	13.0
9. Line 7 Minus Line 8 Equals Effective Masking at 0 dB on Dial											

Fig. 8.5. Worksheet for computation of effective masking level. (*) Bandwidth of masker through transducer. (**) LPC = level per cycle. (***) critical bandwidth from Fletcher (1953).

the calibration we found that the increments were precisely 1 dB and not louder as we had anticipated; however, the oscilloscope showed that when the increment was introduced there was a change in the wave form which resembled peak clipping. The SISI signal appeared to change in pitch when each increment was introduced. Patients are unlikely to differentiate between a slight pitch change as opposed to a slight loudness change. If a properly damped graphic level recorder is not available it is possible to check the increment size on a measurement device such as a spectrometer. The ballistics of the VU meter on the spectrometer must accurately represent the rapidly interrupted signals without overshoot or undershoot.

On checking the calibration of the SISI unit, one will note that some units add the increment to the original background signal (20 dB plus 1 dB = 21 dB), while other units attenuate the background signal and then add the increment back on (20 dB minus 1 dB then plus 1 dB = 20 dB) (Fig. 8.6). Since there is no present standard for SISI units the examiner should simply check to see what his instrument does.

AUTOMATIC AUDIOMETERS

A calibration check of automatic (or Bekesy) audiometers begins with frequency, intensity,

cross-talk and other aspects described for manual pure tone audiometers. In addition, the attenuation rate and interruption rate for pulsed signals should be checked. The attenuation rate may be measured quite easily with a stopwatch. After starting the motor, one starts the marking pen on the chart and at the same instant starts a stopwatch. One reads the chart to determine how far the signal was attenuated, or conversely increased, during the measured time interval. By dividing the time duration into the dB change in intensity one can find the dB per second attenuation rate. The

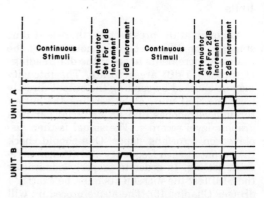

Fig. 8.6. SISI signals for two different types of SISI units.

proposed standard for audiometers suggests that the preferred rate of change will be 2.5 dB per second. Other alternatives, however, are listed. One should check the audiometer both when the signal is being attenuated, and separately when it is being increased. To check the pulsed stimulus duration one may go from the "scope sync" position on the back of the audiometer to an electronic counter, or, if this is not available, one may bridge across the terminals of the timing mechanism inside the audiometer. It is difficult to check the pulse speed on a graphic level recorder although it is sometimes possible to use an oscillograph or storage oscilloscope for that purpose. It is not difficult to estimate if there is roughly a 50% duty cycle (half on and half off), but it is quite difficult to judge whether the signal is on for 200 msec versus 210 msec. The proposed standard calls for a pulse duration of 200 msec on and 200 msec off. There is no indication of the tolerance that will be allowed. If one cannot use a scope sync output or bridge across the terminals of the electronic switch inside the audiometer, it is possible to connect the output of the audiometer directly to a storage oscilloscope to check the pulse rate.

It is important to check the relative intensity of the pulsed and continuous signals. If they are not equal this should be corrected. The relative intensities can be compared by observing the envelope of the wave form on an oscilloscope or by recording the output with a graphic level recorder. The attenuation rate and pulse rate should be checked annually unless there is reason to suspect a problem sooner. If there is an attenuator pad its characteristics should be measured during the routine output calibration check.

IMPEDANCE/ADMITTANCE MEASURING DEVICES

As of this writing there is no ANSI standard for acoustic impedance (or otoadmittance) measurement devices. However, an ANSI Working Group has been formed to study the problem and it is expected that within the next few years such a standard will exist. Despite the lack of an official standard there are certain parameters which should be measured by the clinician.

The clinician should determine the precise air pressure which is emitted from the air pressure probe on any of the electroacoustic bridges which use this parameter. Standard manometers are commercially available. By using either a direct connection or a piece of rubber tubing the probe from the impedance/admittance bridge may be connected to a manometer or "U" tube. One may then read directly the output in millimeters of water pressure (wp). At + 200 the gauge should read + 200; at 0 it should read 0 and at − 200 one should see − 200. It is recommended if pressure variations exceed 25 mm/wp the impedance/admittance device should be adjusted. Variations from listed values will affect the absolute acoustic impedance measurement and to a lesser extent the tympanogram.

In our facility bridges have been measured which were off by more than 100 mm/wp. This can dramatically change acoustic impedance estimates since the hearing mechanism has not been subjected to its initial standard stiffening.

The next parameter which should be measured is the decibel output. Each bridge indicates in its manual the output which should be expected at a given (usually 2-cc) volume setting. By attaching the probe to a 2-cc coupler or Hearing Aid Type I or Type II coupler and attaching that coupler to a sound level meter, one can directly read the output from the bridge. One should set the bridge to the appropriate volume and then read the output on the sound level meter. This measurement parameter can usually be adjusted internally and the clinician should refer to the schematic of his particular instrument for this adjustment. Although there is no standard, this measurement should probably be within ± 3 dB of its stated output. The frequency of the probe tone may be checked in the standard manner by either reading directly from the machine or by attaching the probe to the coupler thence to a sound level meter and finally to an electronic counter. The frequency should probably be within 5% of the stated test frequency. Care should also be taken to ensure that any attached XY plotter has readings which correspond to the parameters on the particular impedance/admittance measuring device.

If there is a built-in acoustic reflex stimulator this should be calibrated in the same manner as described earlier for pure tone audiometers. Attention should be paid to the frequency, intensity and rise-fall time of the reflex stimulus. If an ipsilateral reflex can be measured this circuit should also be checked by attaching a probe to the 2-cc coupler and then monitoring its output through use of a sound level meter or other appropriate device. In order to note any timing differential between the cessation of a probe tone and the initiation of a reflex eliciting stimulus, one should use a storage oscilloscope.

We have also found it helpful to check acoustic reflex systems by affixing the probe to a standard closed 2-cc coupler to make sure that there is no apparent reflex elicited in the cavity. In some instances when there is electronic crossover one will see a deflection on the meter which might suggest the presence of a reflex. Clearly a closed metal cavity cannot have an acoustic reflex. This false deflection indicates a problem within the machine which must be corrected.

If the impedance bridge or otoadmittance meter reads in equivalent volume one may use a hypodermic syringe which is calibrated in cubic centimeters or one may obtain a commercially available cubic centimeter cavity device which has different cubic centimeter readings. To calibrate the various positions on the bridge, one should achieve a balance reading at 2 cc when the probe is inserted into a 2-cc cavity, 4 cc should achieve a balance when the probe is inserted into a 4-cc closed cavity, and so on. There are usually internal adjustments which will allow one to compensate for any errors in measurement. When a hypodermic syringe is used for this calibration one must be extremely careful to make sure that there is an airtight seal and no leak of air when the connection is made. One may notice differences in the volume readings depending upon whether a long or broad volume device is used because there is some difference in the impedance of the air in the two size cavities. This is not strictly a volume measurement and thus the compliance of the air can be affected in some cases by the dimensions of the cavity. Until a standard cavity has been developed and approved it is recommended that the owner use the same cavity on all of his measuring devices and that he be able to describe this cavity when making comparisons between facilities.

Impedance/admittance measuring devices should be calibrated as carefully as any pure tone audiometer. Failure to do so may lead to variability which will make the impedance measurement invalid.

AUDITORY TRAINERS

Auditory trainers may be checked in the same manner as speech audiometers. Pure tone signals are presented into the microphone jack input (or directly through the microphone if an anechoic chamber is available) and the output is measured (e.g., frequency response, attenuator linearity). Harmonic characteristics of an auditory trainer are especially important. Unfortunately there are no standards for auditory trainers at the present time. It appears realistic to expect that the harmonic distortion of auditory trainers should be less than 6% and their output should be capable of being flat (± 3 dB) within the speech range. If output levels are specified in dB it is reasonable to expect these outputs to be accurate within 5 dB. If the auditory trainer uses a loop system, one should check the output through the child's receiver in various parts of the room. Matkin

and Olsen (1970) reported differences of 22 dB from one part of a room to another when they made such measurements. If this is true in the system under test the user should at least be aware of the problem.

CONCLUSION

With all audiometric equipment the clinician must first learn to listen to the output since there are many potential problems which can be detected by a trained human ear. To determine the precise characteristics of the instrument routine electronic calibration checks must be carried out since it is important to remember the human listener is simply not adequate to check the auditory equipment with the precision which is needed to ensure its proper working. The test result is no more accurate than the equipment on which it is performed. The ultimate responsibility for the accuracy of the test rests with the audiologist and, therefore, the audiologist must make sure that the equipment is working properly by having regular calibration checks.

REFERENCES

American Medical Association. Specifications of the council on physical medicine and rehabilitation of the American Medical Association. *J.A.M.A.*, **146**, 255–257, 1951.

American National Standards Institute. Volume measurements of electrical speech and program waves. ANSI C16.5-1954 (R 1961), American National Standards Institute, Inc., New York, 1961.

American National Standards Institute. Weighted peak flutter of sound recording and reproducing equipment. ANSI S4.3-1972, American National Standards Institute, Inc., New York, 1972.

American National Standards Institute. Specifications for audiometers. ANSI S3.6-1969. American National Standards Institute, Inc., New York, 1970.

American National Standards Institute. Artificial head-bone for the calibration of audiometer bone vibrators. ANSI S3.13-1972, American National Standards Institute, Inc., New York, 1972.

Benson, R., Charan, K., Day, J., Harris, J., Niemoller, J., Rudmose, W., Shaw, E., and Weissler, P., Limitations on the use of circumaural earphones. *J. Acoust. Soc. Am.*, **41**, 713–714, 1967.

Burkhard, M. D., and Corliss E. L. R., The response of earphones in ears and couplers. *J. Acoust. Soc. Am.*, **26**, 679–685, 1954.

Corliss, E. L. R., and Burkhard, M. D., A probe tube method for the transfer of threshold standard between audiometer earphones. *J. Acoust. Soc. Am.*, **25**, 990–993, 1953.

Fletcher, H., *Speech and Hearing in Communication*. Princeton, N. J.: D. Van Nostrand Co., Inc., 1953.

Hawley, M. S., An artificial mastoid for audiophone measurements. *Bell Lab. Rec.*, **18**, 73–75, 1939.

International Electrotechnical Commission. Magnetic tape recording and reproducing systems: Dimensions and characteristics, including amendment I and supplement 94A (1972) IEC-94 1968, American National Standards Institute, Inc., New York, 1972.

International Electrotechnical Commission. An IEC artificial ear, of the wide band type, for the calibration of earphones used in audiometry. IEC-318 1970, American National Standards Institute, Inc., New York, 1970.

International Electrotechnical Commission. An IEC mechanical coupler for the calibration of bone vibrators having a specified contact area and being applied with a specified static force. IEC-373-1971. American National Standards Institute, Inc., New York, 1971.

International Standards Organization. Standard reference zero for the calibration of pure-tone audiometers. ISO Recommendation R389. American National Standards Institute, Inc., New York, 1964.

Lybarger, S., Interim bone conduction thresholds for audiometry. *J. Speech Hear. Res.*, **9**, 483–487, 1966.

Martin, M. C., The routine calibration of audiometers. *Sound*, **2**, 106–109, 1968.

Matkin, N., and Olsen. W., Induction loop amplification systems classroom performance. *ASHA* **12**, 239–244, 1970.

Olsen, W. O., Personal communication, 1975.

Olsen, W., Jabaley, T., and Pappas, N., Interaural attenuation for a TDH-39 earphone in an MX-41/AR cushion and for an insert receiver. Paper presented at American Speech and Hearing Association Convention, Chicago, 1967.

Proposed American National Standard for Audiometers, April 1975.

Roach, R., and Carhart, R., A clinical method for calibrating the bone-conduction audiometer. *Arch. Otolaryngol.*, **63**, 270–278, 1956.

Rudmose, W., Concerning the problem of calibrating TDH-39 earphones at 6 kHz with a 9 A coupler. *J. Acoust. Soc. Am.*, **36**, 1049 (A), 1964.

Shaw, E. A. G., and Thiessen, G. J., Acoustics of circumaural earphones. *J. Acoust. Soc. Am.*, **34**, 1233–1246, 1962.

Sivian, L. J., and White, S. D., On minimum audible sound fields, *J. Acoust. Soc. Am.*, **4**, 288–321, 1933.

Stein, L., and Zerlin, S., Effect of circumaural earphones and earphone cushions on auditory threshold. *J. Acoust. Soc. Am.*, **35**, 1744–1745, 1963.

Stewart, K. C., and Burgi, E. J., Loudness balance study of selected audiometer earphones. *National Center for Health Statistics*, Series 2, Number 40, U.S. Dept. of Health, Education and Welfare, (Rockville, Maryland), December 1970.

Stream, R. W., and Dirks, D. D., Effect of loudspeaker position on differences between earphone and free-field thresholds (MAP and MAF) *J. Speech Hear. Res.*, **17**, 549–568, 1974.

Studebaker, G., Intertest variability and the air-bone gap. *J. Speech Hear. Disord.*, **32**, 82–86, 1967.

Thomas, W. G., Preslar, M. J., Summers, R., and Stewart, J. L., Calibration and working condition of 100 audiometers. *Public Health Rep.*, **84**, 311–327, 1969.

Tillman, T. W., and Gish, K. D., Comments on the effect of circumaural earphones on auditory threshold. *J. Acoust. Soc. Am.*, **36**, 969–970, 1964.

Tillman, T., Johnson, R., and Olsen, W., Earphone *versus* soundfield threshold sound pressure levels for spondee words. *J. Acoust. Soc. Am.*, **39**, 125–133, 1966.

Walton, W. K., Williams, P., and Labiak, J., Stability of routinely serviced public school audiometers. Paper presented American Speech and Hearing Convention, 1971.

Weiss, E., An air-damped artificial mastoid. *J. Acoust. Soc. Am.*, **32**, 1582–1588, 1960.

Weissler, P., International standard reference zero for audiometers. *J. Acoust. Soc. Am.*, **44**, 264–275, 1968.

Wilber, L. A., and Goodhill, V., Real ear *versus* artificial mastoid methods of calibration of bone-conduction vibrators. *J. Speech Hear. Res.*, **10**, 405–416, 1967.

Wilber, L. A., Calibration: Pure Tone, Speech and Noise Signals. In Katz, J. (Ed.), *Handbook of Clinical Audiology*. Baltimore: Williams & Wilkins, 1972a.

Wilber, L. A., Comparability of two commercially available artificial mastoids. *J. Acoust. Soc. Am.*, **52**, 1265–1266, 1972b.

Zwislocki, J. J., An acoustic coupler for earphone calibration. Rep. LSC-S-7, Lab. Sensory Commun., Syracuse Univ., 1970.

Zwislocki, J. J., An ear-like coupler for earphone calibration. Rep. LSC-S-9, Lab. Sensory Commun., Syracuse Univ., 1971.

chapter 9

PURE TONE AIR-CONDUCTION TESTING

David S. Green, Ph.D.

The measurement of pure tone air-conduction thresholds is basic to any consideration of clinical audiology, and it is not surprising that most of the audiology textbooks that have been written include this topic. Its treatment, however, varies as a function of the individual experiences and preferences of the author. In this chapter emphasis will be placed on calibration of the audiologist as well as on testing techniques. Audiologist calibration involves encouraging the tester to become aware of the multifaceted nature of the test situation and to make every effort to take critical variables into account. Audiometer calibration is covered elsewhere in this book along with other important aspects of testing such as masking, testing children and other special testing procedures employing pure tone signals.

THRESHOLD MEASUREMENT

The task of obtaining pure tone threshold measurements that are both reliable and valid is not a simple one. To carry it out effectively, the tester must have a workable definition of the term "threshold," be aware of the variables which influence threshold measurement and be thoroughly versed in the mechanics of testing methodology. Moreover, it is essential that he have knowledge of the complex interactions between tester, patient and audiometer.

Definition of Threshold

In theory, the term threshold as applied to pure tones may be defined as the faintest tone a subject can hear. In clinical practice it is not as simple as that. The tester must give consideration to a number of variables which, if ignored, may affect the stability of threshold measurement. For example, the purpose for which the measurement is made may have an influence on the dB value selected to represent threshold. Absolute versus relative auditory threshold hinges on such a distinction.

In clinical practice, pure tone thresholds are determined for two main purposes: (1) to assist in the diagnosis of ear pathology and (2) to acquire information which may be used in obtaining appropriate habilitation or rehabilitation programs for hearing-impaired persons.

In the sense that clinical audiologists derive thresholds that compare the sensitivity of a hearing-impaired subject with the so-called "normal hearing standard," the clinical threshold may be considered "relative."

On the other hand, scientists who study psychoacoustics under ideal laboratory conditions are likely to view threshold measurement quite differently. In the laboratory the frequency, intensity and duration characteristics of the stimulus can be altered in very small amounts and thresholds are usually defined as a point at which 50% of the subject's responses are positive. On the whole psychoacousticians devote their study to frequency and intensity characteristics of sounds audible to normal rather than abnormal ears, and for this reason are said to pursue the measurement of "absolute" auditory threshold. Despite their slightly more technical orientation, laboratory hearing studies often produce results that have clinical applicability.

Variables Which Influence Threshold

Technique of Measurement. Some testers are inclined to establish threshold by going from an inaudible to an audible stimulus (ascending method), while others approach the threshold point by going from an audible to an inaudible stimulus (descending method). In an unpublished study by Rosenblith and Miller, cited by Hirsh (1952), data are presented which indicate that these two basic methods may not produce the same threshold values. They determined threshold on the basis of observer judgments of the presence or absence of a tone. Threshold was defined as the dB level at which 50% of the judgments were positive. Rosenblith and Miller found that threshold measurements using a descending technique and a 4000-Hz interrupted tone yielded lower (better) thresholds by about 4 dB than those obtained with an ascending technique. Conversely, a 4000-Hz continuous tone yielded higher (poorer) thresholds when a descending rather than an ascending method was used.

The poorer thresholds obtained with a descending compared to an ascending method when continuous tones are used may be explained on the basis of perstimulatory fatigue (see Chapter 17 for discussion of related terminology). It happens that the initial response of the auditory system to a sustained tone is its most vigorous response. This is called the "on-effect." As the tone continues there may be a reduction in responsiveness, varying from a slight lessening in normal ears to an extreme loss of responsiveness in ears with neural pathology. Thus, when establishing threshold with a continuous tone using a descending rather than an ascending method, poorer threshold resulting from neural fatigue may be expected. The effect is most likely to occur when there is strong uninterrupted auditory stimulation immediately preceding ascertainment of threshold. As Rosenblith and Miller noted, when the starting level of their series of descending signals was raised from 20 to 40 dB sound pressure level (SPL), thresholds were more than 12 dB poorer. Ascending and descending techniques yielded approximately equivalent results only when the descending sequence was begun very near threshold.

For general clinical purposes Carhart and Jerger (1959) encouraged the use of an ascending technique employing short duration tones. The Hughson-Westlake ascending procedure which they recommended presents signals for a second or two in duration so as to elicit on-effect responses from the subject. By so doing, variability due to perstimulatory fatigue is minimized and threshold reliability is enhanced. The technique has the added advantages of being simple to perform and of having gained wide acceptance among audiologists. It is also recommended by the Committee on Conservation of Hearing of the American Academy of Ophthalmology and Otolaryngology.

Aware of the findings of Rosenblith and Miller, Carhart and Jerger compared ascending, descending and ascending-descending clinical techniques to determine whether differences noted in laboratory studies pertained also to clinical application of pure tone threshold tests. Carhart and Jerger found that mean thresholds obtained by the descending method were slightly lower than for the other two methods, but that the differences were considerably smaller than the 5-dB intensity interval of most clinical audiometers. While in essence, the three methods yielded clinically equivalent results, Carhart and Jerger recommended the Hughson-Westlake ascending method because of the advantages previously mentioned, as well as the desirability of developing a standard procedure for performing pure tone clinical audiometry.

Instructions to Subject. Another source of variability lies with the instructions given to a subject. If he is told to respond to a stimulus even though it is so faint that he may not be completely certain that he heard it, the subject may give 5-dB better thresholds than if instructed to respond only to tones that he hears for certain. Pollack (1948) plotted thresholds of pure tones having tonal quality and characteristic pitch and also thresholds of audibility where the same observer was told to respond to anything that was different from silence. Thresholds for the latter were better at all test frequencies but threshold discrepancies between the two sets of listening criteria were greatest for the higher frequencies. The difference for example at 4000 Hz was found to be about 7 dB.

Positioning of Earphones. Care must be taken to place the diaphragm of the audiometer earphone squarely over the opening of the external canal. Failure to do so may result in poor test-retest reliability. Auricles come in all sizes and shapes and when covered by an earphone it is often difficult to judge from the exposed portion whether or not the earphone is centered on the canal. If in doubt, the best way to make this determination is by drawing the phone away from the subject's ear and taking a careful look. Threshold variations of 15 dB or more may be demonstrated clinically as a result of poor earphone placement.

Audiometer Limitations. Inherent characteristics in the design and calibration of audiometers have an influence on threshold variability. Assuming that two audiometers meet current calibration standards, it is possible to test a single subject with each one in exactly the same manner and to get different thresholds. At this writing, the sound pressure produced by the earphone at each hearing threshold level (HTL) reading may differ from the indicated value by ±3 dB for frequencies 250 to 3000 Hz inclusive, by ±4 dB for 4000 Hz, and by ±5 dB for frequencies below 250 and above 4000 Hz, and still allow the audiometer to meet current calibration standards (ANSI-1969). This makes it possible for one audiometer with acceptable calibration to deliver a 55-dB 8000-Hz tone with a dial reading of 50 dB HTL, and another with acceptable calibration to deliver only 45 dB of the same tone with a dial reading of 50 dB HTL. If the "true threshold" were 55 dB, the tester would obtain a dial reading of 50 dB on the first audiometer and 60 dB on the second. He would then have to record the thresholds as being 10 dB different when in fact they were the same.

Another possible source of variability is related to the zero reference level of the audiometer. Most pure tone audiometers in use today are calibrated to either ANSI-1969 or to ISO-1964 zero reference levels, both of which are roughly equivalent, although the ANSI-1969 is slightly more stringent and is the standard currently endorsed by the American Speech and Hearing Association. A third and older calibration standard, ASA-1951, may also be in use with a small number of audiometers. This latter calibration standard is significantly less stringent than the previously mentioned ones and will yield thresholds as much as 15 dB better for some frequencies.

One problem with having significantly different zero levels in use is that it is necessary to know to which standard an audiometer is calibrated in order to compare serial audiograms on a given subject. Before current ANSI and ISO zero levels came into use, audiograms did not include information about audiometric calibration. With the advent of the newer standards, proponents suggested that until the transition was complete it would be expedient to note on the audiogram whether the recorded hearing threshold levels were relative to the outdated ASA-1951 or to the current calibration standard. It was also recommended that information for conversion from one scale to another appear on the audiograms. When a subject brings in a copy of an old audiogram and asks whether his hearing has changed, it is important that both the old and the new audiograms be viewed from the same zero reference level.

Another factor which affects the determination of threshold concerns the upper and lower output capability of the audiometer. Audiometers that are calibrated to ANSI or ISO standards commonly have an output range extending from 0 to 110 dB for most frequencies. It is customary when making an audiogram on such an audiometer to indicate lack of response at maximum output by making a downward pointing arrow at the 110-dB point on the graph, or if the maximum output at the test frequency is only 90 dB, the arrow is placed at the 90-dB point.

However, on the low end of the output scale, there appears to be less agreement in recording thresholds. There is no commonly used symbol to indicate that a subject was able to hear a test tone at the lowest output setting of the audiometer. If the lowest dial reading is 0, and the subject responds 100% of the time, his threshold is obviously *less* than 0. Yet in most clinical settings the tester simply records a "threshold" level of 0 dB and lets it go at that.

In a study by Eagles et al. (1963), data were collected on over 4000 Pittsburgh school children aged 5 to 14 years. Testing was performed with specially calibrated audiometers which permitted threshold measurement below the minimum output of most clinical audiometers. These authors found, as might be expected, that the hearing sensitivity of some children was too good to be accurately measured with a standard audiometer.

Subject Variability. Variability in threshold measurements often relate to the person being tested. Aside from the moment to moment changes due to an auditory system in constant flux, three factors that contribute to threshold instability are (1) ear pathology, (2) motivation during the test and (3) ability to cooperate.

Certain kinds of ear pathology are associated with physical discomfort. If the patient has Meniere's disease and is dizzy or nauseated while being tested, thresholds may be poorer than when the subject is physically well.

The type of hearing pathology which produces episodic tinnitus might also affect results. Thresholds obtained during the tinnitus attack may be poorer than during remission, particularly if there is similarity between the tinnitus and the test tone. A pulsed or warbled test tone is often used to provide greater contrast between the tinnitus from within and the test tones from without. This enables the patient to respond more reliably.

Individuals who have been exposed to high levels of industrial noise or to the sound of gunfire may suffer temporary threshold shifts. If so, they will exhibit poorer thresholds immediately after the cessation of noise than after a sufficient interval of quiet.

Thresholds are known to fluctuate during the course of both sensory-neural and conductive ear pathologies. Several of these are worthy of mention.

Sensory-neural hearing losses associated with Meniere's disease, sudden deafness of unknown etiology, certain antibiotic drugs, nerve VIII lesions, excessive aspirin ingestion and menstrual cycle show threshold instability. When the hearing loss is caused by Meniere's disease or by physiologic changes associated with menstruation, thresholds get alternately better and poorer. Hearing loss induced by ingestion of large dosages of aspirin, as prescribed for persons suffering from arthritis, usually disappears when the aspirin is discontinued. Ototoxic drugs such as dihydrostreptomycin and kanamycin make thresholds poorer. Of these, the former has an unusual effect on the auditory system – a delayed loss of hearing sensitivity in which the hearing loss may occur several months after the drug is discontinued. In the case of nerve VIII lesions, thresholds tend to become progressively poorer, whereas in the sudden deafness cases they tend to show spontaneous recovery or remain the same.

Conductive hearing deficits resulting from middle and outer ear lesions are frequently a source of threshold instability. The child, for example, who develops frequent colds that "settle in his ears" may exhibit a conductive hearing loss that fluctuates from one test to another. In an individual who suffers from Eustachian tube malfunction and finds that he can inflate his middle ear by pinching his nostrils and blowing through pursed lips (Valsalva), thresholds obtained before and after this maneuver may vary considerably. I found the following differences (improved hearing after inflation) in one such patient: 0 dB at 250 Hz; 10 dB at 500 Hz; 35 dB at 2000 Hz; 30 dB at 4000 Hz; and 0 dB at 8000 Hz. I have also seen patients with middle ear pathology who claimed that they were able to hear better if, while sitting, they leaned forward and lowered their head between their knees. Surprisingly enough, their claims were substantiated by obtaining two sets of thresholds, one with head up and one with head down. Differences of up to 20 dB were recorded.

Motivation to cooperate is also a factor in test reliability. For example, an individual who is determined to meet the hearing standards which will qualify him for training as a commercial pilot is likely to give his full attention to the listening task. Another individual with similar hearing who is actively trying to avoid military service might not be inclined to listen as carefully.

Some individuals, particularly the elderly and infirm, have limited ability to cooperate. They tire easily and have difficulty in attending to the listening task. Others may not have the intellectual capacity to maintain sustained interest in the test procedure. The tester should be alert to these possibilities and be prepared to modify his approach as circumstances require.

Suggested Test Procedures

Having reviewed some of the sources of test variability, it is desirable at this juncture to give a description of a general testing procedure applicable for clinical use. Appropriate modifications, when made with good cause, are certainly to be encouraged.

Testing should be preceded by a check of the audiometer. After the audiometer has had a suitable warm-up period, the tester should place the earphones on his own ears and listen to various frequencies and intensities of the test tones. He should be familiar enough with his own thresholds to be able to detect gross calibration errors. He should also listen to the masking noise, check for audible clicks in the interrupter switch and for loose connections in the earphone wiring. Once the audiometer is checked out, the testing may begin. The thresholds may be plotted by making an appropriate symbol on a graph as shown in Figure 9.1 or by recording the threshold as a numerical entry in a tabular audiogram as illustrated in Figure 9.2. A standardized set of audiometric symbols has been developed by the ASHA Committee on Audiometric Evaluation (1974) and has been approved by the Executive Board of ASHA.

Informal Preliminaries. The hearing test begins informally when the tester makes his first contact with the patient. During the course of exchanging casual conversation and gathering pertinent case history material, the tester is in a position to observe the patient's response to speech. Is the patient having a relatively easy or difficult time communicating? Does he favor one ear over the other? The ear that is cocked toward the tester is usually the better ear. If he is having difficulty, how does he handle it? Does he ask for repetition when you speak in a normal conversational level or does he simply not answer until your voice level compensates for his hearing loss? Answers to these questions and others provide a useful background for the formal portion of the hearing test.

Before the tones are presented, the patient must be positioned properly and instructed in the listening task. The patient should be seated in an armchair where the control panel of the audiometer is out of his line of vision. A suitable position for the subject's head is a point midway between full left profile and back of head facing tester. It is my opinion that for pure tone audiometry better control can be maintained when the patient and tester are in the same room, rather than in adjacent rooms. Instruction to the subject may vary according to the preference of the individual tester but should follow this general pattern: PROP YOUR ELBOW ON THE ARM OF YOUR CHAIR, MAKE A FIST AND RAISE IT KEEPING YOUR ELBOW IN CONTACT WITH THE CHAIR. WHEN YOU HEAR THE TONE, RAISE YOUR INDEX FINGER, EVEN

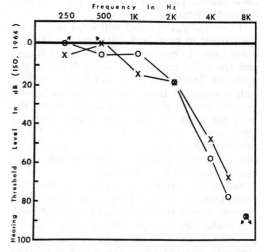

Fig. 9.1. An audiogram used to graph a patient's thresholds at various frequencies in each ear. Note that lack of threshold determination because of audiometric limits are designated by an *arrow attached to the symbol.*

HEARING RECORD

Name								Phone				Age	Referred by:			
Address												Diagnosis:				

			AIR CONDUCTION														
			RIGHT								LEFT						
DATE	TEST ROOM	LEFT MASK	250	500	1000	2000	4000	8000	RIGHT MASK	250	500	1000	2000	4000	8000	AUDIOM.	EXAM
		—	0↑	5	5	20	60	90↓	—	5	0↑	15	20	50	90↓		

Fig. 9.2. A form for tabular collection of audiometric data. *Numbers* rather than symbols are entered in the appropriate boxes.

WHEN THE TONE IS VERY SOFT. HOLD IT UP AS LONG AS YOU HEAR IT. WHEN YOU NO LONGER HEAR IT, BRING YOUR FINGER RIGHT DOWN. UP WHEN YOU HEAR IT, DOWN WHEN YOU DON'T. These instructions are accompanied by appropriate simultaneous gestures illustrating and reinforcing the verbal explanation.

For most patients, the index finger response is preferred to a more gross movement such as a raised hand or a verbal yes-no response. Two reasons for this are (1) the finger-up and finger-down movements give two clear responses for one stimulus and (2) the index finger provides subtle clues about the patient's perception of the stimulus. The second point will be discussed in greater detail later.

Occasionally, the tester will want to instruct the patient to raise both fists and use the left index finger to respond to tones in the left ear, and the right one for tones localized to the right ear. This approach is useful when testing bone conduction in an ear with a conductive hearing loss as it helps the tester assess the need for masking. For some elderly and for some young patients, requiring index finger responses may prove to be too mentally or physically taxing and consequently some other form of response must be accepted.

Before the earphones are placed over the patient's ears, it is customary to remove eyeglasses, hair nets, earrings and chewing gum. It is useful also to inspect the ear canals with a penlight. If the canal opening is small or if it seems to collapse when the pinna is pressed experimentally in a manner which simulates pressure from the earphones, the tester may want to explore the possibility of spurious test results due to earphone placement. Ventry, Chaiklin and Boyce (1961) have reported audiometric air-bone gaps from collapsed canals ranging from 15 to 30 dB for the speech frequencies. When plastic tubes were inserted in the ear canals to keep them open, thresholds improved.

Another technique that may be used to check for a collapsed canal is removing the earphone from the spring headband and holding it loosely against the subject's ear. If he hears better when the earphone is applied in this manner it is likely that a collapsed canal is the source of difficulty.

The earphones should be loosened as fully as possible in the headband before they are placed over the patient's ears. After the center of the earphone is lined up with the center of its assigned ear canal, both earphones should be pressed lightly against the ear and held firmly in place while the headband is tightened with pressure applied by the tester's thumbs.

A routine should be established to place a specific earphone over the left or right ear. If the earphones are marked "left" and "right" the choice is simplified. If they are color coded, red goes on the right and blue on the left in keeping with the traditional air conduction symbols, namely "red O" for the right and "blue X" for the left.

Testing Technique

The "up 5-down 10" method of threshold exploration for the test frequencies is recommended in keeping with the principles of the Hughson-Westlake ascending technique. For most of the testing, tones of short duration should be used in order to elicit thresholds governed by the on-effect.

Although the range of human hearing is roughly 20 to 20,000 Hz encompassing 19,980 individual frequencies, it is not practical to obtain thresholds for each individual frequency. Usually a sample of no more than 10 individual frequencies per ear is tested. Fortunately this small sample has proven to be clinically serviceable, although some audiologists feel that diagnostically significant information is contained in frequencies higher than those capable of being tested on conventional audiometers.

The "up 5-down 10" procedure entails the following steps.

Step 1. Test the better ear first in order to determine the need for masking. It is assumed that appropriate masking will be used as needed.

Step 2. Start with a 1000-Hz tone at a level enough above threshold to allow easy identification of the tone. This tone (1000-Hz) is usually selected because it is an important speech frequency and because the patient is less apt to misunderstand the listening task. Patients have sometimes shown uncertainty when initially presented with a 250-Hz tone because they were not sure whether the tester intended for them to respond to what sounded like a "fog horn."

The tester may wish to start with a 250-Hz tone if he suspects a profound loss. A low frequency is selected as the initial test tone in recognition of the fact that individuals with profound hearing loss often have testable hearing only in the low frequency range.

Step 3. Check the patient's understanding of the listening task by using both short and long duration presentations of the initial test tone. The index finger should be raised immediately on presentation of the tone and dropped as soon as the tone is discontinued. If the finger movements are sluggish, instructions should be repeated and the patient should be encouraged to be more responsive.

Step 4. During the course of testing, the examiner should vary the interval between tone presentations to avoid "telegraphing the stimulus." He should have one hand on the attenuator control and one on the interrupter switch to minimize gross physical movements which might be peripherally observed by the patient. Tones should not be presented while the attenuator dial is being rotated as switching artifacts may contaminate the test signal. As threshold is being approached it is desirable to check informally for abnormal tone decay by sustaining the tone for several seconds longer than usual. If the index finger drops before the tone is discontinued, abnormal tone decay may be suspected.

Step 5. The starting intensity of the test tone is reduced in 10-dB steps following each positive response, until a hearing threshold level is reached at which the subject fails to respond. Then, the tone is raised 5 dB. If the subject hears this increment, the tone is reduced 10 dB; if he does not, the tone is increased in 5-dB steps until it is heard. The essence of the "up 5-down 10" method is that a 5-dB increment is always used if the preceding tone was not heard, and a 10-dB decrement is always used when the tone is heard. For clinical purposes threshold is defined as the faintest tone that can be heard 50% or more of the time and is established after several threshold crossings.

With an audiometer calibrated in 5-dB steps, the hearing level which designates threshold is usually a point at which the tone is heard almost 100% of the time and below which the tone is almost never heard. Only if the steps of attenuation were less than 5 dB would it be feasible to define threshold as the point at which the patient responded correctly 50% of the time.

If there is no response at the maximum output of the audiometer an arrow pointing downward should be attached to the symbol designating the test ear and placed on the audiogram at the hearing threshold level coinciding with the maximum output for the test frequency. If the tone is heard at the minimum level, the audiogram should be marked in similar fashion but should have the arrow pointing upward.

Step 6. After the threshold for 1000 Hz has been established in the better ear, the procedure is repeated for the other audiometric frequencies including 2000, 4000, 8000, 500 and 250 Hz in that order. If the thresholds show significant rising or dropping between octaves, thresholds for 125 Hz and for the half octaves 750, 1500, 3000 and 6000 Hz may be explored to get a more complete assessment of the overall hearing configuration.

Step 7. Testing in the second ear should begin with the last frequency used to test the first ear. There is no need to start again with a 1000-Hz tone because if one side of the head has learned the listening task the other side knows it as well. The test is terminated after all desired frequencies have been examined.

INTERPRETATION OF AIR-CONDUCTION HEARING TESTS

Air-conduction thresholds alone, no matter how valid or reliable they may be, provide insufficient information for diagnostic and rehabilitative purposes. An adequate diagnosis can only be made as a result of complete audiometric, case history and medical appraisals. With only air-conduction testing one cannot even draw the basic distinction between conductive and sensory-neural hearing loss. While it is true that certain audiometric patterns have come to be associated with specific ear pathologies, there are far too many exceptions to risk using these configurations for diagnosis.

When there is a hearing loss present, the air-conduction threshold represents cumulative deficits from the outer, middle, inner ear and retrocochlear system of a subject. Bone conduction (see Chapter 10) is used in conjunction with air conduction to determine whether the hearing problem should be classified as conductive, sensory-neural or mixed. When air-conduction thresholds are 10 dB or more poorer than bone conduction, a "conductive element" is said to be present. If there is a conductive element with audiometrically normal bone-conductive thresholds, the hearing problem is conductive. If there is a conductive element but the bone-conduction thresholds are poorer than normal, the loss is characterized as mixed. A sensory-neural hearing deficit exists when the air- and bone-conduction thresholds are approximately equal to each other but poorer than normal.

Conductive hearing loss, which results from pathology in the outer or middle ear, is qualitatively different than sensory-neural loss associated with pathology of the inner ear. Generally the conductively impaired ear suffers a loss of sensitivity (sounds have to be louder to be heard) but does not lose the ability to hear speech clearly when it is made sufficiently loud. The ear with sensory-neural impairment suffers both a loss of sensitivity and a loss of clarity (even after speech is made sufficiently loud, the words may not sound clear). Because of the clarity factor, two persons with the same degree of hearing loss by air conduction may have dissimilar problems. All things being equal, the individual with a conductive loss has less of a communication problem than someone with the same degree of sensory-neural loss.

Categorizing Air-Conduction Hearing Threshold Levels

The speech frequencies are 500, 1000 and 2000 Hz. Studies have shown that the dB average of these three frequencies serves quite well in predicting the threshold for understanding speech. This relationship highlights an important application of the air-conduction audiogram, namely, that it provides a means of predicting the loss of sensitivity for speech. If this prediction is made, the audiologist will have an idea of the degree of disability present as well as an appreciation of the magnitude of rehabilitative needs. Goodman (1965) adapted material from Silverman (1960) to prepare a guide relating hearing threshold levels and degree of hearing impairment. Table 9.1 contains hearing threshold level categories based on both ASA-1951 and ANSI-1969 (or ISO-1964) reference standards and provides a scale of terms commonly used to describe the severity of hearing impairment. Table 9.2, in similar fashion, groups categories of hearing threshold level in terms of probable handicap and needs. Goodman wisely cautioned against too literal an interpretation of information contained in the tables. Since the degree of handicap imposed by a hearing loss is clearly not measured in hearing threshold level alone, it is obvious that additional factors are to be considered in making recommendations for education and rehabilitation. In this connection it should be noted that the guidelines fail to make a distinction between categories of hearing threshold level associated with conductive as compared to sensory-neural deafness. The importance of this distinction is illustrated by patients with nerve VIII tumors, a significant number of whom show mild hearing loss for pure tones with almost complete loss of ability to understand speech at any level.

Categorizing Qualitative Test Factors

At the beginning of this chapter, it was stated that emphasis would be placed on calibration of the audiologist. As a background for this, a number of variables which are known to influence the measurement of threshold have been reviewed, and a technique of threshold testing described. Throughout the chapter there has been an attempt to foster an attitude of scientific and clinical curiosity on the part of the reader. In so doing, certain material which has been treated more traditionally elsewhere has been touched upon only lightly here. While it is hoped that the reader will absorb the information and attitudes which this chapter has meant to convey, he is encouraged at the same time to supplement this and to expand his knowledge of audiology with references to other available textbook material.

In a paper presented at a meeting of the Audiology Study Group of New York (Green, 1969), the author attempted to stress the importance of enlightened observation. A modification of this paper is offered here (*lingua in bucca*) for the purpose of conveying what is meant by "audiologist calibration."

The paper's basic premise is that clinical observations of behavior contribute useful, and often vital information about the hearing of an individual who is being tested. It advises the inexperienced tester that a good hearing test involves something more than a linked series of Xs and Os on an audiogram blank. The additional something is a calibrated audiologist.

TABLE 9.1. *Scale of Hearing Impairment**

Hearing Threshold Level†		Descriptive Term
1951 ASA reference	1969 ANSI reference‡	
dB	dB	
−10 to 15	−10 to 26	Normal limits
16–29	27–40	Mild hearing loss
30–44	41–55	Moderate hearing loss
45–59	56–70	Moderately severe hearing loss
60–79	71–90	Severe hearing loss
80 plus	91 plus	Profound hearing loss

* After Goodman (1965).
† Average of hearing threshold levels from 500, 1000 and 2000 Hz.
‡ Equivalent to ISO-1964 reference.

TABLE 9.2. *Relations between Hearing Threshold Level and Probable Handicap and Needs**

Hearing Threshold Level		Probable Handicap and Needs
1951 ASA reference	1969 ANSI reference	
dB	dB	
<30	<40	Has difficulty hearing faint or distant speech; needs favorable seating and may benefit from lip reading instruction. *May also benefit from hearing aid.*
30–45	40–55	Understands conversational speech at a distance of 3 to 5 feet; needs hearing aid, auditory training, lip reading, favorable seating, speech conservation and speech correction.
45–60	55–70	Conversation must be loud to be understood and there is great difficulty in group and classroom discussion; needs all of above plus language therapy and maybe special class for hard of hearing.
60–80	70–90	May hear a loud voice about 1 foot from the ear, may identify environmental noises, may distinguish vowels but not consonants; needs special education for deaf children with emphasis on speech, auditory training and language; may enter regular classes at a later time.
>80	>90	May hear loud sounds, does not rely on hearing as primary channel for communication; needs special class or school for the deaf; some of these children eventually enter regular high schools.

* After Goodman (1965).

Here then, at the risk of losing his literary license, the author offers the aforementioned, clinically oriented, treatise which follows.

USEFUL FINGER OBSERVATION (UFO) IN PURE TONE THRESHOLD AUDIOMETRY

Sightings of UFOs are most often reported when the viewer has fixed his gaze intently upon the index finger of a person having his hearing tested. These observations require no special locale. They may be made wherever pure tone audiometry is practiced.

As a longtime exponent and practitioner of the art of index finger response analysis in clinical audiometry, I have come to observe that the behavior of an individual's finger is often characteristic of the total organism's response to sound stimuli. Experience has taught that while finger behavior may appear capricious to the casual observer, in actuality it follows lawful and predictable patterns.

Thus far, six basic categories of finger behavior have been identified. Each category has its own distinct symptomatology, each has its own test profile and each is associated with characteristic pathology.

Most standard audiology texts fail to mention the existence of these diagnostic categories, leaving their discovery to chance. They are identified here to avoid such haphazard treatment of this important clinical material.

Before the search for UFOs can begin, it is necessary that the subject be instructed to raise his index finger when he hears a tone and to lower it as soon as he no longer hears it.

It is important to remember that the finger categories described in the following paragraphs are neither mutually exclusive nor necessarily complete. It is well for the audiologist to remain on the constant alert for rare sightings which may herald the discovery of a new category.

The Halfup Finger

The halfup finger rarely occurs in the company of an ear suspected of a sensory-neural hearing loss. For this reason, it is less likely to be sighted in a medical setting and more likely to be seen in the public schools, among university students or other groups who practice giving hearing tests to each other. The halfup finger reflects uncertainty in the mind of the subject regarding the presence of tonal signals and occurs when there is a normal sensory-neural level. Unlike the fallsalarm finger (described later), which also shows uncertainty regarding the presence of test ones, the halfup finger is seldom in error. From its inimitable semierect slouch it unerringly fingers its own true threshold. As to the uncertainty of the finger, it can be simply dispelled by raising the intensity of the test tone by 5 dB. When this is done, the halfup finger stands all the way up, straight and tall. It is probably a good idea for the beginning audiologist to keep this in mind and, when necessary, to boost the sagging ego of a halfup finger by giving it a 5- or 10-dB above threshold increment. This should be given as the last signal in a series for a given tone. For instance, let us suppose that the halfup finger was consistently sighted at 40 dB at 1000 Hz in a conductively impaired ear. After several threshold crossings, the tester may suddenly become aware that his subject has begun to fidget, sweat and show other signs of anxiety. These signs are related to trying to find the softest tone that will elicit a response 50% or more of the time. As soon as the threshold is established at 40 dB the examiner should mark it on the audiogram, and then present a 45- or 50-dB tone to reassure the subject before turning attention to the next test frequency.

The Allernone Finger

With impressive sure-fingeredness the allernone finger makes unhesitating choices about the audibility of test tones. Lest one become overly impressed with this finger feat, be warned that the pseudoalertness may be related to a cochlear lesion and the recruitment of loudness associated with such a lesion. The allernone finger is not necessarily more alert than the next finger, although it may give that appearance. Why it responds as it does is not precisely known. Many experts agree, however, that the finger's response is in some way related to a supersensitivity generated by a premature loss of hair. This baldness in the hair cells of the cochlea has the effect of making incoming tones either inaudible or equivalent in loudness to a tone 10 to 20 dB above normal threshold. This either-or effect makes the choice between audibility and inaudibility an easy one for the allernone finger.

The Body Finger

This finger is usually ankylosed to a worn nervous system which has lost some of its ability to selectively inhibit motor responses. Thus when the body finger is induced to respond, a response may also be expected from a number of other extremities as well. The latter may be discounted as being redundant, but the multiresponse configuration should alert the beginning clinician that somewhere underneath the body finger he is likely to find an ear with presbycusis. Sightings are frequently made with geriatric patients.

The Malingafingers

Malingafingers come in all sizes. Frequently they are attached to small hands and have been sighted in school hearing tests but have gone unrecognized. Malingafingers also are attached to larger hands whose fingers frequently itch for illicit monetary gain. Large malingafingers occasionally become sore when they are sighted and recognized. The diagnosis of malingafinger, although often suspected, can only be confirmed in the presence of a self-incriminating admission. Whether faced by large or small malingafingers, beginning clinicians will do well to remain on their guard against their misleading responses.

Clinicians should be particularly alert to sightings of the "delayed reaction" finger and the finger known as the "inflation index," two of the more salient types of malingafinger. On the one hand, the "delayed reaction" finger can be recognized by the fact that it does not respond unless the tone remains on for longer than usual. The "inflation index" finger, on the same hand, can be recognized by the fact that it will only respond to progressively greater increments of tonal intensity. For example, the "inflation index" finger might respond as follows to a test tone:

Hearing Threshold Level (dB)	Response
40	Yes
30	No
35	No
40	No
45	Yes
35	No
40	No
45	No
50	Yes

Once a malingafinger is sighted, regardless of type, special techniques must be brought into play if valid thresholds are to be obtained.

The Fallsalarm Finger (Reverse Malingafinger)

The fallsalarm finger is usually attached to an individual who is very difficult to test. Its action is frequently independent of the action of the tester and is often marked by five or six positive finger responses in the interval between placement of the earphones and initial presentation of the tone. The fallsalarm finger is moved by tinnitus or the suggestibility associated with certain forms of pre- and postoperative anxieties. Whatever else moves the finger, one can be relatively certain that it is not moved by the impulse to malinger (Chaiklin and Ventry, 1965).

The Tired Finger

Tired finger may be confused with dumb finger by the beginning clinician. Dumb finger is a category of questionable authenticity since it discourages the pursuit of more valid diagnostic UFO categories. After repeated instructions, the finger still responds initially, but then drops before the tone is discontinued. To label the finger "dumb" on this basis is to commit an error that may be fraught with serious consequences. Tired finger may be the first sign of a brain tumor or other retrocochlear lesion. While the tired finger is capable of responding to the "on-effect" of a tone, the damaged nerve fibers in the hearing mechanism rapidly become fatigued and the response cannot be maintained. Occasionally the tired finger may waver, but not fall. Questioning the finger's owner may reveal that the initial test stimulus had a tonal quality, but as the duration of the stimulus was extended the tonality was replaced by a "buzz," "hum," "hiss" or other nontonal sound (Green, 1963). Whether the whole stimulus is lost or just the tonality, the audiologist should plan further exploration for a possible retrocochlear lesion.

Summary

The existence of UFO categories in pure tone threshold audiometry is not really a controversial question in the mind of the experienced audiologist. This paper takes the position that UFOs exist in pure tone threshold audiometry and furthermore, that they can be divided into at least six major and two minor diagnostic categories. Descriptive information about each has been offered to the audiologist who may wish to participate in future sightings. The point has been stressed that fingers behave in different ways not through caprice, but for reasons of cause and effect. While, at first, the differences seem inconsistent, greater understanding of the nature of the sound, as heard by members of each category, brings order to the apparent chaos (Simmons and Dixon, 1964).

Table 9.3 presents a quick summary of the finger categories, their symptomatology, their test results and their associated pathology.

The beginning audiologist is encouraged to waste no time in learning to assign finger responses to their appropriate categories. This sense of urgency is dictated by the fact that diagnostic opportunity may knock but once for a given finger.

> The Moving Finger writes; and, having writ,
> Moves on: nor all your Piety nor Wit
> Shall lure it back to cancel half a Line,
> Nor all your Tears wash out a Word of it.
> Omar Khayyam (*Rubaiyat*)

CONCLUSION

The audiologist is a vital link in the total process that results in valid and reliable pure tone threshold measurements. Starting with basic skills, he progresses through a dynamic process of growth to shape his powers of observation and to apply his knowledge with ever increasing efficiency. He becomes skillful in minimizing variables associated with test instrumentation, the person being tested and the testing methodology. He learns to be on the lookout for the fleeting furrow in the brow which signifies a puzzling auditory experience, and then pursues this observation by finding out what the subject heard.

In testing children he often finds it necessary to structure the test situation in a manner that may seem threatening to the child. It will be advantageous to the audiologist if he can perceive clues which help him to identify the child's reaction to this type of pressure. In that crucial instant before the child's tears become a torrent, swift counteraction may prevent test breakdown.

Children give other indications that a test may be about to deteriorate. The child's "bathroom dance" deserves and receives a quick response from the audiologist familiar with its universal choreography. At first sign of discom-

TABLE 9.3. *Summary of Symptomatology, Test Results and Associated Pathology for Six Finger Categories*

Finger Category and Symptomatology	Special Hearing Tests				Associated Pathology
	ABLB	SISI	Bekesy	Tone decay	
1. The Halfup Finger Uncertainty marks this finger. Torn by self-doubt it points accusingly at itself and asks, "Am I really responding to tone or just confusing the tester?"	Neg	Neg	I	Neg	No lesion or conductive lesion
2. The Allernone Finger Exuding great self-confidence, this finger reacts with enormous vitality, but only when it is appropriate to do so.	Pos	Pos	II	Mild (high frequencies)	Cochlear lesion
3. The Body Finger This finger, once the essence of dexterity and unfettered action, has failed to withstand the rigors and ravages of time. Gone now are freedom and independence of movement. When this finger is raised, all body extremities are thrown into turbulent activity.	Pos or Neg	Pos or Neg	I or II	?	Presbycusis may have either cochlear or neural lesion.
4. The Malingafingers a. Delayed action b. Inflation index Malingafingers are often attached to greedy hands. They are either slow to respond or else only respond to ever increasing intensities of sound.	Neg	Neg Unless there is true organic loss	V	Neg	Often nonorganic loss superimposed on organic one (malingering likely)
5. The Fallsalarm Finger Fallsalarm finger is often up, even when there is no tone being presented. It is also known as "Good Man Finger" because it's hard to keep a good man down.	?	?	?	?	Psychogenic pre or post operative anxiety sometimes associated with tinnitus (malingering unlikely)
6. The Tired Finger A finger with a short attention span rapidly loses interest in low intensity tones and tones presented at a fixed intensity.	Neg	Neg	III or IV	Moderate to severe (high and low frequencies)	Retrocochlear lesion

fort, a casual offer is made to show the child to the bathroom.

Whether dealing with child or with adult, the nonauditory clues become known through experience. Recognition of these signs can be helpful in the performance of accurate clinical testing.

REFERENCES

ASHA Committee on Audiometric Evaluation, Guidelines for Audiometric Symbols. *ASHA*, 16, 260–264, 1974.

Carhart, R., and Jerger, J., Preferred method for clinical determination of pure tone thresholds. *J. Speech Hear. Disord.*, 24, 330–345, 1959.

Chaiklin, J., and Ventry, I., Multidiscipline study of functional hearing loss. V. Patient errors during spondee and pure tone threshold measurements. *J. Auditory Res.*, 5, 219–230, 1965.

Eagles, E., Wishik, S., Doerfler, L., Melnick, W., and Levine, H., Hearing sensitivity and related factors in children. *Laryngoscope*, Monograph Supp., June 1963.

Goodman, A., Reference zero levels for pure-tone audiometer. *ASHA*, 7, 262–263, 1965.

Green, D. S., The modified tone decay test (MTDT) as a screening procedure for eighth nerve lesions. *J. Speech Hear. Disord.*, 28, 31–36, 1963.

Green, D. S., UFOs (useful finger observations) in pure tone audiometry. Paper presented at Audiology Study Group of New York, New York, March, 1969.

Hirsh, I., *The Measurement of Hearing* pp. 103–105. New York: McGraw-Hill, 1952.

Pollack, I., The atonal interval. *J. Acoust. Soc.* *Am.*, 20, 146–149, 1948.

Silverman, S. R., Hard of hearing children. In H. Davis (Ed.), *Hearing and Deafness*, Ch. 17. New York: Holt Rinehart & Winston, 1960.

Simmons, F., and Dixon, R., On the importance of the question: What do you hear? *Arch. Otolaryngol.*, 80, 167–169, 1964.

Ventry, I., Chaiklin, J., and Boyce, W., Collapse of the ear canal during audiometry. *Arch. Otolaryngol.*, 73, 727–731, 1961.

chapter 10

BONE-CONDUCTION TESTING

Donald D. Dirks, Ph.D.

As Hood (1962) observed, no specific physiologically useful purpose has been attributed to the bone-conduction system in man. According to Barany (1938) and Bekesy (1939) the ossicular chain in man appears to be balanced to diminish bone conduction by the development of relatively substantial masses above the chain's axis of rotation. While this design is not optimal for air-conduction transmission, it does minimize the effect of bone conduction. Thus the potential annoyance from body noises such as breathing, chewing, blood flow and creaking of joints is reduced.

Except for certain theoretical considerations, the principal interest in bone-conduction measurements has been its usefulness as a diagnostic tool in determining the presence or absence of a middle ear or conductive hearing loss. In the range of hearing encompassing frequencies necessary for speech reception, bone-conduction thresholds from airborne sound are not obtained until the sound pressure level is approximately 60 dB above the air-conduction threshold. This relatively poor threshold is a result of the impedance mismatch between the skull and the surrounding air. Bekesy (1932) was the first investigator to demonstrate clearly that the mode of excitation of the cochlear receptors was identical for both air- and bone-conducted signals. He applied a 400-Hz bone-conducted tone at a level of 57 dB above threshold to the forehead simultaneously with an air-conducted tone of the same frequency. By adjusting the intensity and phase of the air-conducted signal he was able to cancel the bone-conducted signal. Bekesy concluded that the vibrations of the basilar membrane are produced by movements of the fluid near the stapes, and thus the two modes of transmission must excite the sensory cells in the same manner. This experiment was a key contribution to bone-conduction theory. It also provided fundamental information for the clinical use of bone-conduction thresholds to estimate the integrity of the sensory-neural system.

Bone-conduction measurements have been the most frequently used auditory clinical procedure next to air-conduction pure tone measurements. In spite of the importance and extensive use of bone-conduction measurements, the clinical assessment has been plagued by numerous inherent problems. These difficulties are related to (1) the participation of the middle ear in the total bone-conduction response, (2) the lack of a reliable and valid method of specifying the vibrational output of a bone-conduction testing system, (3) difficulties and limitations of masking the nontest ear and (4) other equipment and procedural variables which substantially influence the outcome of the test such as the type of vibrator, the placement of the vibrator and the force of vibrator application. Prior to discussing some of the problems associated with the clinical measurement of bone conduction, a brief review of the mechanism of bone conduction is provided.

MECHANISM OF BONE CONDUCTION

Most of the currently accepted concepts regarding bone conduction have evolved from the investigations and theoretical explanations of Herzog and Krainz (1926), Bekesy (1932), Barany (1938), Kirikae (1959), Huizing (1960) and Groen (1962). While each of the mechanisms stressed by the various investigators plays a major or minor role depending on the conditions of the experiment, two modes of stimulation, compression and inertia, are the most commonly accepted concepts among the early theorists.

According to Herzog and Krainz (1926), in compression bone conduction, the vibratory energy reaching the cochlea causes alternate compressions and expansions of the cochlear shell. The incompressible cochlear fluid must yield under the influence of these opposite movements and produce a displacement of the basilar membrane. If the elastic characteristics of the cochlear scalae were equal, then a compression of the cochlea would not produce fluid displacement. This condition is illustrated in Figure 10.1A. A compensatory mechanism, as shown in Figure 10.1B, would be required to produce volume changes of the cochlear spaces. Such a mechanism is possible since the round window is more compliant than the oval window. In addition, the presence of semicircular canals and vestibule in the region of the stapes (Fig. 10.1C) enhance further a displacement of the fluid from scala vestibuli to scala tympani. The contribution of compressional bone conduction is greatest at high frequencies where the skull no longer moves as a rigid body but rather is compressed and expanded segmentally in response to an alternating vibration (Bekesy, 1932).

The second mode is referred to as inertial bone conduction since it arises from the inertia of the ossicular chain. According to Bekesy (1932) and Barany (1938), the inertia of the

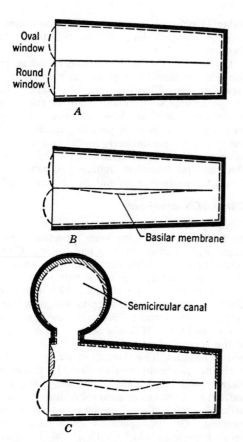

Fig. 10.1. Compression of the inner ear and the displacement of the basilar membrane. The *broken lines* indicate the position of the various membranes during compression. *A* shows a hypothetical case of equal yielding at both windows, symmetrical compression and no movement of the basilar membrane. The round window actually yields more than the oval window (*B*), and the compression is nonsymmetrical, leading to a downward displacement of the basilar membrane. Since the semicircular canals are also compressed (*C*), more fluid is forced into the upper canal, and the basilar membrane is forced downward even more. From G. Bekesy and W. A. Rosenblith. In Stevens, S. S. (Ed.), *Handbook of Experimental Psychology*, p. 1110, Ch. 27, New York: John Wiley & Sons, 1951.

ossicles during forced vibrations of the skull sets up a relative motion between the stapes and the oval window. This motion leads to cochlear stimulation in the same manner as that produced by an air-conducted signal.

The most significant recent contributions to the theory of bone conduction are by Tonndorf (1966, 1972). Tonndorf stresses the futility of accounting for all bone-conduction phenomena by a single mechanism. Among the factors contributing to the total bone-condution response are three major mechanisms: (1) the reception of sound energy radiated into the external canal, (2) the inertial response of the middle ear ossicles and inner ear fluid and (3) the compressional response of the inner ear spaces.

Tonndorf observed that when a vibrating signal is applied to the skull, energy is produced by the walls of the external canal and transmitted to the tympanic membrane. This mode may be increased or decreased by closing or opening the external canal, or by changing the canal resonance or the impedance of the tympanic membrane. An impairment of the middle ear may eliminate or reduce the transmission of the sound energy developed in the external canal.

The inertial response, according to Tonndorf, is primarily a result of the impedance of the middle ear ossicles and the inertia of the inner ear fluids. The response of the ossicular chain can be modified by the air column within the external canal and by the air enclosed in the middle ear.

The compressional response is a product of the distortional vibrations of the cochlear shell and may be independent of the cochlear openings. The response, however, is modified by the oval and round window release as well as by the "third" window release of the cochlear aqueduct. The normal ear integrates these components according to their amplitude and phase relationships. The clinical orientation of this chapter does not permit further formal discussion of theory but the student or clinician interested in the purely theoretical aspects of bone conduction will find ample references throughout the chapter. Tonndorf's (1972) recent contribution is of considerable importance in understanding the basic mechanisms involved in bone conduction.

EFFECT OF MIDDLE EAR ON BONE-CONDUCTION RESPONSE

Clinical bone-conduction thresholds are used primarily to ascertain the presence or absence of an external or middle ear lesion and to determine quantitatively the magnitude of the conductive hearing impairment. The usefulness of the difference between the air- and bone-conduction threshold (air-bone gap) is based on two assumptions: first, that the threshold for bone-conducted signals is a measure of the integrity of the sensory-neural system, and second, that the air-conduction threshold reflects the function of the total hearing system both conductive and sensory-neural.

As a result, the discrepancy between the air- and bone-conduction thresholds is often assumed to indicate the magnitude of the conductive component. Theoretically, in a purely conductive loss, the bone-conduction thresholds should be normal. However, the fact that bone-conduction sensitivity is not independent of the state of the middle ear has been repeatedly demonstrated in both animal and human experiments. It is instructive to review some of the literature on this problem.

Experimental Results in Animals

Various investigators have demonstrated both increased and decreased bone-conduction responses in animals following alterations of the external and middle ear systems. Particularly good examples can be found in experiments where the tympanic membrane was weighted down (loaded) or various middle ear structures were selectively removed or fixated.

Most experimenters report improvements in bone-conduction responses after loading the eardrum with water, mercury, pieces of metal or other materials (Barany, 1938; Rytzner, 1954; Kirikae, 1959; Legouix and Tarab, 1959; Allen and Fernandez, 1960; Abu-Jaudeh, 1964; Brinkman, Marres and Tolk, 1965). Tonndorf (1966) demonstrated that a loaded tympanic membrane caused the resonance frequency of the ossicular system to shift downward. Thus, the bone-conduction responses were elevated at frequencies above the newly established resonant point but improved at frequencies below this resonant point.

Tonndorf has also reported changes in bone-conduction responses (as determined from changes in the amplitude and phase of cochlear microphonics) following certain alterations of the middle ear system, such as, disarticulation of the incudostapedial joint, severing of the stapedial tendon, removal of the stapes superstructure, stapedectomy, occlusion of the oval or round window and fixation of the stapes. Among seven specific components which Tonndorf identified as contributing to the total bone conduction response, four (middle ear inertia, middle ear cavity compliance, round window, and oval window pressure release) were directly related to participation of the middle ear.

Smith (1943) fixated the stapes in cats by means of a thread attached to one stapedial crus. Essentially, no mass was added to the stapes by this method, although the fixation was probably not very firm. The results indicated a reduction in the bone-conduction response, especially in the frequency range around 500 to 1000 Hz. In other experiments of stapes fixation, amplitude losses centering around 500 Hz were reported by Tonndorf and

Tabor (1962) and Tonndorf (1966). The magnitude of the loss depended on the degree of fixation.

Tonndorf further demonstrated elevation in the bone-conduction responses in various species of animals following removal of the middle ear structures or immobilization of the tympanic membrane. In these instances the loss was due to the total or partial elimination of the ossicular inertial component, and the frequency region of maximal loss was related to the ossicular resonant frequency characteristics of the particular animal species examined.

Clinical Observations

Numerous examples of changes in bone-conduction thresholds have been reported in humans with various middle ear lesions. Clinically, patients with otosclerosis often show a loss in bone-conduction thresholds in the frequency region around 2000 Hz. This notch in the bone-conduction audiogram was described originally by Carhart (1950) and now bears his name. In Figure 10.2, *Curve A* is an example of the bone-conduction loss resulting from stapedial fixation. The Carhart notch is present with the maximum loss at 2000 Hz. *Curve B* shows bone conduction levels for the same patient 8 months after successful stapedial mobilization with almost perfect restoration of hearing. The postoperative bone-conduction levels have improved by 5 dB at 500 Hz, 10 dB at 1000 Hz, 15 dB at 2000 Hz and 5 dB at 4000 Hz. These improvements in the postoperative bone-conduction levels correspond closely to the average shifts in the bone-conduction responses due to stapedial fixation as described by Carhart. Obviously the improvement is due to mechanical changes in the ossicular system and not to cochlear modification.

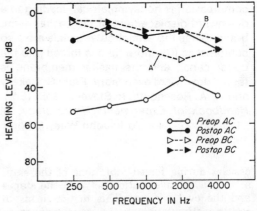

Fig. 10.2. Pre- and postoperative air (*AC*) and bone conduction (*BC*) audiogram for a patient with otosclerosis.

Fournier (1954), Hirsh (1952) and Carhart (1962) have commented upon the incompatibility of the bone-conduction loss due to stapedial fixation with the theory of inertial bone conduction. They suggest that since the head moves as a whole with no compression waves at low frequencies, inertia is the dominant mode of bone conduction, while compression bone conduction is the dominant feature at high frequencies. It might be anticipated from classical theory that stapedial fixation should impair inertial bone conduction with a loss primarily in the low and not the high frequencies. Tonndorf (1966) explains and demonstrates that it is essentially the missing ossicular inertial component which determines the frequency value of the maximal loss by bone conduction due to stapedial fixation. He suggests that the middle ear contribution is not confined to low frequencies as classical theory suggests. Rather the ossicular vibrating system has a resonant frequency which varies from species to species. When responding to vibratory stimulation, the resonant frequency of the ossicular chain in man is found at 1500 to 2000 Hz. If the participation of the ossicular chain is eliminated or reduced due to stapedial fixation, the maximal bone-conduction loss should also correspond closely to this frequency area.

Other types of middle ear impairment, which influence the bone-conduction thresholds, have been reported among clinical cases. Bekesy (1939) and Tonndorf (1966) have each described a case in which bone-conduction thresholds were altered following radical mastoidectomy. Reduction in hearing by bone conduction was noted especially in the frequencies around 2000 Hz, the frequency area of ossicular resonance in man. Goodhill (1965) reported a Carhart-type notch extending into the higher frequencies for a patient with surgically confirmed mallear fixation. Subsequently, a patient with surgically confirmed mallear fixation was reported by Dirks and Malmquist (1969). Figure 10.3 shows the results of air conduction, pre- and postoperatively, and preoperative bone-conduction thresholds at the mastoid process and frontal bone.

The audiometric results in Figure 10.3 must be reviewed rather carefully since there is also a sensory-neural component. The question is, how large is the sensory-neural component? The bone-conduction thresholds obtained at the frontal bone suggest considerably less sensory-neural involvement than do the measurements at the mastoid process. The largest difference between the measurements is 20 dB at 2000 Hz. A large difference is also present at 4000 Hz. The difference is gradually reduced as the test frequency is lowered and becomes nonexistent at 250 Hz. The discrimination score for

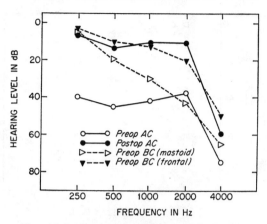

Fig. 10.3. Pre- and postoperative air conduction (AC) and preoperative bone conduction (BC) audiogram for a patient with mallear fixation.

phonetically balanced (PB-50) words was 80%. It is important to note that the postoperative air-conduction curve interweaves with the pre-operative frontal, but not the mastoid measurements. While there was an overclosure of the air-bone gap relative to bone-conduction measurements at the mastoid process, it would appear that bone-conduction thresholds at the frontal bone were the better predictor of surgical gain in this case. These results are instructive for two reasons: first, they demonstrate clearly the substantial effect that a middle ear lesion may have on bone conduction responses and, second, they illustrate that bone-conduction thresholds may be affected differently depending on the location of vibrator placement.

Hulka (1941) described a gain in the low and a loss in the high frequency areas for patients with otitis media. Palva and Ojala (1955), however, did not find a shift in bone-conduction thresholds in similarly diagnosed cases. Naunton and Fernandez (1961) reported results of bone-conduction tests at the forehead for three individuals during and following attacks of bilateral secretory otitis. When fluid was present in the middle ears of these patients, there was an improvement in bone-conduction responses at the low frequencies and a slight loss in the high frequencies. Huizing (1960) has also reported bone-conduction threshold changes in patients with otitis media, tubotympanitis and chronic inflammatory processes. One patient with secretory otitis media was followed in our laboratory over a period of 7 months. Figure 10.4 illustrates the pre- and posttreatment air- and bone-conduction audiograms. Notice the depression in the bone-conduction thresholds especially around 2000 Hz when the patient was initially tested. Following medical

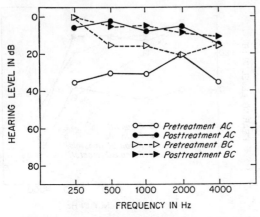

Fig. 10.4. Pre- and post-treatment air (AC) and bone conduction (BC) audiogram for a patient with secretory otitis media.

treatment there was no air-bone gap and the thresholds returned to normal levels.

The results of numerous investigations, primarily involving individuals with normal auditory systems, have demonstrated that bone-conduction responses can be altered experimentally by (1) air pressure changes in the external auditory canal (Fowler, 1920; Loch, 1942; Barany, 1938; Kirikae, 1959; Allen and Fernandez, 1960; Huizing, 1960); (2) loading of the tympanic membrane (Barany, 1938; Kirikae, 1959; Allen and Fernandez, 1960); and (3) the occlusion of the external auditory canal (Pohlman and Kranz, 1926; Bekesy, 1932; Kelley and Reger, 1937; Watson and Gales, 1943; Sullivan, Gotlieb and Hodges, 1947; Onchi, 1954; Allen and Fernandez, 1960; Huizing, 1960; Elpern and Naunton, 1963; Goldstein and Hayes, 1965; Hodgson and Tillman, 1966; Dirks and Swindeman, 1967). Details of the specific gains or elevation of the bone-conduction thresholds during these conditions require a more extensive search into the literature by the interested reader. In these experimental conditions it was the modification of either the external or middle ear system which produced changes in the bone-conduction response.

Substantial data have accumulated demonstrating that bone-conduction thresholds do not represent a pure estimate of "cochlear reserve." Surely this is a serious shortcoming when bone-conduction audiometry is employed as a quantitative measure of sensory-neural sensitivity. Such a limitation is not reported here to discourage the clinician from attempting to estimate the magnitude of the conductive hearing loss with bone-conduction tests. Rather, it is mentioned to impress on the clinician the practical limitations of bone-conduction thresholds so that a more realistic use of the measurement may evolve.

CALIBRATION OF BONE-CONDUCTION TESTING SYSTEMS

A major problem in the measurement of bone-conduction thresholds has been the absence of a reliable and objective method for specifying the vibrational output of bone-conduction testing systems. Stable acoustic devices, such as the 2 cubic centimeters (2-cc) and 6-cc couplers, have been developed for calibration of air-conduction receivers, but no comparable instruments are available for bone vibrator calibration. Recently, the possibility for objective calibration of bone-conduction vibrators has been enhanced by the development of artificial mastoids, which are essentially immune to aging and can be manufactured within acceptable tolerance limits.

Formerly calibration of bone-conduction testing systems was performed by testing a group of normal listeners or individuals with sensory-neural hearing loss, using a technique described by Carhart (1950) and Roach and Carhart (1956). The rationale for the method is based principally on the theory that air- and bone-conduction thresholds are essentially equivalent among persons with normal hearing or among patients with "pure" sensory-neural losses. While this method of calibrating bone-conduction systems has been extremely valuable, variability of procedures and among listeners requires that either a large group of individuals be tested or that the measured thresholds be corrected by the amount that the air-conduction sensitivity of the group varies from audiometric zero.

Some of the difficulties encountered in using small groups of listeners for calibration purposes have been described by Wilber and Goodhill (1967). In some instances, calibration procedures have been performed with only a small number of normal listeners or by one individual with a so-called golden ear. As a result, values utilized for normal threshold by bone conduction have varied substantially among manufacturers, clinics, and laboratories.

In early attempts to develop an artificial mastoid, Hawley (1939), Carlisle and Mundel (1944), and Carlisle and Pearson (1951) used a viscoelastic pad to simulate the mechanical impedance of the skin and headbones. Since relatively little information concerning the impedance of the human mastoid was available at that time, these artificial mastoids represented only a first-order approximation to the human mastoid. The viscoelastic pads also varied with temperature and humidity and were susceptible to aging.

In 1955, Corliss and Koidan of the National Bureau of Standards developed a method for determining the resistive and reactive components of the impedance of the human head and mastoid. Similar data were also published by Dadson (1954), and Dadson, Robinson and Greig (1954) at the National Physical Laboratory in England. These studies were a first step leading to the design and development of stable artificial headbones or mastoids for the reliable and valid physical calibration of bone vibrators.

During the 1960s two reliable artificial mastoids, the Beltone 5A (Weiss, 1960) and the Bruel and Kjaer 4930 (Stisen and Dahm, 1969), became commercially available. However, there was no international agreement for standardization of either the exact physical characteristics for aritificial mastoids or for the normal threshold of hearing by bone conduction. In the United States, the Standards Committee of the Hearing Aid Industry Conference (HAIC) compiled data for the purpose of developing interim norms for use until international deliberations on standards were completed. As a result, the HAIC Interim Bone Conduction Norm for Audiometry was established in 1965 and reported by Lybarger (1966). Further calibration data from measurements at the mastoid process and/or the frontal bone also became available in publications by Sanders and Olsen (1964), Weston et al. (1967), Wilber and Goodhill (1967), Studebaker (1967), Dirks et al. (1968) and Olsen (1969).

Recently, both the International Electrotechnical Commission (IEC Recommendation 373, 1971) and the American National Standards Institute (ANSI S3.13-1972) have issued documents recommending identical mechanical impedance characteristics for an artificial mastoid. These artificial mastoid specifications were intended for use with bone vibrators that have a circular contact tip area of 1.75 sq cm and are coupled to the skull with a static force of 5.4 Newtons (N) or approximately 550 g weight (1 N = 102 g).

Until recently, bone vibrators available for general clinical use did not conform in size to the tip contact area suggested by the IEC 373 recommendation or ANSI S3.13-1972. Also, headbands used to couple the vibrator to the skull resulted in average static force levels of ~3.0–3.4 N (Studebaker, 1967) on an adult head rather than the recommended 5.4 N. Fortunately, new bone vibrators are now available and incorporate circular contact tip areas of 1.75 sq cm. Furthermore, headband assemblies have also been developed for the purpose of coupling these bone vibrators to an adult head with an average application force of 5.4 N. The physical characteristics of two of the new vibrators (Radioear B-71 and B-72) have been reported (Dirks and Kamm, 1975) together with behavioral thresholds. Figure 10.5 shows a comparison of the mean frequency responses from three bone vibrators, the Radioear B-70A

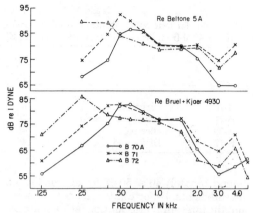

Fig. 10.5. Mean frequency response of three bone vibrators in dB *re* 1 dyne referenced to either the Beltone 5A (*upper*) or the Bruel & Kjaer 4930 (*lower*) artificial mastoid.

(used previously in many clinics) and the B-71 and B-72 vibrators referenced to the Beltone 5A and Bruel and Kjaer 4930 artificial mastoids.

Close comparison of the upper and lower portions of Figure 10.5 demonstrates that, with input voltage to the bone vibrators held constant, the Bruel and Kjaer artificial mastoid yields consistently lower force levels than the Beltone 5A. These differences in artificial mastoid output, which vary with frequency and vibrator type, are due, at least in part, to differences in the mechanical impedance of the artificial mastoids and to interactions between the bone vibrators and the artificial mastoids.

Behavioral thresholds on normal listeners were also described in the Dirks and Kamm (1975) report for the three vibrators. These results together with those (Olsen, 1975) on six normal listeners with an Oticon A-20 bone vibrator are summarized in Table 10.1. There is reasonable agreement between the results from the two laboratories using the A-20 and B-71 vibrators. The contact area of the vibrators is the same and the frequency responses are similar. These data should provide diagnosticians with a first approximation of the threshold for normal hearing by bone conduction with vibrators meeting standard requirements in terms of contact tip area. However, further collection and reporting of thresholds with the new vibrators referenced to one of the available artificial mastoids is necessary in order to establish a standard for normal hearing by bone conduction.

MASKING

When earphones encased in supra-aural cushions are used, the mass of the head provides an average interaural attenuation factor

TABLE 10.1. *Mean Bone-Conduction Thresholds*

Thresholds for four bone vibrators (Radioear B-70A, B-71, B-72 and Oticon A-20) referenced to the Bruel and Kjaer 4930 from two laboratories (Dirks and Kamm, 1975; Olsen, 1975).

		Frequency in Hz				
		250	500	1000	2000	4000
				dB		
B-70A	Dirks and Kamm	47.7	38.5	24.0	11.5	14.5
B-71	Dirks and Kamm	47.5	38.9	23.5	10.1	13.4
A-20	Olsen	46.9	37.8	28.2	21.9	18.9
B-72	Dirks and Kamm	47.0	38.3	22.5	8.1	6.8

of approximately 40 or 50 dB for air-conduction measurements. Unfortunately for bone conduction, the interaural attenuation factor is almost negligible regardless of the position of the vibrator on the skull. Hence, it is necessary to exclude the nontest ear by an adequate air-conducted masker when obtaining bone-conduction thresholds. There are instances such as bilaterally symmetrical sensory-neural losses when masking may not be necessary (Naunton, 1963), but these cases should be the exception and not the general rule. Studebaker (1964) suggests that a more efficient rule is to apply a masker to the nontest ear whenever an air-bone gap appears.

The specific procedure for masking when testing for bone-conduction thresholds will be described in a complete manner in Chapter 11. However, a few brief statements concerning masking are appropriate. Although masking may theoretically be accomplished by almost any sound, it is generally accepted that narrow bands of noise centered around the test frequency provide the greatest shift in the nontest ear threshold with a minimum of sound energy (Fletcher, 1940; Zwislocki, 1951; Denes and Naunton, 1952; Hood, 1957; Liden, Nilsson and Anderson, 1959; Hood, 1962; Konig, 1963; Studebaker, 1964; Sanders and Rintelmann, 1964).

The results of Zwislocki (1953), Littler, Knight and Strange (1952) and Studebaker (1962) have demonstrated that the interaural attenuation factor can be increased as the area of the head exposed to the transducer is decreased. This may be accomplished by introducing the masking signal via an insert receiver rather than by the standard earphone encased in either a supra-aural or circumaural cushion. There are still some calibration problems associated with the use of insert receivers and their coupling to the ear. Nevertheless, the introduction of narrow bands of noise delivered to the nontest ear via an insert receiver is highly desirable when measuring bone conduction thresholds.

The least complex but most accurate method for masking in bone conduction testing has been detailed by Hood (1962). Studebaker (1964) also describes a method of masking similar to

the procedure suggested by Hood (see Chapter 11).

Regardless of the method, there are numerous instances in which sufficient masking is unavailable and therefore the responses obtained cannot be assumed to be a measure of the desired test ear. The limitations of masking in clinical audiometry have received a rigorous appraisal by Konig (1963). These difficulties and limitations should encourage the clinician to perform additional auditory tests to determine the presence or absence of a conductive component when problems of insufficient masking or overmasking arise.

EQUIPMENT AND PROCEDURAL VARIABLES

Bone-Conduction Vibrators

The requirements for the physical characteristics of an idealized bone receiver were generally well described by Lierle and Reger (1946). They suggested a "mechanical design that will stand up under continued and rough usage without change in calibration, extension of the frequency range to values near or coincident with the normal upper limits of audibility, freedom from overtones, freedom from the effects of differences in pressure when the vibrator is held against the head and a wide a.c.-b.c. differential" (p. 221).

In the early days of clinical bone conduction audiometry, bone vibrators were often held by hand against the mastoid process. It was important, therefore, that the housing of the vibrator be isolated from the vibration system itself. Such units were large and cumbersome and are not in general clinical use today. Grossman and Malloy (1943) compared the physical characteristics of vibrators commonly designed as hearing aids with some of the older bone-conduction receivers which were composed of a rod connected to an electromagnetically excited driving system. They concluded that the older bone vibrators were probably more advantageous from a physical point of view than the hearing aid-type vibrators. In particular, the investigators reported more variability in the response of the hearing aid-type receiver than in the older grenade-type vibrators. Furthermore, the harmonic distortion of the hearing aid-type vibrator was found to be large, especially at low frequencies.

Sanders and Olsen (1964) and Wilber and Goodhill (1967) have also reported undesirable harmonic distortion at low frequencies for a hearing aid-type vibrator. Their results were obtained from measurements of the vibrational output of a vibrator with the receiver placed on the mass of an artificial mastoid. In addition, Sanders and Olsen's data indicate that the intensity output of the second and third harmonics grows disproportionately to the input.

Another practical problem with the hearing aid-type vibrator is that the entire case vibrates. As a result, there is always the unfortunate possibility that some part of the vibrator mechanism, when located on the mastoid process, might touch the pinna and transmit sound into the external auditory canal. In addition, any holding device must grip the hearing aid-type vibrator at some location on its vibrating case, thereby increasing the possibility of a change in the frequency response characteristics of the vibrator.

One of the greatest difficulties in the construction of a bone-conduction vibrator is in preventing the radiation of aerial sound waves. Jones and Knudsen (1936) reduced the aerial sound by enclosing a bone vibrator in a metal case surrounded with felt and having only the vibrating rod exposed to the outside. A metal ring holding a pair of rubber rings was fastened to the outside of the case. When the vibrating rod was applied to the skull the rubber rings also made contact with the head and formed an airtight juncture. A similar arrangement was used in some of the older piston-rod-type vibrators in order to minimize the aerial radiation of sound waves. Disturbing acoustic radiations can also be demonstrated for the hearing aid-type vibrator especially at the higher test frequencies. Systematic investigation is needed to define precisely the extent of the problem.

In summary, the commonly used hearing aid-type vibrator is, no doubt, more convenient to use than the older grenade-shaped bone receiver containing a vibrating rod. However, the convenience of adjusting the modern vibrator to the skull may not outweigh the loss of certain desirable physical characteristics found in some of the older bone vibrators.

Vibrator Placement

Traditionally, clinical bone-conduction measurements have been performed with the vibrator or the tuning fork located on the mastoid process. The preference of the site on the skull was perhaps based on the erroneous assumption that the ear under examination could be tested more or less independently of the nontest ear. Unfortunately, there is generally little, if any, interaural isolation by bone conduction and, hence, both cochleas may participate in the response.

The question of the placement of the bone vibrator for the clinical determination of the bone-conduction threshold has not as yet been completely resolved. Although the vertex (Barany, 1938; Studebaker, 1962) of the skull and the teeth have been considered, the mastoid process and frontal bone have received the most attention. Three major arguments have been advanced in favor of placement of the vibrator on the frontal bone rather than on the mastoid process.

First, it has been suggested that there is an increase in the test-retest reliability of bone-conduction measurements at the frontal bone. These observations were based originally on the report by Bekesy (1932) that the displacement of the vibrator away from the middle of the forehead gives rise only to relatively small fluctuations in bone conduction thresholds, whereas similar variations in placement at the mastoid process result in changes of 10 dB or more. Results of five repeated measurements by Hart and Naunton (1961) indicated that there was less variation when tests were performed on the frontal bone as compared to the mastoid process. It may be noteworthy that these observations were made with vibrators containing vibrating tips which covered only a small contact area. The comparative results of more recent investigations (Studebaker, 1962; Dirks, 1964) using hearing aid-type vibrators with large contact areas have not demonstrated test-retest differences between mastoid and frontal bone placement that were of great practical advantage.

The second argument favoring frontal bone placement is concerned with intersubject variability. At the frontal bone, the tissues seem to be more homogeneous over the general test area than at the mastoid process, and, thus, the difference in bone-conduction thresholds among the individuals should be reduced. The results of Studebaker (1962) and Dirks (1964) seem to verify this contention. The differences in intersubject variability between the two sites, however, were small.

A third advantage of forehead placement was evolved primarily from the classical investigation by Barany in 1938. He suggested that bone-conduction tests at the frontal bone reduce the participation of the middle ear more effectively than those performed at the mastoid process. Experimental results by Link and Zwislocki (1951) on patients with otitis media demonstrated less hearing loss from measurements at the frontal bone than at the mastoid process. Studebaker (1962) and Dirks and Malmquist (1969) made similar comparisons on individuals with middle ear impairments and observed less hearing loss (*re* normal hearing at each placement site) when measurements were obtained at the forehead than at the mastoid process. However, the average threshold difference at the test frequencies was only about 5 dB. In the Dirks and Malmquist data, however, average threshold differences of over 10 dB favoring the frontal bone were observed in a selected group of cases with middle ear impairments.

The principal disadvantage to testing bone-conduction thresholds at the frontal bone is that more intensity is required to reach threshold than for comparable mastoid measurements. The decibel differences between thresholds at the frontal bone and those at the mastoid process from various investigations are summarized in Table 10.2. These comparisons are of current clinical interest since commercially available hearing aid-type bone vibrators were employed in each experiment.

While the difference in thresholds at the two locations averages approximately 10 dB, the results from six investigations cited in Table 10.2 indicate that the difference appears to be frequency-dependent. The largest average differences (14.6 and 14.3 dB) are found in the lower test frequencies at 250 and 500 Hz and the smallest difference of 5.5 dB is observed at 4000 Hz. Since more energy is required to reach threshold at the frontal bone than at the mastoid process, the range of measurable hearing is reduced when testing at the frontal bone because of the power handling limitations of commercially available vibrators. The requirement of greater vibrational output to reach

threshold at the frontal bone may become a practical problem when testing patients whose bone-conduction thresholds are more than moderately reduced from normal.

Vibrator Application Force and Surface Area

Another source of variability in bone-conduction measurement is the force of application of the bone vibrator on the skull. In general, as vibrator application force is increased, less energy is required to reach threshold by bone conduction. There are, however, certain limitations and modifications to this general principle. Bekesy (1939) and Konig (1957) investigated the variation of bone-conduction thresholds over a wide range of static forces. Their findings suggest that the largest changes in bone-conduction thresholds are observed at forces below 750 g. While some changes could still be observed between 1000 and 1500 g in Konig's results, they were small. Konig suggested that it would be desirable to employ a coupling force of approximately 1000 g in clinical audiometry so that variability would be minimal.

Harris, Haines and Myers (1953) investigated the effects of increased application force from 100 to 400 g at the test frequencies of 250, 1000 and 8000 Hz. The greatest change in threshold was found at 250 Hz while little change was observed at 1000 and 8000 Hz. They suggested that bone-conduction receiver application force be standardized somewhere between 200 and 400 g. In the ranges of application force where Harris et al. and Konig's measurements overlap, the results from the two experiments do not agree. Konig's results indicate that thresholds continue to change as force is increased above 400 g whereas Harris

TABLE 10.2. *Differences between Mean Thresholds Measured at Forehead and Mastoid for Six Investigations in which Hearing Aid-type Vibrators Were Used*

Investigation	Vibrator	N	Static Force	Masking	Frequency in Hz				
					250	500	1000	2000	4000
			g				*dB*		
1. Studebaker (1962)	Sonotone B-9	20	300–400	Narrow bands	15.2	16.0	10.0	12.9	9.7
2. Dirks (1964)*	Sonotone B-9	24	300–400	Narrow and widebands	10.0	9.4	6.1	8.7	5.2
3. Whittle (1965)	BV 11	22	350	Narrow bands	14.5	17.1	11.9	5.1	−3.0
4. Weston et al. (1967)	Radioear B-70-A	10	400–600	Narrow bands	16.7	15.2	3.9	7.0	6.9
5. Studebaker (1967)	Radioear B-70-A	132	300–500	White noise	13.4	16.6	12.0	10.0	8.6
6. Dirks et al. (1968)†	Radioear B-70-A	83	Varied by study	Narrow bands	14.9	13.4	10.6	13.5	7.7
Mean [1–6]					14.6	14.3	9.2	9.5	5.5
SD [1–6]					2.2	2.8	3.3	3.2	4.5

* Average of two studies.
† Average of eight studies.

et al. results suggest that thresholds do not change substantially once 400 g is reached.

Goodhill and Holcomb (1955) studied the changes in cochlear microphonics produced by bone-conducted signals with the vibrator placed on the skull of cats. Erratic responses were reported when the force was less than 200 g, but little change was observed as force was modified between 300 and 600 g.

Whittle (1965) recorded bone-conduction thresholds on normal listeners at forces of 250, 350 and 750 g. For two bone vibrators, thresholds were compared at forces of 350 and 750 g. While there was a tendency for the average thresholds to be elevated with the greater force, intersubject variations were as large at a force of 750 g as the lowest application forces used.

The surface area under the vibrator may constitute another source of variability, but its influence on bone-conduction thresholds has not been studied in depth. Watson (1938) reported that thresholds varied only negligibly at low frequencies but improved with larger surface areas for frequencies between 3000 and 7000 Hz. Goodhill and Holcomb (1955) on the other hand suggest that bone-conduction thresholds were more consistent with a vibrator surface area of 1 sq cm than for a comparative vibrator with a surface area of 3.2 sq cm. Nilo (1968) observed that vibrator surface area had no influence on bone-conduction thresholds at frequencies up to 2000 Hz. At 2000 Hz, the bone-conduction thresholds improved as the surface increased from 1.125 to 4.5 sq cm. The investigator noted that in a subsequent study threshold levels were improved at 4000 Hz as the vibrator surface area increased.

In summary, investigators have generally demonstrated that increasing application force produces a decrease in bone-conduction thresholds. Most experimenters have observed a ceiling or limit to the magnitude of force evoking threshold variations. The ceiling has been placed anywhere from 400 to 1000 g.

Other Clinical Procedures

Occlusion of the External Auditory Canal. There are several other auxiliary diagnostic procedures involving bone conduction which have received both substantial audiologic and otologic consideration. The first of these is the now familiar method of modifying bone-conduction thresholds by occluding the external auditory meatus. It has been well established that the occlusion of the external auditory canal produces a low frequency enhancement for bone-conducted signals. Numerous references on the effects of occlusion have been listed previously in this chapter.

Clinical interest in the occlusion effect stems from the observation that, in general, the effect is absent in almost all impairments located anywhere along the conductive pathway. Bing, in 1891, was probably the first to use the occlusion of the auditory canal as a method of clinical examination. Briefly, the audiologist can perform the test by obtaining bone-conduction thresholds for low frequency signals with the test ear open and then occluded by an earphone and the supra-aural cushion (MX-41/AR) customarily used in clinical testing. If there is no difference in these thresholds, this suggests the presence of a lesion in the conductive mechanism. If the threshold improves under occluded conditions, it is an indication that the hearing loss is due to a sensory-neural lesion. Especially for the patient with a small air-bone gap, the absence of an occlusion effect will help to assure the clinician that the measured difference between air and bone conduction is not due to variability in the test measurement or patient unreliability, but is, in fact, indicating the presence of a conductive component.

The question often arises of whether bone-conduction tests should be performed routinely with the test ear occluded or open. According to Huizing (1960), some English authors formerly recommended that the external auditory canal be closed for bone-conduction audiometry. This advice was given in order to eliminate the masking effect due to ambient room noise and thereby the supposed real or "absolute" threshold could be measured. Subsequent observations have shown that the presence of the occlusion effect is not based on the elimination of masking. According to Tonndorf (1966), the occlusion effect is more likely due to the elimination of the high pass effect of an open ear canal when the external auditory meatus is occluded.

The clinical utility of performing bone-conduction thresholds under occluded conditions also rests upon the reliability and consistency of the occlusion effect. Elpern and Naunton (1963) reported that the reliability of the occlusion effect was poor from subject to subject and from test to retest. Earlier results (Carhart and Hayes, 1949; Roach, 1951; Studebaker, 1962; Dirks, 1964) demonstrated that unoccluded bone-conduction thresholds may be highly consistent from test to retest when sufficient controls are employed. Thus it might be conjectured that the prime source of variability in the Elpern and Naunton data was a result of the introduction of the occluding device. However, Malmquist and Jerger (1966) and Dirks and Swindeman (1967) found that bone-conduction thresholds obtained during occluded conditions were as reliable as those obtained with the ear open. Hodgson and Tillman (1966) observed a positive correlation between the application force of an occluding earphone and the magnitude of the occlusion effect. They suggested that the common failure to control the force of the earphones against the head adds an important source of variability to occluded bone-conduction measurements.

The basis for deciding whether the clinician should perform bone-conduction tests with the ear open or occluded will probably depend upon the final and complete explanation of the effect. Practically, it will also depend upon whether or not the clinician performs bone-conduction tests at the forehead or at the mastoid process. If the vibrator is placed on the mastoid process, it is difficult to occlude the test ear properly without the earphone and cushion touching the bone vibrator.

It is also important to remember that the masking signal is delivered to the nontest ear through an earphone and cushion which also produces an occlusion effect. Care must be taken to ensure that the intensity level of the masker is sufficient to eliminate the resultant improved bone conduction threshold in the nontest ear.

Weber Test. Clinical interest in the Weber test stems from the general observation that various impairments of the middle ear produce lateralization of a bone-conducted signal to the involved ear or to the ear with the greater conductive component. The patient is asked to determine the location of the sound following stimulation by a bone-conducted tone with the vibrator located at the forehead.

Various explanations have been offered for the lateralization of the sound during the Weber test. These explanations fall into two general categories. It has been suggested, first, that the tone lateralizes to the conductively impaired ear because the effective amplitude in the cochlea is greater on that side, and second, that the lateralization is based on a phase lead at the ear with a conductive loss. Several investigators (Christian and Roser, 1957; Legouix and Tarab, 1959; Allen and Fernandez, 1960) report findings favoring the phase lead explanation. Others (Spoor, Schmidt and Van Dishoeck, 1957; Groen and Hoogland, 1958; Naunton and Elpern, 1964) present evidence which suggests that interaural intensity differences play a relatively major role in the lateralization of the signal in the Weber test.

Groen (1962) presented an extensive review of the Weber Test. He reported that the Weber test is a reliable procedure in frequency areas below 1000 Hz and above 3000 Hz. Somewhat unreliable results appeared in the area around 2000 Hz. The investigator suggested that around 2000 Hz, lateralization frequently occurred toward the side of the uninvolved ear. Tonndorf (1966) reports that the lateralization toward the involved ear depends upon the particular middle ear problem; in some instances, interaural intensity differences play the major role, and, in others, interaural phase differences account for the lateralization.

CONCLUSION

Important features of this chapter may be summarized by the following statements.

1. Regardless of whether bone-conduction measurements are made at the forehead or mastoid process, the result will be influenced by the status of the external and middle ear. As a result, the clinician must use considerable restraint in the acceptance of any bone-conduction threshold as a pure measure of "cochlear reserve." There are sufficient examples of changes in bone-conduction thresholds due to middle ear impairments, and this limitation should be well understood.

2. In bone-conduction audiometry, the sound applied to one mastoid will pass to the other mastoid process with little or no attenuation. As a result, a masking signal must be carefully employed to exclude participation of the nontest ear. Although there may be instances in which the clinician may dispense with masking, the more conservative general rule is to use masking routinely for bone-conduction measurements. There is no shortcut to masking procedures, and it is incumbent upon the clinician to understand the physical characteristics of the noise, the procedure and the limitations of the masker. This requires study and additional clinical time; however, for the sake of accuracy the effort is well spent.

3. Both the International Electrotechnical Commission (IEC Recommendations 373, 1971) and the American National Standards Institute (ANSI S. 3. 13-1972) have issued documents recommending mechanical impedance characteristics for an artificial mastoid. These specifications are intended for use with bone-conduction vibrators that have a circular contact tip area of 1.75 sq cm and are coupled to the skull with a static force of 5.4 Newtons. Several new bone vibrators and headband arrangements that conform to these requirements are now available. The establishment of bone-conduction threshold norms with the new vibrators is an acute clinical need.

4. Various locations of the vibrator on the skull have certain assets and limitations. If one were compelled to choose only one site on the skull for vibrator placement, it should probably be the frontal bone. The forehead offers advantages over mastoid or vertex placement, such as slightly greater reliability, comparatively less influence from the status of the external and middle ear and ease of vibrator placement. The reduction in the dynamic range of measurement when testing from the fore-

head is unfortunate, but the problem may be reduced in importance if a bone vibrator were developed which would allow for greater undistorted vibrational output than is afforded in presently available hearing aid-type vibrators.

5. For many years, the results of bone-conduction measurements have provided useful clinical information both for determining presence or absence of a conductive lesion and for making decisions concerning the therapeutic or surgical management of the patient. Within the past two decades, diagnosis of conductive lesions has been enhanced by the clinical measurements of static acoustic impedance at the eardrum, tympanometry and the determination of the presence of a reflex from middle ear muscle contraction. From the results of these impedance measurements, both an objective diagnosis of the presence of a middle ear lesion and differential diagnostic information can be obtained. Because of the great potentials offered by the impedance procedures, the historic role of bone conduction as the primary tool for identifying middle ear lesions will most likely change.

Once the presence of a conductive lesion has been established, the determination of sensory-neural level is of importance as a guideline in making decisions concerning surgery and the potential hearing improvement which might be anticipated. In particular patients, when confirmation of a middle ear lesion is needed, the clinician may use modified Rainville procedures (Rainville, 1959) such as SAL (Jerger and Tillman, 1960), the occlusion test, or Weber test. The combined effects of several of the aforementioned measurements may provide a more thorough evaluation of the hearing loss, especially when routine examination leaves the precise diagnosis in doubt.

REFERENCES

Abu-Jaudeh, C. N., The effect of simultaneous loading of the tympanic membrane of the external auditory canal on bone conduction sensitivity of the normal ear. Ann. Otol., 73, 934–947, 1964.

Allen, G. W., and Fernandez, C., The mechanism of bone conduction. Ann. Otol., 69, 5–29, 1960.

American National Standards Institute, Specification for an Artificial Head-bone. ANSI S3.13-1972, American National Standards Institute, Inc. New York, 1972.

Barany, E., A contribution to the physiology of bone conduction. Acta Otolaryngol., Suppl. 26, 1–223, 1938.

Bekesy, G. V., Zur theorie des hörens bei der schallaufnahme durch knochenleitung. Ann. Physik., 13, 111–136, 1932.

Bekesy, G. V., Über die piezoelectrische messung der absoluten hörschwelle bei knochenleitung. Akust. Z., 4, 113–125, 1939.

Bing, A., Ein neuer stimmgabelversuch. Beitrag zur differential-diagnostik der Kranheiten des mechanischen schallleitungs- und nervösen hörapparates. Weiner med. Blätter, No. 41, 1891. Cited by Tonndorf, J. Bone conduction. Acta Otolaryngol., Suppl. 213, 1966.

Brinkman, W. F. B., Marres, E. H. A. M., and Tolk, J., The mechanism of bone conduction. Acta Otolaryngol., 59, 109–115, 1965.

Carhart, R., Clinical application of bone conduction. Arch. Otolaryngol., 51, 789–807, 1950.

Carhart, R., Effect of stapes fixation on bone conduction. In Schuknecht, H. F. (Ed.), International Symposium on Otosclerosis. Ch. 13. Boston: Little, Brown & Co., 1962.

Carhart, R. C., and Hayes, C., The clinical reliability of bone conduction audiometry. Laryngoscope, 59, 1084–1101, 1949.

Carlisle, R. W., and Mundel, A. B., Practical hearing aid measurements. J. Acoust. Soc. Am., 16, 45–51, 1944.

Carlisle, R. W., and Pearson, H. A., A strain-gauge type artificial mastoid. J. Acoust. Soc. Am., 23, 300–302, 1951.

Christian, W., and Roser, D., Ein beitrag zum richtungshoren. Z. Laryngol. Rhinol. Otol., 36, 432–445, 1957.

Corliss, E. L. R., and Koidan, W., Mechanical impedance of the forehead and mastoid. J. Acoust. Soc. Am., 27, 1164–1172, 1955.

Dadson, R. S., The normal threshold of hearing and other aspect of standardisation in audiometry. Acustica, 4, 151–154, 1954.

Dadson, R. S., Robinson, D. W., and Greig, R. G. P., The mechanical impedance of the human mastoid process. Br. J. Appl. Physiol., 5, 435–442, 1954.

Denes, P., and Naunton, R. F., Masking in pure-tone audiometry. Proc. R. Soc. Med., 45, 790–794, 1952.

Dirks, D., Factors related to bone conduction reliability. Arch. Otolaryngol., 79, 551–558, 1964.

Dirks, D., and Kamm, C., Bone-vibrator measurements; physical characteristics and behavioral thresholds. J. Speech Hear. Res., 18, 242–260, 1975.

Dirks, D., and Malmquist, C., Comparison of frontal and mastoid bone conduction thresholds in various conduction lesions. J. Speech Hear. Res., 12, 725–746, 1969.

Dirks, D., Malmquist, C., and Bower, D., Toward the specification of normal bone conduction threshold. J. Acoust. Soc. Am., 43, 1237–1242, 1968.

Dirks, D., and Swindeman, J., The variability of occluded and unoccluded bone conduction thresholds. J. Speech Hear. Res., 10, 232–249, 1967.

Elpern, B. S., and Naunton, R. F., The stability of the occlusion effect. Arch. Otolaryngol., 77, 376–384, 1963.

Fletcher, H., Auditory patterns. Rev. Mod. Phys., 12, 47–65, 1940.

Fournier, J. E., The "false-Bing" phenomenon; Some remarks on the theory of bone conduction. Laryngoscope, 64, 29–34, 1954.

Fowler, E. P., Sr., Drum tension and middle ear pressure, their determination, significance and effect upon the hearing. Ann. Otol., 29, 688–694, 1920.

Goldstein, R., and Hayes, C., The occlusion effect in bone conduction hearing. *J. Speech Hear. Res.*, 8, 137–148, 1965.

Goodhill, V., *Trans. Am. Acad. Ophthalmol. Otolaryngol.*, 69, 797, 1965. (Abstract).

Goodhill, V., and Holcomb, A. L., Cochlear potentials in the evaluation of bone conduction. *Ann. Otol.*, 64, 1213–1234, 1955.

Groen, J. J., The Value of the Weber Test. In Schuknecht, H. F. (Ed.), *International Symposium on Otosclerosis*. Ch. 14. Boston: Little Brown & Co., 1962.

Groen, J. J., and Hoogland, G. A., Bone conduction and otosclerosis of the round window. *Acta Otolaryngol.*, 49, 206–212, 1958.

Grossman, F., and Malloy, C., Physical characteristic of some bone oscillators used with commercially available audiometers. *Arch. Otol.*, 40, 2–17, 1943.

Harris, J. D., Haines, H. L., and Myers, C. K., A helmet-held bone conduction vibrator. *Laryngoscope*, 63, 998–1007, 1953.

Hart, C., and Naunton, R., Frontal bone conduction tests in clinical audiometry. *Laryngoscope*, 71, 24–29, 1961.

Hawley, M. S., Artificial mastoid for audiophone measurements. *Bell Lab. Rec.*, 18, 73–75, 1939.

Herzog, H., and Krainz, W., Das Knochenleitungsproblem. *Z. Hals Usw. Heilk.*, 15, 300–306, 1926. Cited by Tonndorf, J., Bone Conduction. *Acta Otolaryngol.*, Suppl. 213, 1966.

Hirsh, I. J., *The Measurement of Hearing*. New York: McGraw-Hill Book Co., 1952.

Hodgson, W. R., and Tillman, T., Reliability of bone conduction occlusion effects in normals. *J. Aud. Res.*, 6, 141–153, 1966.

Hood, J., The principles and practice of bone conduction audiometry: A review of the present position. *Proc. R. Soc. Med.*, 50, 689–697, 1957.

Hood, J. D., Bone conduction: A review of the present position with especial reference to the contributions of Dr. Georg von Bekesy. *J. Acoust. Soc. Am.*, 24, 1325–1332, 1962.

Huizing, E. H., Bone conduction—The influence of the middle ear. *Acta Otolaryngol.*, Suppl. 155, 1–99, 1960.

Hulka, J., Bone conduction changes in acute otitis media. *Arch. Otolaryngol.*, 33, 333–346, 1941.

International Electrotechnical Commission, An IEC mechanical coupler for the calibration of bone vibrators having a specified contact area and being applied with a specified static force, IEC-373, 1971.

Jerger, J., and Tillman, T., A new method for the clinical determination of sensorineural acuity level (SAL). *Arch. Otolaryngol.*, 71, 948–953, 1960.

Jones, I. H., and Knudsen, V. O., Audiometry and the prescribing of hearing aids. *Laryngoscope*, 46, 523–536, 1936.

Kelley, N. H., and Reger, S. N., The effect of binaural occlusion of the external auditory meati on the sensitivity of the normal ear for bone conducted sound. *J. Exp. Psychol.*, 21, 211–217, 1937.

Kirikae, I., An experimental study on the fundamental mechanism of bone conduction. *Acta Otolaryngol.*, Suppl. 145, 1–111, 1959.

Konig, E., Les variations de la conduction osseuse en fonction de la force de pression excercee sur le vibrateur, 11 Congres, *Societe Internat. d'Audiologie*, Paris. 1955. Cited from its English translation edited by the Beltone Institute for Hearing Research, No. 6, May 1957.

Konig, E., The use of masking noise and its limitations in clinical audiometry. *Acta Otolaryngol.*, Suppl. 180, 1–64, 1963.

Legouix, J. P., and Tarab, S., Experimental study of bone conduction in ears with mechanical impairment of the ossicles. *J. Acoust. Soc. Am.*, 31, 1453–1457, 1959.

Liden, G., Nilsson, G., and Anderson, H., Narrow band masking with white noise. *Acta Otolaryngol.*, 50, 116–124, 1959.

Lierle, D., and Reger, S., Correlations between bone and air conduction acuity measurements over wide frequency ranges in different types of hearing impairments. *Laryngoscope*, 5, 187–224, 1946.

Link, R., and Zwislocki, J., Audiometrische knochenleitungsuntersuchungen. *Arch. Klin. Exp. Ohr Nas Kehkopfheik*, 160, 347–357, 1951.

Littler, T. S., Knight, J. J., and Strange, P. H., Hearing by bone conduction and the use of bone conduction hearing aids. *Proc. R. Soc. Med.*, 45, 783–790, 1952.

Loch, W. E., Effect of experimentally altered air pressure in the middle ear on hearing acuity in man. *Ann. Otol.*, 51, 995–1006, 1942.

Lybarger, S. F., Interim bone conduction thresholds for audiometry. *J. Speech Hear. Res.*, 9, 483–487, 1966.

Malmquist, C. W., and Jerger, J. R., Some aspects of the normal occlusion effect. Paper presented at the Annual Convention of the American Speech and Hearing Association, Washington, D.C., 1966.

Naunton, R. F., The Measurement of Hearing by Bone Conduction. In Jerger, J. F. (Ed.)., *Modern Developments in Audiology*. New York: Academic Press, 1963.

Naunton, R. F., and Elpern, B. S., Interaural phase and intensity relationships; the Weber test. *Laryngoscope*, 75, 55–63, 1964.

Naunton, R. F., and Fernandez, C., Prolonged bone conduction; observations on man and animals. *Laryngoscope*, 71, 306–318, 1961.

Nilo, E. R., The relation of vibrator surface area and static application force to the vibrator-to-head coupling. *J. Speech Hear. Res.*, 11, 805–810, 1968.

Olsen, W. O., Comparison of studies on bone conduction thresholds and the HAIC interim standard for bone conduction audiometry. *J. Speech Hear. Dis.*, 34, 54–57, 1969.

Olsen, W. O., Personal communication, 1975.

Onchi, Y., The blocked bone conduction test for differential diagnosis. *Ann. Otol.*, 63, 81–96, 1954.

Palva, T., and Ojala, L., Middle ear conduction deafness and bone conduction. *Acta Otolaryngol.*, 45, 135–142, 1955.

Pohlman, A. G., and Kranz, F. W., The influence of partial and complete occlusion of external auditory canals on air and bone transmitted sound. *Ann. Otol.*, 35, 113–121, 1926.

Rainville, M. J., New method of masking for the determination of bone conduction curves. *Trans. Beltone Inst. Hearing Res.*, No. 11, 1959.

Roach, R. E., A study of reliability and validity of bone conduction audiometry. Unpublished Ph.D. dissertation, School of Speech, Northwestern University, 1951.

Roach, R. E., and Carhart, R., A clinical method for calibrating the bone conduction audiometer. *Arch. Otolaryngol.*, **63**, 270–279, 1956.

Rytzner, C., Sound transmission in clinical otosclerosis. *Acta Otolaryngol.*, Suppl. 117, 1–137, 1954.

Sanders, J. W., and Olsen, W. O., An evolution of a new artificial mastoid as an instrument for the calibration of audiometer bone conduction systems. *J. Speech Hear. Dis.*, **29**, 247–263, 1964.

Sanders, J. W., and Rintelmann, W. F., Masking in audiometry; a clinical evaluation of three methods. *Arch. Otolaryngol.*, **80**, 541–556, 1964.

Smith, K. R., Bone conduction during experimental fixation of the stapes. *J. Exp. Psychol.*, **33**, 96–107, 1943.

Spoor, A., Schmidt, P. H., and Van Dishoeck, H. A. E., The location on the skull of a bone conduction receiver and the lateralization of the sound impression. *Acta Otolaryngol.*, **48**, 594–597, 1957.

Stisen, B., and Dahm, M., Sensitivity and mechanical impedance of artificial mastoid type 4930, Bruel & Kjaer Technical Information, 1969.

Studebaker, G. A., Placement of vibrator in bone-conduction testing. *J. Speech Hear. Res.*, **5**, 321–331, 1962.

Studebaker, G. A., Clinical masking of air- and bone-conducted stimuli. *J. Speech Hear. Dis.*, **29**, 23–35, 1964.

Studebaker, G. A., The standardization of bone-conduction thresholds. *Laryngoscope*, **77**, 823–835, 1967.

Sullivan, J. A., Gotlieb, C. C., and Hodge, W. E., Shift of bone conduction thresholds on occlusion of the external ear canal. *Laryngoscope*, **57**, 690–703, 1947.

Tonndorf, J., Bone conduction; studies in experimental animals. *Acta Otolaryngol.*, Suppl. 213, 1–132, 1966.

Tonndorf, J., Bone Conduction. In Tobias, J. V. (Ed.), *Foundation of Modern Auditory Theory*, Ch. 5. New York: Academic Press, 1972.

Tonndorf, J., and Tabor, J. R., Closure of the cochlear windows; its effect upon air- and bone-conduction. *Ann. Otol.*, **71**, 5–29, 1962.

Watson, N. A., Limits of audition for bone-conduction. *J. Acoust. Soc. Am.*, **9**, 294–300, 1938.

Watson, N. A., and Gales, R. S., Bone conduction threshold measurements; effects of occlusion, enclosures, and masking devices. *J. Acoust. Soc. Am.*, **14**, 207–215, 1943.

Weiss, E., An air damped artificial mastoid. *J. Acoust. Soc. Am.*, **32**, 1582–1588, 1960.

Weston, P. B., Gengel, R. W., and Hirsh, I. J., Effects of vibrator types and their placement on bone-conduction threshold measurements. *J. Acoust. Soc. Am.*, **41**, 788–792, 1967.

Whittle, L. S., A determination of the normal threshold of hearing by bone conduction. *J. Sound Vibration*, **2**, 227–248, 1965.

Wilber, L. A., and Goodhill, V., Real ear *versus* artificial mastoid methods of calibration of bone conduction vibrators. *J. Speech Hear. Res.*, **10**, 405–417, 1967.

Zwislocki, J., Eine verbesserte vertäubungsmethode für die audiometrie. *Acta Otolaryngol.*, **39**, 338–356, 1951.

Zwislocki, J., Acoustic attenuation between the ears. *J. Acoust. Soc. Am.*, **25**, 752–759, 1953.

chapter 11

MASKING

Jay W. Sanders, Ph.D.

Of all the clinical procedures used in auditory assessment, masking is probably the most often misused and the least understood. For some clinicians the approach to masking is a haphazard, hit-or-miss bit of guess work with no basis in any set of principles. Yet, there are principles of masking readily available, developed from an extensive array of careful research. Attesting the extent of research in masking, Studebaker (1967) surveyed 56 different investigations of masking in audiometry.

The importance of appropriate and accurate masking cannot be overemphasized. Without correct masking, it is very possible to obtain pure tone thresholds indicative of a moderate conductive impairment in an ear with a profound sensory-neural loss, a reasonably good word discrimination score in an ear with severely impaired speech discrimination or moderate tone decay in an ear with highly abnormal auditory adaptation. The purpose of this chapter is to discuss the principles of auditory masking and to propose clinical masking procedures based on those principles.

THE PROBLEM

The problem is posed by the patient with a unilateral hearing loss or with an asymmetrical bilateral loss. When a test signal is presented to the poorer ear of a patient, the intensity may be raised to such a level that it is transmitted across the skull and heard in the better ear before it reaches threshold level in the ear under test. A number of investigators (Zwislocki, 1951, 1953; Liden, 1954; Liden, Nilsson and Anderson, 1959a) have shown that a pure tone presented by air conduction may be heard in the nontest ear when the signal intensity is 50 to 60 dB above sensory-neural sensitivity in the nontest ear. This intensity reduction of 50 to 60 dB from the test ear across the skull to the nontest ear has been called interaural attenuation. When the signal is presented by bone conduction, however, interaural attenuation is essentially zero. Indeed, it is possible to obtain a false bone-conduction threshold in the test ear at a *better* hearing threshold level (HTL) than the actual bone-conduction threshold in the nontest ear. This possibility was suggested by Studebaker (1964) and demonstrated in a case reported by Sanders and Rintelmann (1964). Thus, it is possible to

obtain a response to a bone-conduction signal at the 0 dB HTL in an ear with a profound sensory-neural loss, if the opposite ear has normal sensitivity.

False air-conduction thresholds at the 50- to 60-dB HTL can be obtained in a "dead" ear when there is a conductive loss of equal severity in the better ear. In this instance, the test tone presented to the poorer ear by air conduction has reached sufficient intensity to stimulate the nontest ear by bone conduction.

From the foregoing it can be seen that without proper masking a patient with a profound sensory-neural loss in one ear may give a variety of results for that ear. Responses might be obtained by air conduction at hearing threshold levels as low as 50 dB and by bone conduction as low as 0 dB. In addition, without proper masking, false results may be obtained in other areas of auditory assessment, such as speech audiometry and special diagnostic tests.

FUNDAMENTAL QUESTIONS IN MASKING

The solution to the problem posed by the patient whose ears differ in sensitivity is to ensure that response is from the ear under test by eliminating the possibility of response from the nontest ear. This can be accomplished through the use of a masking noise in the nontest ear. Masking has been defined variously, but for clinical purposes it can be regarded as the elevation in threshold for one signal (the test tone) by the presence of a second signal (the masking noise). Delivering masking to the better ear shifts its sensitivity to a higher hearing threshold level, permitting the test signal to be presented at higher intensities to the poorer ear without crossover. The extent of threshold shift in the masked ear is dependent upon the nature and intensity of the masking noise.

The use of a masking noise, however, introduces a new problem. Just as the test signal may cross the skull and be heard in the nontest ear given sufficient intensity, so may the masking noise presented to the nontest ear cross over and elevate threshold in the test ear. This situation is known as overmasking.

Before the clinician can make effective use of masking, he needs answers to three fundamental questions:

1. When should masking be used?
2. What kind of masking noise should be used?
3. How much masking should be used?

The following sections will answer these questions through a discussion of the principles of masking based on experimental evidence.

WHEN TO MASK

The question of when to mask is answered most simply by saying that masking should be used whenever there is any danger of the test tone being heard in the nontest ear. The danger occurs whenever the test signal is presented with enough intensity to cross the skull and stimulate the opposite ear. Thus, the important considerations for when to mask are the intensity of the test signal, threshold sensitivity in the nontest ear and the interaural attenuation. Since this last factor varies in air and bone conduction testing, these two clinical procedures will be considered separately.

Air Conduction

It is important to recognize that a determination of when to mask should be based on sensory-neural sensitivity in the nontest ear, not on the air-conduction thresholds. Even when the test signal is presented by air conduction, it will cross the skull by bone conduction whenever its intensity at the test ear is about 50 dB greater than the bone-conduction threshold of the nontest ear, regardless of air-conduction threshold in the nontest ear. With no masking in the nontest ear, false air-conduction thresholds of 50 to 60 dB will be obtained for an ear with severe sensory-neural loss, even with air-conduction thresholds in the nontest ear of 50 to 60 dB, as long as bone conduction in that ear is normal. Thus, in air-conduction testing, interaural difference refers to the difference between the intensity level of the test signal and bone-conduction sensitivity of the nontest ear.

Investigation has shown that for an air-conducted signal presented through a standard audiometer earphone (TDH-39 set in an MX-41/AR cushion), interaural attenuation ranges from 40 to about 80 dB, varying with test frequency and with subject (Zwislocki, 1953; Liden et al., 1959a). Zwislocki has shown that if a larger cushion, such as the doughnut type, is used, resulting in a larger contact area between skull and cushion, interaural attenuation is actually decreased.

In view of the wide variability in interaural attenuation, it seems wise to follow Studebaker's (1967) principle that whenever variability is a result of intersubject differences, the safest course is to adopt the extreme value, in this case the smallest observed interaural attenuation. On this basis, the rule for when to mask in air-conduction testing becomes:

In air-conduction testing, the nontest ear should be masked whenever the signal presented to the test ear exceeds bone conduction sensitivity in the nontest ear by more than 40 dB.

This rule may occasionally lead to unnecessary masking, but it will prevent failure to mask in those cases where it is required.

Bone Conduction

Clinical observation and research evidence (Zwislocki, 1951; Liden et al., 1959a; Feldman, 1961; Studebaker, 1964; Sanders and Rintelmann, 1964) suggest that interaural attenuation for a signal presented by bone conduction is negligible and should be considered as zero. Although attenuation on the order of 10 dB may be observed in some subjects for the higher frequencies, the value varies from one subject to another and cannot be regarded as dependable. Indeed, as pointed out earlier, it is possible to obtain a false bone conduction threshold response at a *better* hearing level than the bone conduction threshold of the nontest ear.

Since no interaural attenuation is expected, it has been proposed that masking always be used in bone-conduction testing (Glorig, 1965; O'Neill and Oyer, 1966). Objecting to this, Studebaker (1964) pointed out that whenever bone-conduction thresholds in the test ear are at the same hearing threshold levels as air-conduction thresholds without masking, the use of masking in the nontest ear should not affect those results.

Complicating the picture of when to mask in bone-conduction testing is the effect of "central masking." Central masking is defined as an elevation in threshold in the test ear as a result of the introduction of a masking noise in the nontest ear, even though the noise is not of sufficient intensity to cross the skull to the test ear. According to Liden et al. (1959b), central masking is probably mediated by the efferent pathways. Whatever its mode of transmission, the effect has been clearly demonstrated. Zwislocki (1953) suggested that the threshold shift as a result of central masking does not exceed about 5 dB, but Liden et al. (1959b) observed shifts up to 15 dB. Studebaker (1962), Dirks (1964) and Dirks and Malmquist (1964) have pointed out that the central masking effect increases with increased intensity of the masking noise and may be as great as 10 to 12 dB. The point here is that bone-conduction thresholds obtained with no masking in the opposite ear will be 5 to 10 dB better than those obtained with masking even when masking is not required to prevent crossover of the test signal. Since the bone-conduction system of an audiometer is usually calibrated according to normal ear responses with masking in the opposite ear, unmasked bone-conduction thresholds will underestimate sensory-neural loss. Lybarger (1966) has suggested that masking always be used in bone-conduction testing with an audiometer calibrated according to the interim thresholds with the Beltone artificial mastoid, since these thresholds are on the basis of masking in the nontest ear of the normal hearers tested.

Because of the central masking effect on the normative data used in calibration of a bone-conduction system, the test ear should always show an air-bone gap if bone-conduction thresholds are obtained without masking the nontest ear. Thus, we can accept Studebaker's (1964) rule for masking in bone-conduction testing and state that:

In bone-conduction audiometry, the nontest ear should be masked whenever the test ear exhibits an air-bone gap.

MASKING NOISES

The question of what kind of masking noise to use requires a consideration of the kinds of noise available and of the masking effectiveness of each. The amount of threshold shift produced by a masking noise depends not only on the intensity but also on the nature of the sound. Although Wegel and Lane (1924) demonstrated that masking can be accomplished with a pure tone, their results suggested that masking is more effective with a noise composed of a number of frequencies. Consequently, the masking signal provided on audiometers is usually a broad band noise. Some audiometers are equipped with white noise, some with complex noise and some with both types. In some cases, the audiometer purchaser has a choice of either complex or white noise. In recent years narrow band noise also has become available to the clinician. Narrow band noise has been produced and used in the laboratory for some time (Egan and Hake, 1950;

Zwislocki, 1951; Denes and Naunton, 1952; Liden et al., 1959a; Jerger, Tillman and Peterson, 1960; Koenig, 1962b; Studebaker, 1962; Dirks, 1963; Sanders and Rintelmann, 1964).

An important factor in choosing among the available masking noises should be the relative masking efficiency of the noise. Masking efficiency, as described by Zwislocki (1951), Denes and Naunton (1952) and others, refers to the ratio of the masking obtained relative to the intensity of the noise. That is, the most efficient masking noise would be one that produces the greatest shift in threshold with the least overall intensity. On this basis, several investigators (Zwislocki, 1951; Denes and Naunton, 1952; Liden et al., 1959a; Studebaker, 1962; Sanders and Rintelmann, 1964) have demonstrated a clear superiority for narrow band noise.

Since the clinician may be faced with a choice, or may be limited by his equipment to one of the three kinds of noise in current use, it is worthwhile to consider the nature and the masking efficiency of each of the noises.

Complex Noise

Although technically there are differences, the term complex noise has come to mean any masking noise composed of a low frequency fundamental plus the multiples of that fundamental. Figure 11.1 shows the acoustic spectrum of such a noise. The fundamental frequency for this particular noise is 78 Hz. The additional frequencies present are multiples of the fundamental (156 Hz, 234 Hz and so on). To understand this noise as a masking signal it is important to note two facts from the line spectrum shown in the figure. First, acoustic energy is present *only* at the discrete frequencies designated by the *vertical lines* and is not spread continuously across the range from 78

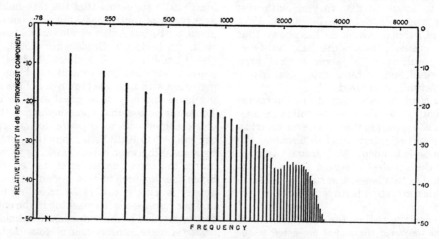

Fig. 11.1. Acoustic spectrum of a sawtooth noise through a PDR-8 earphone. From J. W. Sanders and W. F. Rintelmann, *Archives of Otolaryngology*, **80**, 541–556, 1964.

to 4000 Hz. That is, there is no energy present at the frequencies between 78 and 156 Hz or between 156 and 234 Hz. This poses a potential problem in masking. Since complex noise is composed of discrete frequencies, it is possible for a given component of the noise to be within 3 or 4 cycles of a test tone, producing a "beat" or pulsing phenomenon in the ear of the listener between that component and the test tone. As Liden et al. (1959a) have pointed out, the fifth harmonic of a 50-Hz fundamental will beat with a test tone of 254 Hz. A tone of 254 Hz is well within the ±3% variability specification for the 250-Hz tone.

The second important fact regarding complex noise is that energy decreases as frequency increases. Note in Figure 11.1 that the energy present near 1000 Hz is about 23 dB less than the intensity level at 78 Hz. By 4000 Hz the energy drop off is greater than 50 dB.* Although the noise spectrum may vary somewhat from one complex noise generator to another, two limitations are generally characteristic of masking noise labeled "complex"—energy is present only at discrete frequencies and intensity decreases with frequency increase. Because of its limitations, complex noise is seldom included on newer clinical audiometers and has even been replaced by white noise on most portable models now available.

White Noise

White noise, sometimes called thermal noise, is defined as a signal containing energy at all frequencies in the audible spectrum at approximately equal intensities. Figure 11.2 shows that the acoustic spectrum is limited, however, by the frequency response of the transducer. Through the TDH-39 earphone, the acoustic spectrum is essentially flat (equal intensity across frequency) to 6000 Hz but drops off rapidly beyond that point. The acoustic spectrum of white noise is constant from one audiometer to another, providing the same type of earphone is used as a transducer. As opposed to complex noise, in white noise the energy is continuous across the spectrum, and there is no significant intensity decrease with increased frequency until about 6000 Hz.

Narrow Band Noise

Narrow band noise is actually not a third kind of noise but is rather white noise in restricted frequency bands produced by selective filtering. For pure tone audiometry, the filters are set to produce a band of frequencies

---

* In at least one audiometer described as a clinical and research instrument, the manufacturer has overcome this problem with additional circuitry to boost the noise output in the higher frequencies.

with the test tone at the center of the band. A 1000 Hz narrow band signal would be white noise in a limited band of frequencies with 1000 Hz at its center. A narrow band noise masking generator produces a separate noise band for each test frequency. A given noise band is described in terms of its center frequency, its band width (the span of frequencies whose energies are no more than 3 dB below that of the peak component) and its rejection rate (the decrease in intensity over a one octave range on either side of the band). The acoustic spectra of three narrow bands of noise are shown in Figure 11.3.

Since the band widths and rejection rates are a product of the filter characteristics and of the transducer used, the acoustic spectra of narrow band noise may vary from one generator to another. For use in clinical masking, the narrow band noise generator is equipped with a frequency dial to permit selection of a band appropriate to the test tone. Since narrow band noise is filtered white noise, the signal is continuous within the frequency band, and intensity is essentially equal across the band.

RELATIVE MASKING EFFICIENCY

As pointed out earlier, the masking efficiency of a noise is the relationship between its overall intensity level and the magnitude of the threshold shift produced by that noise. Thus, if our three noises were presented to an ear at equal overall sound pressure levels, the noise producing the greatest threshold shift in that ear could be regarded as the most efficient. Before actually measuring the threshold shift obtained with each masking noise, let us consider the way in which masking noise affects auditory sensitivity and a method for predicting masking efficiency.

The Critical Band Concept

The concept of masking effect relative to a band of frequencies of a critical width has developed from the work of Fletcher (1940) and Fletcher and Munson (1937). Elaboration of the concept was provided by later investigations (Hawkins and Stevens, 1950; Egan and Hake, 1950). The concept may be stated in two parts:

In masking a pure tone with a broad band noise, the only components of the noise having a masking effect on the tone are those frequencies included in a restricted band with the test tone at its center.

When the pure tone is just audible in the presence of the noise, the acoustic energy in the restricted band of frequencies is equal to the acoustic energy of the test tone.

The width of the restricted band of frequencies responsible for masking a pure tone is critical.

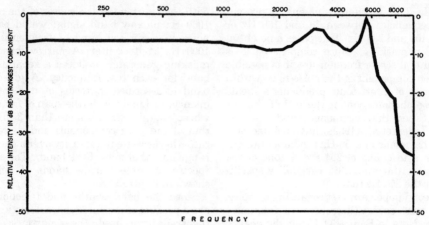

Fig. 11.2. Acoustic spectrum of a broad band white noise through a THD-39 earphone. From J. W. Sanders and W. F. Rintelmann, *Archives of Otolaryngology,* **80,** 541–556, 1964.

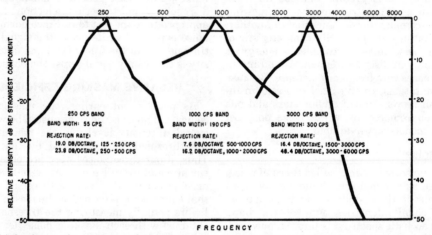

Fig. 11.3. Acoustic spectra of three narrow bands of noise through a hearing aid type receiver. From J. W. Sanders and W. F. Rintelmann, *Archives of Otolaryngology,* **80,** 541–556, 1964.

If a band is narrowed to less than the critical width without adding to the energy within the band, its masking *effect* is decreased. If the band is widened beyond critical width, its masking *efficiency* is decreased, in that the noise is increased in overall intensity without further shift in threshold. For example, the critical band width for a 1000-Hz tone is 64 Hz. Thus, according to the first part of the critical band concept, if we mask a 1000-Hz pure tone with white noise, the only energy in the noise having a masking effect on the tone is that included in the band of frequencies from 968 to 1032 Hz, inclusive. The acoustic energy in the white noise below and above that band of frequencies could be removed without changing the masking effect produced by the noise.

From the second part of the concept we see that the intensity level within the critical band

rather than the overall intensity determines the effectiveness of the masking, since the overall level includes the energy above and below the critical band which has no masking effect. Thus, in determining the relative efficiency of several masking noises, the intensity level of concern to us is the spectrum level within the critical band, often referred to as the level per cycle—the intensity of each individual cycle. The critical band concept can be used to evaluate masking noises used for clinical purposes.

Application of the Critical Band Concept

It should be noted that the critical band concept will not hold entirely true for complex noise, since the concept is specific to a noise of continuous and flat spectrum. Complex noise, it will be recalled, is neither flat nor continuous. We can, nevertheless, make a general application, since the component frequencies of a complex noise will, in effect, combine their acoustic energies in masking.

It should be clear by this point that both broad band noises, complex and white, are to some extent inefficient, since for any given pure tone both noises will include considerable energy outside the critical band. Of these two noises, however, white noise should have greater masking efficiency, at least in the middle and higher frequencies, since its spectrum is essentially flat; whereas energy in the complex noise is concentrated in the lower frequencies with a rapid drop off of energy in the middle and higher frequencies.

Of the three masking noises, narrow band noise clearly should have the greatest masking efficiency if the important factor in terms of intensity is the level per cycle in the critical band rather than the overall intensity. If we examine the three noises at an overall sound pressure level (SPL) of 80 dB, the level per cycle should be highest in the narrow band noise, since the 80 dB are concentrated in the critical band and the region immediately around it; whereas in the broad band noises the sound pressure is spread across a much wider range of frequencies. This can be demonstrated for white noise and narrow band noise, since it is possible to compute level per cycle for a noise of continuous, flat spectrum. The level per cycle (energy in each individual cycle) is the overall sound pressure divided by the number of cycles. For the white noise in our example, this would be 80 dB divided by 6000 Hz (band width of the white noise through a TDH-39 earphone). In order to carry out the computation, however, the latter value must be converted to its logarithm, and the function then becomes one of subtraction.

Level per cycle = overall intensity minus 10 times the logarithm of the band width

Since the logarithm of 6000 is 3.78, the formula for determining the level per cycle (LPC) of a white noise of 80 dB would be

$$LPC = OA\ SPL - 10 \log BW$$

$$LPC = 80 - 37.8$$

Therefore, the level per cycle would be 42.2 dB SPL.

Applying the same formula to a narrow band of noise with a band width (BW) of, let us say 200 Hz (log 200 = 2.3), the computation would be

$$LPC = OA - 10 \log BW$$

$$LPC = 80 - 23$$

The level per cycle would be 57 dB SPL, 14.8 dB greater than that for the white noise. Thus, at equal overall intensity we would expect a 15 dB greater threshold shift from the narrow band noise. Looking at it from another point of view, for a given threshold shift the overall intensity would be less for the narrow band noise.

The foregoing computations suggest that the narrow band noise will approach maximum masking efficiency as its band width approaches the critical band width. The narrower the band, the greater the masking efficiency, providing it is no less than the critical width. Since the band width is a result of the filtering characteristics of the noise generator, the efficiency of narrow band masking may vary from one generator to another.

Experimental Verification

Computations concerning relative masking efficiency are subject to verification through actual threshold measurement. Noise can be mixed electronically with a pure tone in the same earphone and threshold determinations made at various noise levels. A number of investigators (Denes and Naunton, 1952; Liden et al., 1959a; Studebaker, 1962; Sanders and Rintelmann, 1964) have carried out this kind of measurement with essentially the same results. Figure 11.4 presents typical data. The masked thresholds shown are the average thresholds in hearing level (according to ASA-1951 standards) for 10 normal hearers in the presence of each of three masking noises at three different overall sound pressure levels. The acoustic spectra of the noises are shown in Figures 11.1 to 11.3. Figure 11.4 shows real ear support for the critical band concept. For a given noise intensity level, narrow band noise shows the greatest masking efficiency. Of the two broad band noises, white noise showed greater masking efficiency than did the complex (sawtooth) noise, at least in the middle and higher frequencies. Note that for the complex noise, threshold shift at 2000, 3000 and 4000 Hz is less than 20 dB even when the overall noise level is at 90-dB sound pressure level.

Two additional observations from Figure 11.4 are of interest. First, for both white and narrow band noise, masking is least effective in the lower frequencies. This is because the human ear requires greater sound pressure to reach threshold in this frequency range. Second, for both white and narrow band noise, the relationship between masking effect and noise level is linear. That is, beyond a certain minimum level, each additional dB of masking noise produces an additional dB of threshold shift for

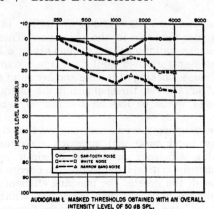

AUDIOGRAM 1. MASKED THRESHOLDS OBTAINED WITH AN OVERALL INTENSITY LEVEL OF 50 dB SPL.

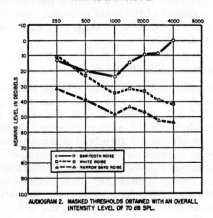

AUDIOGRAM 2. MASKED THRESHOLDS OBTAINED WITH AN OVERALL INTENSITY LEVEL OF 70 dB SPL.

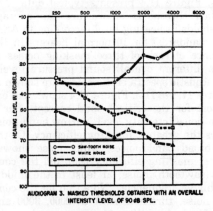

AUDIOGRAM 3. MASKED THRESHOLDS OBTAINED WITH AN OVERALL INTENSITY LEVEL OF 90 dB SPL.

Fig. 11.4. Masking audiograms obtained with three types of masking noise at three intensity levels. From J. W. Sanders and W. F. Rintelmann, *Archives of Otolaryngology*, **80**, 541–556, 1964.

any given pure tone. This linearity is not obtained with complex noise.

What Kind of Masking Noise to Use

The foregoing discussion has provided us with an answer to our second question, "What kind of masking noise should be used?" If the audiologist has a choice among the three masking noises generally available, he should select narrow band noise for its superior masking efficiency. If he is limited to either white or complex noise, his choice should be white noise. Although not as efficient as narrow band noise, white noise enjoys considerable superiority over complex noise and will provide adequate masking in most cases if the maximum output of the generator is sufficiently high.

HOW MUCH MASKING?

After deciding on the kind of masking noise and that masking of the nontest ear is required, the clinician is faced with the problem of how much masking noise to use. To what number should the masking dial be set to ensure appropriate masking? First of all, the intensity must be great enough to effect the needed threshold shift in the masked ear. The least amount required to do this has been called the minimum effective masking level (Liden et al., 1959b) or the minimum masking level (Studebaker, 1962) and defined as the masking noise level just sufficient to mask the test signal in the masked ear. Secondly, the masking intensity must not be so great as to shift threshold in the test ear by crossover from the masked ear. This level, the maximum effective masking level or maximum masking level, is defined as the intensity just insufficient to mask the test signal in the *test* ear (Studebaker, 1967). Several investigators have proposed mathematical formulae for determination of the minimum and maximum levels.

The Formula Approach

A formula approach to determine minimum and maximum masking levels has been proposed by a number of investigators. The following formulae (Liden et al., 1959a) were suggested for bone conduction testing:

$$M_{min} = B_t + (A_m - B_m)$$

$$M_{max} = B_t + 40, \text{ provided } M_{max} \text{ is less than } D$$

That is, minimum masking equals bone conduction threshold in the test ear plus the difference between air and bone conduction thresholds in the masked ear. The maximum level equals the bone conduction threshold in the test ear plus the attenuation factor (40), provided the maximum level does not exceed the patient's discomfort level (*D*).

For masking in air conduction testing, the following formulae were proposed:

$$M_{min} = A_t - 40 + (A_m - B_m)$$

$$M_{max} = B_t + 40, \text{ provided } M_{max} \text{ is less than } D$$

Minimum masking is equal to the air-conduction threshold in the test ear minus the attenuation factor plus the difference between the air- and bone-conduction thresholds in the masked ear. The maximum level is equal to the bone-conduction threshold in the test ear plus the attenuation factor, provided the maximum level does not exceed the patient's discomfort level.

Two problems are apparent in the formula approach. In this instance, the clinician would be required to work out four formulae for each patient at each test frequency in order to obtain air and bone conduction thresholds in one ear. Further, the formulae assume that the masking dial is calibrated in effective masking level. Studebaker (1964) simplified the problem somewhat by combining air and bone conduction testing into a single formula and by providing methods for determining effective levels. He recognized the problems involved in a formula approach to masking, however, and suggested that this method, while perhaps desirable in laboratory research, was not suited to clinical audiometry.

The Audiometer Masking Dial

Whatever masking approach the clinician adopts, he must know the relationship between the masking effect and each marking on the audiometer dial that controls the intensity of the masking noise. In the past there has been no consistency among audiometers as to the meaning of the numbers on the dial, as shown by a survey of the noise output of eight different audiometers (portable, clinical and research models). With the dial of each set on "60," the masking noise output ranged from 60 to 120 dB SPL. Any assumptions concerning numbers on the masking dial of these instruments would be precarious at best.

As a note of caution, some clinical audiometers producing white noise as a masker provide a set of numbers on the dial labeled "effective masking." The numbers may be approximately correct for one or two frequencies, probably in the area of 1000 Hz, but cannot apply to all test frequencies, since the sound pressure level necessary for effective masking varies with the frequency of the test tone.

Since the narrow band masking requires a different noise band for each test frequency, the masking dial can be calibrated in effective masking. The newer audiometers that contain narrow band masking noise are calibrated in effective masking level. For instruments that are not calibrated in true effective masking levels, the audiologist can at least determine the relationship between the dial numbers and their masking effect.

Effective Masking Level

The most practical and useful calibration of the audiometer masking dial is in effective level according to the normal ear for the different test frequencies. This calibration is applicable with white noise and narrow band noise and, with some qualifications, with complex noise. The following discussion will apply, however, only to white and narrow band noise.

Effective level is defined as the number of dB that the total energy in the critical band is above the threshold energy for a pure tone whose frequency is at the center of the band. Effective level can also be regarded as the threshold shift in decibels produced in the masked ear by a given amount of noise. Thus, if we determine effective level according to the normal ear and express it in decibels on the hearing threshold level scale, we can interpret it as the hearing threshold level to which an ear will be shifted by a given amount of noise. If we relate these effective levels to the numbers on the audiometer masking dial for each frequency, we can predict the masked threshold that will be produced by each setting of the dial.

Determining Effective Masking Level

Two methods may be used for determining effective masking levels and relating them to the dial readings for either white noise or narrow band noise. The first method is through computation with the critical band data.

Effective Level through Computation. From our earlier discussion of the critical band concept, it will be recalled:

When the pure tone is just audible in the presence of the noise, the acoustic energy in the restricted band of frequencies is equal to the acoustic energy of the test tone.

If we can determine the acoustic energy in the critical band, we can predict the masking effect. The level per cycle can be computed from knowledge of the overall sound pressure level and the band width. If we also know the width of the critical band, we can determine the total energy in the critical band. The critical band widths from the data of Hawkins and Stevens (1950) are shown in Table 11.1. Each band width is stated in frequency and in 10 times its logarithm. The total energy in the critical band is the level per cycle (the energy in each individual cycle) multiplied by the number of cycles in the critical band. In masking a 1000 Hz tone, if the energy in each cycle of white noise is 42.2 dB (see example given above), and we have a frequency band that includes 64 cycles (critical band width (CBW) at 1000 Hz), the total energy in the critical band would be 42.2 multiplied by 64. Here again we must convert the band width to a logarithmic value, and the function then becomes one of addition.

Energy in the critical band = level per cycle plus 10 times the logarithm of the critical band width

If we take an overall intensity of 80 dB of white noise and the critical band at 1000 Hz, the computation is as follows:

$$E \text{ in CB} = \text{LPC} + 10 \log \text{CBW}$$

$$E \text{ in CB} = 42.2 + 18$$

$$E \text{ in CB} = 60.2 \text{ dB SPL}$$

TABLE 11.1. *Critical Band Widths* for Eleven Test Frequencies*

Center Frequency	Critical Band Width (CBW)	
	In Hz	10 log CBW
125	70.8	18.5
250	50	17
500	50	17
750	56.2	17.5
1000	64	18
1500	79.4	19
2000	100	20
3000	158	22
4000	200	23
6000	376	25.75
8000	501	27

* Hawkins and Stevens (1950).

The total energy in the critical band is 60.2 dB SPL. The difference between that level and the level necessary to reach threshold at 1000 Hz in a given ear is the effective level of the noise at that frequency in that ear. Thus, effective level often designated as Z, can be computed as follows:

$$Z = \text{LPC} + 10 \log \text{CBW} - \text{threshold in quiet}$$

In this computation, threshold in quiet must be expressed in decibels sound pressure level (0 dB according to ANSI-1969 = 7 dB at 1000 Hz). As an example of this computation, the effective level of 80 dB of white noise in a TDH-39 earphone at 1000 Hz in a normal ear would be

$$Z = 42.2 + 18 - 7$$

$$Z = 53.2 \text{ dB}$$

With an effective level of 53.2 dB, we would expect 53.2 dB of masking in the normal ear for the 1000-Hz tone.

Since our prediction is based entirely on computation with the critical band data, we might well ask at this point for verification. Does 80 dB of white noise actually produce 53.2 dB of threshold shift for a 1000-Hz tone in a normal ear? The relationship of predicted masking (effective level) and the masking actually obtained with white noise at three different sound pressure levels in 10 normal hearers is shown in Figure 11.5. Figure 11.6 reports

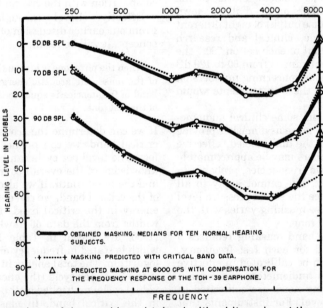

Fig. 11.5. Comparison of the masking obtained with white noise at three different intensity levels for 10 normal hearing subjects and the masking predicted with the critical band data of Fletcher (1940). From J. W. Sanders and W. F. Rintelmann, *Archives of Otolaryngology,* **80,** 541–556, 1964.

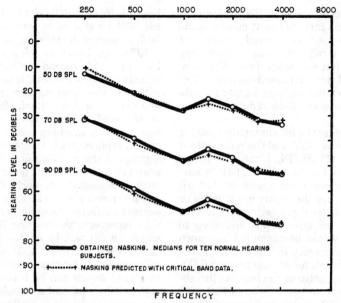

Fig. 11.6. Comparison of the masking obtained with narrow bands of noise at three different intensity levels for 10 normal hearing subjects and the masking predicted with the critical band data of Fletcher (1940). From J. W. Sanders and W. F. Rintelmann, *Archives of Otolaryngology*, **80**, 541–556, 1964.

the same relationship (predicted to obtained masking) for narrow band noise. In these figures, for a given overall intensity level of the masking noise, one curve shows the masked thresholds predicted with the critical band data and the second curve shows the hearing threshold levels (according to ASA-1951) to which the 10 normal ears were actually shifted. Converting the measured and predicted masked thresholds to hearing thresholds levels *re* the ANSI-1969 standard would not, of course, change the relationship shown.

The results shown in Figures 11.5 and 11.6 indicate that, beyond a certain minimum level, there is indeed a direct, one-to-one relationship between effective level and threshold shift and that if the overall intensity of the noise (white or narrow band) is known, it is possible to predetermine the hearing threshold levels to which an ear will be shifted by a given noise intensity. With this information, it is possible to construct a table of effective masking levels to be posted on the audiometer.

Effective Masking Table. The purpose here is to provide the clinician with a predetermined set of effective masking levels according to the dial settings of his audiometer. The first step is to measure the acoustic output of the masking noise in sound pressure level. This must be done with an artificial ear. If the clinician does not have that equipment, it should be possible to get this measurement made by the people

who service and calibrate the audiometer. For the maximum noise output, the level per cycle and the energy in the critical bands can be determined with the formulae given, using the critical band data from Table 11.1. Finally, the effective levels according to audiometric zero can be determined by subtracting the appropriate sound pressure level values representing audiometric zero (ANSI-1969) from the energy in the critical bands. The resulting values are the effective levels according to normal hearing at each test frequency for the maximum output of the masking noise.

The next step is to check the linearity of the masking dial. That is, does a 10-dB change on the dial bring about a 10-dB change in output. Most clinical audiometers are equipped with attenuators that should provide satisfactory linearity. Some older audiometers, however, and most portables are equipped with potentiometers which do not provide linear control. The linearity check can be done with the artificial ear, but it is done more satisfactorily with a vacuum tube voltmeter. Connect the voltmeter across the leads to the earphone. Set the masking dial to maximum and then decrease in 10-dB steps, noting whether the voltmeter shows a corresponding 10-dB decrease in output. If the dial departs from linearity by more than 1 or 2 dB per 10-dB step, or if the cumulative error is greater than 4 or 5 dB, use the voltmeter to determine 10-dB steps and mark those points on the dial. If a voltmeter is not available, this measurement can be made by the people who service the audiometer or it can be made by a radio-television repair shop if you explain what you want done. With dial linearity assured, you can now determine effective level for each dial setting simply by subtracting 10 dB for each 10-dB reduction on the dial.

Example. Suppose the maximum dial setting on an audiometer is "100" and the noise output at that setting is 110 dB SPL. If the audiometer is equipped with the standard TDH-39 earphone, the level per cycle would be 110 dB minus 37.8 (10 times the logarithm of 6000) or 72.2 dB. With this level per cycle and the data from Table 11.1, effective levels according to normal hearing would be computed as shown for three test frequencies in Table 11.2. These are the effective levels for normal hearers (HTL = 0 dB) and thus constitute the hearing threshold levels to which an ear will be shifted with a dial setting of 100 on this audiometer. These levels, rounded off to the next lower 5-dB level, would be entered in the table of effective masking opposite the dial setting of 100, as shown in Table 11.3. Table 11.3 is a sample effective masking table, showing the levels for the three frequencies computed in Table 11.2. The table would include effective levels for all test frequencies.

Next, if the masking dial is linear, effective levels can be entered for each dial setting by subtracting 10 dB from the maximum effective level for each 10-dB reduction on the dial. The table now tells us for each test frequency the

hearing threshold level to which the masked ear will be shifted by our masking noise at each setting of the masking dial.

Effective Level by Measurement. Let us turn now to a second method of determining effective masking levels. If the actual acoustic output of the masking generator is unknown and cannot be determined, effective levels can be obtained through actual measurement. In this method, masking noise is mixed in the same earphone with the test tone. At several settings of the masking dial, thresholds in the presence of the noise are determined for 8 or 10 normal hearers. For each dial setting, the mean threshold value at each frequency represents the effective level for normal hearers and thus represents the hearing threshold level to which an ear will be shifted by noise at each dial setting. If the masking dial is linear, effective levels for those dial settings not used in measurement can be interpolated from the obtained results, and a complete table of effective masking levels according to dial settings can be constructed. If the dial is not linear, the alternatives are to mark linear points on the dial as described above or to measure masking in the normal hearers at all dial settings.

This method is based on the assumption that the noise and tone can be mixed into the same earphone. This is not possible on most one channel audiometers, but the same thing can be accomplished through construction of a simple mixing network described by Studebaker (1967) and shown in Figure 11.7. If the clinician lacks the facilities or the know-how to construct the network, he can have it made in a radio-television repair shop.

Effective Masking and Complex Noise. It should be evident by now that complex noise is not highly regarded as a masking source. If the clinician has no choice, however, he should be fully aware of the limitations of complex noise. First, masking with complex noise is not linear. That is, each additional dB of noise

TABLE 11.2. *Illustration of Computation of Effective Masking Levels at Three Test Frequencies*

Frequency	Computation	Effective Level
250	Z = 72.2 + 17 − 25.5* =	63.7
1000	Z = 72.2 + 18 − 7* =	83.2
4000	Z = 72.2 + 23 − 9.5* =	85.7

* Audiometric zero according to the ANSI-1969 standards.

TABLE 11.3. *Illustration of Effective Masking Table*

Dial Setting	Effective Levels		
	250	1000	4000
20			5
30		10	15
40		20	25
50	10	30	35
60	20	40	45
70	30	50	55
80	40	60	65
90	50	70	75
100	60	80	85

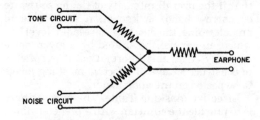

ALL RESISTORS 3.3 OHMS, 1/4 WATT

Fig. 11.7. Combining network for mixing the pure tone and the masking noise into the same earphone. From G. A. Studebaker, *Journal of Speech and Hearing Disorders,* **32,** 360–371, 1967.

does not necessarily produce an additional dB of masking. Further, the critical band data cannot be applied to complex noise because the spectrum is neither continuous nor flat. This means that the only approach to determination of effective masking levels is by actual measurement with normal hearers and that measurement must be made at each setting of the masking dial. Even with a table of effective levels, the clinician must exercise great care because of the previously mentioned possibility of a beat phenomenon between a component of the noise and a test tone.

Using the Effective Masking Table

After the effective masking table has been constructed by whatever method, it should be posted in a readily accessible spot on or near the audiometer. The clinician now has in front of him an immediate indication of the hearing threshold level to which an ear will be shifted by each setting of his masking dial for each test frequency. To use the table accurately, however, the clinician must be aware of several additional factors.

Effective Levels Refer to Any Ear. The values in our table are effective levels, defined as the number of decibels that the total energy in a critical band is above the threshold energy for a tone whose frequency is at the center of the band. Beyond a certain minimum level, there is a one-to-one relationship between the effective level of a noise and threshold shift in the presence of that noise. Since the values in the table are effective levels according to normal hearing (audiometric zero), they can be interpreted as the hearing threshold levels to which the ear will be shifted. Finally, we can see that this is true for any ear, not just the normal ear. For example, going back to the illustration we used under "Computation of Effective Level," we saw that white noise at an overall intensity of 80 dB gave us an effective level in the normal ear of 53.2 dB at 1000 Hz. A threshold shift of 53.2 dB re 0 dB hearing threshold level would produce, of course, a hearing threshold level of 53.2 dB. Now then, if we apply that white noise (overall intensity of 80 dB) to an ear with a hearing loss (e.g., 40 dB hearing threshold level), the effective level and threshold shift would be smaller than in the normal ear, but the hearing threshold level to which the ear would be shifted would be the same (53.2 dB). Remember that the computation of effective level for a given ear requires us to subtract that ear's threshold in quiet, expressed in sound pressure level, from the total energy in the critical band. Computation for determining effective level in the ear with a 40 dB hearing loss would be:

$$Z = 42.2 + 18 - 47$$

$$Z = 13.2 \text{ dB}$$

The value of 47 in the computation is a hearing loss of 40 dB for a 1000 Hz tone expressed in sound pressure level (7 dB at audiometric zero plus the 40 dB loss). Effective level in this ear, and thus the threshold shift, would be 13.2 dB. A threshold shift of 13.2 dB from a hearing threshold level of 40 dB would be to a hearing threshold level of 53.2 dB. Thus, we can interpret the effective levels according to the audiometric zero in our table as the hearing threshold levels to which an ear will be shifted, regardless of hearing loss in the ear. This assumes that the pathologic ear will show the same linear response to masking noise as the normal ear. While clinical experience suggests that undermasking with the effective level method is generally not a problem, there may be instances where masking an ear with sensory-neural impairment produces questionable results. In such cases, the clinician should combine the effective level approach with the Hood technique to be described later.

Effective Level Is by Air Conduction. It is important to remember that when we talk about the effective levels in our table as the hearing threshold levels to which an ear will be shifted, we mean by *air conduction*, not by bone conduction. The introduction of masking noise into an ear does not change the air-bone relationship in that ear. For example, if we introduce an effective level of 50 dB from our table into an ear with an air-conduction threshold of 40 dB and a bone-conduction threshold at 0 dB HTL, the air-conduction threshold in that ear will be shifted 10 dB to the 50-dB HTL, but the bone-conduction threshold in that ear will be shifted to only 10 dB HTL, a 10-dB change. If we now increase our effective level to 60 dB, the air-conduction threshold will shift to 60 dB HTL, but the bone threshold will shift to only 20 dB HTL. The air-bone gap in that ear remains the same. In effect, in masking an ear with a 40-dB air-bone gap, we are losing 40 dB of effective masking in our attempt to shift bone-conduction threshold in that ear. This is why in the formula approach cited in this chapter for determining minimum effective masking levels Liden et al. (1959a) included subtraction of the air-bone gap in the masked ear. Since our concern in masking is with bone-conduction sensitivity in the masked ear, awareness of this loss of effective masking due to an air-bone gap is of great importance.

Occlusion Effect. The occlusion effect, described by Liden et al. (1959b), Feldman (1961), Studebaker (1962), Dirks and Swindeman (1967) and others, is an improvement in bone-conduction responses in an ear that is covered (occluded) by an earphone. The improved responses are a result of sound pressure generated in the closed external auditory canal and transmitted through the conductive mechanism. True sensitivity is not changed, but response is obtained at better hearing threshold levels because of the additional energy reaching the cochlea. Since the additional energy is transmitted through the conductive mechanism, the effect does not occur in the ear with conductive impairment. The effect might be as great as 25 dB (Dirks and Swindeman, 1967) but is limited to the lower frequencies, primarily 125, 250 and 500 Hz. Because of the occlusion effect, 30 dB of effective masking must be added to the minimum effective level when testing at these frequencies, unless the masked ear is known to have a conductive impairment.

Some Illustrative Cases. The following cases are presented to illustrate the use of an effective masking table. For effective levels in these cases we will use the example given earlier (Table 11.3) as our effective masking table, assuming that the white noise generator has been calibrated in effective levels and that these values are given in Table 11.3. The five illustrative cases are shown in Figure 11.8.

Case A. In this case we obtain air-conduction threshold responses at a hearing threshold level of 60 dB in the right ear after ascertaining that air- and bone-conduction thresholds in the left ear are at 0 dB HTL. As we have already seen in our discussion of when to mask, the right ear response must be checked with masking in the left ear. The minimum effective masking level we can use in this case is 10 dB. If the right ear response is actually due to crossover of the test signal to the left ear, a 10-dB threshold shift in the left ear should cause the response to disappear. In this case,

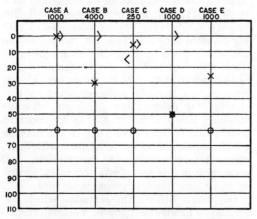

Fig. 11.8. Five hypothetical cases illustrating the application of effective masking.

however, we can use an effective level greater than the minimum without danger of overmasking. An effective level of 40 dB in the left ear would produce a substantial threshold shift in that ear without danger of masking crossover to the right ear, even if bone-conduction threshold in the right ear is at 0 dB. In this case, we set the masking dial to 60, shifting threshold in the left ear to a hearing threshold level of 40 dB. With this level of masking noise present in the left ear, we redetermine threshold in the right ear. If the response continues at 60 dB, we can accept it as a true threshold, since the difference between the test signal and bone-conduction sensitivity in the masked ear is now only 20 dB. Disappearance of the response at 60 dB, however, does not guarantee that it was a result of crossover, since it could disappear as a result of central masking. If the redetermined threshold is at 70 dB, this can be accepted as correct, since with the left ear at 40 dB HTL, the interaural difference is only 30 dB and insufficient for crossover. If, on the other hand, the redetermined threshold is at 85 dB or higher (interaural difference of 45 dB or more), masking must be increased and threshold search continued until a stable threshold response is obtained with an effective level in the left ear that is no more than 40 dB below presentation level in the right ear. In some instances, of course, this might never occur. If, for example, threshold in the right ear is actually so poor as to be beyond the limits of the audiometer, we would eliminate the response entirely in that ear with increasing levels of masking and thus demonstrate the profound nature of the hearing loss. In still another instance, if our masking output were limited to an effective level no greater than 60 dB, we might continue to obtain a right ear response at 105 or 110 dB HTL that does not meet our criterion of acceptability. Under these circumstances we would have to conclude that actual threshold is at least as poor as and probably poorer than the last obtained response.

Case B. Air-conduction responses are obtained for a 4000-Hz tone at 60 dB HTL in the right ear with left ear thresholds established at 30 dB by air and 0 dB by bone conduction. Here again we recognize the need to check the right ear response with masking in the left ear, since the difference between the presentation level in the test ear and bone-conduction sensitivity in the nontest ear is 60 dB, considerably greater than the expected interaural attenuation of 40 dB. As in Case A, the minimum threshold shift in the masked ear is 10 dB. We cannot use an effective level of only 10 dB in this case because of the air-bone gap. In order to shift the bone-conduction sensitivity in the left ear to a hearing threshold level of 10 dB, we must use an effective level of 40 dB (dial setting of 55), shifting air-conduction threshold to 40 dB and thus shifting bone conduction to 10 dB. With a 40-dB interaural attenuation for the masking noise, an effective level of 40 dB would not result in overmasking, even if bone conduction threshold in the right ear is at 0 dB. If the right ear response continues at 60 dB with masking at an effective level of 40 dB in the left ear, it can be accepted as threshold. If it disappears, the procedure outlined for Case A must be followed until a response that meets our criterion of acceptability is obtained. The chances of failure to meet criterion because of insufficient masking noise output are increased in this case by the presence of the air-bone gap in the masked ear, remembering that our masking effect is decreased by an amount equal to the difference between air- and bone-conduction thresholds in the masked ear.

Case C. In this case, bone-conduction threshold responses are obtained for a 250-Hz tone in the right ear at a hearing threshold level of 15 dB, with air-conduction threshold in that ear already established at 60 dB and air- and bone-conduction thresholds in the left ear established at 5 dB. Since no interaural attenuation is expected for a tone presented by bone conduction, and since the test ear exhibits an air-bone gap greater than 10 dB, the right ear bone response must be checked with masking in the left ear. In this case a shift of 10 dB is not sufficient as a minimum. With the test signal at a low frequency, we must add 30 dB to compensate for the occlusion effect in the masked ear, making our minimum effective level 45 dB (dial setting 85). In this case, however, we can exceed the minimum level by 10 dB without danger of overmasking, since an effective level of 55 dB is only 40 dB above the bone conduction response level of the test ear.

Case D. An air-conduction response at a 50 dB HTL is obtained in the right ear for a 1000-Hz tone with previously obtained responses (unmasked) for the left ear indicating an air-conduction threshold at 50 dB and a bone-conduction threshold at 0 dB. The need for checking the right ear response with masking in the left ear is apparent. In order to bring about a minimum shift of 10 dB in bone-conduction sensitivity in the left ear, we must use an effective masking level of 60 dB (to overcome the air-bone gap). However, if bone-conduction threshold in the right ear is actually at 0 dB or even at 5 dB, an effective level of 60 dB would be overmasking since the noise level in the masked ear would exceed that hypothetical cochlear sensitivity in the test ear by more than 40 dB. If we attempt to establish a bone-conduction threshold for the right ear, we face the same masking problem. Enough masking in the left ear to produce a minimum shift of 10 dB in that ear would also eliminate a true bone-conduction response at 0 dB in the right ear. Further, if we obtain an unmasked bone-conduction threshold at 0 dB in the right ear, we have no way of knowing whether 0-dB thresholds by bone are correct in both ears or correct in one and due to crossover in the other. If one is due to crossover, we cannot tell which. Finally, the same is true for air-conduction responses. Responses in one ear might be due to crossover, and, as with the bone responses, we

cannot tell which. This problem, described by Carhart (1960) and by Feldman (1961) and labeled a "masking dilemma" by Naunton (1960), cannot be solved with standard masking procedures. The only masking approach to the problem is to increase the interaural attenuation for the masking noise. As Zwislocki (1953) and Koenig (1962a) have pointed out, this can be done by transducing the masking noise in an insert type receiver (a small hearing aid-type receiver fitted with an insert covered with a soft, rubber tip). Since this involves a much smaller area of contact between the transducer and the skull, interaural attenuation may be increased to as much as 70 to more than 90 dB.

In cases like this in which adequate masking poses problems, an excellent method for determining the true nature of the hearing loss is acoustic impedance measurement. This procedure is discussed in another chapter.

Case E. In Cases A, B and C, we considered the amount of masking to be used when air- and bone-conduction thresholds are known for the nontest ear. This is frequently not the case, since clinicians usually complete air-conduction threshold measurement for both ears before testing by bone conduction. In Case E, then, air-conduction responses are obtained at 60 dB in the right ear with air-conduction threshold previously established for the left ear at 25 dB. Since the bone-conduction threshold for the left ear might be at 0 dB HTL, the right ear response cannot be accepted without masking. In this situation the clinician has two alternatives. First, he can accept the right ear response at 60 dB temporarily and make a final decision as to the need for masking after bone-conduction testing. His second alternative is to assume a bone-conduction threshold of 0 dB in the left ear and mask accordingly.

The illustrative cases presented here were not intended to cover every possible problem in masking. They should, however, present the principles of effective masking in a manner representative enough to permit the clinician to reason from them to specific problems not covered here.

The Hood Technique

Another procedure for ensuring sufficient masking without overmasking is a technique described by Hood (1960) and referred to by various names such as the plateau method, the threshold shift method or the shadowing method. In this procedure, a threshold is obtained initially without masking. Masking is then introduced at a minimum level and increased in 10-dB steps with a redetermination of threshold at each noise level until a plateau of threshold response is reached—a level at which threshold shows no further increase with increase in masking over a range of at least 20 to 30 dB of masking noise. This method is demonstrated with two illustrative cases in Table 11.4 and Figure 11.9. In Case 1, left ear air- and bone-conduction thresholds have been established at 0 dB. Air-conduction threshold responses have been obtained at 50 dB in the right ear although, unknown to the clinician, the ear actually has a sensory-neural loss with threshold at 80 dB. Since the response at 50 dB in the right ear is actually due to crossover to the left ear, the presence of masking at a minimum effective level of 10 dB in the left ear would shift right ear response to 60 dB, as shown in Table 11.4. This response could not be accepted, of course, since the difference between presentation level to the right ear and masked threshold level of 10 dB in the left ear exceeds 40 dB. The next step would be to increase masking by 10 dB to an effective level of 20 dB. At this masking level, response in the right ear would shift to 70 dB, also unacceptable since the difference still exceeds 40 dB. Continuing the procedure of increasing masking in 10-dB steps with threshold redetermination at each step, however, would bring us to a threshold response at 80 dB. At this point we would observe no further increase in hearing threshold level response with increase in masking level in this patient, since the response is no longer due to crossover but rather is the true right ear threshold. Further shifts in left ear threshold with masking will not affect the response.

Case 2 presents a somewhat different situation. Left ear thresholds by air and bone conduction have been established at 0 dB. In the right ear, air-conduction responses are obtained at 50 dB. These responses are due to crossover, since, again unknown to the clinician, the ear actually has an air-conduction threshold at 70 dB and a bone-conduction threshold at 20 dB. Applying the Hood technique in this case, we would observe a response plateau at a 70-dB HTL in the test ear. In this case, however, if we continue to increase masking noise level, we will eventually observe a

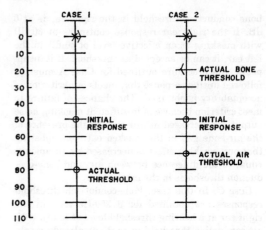

Fig. 11.9. Two hypothetical cases illustrating application of the Hood technique in masking.

further increase in threshold response. As shown in Table 11.4, at an effective level of 70 dB, threshold response would shift to 80 dB, since at this point the masking noise is more than 40 dB greater than bone conduction sensitivity in the test ear and overmasking is occurring. The masking noise is now crossing over to the cochlea of the test ear and shifting sensitivity in that ear beyond its actual level.

MASKING IN SPEECH AUDIOMETRY

Although a considerable amount of attention has been given in the literature to the subject of masking, most of that attention has been directed to masking in pure tone audiometry with little said about the equally important need for and use of masking in speech audiometry. Although the signal and the task are different in speech audiometry, since we are asking for recognition of spoken language rather than the detection of a pure tone, we still face the possibility of response from the nontest ear. Indeed, as pointed out by Studebaker (1967), the danger is increased in word discrimination testing, since we present the signal to the test ear at a suprathreshold level. It is important, then, that we direct attention to masking in speech audiometry.

First of all, it seems clear that of the generally available masking noises, white noise is the most efficient for masking in speech audiometry. Narrow bands of noise, such as those used in pure tone audiometry, are too limited in frequency response for the relatively broad spectrum speech signal (Miller, 1947; Hirsh and Bowman, 1953). Complex noise suffers from the same deficiency it exhibits as a pure tone masker (energy concentration in the lower frequencies). Although speech noise (white

TABLE 11.4. *Two Illustrative Cases of Hood Technique of Masking*

Threshold response	Effective level	Threshold response	Effective level
50	0	50	0
60	10	60	10
70	20	70	20
80	30	70	30
80	40	70	40
80	50	70	50
80	60	70	60
		80	70
		90	80

noise filtered to a low and middle frequency spectrum) is somewhat more efficient than broad band white noise, it is available only on certain audiometers. It can be used, however, in the same way as will be described for broad band white noise.

Hawkins and Stevens (1950), Liden (1954) and Liden et al. (1959b) have shown that the relationship between white noise intensity level and threshold for speech is a linear, one-to-one function. That is, beyond a certain minimum level, each additional dB of noise produces an additional dB of shift in threshold for speech.

Hawkins and Stevens (1950) demonstrated the linearity by obtaining speech thresholds in normal hearers at three different noise intensity levels. They also showed that there is good agreement between masked speech thresholds and masked pure tone threshold averages (average of the masked pure tone thresholds at 500, 1000 and 2000 Hz). These results, shown in Table 11.5, are compared with the masked speech thresholds in normal hearers obtained by Lizar et al. (1969). The table also includes masked pure tone averages derived from the results reported by Sanders and Rintelmann (1964) and shown in Figure 11.4. It should be pointed out that the masked thresholds obtained by Sanders and Rintelmann were in hearing level according to the 1951 ASA standards; whereas the pure tone thresholds of Hawkins and Stevens were sensation levels above their subjects' thresholds in quiet. Since the thresholds in quiet were within ±1 to 2 dB of the 1969 ANSI standards, the data of Sanders and Rintelmann were converted to the newer standards for presentation here.

The data in Table 11.5 show excellent agreement among the studies and demonstrate the linear nature of speech masking with white noise as well as the close agreement between

TABLE 11.5. *Masked Speech and Pure Tone Thresholds in Normal Hearers Obtained with White Noise at Three Intensity Levels Expressed in Level per Cycle*

Measures	Level per Cycle		
	40	50	60
Average TD and TI*	50.9	60.4	69.8
Pure tone average*	51.0	60.8	69.7
Speech reception threshold†	49.8	59.8	69.8
Pure tone average‡	49.2	59.0	69.0

* Hawkins and Stevens (1950). TD was threshold of detectability. TI was least intensity at which subject was able to get the meaning of almost every sentence in running speech.

† Lizar et al. (1969).

‡ Sanders and Rintelmann (1964).

masked hearing for speech and for the pure tones (500, 1000 and 2000 Hz). Thus, we can develop a table of effective masking for speech on a particular audiometer with either of two approaches.

First, effective masking levels for speech can be derived from the table of effective masking for pure tones by averaging the effective levels at 500, 1000 and 2000 Hz for each dial setting. Secondly, effective levels can be obtained through actual measurement with a group of normal hearers. The speech signal and masking noise are mixed into the same earphone and speech reception thresholds are determined at three different settings of the masking noise dial. If the dial is linear, the average thresholds obtained will show a linear relationship, and effective levels at additional dial settings can be interpolated to derive a complete table. Just as with the effective masking table for pure tone audiometry, the values in the table represent the hearing threshold levels for speech to which the masked ear will be shifted by air conduction with masking noise at the corresponding dial setting.

Liden (1954) and Liden et al. (1959b) have indicated that the interaural attenuation for speech is 50 dB. In determining when to mask, however, it is important to remember that interaural difference should be determined as the difference between presentation level to the test ear and bone conduction sensitivity in the nontest ear. If an air-bone gap is present in the nontest ear, the need for masking must be determined on the basis of the pure tone average by bone conduction in that ear. If the nontest ear does not have a conductive loss, masking can be based on the speech reception threshold or on the air conduction pure tone average if the speech reception threshold (SRT) has not been obtained. Finally, if masking is based on the pure tone average in the nontest ear, the effective level employed should be greater than the minimum level if the audiogram is irregular in configuration. In such cases the clinician can use either the 500 to 1000 Hz average or just the pure tone threshold at either 500 or 1000 Hz, whichever is better. Carhart (1971) has reported correlation coefficients between SRT and pure tone thresholds of 0.90 for 500 Hz and 0.92 for 1000 Hz. The correlation coefficient between SRT and pure tone threshold at 2000 Hz was 0.78.

MASKING IN NONTHRESHOLD AUDIOMETRY

This chapter would not be complete without at least a brief mention of the importance of masking in hearing tests other than pure tone and speech threshold audiometry. The need for masking in word discrimination testing has already been discussed. In addition, such tests as the short increment sensitivity index, the tone decay test and Bekesy audiometry frequently must be done with masking in the nontest ear if accurate results are to be obtained. This is especially true in procedures such as the tone decay test that involve signal presentation at suprathreshold levels. Without appropriate masking, it is possible to obtain a pattern of special auditory test results consistent with cochlear pathology in an ear with sensory-neural loss actually due to nerve VIII lesion. Whatever the nature of the auditory test, the safe rule to follow is that masking must be used any time there is a possibility of response from the nontest ear.

REFERENCES

Carhart, R., Assessment of sensorineural response in otosclerosis. *Arch. Otolaryngol.*, **71**, 141–149, 1960.

Carhart, R., Observations on relations between thresholds for pure tones and for speech. *J. Speech Hear. Disord.*, **36**, 476–483, 1971.

Denes, P., and Naunton, R. F., Masking in pure tone audiometry. *Proc. R. Soc. Med.*, **45**, 790–794, 1952.

Dirks, D., Factors related to reliability of bone conduction. Ph.D. dissertation, Northwestern University, 1963.

Dirks, D., Bone-conduction measurements. *Arch. Otolaryngol.*, **79**, 594–595, 1964.

Dirks, D., and Malmquist, C., Changes in bone-conduction thresholds produced by masking in the nontest ear. *J. Speech Hear. Res.*, **7**, 271–278, 1964.

Dirks, D., and Swindeman, J. G., The variability of occluded and unoccluded bone-conduction thresholds. *J. Speech Hear. Res.*, **10**, 232–249, 1967.

Egan, J. P., and Hake, H. W., On the masking pattern of a simple auditory stimulus. *J. Acoust. Soc. Am.*, **22**, 622–630, 1950.

Feldman, A. S., Problems in the measurement of bone conduction. *J. Speech Hear. Disord.*, **26**, 39–44, 1961.

Fletcher, H., Auditory patterns. *Rev. Mod. Physics*, **12**, 47–65, 1940.

Fletcher, H., and Munson, W. A., Relation between loudness and masking. *J. Acoust. Soc. Am.*, **9**, 1–10, 1937.

Glorig, A., *Audiometry: Principles and Practices*. Baltimore: Williams & Wilkins Co., 1965.

Hawkins, J. E., and Stevens, S. S., Masking of pure tones and of speech by white noise. *J. Acoust. Soc. Am.*, **22**, 6–13, 1950.

Hirsh, I. J., and Bowman, W. D., Masking of speech by bands of noise. *J. Acoust. Soc. Am.*, **25**, 1175–1180, 1953.

Hood, J. D., Principles and practice of bone conduction audiometry. *Laryngoscope*, **70**, 1211–1228, 1960.

Jerger, J. F., Tillman, T. W., and Peterson, J. L., Masking by octave bands of noise in normal and impaired ears. *J. Acoust. Soc. Am.*, **32**, 385–390, 1960.

Koenig, E., On the use of hearing-aid type earphones in clinical audiometry. *Acta Otolaryngol.*, **55**, 131–143, 1962a.

Koenig, E., The use of masking noise and its limitations in clinical audiometry. *Acta Otolaryngol.*, Suppl. 180, 1, 1962b.

Liden, G., Speech audiometry. *Acta Otolaryngol.*, Suppl. 114, 72–76, 1954.

Liden, G., Nilsson, G., and Anderson, H., Narrowband masking with white noise. *Acta Otolaryngol.*, **50**, 116–124, 1959a.

Liden, G., Nilsson, G., and Anderson, H., Masking in clinical audiometry. *Acta Otolaryngol.*, **50**, 125–136, 1959b.

Lizar, D., Peck, J., Schwartz, A., and Stockdell, K., Masking in speech audiometry. Unpublished report, Vanderbilt University, 1969.

Lybarger, S. F., Interim bone conduction thresholds for audiometry. *J. Speech Hear. Res.*, **9**, 483–487, 1966.

Miller, G. A., The masking of speech. *Psych. Bull.*, **44**, 105–129, 1947.

Naunton, R. F., A masking dilemma in bilateral conduction deafness. *Arch. Otolaryngol.*, **72**, 753–757, 1960.

O'Neill, J. J., and Oyer, H. J., *Applied Audiometry*. New York: Dodd, Mead & Co., 1966.

Sanders, J. W., and Rintelmann, W. F., Masking in audiometry; a clinical evaluation of three methods. *Arch. Otolaryngol.*, **80**, 541–556, 1964.

Studebaker, G. A., On masking in bone-conduction testing. *J. Speech Hear. Res.*, **5**, 215–227, 1962.

Studebaker, G. A., Clinical masking of air- and bone-conducted stimuli. *J. Speech Hear. Disord.*, **29**, 23–35, 1964.

Studebaker, G. A., Clinical masking of the nontest ear. *J. Speech Hear. Disord.*, **32**, 360–371, 1967.

Wegel, R. L., and Lane, C. E., Auditory masking of one pure tone by another and its probable relation to dynamics of inner ear. *Phys. Rev.*, **23**, 266–285, 1924.

Zwislocki, J., Eine verbesserte vertaubungsmethode fur die audiometrie. *Acta Otolaryngol.*, **39**, 338–356, 1951. Translations: Beltone Institute for Hearing Research, No. 19, April, 1966.

Zwislocki, J., Acoustic attenuation between ears. *J. Acoust. Soc. Am.*, **25**, 752–759, 1953.

chapter 12

SPEECH RECEPTION THRESHOLD

Norma T. Hopkinson, Ph.D.

What is speech reception threshold (SRT)? There are several answers to that question, because there are different hearing measures which could be called SRT. The audiologist typically uses SRT to refer to the threshold of intelligibility. The threshold of intelligibility is the level (in dB) at which the listener is able to identify approximately 50% of spondaic words.

Other measures which are similar to the threshold of intelligibility are the thresholds of detectability and perceptibility. The threshold of detectability is simply the level at which the listener is able to detect the presence of a speech signal about one-half of the time. The threshold of perceptibility is obtained by using a sample of continuous discourse and is defined as the level at which the listener is just able to understand the message with effort (Egan, 1948).

Although these hearing tests are quite similar, the average performance for listeners on these three procedures varies somewhat. The threshold of detectability requires the least amount of intensity, perceptibility requires an additional 8 dB and the threshold of intelligibility requires 4 dB more than the latter (or 12 dB more than detectability) (Egan, 1948).

The second leading question is why do you want to obtain an SRT? Is it for research or diagnostic purposes or perhaps to determine residual hearing? For research purposes as an indicator of the level of hearing sensitivity, you might choose to use a specific prescribed method presenting the speech signals and recording the response.

The SRT by itself is rarely used to identify the site of lesion but it is often used in differentiating true hearing loss from nonorganic hearing loss and as a measure of residual hearing. The SRT may provide the audiologist with important insight into how well a particular patient is utilizing the information that he hears. We will be primarily concerned with SRT in this chapter. Terms that are now used to describe SRT are: spondaic word threshold,

The work reported in this chapter was supported in part by grants NS 04105 and NS 12501 CDR from the National Institutes of Neurological Diseases and Stroke of the United States Public Health Services.

threshold for spondaic words, or just spondaic threshold.

HISTORY OF SPEECH THRESHOLD TESTING

Historically, speech threshold testing dates back to the times when specialists obtained estimates of a patient's hearing empirically by using spoken and whispered voice tests at various distances from the listener. Fletcher (1929) devised a table showing hearing loss categories as a function of the distance between speaker and listener. Because intensity levels could not be validated in each instance where whispered voice was used, a quantity of hearing impairment for speech was difficult to specify. As a result of attempts to quantify hearing for speech, more controlled and reliable measures were initiated.

The first widely used recorded auditory test for measuring hearing loss for speech was developed at Bell Telephone Laboratories in 1926. The test called Western Electric 4A (later 4C) was a recording of spoken digits (Fletcher and Steinberg, 1929). For many years the phonograph records were the standard recorded materials used in the group testing of school children (Hirsh, 1952).

Three requirements were indicated for measurement of hearing impairment for speech: (1) adequate test materials, (2) suitable equipment and (3) a baseline of speech thresholds for a group of normal listeners (Hudgins et al., 1947). The recorded materials that were developed at Harvard Psychoacoustics Labs included attenuated auditory tests No. 9 and No. 12 and spondaic constant level, No. 14. Tests No. 9 and 14 were composed of the same list of spondaic words. No. 12 was a list of sentences which was in the form of questions. The spondaic words were selected to be (1) familiar to the listeners, (2) dissimilar in phonetic construction, (3) a normal sampling of English speech sounds and (4) homogeneously audible. Homogeneous audibility refers to a narrow range of intensity levels at which all of the words become identifiable. Thus, we see a sharp increase in the curve showing the relationship of intensity levels to the percentage of words correct (Hudgins et al., 1947). Additional tests were developed at the Central Institute for the Deaf (CID). The purpose was to restrict vocabulary level to suit a general clinical population. Speech reception tests W-1 and W-2 were developed as the CID recorded versions of auditory tests No. 14 and No. 9, respectively (Hirsh et al., 1952).

Speech thresholds have been obtained for various speech materials such as monosyllabic words, sentences and connected discourse; however, these materials are used less frequently than spondees (Harris, 1965). One usually assumes that the threshold of intelligibility has been used as the method and spondaic words as the materials in clinical audiology. When this is not the case the variation should be carefully noted.

Materials such as nonsense syllables or synthetic sentences (Jerger, Speaks and Trammell, 1968) will be the source of some investigation in the future, especially as they might be appropriate to measure threshold of detectability or an awareness of speech. In these materials, meaningful context is limited as a variable but it would appear they will not be in widespread clinical use very soon.

PURPOSE OF SPEECH RECEPTION TESTING

The speech reception threshold is used as the basis for setting a level for speech discrimination testing. That is, a level which is most comfortable and provides the highest discrimination scores which can be tested in a more time-consuming manner or simply approximated with the use of SRT.

The SRT serves as a check on the relationship between pure tone thresholds for test frequencies associated with the understanding of speech and an actual measure of the listener's ability to hear speech. While we would expect a close relationship between SRT and the thresholds for certain pure tones there are many factors which might interfere with this close relationship. Two of these factors are the shape of the audiogram within the speech frequencies and the degree of nonorganicity the patient might have shown on pure tone testing. SRTs can be compared with special tests of nonorganic hearing loss such as the speech Stenger and the Doerfler-Stewart among others.

The SRT can be used in categorizing hearing impairment, or for considering a hearing aid, as well as for other habilitative and rehabilitative needs. The SRT is used in hearing aid evaluation to judge the amount of gain needed by the patient in the relative benefits of amplification over unaided performance.

DEFINITION OF SPEECH RECEPTION THRESHOLD

For practical, clinical purposes we can define SRT as the faintest intensity at which the listener correctly repeats approximately 50% of the spondaic words. Spondees are simple two-syllable compound words which have equal stress on each monosyllable.

The SRT is a highly reliable threshold and is relatively rapid to administer. It is not as subject to criticisms of instability as are other threshold measures (Hirsh, 1952; Swets, 1961). To date, decision theory and forced choice techniques have not replaced the more traditional SRT in audiology clinics. This may be because the SRT is a simple procedure which is rapid, requires little preparation of the patient, is widely applicable, is reliable and offers practical information for the clinical audiologist. There is no indication that the basic SRT procedure will be changed in audiology clinics in the last half of the 1970s.

The threshold of intelligibility for speech is obtained using spondaic words spoken with equal emphasis on each syllable. With either a live voice or recorded speech procedure the intensity levels are varied systematically to find the threshold value.

In order to determine the typical SRT value, thresholds were established independently of response to pure tone signals (ASA-1953). A statistical average SRT was computed based on the results of normal listeners. The result was 22 dB sound pressure level (SPL) re 0.0002 microbar (20 μPa) and that level was used as a basis for 0 dB in most commercially available speech audiometers (ASA-1953). The standard for intelligible speech has been revised as 19 dB above 0.0002 microbar (20 μPa). The standard reference threshold sound pressure level applies to the use of Western Electric Type 705-A earphones, in the National Bureau of Standards 9-A coupler (ANSI-1970).

If the Telephonics TDH-39 earphone is used, the reference threshold sound pressure level should be 20 dB above 0.0002 microbar. The TDH-39 earphone is that most often supplied by manufacturers of speech audiometers in the United States.

SRT AND PURE TONE AVERAGE

When the ISO-1964 standard for pure tones was instituted, some discussion followed over a reference level for speech that would correspond to the threshold for pure tone signals. The correspondence would appear to have face validity; however, an independent standard based on the response of normal ears to speech was used. The interdependence of the reception of speech signals and the detection of pure tone signals within the range of speech frequencies cannot be overlooked. The relationship was studied systematically as far back as the 1920s (Fletcher, 1929), and is even supported in masking studies (Hawkins and Stevens, 1950). Masking noise within the speech frequencies effectively masks speech.

The relationship between pure tone and SRT can vary somewhat depending on the following: (1) the kind of speech threshold investigated, (2) the speech materials used and (3) the method of testing (Jerger et al., 1959). The major concern here is with the threshold of intelligibility using spondaic words.

The average pure tone result for 500, 1000, and 2000 Hz has been the most popular method for predicting a relationship between pure tone and speech thresholds. The average of the two smallest threshold levels among the three speech frequencies is another method used clinically (Fletcher, 1950; Carhart and Porter, 1971). In general, these methods cannot predict without error the complex effects of frequency and energy in speech dynamics nor can the effects of distortion and perception be eliminated from this measurement. French and Steinberg (1947) have shown that certain frequency ranges are more important to accurate speech discrimination than others. To some extent the configuration of the hearing pattern and the specific spondees will also influence the SRT. Time is another factor which is not considered in the speech average. Speech is a rapid series of sounds, whereas pure tone thresholds are obtained by a comparatively slow series of long constant tones.

ARTICULATION FUNCTION FOR SPONDEES

Figure 12.1 shows how rapidly the intelligibility of spondaic words rises as a function of intensity (Hudgins et al., 1947). Threshold for spondees can be reached more precisely because of the steepness of the articulation function. The average slope for selected spondees is 10% per dB over the range between 20 and 80% correct.

Between the 50% correct point and the 66% point on the *ordinate* in Figure 12.1, required increase in intensity is a little over 1 dB on the

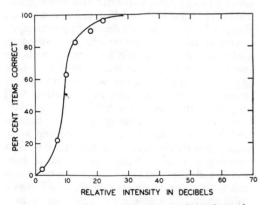

FIG. 12.1. The articulation function for spondaic words based on a figure in Hudgins et al. (1947). The steep rise of the percentage correct score is shown as a function of intensity.

abscissa. As long as methods and materials are used that satisfy the criterion of a steep rise in intelligibility, other factors in speech reception testing become less critical.

SRT METHOD

SRT is a stable measure, provided the patient is cooperative, well motivated and well informed. The results can be repeated on retest within 5 dB. SRT was found to be highly reliable on both normals and patients when it was first studied (Hudgins et al., 1947).

SRT can be administered quickly with a minimum of instruction. The patient needs only to hear examples of test words. When he hears the initial words loudly enough to identify them, he usually will generalize quickly to such words at lower intensities.

Presentation of spondees can be flexible. The clinician may improvise the presentation of words to suit the patient's clinical needs. He is not compelled to follow a rigid structure of testing, and may be guided in his presentation by the responses of the patient. If a patient always misses the word "hothouse" even at high levels of presentation, while he repeats correctly all of the other spondees at the same levels, he must be assumed to have a set against repeating "hothouse." The clinician will be wise to omit the word in the remainder of the test.

In studies of speech reception and word discrimination testing, a carrier phrase has been used. In word discrimination testing the phrase has been used to aid the speaker to monitor some sample of speech so that the final word may be emitted naturally. The reasons for using a carrier phrase preceding spondees cannot be the same, since the spondee itself is monitored with equal emphasis on each syllable; however, the phrase may make the speaker's work easier in the recording of materials. At one time it was thought that the carrier phrase prepared the patient for listening (Egan, 1948). The carrier phrase was used, when the carbon button microphone was in use, to "agitate the particles of carbon and reduce the variability inherent in such microphones" (Egan, 1948). Martin and Pennington (1971) reported that common usage of the carrier phrase is favored by 50% of the respondents to the questionnaire and the other 50% do not use the carrier phrase.

Recorded or Live Voice Presentation

There appears to be little difference between live voice and recorded SRTs (O'Neill and Oyer, 1966). Continued research studies have supported what started as a clinical observation (Beattie, Edgerton, Svihovec, 1975a; Beattie,

Svihovec, Edgerton, 1975b; Beattie, Forrester, Ruby, 1977). Of course recorded tests provide greater standardization from test to test and from center to center. The recorded tests include the calibration tone to properly set the sensitivity gain (Harris, 1965; O'Neill and Oyer, 1966; Newby, 1972).

The most commonly used recorded versions are the CID W-1, a constant level recording, and the CID W-2 recording on which the presentation level is decreased by 3 dB after every 3 words. A 1000-Hz calibration tone was recorded on each record and a carrier phrase preceded each word. These two tests are available in either 78.26 rpm or 33.33 rpm.

Although the recordings are available commercially, and receive widespread use, some clinicians choose to make magnetic tape recording of their own voices for speech testing. If that is done, the carrier phrase and test words can be recorded at the same level, rather than at different levels as done on the commercially available W-2 disc recordings. The first discs were recorded with the first nine carriers at the level of the first three words. The remainder of the carriers decreased 3 dB after every set of three carrier phrases, so that they remained 6 dB above the word that followed (Hirsh et al., 1952). The advantage of the increased level of the carrier phrase is apparent when the spondees reach a level of poorer intelligibility. The listener is then able to identify the space in which the word occurred (Hirsh et al., 1952).

Detailed instructions on how to use the W-1 and W-2 tests effectively are provided with copies of the records.* Between 1956 and 1958 the shape of the groove was changed in cutting the recordings, so that, since 1959, a 1.0-mil stylus has been appropriate. The tone arms on many speech audiometers were equipped with larger 2.5-mil styli at one time and are inappropriate for use with the more recent recordings (Lilly and Franzen, 1968).

Recorded speech reception tests are more standardized than live voice tests but are more difficult to vary. The flexibility of live voice testing that allows the clinician to fit the test to the patient's needs is missing in the recorded method.

Speech reception testing is very effective using a live voice method. Harris (1946) found a close relationship between auditory test No. 9 and pure tone thresholds, whether the test was presented from a recording or by live voice.

Several factors may militate against the use of recordings to measure speech threshold. One

of these is the age of the patient, another is whether the patient "thinks" in English, and whether any disability deters a rather rapid response. An adult whose first language was not English, generally, will be able to repeat spondees acceptably well. Depending on many other factors, a monitored live voice presentation rather than recorded presentation may be necessary, as well as improvisation of materials. In a clinical setting speech reception measures can be modified to meet the needs of each patient.

In either method, to make sure that the patient understands the task, the clinician may ask the patient, in a face-to-face situation, to repeat several spondees after him. The clinician may provide the patient with a printed list of the words (Jerger et al., 1959; Chaiklin, 1959), which is appropriate for those with reasonable proficiency in reading English.

A descending, ascending, descending technique has been recommended for both recorded and live voice procedures. Large steps up or down would not be possible if the attenuated recordings were being used (Harris, 1965; Newby, 1972). Definition of the 50% point of intelligibility varies depending on the procedure used (O'Neill and Oyer, 1966; Newby, 1972). As long as the major criterion of a rapid rise from 0 to 100% intelligibility is satisfied, these other factors remain a matter of the clinician's preference.

Descending vs. Ascending Method

In a report of most commonly used methods, more of the responding audiologists used bracketing to establish SRTs than any other method. The second largest group used descending steps and only one-fifth of a total of 290 respondents used ascending steps (Martin and Pennington, 1971). The CID W-1 and W-2 versions are also designed incorporating a descending technique.

One of the arguments for using an ascending technique is to maintain consistency with the commonly proposed method for pure tone testing. A few investigations which were mainly concerned with a method incorporating 5-dB steps or 2-dB steps in the SRT, also dealt with a descending or ascending method. Chaiklin and Ventry (1964) using a descending technique showed no significant difference in SRT between a 2- and a 5-dB step. Chaiklin, Font and Dixon (1967) using an ascending technique and 5-dB steps demonstrated that SRT was a valid and reliable procedure. The same authors point out that there are patients for whom a descending procedure may be preferable, among those young children and persons who do not take instructions well. In summary, on the basis of available research there is no

---

* Technisonic Studios, 1201 South Brentwood Blvd., Richmond Heights, Missouri 63117.

clinically significant difference in SRT obtained in using either a live voice or recorded procedure, in ascending or descending technique, or 2- or 5-dB increments.

Proposed Methods

There may be as many different methods of testing SRT as there are clinical audiologists. These methods may be appropriate to the patients and effective for the clinicians using them. Much has been written about recorded SRT methods (Jerger et al., 1959; Chaiklin, 1959). Very little has been written on a live voice technique; consequently, the following section includes a suggested procedure using live voice as well as a procedure for a recording.

First, we will briefly review the W-1 recorded procedure. The test material in W-1 is a list of 36 spondaic words. Six lists of W-1 are available, each list being a different scrambling of the same 36 words. Identification of the list is provided at the beginning of each recorded test, for example; "This is CID auditory test W-1, list A . . . Are you ready?" The carrier phrase is "Say the word."

Auditory test W-1 is the "constant level" test referred to earlier. The carrier phrase has been recorded approximately 10 dB above the average level of the words. If you have set the calibration tone to the reference point on your meter, the carrier phrase will monitor close to the reference point but the words will monitor 10 dB below it. The test is designed for use with the step attenuator to obtain the greatest possible flexibility and speed in finding speech thresholds.

The familiarity procedure is to show the listener an alphabetical list of the words that he is to hear. The listener is instructed to repeat as many of the words as he can and to guess when he is not sure of a word. Next, the calibration tone of the W-1 recording should be set to the reference level on your meter. Begin with the setting of the attenuator such that the listener easily understands the first two or three words presented to him in the ear under test. Reduce the intensity of the words until the listener can just hear the carrier phrase but cannot repeat the test words correctly. The instructions presented with the W-1 record state that the intensity should be increased until he repeats correctly some but not all of the test words presented to him. If the listener repeats approximately half of the words correctly the setting of the attenuator represents his threshold. Not more than three or four words should be needed at each dial setting. The difference between the attenuator reading and the reading for the normal threshold established for your apparatus represents the hearing loss for speech. If the obtained threshold is to be compared with the dial reading you must subtract 10 dB to compensate for the fact that the spondees were 10 dB below the calibration tone.

The method described next is one using live voice. The purpose of this clinical approach is to capitalize on the way in which each patient responds, to determine just how many of the cues in everyday speech he or she might be able to identify and put to good use for communication. More rigid procedures can be saved for the tests which provide more diagnostic information than SRT.

Suggested Procedure

Introduction. The patient brings a different mechanism to the test situation than the subject with normal hearing. He brings a different set for hearing and listening and, therefore, different criteria. These subtleties will depend on numerous other factors as disparate as hearing losses and personality traits themselves. Many parts of the procedure are based on the assumption that patients, although not classifiable as nonorganic, have imprecise criteria for listening. The patient's criteria for listening in combination with a belief that he is handicapped affect his approach to the task. The following procedure attempts to structure the SRT so that the effects of criterial factors are minimized.

Instructions. Instructions can be designed to counter the patient's lack of sophistication in listening tasks. By using specific, carefully chosen instructions the audiologist can reduce the variability due to imprecise criteria. Too much and too little instruction have the same effect. In fact, a patient may be less confused by re-instruction than he is by excessive direction before the test is begun.

The method proposed here assumes the use of a calibrated speech audiometer that meets ANSI-1969 specifications and an adequate sound test environment. Instructions are given face-to-face as follows: "I am going to say some words to you that have two parts; words like airplane, baseball, mushroom, eardrum. My voice will get softer and softer. Just repeat the words after me. If you are not sure of a word, do not be afraid to guess."

If the patient seems to have difficulty with English, ask him to repeat the examples as you say them in the instructions. The printed list of words should be presented to him if he has extreme difficulty in verbal communication. The list should not be kept by the patient during the test. All recent SRT methods concerned with providing a standardized approach utilize familiarization with the printed list.

Better Ear. Earphones are placed so that the clinician is aware of which phone is on which ear. The better ear is tested first. With a knowledge of the pure tone air-conduction responses the clinician will be able to choose a level to begin the test at approximately 20 dB above the threshold at 1000 Hz. The audiologist speaks one spondee for each of 2-dB or 5-dB decrease (Chaiklin and Ventry, 1964). The audiologist monitors his voice on the volume unit (VU) meter to 0 dB (± 2 dB) with equal stress on each syllable. As the patient begins to show signs of having trouble responding to the words, more words are spoken at each decrease. The speech reception score is recorded as the level 2 dB above which the patient cannot repeat any more words correctly. The derived SRT will be 2 to 8 dB above the speech detection threshold and therefore provide an excellent estimate of the SRT without the laborious exercise of finding the 50% point.

The speech reception score is used as reference for the sensation level of the recorded word discrimination test. If the clinician wishes to save time he may administer the speech discrimination test at this point to the better ear.

Poorer Ear. Whether or not the discrimination testing was done in the better ear the intensity is set at 20 dB above the SRT in the better ear. The poorer ear is approached without calling this to the patient's attention. Spondaic words are spoken as they were to the better ear. If the patient responds, a speech reception score is obtained. The audiologist may follow this by word discrimination testing for that ear.

When the poorer ear is approached in the manner described above, if the patient does not respond after a few repetitions of a spondee he has repeated before, the following method is recommended: If a window is available, the clinician will look into the room at the patient without changing the attenuator setting. He asks, while allowing the patient to see his lips and face, whether or not the patient hears anything. It is probable that the patient will respond negatively. The audiologist does not permit the patient to see him as he says into the microphone, "All right, now we shall make the sound louder." The clinician increases the intensity 5 dB and says one spondee, which he repeats if there is no response. He continues to raise intensity then in 5-dB steps, saying spondees until the patient repeats the word. When the patient has responded, the descent is begun. When a score is obtained, if it is less than 30 dB greater than the score for the better ear (provided that there is no air-bone gap), it should be recorded as the speech reception score for the poorer ear.

If the patient responds at 30 dB or more above the speech reception score (or bone conducted responses) for the better ear, that number should be kept as an unmasked score for reference purposes. And at that same level, the audiologist will direct his next instructions to the better ear and allow the patient to see his face. "I am going to put a noise in your better ear. Just ignore it and say the words as best you can, in spite of the noise."

The level of the contralateral masking noise should be checked for calibration and directed to the better ear. The audiologist maintains the same level of intensity in the poorer ear at which he left it, and asks the patient, "Do you hear the noise?" The patient is not able to see the audiologist during this part of the procedure. If there is no response, the intensity is raised 5 dB and the question is asked again. This method is continued until the patient answers that he hears the noise. Immediately, the descent should begin as described in the SRT procedure for the better ear. The masked score is recorded as SRT for the poorer ear. The recorded word discrimination test is then conducted for the poorer ear.

Discussion. On the basis of clinical experience the SRT should correspond to the best of the three pure tone speech frequencies by minus 8 to plus 6 dB. The suggested procedure can be analyzed for the reasoning behind its parts. Although the value of familiarizing the patient with spondaic words before the test has been well documented (Jerger et al., 1959), the method of familiarization varies. Standard practice is to present the listener with a printed list. The practice of emphasizing a few typical spondees using live voice or of having the patient repeat examples face-to-face seems superior in the clinical situation. The majority of patients deal well with the limited set of examples and they generalize quickly to other spondaic words.

Major departures from other recommended procedures are the use of monitored live voice presentation and the omission of a carrier phrase. Since SRT is an estimate at best, and one that is taken to task only if it is seriously disparate from other threshold measures, the most efficient method would seem to offer the greatest return for the least time investment. This is so particularly since so many other procedures in the clinical audiologic test battery are necessarily time consuming. The writer has used both the recorded and live voice procedures extensively, and finds no clinical advantage provided by the former. This judgment applies only to SRT not to discrimination testing.

The flexibility of monitored live voice testing is its greatest advantage. Flexibility is demonstrated in the following abilities: (1) to control length of time between presentations, (2) to prod a reticent patient to respond, and (3) to demonstrate to the patient that the audiologist is in full control of the test. These features reinforce the clinical efficiency of monitored live voice testing. In addition, the audiologist has learned something about how well the patient is motivated to use his residual hearing to identify cues in familiar speech. He may get the same information from the recorded test but, in general, he has less control of the sequence of words and the time for presentation.

Another departure from recommended procedures (O'Neill and Oyer, 1966; Newby, 1972), is the testing of the better ear for both speech reception and word discrimination before the approach to the poorer ear. The reasoning is that the patient is probably expecting the poorer ear to be investigated with the same spondaic words. The patient's criteria for listening with that ear may be affected by his own thoughts that he either has no hearing in the ear or he is extremely hard-of-hearing. His attention is diverted from the poorer ear until he has had "louder" signals presented to the better ear. The PB words are such that he will either have to listen carefully to identify their elements or he will feel that they were louder and therefore, he had more success with them.

The patient is not made aware that his poorer ear is under test until he may have already responded to several words. The transition from a higher sensation level (SL) to 20 dB SL (with the better ear as the reference ear for the level) followed by immediate presentation of spondees to the poorer ear guards against the patient establishing a specific loudness-listening criterion in the poorer ear.

The approach to the poorer ear also provides an unmasked speech score that can be of significance to the clinical audiologist when he makes decisions about the patient's consistency of response. The value of this method depends somewhat on the same information obtained by pure tone, air conduction testing of the poorer ear before the use of a contralateral masking noise. When the hearing threshold levels in one ear show significantly greater loss than the other (at 500 to 2000 Hz), a record of the responses should be kept so that "crossover" levels among tests may be compared. These same crossover responses can be related to the levels obtained on the speech Stenger test and the pure tone Stenger test. Intertest consistency among crossover levels should not be overlooked.

During the masking procedure the question, "Do you hear the noise?" is not designed to find out if the patient hears the noise. The audiolo-gist is certain that he hears the noise in his better ear. It is a catch question to determine when the patient begins to hear in the poorer ear, without his attention being called to that ear.

In many cases where the patient has a 65- to 70-dB monaural loss, he describes the ear as deaf or "dead." The patient often does not attempt to use the hearing in such an ear even under test conditions. Under these circumstances, the procedure described for approaching the poorer ear without the masking noise in the better ear has provided excellent results. Because there is no sure way of knowing beforehand that the patient may behave as described, the technique is used in every case where masking finally is indicated.

SPECIAL CONSIDERATION

The spondee is appropriate to measure speech threshold for nearly every kind of patient who has reached the age at which he is able to imitate or repeat words. Adults with aphasia or other organic speech problems may be unable to make the required response. Very young children may not know some of the words especially if a hearing loss or deafness has deprived them of the stimulation of language. In these instances, single syllable numbers given in pairs by monitored live voice may be used to obtain an estimate of speech threshold. Picture cards of selected spondees may also be used so that the patient who is not able to speak intelligibly can identify the words by picking out the picture.

It may be necessary to obtain a threshold of detectability or awareness in cases of aphasia. When earphones cannot be used, or before earphones are placed on a young child, a speech awareness measure may be estimated by conversing with him, or by calling his name, using a loudspeaker and sound field system. These methods are described in greater detail in Chapter 33 on testing infants and young children.

COMMENTS

The American Speech and Hearing Association has a committee working on guidelines for SRT among other clinical procedures. That committee has grappled for several years with a number of problems associated with standardizing the test. A few of the problems are as follows: (1) use of recorded or live voice presentation, (2) use of an ascending or descending series and (3) familiarization technique and number of words (Tillman and Jerger, 1959). At this time there has been insufficient input from the clinical consumers of speech reception testing to determine what the final output of the committee will be, so it would be premature to attempt to describe any method proposed by the committee.

Tillman and Olsen (1973) and Wilson, Morgan and Dirks (1973) have proposed procedures for SRT which are very reasonable and could be readily adopted as standardized clinical methods. Both are relatively conventional methods.

Inferences about practical performance are difficult to make from the measurement of speech reception in a noise background. This method has been used as an informal clinical tool in some settings to make predictions about the patient's use of a hearing aid. The prediction has been generally inadequate because the thresholds obtained under circumstances using simulated environmental noise do not account for the variety of problems that will be encountered by the patient.

REFERENCES

American National Standards Institute Specifications for Audiometers. ANSI S3.6-1969. New York: American National Standards Institute, Inc., 1970.

American Standards Association. Specifications for Speech Audiometers. *American Standard Association Bulletin*, ASA Z24.13-1953. New York, 1953.

Beattie, R. C., Edgerton, B. J., and Svihovec, D. V., An investigation of the Auditec of St. Louis recordings of the Central Institute for the Deaf spondees. *J. Am. Audiol. Soc.*, 1, 97-101, 1975a.

Beattie, R. C., Svihovec, D. V., and Edgerton, B. J., Relative intelligibility of the CID spondees as presented via monitored live-voice. *J. Speech Hear. Disord.*, 40, 84-91, 1975b.

Beattie, R. C., Forrester, P. W., and Ruby, B. K., Reliability of the Tillman-Olsen procedure for determination of spondee threshold using recorded or live voice presentations. *J. Am. Audiol. Soc.*, 2, 159-162, 1977.

Carhart, R., and Porter, L. S., Audiometric configuration and prediction of threshold for spondees. *J. Speech Hear. Res.*, 14, 486-495, 1971.

Chaiklin, J. B., The relation among three selected auditory speech thresholds. *J. Speech Hear. Res.*, 2, 237-243, 1959.

Chaiklin, J. B., and Ventry, I. M., Spondee threshold measurement; a comparison of 2- and 5-dB methods. *J. Speech Hear. Disord.*, 2, 47-59, 1964.

Chaiklin, J. B., Font, J., and Dixon, R. F., Spondee thresholds measured in ascending 5-dB steps. *J. Speech Hear. Res.*, 10, 141-145, 1967.

Egan, J. P., Articulation testing methods. *Laryngoscope*, 58, 955-991, 1948.

Fletcher, H., *Speech and Hearing*. New York: Van Nostrand Co., 1929.

Fletcher, H., A method of calculating hearing loss for speech from an audiogram. *J. Acoust. Soc. Am.*, 22, 1-5, 1950.

Fletcher, H., and Steinberg, J. C., Articulation testing methods. *Bell Syst. Tech. J.*, 8, 806-854, 1929.

French, N., and Steinberg, J., Factors governing the intelligibility of speech sounds. *J. Acoust. Soc. Am.*, 19, 90-119, 1947.

Harris, J. D., Studies on the comparative efficiency of the free voice and the pure tone audiometer for routine testing of auditory acuity. *Arch. Otolaryngol.*, 44, 452-467, 1946.

Harris, J. D., Speech Audiometry. In Glorig, A. (Ed.), *Audiometry: Principles and Practices*, Ch. 7, pp. 151-169. Baltimore: Williams & Wilkins Co., 1965.

Hawkins, J. E., Jr., and Stevens, S. S., The masking of pure tones and of speech by white noise. *J. Acoust. Soc. Am.*, 22, 6-13, 1950.

Hirsh, J. J., *The Measurement of Hearing*. New York: McGraw-Hill Book Co., 1952.

Hirsh, J. J., Davis, H., Silverman, S. R., Reynolds, E. G., Eldert, E., and Benson, R. W., Development of materials for speech audiometry. *J. Speech Hear. Disord.*, 17, 321-337, 1952.

Hudgins, C. V., Hawkins, J. E., Karlin, J. E., and Stevens, S. S., The development of recorded auditory tests for measuring hearing loss for speech. *Laryngoscope*, 57, 57-89, 1947.

International Studies Organization Technical Committee 43-Acoustics Standard reference zero for calibration of pure-tone audiometers, 1964, no. 554. New York: American Standards Association, 1965.

Jerger, J. F., Carhart, R., Tillman, T. W., and Peterson, J. L., Some relations between normal hearing for pure tones and for speech. *J. Speech Hear. Res.*, 2, 126-140, 1959.

Jerger, J. F., Speaks, C., and Trammell, J. L., A new approach to speech audiometry. *J. Speech Hear. Disord.*, 33, 318-328, 1968.

Lilly, D. J., and Franzen, R. L., Reproducing styli for speech audiometry. *J. Speech Hear. Res.*, 11, 817-824, 1968.

Martin, F. N., and Pennington, C. D., Current trends in audiometric practices. *ASHA*, 13, 671-678, 1971.

Newby, H. A., *Audiology*, Ed. 3. New York: Appleton-Century-Crofts, 1972.

O'Neill, J. J., and Oyer, H. J., *Applied Audiometry*. New York: Dodd, Mead, & Co., 1966.

Swets, J. A., Is there a sensory threshold? *Science*, 134, 168-177, 1961.

Tillman, T. W., and Jerger, J., Some factors affecting the spondee threshold in normal hearing subjects. *J. Speech Hear. Res.*, 2, 141-146, 1959.

Tillman, T. W., and Olsen, W. O., Speech Audiometry. In Jerger, J. (Ed.), *Modern Developments in Audiology*, Ed. 2, Ch. 2, pp. 37-74. New York: Academic Press, 1973.

Wilson, R. H., Morgan, D. E., and Dirks, D. D., A proposed SRT procedure and its statistical precedent. *J. Speech Hear. Disord.*, 38, 184-191, 1973.

chapter 13

WORD DISCRIMINATION TESTING

Cornelius P. Goetzinger, Ph.D.

Precision in the measurement of hearing sensitivity at threshold gained impetus as a result of the development of the Western Electric pure tone vacuum tube audiometer in the early 1920s (Glorig, 1965). A number of studies were carried out to establish the threshold sensitivity of the human ear for pure tones as a function of frequency (Stevens and Davis, 1938). In addition, research at the Bell Laboratories focused on the intelligibility of speech as it pertained to communication over the telephone. The purpose of this chapter is (1) to acquaint the reader with the development of suprathreshold auditory discrimination testing in the United States; (2) to discuss some of the parameters, both physical and linguistic, which have a bearing on the measurement of speech discrimination; (3) to describe some of the currently used tests and (4) to present examples of the clinical use of such tests.

HISTORICAL BACKGROUND

The research of Fletcher (1929; 1953) at the Bell Laboratories during the 1920s was concerned with speech perception and discrimination as related to communication over the telephone. The articulation scores method which pertains to auditory discrimination as a function of intensity was developed and provides data on the intelligibility of the units of speech such as vowels and consonants, nonsense syllables, words and sentences. Other parameters which affect speech production and reception as voice quality, fidelity of equipment, speech-in-noise, the average speech spectrum and so forth, were also investigated with a precision not possible prior to the development of electronic equipment.

The beginning of World War II gave impetus to the study of speech in many institutions. In particular, the Psychoacoustic Laboratories (PAL) at Harvard University conducted studies pertaining to the development of tests, many of which were utilized in research and in the clinical evaluation of hearing impairment. Among them were the PAL No. 9 and No. 14 spondaic word and the No. 12 sentence tests to determine the speech reception threshold, and the PAL phonetically balanced (PB) monosyllabic word lists to evaluate auditory word dis-

crimination. Multiple choice versions of the monosyllabic word discrimination tests were likewise devised (Haagen, 1946; Black, 1957) but were used principally in research (Hirsh, 1952; Davis and Silverman, 1960, 1970; Newby, 1964; Glorig, 1965; O'Neill and Oyer, 1966). Later, Fairbanks (1958) developed the rhyme test, which was modified by House et al. (1965). Also, Lynn (1962) published a paired PB-50 test.

Hirsh (1952) recognizing several limitations in the PAL test, developed the CID (Central Institute for the Deaf) W-1 and W-2 spondaic word tests for threshold measurement, and the CID W-22 monosyllabic word lists to assess speech discrimination ability. These tests are used extensively in clinics in this country. Phonetically balanced word tests were also generated by Lehiste and Peterson (1959), Tillman, Carhart and Wilber (1963), and Tillman and Carhart (1966). Furthermore, Haskins (1949) constructed PB lists for testing children.

Bocca and Calearo (1963) in Italy noted that conventional type auditory tests were not sufficiently sensitive for the diagnosis of centrally located auditory lesions. These investigators developed word and sentence tests designed to tax the central auditory processes. Jerger (1960), Katz (1962) and others published similar tests in this country. A great deal of research has been conducted during recent years toward a better understanding of the nature of dichotic and monotic listening in normal subjects and subjects with central auditory nervous systems disorders (Kimura, 1961, 1967; Shankweiler and Studdert-Kennedy, 1967; Lowe et al., 1970; Zurif and Sait, 1970; Berlin et al., 1972; Jerger and Jerger, 1975).

SOME PHYSICAL AND LINGUISTIC PARAMETERS OF SPEECH

The articulation score method has been used by most investigators in studying the physical parameters of speech. The method involves the plotting of the percentage of speech units correctly identified by a listener as a function of the intensity of the speaker's voice. Figure 13.1, modified from Davis and Silverman (1970), shows the articulation functions for normal hearing subjects for CID spondaic words, the CID W-22 monosyllabic words and the Rush Hughes recordings of the PAL monosyllabic words.

As shown in the figure, 100% of the spondees are identified correctly at a sound pressure level (SPL) of 30 dB, as compared to about 53 dB SPL for the W-22 words. The Rush Hughes recordings of the Harvard PB-50 monosyllabic

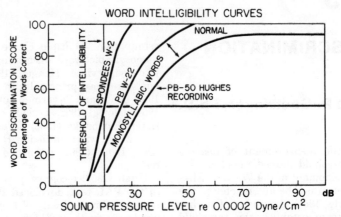

Fig. 13.1. Articulation functions for the spondee, W-22 and Rush Hughes tests. The thresholds for the tests are, respectively, 20, 27 and 33 dB SPL. The Rush Hughes test reaches a maximum at 92% intelligibility in contrast to 100% for the other two tests. (Modified from Davis and Silverman, (1970.))

words reach a maximum of 92% at an intensity of approximately 70 dB SPL. Furthermore, 50% of the spondaic words are heard correctly at a 20-dB SPL level, whereas the sound pressure must be increased to 27 and 33 dB, respectively, for the monosyllabic W-22 and PB-50 words.

These observations emphasize several factors associated with word discrimination. First, less intensity is required to reach the 50% correct threshold for the spondaic than for the monosyllabic words; second, maximum discrimination for spondees requires less intensity than for either the W-22 or the Rush Hughes recordings of the PB-50 monosyllabic words; third, spondaic words are more homogeneous in discriminability than monosyllabic words as may be deduced by the steeper slope of their articulation function; and fourth, maximum discrimination on Rush Hughes recordings of the Harvard lists reaches a plateau at 92%.

The final point focuses upon the effects of distortion either of the equipment or of the speaker's articulation upon the scores, for as Davis and Silverman (1960, p. 190) maintain, "For normal ears under good listening conditions, the plateau of the articulation curve is at 100% of words correctly understood."

The difference in sound pressure which is required to discriminate the words of the W-22 recordings as compared to the Rush Hughes PB-50 records is ascribed to word familiarity and speaker intelligibility by Davis and Silverman (1960). Although the PB-50 words are reasonably familiar, the lists do not contain as many common words as the W-22 tests. Furthermore, the articulation of the speaker (Ira Hirsh) on the W-22 records is superior to that of his counterpart (Rush Hughes) on the Harvard recordings.

Speech discrimination tests cover a wide range of difficulty which may be dependent upon the test material as well as the type of test. At one end of the spectrum, aside from isolated phonemes, are nonsense syllables followed by monosyllabic words, words of two syllables or more and sentences. Nonsense syllables, being devoid of meaning, contain no semantic cues to assist in discrimination. Monosyllabic words, as meaningful linguistic units of speech, are not as difficult as nonsense syllables. In addition, monosyllabic words in sentences are more discriminable than in isolation because of contextual cues (Miller, Heise and Lichten, 1951). Words of two syllables or more afford more cues for discrimination than monosyllabic words. Sentences are generally easier to discriminate than words. Furthermore, the percentage of words discriminated correctly, plotted relative to the signal-to-noise ratio, varies inversely with the number of items included in the list. The data of Miller et al. (1951) showed that at a signal-to-noise ratio of −9 dB (the overall level of the noise was 9 dB more intense than the words) less than 30% of a list containing 250 words was discriminated correctly as compared to about 60% of a list of 32 words if the lists were known beforehand.

Another parameter of importance in word discrimination is frequency range. Fletcher (1929) studied articulation curves as a function of intensity and frequency for many of the elementary sounds of speech (consonants and vowels). Later, French and Steinberg (1947), using a number of high and low pass filters, plotted articulation functions for consonant-vowel-consonant syllables and demonstrated the importance of frequency range to discrimination. Their curves were generated with reference to the orthotelephonic gain which is " . . . merely the transmission of a system relative to that of a standard system consisting of a talker and a listener who face one another at a distance of 1 meter in open air. For normal conversational levels, the O-dB orthotelephonic gain corresponds to approximately 65-dB SPL at a distance of 1 meter in front of a talker" (Licklider and Miller, 1951, p. 1052).

Figure 13.2 constructed from the curves of French and Steinberg (1947), shows the relation between maximum discrimination and frequency for their low and high pass filtering conditions. In Figure 13.2A, 98% of the syllables were articulated correctly at full band width of 7000 Hz. In contrast, syllable discrimination decreases progressively with each succeeding cut-off of the high frequencies. For example, only 50% of the syllables were repeated correctly when the frequencies above 1500 were filtered out. Figure 13.2B provides the same kind of information when the low instead of the high frequencies are rejected progressively. It is evident from Figure 13.2A and B, that the frequencies below 500 Hz do not contribute substantially to the auditory discrimination of syllables (about 5%). Furthermore, that equal discriminability for syllables is attained when either the lower or higher frequencies are rejected at about 1900 to 1950 Hz with the scores being 68 to 69%. Also, approximately 77% of the syllables are repeated correctly when the frequency band 500 to 2450 Hz is passed. Clearly, frequency range affects syllable discrimination. However, variables such as familiarity of the material, the recording, the speaker's articulation, the rapidity of speech and so forth may markedly influence auditory discrimination. Figure 13.3 illustrates this point.

Figure 13.3 shows that frequency cut-off is highly detrimental to the Rush Hughes test in contrast to continuous discourse. The CID sentences (recorded on tape) and the W-22 test occupy intermediate positions with the former being more discriminable. The difference between the W-22 and the Rush Hughes tests is attributable to speaker articulation and word familiarity. Another important factor is probably stylus size of the cartridge. Speech audiometers were equipped with 2.5-mil styli as

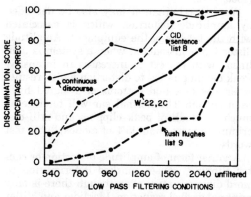

Fig. 13.3. Comparisons among continuous discourse, sentences, W-22 and Rush Hughes tests in terms of percentage of items correct for seven filtering conditions. The curves for continuous discourse, the W-22 and the Rush Hughes are from the data of Giolas and Epstein (1963); the curve for the sentence test is from Giolas (1966).

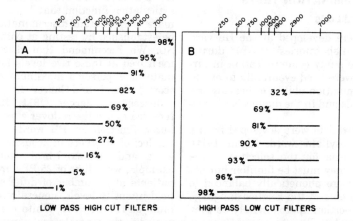

Fig. 13.2. Maximum discrimination for syllable articulation for low and high pass filter conditions as related to the cut-off frequency. The discrimination scores were derived from the curves of French and Steinberg (1947) at an orthotelephonic gain of +10 decibels (75 dB SPL).

recommended by the American Standards Association (ASA, 1953). Between 1956 and 1958 Technisonic Studios of St. Louis, Missouri, changed to universal microgroove for their recordings (Lilly and Franzen, 1968). Since the conversion to 1-mil styli in our clinic a number of years ago, the Rush Hughes recordings have not proven to be as difficult as formerly. Hall (1970) used the Rush Hughes No. 9 recording with normal subjects. The mean discrimination score for these normal listeners using the 1-mil stylus was 91.6%. This finding is in agreement with the 92% plateau for the Rush Hughes records as reported by Davis and Silverman (1960, 1970).

Word discrimination may also be degraded by amplitude distortion which is associated with the fidelity of the equipment. Amplitude distortion is introduced when a system is nonlinear with respect to increases in intensity. Peak clipping refers to distortion which results when the tops and bottoms of a signal have been cut off. The normal ear will tolerate as much as 24 dB of peak clipping and still discriminate more than 95% of monosyllabic test words.

Another form of amplitude distortion or center clipping, causes marked deterioration in word discrimination even though there is only minimal decibel reduction. Licklider and Miller (1951) showed that clipping of 6 dB reduces word discrimination to 30% or so because of its effect upon the consonants.

Other factors which affect word discrimination are noise, room reverberation (Chapter 38), interruption rate of speech, compression and expansion of speech.

DESCRIPTION OF VARIOUS DISCRIMINATION TESTS

PAL PB-50 Word Lists

These lists were developed at the Harvard Psychoacoustic Laboratories (PAL) during World War II to study communication in aircraft. The lists were used eventually to evaluate word discrimination ability of hearing impaired individuals and in the diagnosis of hearing problems.

The PB-50 word lists were developed from a pool of 1200 monosyllabic words (Egan, 1944). The general criteria for the selection of the words were that they must be familiar but not easy. The lists were phonetically balanced to contain the elements of the English language in the same proportion approximately as they occur in the language. Twenty lists of 50 words each were compiled relative to the following criteria: (1) monosyllabic structure, (2) equal average difficulty, (3) equal range of difficulty, (4) equal phonetic composition, (5) representative of English and (6) words in common usage (Egan, 1948). Later, eight of the lists (5, 6, 7, 8, 9, 10, 11 and 12) were recorded at Central Institute for the Deaf (CID) by Rush Hughes, a professional announcer in St. Louis at that time (Eldert and Davis, 1951). The articulation function shown in Figure 13.1, was generated using the Rush Hughes recordings of the PAL PB-50 lists. A study by Eldert and Davis (1951) indicated that the 8 recorded Rush Hughes tests were not equal in difficulty. Lists 5, 6, 7, 9 and 10 were equivalent. Test 8 was the most difficult and tests 11 and 12 the easiest. They recommended that 2% be added to the PB maximum score for test 8, and that 2% be subtracted for tests 11 and 12 when they were used with conductive and mixed (predominantly sensory-neural) hearing loss cases.

Davis (1948) recommended that the tests be administered routinely at 110 dB SPL for hearing losses of 55 dB or less, and at 120 dB SPL for hearing losses greater than 60 dB unless the latter causes discomfort. He stated, "The exact intensity at which the minimum discrimination loss (or the 'PB maximum score') is measured is not critical. It is only necessary that it be at least 35 dB above the patient's threshold for the Test No. 9" (Davis, 1948, p. 772). Carhart (1951-1952) recommended that the Rush Hughes test be administered at a 35-dB level. However, it is apparent now that there is no one fixed level above threshold at which the PB Max can be determined for all pathologic ears (Carhart, 1965).

Clinicians as well as researchers have long been aware that some patients exhibit rollover in the articulation function (Davis and Silverman, 1960). Clemis and Carver (1967) as a result of their research on subjects with Meniere's disease concluded that " . . . a reliable estimate of maximum discrimination ability can be established by testing at both 32 and 40 dB SL. We recommend that discrimination be measured at these two levels for a valid estimate of a person's maximum discrimination score." (Clemis and Carver, 1967, p. 618).

Jerger and Jerger (1971, 1975) have attempted to use the rollover effect of the articulation function for PB words to differentiate the loci of disorders in acoustic tumors and in extra- and intra-axial brain stem insults. For example, word lists of 25 PBs are presented to patients at a number of different suprathreshold intensity levels, generally, up to a maximum of 110 dB SPL. White noise masking is routed to the contralateral ear when the words are given loud enough to crossover to this nontest ear. In acoustic tumors the rollover effect will occur in the affected ear. Similarly, in extra-axial lesions, the rollover phenomenon is observed in the ear which is ipsilateral to the disorder. However, in intra-axial lesions the rollover effect may be manifested either bilaterally or contralaterally. After intensive study Jerger and Jerger (1975, p. 107) concluded that, "The rollover phenomenon did not reliably differentiate the two brain stem groups."

CID W-22 Word Lists

Hirsh et al. (1952) undertook a modification of the PAL PB-50 lists because of the lack of familiarity of many of the test words, and the poor standardization of the recordings. From a pool of 1000 PB-50 words, they selected 120 and added 80 new words. All but one of the words appear in Thorndike's list of 20,000 familiar words. The criteria for selecting the words included: (1) monosyllables, (2) familiarity and (3) phonetic composition corresponding to that of the English language.

The 200 words were arranged into four phonetically balanced lists of 50 words each. The criteria for phonetic balance were derived from Dewey's phonetic analysis of written language and the Bell phonetic study of New York business telephone calls. There are six recorded scramblings of each of the four lists.

Hirsh, in the test manual, recommends that the test be administered at an 80-dB SPL for subjects with hearing levels of 20 dB or less, and at a 40-dB sensation level relative to the hearing loss when the impairment exceeds 40 dB as measured by spondees. Clinicians generally recommend that word discrimination tests be administered between 25 and 50 dB sensation level in most cases for a maximum score (PB Max). A recent study by Northern and Hattler (1974) is pertinent to this problem. Data from their study are shown in Figure 13.4.

Figure 13.4 shows word discrimination for the normal hearing subjects on the W-22 test increases from 74% at a SL of 10 dB (*re* SRT) to 97% approximately at 50 dB SL. In contrast, the Rush Hughes test increases from about 34% to 87% over the 10- to 50-dB SL range. However, the results for the subjects with sensory-neural hearing loss are markedly different with discrimination increasing about 20% for the W-22 (from 50% to 70%) and about 9% (32% to 41%) for the Rush Hughes PB-50 over the 10- to 50-dB range. The PB Max is reached on both tests at 40 dB SL. The curve for the sensory-neural subjects on the W-22 test parallels essentially the normal function. Nevertheless, there is a pronounced difference between the normal and sensory-neural articulation functions for the Rush Hughes test. Apparently, the distortion in this recorded version of the test is too severe for the defective ear to

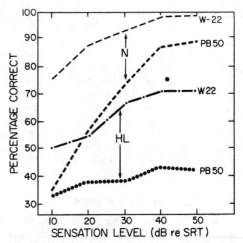

Fig. 13.4. Mean articulation scores as a function of SL for 25 normal hearing and 100 sensory-neural hearing loss subjects. There were 5 normal and 20 sensory-neural subjects at each sensation level. The "clinic" live voice discrimination score at 40 dB SL was 72% as compared with the Rush Hughes score of 44% for the same subjects at the same SL. (From the data of Northern and Hattler, 1974.)

integrate fully as a function of increasing sensation level. Some support for this position may be deduced from Figure 13.4. As noted in the caption the "clinic" live voice word discrimination average at 40 dB SL is 72% in contrast to the Rush Hughes score of 44% at the same SL for the same subjects. Although the response to the live voice test was vocal as compared to the Rush Hughes which was written, nevertheless, it is not likely that this difference explains completely the large difference in results (Northern and Hattler, 1974). As a result of their study Northern and Hattler (1974) recommended that a 40-dB+ SL be used either for the W-22 or Rush Hughes test when a single level of word discrimination testing is used. One should keep in mind the recommendation of Clemis and Carver (1967) that 32 and 40 dB SL should be used when the results from a discrimination test appear to be questionable. In our clinic, when there is a discrepancy between ears in word discrimination, we retest the poorer ear at two or three sensation levels.

In the clinical administration of the recorded PB tests (W-22 and Rush Hughes) we have found it to be expedient to use a practice period of several words (usually five) from another recorded list to prepare the patient for the test. Furthermore, the responses of the patient are monitored through lip reading in addition to the auditory to minimize tester error. Merrell and Atkinson (1965) have provided evidence of the frequency of auditor error during testing.

There are 50 words in each of the PB mono-syllabic word lists. In scoring the test two percentage points are credited for each correct response. Therefore, the patient who repeats the 50 words correctly is credited with a word discrimination score of 100%. In like manner, one who gets 35 of the words correct receives a score of 70%. As a time-saving device some clinicians have advocated the use of half lists (Elpern, 1961; Resnick, 1962). This practice is debatable (Jirsa, 1970).

NU Auditory Test Lists 4 and 6

During the intervening years, a number of researchers questioned the adequacy of the PAL PB-50 as well as the CID W-22 lists. Generally, the PAL lists include many unfamiliar words, and their phonetic balance has been challenged. The W-22 words, although highly familiar, are regarded as too easy for fine differential diagnosis. Lehiste and Peterson (1959), cognizant of the inadequacies in the phonetic balance of the PB-50 lists, developed a new monosyllabic word test.

In the construction of the test 1263 monosyllabic words of the consonant-nucleus-consonant type (CNC) were selected with a frequency count of one time or more per million words from the Thorndike list. The frequency of occurrence of each initial consonant, vowel nucleus and final consonant was determined, and incorporated into the construction of 10 lists of 50 words each. The purported advantages of the lists are: (1) only CNC words are used, (2) each list matches the phonetic balance of the parent list of 1263 words rather than English, generally, and (3) the lists consist of familiar words. However, data related to the reliability of the 10 lists are lacking (Tillman, Carhart and Wilber, 1963).

Tillman et al. (1963) using the Lehiste and Peterson lists developed the Northwestern University (NU) auditory test No. 4. They selected 95 of the 500 words comprising the ten 50-word lists of Lehiste and Peterson and added 5 more to construct lists I and II of the NU test No. 4. Research with the two lists has shown them to be interchangeable.

Later, Tillman and Carhart (1966) developed another test which they labeled the NU test No. 6. The test consists of four lists, each with 50 words. They selected 185 words from the parent list of 1263 words of Lehiste and Peterson and 15 from outside sources. The four lists were randomized four times. Research with normal hearing and sensory-neural hearing loss subjects indicated the intertest reliability to be high. Neither NU No. 4 nor NU No. 6

has had extensive clinical use. In addition, there are neither commercial recordings nor tapings of these tests. Whether or not the phonetic balance as used in the new tests (Lehiste and Peterson, 1959, and Tillman and Carhart, 1966) as compared to that of the PAL PB-50 and CID W-22 words will induce significant changes in clinical interpretation is yet to be determined. Carhart noted " . . . we have found in our laboratory that discrimination scores are not changed importantly by shift from the PB-50 to the Lehiste-Peterson criterion of phonetic balance. In general, as long as the test items are meaningful monosyllables for the patient and their phonetic distribution is appropriately diversified, one 50 word compilation is relatively equivalent to another" (Carhart, 1965, p. 254).

Rhyme Tests

Fairbanks (1958) developed the rhyme test as a more specific measure of the locus of difficulty in word discrimination problems. The test is of the multiple choice type and affords information about phonetic confusions. Kopra, Blosser and Waldron (1968) did not find any significant differences in diagnostic capability between the rhyme and the W-22 tests. The rhyme test was not as effective as the PB-50's in differentiating pathologic discrimination cases (Kryter and Whitman, 1965). Northern and Hattler (1974) administered the modified rhyme test as described by Kreul et al. (1968) and obtained essentially the same results.

Children's Lists

Phonetically balanced word lists have been constructed for children. Haskins (1949) developed four PB word lists in which the test items were within the speaking vocabularies of young children. These so-called PBK lists (phonetically balanced kindergarten) have had wide applicability in clinics throughout this country.

For children with speech defects and expressive problems several multiple choice picture identification tests have been devised. One of these tests by Ross and Lerman (1971) is used extensively in clinics.

Synthetic Sentences

Jerger, Speaks and Trammell (1968) in describing a new approach to speech audiometry, pointed out that single words as test material do not provide sufficient information on the capacity of individuals "to manipulate a crucial parameter of ongoing speech, its changing pattern over time" (Jerger et al., 1968, p. 319). Therefore, it is necessary to develop longer samples of speech. They also take note of the problems of scoring inherent in the open message set method (e.g., tester error) and the linguistic variables to which the method is vulnerable.

Jerger et al. constructed a number of lists of 10 third order approximations to real sentences. Third order synthetic sentences are characterized by the dependency of any word on the two words which precede it. An example of a third order synthetic sentence is, "Go change your car color is red." In their test Jerger et al. used a closed message set paradigm.

Jerger and his co-workers found early in their research that synthetic sentences presented in quiet were not difficult enough to reveal problems in the understanding of speech. They subsequently used an ipsilateral competing message of continuous discourse at a signal-to-noise ratio of 0 dB to make message identification more difficult (see Chapter 22).

In using the sentences diagnostically a performance intensity (PI) function (like an articulation function) is generated. The area under the curve is calculated. The area for the sentences is compared to one for PB words. Information concerning the functional state of the ear appears to be emerging from these comparisons. The use of sentence-like material appears to be necessary to get at variables in the time domain which affect auditory identification. Northern and Hattler (1974) included the synthetic sentence identification (SSI) test in their study of normal hearing subjects and subjects with sensory-neural hearing loss. They found the test to yield low intertest variability for the normal but high intertest variability for the hearing loss subjects. This is a desirable feature of a test in the view of some investigators.

Monitored Live Voice Versus Recorded Materials

The question of monitored live voice testing versus the use of recordings has been a lively issue ever since the advent of speech audiometry. Proponents of the recorded tests have stressed the point that speakers differ. Therefore, results are not comparable among clinics or laboratories unless speaker equivalence can be demonstrated. But as Carhart has noted: "There may be as much difference between one recording and another as between two live-voice talkers" (Carhart, 1965, p. 254). This would appear to imply the need for standardized recorded versions of the word discrimination tests. Moreover, standardization of equipment is imperative. Irrespective of one's proclivity in the matter, no one seriously questions the need for both methods in a clinic setting. For example, the use of monitored live voice testing with very young children and with

many aged persons often provides information quickly which otherwise might require a considerable period of conditioning or else be unattainable.

CLINICAL APPLICATION

Speech audiometry has become an integral part of the audiologic and otologic diagnosis of hearing impairment during the last 25 years. Speech is used to measure auditory sensitivity, to evaluate the functional state of the auditory system at suprathreshold levels, to contribute to the localization of specific lesions of the auditory tracts, to predict the outcome of otologic surgery, to assess the value of therapeutic procedures such as lip reading and auditory training and in the selection of hearing aids. Therefore, the application of speech audiometry, with emphasis upon word discrimination, will be discussed relative to diagnosis and prediction.

The relationship of word discrimination scores to social adequacy is not well defined. The social adequacy index as suggested by Walsh and Silverman (1946), and refined by Davis (1948), has not proven to be as effective as anticipated. The research of Jerger et al. (1968) with synthetic sentences in conjunction with word discrimination scores may increase the accuracy of tests to predict the social adequacy of hearing deficit. A general guide for evaluating word discrimination ability is as follows:

1. 90 to 100% – normal limits
2. 75 to 90% – slight difficulty, comparable to listening over a telephone
3. 60 to 75% – moderate difficulty
4. 50 to 60% – poor discrimination, difficulty in following conversation
5. Below 50% – very poor discrimination, difficulty in following running speech.

Conductive Impairment

Word discrimination scores in conjunction with bone-conduction thresholds have been used for many years to predict the outcome of surgery in otosclerosis. Unless the word discrimination scores are reasonably high, the likelihood is strong of other complications which may contraindicate surgery. Figure 13.5, *A* and *B*, illustrates preoperative conductive hearing loss with very good bone conduction and word discrimination of the right ear, and postoperative successful results.

Cochlear

Hearing impairment due to inner ear or cochlear pathology ranges from slight to total loss of hearing. Diseases such as measles, mumps, maternal rubella, viral labyrinthitis, Meniere's as well as noise exposure and acoustic trauma may induce inner ear hearing loss. Since the cochlea is the peripheral analyzer of sound it follows that lesions of cochlear origin may be expected to cause distortion in the transmission of speech. In general, there is a relationship between the degree of hearing loss and decrease in word discrimination. However, the relationship is not as high as would be desired. Figure 13.5C illustrates a decrease in word discrimination of the left ear (70%) which has greater hearing loss as compared to the right ear (84%).

The deleterious effects of high frequency filtering upon the auditory discrimination of normal hearing subjects using various types of speech material were discussed previously. It is clear that isolated words are more affected than continuous discourse. Therefore, generalizations based on word discrimination tests must be interpreted with caution. In short, patients with precipitous hearing losses in the higher frequencies are not as seriously handicapped in general conversation (in quiet) as the word discrimination scores indicate. However, variables such as age, lip reading skill,

age at onset of hearing impairment, educational and psychological factors and the acoustic environment must be taken into consideration in diagnosis and in therapy in addition to the quantitative scores. In addition, the skill of the listener in interpreting the nonverbal aspects of communication as awareness of body movements, tone of voice, phrase emphasis of the speaker, contribute to one's ability to communicate effectively, regardless of the type of hearing loss.

Retrocochlear Hearing Impairment

Schuknecht (1955) demonstrated degenerative changes in the cochlea, spiral ganglion and neural pathways in presbycusis from histologic studies of animal and human temporal bones. Neural atrophy beginning late in life is superimposed on epithelial atrophy of the cochlear structures and is observed in degeneration of the spiral ganglion cells as well as in the higher auditory pathways. It is manifested by poor auditory discrimination and high frequency hearing loss.

Even more specific to retrocochlear hearing impairment as defined here, are tumors of cranial nerve VIII which may have a profound

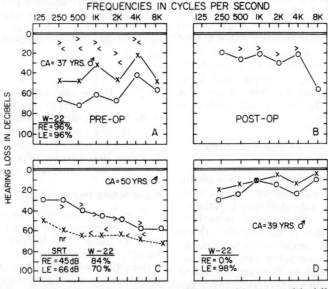

Fig. 13.5. (A) Preoperative audiogram of a 37-year-old man with bilateral conductive hearing loss which was diagnosed as otosclerosis. Word discrimination in both ears was excellent. (B)Postoperative result of the right ear demonstrates marked improvement in hearing threshold. (C) Example of bilateral sensory-neural hearing loss. Word discrimination is poorer in the ear with the greater hearing loss. (D) Case of a patient with a surgically verified acoustic tumor of the right ear. Word discrimination in the right ear was 0% even though the tonal threshold was within normal limits. There was also profound tone decay and a type III Bekesy of the right ear. (Bone conduction thresholds for the right ear are shown as > and those for the left ear shown as <).

effect upon word discrimination scores and understanding of speech, even though hearing sensitivity for pulsed pure tones is normal or near normal. Figure 13.5D is an example (Goetzinger and Angell, 1965). Therefore, when word discrimination scores are abnormally poor compared to threshold sensitivity, the audiologist is alerted at once to the possibility of a tumor. Acoustic tumors are usually unilateral, but may be bilateral in 10 to 20% of the cases.

Hearing Aid Evaluation

Word discrimination tests have been used in audiology clinics in the evaluation of hearing aids for the past three decades. Generally, there is no question of the effectiveness of word discrimination tests in demonstrating differences among hearing aids when they have marked variations in important physical characteristics such as width of frequency response and degree of harmonic distortion. However, the word discrimination tests appear to be ineffective when the physical differences are small. Part of the problem may be related to the effect of the earmold in the external canal upon the frequency response of an instrument in comparison to the frequency response of the same hearing aid as measured in the standard 2-cc coupler. Research on the effects of earmolds upon word discrimination has been revived recently (McClellan, 1967; Northern and Hattler, 1970). Likewise, there is interest in the new Zwislocki artificial ear. The Sachs and Burkhard (1972) data imply that there is preservation of the high pass filter effect even when there is occlusion with a standard earmold.

SUMMARY

This chapter reviewed the history, development, administration and interpretation of word discrimination tests with specific reference to their use in audiology. These tests have augmented the clinical armamentarium of the audiologist by contributing to the diagnosis of hearing impairment and to the understanding of the patient's ability to follow speech in social situations.

REFERENCES

American Standards Association. Specifications for speech audiometers. ASA, Z24.13-1953, New York: U. S. A. Standards Institute, 1953.

Berlin, C. I., Lowe-Bell, S. S., Jannetta, J. J., and Kline, D. G., Central auditory deficits after temporal lobectomy. Arch. Otolaryngol. 96, 4–10, 1972.

Black, J. W., Multiple-choice intelligibility test. J. Speech Hear. Disord., 22, 213–235, 1957.

Bocca, E., and Calearo, C., Central Hearing Processes. In Jerger, J. (Ed.), Modern Developments in Audiology. New York: Academic Press, 1963.

Carhart, R., Instruments and materials for speech audiometry. Acta Otolaryngol., 40, 313–323, 1951-1952.

Carhart, R., Problems in the measurement of speech discrimination. Arch. Otolaryngol., 82, 253–260, 1965.

Clemis, J. D., and Carver, W. F. Discrimination scores for speech in Meniere's disease. Arch. Otolaryngol., 86, 614–618, 1967.

Davis, H., The articulation area and the social adequacy index for hearing. Laryngoscope, 58, 761–778, 1948.

Davis, H., and Silverman, S. R., Hearing and Deafness, Rev. Ed. New York: Holt, Rinehart & Winston, Inc., 1960.

Davis, H., and Silverman, S. R. Hearing and Deafness, Ed. 3. New York: Holt, Rinehart & Winston, Inc., 1970.

Egan, J. P., Articulation testing methods. II. OSRD Report 3802, 1944.

Egan, J. P., Articulation testing methods. Laryngoscope, 58, 955–991, 1948.

Eldert, M. A., and Davis, H., The articulation function of patients with conductive deafness. Laryngoscope, 61, 891–909, 1951.

Elpern, B. S., The relative stability of half-list and full list discrimination tests. Laryngoscope, 71, 30–36, 1961.

Fairbanks, G., Test of phonemic differentiation; the rhyme test. J. Acoust. Soc. Am., 30, 596–601, 1958.

Fletcher, H., Speech and Hearing. New York: D. Van Nostrand Co., 1929.

Fletcher, H., Speech and Hearing in Communication. New York: D. Van Nostrand Co., 1953.

French, N. R., and Steinberg, J. C., Factors governing the intelligibility of speech sounds. J. Acoust. Soc. Am., 19, 90–119, 1947.

Giolas, T. G., Comparative intelligibility scores of sentence lists and continuous discourse. J. Auditory Res., 6, 31–38, 1966.

Giolas, T. G., and Epstein, A., Comparative intelligibility of word lists and continuous discourse. J. Speech Hear. Res., 6, 349–358, 1963.

Glorig, A., Audiometry: Principles and Practices. Baltimore: Williams & Wilkins Co., 1965.

Goetzinger, C. P., and Angell, S. N., Audiological assessment in acoustic tumors and cortical lesions. Eye Ear Nose Throat Mon., 44, 39–49, 1965.

Haagen, C. H., Intelligibility measurement. Speech Mongr., 13, 4–7, 1946.

Hall, L. W., A study of the speech discrimination ability for normal hearing and sensorineural subjects on three tests employing a 1 mil stylus. Unpublished master's thesis, University of Kansas, 1970.

Haskins, H., A phonetically balanced test of speech discrimination for children. Unpublished master's thesis, Northwestern University, 1949.

Hirsh, I. J., The Measurement of Hearing. New York: McGraw-Hill Book Co., 1952.

Hirsh, I. J., Davis, H., Silverman, S. R. Reynolds, E., Eldert, E., and Benson, R. W., Development of materials for speech audiometry. J. Speech Hear. Disord., 17, 321–337, 1952.

House, A. S., Williams, C. E. Hecker, M. H., and Kryter, K. D., Articulation testing methods; consonantal differentiation with a closed-response set. *J. Acoust. Soc. Am.*, 37, 158–166, 1965.

Jerger, J., Observations on auditory behavior in lesions of the central auditory pathways. *Arch. Otolaryngol.*, 71, 797–806, 1960.

Jerger, J., and Jerger, S., Diagnostic significance of PB word functions. *Arch. Otolaryngol.*, 93, 573–580, 1971.

Jerger, J., Speaks, C., and Trammell, J. L., A new approach to speech audiometry. *J. Speech Hear. Disord.*, 33, 318–328, 1968.

Jerger, S., and Jerger, J., Extra- and intra-axial brain stem auditory disorders. *Audiology*, 14, 93–117, 1975.

Jirsa, R., The study of effects of harmonic distortion in hearing aids on the intelligibility of four discrimination tests in normal and hearing impaired listeners. Unpublished doctoral dissertation, University of Kansas, 1970.

Katz, J., The use of staggered spondaic words for assessing the integrity of the central auditory nervous system. *J. Auditory Res.*, 2, 327–337, 1962.

Kimura, D., Some effects of temporal lobe damage on auditory perception. *Can. J. Psychol.*, 15, 156–165, 1961.

Kimura, D., Functional asymmetry of the brain in dichotic listening. *Cortex*, 3, 163–178, 1967.

Kopra, L., Blosser, D., and Waldron, D., Comparison of Fairbanks rhyme test and CID auditory test W-22 in normal and hearing impaired listeners. *J. Speech Hear. Res.*, 11, 735–739, 1968.

Kreul, E. J., Nixon, J. C., Kryter, K. D., Bell, D. W., Lang, J. S., and Schubert, E. D., A proposed clinical test of speech discrimination. *J. Speech Hear. Res.*, 11, 536–552, 1968.

Kryter, K., and Whitman, E., Some comparisons between rhyme and PB word intelligibility tests. *J. Acoust. Soc. Am.*, 37, 1146, 1965.

Lehiste, I., and Peterson, G. E. Linguistic considerations in the study of speech intelligibility. *J. Acoust. Soc. Am.*, 31, 280–286, 1959.

Licklider, J. C., and Miller, G. A., The Perception of Speech. In Stevens, S. S. (Ed.), *Handbook of Experimental Psychology*. New York: John Wiley & Sons, 1951.

Lilly, D. J., and Franzen, R. L., Reproducing styli for speech audiometry. *J. Speech Hear. Res.*, 11, 817–824, 1968.

Lowe, S. S., Cullen, J. K., Berlin, C. I., Thompson, C. L., and Willett, M. E., Perception of simultaneous dichotic and monotic monosyllables. *J. Speech Hear. Res.*, 13, 812–822, 1970.

Lynn, G., Paired PB-50 discrimination test; a preliminary report. *J. Auditory Res.*, 2, 34–37, 1962.

McClellan, M., Aided speech discrimination in noise with vented and unvented earmolds. *J. Auditory Res.*, 7, 93–99, 1967.

Merrell, H. B., and Atkinson, C. J., The effect of selected variables upon discrimination scores. *J. Auditory Res.*, 5, 285–292, 1965.

Miller, G. A., Heise, G., and Lichten, W., The intelligibility of speech as a function of the context of the test materials. *J. Exp. Psychol.*, 41, 329–335, 1951.

Newby, H. A., *Audiology*. New York: Appleton-Century-Crofts, 1964.

Northern, J. L., and Hattler, K. W., Earmold influence on aided speech identification tasks. *J. Speech Hear. Res.*, 13, 162–172, 1970.

Northern, J. L., and Hattler, K. W., Evaluation of four speech discrimination test procedures on hearing impaired patients. *J. Auditory Res.*, Suppl. 1, 37, 1974.

O'Neill, J., and Oyer, H., *Applied Audiometry*. New York: Dodd, Mead & Co., 1966.

Resnick, D., Reliability of the twenty-five word phonetically balanced lists *J. Auditory Res.*, 2, 5–12, 1962.

Ross, M., and Lerman, J., *Word Intelligibility by Picture Identification*. Pittsburgh: Stanwix House Inc., 1971.

Sachs, R. M., and Burkhard, M. D., Zwislocki coupler evaluation with insert earphones. Report No. 20022-1 (for Knowles Electronics, Inc.), Industrial Res. Products, Inc., November 1972.

Schuknecht, H. F., Presbycusis. *Laryngoscope*, 65, 402–419, 1955.

Shankweiler, D., and Studdert-Kennedy, M., Identification of consonants and vowels presented to left and right ears. *Q. J. Exp. Psychol.*, 19, 59–63, 1967.

Stevens, S. S., and Davis, H., *Hearing*. New York: John Wiley & Sons, 1938.

Tillman, T. W., and Carhart, R., An expanded test for speech discrimination utilizing CNC monosyllabic words (Northwestern University Auditory Test No. 6). Technical Report, SAM-TR-66-55, USAF School of Aerospace Medicine. Aerospace Medical Division, (AFSC) Brooks Air Force Base, Texas, 1966.

Tillman, T. W., Carhart, R., and Wilber, L., A test for speech discrimination composed of CNC monosyllabic words. (Northwestern University Auditory Test No. 4), Technical Report, SAM-TDR-62-135, USAF School of Aerospace Medicine, Aerospace Medical Division (AFSC), Brooks Air Force Base, Texas, 1963.

Walsh, T. E., and Silverman, S. R., Diagnosis and evaluation of fenestration. *Laryngoscope*, 56, 536–555, 1946.

Zurif, E. B., and Sait, P. E., The role of syntax in dichotic listening. *Neuropsychologica*, 8, 239–244, 1970.

Differentiating Cochlear and Retrocochlear Dysfunction

chapter **14**

THE TEST BATTERY APPROACH

Philip E. Rosenberg, Ph.D.

Gone are the days when a hearing examination was based on a tuning fork in the doctor's noisy office. Gone, too, are the days when the pure tone audiogram represented the ultimate in examining the auditory system. The audiologist's horizons have broadened and his task is both more precise and complex than ever before. He asks many questions about the auditory system which he had not contemplated in the past. His view of the auditory system is more complete than ever before and he is increasingly aware of its incredible complexity. At the same time there has been a proliferation of audiologic test procedures.

THE AUDIOLOGIC TEST BATTERY

Why Is It Needed?

The audiologist is called upon to make statements concerning the hearing of his patients. Not only must he ascertain the existence of a hearing impairment, but he must also make judgments concerning its severity, its influence upon the patient's life, the locus of the lesion or lesions responsible for the pathology and possible areas of remediation of the disorder. Obviously, no single test yields sufficient information to answer all of these questions. Some tests are designed specifically to assist in pinpointing the site of the lesion while others have as their primary purpose the determination of the existence of an auditory deficit. Thus, an extensive battery of audiologic tests must be available to the audiologist to fulfill the demands made upon him.

The rule of paradoxical findings has been extant in the audiologic profession for many years. The audiologist neither expects nor gets complete agreement on all the different tests he performs. Individual variability, peculiarities of different audiologic pathologies and other incidental factors have an effect upon the consistency of audiologic findings. The utilization of a large number of tests, therefore, renders clarity to an otherwise muddy series of events. By performing numerous overlapping examinations, a picture eventually emerges that is a great deal clearer than that presented by any single examination finding. The paradoxes are smoothed out by the use of a test battery and frequently disappear altogether in light of the totality of the examination findings.

There is also a statistical advantage to the test battery approach when compared with the utilization of but a single examination finding. The multiplicity of judgments in the test battery renders the entire examination more reliable and valid. Statistically, a single judgment is worth but little whereas hundreds of judgments lend statistical safety to the interpretation of raw data. It is possible for one individual patient to provide sufficient data to ensure statistical confidence concerning his auditory behavior. Both multiple judgments and different approaches to the study of the same aspect of behavior lend credence to its interpretation.

What Should It Include?

The basic hearing test is, by itself, a test battery. No self-respecting audiologist in a clinical situation should consider an "audiogram" an adequate basic test of hearing. Most clinicians today feel that an irreducible minimum audiologic examination consists of pure tone testing by air and bone conduction with adequate masking, speech reception threshold tests, the examination of auditory discrimination at suprathreshold levels, tympanometry, and the elicitation of the acoustic reflex. One rarely does less than this and, frequently, much more.

The initial basic examination, then, is not a single test at all but rather the utilization of many different examinations in order to make a simple basic statement concerning hearing. Appended to this statement can be an infinite variety of additional statements each yielding information of value concerning some aspect of the patient's problem.

One very important contribution which the audiologist can make is the determination of the locus of the pathology of the auditory system, that is, the site of the lesion.

Tests for cochlear pathology have been extant for a long time and have undergone a substantial history of refinement and improvement. Certain behavior on auditory tests correlates highly with pathology of the hair cells of the organ of Corti. Histologic examination of temporal bones, particularly with scanning electron microscopy, has validated our procedures. Those tests of cochlear pathology which have stood the test of time and are most widely used today include the alternate binaural loudness-balance test of Fowler, the monaural loudness-balance test of Reger (see Chapter 15), the short increment sensitivity index (see Chapter 16), the observation of a Type II Bekesy audiogram (see Chapter 18), and the measurement of middle ear reflex thresholds (see Chapters 29 and 30). At least two of these tests should be included in any battery concerned with the determination of a cochlear site of lesion. It must be borne in mind that the primary purpose of these tests is the determination of hair cell integrity within the organ of Corti.

Tests for retrocochlear pathology are almost always used to investigate the possibility of a space-taking lesion in the cerebellopontine angle or lower brain stem. Tests for this purpose include the various measurements of abnormal adaptation, the tone decay tests as originally described by Carhart and the many subsequent modifications of this technique (see Chapter 17). A Type III Bekesy audiogram illustrates most elegantly the same essential examination finding. Decay of the middle ear reflex can be recorded from the probe on the side of the poor ear or tone decay can be measured by recording the decay of the reflex on the side of the better ear with the earphone and tonal stimulus on the bad ear. While this group of tests looks only at one portion of the neural mechanism of audition, a substantial patient population suffers from lesions of cranial nerve VIII and brain stem. There is no question but that truly positive findings on these tests are powerful indicators of the existence of such a lesion. Due to the simplicity and ease of administration of these tests, they are frequently included routinely in any audiologic test battery.

The audiologist is increasingly called upon to determine the presence or location of brain pathology. He has within his armamentarium the necessary tools to examine for lesions in various parts of the brain. The tests originally suggested by Bocca and subsequently modified beyond recognition serve this purpose quite well. By "stressing" the auditory stimulus for the discrimination task, one is able to determine by a dramatic reduction in auditory discrimination a lesion of the contralateral temporal lobe. This "stressing" of the stimulus can be accomplished through acoustic filtering, rapid interruption of the stimulus, and binaural competition. Recent research in the area of dichotic listening has provided exciting and challenging speculation concerning the utilization of these listening tasks in clinical application. Inferences drawn from such test results bear not only upon specific auditory behavior but upon the integrity of the entire organism in ways we are only now beginning to understand. Certainly, tests involving dichotic listening shall be added to clinical batteries as they emerge from the laboratory. Tests of central function should be available for use when such a lesion is suspected (see Chapters 20 to 23).

Most of the audiologic tests described thus far are designed to assist in the determination of the pathology in the auditory system and in localizing that particular pathology to one or more specific areas. There are, however, many other special tests utilized by the audiologist for other purposes.

Hearing impairment is frequently the cause of litigation. Perhaps as a result of trauma or accident, a lawsuit is initiated which involves a precise determination of the auditory function. This type of evaluation requires a highly specialized test battery in which the audiologist is concerned with the description and determination of the physiologic hearing levels rather than precise determination of the site of the lesion (Chapters 24, 25 and 26). The audiologist must first decide whether or not the hearing loss is indeed organic. If this decision is affirmative, he must then determine the severity of the deficit through both volitional and nonvolitional examinations. This test battery includes the Stenger test, the Lombard test, delayed feedback tests, and electrodermal audiometry. Recent additions to this classic list include the use of the electroencephalogram through evoked response audiometry (Chapter 27) and the direct electrical measurement of cochlear microphonics and cranial nerve VIII action potentials through the use of cochleography using either transtympanic or extratympanic recording (Chapter 28). Some of these tests are designed merely to give an indication of the possibility of nonorganicity, while others have, as their primary purpose, the precise determination of peripheral auditory thresholds without the conscious cooperation of the patient. The audiologist must become proficient in the administration and interpretation of these tests, since he may be called upon to testify in court and to explain the auditory test findings to a judge and jury. As in other cases, any single test selected from this test battery is inadequate. It is necessary to perform several tests in this particular battery in order to state with any certainty the condition of the auditory system.

The audiologist is often called upon for statements concerning otoaudiologic pathology as revealed by special examination. The otologic surgeon, for example, may well require information concerning the integrity of the middle ear which is not supplied by the standard audiogram. The measurement of the acoustic impedance of the middle ear (Chapters 29 and 30) and the integrity of the stapedius acoustic reflex certainly fall within the audiologist's domain and have become an integral part of his armamentarium.

Interpretation of the Audiologic Test Battery

Once the test battery has been administered, the audiologist must interpret the raw data and make a statement concerning the meaning of his examination results. Simple presentation of test results will not suffice. Such a presentation invites confusion and misinterpretation. It is the audiologist's responsibility, therefore, to summarize his examination findings into a coherent statement of the problem as he sees it. In order to do this, he has to look at the information in two different ways. First, he must examine the results of single tests. Second, he must be able to obtain the feeling of the "gestalt" of the entire examination. This has proven to be one of the greatest stumbling blocks in the use of the audiologic test battery. Many audiologists have felt the presence of "paradoxical" findings disturbing. They have been unwilling to accept combinations of single tests which do not agree or which seem to point in different directions. This is most unfortunate since actual paradoxes are rare and most of the seeming conflicts can be explained easily. A major maxim of audiologic practice should be, "Believe your test results." If any test or subtest is rigorously administered and scrupulously interpreted the audiologist should accept the findings of that test as fact. For example, many audiologists express concern about the "discrepancy" of finding both loudness recruitment and substantial abnormal adaptation in the same ear. If one accepts each single test in the battery as meaningful, then the problem simply disappears. That is, loudness recruitment *means* damage to the hair cells of the organ of Corti and abnormal adaptation *means* retrocochlear pathology. The concurrence of these two pathologic conditions is not at all unusual either from dependent or independent causes. Indeed, it is not at all uncommon for two or even three or more pathologic entities to coexist in a single ear. One patient who had a cerebellopontine angle tumor had a prior history of noise-induced hearing impairment, endolymphatic hydrops, clinical otosclerosis and chronic otitis media.

If the comparison between the air and bone conduction pure tone tests demonstrates a conductive lesion, believe it. If the tests for cochlear pathology indicate hair cell damage, believe it. If the tests for retrocochlear pathology indicate damage to cranial nerve VIII, believe it. If the test battery suggests all three pathologic entities, *believe them all*. It is important that the audiologist not force himself into an "either/or" dichotomy. The ear, as any other body system, simply does not work that way. Furthermore, the test battery should be utilized for all of the information it can yield, not as a forced choice device. Each test, therefore, must be analyzed separately before the whole battery can be put together as any meaningful diagnostic entity.

There are cases, of course, where specific test conflicts do occur. In this case, the knowledgeable audiologist will accept the evidence of the stronger test. A situation may arise where the alternate binaural loudness-balance (ABLB) test is strongly positive when the short increment sensitivity index (SISI) is entirely negative. Since the SISI test requires a greater cochlear hearing loss for positive results, there may be no conflict at all. In such an instance the audiologist should accept the evidence of the ABLB as well as the contradictory suggestion of the SISI.

The statistics of decision are strongly aided by the inclusion of numerous subtests in the audiologic battery. The more evidence one has upon which to base a decision, the more reliable and valid that decision is apt to be.

THE EXTRA AUDIOLOGIC TEST BATTERY

The audiologic test battery, in itself, is rarely definitive. Often the audiologic work-up is an adjunct to other examinations, or other areas of investigation are needed to confirm the audiologic test findings. It is incumbent upon the audiologist to recognize the need for these other tests and to participate to some degree in their administration and interpretation. He must be cognizant of the potential contributions of many other specialties to the total handling of any individual audiologic problem. The audiologist also bears the responsibility for knowing the availability of ancillary areas of investigation and properly channeling or referring the patient to them.

The Otologic Test Battery

The otolaryngologic examination frequently, although not invariably, precedes the audiologic evaluation. Detailed audiologic testing without an equivalent otolaryngologic or neurologic examination is unthinkable. Careful and expert examination of the ears, nose, throat, and accessory structures should be combined with the audiologic test findings to make a reasonable interpretation. A careful otoscopic examination and description of the external ear, the ear canal, and the tympanic membrane should, if possible, precede audiologic investigation. A statement concerning nasopharyngeal integrity and Eustachian tube function should also be obtained. Skillful administration of tuning fork tests frequently serves as confirmatory evidence of the audiologic findings. Physical examination of the head, the face, the temporomandibular joint, and the neck may often reveal pathologic conditions which subsequent audiologic evaluation can support. It is wasteful indeed to complete an extensive audiologic test battery only to find upon subsequent examination that the ears are solidly occluded by cerumen. For a more complete presentation of the interrelationship of both otology and audiology see Chapter 2.

The Vestibular Battery

Although the vestibular examination is listed as part of the extra audiologic test battery, the audiologist often participates directly in the administration of vestibular tests. It is foolish for the audiologist to concern himself exclusively with one-half of a complex system. He must be aware of the examination of the balance mechanism and the influence of vestibular pathology upon his test findings. The advent of electronystagmography is to the vestibular examination what audiology was to the hearing examination (Chapter 31). Electronystagmography can quantify and demonstrate pathology of the vestibular system with great precision. Standard techniques for examination have evolved utilizing rotation as well as bithermal caloric stimulation of known and controlled intensity and duration with electronystagmography as the recording medium of the response. Many audiologists are engaged in vestibular testing and all should be familiar with aberrant responses. Not only evoked nystagmus through caloric or galvanic stimulation, but spontaneous and positional nystag-

mus should also be noted by the audiologist and, if possible, interpreted based upon extensive knowledge of the vestibular system.

The Radiologic Battery

The contribution of radiology to the audiologist's practice is relatively recent. In the past, standard skull films and mastoid x-rays yielded little to the audiologist. These films were and are most meaningful to the otolaryngologist and assisted him greatly in the diagnosis and treatment of his patient. Newer radiologic techniques have been of inestimable value in the visualization of both cochlear and retrocochlear pathology. Specifically, the advent of plesiosectional tomography and its subsequent development and refinement has opened new vistas to all concerned. It is now possible to visualize a grossly aberrant cochlea or to see the widening and trumpeting of one internal auditory meatus as a result of an acoustic tumor. While tomography is not foolproof or ideally definitive, its utilization was a great leap forward in the diagnosis of certain difficult pathologies. Still, more recently, the use of dye contrast media such as pantopaque in encephalography has enlarged yet further the visibility of hidden and remote structures. These techniques are able to delineate with great specificity the boundaries of space-taking lesions within the subarachnoid spaces. Such delineation certainly eases the surgeon's task and may offer the audiologist rapid and direct confirmation of his diagnostic findings.

The Neurologic Battery

The ear functions as a portion of a total neurologic unit within the central nervous system. The audiologist, therefore, must have some awareness not only of the hearing sense but of the entire framework within which it operates. He must be familiar with the contributions the neurologist can make to the definition of the auditory system and its interrelationships with other portions of the central nervous system. The description of the integrity of all 12 pairs of cranial nerves yields information of value to the audiologist. Both peripherally and centrally cranial nerve VIII interacts or intertwines with many others and specific areas of pathology can be determined by comparing coexisting pathologies of the cranial nerves. The electroencephalogram can also prove of great value in explaining brain pathology which may involve audition. While the audiologist need not be competent in the administration of the electroencephalogram, he should be familiar with its interpretation and its relevance to his particular field. The neurologist can also determine diffuse central nervous system pathology such as multiple sclerosis which often has peculiar manifestations in the auditory system. As a matter of fact, recent research has suggested that certain pathologic manifestations of auditory behavior may well be among the first indicators of multiple sclerosis. The neurologist and the audiologist can serve each other well by understanding one another's capabilities and techniques. A more complete discussion of this is found in Chapter 3.

The Psychological Battery

Few specialities are as important to the audiologist as that of psychology. The clinical psychologist, through his interpretation of human behavior, can often be of substantial help to the audiologist in the delineation of the patient's problem. Specification of mental capacity, indications of emotional disorder and mental disease, suggestions of diffuse brain injury all fall within the realm of the clinical psychologist. The psychologist's skills are required particularly in the evaluation and management of the young child. Again, the audiologist must be familiar with the language used by this specialist and with the techniques he employs. He must know when to make a knowledgeable referral and to whom.

CONCLUSION

The use of a single test for the assessment of human hearing is a thing of the past. Even the most basic audiologic examination includes a battery of hearing tests. As more complex questions concerning the auditory system are asked, additional test items are added to the battery. Tests specifically designed to investigate the locus of pathology of the auditory system beyond those used in the standard examination include tests for cochlear pathology, retrocochlear pathology and brain pathology. More than one test in each area should be employed.

Other special test batteries may be used for medicolegal or compensation problems and for special diagnostic investigations.

Test battery interpretation includes not only the evaluation of each test individually but an analysis of the "gestalt." If the tests are rigorously administered, the audiologist is obliged to believe his test results. Truly paradoxical findings within the test battery are rare although seeming discrepancies occur quite frequently. These discrepancies are not usually contradictory at all if one accepts the test findings as valid. Findings on any individual patient may well reflect a number of different pathologic conditions which can and do occur with considerable frequency. The decision making process is facilitated by using a number of different procedures and the reliability of the examination is enhanced by the increased number of patient judgments.

It is also incumbent upon the audiologist to familiarize himself with ancillary examinations and those test batteries employed by other specialists. The audiologist should recognize the need for these further examinations, know where they may be obtained, and be reasonably competent in integrating these data with his own. These other areas include the otologic, vestibular (including electronystagmography), radiologic, neurologic and psychological test batteries.

Additional tests, both audiologic and extra audiologic, do not confuse the diagnostic process at all but, rather, clarify and enhance the quality of audiologic investigation of the patient.

chapter 15

LOUDNESS BALANCE PROCEDURES

William F. Carver, Ph.D.

Abnormally rapid loudness growth has been the subject of interest and investigation for many years. Early reports indicated that in some persons with hearing loss the threshold deficit "disappeared" at higher intensity levels (Pohlman and Kranz, 1924; Fowler, 1928). Clinical interest in abnormal loudness growth, which was labeled recruitment by Fowler (1937), began with his report and description of the alternate binaural loudness balance (ABLB) test (Fowler, 1936). Eight years before Fowler first described the ABLB procedure, his interest in loudness perception was shown in a report of recruitment (although he did not call it recruitment at that time) in an individual with a 4000-Hz notch. It is interesting to note that Fowler devised and originally used this method believing it would help him diagnose early subclinical otosclerosis (Fowler, 1936). The ABLB did not provide the hoped for information, but did demonstrate vividly in some unilateral sensory-neural hearing loss cases that loudness grows more rapidly in the abnormal ear. Because recruitment was not seen in conductive hearing losses, it was assumed that abnormal loudness growth was symptomatic of sensory-neural hearing loss. Lorente de No (1937) commenting on Fowler's 1937 paper on recruitment theorized that recruitment was due to either hair cell damage or nerve fiber loss.

There is, at present, some disagreement on the diagnostic significance of recruitment (Coles, 1972; Priede and Coles, 1974). However, the measurement of loudness growth remains a valuable part of diagnostic audiology.

DEFINITION OF RECRUITMENT

Recruitment is usually defined as an abnormally rapid growth of loudness as intensity is increased. Although, an increasingly intense signal is perceived as increasing in loudness, the ear which exhibits recruitment shows a more rapid increase in loudness than would normally be expected. Perhaps the phenomenon can be visualized by this example. If one ear is impaired, having a hearing threshold level (HTL) of 40 dB, and the other ear is normal with a threshold of 0 dB, then one could say that it requires 40 dB in the impaired ear to sound as loud (really just perceptible) as

a 0 dB signal in the good ear. Then, when the good ear is stimulated at 20 dB, it would appear that an equal increment of 20 dB would be required in the poor ear (i.e., 60 dB HTL) to sound equal in loudness to the 20 dB signal in the good ear. In a nonrecruiting ear this is true. On the other hand, if the poor ear only requires a 5-dB increment (45 dB HTL) to appear equal in loudness to the 20-dB signal in the good ear, then loudness has grown more rapidly in the poor ear. That is for a 20-dB change in the good ear only a 5-dB change was required in the poor ear for the same increase in loudness. Therefore, the poor ear is exhibiting loudness recruitment.

THE MEASUREMENT OF RECRUITMENT

One must always keep in mind that loudness is the subjective experience of the physical intensity of sound. Essentially, as the intensity of sound increases it becomes louder. We measure intensity directly, but the psychological experience of loudness cannot be measured "objectively." Nevertheless, loudness experiences have been quantified.

A great deal of research has been done with loudness in both the normal and abnormal ear. The scientist has quantified loudness perception through a variety of psychophysical methods with normal listeners, thus much is known about loudness in the normal ear, but not as much is known of loudness growth in the abnormal ear.

The psychophysical methods which have been used extensively with the normal have not been widely used clinically. The phenomenon of recruitment is almost always measured by having the patient compare the loudness of the tone which is heard within normal limits with a tone for which the patient has an impaired threshold. These loudness comparisons are performed at suprathreshold levels and the patient is required to "balance" or match the loudness of these two tones. The tones are made to alternate so that the patient may listen to each tone alone and make judgments on the relative loudness of the two tones. This may be accomplished in the same ear, using different tones in the monaural loudness balance or MLB (Reger, 1936) or between ears with the same frequency tone in the alternate binaural loudness balance or ABLB (Fowler, 1936).

The ABLB and the MLB are two clinical tests for recruitment. The choice is dictated by the hearing loss; if the loss is unilateral, then the balances are made between ears at the same frequency (ABLB), if, on the other hand, the loss is bilateral, then the comparisons are made in the same ear but at different frequencies (MLB). In each case the thresholds of one tone must be within normal limits. There may be some difference of opinion regarding the requirement of normality of one tone, but it is believed that if both tones are heard abnormally, the results may be confounded by the contribution of two unknown loudness growth patterns.

One of two psychophysical methods is usually employed with either the ABLB or the MLB. These are the method of limits or the method of adjustment. There is no unanimity among clinicians regarding the method of choice (Jerger, 1962; Hood, 1969). The selection of a method is often dictated by the available apparatus and the time alloted.

Both methods will be discussed as they apply to the ABLB test. Most of the information is applicable to the MLB as well. For instance, where "reference and variable ears" are discussed, the MLB equivalent would be "reference and the variable tones."

With the MLB test, the task for the patient is complicated by the fact that he must equate loudness with two tones which differ in pitch. The task is difficult and becomes even more so with greater frequency separation (Graham, 1967). At the same time, however, the test is not impossible and should be used more frequently.

Method of Limits

Perhaps the most widely used psychophysical method is the method of limits. This procedure requires that the examiner manipulate the intensity of the signal while the patient judges its relation to a criterion (Stevens, 1951).

The equipment must be such that the same frequency tones can be alternated between the ears with separate attenuators for each ear. Many "clinical" audiometers have this capability. Some will automatically alternate the tones while others require manual tone presentations. If this type of audiometer is not available, two pure tone audiometers could be used, as long as the test frequencies are reasonably well matched.

In any case, one ear, usually the better ear, is established as the reference (fixed) ear, while the opposite ear (the poorer ear) is made the variable ear. The patient is carefully instructed to listen to the tones as they alternate between the ears and to report which is louder (or softer) or if they are equal. Frequently, diplacusis will exist and the tones will appear to be of different pitch and often of different quality. The patient is asked to ignore any pitch or quality differences and to make his judgments solely on the relative loudness of the two tones.

The examiner sets the reference tone attenuator to some predetermined level above threshold and leaves it there. The variable ear attenuator is set to an arbitrary level and the test begun. If the equipment requires manual tone presentations, the tester must try to make each stimulus equal in duration. The duration should be about $1/2$ sec. Allow the tones to alternate until the patient has made his judgment. The tester then sets the variable attenuator to a different level and turns on the tones again. Each variable attenuator setting should be made in such a manner as to bracket the equal loudness point, that is, if the patient reports variable ear softer, the next presentation should be at a higher level, high enough to cause a "louder" response. Initially, fairly large intensity changes should be made, but then, while continuing to bracket, the tester "closes in" on the equal loudness point. Several trials should be done at each reference level for increased accuracy.

Method of Adjustment

In the method of adjustment, the patient adjusts the stimulus until it is subjectively equal to a criterion (Stevens, 1951). This method requires a modification of most commercially available audiometers, but many believe the results obtained are far superior to the method of limits as it is usually applied clinically (Jerger, 1962). Hood (1969) disagrees; he believes the examiner must maintain "control" by employing the method of limits. In the method of limits, the tester might "expect" a particular result and thus lead his patient to say "equal" at the level the tester expects, or the result of the first trial can too easily lead the tester to "force" the patient to the same response on the following trials. Figure 15.1 is a block diagram of one way to modify a two-channel or split channel audiometer for the psychophysical method of adjustment. Another method would be to link the variable attenuator mechanically to a driving rod and an unmarked knob for the patient to adjust.

For the ABLB, a tone (the reference tone) to one ear is fixed at a specified intensity level above threshold. The subject adjusts the loudness of the same frequency tone (the variable tone) to the other ear with his attenuator so that its loudness is equal to the loudness of the reference tone. If a set-up similar to that described in Figure 15.1 is used, the *audiometer* attenuator controlling the level to the *patient* attenuator must be set at a very high level, since the subject will be attenuating (reducing) the level with his own attenuator. The final hearing level (balance point) is equivalent to the audiometer hearing level minus the amount of attenuation the patient has inserted with his attenuator plus the constant inherent

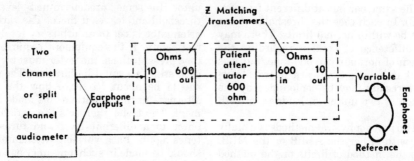

Fig. 15.1. Block diagram of one way to adapt a two channel audiometer for the method of adjustment. The system *within the dotted lines* is inserted *between* the audiometer output (variable ear channel) and the earphone (variable earphone). Impedance matching transformers are used because the output impedance in most audiometers is a nominal 10 ohms while most attenuators have an impedance of 600 ohms. Direct coupling will result in a large voltage loss and distortion. Note that the two transformers and the attenuator will insert approximately a 3-dB loss which must be taken into account when the data are analyzed.

loss of the transformers and patient attenuator. For example, if the audiometer hearing threshold level is set at 90 dB, the patient attenuator at 22 dB, then, with a system loss of 3 dB, the hearing level would be equal to 71 dB ([90 − 22] + 3 = 71).

A patient bias which must be avoided is patient attenuator positional clues. That is, if no changes are made in setup between trials, the patient will tend to return to the same place on his attenuator dial for each trial. To avoid this bias the hearing threshold level dial on the audiometer controlling the level to the variable ear must be changed between each trial. For example, if the audiometer is set at 90 dB for the first trial, it should be moved to other levels for the second and subsequent trials, say 102 dB for the second and 84 dB for the third. This should force the patient to attenuate to different positions on his attenuator.

In all cases, instructions to the patient are very important. Good instructions save time and keep the patient motivated. For the method of adjustment the patient should be aware of the following: (1) the tones will be alternating between his ears, (2) he will be controlling the loudness of the tone in one ear (the variable ear), (3) he must make the tone in his variable ear equal in loudness to the tone in his opposite ear (the reference ear), (4) he must ignore any difference in pitch or quality and make his judgments only on the loudness of the tones, (5) he must first bracket the equal loudness point by alternately making the variable tone definitely louder, then definitely softer, then barely louder, then barely softer and finally equal and (6) he is not expected to arrive at the same spot on his control dial with each trial.

Some clinicians find that if patients do not at first bracket the equal loudness point, they tend to be biased by the starting intensity. In other words, if the patient is not instructed to bracket, when he begins his loudness matching with the initial intensity of the variable tone higher than equal loudness, he will often tend to underestimate the loudness of the variable tone and end up with the variable tone louder than the reference tone. When the variable tone is begun softer than the reference tone, the reverse is often observed. Bracketing tends to minimize this bias. To further compensate for this type of bias, it is wise to begin some trials with the variable ear louder and some softer than the reference tone. This is accomplished by asking the patient to turn his attenuator to one end before trial No. 1 and to the other end for the next trial and so on.

The Tracking Method

In 1964, Miskolczy-Fodor reported a modification of the ABLB procedure. It differs from the more standard procedure in that during the tests the reference signal varies over time. Using the Bekesy tracking method, the patient continuously bracketed the equal loudness point by adjusting the intensity of the tones in his opposite ear to be alternately just louder and just softer than the reference tone. This procedure provides a loudness growth function in a relatively short period. Miskolczy-Fodor presented some clinical cases which illustrated that recruitment of loudness could be observed by this method. However, a study of this procedure on normals (Carver, 1970) indicates that subjects tend to lag behind the changing reference tone so that the entire function (that is, ascending reference and descending reference tone) often describes a hysteresis loop. Some unpublished data on a few abnormals (Carver) also indicate that recruitment is evidenced by the tracking method, but again it was observed that the patients tended to lag behind the reference tone. It may be, however, that by using an ascending and descending reference tone and averaging the two, that a more accurate function may be realized.

Reference Attenuator Levels

The usual reference ear levels tested are 20, 40, 60, 80 and perhaps 100 dB sensation level (SL). However, if time is a factor, several trials at each level are probably more important than measuring at many different increments. Instead 30- or perhaps 40-dB steps should be considered.

Mode of Tone Alteration

There is not general agreement about the mode of tone alteration (Hood, 1969; Jerger, 1962). However, the author agrees with Jerger's (1962) recommendation that the tones alternate at a 50% duty cycle with a period of 1 sec. Thus, the duration to each ear would be 500 msec. He also recommends 50-msec rise and decay times.

CHARTING METHODS AND CRITERIA

The data obtained should then be recorded in a manner which will illustrate the growth of loudness in the impaired ear as it compares with the reference ear.One of two kinds of illustration is usually drawn. One is called a laddergram (Fig. 15.2). Note that it looks like an abbreviated audiogram. The rung (of the ladder) at the top is equivalent to 0-dB hearing threshold level. The successive rungs represent higher and higher hearing levels. Thresholds are plotted as illustrated and then the average variable ear loudness levels for the several trials at each reference (fixed) level are plotted as on an audiogram. To facilitate viewing the results, the variable level plot is connected by a straight line to its corresponding reference level plot.

The other method used to illustrate loudness growth is a graph as shown in Figure 15.3. Here the poorer ear (or tone) data are plotted from the *abscissa* and the better ear (or tone) from the *ordinate*. Again, the numbers represent hearing threshold level. The 45° line represents equal loudness growth for two normal ears. In this illustration (Fig. 15.3) the data are the same as in Figure 15.2. The points which are plotted are usually connected by a curve of best fit.

For the ABLB test, one ear, usually the reference ear, must be within normal limits at

the frequency of interest, while in the MLB test one frequency must be within normal limits in the test ear. The comparison tone, the variable tone, in both cases, must have from 20 to 50 (or 60) dB poorer threshold than the reference tone threshold. If masking is not used with greater than 50 dB or more difference between ears, the results may be contaminated

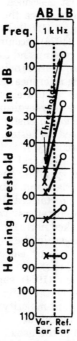

Fig. 15.2. Laddergram method of plotting loudness balances.

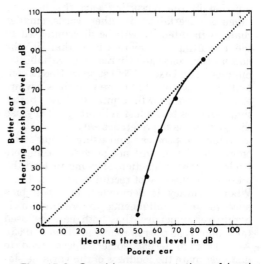

Fig. 15.3. Graphic representation of loudness balances. The data are the same as the data in Figure 15.2.

by the lateralization of the tone (Reger, 1965). However, the effect of lateralization in the ABLB test has not been investigated thoroughly. The question that must be answered is, how much loudness does the lateralized tone add to the total loudness? The effect might very well be minor, but masking should be used until more definitive studies are done on the effect of lateralization.

Since Fowler first described the ABLB, the practice has been to make the better ear the reference ear. Jerger (1962), Reger (1965) and Priede and Coles (1974) recommend the opposite, that is, they recommend that the poor ear be the reference ear. Jerger believes that using the poor ear as the reference ear will result in a faster and more accurate establishment of recruitment versus no recruitment, since only one or two reference intensity levels (i.e., 20 and 40 dB SL) need be tested. Jerger recommends that for accuracy it is better to spend more time obtaining several balances at fewer levels rather than spending the time at more levels with fewer trials and, consequently, less accuracy. Jerger and Harford (1960) found with four experienced listeners with unilateral losses and ten masked normals, that there was no difference between loudness matches when either the good or poor ear was made the reference ear (fixed ear).

Priede and Coles (1974) suggest that the poorer ear serve as the reference primarily because, "a significant majority of patients preferred the Jerger technique. . . . " Hood (1969) objects (Fig. 15.4) to the use of the poor ear as the reference ear. He states that the range of uncertainty is reduced by making the poor ear variable. That is, the steeper the loudness function in the recruiting ear, the less the range of uncertainty. In other words, smaller changes in intensity will be discriminated in the recruiting ear more easily than in the normal ear, consequently reducing variability. Simmons and Dixon (1966) support Hood's contention. They note that those who show asymptotic loudness growth typically show "better than average test-retest reliability." They use the good ear as the reference ear.

Fixing the poor ear and using Jerger's recommended levels will not provide a complete loudness growth function; showing instead the presence or absence of recruitment (Fig. 15.4). When accuracy is demanded, or when bias appears to be influencing the results, it is highly recommended that both ears be used (alternately) as the reference ear (Reger, 1965). At very high levels, some subjects tend to underestimate the loudness of the variable signal (Hellman and Zwislocki, 1964). Reversing reference and variable ears should compensate for this bias.

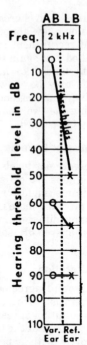

Fig. 15.4. Laddergram illustrating recruitment as measured by Jerger's (1962) recommendation where the poorer ear is fixed (reference) at 20 dB and 40 dB SL.

The Problem of Adaptation

Some controversy surrounds the basic procedures for performing the ABLB test. The basic argument revolves around the mode of the alternating tones. Hallpike and Hood (1951) and Hood (1951; 1969) believe that there must be a comparatively large rest period between tone presentations to avoid differential adaptation. That is, they require that ear 1 be stimulated for approximately 300 msec, then the tone is off about 600 msec before ear 2 is stimulated. Then another 600-msec silent period intervenes before ear 1 is again stimulated. This is accomplished by manual switching of the tone. Hood (1969) states that a shorter or no rest period will bring about adaptation and supports his contention with the results of his studies on perstimulatory adaptation (Hood, 1950). His data indicate that a significant degree of adaptation occurs with suprathreshold continuous stimulation. In addition, Hallpike and Hood (1951) show, using Hood's (1950) simultaneous balance procedure, that the abnormal ear, specifically an ear affected by Meniere's disease, adapts more rapidly than the normal ear.

They believe that loudness is essentially a function of the "on-effect" alone, and argue that the on-effect is diminished or even extinguished when there is insufficient rest period between stimulus presentations. These arguments are based on a study by Matthews (1931) on the action potential (AP) of the stretch receptors of muscles. Matthews observed (1) that there is a rapid negatively accelerated reduction in the number of APs seen when a muscle is stretched, (2) that the recovery of the on-effect (the large number of initial AP responses) is rapid and (3) that recovery is not complete if the stimulus is reapplied after a rest period of less than 1 sec but more than 0.2 sec. In other words if the rest period was greater than 1 sec, the on-effect was observed to be normal, if less than 0.2 sec, it was absent, and for periods in between, it was diminished. Hood also considered the studies of Derbyshire and Davis (1935) on equilibration of the auditory nerve of cats. Derbyshire and Davis reported on the amplitude of the whole nerve response to continuous stimulation (1500 Hz). They noted that the response diminished rapidly with time and reached an asymptote at about $3^{1}/_{2}$ min. Since the time courses of perstimulatory adaptation, equilibration and stretch receptor adaptation are similar (according to Hood), he postulated that the identical process is occurring in the ear. Therefore, since the stretch receptor requires at least 1 sec of rest in order to recover its on-effect completely, the same rest period must be allowed the cochlear end organ. If a rest period is not allowed, Hood believes that the on-effect will adapt and loudness will decrease.

On the other hand, Jerger (1962) recommends that the tones alternate automatically with a 50% duty cycle and a period of 1 sec. Thus each ear is stimulated for 500 msec and rested for 500 msec. Jerger apparently does not believe that the short repetitive stimulus presentations will cause a significant adaptation. However, to avoid any *differential* adaptation, Jerger strongly recommends automatic alternation so that the duration to each ear will be identical.

Hood (1969) criticizes Jerger's recommended procedure on almost all points, but the most important and most critical is Hood's contention that Jerger's method will result in adaptation and that the adaptation rates of the two ears will be different.

The literature is replete with studies on adaptation (Small, 1963). The results of these investigations indicate that loudness does diminish with continuous acoustic stimulation. However, there is a lack of agreement among these various studies concerning the magnitude of adaptation for a specific stimulus. This disagreement hinges primarily upon the method of measurement. Many of these investigations do

not support Hood's data. Recall that Hood bases his disagreement with Jerger's recommended procedure on his work on perstimulatory adaptation as well as the studies of equilibration and AP adaptation of stretch receptors. Recall also that Hood's method requires the measurement of perstimulatory adaptation *during* the process of adaptation, therefore requiring simultaneous balances. Other investigators have attempted to look at adaptation in ways which will avoid certain difficulties inherent in simultaneous balancing procedures. The problems include (1) median plane localization clues with loudness clues (Jerger and Harford, 1960; Small, 1963; Petty, Fraser and Elliott, 1970), (2) adaptation of the comparison ear during balance (Small, 1963) and (3) binaural interaction (Fraser, Petty and Elliott, 1970). When experimenters attempted to avoid these problems by different experimental approaches, the amount of adaptation is seen to be reduced drastically. However, some adaptation to continous stimulation does appear to exist. Therefore, the question relating to Jerger's loudness balance procedure still remains. That is, is there enough silent period between presentations to allow complete recovery from any adaptation that may take place?

There is evidence which indicates that sufficient rest is allowed. First, Sergeant and Harris (1963) looked at perstimulatory adaptation with interrupted tones, using Hood's simultaneous balance procedure. Recall that it is this method in which the greatest degree of adaptation is observed. Sergeant and Harris used, among others, an adapting stimulus duration of 300 msec and a similar rest (which was the closest to Jerger's 500-msec duration). They noted, with normals, that the magnitude of adaptation during a 5-min run was no greater than about 2.5 dB and, at the end of 5 min, adaptation was approximately 1 dB. Second, Jerger and Jerger (1966) investigated critical off times (COT) during threshold measurements of persons with abnormal threshold tone decay. They showed that very little threshold adaptation occurs with COTs of greater than 200 msec. Third, Dallos and Tillman (1966) and Tillman (1966) discussed patients with acoustic neuromas. Here Type III discrete Bekesy tracings were shown. At each frequency tested, the patients adapted, often to the limit of the audiometer, on continuous stimulation, but *recovered* at a pulse rate of 250 msec on, 250 msec off. In other words, in patients with extreme threshold adaptation, a 250-msec silent period is sufficient for complete recovery from adaptation. This phenomenon has been observed many times by this author, not only in patients with Type III Bekesy tracings but with Types II and IV as well.

Interpretation

These data must now be interpreted. The four categories in which a patient may fall are no recruitment, partial recruitment, complete recruitment and decruitment (abnormally slow loudness growth).

Jerger (1962) has established criteria for the first three (Table 15.1), decruitment has been added to this table. Figure 15.5 shows these relationships graphically.

Note that Jerger allows a tolerance of ±10 dB. Hood (1969), on the other hand, does not allow a tolerance of ±10 dB for complete recruitment. However, most clinicians familiar with ABLB measurements in a clinical population will attest to the rather disappointingly large variability of many patients' judgment of equal loudness. For this reason, this author prefers to allow a ±10-dB tolerance for all categories.

For purposes of illustration, two patients with unilateral hearing losses are shown in Figures 15.6 and 15.7. The patient shown in Figure 15.6 had a diagnosis of Meniere's disease. The ABLB results are shown and exhibit complete recruitment. The patient in Figure 15.7, on the other hand, had a surgically proven acoustic neuroma. Here no recruitment was observed.

THEORY

Lorente de No (1937) postulated that recruitment was caused by either cochlear or nerve fiber pathology. It was Dix, Hallpike and Hood (1948) who demonstrated that recruitment may point to a cochlear lesion. They noted that recruitment very seldom occurred in persons with cranial nerve VIII tumors, while recruitment was typically seen in patients with Meniere's disease. This report again heightened interest in recruitment as an interesting suprathreshold phenomenon, which, when pres-

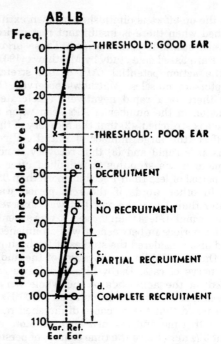

Fig. 15.5. Laddergram illustrating the interpretation of loudness balance results. Decruitment has been added. From J. Jerger: *ASHA*, **4**, 139–145, 1962.

ent, pointed to the cochlea as the locus of the hearing loss.

The opposite of recruitment, that is abnormally slow growth of loudness, has received much less attention in the literature. First noted by Dix et al. (1948) in one patient with a nerve VIII tumor, decruitment may well be a part of the symptomatology of retrocochlear or nerve VIII pathology (Simmons and Dixon, 1966; Tillman, 1969). The patient who exhibits decruitment which Simmons and Dixon call loudness decrement will report little or no change in loudness for a pulsed tone as intensity is increased. In those cases where recruitment is observed in nerve VIII losses, Hallpike and Hood (1951) believe that the tumor has reduced the blood supply to the cochlea (by pressure) thereby producing a cochlear loss and concomitant recruitment.

Cochlear pathologies are complex and recruitment is not necessarily pathognomonic of cochlear lesions. Simmons and Dixon (1966), discussing loudness recruitment, carefully outline two principles which may be operating in recruiting (or decruiting) ears. The first is the "place principle." Assuming the outer hair cells require less intense mechanical agitation to produce an adequate stimulus (threshold is more sensitive) than the inner hair cells, when

TABLE 15.1. *Criteria for Interpretation of Loudness Balance Result*

Classification	ABLB or MLB Results*
No recruitment	Equal loudness at equal *sensation levels* ± 10 dB
Complete recruitment	Equal loudness at equal *hearing threshold levels* (or intensities) ± 10 dB
Partial recruitment	Equal loudness between complete recruitment and no recruitment
Decruitment	Equal loudness with 10 dB or greater sensation level in the poor ear than in the good ear

* ABLB = alternate binaural loudness balance; MLB = monaural loudness balance.

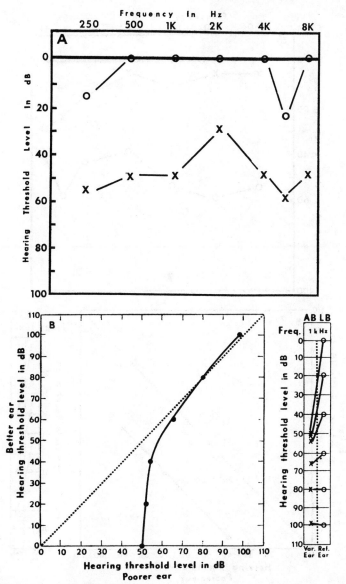

Fig. 15.6. Audiogram (A) and ABLB (B) results of a patient with a diagnosis of Meniere's disease. The bone-conduction thresholds were equal to air-conduction. Complete recruitment is observed, the function is asymptotic.

the outer hair cells are damaged, thresholds are elevated. Then, when the stimulus intensity is increased, the inner hair cells are excited with a concomitant rapid increase in loudness.

The second principle is the "summation" principle or the total number of cells excited. As intensity increases, larger and larger areas of the basilar membrane are stimulated and, importantly, the spread of energy is primarily toward the basal (high frequency) end of the cochlea. They suggest that in sensory-neural losses where the loss is greatest in the low

frequencies, recruitment can almost certainly be demonstrated no matter what the cause. When recruitment is measured in the damaged low frequency area, the spread of energy is out of the damaged area into the normal area where loudness growth (as intensity increases) would suddenly be normal, therefore, going from an impaired threshold to close to normal loudness suprathreshold.

On the other hand, Simmons and Dixon note that the phenomenon of decruitment (abnormally slow loudness growth) can be seen where

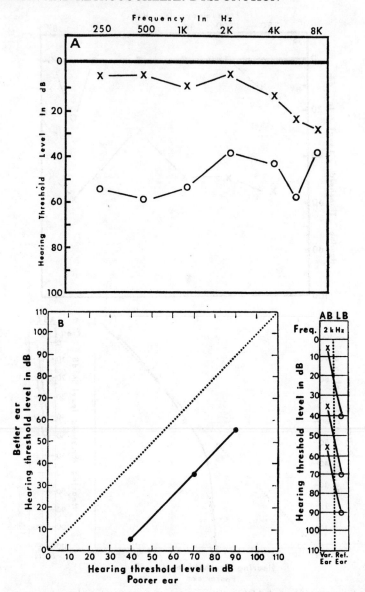

Fig. 15.7. Audiogram (A) and ABLB (B) results of a patient with a surgically confirmed acoustic neuroma. The bone-conduction results were equal to air-conduction. No recruitment is observed.

hearing is normal, but adjacent to an impaired higher frequency. Assume that there has been hair cell damage or nerve supply reduction (intracochlear) near the basal end, then, when the ear is stimulated at a frequency lower than the damaged area or apical (toward the low frequency end) to the damaged area, thresholds would be normal. However, as intensity is increased the spread of energy, which is primarily toward the basal end, would extend into the damaged area. Since there is hair cell damage or a reduction in the nerve supply in this area, there would be no summation and a loudness decrement would result. Simmons and Dixon call this a "summation deficit."

Priede and Coles (1974) have stated that the "mere presence of recruitment" is of little meaning diagnostically. They present data comparing ABLB results on patients with cochlear and nerve VIII lesions. These data, as presented, show that all categories of recruitment (i.e., "over," "complete" according to

Hood, "complete" according to Jerger, and "partial") do not differentiate well between cochlear and neural lesions.

Priede and Coles' data show that, if partial recruitment is ignored, complete recruitment (as defined by Jerger) is a good indicator of cochlear lesion, while no recruitment is an excellent indicator of neural lesion in a patient with a sensory-neural loss. Also, decruitment (loudness reversal) did not occur in any of Priede and Coles' patients with cochlear lesions, only in those with neural lesions.

Table 15.2 reproduces the Priede and Coles' data somewhat differently. When one combines categories, it becomes obvious that the presence of complete recruitment (Jerger's criteria) occurs primarily in cochlear lesions somewhat over two-thirds of the time, but in only 14% of those with neural lesions. More revealing, however, is that no recruitment and decruitment are good predictors of neural lesions. Incomplete or partial recruitment appears to be a poor indicator of site of lesion from these data.

Generally the ABLB or the MLB are performed when one ear or one frequency is poorer than the other. However, in some cases information can be gained with equal or nearly equal thresholds which are within normal limits. Decruitment is often seen in patients with acoustic neuromas. An interesting example where both ears are within normal limits is shown in Figure 15.8. This figure displays the audiogram and loudness balance results for a patient with a surgically confirmed acoustic neuroma. Note the obvious loudness decrement which occurs in an ear which is within normal limits for pure tones.

CLASSIFICATION OF RECRUITMENT

Early studies of the recruitment phenomenon led to the classification of growth patterns. That is, loudness growth functions appear to have several different configurations. Harris, Haines and Myers (1952) describe four distinct types of loudness growth; asymptotic, straight line, delayed and delayed-asymptotic. Stylized representations of these four types are presented in Figure 15.9. Other investigators differ in regard to the number of different types of recruitment functions. Clinically, there appears to be no end to the number of different patterns. Reger (1965) mentioned all four but described only two. Simmons and Dixon (1966) discussed only two types of loudness growth. On the other hand, Stevens (1966) postulated that there may be but one function.

There is evidence that certain clinical entities will tend to show a specific type of loudness growth pattern (Harris, 1953; Harris et al., 1952; Hickling, 1967; Reger, 1965; Simmons and Dixon, 1966). For instance, it is fairly well agreed that asymptotic growth is seen in persons with hair cell damage (Simmons and Dixon's place principle), such as that produced by noise. Also, recruitment seen in Meniere's disease is often described as asymptotic. Hood (1969) on the other hand, claims that recruitment in Meniere's disease is linear or straight line. Carver (1972) found straight line recruitment in 13 of 17 patients with Meniere's disease, the 4 others were asymptotic. The other types are less well established. Simmons and Dixon indicate that loudness growth patterns associated with the summation principle will be delayed or slow and sometimes incomplete. They suggest that one cannot assign specific tissue damage to this type of loudness growth pattern.

Stevens (1966) contends that there may be but one type of abnormal loudness growth which can best be described as two straight lines in log-log plot. This is based on the type of loudness growth seen in masked normals.

When loudnesses are compared between normal ears by the ABLB procedure and the results plotted on dB coordinates (log-log), the slope would be 1.0. On the other hand, when one ear is masked the function changes. The early part of the function describes a slope

TABLE 15.2. *Alternate Binaural Loudness Balance (ABLB) Test Results in Series of Sensory-Neural Hearing Loss Cases**

	Known Cochlear Cases		Known Neural Cases	
	N	%	N	%
Over recruitment	8	7	1	2
Complete recruitment (Hood's criteria)	11	10	2	4
Complete recruitment (Jerger's criteria, excluding above)	59	53	4	8
Total "complete recruitment" (includes all above)	(78)	(70)	(7)	(14)
Incomplete recruitment (Jerger's criteria)	31	28	25	48
No recruitment (Jerger's criteria)	2	2	14	27
Loudness reversal	0	0	6	12
Total no recruitment and loudness reversal	(2)	(2)	(20)	(39)

* Adapted from Priede and Coles (1974).

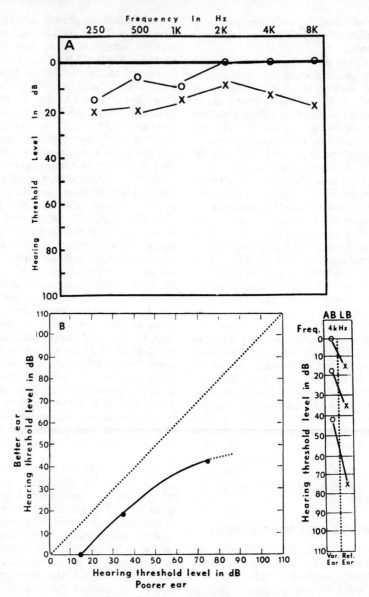

Fig. 15.8. Audiogram (*A*) and ABLB (*B*) results of a patient with a surgically confirmed acoustic neuroma. Bone-conduction results were equivalent to air-conduction. This case illustrates decruitment in an ear which is within normal limits for pure tones.

which is considerably greater than 1.0, while the latter part returns to 1.0. Stevens postulates that there is a power transformation which takes place at the intersect of these two functions. Figure 15.10 shows some experimental data which illustrates where and how this power transformation might occur, but these data neither prove nor disprove his thesis. In practice, the function would most likely be more complex (probably asymptotic) because the averaging process would tend to obliterate

the sharp knee at the point of transformation (Fig. 15.11).

At the present time, the primary interest in recruitment measurement appears to be in relation to its usefulness as part of a battery of tests used in the differential diagnosis of unilateral sensory-neural hearing loss (Dix et al., 1948; Jerger, 1962; Tillman, 1969). This is not to say that recruitment in bilateral sensory-neural losses is not of interest; however, the difficulties encountered in measuring recruit-

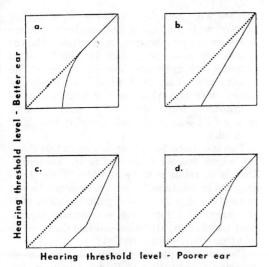

Fig. 15.9. Stylized types of loudness growth functions. *a*, asymptotic; *b*, straight line; *c*, delayed; *d*, delayed-asymptotic. From J. D. Harris, H. L. Haines, and C. K. Myers, *Archives of Otolaryngology*, **55**, 107–133, 1952.

ment in bilateral hearing losses are great and, with the usual methods, sometimes impossible.

Tests for differential sensitivity (DL) are not measures of recruitment. Recruitment is defined as an abnormally rapid growth of loudness. The difference limen (DL) and the SISI tests tell us about differential sensitivity, not necessarily loudness growth (Hirsh, Palva and Goodman, 1954).

RESEARCH NEEDS IN LOUDNESS GROWTH

Abnormal loudness growth has been measured primarily by comparison between two tones, one heard normally, the other heard abnormally. When thresholds for both ears are raised and no one frequency remains normal for comparison, so-called "indirect" tests for recruitment may be used. Since there are many more bilateral hearing losses than unilateral, it is perhaps for this reason that little has been accomplished toward more carefully defining the configurations of loudness growth and their meaning.

There are psychophysical methods available by which one could study loudness growth in

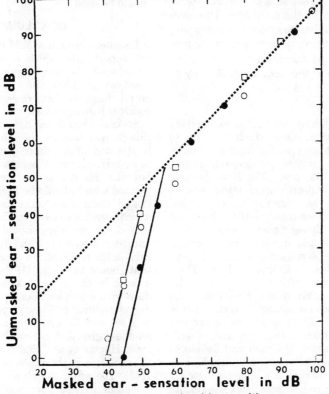

Fig. 15.10. Loudness matches of three normal subjects with one ear masked. Illustrates Steven's theory of power transformation, that is, the functions could be described by two straight line segments. From S. S. Stevens, *Journal of the Acoustical Society of America*, **39**, 727, 1966.

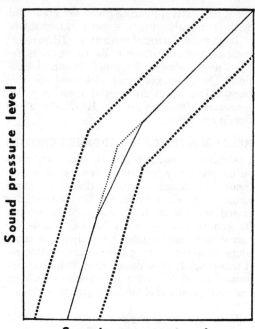

Sound pressure level

Fig. 15.11. The *dashed lines* represent the assumed locus of two sets of values whose average is shown by the *solid line*. This simplified diagram illustrates how the averaging of variable data tends to decrease the sharpness of angles of curvatures. From S. S. Stevens, *Journal of the Acoustical Society of America*, **39**, 727, 1966.

these cases. They have been used extensively on normal listeners. One which appears to have promise is known as the method of magnitude estimation and its counterpart, magnitude production (Stevens, 1966; Hellman and Zwislocki, 1963). Another interesting method is cross-modality matching (Stevens, 1959). With a few exceptions these methods have not been used with pathologic populations.

A few studies employing these psychophysical methods have been used on pathologic populations (Scharf and Hellman, 1966; Thalmann, 1965; Carver, 1972; Carver and Brady, 1973). One study (Scharf and Hellman, 1966) used the magnitude estimation procedure while another (Carver, 1972) used the combined method of magnitude estimation and magnitude production which Hellman and Zwislocki (1968) labeled psychological magnitude balance. Apparently magnitude balance methods require sophisticated listeners, since the results with pathologic patients were somewhat disappointing.

Thalmann (1965) and Carver and Brady (1973) employed the cross-modality matching

method with pathologic subjects. This method appears more promising. Both authors matched loudness with vibratory magnitude. Carver and Brady used the method of adjustment in patients with unilateral Meniere's disease. The results were compared with the results obtained with the ABLB in the same patients. Recruitment was observed in all subjects, both by the ABLB and the cross-modality matching method.

Two questions have been raised in this chapter which have not been directly answered. One is in relation to adaptation. While I attempted to refute with indirect evidence Hood's contention that Jerger's recommendation of 1-sec period, 50% duty cycle, would cause significant adaptation, studies should be designed to test this controversy directly.

The second question relates to the use of masking during the ABLB test. I believe that masking is probably not necessary, but certainly at high intensities, lateralization of the tone to the contralateral (better) ear will occur. The question is, what is the contribution of the contralateral ear to loudness perception in the ipsilateral ear? This problem should be investigated, but, until it has been, masking probably should be used.

CONCLUSION

Loudness growth should be measured at every opportunity which presents itself to the audiologist. The presence or absence of recruitment can often help the otologist make a differential diagnosis between cochlear and retrocochlear hearing losses.

Several procedures have been discussed in this chapter because there has been little done in the way of standardization. There is much to be learned, not only about loudness growth, but also about the most reliable and precise method which should be used. For the present, the clinician must make several decisions: (1) which psychophysical method should be employed, (2) which ear should be made the reference ear (fixed ear) and which the variable ear, (3) the levels above reference ear threshold that should be tested (4) the number of trials at each level, (5) whether Hood's (1969) procedure with a rest between tone presentations or Jerger's (1962) 50% duty cycle method should be used and (6) whether one desires to plot a loudness growth function (Fowler, 1936; Hood, 1969; Harris et al., 1952) or merely establish the presence or absence of recruitment (Jerger, 1962). Too often the choice of many of these variables will be governed by the equipment available and the testing time allotted.

I believe that (1) the method of choice is the method of adjustment, (2) the reference ear should be the better ear (with some exceptions),

(3) the number of levels tested should be sufficient to define a function, (4) at least three trials should be completed at each level and more if there is too much variability, (5) Jerger's 50% duty cycle method should be used and (6) a function should be plotted, not because it is presently diagnostic but because the more careful defining of configurations of abnormal loudness growth may not only help in the differential diagnosis of cochlear lesions but may also help the investigator define how the ear works.

REFERENCES

Carver, W. F., The reliability and precision of a modification of the ABLB test. *Ann. Otol. Rhinol. Laryngol.*, 79, 398–412, 1970.

Carver, W. F., The psychological numerical magnitude balance method with unilaterally impaired listeners. Presented at the American Speech and Hearing Association Convention, San Francisco, 1972.

Carver, W. F., and Brady, J., Cross-modality matching in Meniere's disease, unpublished study, 1973.

Coles, R. R. A., Can present day audiology really help in diagnosis? An otologist's opinion. *J. Laryngol. Otol.*, 86, 191–224, 1972.

Dallos, P. J., and Tillman, T. W., The effects of parameter variations in Békésy audiometry in a patient with acoustic neurinoma. *J. Speech Hear. Res.*, 9, 557–572, 1966.

Derbyshire, A. J., and Davis, H., The action potentials of the auditory nerve. *Am. J. Physiol.*, 113, 476–504, 1935.

Dix, M. R., Hallpike, C. S., and Hood, J. D., Observations upon the loudness recruitment phenomenon, with especial reference to the differential diagnosis of disorders of the internal ear and VIII nerve. *Proc. R. Soc. Med.*, 41, 516–526, 1948.

Fowler, E. P., Marked deafened areas in normal ears. *Arch. Otolaryngol.*, 8, 151–155, 1928.

Fowler, E. P., A method for the early detection of otosclerosis. *Arch Otolaryngol.* 24, 731–741, 1936.

Fowler, E. P., The diagnosis of diseases of the neural mechanism of hearing by the aid of sounds well above threshold. *Trans. Am. Otol. Soc.*, 27, 207–219, 1937.

Fraser, W. D., Petty, J. W., and Elliott, D. N., Adaptation; central or peripheral? *J. Acoust. Soc. Am.*, 47, 1016–1021, 1970.

Graham, A. B. (Editor), Alternate loudness balance techniques. In *Sensorineural Hearing Processes and Disorders*, pp. 245–257. Boston: Little, Brown & Co. 1967.

Hallpike, C. S., and Hood, J. D., Some recent work on auditory adaptation and its relationship to the loudness recruitment phenomenon. *J. Acoust. Soc. Am.*, 23, 270–274, 1951.

Harris, J. D., A brief critical review of loudness recruitment. *Psychol. Bull.*, 50, 190–203, 1953.

Harris, J. D., Haines, H. L., and Myers, C. K., Loudness perception for pure tones and speech.

Arch. Otolaryngol., 55, 107–133, 1952.

Hellman, R. P., and Zwislocki, J. Monaural loudness function at 1000 cps and interaural summation. *J. Acoust. Soc. Am.*, 35, 856–865, 1963.

Hellman, R. P., and Zwislocki, J., Loudness function of a 1000 cps tone in the presence of a masking noise. *J. Acoust. Soc. Am.*, 36, 1618–1627, 1964.

Hellman, R. P., and Zwislocki, J. J., Loudness determination at low sound frequencies. *J. Acoust. Soc. Am.*, 43, 60–64, 1968.

Hickling, S., Hearing test patterns in noise induced temporary hearing loss. *J. Aud. Res.*, 7, 63–76, 1967.

Hirsh, I. J., Palva, T., and Goodman, A., Difference limen and recruitment. *Arch. Otolaryngol.*, 60, 525–540, 1954.

Hood, J. D., Studies in auditory fatigue and adaptation. *Acta Otolaryngol.*, Suppl. No. 92, 1950.

Hood, J. D., Auditory adaptation and its relationship to clinical tests of auditory function. *J. Laryngol.*, 65, 530–544, 1951.

Hood, J. D., Basic audiological requirements in neuro-otology. *J. Laryngol.*, 83, 695–711, 1969.

Jerger, J., Hearing tests in otologic diagnosis. *ASHA*, 4, 139–145, 1962.

Jerger, J. F., and Harford, E. R., The alternate and simultaneous balancing of pure tones. *J. Speech Hear. Res.*, 3, 15–30, 1960.

Jerger, J., and Jerger, S., Critical off-time in VIIIth nerve disorders. *J. Speech Hear. Res.*, 9, 573–583, 1966.

Lorente de No, R., Discussion of Fowler, E. P., The diagnosis of diseases of the neural mechanism of hearing by the aid of sounds well above threshold. *Trans. Am. Otol. Soc.*, 27, 219–220, 1937.

Matthews, B. H. C., The response of a single end organ. *J. Physiol.*, 71, 64–110, 1931.

Miskolczy-Fodor, F., Automatically recorded loudness balance testing. *Arch. Otolaryngol.*, 79, 355–365, 1964.

Petty, J. W., Fraser, W. D., and Elliott, D. N., Adaptation and loudness decrement; a reconsideration. *J. Acoust. Soc. Am.*, 47, 1074–1082, 1970.

Pohlman, A. G., and Kranz, F. W. Binaural minimum audition in a subject with ranges of deficient acuity. *Proc. Soc. Exp. Biol. Med.*, 20, 335–337, 1924.

Priede, V. M., and Coles, R. R. A., Interpretation of loudness recruitment tests–some new concepts and criteria. *J. Laryngol. Otol.*, 88, 641–662, 1974.

Reger, S. N., Differences in loudness response of normal and hard-of-hearing ears at intensity levels slightly above threshold. *Ann. Otol. Rhinol. Laryngol.*, 45, 1029–1039, 1936.

Reger, S. N., Pure Tone Audiometry. In Glorig, A. (Ed.), *Audiometry: Principles and Practices*, pp. 108–150. Baltimore: The Williams & Wilkins Co., 1965.

Scharf, B., and Hellman, R. P., Model of loudness summation applied to impaired ears. *J. Acoust. Soc. Am.*, 40, 71–78, 1966.

Sergeant, R. L., and Harris, J. D., The relation of perstimulatory adaptation to other short-term threshold-shifting mechanisms. *J. Speech Hear.*

Res., 6, 27–39, 1963.

Simmons, F. B., and Dixon, R. F., Clinical implications of loudness balancing. *Arch. Otolaryngol.*, 83, 449–454, 1966.

Small, A. M., Jr., Auditory Adaptation. In Jerger, J. (Ed.), *Modern Developments in Audiology*, pp. 287–336. New York: Academic Press, 1963.

Steinberg, J. C., and Gardner, M. B., The dependance of hearing impairment on sound intensity. *J. Acoust. Soc. Am.*, 9, 11–23, 1937.

Stevens, S. S. (Ed.), Mathematics, Measurement and Psychophysics. In *Handbook of Experimental Psychology*, pp. 1–49. New York: John Wiley & Sons, Inc., 1951.

Stevens, S. S., Cross-modality validation of subjective scales for loudness, vibration and shock. *J. Exp. Psychol.*, 57, 201–209, 1959.

Stevens, S. S., Power-group transformations under glare, masking and recruitment. *J. Acoust. Soc. Am.*, 39, 725–735, 1966.

Thalmann, R., Cross-modality matching in the study of abnormal loudness functions. *Laryngoscope*, 65, 1708–1726, 1965.

Tillman, T. W., Audiologic diagnosis of acoustic tumors. *Arch. Otolaryngol.*, 83, 574–581, 1966.

Tillman, T. W., Special hearing tests in otoneurologic diagnosis. *Arch. Otolaryngol.*, 89, 25–30, 1969.

chapter 16

THE SISI TEST

Frederick N. Martin, Ph.D.

As new auditory tests are developed and old ones refined the audiologist finds himself with more methods at his disposal for the determination of the locus of an auditory lesion. The short increment sensitivity index (SISI) test continues to be a widely used method for determining the likelihood of cochlear pathology. The present chapter is devoted to the background and application of this procedure.

THE DIFFERENCE LIMEN FOR INTENSITY

For reasons that will become apparent later in this chapter it seems illogical to discuss the SISI test without mentioning that phenomenon of abnormal loudness growth called recruitment. Since the observations of Dix, Hallpike and Hood (1948) relating loudness recruitment to cochlear pathology, the audiologist has been able to determine with some degree of certainty that the presence of recruitment implies a cochlear disorder.

The difference limen for intensity (DLI) is the smallest change in the intensity of a pure tone which can just be detected. It is usual for persons with normal hearing to have difficulty in detecting small changes in intensity close to threshold. As intensity is increased the DLI decreases. There appears to be a strong relationship between the ability to detect small intensity changes at relatively low sensation levels (SL) and the presence of loudness recruitment. Many clinicians have assumed that a small DLI is an indirect indication of recruitment, and other have assumed that the DLI and direct tests for recruitment measure related pathologic phenomena.

Luscher and Zwislocki (1949) developed a DLI test which enjoyed popular use for a time. In this test the patient listened to a pure tone presented 40 dB above threshold and was asked to indicate when amplitude modulation of the steady-state signal resulted in a pulsating sound. Those patients who could detect small intensity changes (a small DLI) were assumed to have cochlear lesions. The Luscher-Zwislocki test was therefore a test of loudness discrimination. Lund-Iverson (1952), using the Luscher-Zwislocki technique, concluded that it did indeed reveal recruitment.

In a test procedure developed by Denes and Naunton (1950) patients were required to report a difference in the loudness of two similar tones presented one after the other. This was in part a test of loudness memory. The signal presentation levels were 4 dB SL and 44 dB SL. The point of interest in this test was not the size of the DLI (in dB) but the difference in the DL sizes between the two levels. Normal hearing subjects had large differences between the two levels while those with cochlear lesions showed very small differences between their two difference limens (DLs).

In his modification of the Luscher-Zwislocki DLI test Jerger (1952) used a 15-dB SL presentation. He found that this showed good differentiation between recruiting and nonrecruiting ears. Jerger's (1953) second DLI test was similar to Denes and Naunton's but compared the size of the DLs at 10 and 40 dB SL. The signal used was one which modulated in intensity, requiring the patient to indicate the smallest level at which intensity changes could be detected. This Jerger called the difference limen difference (DLD) test. By allowing each subject to serve as his own norm the DLD test eliminated some of the difficulties imposed by intersubject variability in the DLI task.

Comparing the results of the Luscher-Zwislocki test to the alternate binaural loudness balance test for recruitment Konig (1962) found that the two tests provided identical information in most cases regarding the presence or absence of loudness recrutiment. It is interesting in light of the above findings that Hirsh, Palva and Goodman (1954), using a modification of the Denes-Naunton test, obtained results contrary to those of other researchers, finding no clear differences between recruiting and nonrecruiting ears with respect to their ability to judge small changes in intensity. The reasons for these different findings are not completely clear.

One indicant of the interest in the DLI test in the 1950s is suggested by the number of commercial audiometers then available which allowed performance of this test by varying the degree of intensity modulation of a tone. In the late 1950s the use of the DLI test began to wane due to difficulties in administrating and taking the test. Harris (1963) suggested that some subjects require considerable time in learning the DL task. Many subjects cannot get the notion of a tone which is to change slightly in loudness while others imagine these changes when they do not exist. Undoubtedly internal criteria set up by the individual have confounding effects on this test.

INTRODUCTION OF THE SISI TEST

In 1959 Jerger, Shedd and Harford introduced the short increment sensitivity index (SISI) as another approach to the measurement

179

of the ear's ability to detect small intensity changes. On this test a pure tone is presented to the patient at an SL of 20 dB and a small increase in intensity is superimposed upon the steady-state tone at periodic intervals. The size of this increment is varied from 5 to 1 dB. Jerger, Shedd and Harford found that the ability to detect the 1-dB increments was largely restricted to patients with cochlear pathology. Conversely, this ability was absent in patients with normal hearing or with conductive or retrocochlear hearing losses. Most importantly, the test was easy to administer and was less confusing than DLI tests for most patients.

The SISI procedure obviously differs from the classical DLI tests in that the patient's precise DLI is not explored. The 1-dB increment tests the cochlea's ability to respond to a transient signal of small amplitude. It would appear that pathologic cochleas give rise to this ability while lesions elsewhere in the auditory system do not. Findings on such diagnostic tests for cochlear function as alternate binaural loudness-balance (ABLB), DLI, acoustic reflex, Bekesy audiometry, performance intensity functions for phonetically balanced (PB) words, as well as the SISI test, may correlate highly with each other in cases of cochlear lesion. This does not mean that these tests are necessarily measuring the same phenomenon.

ADMINISTRATION OF THE SISI TEST

In their original report Jerger et al. (1959) recommended that the carrier tone be introduced into the patient's ear at an SL of 20 dB. Every 5 sec a short increment is superimposed, starting with 5-dB increments. The signal has an on-off time of 50 msec and 5 sec elapse between increments (Fig. 16.1). The patient is instructed to indicate that he has heard a brief "jump" in the loudness of the tone. After approximately five such jumps the size of the increment is lowered to 1 dB, marking the

beginning of scoring for the SISI test. Twenty 1-dB increments are introduced and the subject is required to indicate when he has heard each increment. If a number of consecutive increments are heard (about five in a row) the examiner is advised to delete several increments so that it can be ascertained that the subject is responding to the change in intensity rather than to a learned time interval. If the patient fails to respond to several increments in a row the increment size can be increased for retraining to allow the opportunity to focus in on the task again before testing 1-dB increments. Thus, false positive and false negative responses to the SISI can be minimized.

The abrupt change from 5 dB directly to 1 dB is often too sudden to allow proper patient adjustment to the assigned task. The procedure recommended by many clinicians (Harford, 1967), which is in common clinical practice, is to begin with 5-dB increments and, having obtained responses, lower the increment size to 4, 3, 2 and then to the 1-dB increment before the test scoring is begun. One such approach to the SISI procedure is illustrated in the form of a flow chart in Figure 16.2.

There are times when a patient may fail to respond to the first several 1-dB increments and then suddenly begin to signal that he has heard the remainder of the 20 presentations. In such cases, the examiner may elect to disregard the initial lack of response and may allow the patient the opportunity to get a higher score by adding the number of increments missed initially to the end of the test (Harford, 1967). Like most tests, the SISI is best performed after practice and experience.

The SISI score is derived by determining the number of correct identifications of the 1-dB increment out of 20 presentations. This number, multiplied by five, yields the SISI score in percent. Jerger et al. (1959), recommended that SISI scores of 0 to 70% should be considered

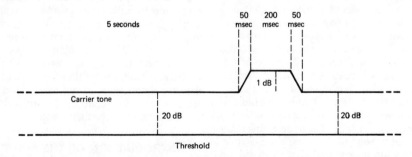

Fig. 16.1. Diagram of the signal for the short increment sensitivity index. The carrier tone is presented at 20 dB above the patient's threshold for the test frequency. Every 5 sec an increment is superimposed that rises to maximum in 50 msec, remains at that level for 200 msec, and then returns to the 20-dB SL in 50 msec (Martin, 1975).

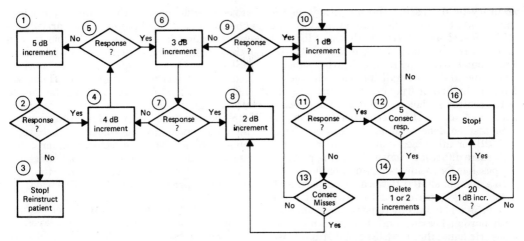

Fig. 16.2. Flow Chart for performance of the short increment sensitivity index.

negative, indicating normal hearing or a non-cochlear lesion, while scores between 70 and 100% should be considered positive, indicating the presence of a cochlear lesion. A survey of certified American audiologists (Pennington and Martin, 1972) showed that of 250 respondents, 121 (48.4%) stated that they consider scores of 80 to 100% as "high." Of 249 respondents, 139 (55.8%) consider scores of 0 to 20% as "low." The range from 25 to 75% should be considered as not strongly diagnostic either way.

The SISI test shows good relative consistency across standard test frequencies with the exception of 250 Hz (Jerger, 1962a). Recently Jerger (1973) reviewed the frequency dependence of the SISI test stating that, in cases with cochlear disorders, scores are low at 250 and 500 Hz (0 to 20%); questionable at 1000 Hz (40 to 60%); and very high at 2000, 3000 and 4000 Hz (80 to 100%). There is general agreement that in the higher frequencies the SISI test appears to effectively differentiate patients with normal hearing from those with sensory-neural hearing loss of cochlear origin when the test is performed at 20 dB SL. Jerger (1962b) found that the ability to detect small changes in loudness is peculiar to disorders of the cochlea.

The strong tendency toward an all-or-none type of response on the SISI test led Owens (1965) to conclude that the test may be justifiably shortened to the use of 10 increments, allotting a credit of 10% to each increment. Other researchers (Griffing and Tuck, 1963; Yantis and Decker, 1964) also found a tendency for SISI scores to cluster at extremes of the continuum and concluded that the test may be reduced to 10 increments in many cases. Clinical experience supports the above findings. If the scores are in the 0 to 10% range or the 90 to 100% range, one may justifiably present only 10 increments. For scores falling outside of these extremes the full 20 increments should be employed to increase the accuracy of the procedure.

It goes without saying that unless the SISI increment is precisely 1 dB the entire procedure is less than useful. A section of Chapter 8 has been devoted to calibration of the SISI unit. There is no way of knowing the frequency or accuracy with which this calibration takes place in individual audiology centers. One might suppose that such calibration checks are achieved with less regularity than sound level checks for air and bone conduction or for speech, and that there is reason to suppose that this is not often enough in many centers. In their original work, Jerger et al. (1959) maintained the carrier tone at a specific level and superimposed the increments above this level. While many examiners probably believe this to be true of their own equipment many audiometers actually attenuate the level of the carrier tone so that the maximum level of the increment is the same, regardless of the increment size. In other words, instead of increasing level for the increment, an audiometer may decrease the carrier tone by the size (in dB) of the increment selected. A change in the level of the carrier tone when switching from one increment size to another may evoke a response from the patient before the increment is presented. The clinician should be familiar with the equipment to be used and be knowledgeable about its proper calibration procedures. There seems to be evidence that decreasing the level of the carrier tone by 1 dB has no effect on SISI scores.

VARIATIONS OF INCREMENT SIZE

The popularity of the SISI procedure led to investigations into methods of sharpening its accuracy by decreasing the magnitude of the increment. For example, Hanley and Utting (1965) tested 48 subjects with the SISI test using increment sizes of 1.0, 0.75 and 0.5 dB. They found that many normal hearing subjects were able to detect small intensity changes of 1 dB in the higher frequencies. Many subjects with cochlear pathology could hear changes as small as 0.5 dB. They recommended that the SISI test be done with an increment size of 0.75 dB for all subjects in order to make the task more difficult for normal hearing persons, yet possible for cochlear-impaired patients.

In a manner similar to the above experiment, Sanders (1966) performed the SISI test using 1.0-, 0.75- and 0.5-dB increments on 24 subjects with normal hearing and 9 with cochlear lesions. He found that the SISI test distinguished the two groups more consistently with a 1-dB increment than with either of the smaller sizes. The major conclusion of this study was that the SISI test should be carried out using 1-dB increments. This is apparently the present consensus among audiologists (Pennington and Martin, 1972).

MODIFIED SISI TESTS

Several modifications of the SISI procedure have been suggested for use in determining pathology which is central to the cochlea. Jerger et al. (1969) suggested that the SISI equipment may be used to perform psychometric functions for intensity discrimination, that is, the percentage correct vs. increment size. The curves for the two ears may differ in lesions of the central auditory pathways. When these functions differ it may be concluded that poor intensity discrimination results at the ear opposite the affected side of the brain.

Two cases with surgically confirmed acoustic neuromas without any appreciable loss of hearing in the test ear are reported by Thompson (1963). The SISI test was administered at 1000 Hz using 1-dB increments at 20 dB SL and then again at 75 dB hearing threshold level (HTL). In each case the patient's normal ear served as a control against which the affected ear was compared. At high levels of stimulation both patients were able to detect small increments in the normal ear but not in the affected ear. It appears that an ear with a retrocochlear lesion is incapable of normal reaction to small intensity increments even at high sensation levels. Hodgson (1967) cited a patient with a unilateral hemispherectomy who showed reduced SISI scores at high intensity levels on the ear opposite the affected side of the brain.

Koch, Bartels and Rupp (1969) compared a normal hearing group with a sensory-neural group on the SISI test at the standard 20 dB SL and at several higher levels. The normal subjects and those with cochlear pathology showed elevated SISI scores as the carrier tone was increased in intensity. Five subjects with retrocochlear lesions continued to have low SISI scores even at high levels. The work of Koch et al. supports the findings of Thompson (1963) that a modified SISI test may be carried out at high sensation levels. Thus, by using both the standard and modified SISI tests we can obtain not only information which separates cochlear from noncochlear lesions, but also precochlear from retrocochlear lesions.

The above research suggests that the SISI test may be performed in at least five ways:

1. One-dB increments at 20 dB SL (the classical SISI test) — high scores suggest a cochlear lesion.
2. Two- to 5-dB increments at 20 dB SL — low scores suggest a retrocochlear lesion.
3. One-dB increments at high sound levels (e.g., 75 dB HTL) — low scores suggest a retrocochlear lesion.
4. Increment sizes varied from 1 to 5 dB at 20 dB SL — poorer scores in one ear than the other (when thresholds are approximately equal) suggest a central lesion opposite the ear with the lower scores.
5. One-dB increments at SLs ranging from 20 dB to high levels (about 75 dB HTL) in 10-dB steps for both ears — difference in the rate at which scores increase suggests a retrocochlear lesion. The disorder is located on the same side as the ear which has not shown normal increases in intensity discrimination with increased loudness.

EXPLANATIONS FOR THE SISI PHENOMENON

The original explanation of the SISI test was based on the premise that the damaged cochlea gives rise to the faculty for detection of small intensity changes. This increased discriminability is not found in precochlear and retrocochlear lesions. Other theories have been suggested to explain the SISI results obtained in patients with various conductive and sensory-neural lesions. Some of these explanations are discussed below.

Swisher (1966) used the SISI procedure to determine the DLI for a 2000-Hz tone at levels ranging from 0 to 100 dB HTL. Subjects for her study included 20 normal hearing individuals and 20 subjects with hearing losses of cochlear origin. SISI scores were much higher in the cochlear disorder group when the data were calculated as a function of SL. Median SISI scores for the pathologic group were quite high even when the presentation level was close to threshold but the group with normal hearing required higher SLs to get comparable scores. However, when the median scores were plotted by HTL the results for the normal and cochlear cases were quite similar.

A physiologic explanation offered for Swisher's findings is based upon the knowledge that neurons with low thresholds increase in their rate of nerve impulses more slowly with increased sound pressure level (SPL) than do neurons with high thresholds. Swisher referred to the work of Davis (1957) and suggested that once the threshold of the inner hair cells of the cochlea is reached, the ear's ability to detect small changes in intensity is markedly improved. This dual excitation theory would suggest that in cochlear lesions showing high SISI scores the inner hair cells are not damaged. Histologic evidence in several cases of Meniere's disease (Hallpike and Hood, 1959) showed no specific sparing of inner hair cells.

Two experiments were conducted which were concerned with the relationship between the hearing level of a standard tone and the sensitivity to an intensity change on the SISI test (Swisher, Stephens and Doehring, 1966). In the first experiment, SISI scores were plotted as a function of the standard SL of 20 dB at which the SISI test is normally performed. In the second experiment, measurements were made on patients with sensory-neural hearing losses in relation to their SISI scores and to the score variability in a group of normal hearing subjects. The results indicated that the SISI score is influenced by both the HTL of the carrier tone and normal variability in differential sensitivity.

Since the DLI was considered by many to be an indirect test for recruitment, and since the SISI is a modification of the DLI tests, the assumption became widespread that the SISI is an indirect test for recruitment. To clarify the relationship between loudness and SISI scores Martin and Salas (1970) conducted a study on subjects with unilateral cochlear pathology. A level in the normal ear equal in loudness to 20 dB SL in the abnormal ear was selected for the SISI test. The two ears produced different SISI scores. Reversing this approach, a level in the poorer ear equal in loudness to 20 dB SL at the better ear was determined and SISI scores obtained at the two ears, again with different results. However, when the same SPLs were used in each ear (equal to 20 dB at the poor ear) equal SISI scores resulted. The conclusion drawn was that when the SISI test is performed at 55 to 65 dB SPL in either normal or cochlear impaired ears, a high score results at 4000 Hz, regardless of the sensation of loudness. This study effectively demonstrates that the SISI test is *not* an indirect test for recruitment.

Further evidence of the effects of sound intensity are shown by Harbert, Young and Weiss (1969) who performed the SISI test at several SPLs in normal and recruiting ears.

Pure tones of 60 dB SPL or greater yielded positive SISI scores in both groups. This study showed that individuals with normal and recruiting ears perceived equal increments at equal SPLs.

A physiologic explanation of the SISI phenomenon may be derived from the work of Eggermont and Odenthal (1974). They concluded that the compound cochlear action potential is comprised of synchronous firings of simultaneous single nerve fibers with the action potential actually having two peaks. This apparently means that there are two separate populations of neural units, one having a longer latency period than the other. The population with the shorter latency has a higher threshold than the population with the longer latency. The dynamic ranges of the two populations are different. These authors postulate that the population with the shorter latency has about 10 times as many nerve fibers as the population with the longer latency. Since amplitude-modulated stimuli produce compound action potentials, the amplitude of these potentials depends in part upon the amount of the intensity increment but primarily upon the level of the continuous tone. If the SISI carrier tone lies in the area below the threshold value for the shorter latency fibers the increment will not be detected. If the area stimulated is in the steep part of the input-output curve the shorter latency fibers are stimulated, producing a greater action potential, resulting in detection of small increments. This means that the intensity of the carrier tone determines the areas of the cochlea stimulated and if a high enough level is reached (e.g., 60 dB SPL) a high SISI score results. Similar conclusions may be drawn from the report of Yoshie (1968).

SISI AND THRESHOLD TONE DECAY

When an ear demonstrates abnormal tone decay the auditory threshold is elevated. Therefore, the 20-dB SL of the SISI test is lowered in proportion to the degree of adaptation. The effects of tone decay on SISI scores were studied by Bartholomeus and Swisher (1971) who found that even with slight adaptation (5 to 20 dB) the SISI scores may be reduced. Therefore, lower SISI scores may result even in the absence of retrocochlear lesions. Ward (1973) also reported that if the sustained stimulus decreases in loudness the SL gets lower and the DLI gets larger, decreasing the likelihood of the detection of the 1-dB increment on the SISI test.

The SISI test follows the same rules as the DLI with regard to the increased ability to detect small intensity changes as a function of increased intensity. Young and Harbert (1967) found that if the cochlea receives an audible signal of 60 dB SPL or greater, a high percentage of correct identifications of the 1 dB increment on the SISI test will result unless the ear is subject to pathologic adaptation. Lack of SISI responses was noted in cases with abnormal adaptation regardless of the intensity of the carrier tone. High scores indicate that the ear is functioning as a normal ear would with an equivalent SPL. A low percentage of responses indicates abnormal adaptation, in the view of Young and Harbert.

Hughes (1968) discussed 18 subjects with such abnormal adaptation that the carrier tone of the SISI quickly faded to inaudibility. The 1-dB increment was detected as a burst of tone which seemed to emerge from silence. His conclusion was that the SISI test retains its validity in cochlear cases even with unusual pathologic adaptation.

The literature is inconsistent regarding the effects of rapid perstimulatory adaptation on SISI scores. Nevertheless, if the SISI test is considered necessary in a particular case it should not be abandoned because of positive findings on the tone decay test. If the scores are high this will provide valuable information. If the scores are low the interpretation may not be clear since the lack of response may be due to the adaptation of the carrier tone and not a result of retrocochlear pathology.

THE SISI TEST AND CONTRALATERAL MASKING

One consideration of SISI test administration which has been of particular concern to this writer is the use or nonuse of contralateral masking. It is appropriate to mask during any auditory test when there is a danger of cross-hearing of the signal. There is a chance that the signal may be heard in the nontest ear when the carrier tone of the SISI, minus the interaural attenuation for the test frequency, is equal to or above the bone-conduction threshold of the nontest ear. It is natural to wonder whether contralateral masking has an effect on SISI scores since masking is used for this procedure only in selected cases.

Blegvad and Terkildsen (1966) found that masking the nontest ear exerts an influence on auditory procedures when a sustained stimulus is involved. In the case of the SISI test the scores tended to increase in the high frequencies. These investigators (Blegvad and Terkildsen, 1967) later tested 10 normal hearing subjects at 250, 1000 and 4000 Hz with contralateral noise at 0, 50, 70, and 90 dB SPL. Their results showed no effects of contralateral masking at 1000 Hz, improved discrimination for the increments at 4000 Hz and poorer discrimination at 250 Hz. The results at 4000 Hz were explained

by neural interaural interdependence. The increased difficulty at 250 Hz may have been due to middle ear muscle reflexes, since this could effectively reduce the SL of the carrier tone.

Auditory intensity discrimination at 2000 Hz for normal subjects using carrier tones at levels from 23 to 78 dB SPL was studied by Swisher, Dudley and Doehring (1969). This was done in the presence of contralateral white or sawtooth noise which was varied from 0 to 63 dB SPL. The results showed that intensity discrimination was significantly improved in both ears by the use of contralateral masking when the carrier tones were 38 dB HTL or above. The DLs for the left ear were significantly smaller than the right ear in both quiet and noise. This apparent difference in the ability to detect small changes in loudness between the right and left ears seems to be ignored in clinical practice, in part because of the apparent lack of replication of these results.

Cortical evoked responses were elicited to SISI signals in normal subjects by Osterhammel, Terkildsen and Arndal (1970). With the carrier tone at 20 dB SL, masking noise in the opposite ear enhanced responses to increments of 2, 3 and 5 dB. With the carrier tone at threshold no response was seen with opposite ear masking, not even to 5-dB increments, which is probably due to central masking effects.

Measuring SISI scores on patients with unilateral sensory-neural hearing loss, Blegvad (1969) found that intensity discrimination improved with contralateral masking with test frequencies at 1000 and 4000 Hz. No changes were seen at 250 Hz. Blegvad concluded that no real compromise is seen in the diagnostic value of the SISI when the opposite ear is masked.

In his review of effects of masking on DLs for intensity, Studebaker (1973) states that ". . . only infrequently do circumstances dictate the need for masking with [the] SISI test." It is difficult to agree with this statement since the major concern for site-of-lesion diagnosis occurs in cases of unilateral sensory-neural hearing loss. The fact that the SISI test is performed at suprathreshold levels suggests that it may contralateralize even if threshold-level signals do not, requiring the use of masking to eliminate nontest ear participation in the test.

If the carrier tone of the SISI test can be heard by the nontest ear the audiologist may inadvertently perform a binaural rather than a monaural test. In order to avoid this possibility, masking should be used. A precise procedure should be undertaken which avoids the unfortunate pitfalls of undermasking or overmasking in the majority of cases. The use of minimum effective masking recommended elsewhere (Martin, 1975) appears applicable. The level of effective masking for use in the nontest ear should be equal to the hearing level dial setting of the carrier tone minus the patient's interaural attenuation for the test frequency (40 dB if this is not known) plus any air-bone gap at the masked ear (Table 16.1). This should provide a minimum level of noise which is high enough to avoid contralateral participation on the SISI test.

VALUE OF THE SISI AS A DIAGNOSTIC TEST

The primary reason for performing the SISI test is to help in determination of the site of lesion in the auditory system by determining whether a disorder is cochlear or noncochlear. Reports conflict on just how effectively this goal is achieved using the SISI.

In support of the SISI test's usefulness Jerger (1961) reported on 20 subjects with Meniere's disease, all of whom had positive SISI scores. He also reported on 11 subjects with acoustic neuromas, 10 of whom had negative SISI scores and one showing a questionable score. There are many other statements in the literature to support the contention that high SISI scores indicate cochlear pathology.

In contrast to this apparent high validity in separating cochlear from retrocochlear hearing losses, numerous case studies exist. For example, Johnson (1966) found that of 163 patients with surgically confirmed retrocochlear lesions, 23 had positive SISI scores. Many similar findings of high SISI scores in the presence of retrocochlear pathology appear in the literature (Brand and Rosenberg, 1963; Shapiro and Naunton, 1967; Johnson, 1968).

There are several explanations for positive SISI scores in cranial nerve VIII lesions. Changes in blood supply to the cochlea caused by pressure on the internal auditory artery by an acoustic neuroma may produce cochlear hypoxia with resultant cochlear symptoms on auditory tests (Perez de Moura, 1967). In addition, alterations in the chemistry of the intracochlear fluids caused by a neuroma may also produce cochlear findings (Perez de Moura, 1967; Benitez, Lopez-Rios and Novon, 1967). Cases with surgically confirmed acoustic neuromas, because of their certainty of site of lesion, have been used to illustrate auditory test findings characterized as "typically" retrocochlear. There may (Hitselberger and House, 1966) or may not (Maddox, 1971) be a relationship between the size of the tumor and SISI scores although it is generally expected that larger tumors produce lower scores.

The diagnostic value of the SISI test depends upon the amount of hearing loss a patient may have. Low scores result when testing patients with mild cochlear losses (Harford, 1967; Owens, 1965). Testing 40 normal hearing subjects using three different sensation levels and eight different increment sizes Blegvad (1966) found that at low SLs SISI scores are higher in the high frequencies than in the low frequencies but at 40 dB SL the scores are the same for all frequencies, a finding which might have been predicted by the early work of Riesz (1928) on DLs for intensity. The patient with a cochlear hearing loss of less than 30 or 40 dB HTL will therefore give a low SISI score for the same reason as a person with normal hearing.

It would seem that in certain nerve VIII involvements the symptoms of both cochlear and nerve VIII pathology may be seen. The audiologist should be alerted by the nerve VIII symptoms rather than diverted by the cochlear findings. There are positive tests for cochlear disorders and positive tests for retrocochlear disorders. The SISI belongs in the former category and so negative SISI findings do not necessarily constitute a positive retrocochlear finding, just as positive SISI scores do not exclude the possibility of a retrocochlear disorder. The fallibility of relying on the SISI test as a single diagnostic tool is pointed out repeatedly in the literature (Menzel, 1966; Jerger, 1962c, Sanders, 1965; Tillman, 1966; Hood, 1969; Katinsky, Lovrinic and Buchheit, 1972; Carhart, 1973). Experienced audiologists maintain that the SISI test is useful diagnostically in that it supplements other auditory tests in differentiation of disorders of the middle ear, cochlea or nerve VIII.

TABLE 16.1. *Masking for Short Increment Sensitivity Index (SISI) Test*

When to mask: SISI HTL−IA = BC_{nte}*
Effective masking level:
EM = SISI HTL − IA + ABG_{nte}**

* Mask when the hearing level dial setting for SISI, minus the interaural attenuation (IA) for the test tone is equal to or higher than the bone-conduction (BC) threshold of the nontest ear (nte).
** The effective masking (EM) level is equal to the hearing level dial setting for the SISI, minus the interaural attenuation, plus any air-bone gap (ABG) at the test frequency in the nontest ear.

CONCLUSIONS

Recent years have not shown much in the way of new research on the SISI test. Most reports on this test have been on the order of clinical comments on its diagnostic efficacy. There is surely no unanimity of agreement on this subject.

There is no way of knowing, at the time of this writing, the extent to which newer auditory tests are replacing the SISI as a routine site-of-lesion procedure. I have a tendency to agree with Jerger (1973) that considering the newer and more rapid tests that are now available, the SISI, although valuable, should perhaps remain as a second rank test, to be used in cases of equivocal findings on other, more reliable tests.

Clinical experience and research data are teaching us the extent to which we can rely on any single test procedure. We have learned that the SISI test is not an indirect test for recruitment or for anything else. For whatever reason, it is a direct test of the ear's ability to detect small intensity changes at a suprathreshold level. The SISI procedure remains an easy one to perform but one which must be interpreted with great care in difficult diagnostic circumstances.

REFERENCES

Bartholomeus, B., and Swisher, L., Tone decay and SISI scores. *Arch. Otolaryngol.*, 93, 451–455, 1971.

Benitez, J., Lopez-Rios, G., and Novon, V., Bilateral acoustic neuromas; a human temporal bone report. *Arch. Otolaryngol.*, 86, 51–57, 1967.

Blegvad, B., The SISI test in normal-hearing listeners; an investigation with noncommercial equipment. *Acta Otolaryngol.*, 62, 201–212, 1966.

Blegvad, B., Differential intensity sensitivity and clinical masking. *Acta Otolaryngol.*, 67, 428–434, 1969.

Blegvad, B., and Terkildsen, K., SISI test and contralateral masking. *Acta Otolaryngol.*, 62, 453–458, 1966.

Blegvad, B., and Terkildsen, K., Contralateral masking and the SISI test in normal listeners. *Acta Otolaryngol.*, 63, 557–563, 1967.

Brand, S., and Rosenberg, P.E., Problems in auditory evaluation for neurosurgical diagnosis. *J. Speech Hear. Disord.*, 28, 355–361, 1963.

Carhart, R., Updating special hearing tests in otological diagnosis. *Arch. Otolaryngol.*, 97, 88–91, 1973.

Davis, H., Biophysics and physiology of the inner ear. *Physiol. Rev.*, 37, 1–49, 1957.

Denes, P., and Naunton, R. F., The clinical detection of auditory recruitment. *J. Laryngol.*, 65, 375–398, 1950.

Dix, M. R., Hallpike, C. S., and Hood, J. D., Observations upon the loudness recruitment phenomenon, with especial reference to the differential diagnosis of disorders of the internal ear and VIIIth nerve. *Proc. R. Soc. Med.*, 41, 516–526, 1948.

Eggermont, J. J., and Odenthal, D. W., Action potentials and summating potentials in the normal human cochlea. *Acta Otolaryngol.*, Suppl., 316, 1974.

Griffing, T. A., and Tuck, G. A., Split-half reliability of the SISI. *J. Aud. Res.*, 3, 159–164, 1963.

Hallpike, C. S., and Hood, J. D., Observations upon the neurological mechanisms of the loudness recruitment phenomenon. *Acta Otolaryngol.*, 50, 472–486, 1959.

Hanley, C. N., and Utting, J. F., An examination of the normal hearer's response to the SISI. *J. Speech Hear. Disord.*, 30, 58–65, 1965.

Harbert, F., Young, I. M., and Weiss, B. G., Clinical application of intensity difference limen. *Acta Otolaryngol.*, 67, 435–443, 1969.

Harford, E. R., Clinical application and significance of the SISI test. In Graham, A. B. (Ed.), *Sensorineural hearing processes and disorders*, p. 223–233. Boston: Little, Brown & Co., 1967.

Harris, J. D., Loudness discrimination. *J. Speech Hear. Disord. Monogr. Suppl.* No. 11, 1963.

Hirsh, I. J., Palva, T., and Goodman, A., Difference limen and recruitment. *Arch. Otolaryngol.*, 60, 525–540, 1954.

Hitselberger, W. E., and House, W. F., Classification of acoustic neuromas. *Arch. Otolaryngol.*, 84, 245–246, 1966.

Hodgson, W. R., Audiological report of a patient with left hemispherectomy. *J. Speech Hear. Disord.*, 32, 39–45, 1967.

Hood, J. D., Basic audiological requirements in neuro-otology. *J. Laryngol. Otol.*, 83, 695–711, 1969.

Hughes, R. L. Atypical responses to the SISI. *Ann. Otol. Rhinol. Laryngol.*, 77, 332–337, 1968.

Jerger, J. A difference limen recruitment test and its diagnostic significance. *Laryngoscope*, 62, 1316–1332, 1952.

Jerger, J., DL difference test; improved method for clinical measurement of recruitment. *Arch. Otolaryngol.*, 57, 490–500, 1953.

Jerger, J., Recruitment and allied phenomena in differential diagnosis. *J. Aud. Res.*, 1, 145–151, 1961.

Jerger, J., Comparative evaluation of some auditory measures. *US Air Force Sch. Aerospace Med.*, Report No. 62–26, 1962a.

Jerger, J., The SISI test. *Int. Audiol.*, 1, 246–247, 1962b.

Jerger, J., Hearing tests in otologic diagnosis. *ASHA*, 4, 139–145, 1962c.

Jerger, J., Diagnostic audiometry, In Jerger, J. (Ed.), *Modern Developments in Audiology*, Ed. 2, pp. 75–115. New York: Academic Press, 1973.

Jerger, J., Shedd, J., and Harford, E., On the detection of extremely small changes in sound intensity. *Arch. Otolaryngol.*, 69, 200–211, 1959.

Jerger, J., Weikers, N., Sharbrough, F., and Jerger, S., Bilateral lesions of the temporal lobe; a case study. *Acta Otolaryngol.*, Suppl. 258, 1–51, 1969.

Johnson, E. W., Confirmed retrocochlear lesions; auditory test results in 163 patients. *Arch. Otolaryngol.*, 84, 247–254, 1966.

Johnson, E. W., Auditory findings in 200 cases of acoustic neuromas. *Arch. Otolaryngol.*, 88, 598–603, 1968.

Katinsky, S., Lovrinic, J., and Buchheit, W., Cochlear findings in VIIIth nerve tumors. *Audiology*, 11, 213–217, 1972.

Koch, L. J., Bartels, D., and Rupp, R. R., The use of a "modified" short increment sensitivity index in assessing site of auditory lesion. Paper read at the 45th annual convention of the American Speech and Hearing Association, Chicago, 1969.

Konig, G., Difference limen for intensity. *Int. Audiol.*, 1, 198–202, 1962.

Lund-Iverson, L., An investigation on the difference

limen determined by the method of Luscher and Zwislocki in normal hearing and in various forms of deafness. *Acta Otolaryngol.*, **42**, 219–224, 1952.

Luscher, E., and Zwislocki, J., A simple method for indirect monaural determination of the recruitment phenomenon (difference limen in intensity in different types of deafness). *Acta Otolaryngol.*, **78**, 156–168, 1949.

Maddox, H. E., Progressive audiometric changes in acoustic neuroma — early diagnosis. *Laryngoscope*, **81**, 707–715, 1971.

Martin, F. N., Auditory Tests for Site of Lesion. In *Introduction to Audiology*, p. 173–179. Englewood Cliffs, N. J.: Prentice-Hall, 1975.

Martin, F. N., and Salas, C. R., The SISI test and subjective loudness. *J. Aud. Res.*, **10**, 368–371, 1970.

Menzel, O. J., The short increment sensitivity index (SISI)-Part II. *Eye Ear Nose Throat Mon.*, **45**, 83–84, 1966.

Osterhammel, P., Terkildsen, K., and Arndal, P., Evoked responses to SISI stimuli. Contralateral masking effects. *Acta Otolaryngol.*, Suppl. 263, 245–247, 1970.

Owens, E., The SISI test and VIIIth nerve versus cochlear involvement. *J. Speech Hear. Disord.*, **30**, 252–262, 1965.

Pennington, C. D., and Martin, F. N., Current trends in audiometric practices. Part II. Auditory tests for site of lesion. *ASHA*, **14**, 199–203, 1972.

Perez de Moura, L., Inner ear pathology in acoustic neuromas. *Arch. Otolaryngol.*, **85**, 125–133, 1967.

Riesz, R. R., Differential intensity sensitivity of the ear for pure tones. *Phys. Rev.*, **31**, 867–875, 1928.

Sanders, J. W., Labyrinthine otosclerosis. *Arch. Otolaryngol.*, **81**, 553–563, 1965.

Sanders, J., The effect of increment size on the short increment sensitivity index scores. *J. Speech Hear. Res.*, **9**, 297–304, 1966.

Shapiro, R., and Naunton, R. F., Audiologic evaluation of acoustic neurinomas. *J. Speech Hear. Disord.*, **32**, 29–35, 1967.

Studebaker, G. A. Auditory Masking. In Jerger, J. (Ed.), *Modern Developments in Audiology*, Ed. 2, p. 117–154. New York: Academic Press, 1973.

Swisher, L. P., Response to intensity change in cochlear pathology. *Laryngoscope*, **76**, 1706–1713, 1966.

Swisher, L. P., Dudley, J. G., and Doehring, D. G., Influence of contralateral noise on auditory intensity discrimination. *J. Acoust. Soc. Am.*, **45**, 1532–1536, 1969.

Swisher, L. P., Stephens, M. M., and Doehring, D. G., The effects of hearing level and normal variability of sensitivity to intensity change. *J. Aud. Res.*, **6**, 249–259, 1966.

Thompson, G., A modified SISI technique for selected cases with suspected acoustic neurinoma. *J. Speech Hear. Disord.*, **28**, 299–302, 1963.

Tillman, T. W., Audiologic diagnosis of acoustic tumors. *Arch. Otolaryngol.*, **83**, 574–581, 1966.

Ward, W. D. Adaptation and Fatigue. In Jerger, J. (Ed.), *Modern Developments in Audiology*, Ed. 2, p. 301–344. New York: Academic Press, 1973.

Yantis, P. A., and Decker, R. L., On the short increment sensitivity index (SISI test). *J. Speech Hear. Disord.*, **29**, 231–246, 1964.

Yoshie, N., Auditory nerve action potential response to clicks in man. *Laryngoscope*, **78**, 198–214, 1968.

Young, I. M., and Harbert, F., Significance of the SISI test. *J. Aud. Res.*, **7**, 303–311, 1967.

chapter 17

TONE DECAY

David S. Green, Ph.D.

Abnormal tone decay is a symptom that is associated with retrocochlear lesions. Extreme tone decay can occur even when thresholds for pure tones of short duration are only mildly or moderately elevated. As a result, a cursory evaluation might underestimate the potential seriousness of the condition. The audiologist should bear in mind that abnormal tone decay *may* be caused by pathology which, if untreated, could result in death to the patient. At the same time, one must be wary not to make the spurious assumption that the presence of the symptom is prima facie evidence that a life-threatening lesion exists.

TERMINOLOGY

Tone decay can be measured at threshold or at suprathreshold levels. Threshold tone decay may be defined as the decrease in threshold sensitivity resulting from the presence of a barely audible sound; suprathreshold tone decay is a decrease in threshold resulting from a sound well above threshold. Tone decay may be operationally defined and its magnitude quantified on the basis of the specific technique used to measure it. Several techniques will be described in this chapter.

The literature on tone decay shows considerable variation in terminology. A partial list of terms associated with this phenomenon would include: auditory threshold fatigue, temporary threshold fatigue (Kos, 1955), abnormal adaptation (Carhart, 1957), pathologic relapse (Hood, 1956), temporary threshold shift (Lierle and Reger, 1955), Albrecht effect (Ward, 1963), slow adaptation (Sorensen, 1962b), tone perversion (Parker, Decker and Richards, 1968), perstimulatory auditory adaptation (Palva, 1964), threshold drift (Harbert and Young, 1962, a and b) and pathologic fatigue (Flottorp, 1963).

When encountering these terms in the literature, the reader should not assume that they may be used interchangeably with tone decay as defined earlier. However, if the signal being discussed is at or near threshold, it is a safe assumption that concurrent changes in threshold sensitivity relate to the tone decay phenomenon being considered here.

There is confusion between the terms fatigue and adaptation. While it is beyond the scope of this chapter to treat these topics elaborately, some discussion of terminology is in order.

Hood (1956) asserted that a major distinction between the two is that fatigue effects last longer and can be measured after the fatiguing stimulus is discontinued. Adaptation effects, on the other hand, recover so rapidly that they must be measured before the source of stimulation is interrupted.

Sergeant and Harris (1963) were in general agreement with the Hood definition and classified threshold tone decay as a unique category of adaptation, differing from "fast adaptation" and " perstimulatory adaptation." Basing their classification on threshold recovery period they indicated that since threshold tone decay recovers within a few seconds following the cessation of the signal, the recovery is too slow for the phenomenon to be classed as fast adaptation and too fast to be classed as perstimulatory adaptation.

Palva (1964) also classified threshold tone decay as a type of adaptation. Unlike Sergeant and Harris, he indicated a preference for the term perstimulatory auditory adaptation noting that it can be measured either at suprathreshold levels or at threshold.

Flottorp (1963), on the other hand, suggested that the term fatigue is relevant if one considers that there are two types, namely perstimulatory and poststimulatory fatigue. Flottorp stated his preference for the term perstimulatory fatigue to designate the tone decay phenomenon, and based this opinion on the agreement between *Webster's* definition of fatigue: "Condition of cells or organs which have undergone excessive activity with resulting loss of power or capacity to respond to stimulation," and the clinical manifestations of tone decay. Because the term poststimulatory fatigue is associated with slow recovery of threshold, it was considered inappropriate.

Many of the inconsistencies in terminology can be reconciled by paying careful attention to the method of measurement. This point of view suggests that things measured in the same way by the same tone decay test are equal to each other, no matter what they are called.

HISTORY OF TONE DECAY

There exists a commonly held, but inaccurate, belief that the phenomenon of tone decay has been discovered recently. Observations relating to tone decay were made and reported as far back as the nineteenth century (Rayleigh, 1882; Corradi, 1890; Gradenigo, 1893). The recent interest in tone decay may be characterized better as a rediscovery.

Early History

In an unpublished chapter devoted to the early history of tone decay in the pre-electronic era, Ward (1970) credits Lord Rayleigh with the earliest known demonstration of tone decay. Using a gas-filled balloon to power a bird call device which sustained a high frequency tone, Rayleigh noted that the tone soon disappeared (decayed). However, he also observed that a brief interruption, merely waving the hand in front of the ear, was enough to bring it back into consciousness. Ward also referred to Corradi who in 1890 demonstrated that tone decay occurs in bone conduction. Corradi found that if, after the tone disappeared, the tuning fork was taken off the mastoid and replaced again quickly, certain of his patients were again able to hear it.

Gradenigo observed that patients with acoustic tumors responded to a maximally vibrating tuning fork for only a few seconds. In 1893 he noted that in these cases an initially loud signal quickly disappeared (decayed) (Reger and Kos, 1958).

Dunlap (1904) was one of the first to use electromagnetic aids in a study related to the off-effect frequently noted in tone decay tests. Dunlap had experimental subjects listen to sound "emitted by telephone receiver" at an intensity near threshold. Their task was to indicate when the tone was present and when it was absent. When the subject reported the signal to be inaudible, Dunlap turned it off. He observed that almost half the cases reported "hearing it cease."

Current History

With the regeneration of interest in tone decay, both Bekesy and conventional audiometers were employed to assess it. At first, there was some question as to its primary diagnostic significance but, as clinical and experimental evidence accrued, it became clear that the characteristics of the tone decay could be used to help diagnose retrocochlear lesions.

Bekesy Audiometer Studies. Soon after Bekesy (1947) described his new audiometer Reger and Kos (1952), using Bekesy instrumentation, made the observation that an abnormally rapid temporary threshold shift occurred in an individual with a cranial nerve VIII tumor. This discovery led to increased interest in the assessment of tone decay and to refinements in techniques of measurement with both standard and Bekesy audiometry. Regardless of whether standard or Bekesy audiometry is used, the diagnostic differentiation between retrocochlear and other lesions is based upon the characteristics of the tone decay which the tests illustrate.

Conventional Audiometer Studies. Schubert (1944), using a conventional audiometer, provided an audiometric technique for the measurement of tone decay. This was published in a foreign journal during the hectic era of World War II, which may account for its delayed recognition and application. Following Schubert, a number of investigators applied conventional pure tone audiometry to the measurement of tone decay. In the process of devising an approach to its assessment, they modified existing techniques to conform to their own observations and experience. Today, as a result, there is considerable variation among test procedures from one diagnostic center to another.

Among those who have described conventional audiometry techniques for measuring tone decay are Hood (1956), Carhart (1957), Rosenberg (1958), Sorensen (1962a), Green (1963), Owens (1964), Parker et al. (1968), Bhatia, Sinha and Abrol (1969), Gjaevenes and Sohoel (1969), Olsen and Noffsinger (1974), and Jerger and Jerger (1975). Several of these techniques will be discussed in detail.

TONE DECAY MEASUREMENT PROCEDURES USING CONVENTIONAL AUDIOMETRY

Tone decay measurements are usually made with a conventional pure tone audiometer and can be applied to any available frequency. The quantity of tone decay in dB is usually taken as the difference between the initial threshold and the threshold at which the test is terminated. The frequencies chosen for study will depend on the patient's hearing status and tester preference. Some techniques employ a brief rest period between successive levels of stimulation. Some require a response to "tone only"; others accept a response to "any sound," tonal or not. Because of the variations in procedure, the end results are often not comparable. More systematic studies are needed which compare the end results of the different tests on individual patients with retrocochlear lesions, although some such studies have been recently reported.

Several procedures for measuring tone decay will be described in the following paragraphs. An attempt has been made to include the essential characteristics of each based on what has been reported in the literature.

Schubert Tone Decay Test

It appears that Schubert (1944) was the first to report the use of a conventional audiometer to measure tone decay. In his procedure, the patient was allowed to listen to a 5-dB sensation level (SL) tone until the tone disappeared. Thereafter, the intensity was raised in 5-dB steps without interruption until a plateau was reached or the maximum limit of the audiometer prohibited following the receding tone.

Hood Tone Decay Test

Hood (1956) reported on a more elaborate tone decay procedure which may be described in five steps.

Step 1. Obtain the subject's threshold of hearing for an interrupted tone.

Step 2. Instruct the subject to raise his finger (or push a button or raise his hand) as long as he hears the tone and to lower it if the signal fades into inaudibility.

Step 3. Begin the test by presenting the tone at a level 5 dB above threshold.

Step 4. If the subject signals that the tone is no longer audible, turn off the tone and allow at least 60 sec of rest.

Step 5. Raise the intensity of the tone 5 dB and repeat the procedure until an intensity is reached which produces a sensation of tone "indefinitely."

Carhart Tone Decay Test

In 1957, Carhart reported a procedure for measuring tone decay which was developed at Northwestern University in 1954. Its purpose was "to refine a technique which could be conducted rapidly in the typical office situation with any standard audiometer." Unlike the Hood method, the Carhart technique makes no provision for a rest period between successive levels of stimulation. The test entails the following steps.

Step 1. Obtain the subject's threshold of hearing for an interrupted tone.

Step 2. Instruct the subject to raise his finger as long as he hears the tone and to lower it if the signal fades into inaudibility.

Step 3. Begin the test with the sustained tone below the established threshold and then ascend in 5-dB steps without interruption until the subject responds.

Step 4. As soon as the subject responds begin timing with a stop watch. If the tone is heard for a full minute, terminate the test.

Step 5. If the subject indicates that he no longer hears the tone before the minute criterion is met, raise the intensity of the tone 5 dB *without interrupting the tone*, set the stop watch back to zero, and begin timing for a minute again. A record is kept of the number of seconds the tone is audible at each intensity level.

Step 6. Continue raising the tone in 5 dB steps as indicated until an intensity is reached that allows the subject to perceive the tone for a full minute. To save time, Carhart suggested setting an arbitrary test terminus (i.e., the subject's 30 dB SL) above which the test need not be continued even though the tone had not been perceived for the full minute.

Most testers who use the Carhart procedure begin the test at threshold or at 5 dB above threshold. However, Olsen and Noffsinger (1974) suggested beginning the test at the 20-dB SL. In their study of 20 patients with surgically confirmed nerve VIII tumor, the standard Carhart test and the 20-dB SL technique were equally sensitive in identifying excessive tone decay. They reported that the 20-dB SL test takes less time and presents an easier listening task for the patient. The authors stressed the importance of requiring response to "tonality" as opposed to response to "any sound" during tone decay testing.

Rosenberg One Minute Modification of the Carhart Tone Decay Test

Finding Carhart's method cumbersome and time-consuming in cases exhibiting marked tone decay, Rosenberg (1958) proposed a shortened version of the test. Exploration for any given tone is limited to a total of 60 sec. No record is kept of the number of seconds the tone is audible at each intensity level.

Steps 1 to 4. These steps are similar to Carhart procedure (above).

Step 5. If the subject indicates that he no longer hears the tone before the minute is completed, raise the intensity of the tone 5 dB without interrupting the stimulus and *without stopping the watch*.

Step 6. Continue in like manner raising the tone in 5 dB steps each time the tone becomes inaudible. At the end of a *total* of 60 sec, the tone is turned off and the amount of tone decay in dB is computed.

Green Modified Tone Decay Test (MTDT)

In 1960, Green noticed that some patients with retrocochlear lesions experienced loss of tonality before loss of audibility on the tone decay test. He modified the instructions given with the shortened 1-min version of the Carhart test (Green, 1963). The patient is seated in an armchair and told to maintain elbow contact with the armrest while he is signaling. He is trained to raise his arm perpendicular to the armrest if he perceives the stimulus as tonal, to lower it to a 45° angle if the stimulus loses tonality but remains audible, and to lower his arm to the rest position if the sound becomes completely inaudible. The patient is cautioned against adjusting the earphones or chewing while the test is in progress, as the slightest interruption in the continuity of the stimulus can impair test reliability. Requiring a response to perception of tonality is felt to enhance the sensitivity of the test.

The subjective change in quality of a pure tone to a noise lacking tonality, which was noted by Green, has been called tone perversion by Parker *et al.* (1968). Pestalozza and Cioce (1962), Sorensen (1962a), Flottorp (1963), Harbert and Young (1964b), Johnson (1966), Sung, Goetzinger and Knox (1969), and Olsen and Noffsinger (1974) have also encountered this phenomenon and take it into account when testing for tone decay.

Jerger and Jerger Suprathreshold Adaptation Test (STAT)

Working on the intriguing hypothesis that symptoms of abnormal tone decay first appear only at the highest testable sound intensities, Jerger and Jerger (1975) proposed a simplified suprathreshold tone decay test. The test frequencies are 500, 1000 and 2000 Hz, and the technique incorporates the following steps.

Step 1. The patient is instructed to signal as long as he hears the sound in the test ear. The nontest ear is masked with white noise at a level of 90 dB sound presure level (SPL).

Step 2. A continuous 500-Hz test tone at 110 dB SPL is presented until either the patient indicates that he no longer hears the tone, or until 60 sec have elapsed, whichever comes first.

Step 3. If the patient has responded for the full 60 sec for the test frequency, the test is scored negative.

Step 4. The test is scored positive if the patient has failed to respond for the full 60 sec.

Step 5. To ensure that the patient has grasped the essential nature of the listening task, the test tone is pulsed for 60 sec. If the patient signals that he heard the pulsed but not the continuous tone for 60 sec, it is likely that he is responding to the test in a reliable manner.

Step 6. The tester may then test 1000 Hz and 2000 Hz, as shown in steps 1 to 5 above.

Since most audiometers are calibrated in hearing level (HL) rather than SPL, the 110-dB SPL stimulus levels specified by the authors should be converted to HL to make them consistent with audiometric intensity calibration. Roughly, the hearing levels equivalent to the 110-dB SPL levels are: 500 Hz = 100 dB HL, 2000 Hz = 100 dB HL and 1000 Hz = 105 dB HL.

Other Variations. Sorensen (1962a) reported using a variation of the Carhart procedure which employed a 90-sec criterion for terminating the test rather than 60 sec. Unlike most other investigators, Sorensen confined his exploration for tone decay to a single frequency (2000 Hz).

In 1964, Owens published data on a modification of the Hood technique which incorporated a 20-sec rest period between stimulus presentations. He provided both amount of tone decay (up to 20 dB SL) and the pattern of tone decay (in seconds) at succeeding levels for categorization into normal, cochlear and retrocochlear types. Table 17.1 shows the interpretation of the Owens modification.

INTERPRETATION OF TEST RESULTS

The tone decay test is a powerful diagnostic procedure for retrocochlear pathology. However, it is only one of a battery of audiologic

TABLE 17.1. *Examples of Tone Decay Patterns**

Levels above Threshold	Patterns of Decay						
	Type I	Type II					Type III
		A	B	C	D	E	
dB							
5	60	25	7	12	15	5	14
10		60	34	26	23	14	16
15			60	40	30	18	12
20				60	39	21	14

* Numbers in the table represent seconds of time the tone was heard at the intensity level indicated before fading to inaudibility. A 20-sec rest was given between 5-dB increments. (From E. Owens: *Journal of Speech and Hearing Disorders, 29,* 14–22, 1964.)

and medical tests which are designed to establish this diagnosis. Therefore, the purpose of the tone decay test should be to identify persons with suspected retrocochlear pathology and to permit proper referral for further confirmation and diagnosis.

Classification

Despite the widespread use of tone decay tests, systems of classification appear infrequently in the literature. Rosenberg (1958) devised a clinically useful scale of gradation based on the number of dB of tone decay resulting from application of his procedure. He used the following criteria.

0 to 5 dB – Normal	20 to 25 dB – Moderate
10 to 15 – Mild	30 dB or more – Marked

Rosenberg (1969) indicated that mild to moderate levels of tone decay were frequently seen in pathology involving the organ of Corti, whereas marked tone decay almost always indicated retrocochlear pathology.

Glasscock (1968) using the same testing technique agreed that a positive tone decay test was one in which there were at least 30 dB of decay. Tillman (1969) advocated the longer Carhart procedure but agreed that patients with retrocochlear lesions typically had tone decay exceeding 30 dB.

Owens (1964) derived three major tone decay types.

Type I. There is no evidence of decay. The tone remains audible for 60 sec at 5 dB SL.

Type II. There is progressively slower decay with each 5-dB increment. The amount of decay is measured only up to the 20 dB SL. Five categories (A, B, C, D and E) of Type II tone decay are delineated on the basis of amount and rate of tone decay.

Type III. There is progressive decay with little or no change in rapidity with each 5 dB intensity increment up to 20 dB SL.

Owens stated that Types I and II are characteristic of Meniere's disease and Type III characteristic of a cranial nerve VIII lesion. He reported a strong positive relationship between Types I, II and III tone decay patterns and Bekesy audiometry (Owens, 1965). Owens (1970) further stated that he considered the Type II-E category "atypical" and found it to occur occasionally in both cochlear and retrocochlear involvement. The Owens variation of tone decay testing looks not only at the total amount of decay but at the changes in rapidity with increasing intensity as well.

Morales-Garcia and Hood (1972) used a four type classification system to indicate increasing amounts and rates of tone decay in patients who were given the Carhart tone decay test. The test frequencies were 500, 1000, 2000 and 4000 Hz. Records were kept of amount of decay as a function of time. Tone decay termed Type I was minimal and did not exceed 15 dB. Slightly greater decay was called Type II. Patients were classified as Type III if they had more then 20 dB of decay at 500 Hz, more than 25 dB at 1000 Hz, more than 30 dB at 2000 Hz or more than 35 dB at 4000 Hz. Type IV was distinguished from Type III primarily by rapidity of the decay. Based upon the average amount of decay during the first 3 min of testing, decay of less than 15 dB/min was classified Type III; decay of more than 15 dB/min was called Type IV. Type IV was a characteristic finding in 15 patients with nerve fiber lesions and Type III with a well marked but slow rate of decay, was found in a significant proportion of patients with brain stem lesions, including a number with normal pure tone thresholds.

From this discussion it can be seen that there is no standard system of classification. However, for the Carhart method and its modifications, there appears to be some agreement that a critical point in the differentiation between cochlear and retrocochlear pathology occurs as one approaches the 30-dB decay level. It would be dangerous to assume that everyone with more than 30 dB of tone decay has a retrocochlear lesion or that everyone with less than that amount does not. A more productive way of looking at tone decay that approaches the 30-dB mark is that each dB of decay above 15 dB should raise the index of suspicion that a retrocochlear lesion may exist.

The greater the tone decay and the number of frequencies involved, the greater the possibility of serious pathology. The index of suspicion should also be raised if the rate of decay does not diminish with increased stimulus intensity. Patients with acoustic tumors frequently exhibit extreme, and often complete, tone decay at all frequencies.

Tumor size appears related to the severity of the symptom. In support of this, Johnson (1966), reporting on 73 patients, found a positive relationship between size of tumor and results on the Green MTDT. Partial or complete tone decay was found in 63% of tumors classed as large and in only 14% of the small tumor category.

Site of Lesion Studies. There was some early confusion regarding the diagnostic significance of tone decay. Hallpike and Hood (1951) emphasized the distinction between the initial burst of auditory excitation, known as the on-effect, and the progressive reduction in excitation to sustained stimulation, which was called adaptation. They described patients in whom the on-effect to pure tone stimulus was normal, but in whom adaptation was unusually rapid. Such abnormal adaptation was called "relapse," and when accompanied by a normal on-effect was considered to be associated with loudness recruitment and disordered hair cell function in the organ of Corti. Other investigators have confirmed that patients with cochlear lesions have mild to moderate degrees of tone decay (Palva, 1957; Yantis, 1959; Jerger, 1960; Sorensen, 1962a; Rosenberg, 1969).

When the accumulation of clinical evidence led to the discovery that *marked* tone decay was characteristically found in patients with retrocochlear lesions, the diagnostic value of the test became more significant (Lierle and Reger, 1955; Sorensen, 1962a, Palva, 1964; Johnson, 1966; Rosenberg, 1969). Tone decay tests could be used to help identify patients with retrocochlear pathology, often tumors of the cerebellopontine angle. In most instances, the abnormal tone decay is found on the same side as the major focus of the lesion. However, cases have been reported where a tumor on one side has been associated with symptoms in the contralateral ear (Stroud and Thalmann, 1969; Katinsky and Lovrinic, 1969).

Attention has been focused on electrophysiologic studies on the assumption that site of lesion and the tone decay phenomenon can be studied in laboratory animals. Research by Gisselsson and Sorensen (1959) working with guinea pigs, Kiang and Peake (1960) and Ruben, Hudson and Chiong (1962) with cats has failed to find significant adaptation in the cochlear microphonics with induced nerve VIII lesions. This would tend to suggest that tone decay is not a cochlear phenomenon.

On the other hand, Sorensen (1959) recorded nerve action potentials in the acoustic nerve and found a poststimulatory reduction in their amplitude after stimulation with pure tones and noise of low intensity. Sorensen's data tend to suggest that tone decay is a nerve VIII phenomenon. It is questionable, however, whether the electrophysiologic studies cited here are sufficiently relevant to the tone decay phenomena measured on patients in a clinical setting to warrant their acceptance as final proof. As Palva, Karja and Palva (1967) state:

. . .We are still at a loss to understand clearly what happens electrophysiologically, and where, in cases of pronounced adaptation. None of the studies measuring the cochlear potentials or auditory nerve responses after prolonged stimulation or after slight damage to the nerve have shown more than very minor changes, not comparable to clinical findings. . .

In humans, as well as in laboratory animals, there is evidence that tone decay is associated with nerve VIII pathology. A series of cases seen at the Cleveland Clinic and described by Parker (1970) affords an unusual opportunity to study the relationship between tone decay measurements and nerve VIII lesions in humans. The patients in this series suffered from hemifacial spasm, an involuntary spasm of the facial nerve. Part of the neurosurgical technique was to free nerve VII in the cerebellopontine angle of any adhesions or other abnormalities which may have been present. The neurosurgeons separate nerves VII and VIII and gently retract nerve VIII. Preoperative and postoperative auditory tests, including tone decay, have been collected on a number of these patients. The majority exhibit a range of threshold tone decay, from moderate amounts in the higher frequencies to complete tone decay at all frequencies. Word discrimination scores are roughly proportionate to the tone decay, varying from moderately depressed to 0%. A few have normal pure tone thresholds with severe tone decay at all frequencies and very poor speech discrimination.

Parker indicates that the neurosurgeons are confident that no injury has been done to the pons, cochlea or to the cochlear blood supply. In essence, this appears to be a selective lesion to nerves VII and VIII with the opportunity to evaluate the status before and after surgery.

Explanation of the Tone Decay Mechanism

The explanation of the mechanics of the tone decay mechanism is still in the realm of speculation. However, there is already considerable clinical and research information which may prove valuable as working hypotheses until further information is obtained.

As a point of departure, Green's observations provide a sample of specific phenomena which need to be explained before any eventual theory is accepted. When Green's MTDT is used, patients report experiencing three types of perceptual phenomena associated with the signal: (A) the fatiguing tone loses both tonality and audibility simultaneously, or nearly so, (B) the fatiguing signal loses tonality but remains audible or (C) the fatiguing tone apparently loses both tonality and audibility, but as soon as the tone is discontinued the patient becomes immediately aware that the signal has been withdrawn.

Davis (1962) contended that the mechanism of tone decay was probably analogous to the Wedensky inhibition of peripheral nerves. The essence of the phenomenon is that if a short stretch of nerve is partially narcotized, the first impulse of a series or perhaps an entire series of impulses with long intervals between them will pass through successfully, but a rapid sequence will fail after the first impulse or first few impulses. Assuming a similarity between Wedensky's narcotically induced neural block and the partial dysfunction of a large number of nerve fibers from a retrocochlear lesion, Davis postulated that the gradual slowing of recovery and failure of complete recovery during continued stimulation should cause the progressive failure of more and more of the impaired fibers. This would obtain in any condition of retrocochlear lesion, whether pressure from a tumor, inflammation or atrophy of nerve VIII fibers. The simultaneous loss of tonality and audibility (condition A) would be accounted for on this basis.

Johnson (1970) stated that condition B, the loss of tonality but not audibility, was common among the many confirmed retrocochlear lesions seen by the Otologic Medical Group of Los Angeles (Johnson, 1968). A possible explanation for condition B is that there is less impairment of function when tonality, but not audibility, is lost than when both are lost together. In keeping with the traveling wave and volley theories, one may speculate that if the place of maximal stimulation on the basilar membrane and adjacent areas is "served" by a large number of diffusely interspersed defective fibers, not only will the stimulating tone fail to be sustained, but the adjacent areas to which the signal spreads will also exhibit lack of response and thus tonality and audibility would fatigue out together as in condition A.

However, if there are not quite as many defective fibers serving the basilar membrane, it is conceivable that the initial stimulus could fatigue the nerve cells mediating the test tone, since they are at the point of maximal stimulation, but that the adjacent areas would have sufficient intact reserve fibers to maintain function for an additional period of time. The response from the adjacent areas might very well continue to be perceived as some form of audible noise as in condition B.

Harbert and Young (1964b) cited a case of sudden deafness with complete recovery for whom tone decay data were collected at 1000 Hz during the recovery period. The data supported the thesis that loss of tonality but not audibility indicates less dysfunction than loss of both. Harbert and Young reported that, while the patient was beginning to recover, tone decay tests with the patient responding to "any sound" showed a reduction in the amount of tone decay. However, upon instructions to respond only to signals with a tonal quality, results showed little, if any, reduction in the amount of tone decay. Later, as the patient continued to recover, the loss of tonality due to threshold stimulation ceased and all signs of tone decay disappeared.

Condition C, where the patient perceives the termination of the signal, was considered by Sorensen (1970) to be analogous to one of three effects which can be reproduced in nerve action potentials, namely the off-effect, the on-effect and the sustained response. Thus, the off-effect was assumed to be responsible for the reaction mentioned in conditon C. Harbert and Young (1962a) noted in this connection, that neural off-fibers have been found in the vertebrate eye and ear which are activated when illumination or sound ceases.

While these speculations on the mechanism of tone decay by no means exhaust the possibilities, it is hoped that they will serve to stimulate further thought aimed at establishing a sound theoretical explanation for phenomena observed in the clinical administration of the tone decay test.

CLINICAL APPLICATION OF TONE DECAY

Having discussed some of the historical, technical and theoretical aspects of tone decay, it is time to consider some questions pertaining to its clinical application. What forms of retrocochlear pathology are associated with it? When and how should the test be applied? What are the pitfalls? How will abnormal tone decay affect the outcome of other audiologic tests?

Pathology Associated with Abnormal Tone Decay

Abnormal tone decay can be caused by neural degeneration, inflammation and trauma, as well as by space-occupying lesions such as tumors, which press against nerve VIII. A partial list of causes would include: acoustic neuroma (neurinoma), primary cholesteatoma (epidermoid cyst), nerve VII neuroma, meningioma (Johnson, 1966), thermal injury to nerve VIII (Harbert and Young, 1962a), multiple sclerosis, mumps neuritis, von Recklinghausen's disease, acquired luetic deafness, Ramsay-Hunt syndrome, intracranial aneurysm, head

trauma (Harbert and Young, 1968), nerve VIII atrophy, pinealoma (Kos, 1955), nerve IX neuroma (Naunton, Proctor and Elpern, 1968), cerebellar atrophy (Miller and Daly, 1967), Arnold-Chiari malformation (Rydell and Pulec, 1971) and extra-axial brain stem lesion (Jerger and Jerger, 1974).

The amounts of tone decay associated with most of the causative pathologies tend either to remain constant or to increase. However, exceptions have been noted. Reversible tone decay has been described in nerve VIII neuritis, sudden deafness of unknown etiology, multiple sclerosis, pinealoma and cerebellar tumor (Stroud and Thalmann, 1969).

Such an impressive array of possible etiologies should certainly discourage a hasty diagnostic judgment based solely on positive tone decay findings.

Application of The Tone Decay Test

Use of the tone decay test need not be confined to a medical setting but it must be done with mature clinical judgment whenever it is undertaken. Abnormal tone decay requires proper referral without an emotional reaction.

Since it is recommended that all patients with sensory-neural hearing loss be given a screening test for tone decay, the question arises: Which test should be used? Should it be the Carhart, the Rosenberg, the Green MTDT, the 20 dB SL of Olsen and Noffsinger, the Owens, the Bekesy, or the Jergers' STAT?

Fortunately, since the first edition of this text went to press, several investigators (Parker and Decker, 1971; Sanders, Josey and Glasscock, 1974, and Olsen and Noffsinger, 1974) have studied this problem. They have through their investigations clarified our understanding of the relative efficiency of the various techniques in identifying retrocochlear lesions.

Parker and Decker. Parker and Decker (1971) reported on comparisons of tone decay test results obtained from the same groups of patients using five different tone decay procedures. The authors concluded after comparison of the Carhart, Bekesy sweep frequency and fixed frequency tests, and the Rosenberg and Owens modifications, that the Carhart test gave more diagnostic information about the amount, rate of appearance, and final configuration of abnormal tone decay than the other tests.

The Carhart was compared with the Bekesy sweep in a group of 10 patients with retrocochlear disease. Differences between pulsed and continuous traces were measured and a comparison was made of the amount of decay at each comparable test frequency for the two tests. Success in identifying retrocochlear abnormality was not based on the conventional Bekesy types. Two retrocochlear cases were cited, however, which generated conventional Bekesy Type I or Type II patterns (not retrocochlear), but showed extreme decay (retrocochlear) on the Carhart. In these examples, the Carhart test pointed toward an accurate diagnosis while the Bekesy sweeps did not.

Amount of decay on the Carhart versus fixed frequency Bekesy was studied on 11 randomly selected cases of "strongly positive tone decay." Sixty-eight percent of the frequencies tested yielded more tone decay on the Carhart than on the fixed frequency Bekesy test during the same time period. Two cases were cited which showed little to moderate tone decay by fixed frequency Bekesy, but complete tone decay by the Carhart procedure.

The Carhart and Owens tests were compared by randomly selecting 50 cases of severe tone decay based on the Carhart test and converting the results to the Owens diagnostic cochlear and retrocochlear types. From the 50 cases, a number of examples were chosen which demonstrated conflicting diagnostic information. For example, 9 cases of complete tone decay (retrocochlear) on the Carhart test yielded Owens Type II-D or Type II-E (cochlear patterns). The authors noted that although a review of their Carhart tone decay tests indicated that rapidity of tone decay and total amount of tone decay were directly related in many instances, there were a significant number of cases in which there was a pattern of slow tone decay in the first four or five intensity increments, followed by a more rapid rate of tone decay above this intensity level. In the latter case, discrepancies between the Owens and the Carhart tests occurred, with greater decay abnormalities being shown by the Carhart test.

In like manner, Parker and Decker (1971) also found that the Rosenberg test failed to detect abnormal decay in patients who showed slow initial decay followed by more rapid decay. They cited one case which yielded 85 dB of tone decay on the Carhart test, but only 12$\frac{1}{2}$ dB at the end of 1 min (Rosenberg test). The same patient would have yielded a Type II-D (cochlear pattern) on the Owens test according to the converted data from the Carhart. In a letter to the editor commenting on the Parker and Decker article, Rosenberg (1971) admitted that, in rare instances of delayed tone decay, the 1-min test would miss but that, for the substantial majority of patients with proven retrocochlear pathology, over 30 dB of tone decay could be demonstrated in 1 min.

Sanders et al. Sanders, Josey and Glasscock (1974) tested 24 ears with confirmed acoustic tumors on the Carhart versus the sweep frequency Bekesy test. The Carhart successfully identified 6 out of the 24 retrocochlear ears that were missed by the sweep frequency Bekesy test.

Olsen and Noffsinger. The Carhart, Rosenberg, 20 dB SL modification of the Carhart, and fixed frequency Bekesy tone decay tests were administered by Olsen and Noffsinger (1974) to 20 patients with confirmed nerve VIII tumors. The purpose of the investigation was to compare the results of the more established tone decay tests with their own procedure which followed the Carhart test except that it was begun at 20 dB SL rather than at threshold. It was hypothesized that a tone decay procedure that was initiated at 20 dB SL would be an effective way to screen out persons with cochlear lesions, who commonly manifest as much as 20 dB of decay. At the same time, the authors felt that the test would still be effective in identifying persons with nerve VIII lesions.

In administering the Carhart test, the length of time in seconds was recorded. To score the results for the Rosenberg test, it was only necessary to sum the lengths of time in seconds that the tone was perceived at each level during the Carhart test until 60 sec were reached. The difference between the level that was reached in 60 sec and threshold was taken as the amount of decay measured by the Rosenberg technique. Since the authors required a response to "tonality" as opposed to response to "any sound," the amount of decay shown in 1 min is also equivalent to the Green MTDT, which requires a response to "tonality."

Fixed frequency Bekesy tracings were obtained. They were classified as Type I when the threshold tracings were superimposed for the pulsed and continuous signals, Type II when threshold for the continuous tone was poorer than that for the pulsed by 5 to 20 dB, Type III when the continuous tone threshold steadily worsened until the limits of the audiometer were reached without perception of the tone at the highest level available, and Type IV when the tracings for pulsed and continuous tones were separated by more than 20 dB, but response to the continuous tone was maintained. Types II and IV were based on the recommendation of Hughes, Winegar and Crabtree (1967).

In fairness to Jerger (1960), whose original four Bekesy types were generated on the basis of pulsed versus continuous Bekesy sweeps, it should be mentioned that there is some question as to whether types generated by fixed frequency are equivalent to types generated by sweep frequency testing. Jerger (1965) has indeed gone on record stating that "the type-classification system for Bekesy audiograms was never intended to apply to tracings obtained at single fixed frequencies." Despite this disputed terminology, the comparison of the fixed frequency versus other tone decay techniques appears valid inasmuch as the same frequencies were tested by each of the tone decay techniques. Fixed rather than sweep frequency Bekesy audiometry was selected on the basis of Owens' (1964) reported findings and the clinical experience of Olsen and Noffsinger, that fixed frequency tracings often demonstrated tone decay not apparent in sweep frequency tracings.

For the Carhart, Rosenberg, and 20 dB SL methods, tone decay of 35 dB at one or more frequencies was regarded as indicative of retrocochlear involvement. The fixed frequency Bekesy tests, Type III and Type IV, as designated by the authors, were also considered retrocochlear. The relative accuracy of prediction of retrocochlear site was determined by comparing the number of confirmed retrocochlear patients correctly identified by each of the different tests.

The results of the Olsen and Noffsinger study are worthy of note. Nineteen of the 20 nerve VIII tumor cases were correctly identified through the Carhart procedure and when testing was begun at 20 dB SL. Only one patient, later found to have nerve VIII tumor, revealed 30 dB or less decay by both the Carhart and 20 dB SL procedures.

In contrast, only 13 of the 20 nerve VIII tumor patients were correctly identified by the Rosenberg test. Thus, the Rosenberg procedure failed to detect excess decay in 35% of the retrocochlear patients in this series, compared to the 5% failure rate for the Carhart and the 20 dB SL tests.

Bekesy tracings were classified as retrocochlear Types III or IV in 14 out of 19 nerve VIII tumor patients. (The Bekesy test was not administered to one subject.) This yielded a failure rate slightly lower than the Rosenberg test, but significantly higher than the Carhart and 20 dB SL tests.

The foregoing studies, while not offering a perfect solution to the problem of selecting an appropriate tone decay test, provide the audiologist with enough pertinent information to make a reasonable choice for the present. Further studies of this type will hopefully be carried out to supplement our existing knowledge.

In general, the previously discussed studies lead to the conclusion that the Carhart and 20 dB SL tests are superior to the Owens and to the shortened versions of the Carhart such as the Rosenberg, and the Green MTDT. When initial tone decay starts slowly and then becomes more rapid, the shorter tests appear to be at a disadvantage. The foregoing studies also support the contention that the Bekesy tests are less sensitive in identifying retrocochlear lesions than the Carhart and the 20 dB SL modification.

The procedure of choice, therefore, as viewed by the authors narrows down to the Carhart or to the 20 dB SL test. While further comparative studies between these two tests are needed, the latter appears to have merit as a screening procedure inasmuch as it is a little shorter, appears to be a little easier for the patient to grasp the listening task, and was as effective as the Carhart in identifying retrocochlear lesions.

The STAT test, recently described by Jerger and Jerger, also appears promising but further data would be desirable. A most convincing experimental design is that provided in the Olsen and Noffsinger study where the same subjects were tested with different tone decay tests. Meanwhile, clinicians are urged to administer at least two tone decay procedures on patients with retrocochlear pathology whenever possible, in a continued effort to evaluate diagnostic accuracy.

An otologic examination should be recommended in the presence of early symptoms associated with retrocochlear lesions. The development of unilateral sensory-neural hearing loss, tinnitus or balance disturbance, even in the absence of abnormal tone decay, should be regarded as worthy of diagnostic exploration to rule out the possibility of serious retrocochlear pathology.

Factors which Interfere with Early Diagnosis

Regardless of etiology, early diagnosis of retrocochlear lesions may enhance a more effective treatment program. Balas and Pirkey (1968) emphasized that a low index of suspicion, inconsistency of test results and dual auditory dysfunction are commonly encountered obstacles to early diagnosis. Their last point is worthy of further comment.

Retrocochlear lesions can coexist with acoustic trauma, middle ear pathology, presbycusis, inherited deafness and drug ototoxicity. The audiologist is well aware, for example, that a drop forge operator whose hearing has been damaged by noise has not lessened his chances for developing an acoustic neuroma.

Retrocochlear and middle ear pathologies are not mutually exclusive, as the following patient illustrates. A 50-year-old woman with a history of childhood ear infections was seen by the New Haven Ear Nose Throat and Maxillo Facial Surgery Group. Otological examination showed a large kidney shaped tympanic membrane perforation with a wet middle ear on the left side. The right tympanic membrane was scarred, thin and somewhat retracted. Hearing studies yielded the following averages (ISO) for the speech frequencies:

Air conduction: Right 7 dB Left 48 dB
Bone conduction: Right 3 dB Left 20 dB

These results indicated normal hearing in the right ear and a moderate mixed loss in the left. While administering pure tone audiometry to the left ear the tester observed that the patient's finger dropped before the tone was discontinued. On the chance that the patient had not understood the original instructions, she was again instructed to raise her finger as long as she heard the tone. When the pure tone thresholds were repeated, it became apparent that the patient was experiencing extreme tone decay. This discovery was followed by the administration of the complete battery of special audiologic and medical tests designed to determine site of lesion. All of the tests pointed to a retrocochlear lesion which was subsequently confirmed by surgery. The patient recovered after removal of a large left cerebellopontine angle tumor.

This example illustrates the importance of the tone decay phenomenon in helping to identify retrocochlear lesions even in the presence of other ear pathology. Above all, where tone decay is concerned, it is well to maintain a high index of suspicion and to expect the unexpected.

Interaction of Tone Decay with Other Auditory Tests and Procedures

Abnormal tone decay exhibits an influence on Bekesy audiometry, the short increment sensitivity index (SISI), the alternate binaural loudness balance (ABLB), the measurement of stapedius reflex, evoked response audiometry and word discrimination. Contralateral masking exhibits a surprising influence on tone decay as measured by either conventional or Bekesy audiometry. Awareness of the pertinent interactions is useful in test interpretation.

Conventional Audiometry. The instructions to respond solely to the tonality of the signal rather than to its audibility may influence the results of the tone decay tests by conventional as well as by Bekesy audiometry (Green, 1963; Harbert and Young, 1964a; Blegvad, 1968). When there is a difference, larger amounts of tone decay are shown when the subject is instructed to respond to "tone only."

Contralateral masking during the measurement of tone decay by conventional audiometry can have an important influence on the test outcome. Shimizu (1969) measured tone decay at 500 Hz, 1000 Hz and 2000 Hz in 11 normal hearing subjects and in 34 with moderate unilateral conductive hearing loss. With 40 dB SL of contralateral masking, the amount of tone decay generally increased, particularly for the higher frequencies. For example, without contralateral masking at 2000 Hz, only 7% of the subjects had as much as 10 dB of tone decay, while with masking 77% had 10 to 40 dB of tone decay. Shimizu also cited tone decay data on a patient with a unilateral sensory-neural loss. Without contralateral masking, the poor ear showed 10 dB of tone decay at 1000 Hz. With 40 dB SL noise in the contralateral ear, there was 30 dB of tone decay, and with 60 dB SL, there was 50 dB of decay. Since these levels of masking are presumably low enough to avoid the risk of overmasking, the tone decay observed during contralateral masking is attributed to a central factor.

Because of this effect, contralateral masking must be taken into account whenever a tone decay test is given. The diagnostic significance of the increased tone decay with contralateral masking is not as yet clear and will require further clinical study. Meanwhile the amount and type of masking that is used should be recorded with the test results.

SISI. Occasionally a patient responds to the SISI with a high score but reports that the carrier tone faded away (Jerger, 1955). Because of the decay of the carrier tone, the 1-dB increment pips appear to emerge from silence. However, the 5-sec interval between pulses apparently allows sufficient recovery time to enable response to successive pips. Hughes (1968) studied 18 such patients, 11 of whom had Meniere's disease. There were also 4 who had a sudden onset of sensory-neural loss and 3 with surgically confirmed acoustic neuromas. All of the subjects who exhibited this phenomenon had at least 20 dB of tone decay on the MTDT for the SISI test frequency. Since the carrier tone is usually set 20 dB above threshold and is continuously on, it is not surprising that ears that show moderate amounts of tone decay soon lose perception of the background stimulus.

Decay of the Acoustic Reflex. The presence of abnormal decay of the acoustic reflex, as measured with an electroacoustic impedance bridge, is a sensitive measure of retrocochlear pathology (Sanders et al., 1974; Jerger and Jerger, 1975; Johnson, 1973). Tonal and acoustic reflex decay are commonly obtained in the same patients.

ABLB. When the ABLB recruitment test is performed at a frequency where there is marked tone decay, loudness growth with increasing intensity is less than normal. This result has been termed decruitment (Fowler,

1965; Davis and Goodman, 1966) or reverse recruitment (Dix and Hallpike, 1960; Harbert and Young, 1962b) in contrast to recruitment where loudness growth with increasing intensity is greater than normal.

Evoked Response Audiometry. Shimizu (1968) investigated the configuration of acoustically evoked response in two groups of patients with unilateral hearing impairment. Nine patients had Meniere's disease and 4 had surgically confirmed nerve VIII lesions. In all cases of nerve VIII lesions, every average evoked response on the impaired side revealed longer latency and smaller amplitude than those obtained from the normal side. On the other hand, the Meniere's cases revealed shorter latency or very little difference in latency and increase in amplitude on the impaired side. According to Shimizu, the responses from the Meniere's patients were compatible with the presence of recruitment. By the same token, the responses of the patients with nerve VIII lesions could be thought to indicate the presence of decruitment or reverse recruitment. Shimizu suggested that the responses observed in the patients with nerve VIII lesions probably resulted from the fact that the passage of nerve impulses was disturbed by pressure on, or destruction of, components of the nerve.

Word Discrimination Tests. In cases where there is marked tone decay, presumably from damage to fibers of nerve VIII, word discrimination may be much worse than the pure tone thresholds would ordinarily indicate. Apparently, many more fibers are needed for the effective transmission of complex signals, such as speech, than for retention of thresholds for pure tones. Schuknecht and Woellner (1955) were able to produce both high and low tone losses by selectively sectioning nerve fibers. They found that more than 75% of the fibers to a particular region of the cochlea had to be eliminated before a threshold elevation for the respective tones occurred.

Miscellaneous Effects Related to Tone Decay

Hearing Aids. Occasionally a patient who has been fitted with a hearing aid will complain that after using the hearing aid for a while the instrument loses clarity or that his ear feels "stuffed." After resting for several hours, the aided hearing may once again seem clear and the ear "unstuffed." When encountering such a patient, an attempt should be made to document the complaint with careful testing. It is possible that it is associated with abnormal tone decay (Goldberg, 1964).

In one such patient seen by me, Bekesy studies were completed before and after a 20-min exposure to aided listening. After only 20 min, the patient demonstrated significant threshold shift from which it took several hours to recover.

Language Impairment. Costello and McGee (1967) described 2 patients whose history and evaluative findings were quite similar. Both patients had normal development in all areas until about 3 years of age at which point they experienced gradual speech and language deterioration without any known illness or injury. Associated with these findings was the presence of normal gross pitch discrimination and normal intelligence including normal memory and recall of verbal material. Conventional pure tone thresholds fell within normal limits although word discrimination scores were markedly impaired. One patient had 0% discrimination in both ears and received her education in a school for the deaf. The other had 32% in one ear and 60% in the other and was initially enrolled in a special class for aphasic children but was later transferred to a regular classroom with normal hearing children. The latter patient complained of a speech monitoring problem. Although she could hear herself talk, she could not understand the words she spoke.

The intriguing finding in both patients was abnormal tone decay and poor speech comprehension despite normal pure tone thresholds. Each patient seemed to show the greatest amount of decay in the speech frequencies as measured by both conventional and Bekesy audiometry. A possible explanation for the language disorder is the existence of pathology interfering with the transmission of the neural impulses in the auditory pathways.

CONCLUSION

Tone decay assessment constitutes an important function in the practice of clinical audiology. Much is already known about the phenomenon of tone decay and its application, but much remains to be learned. In particular, comparative information is needed about different tone decay tests when used on the same patient with retrocochlear pathology.

Another area that should be explored further is the demonstration of tone decay in laboratory animals trained to respond to sustained pure tones. Experimentally induced lesions in the auditory systems of such animals could provide precise site of lesion data.

REFERENCES

Balas, R. F., and Pirkey, W. P., Retrocochlear lesions; problems in early diagnosis. *Ann. Otol. Rhinol. Laryngol.*, 77, 78–87, 1968.

Bekesy, G. v., A new audiometer. *Acta Otolaryngol.*, 35, 411–422, 1947.

Bhatia, P. L., Sinha, A., and Abrol, B. M., The tone decay test; a simple and reliable audiological test. *Laryngoscope,* 79, 1879-1890, 1969.

Blegvad, B., Bekesy audiometry and clinical masking. *Acta Otolaryngol.,* 66, 229-240, 1968.

Bosatra, A., Further observations on the mechanism inducing a temporary reduction of threshold hearing; adaptation-fatigue-habituation. *Int. Audiol.,* 2, 267-270, 1963.

Carhart, R., Clinical determination of abnormal auditory adaptation. *Arch. Otolaryngol.,* 65, 32-39, 1957.

Corradi, C., Zur Prufung der Schallperception durch die Knochen. *Arch. Ohrenheilk.,* 30, 175-182, 1890.

Costello, M. R., and McGee, T. M., Language impairment associated with Bilateral Abnormal Auditory Adaptation. In Graham, A. B. (Ed.), *Sensorineural Hearing Processes and Disorders.* Boston: Little, Brown & Co. 1967.

Davis, H., A functional classification of auditory defects. *Ann. Otol. Rhinol. Laryngol.,* 71, 693-704, 1962.

Davis, H. and Goodman, A. C., Subtractive hearing loss, loudness recruitment, and decruitment. *Ann. Otol. Rhinol. Laryngol.,* 75, 87-94, 1966.

Dix, M. R., and Hallpike, C. S., Discussion on acoustic neuroma. *Laryngoscope,* 70, 105-122, 1960.

Dunlap, K., Some peculiarities of fluctuating and inaudible sounds. *Psychol. Rev.,* 11, 308-318, 1904.

Flottorp, G., Pathological fatigue in part of the hearing nerve only. *Acta Otolaryngol.,* Suppl., 188, 298-307, 1963.

Fowler, E. P., Some attributes of loudness recruitment. *Trans. Am. Otol. Soc.,* 53, 78-84, 1965.

Gisselsson, L., and Sorensen, I., Auditory adaptation and fatigue in cochlear potentials. *Acta Otolaryngol.,* 50, 391-405, 1959.

Gjaevenes, K., and Sohoel, Th., The tone decay test. *Acta Otolaryngol.,* 68, 33-42, 1969.

Glasscock, M. E., Acoustic neuroma; recent advances in the diagnosis and treatment. *Rev. Laryngol.* 89, 28-42, 1968.

Goldberg, H., What to do about auditory fatigue. *Hear. Dealer,* 14, 12-13, 1964.

Gradenigo, G., On the clinical signs of the affections of the auditory nerve. Translated by S. E. Alle. *Arch. Otol.,* 22, 213-215, 1893.

Green, D. S. The modified tone decay test (MTDT) as a screening procedure for eighth nerve lesions. *J. Speech Hear. Disord.,* 28, 31-36, 1963.

Hallpike, C. S., and Hood, J. D., Some recent work on auditory adaptation and its relationship to the loudness recruitment phenomenon. *J. Acoust. Soc. Am.,* 23, 270-274, 1951.

Harbert, F., and Young, I. M., Threshold auditory adapatation. *J. Aud. Res.,* 2, 229-246, 1962a.

Harbert, F., and Young, I. M., Clinical application of hearing tests. *Arch Otolaryngol.,* 76, 55-67, 1962b.

Harbert, F., and Young, I. M., Threshold auditory adaptation measured by tone decay test and Bekesy audiometry. *Ann. Otol. Rhinol. Laryngol.,* 73, 48-60, 1964a.

Harbert, F., and Young, I. M., Sudden deafness with complete recovery. *Arch. Otolaryngol.,* 79, 459-471, 1964b.

Harbert F., and Young, I. M., Clinical application

of Bekesy audiometry. *Laryngoscope,* 78, 487-497, 1968.

Hood, J. D. Fatigue and adaptation of hearing. *Br. Med. Bull.,* 12, 125-130, 1956.

Hughes, R. L., Atypical responses to the SISI. *Ann Otol. Rhinol. Laryngol.,* 77, 332-337, 1968.

Hughes, R. L., Winegar, W. J., and Crabtree, J. A., Bekesy audiometry; type 2 versus type 4 patterns. *Arch. Otolaryngol.,* 86, 424-430, 1967.

Jerger, J., Differential intensity sensitivity in the ear with loudness recruitment. *J. Speech Hear. Disord.,* 20, 183-191, 1955.

Jerger, J., Bekesy audiometry in analysis of auditory disorders. *J. Speech Hear. Res.,* 3, 275-287, 1960.

Jerger, J., Bekesy audiometry, a misunderstanding. *J. Speech Hear. Disord.,* 30, 302-303, 1965.

Jerger, J., and Jerger, S., Auditory findings in brain stem disorders. *Arch. Otolaryngol.,* 99, 342-350, 1974.

Jerger, J., and Jerger, S., A simplified tone decay test. *Arch. Otolaryngol.,* 101, 403-407, 1975.

Johnson, E. W., Confirmed retrocochlear lesions. *Arch. Otolaryngol.,* 84, 247-254, 1966.

Johnson, E. W., Auditory findings in 200 cases of acoustic neuromas. *Arch. Otolaryngol.,* 88, 598-603, 1968.

Johnson, E. W., Personal communication, 1970.

Johnson, E. W., Clinical application of special hearing tests. *Arch. Otolaryngol.,* 97, 92-95, 1973.

Katinsky, S., and Lovrinic, J., Paradoxical findings in eighth nerve tumors. Paper presented at American Speech and Hearing Association convention, Chicago, November 1969.

Kiang, N. Y., and Peake, W. T., Components of electrical responses recorded from the cochlea. *Ann. Otol. Rhinol. Laryngol.,* 69, 448-458, 1960.

Kos, C. M., Auditory function as related to the complaint of dizziness. *Laryngoscope,* 65, 711-721, 1955.

Lierle, D. M., and Reger, S. N., Experimentally induced temporary threshold shifts in ears with impaired hearing. *Ann. Otol. Rhinol. Laryngol.,* 64, 263-277, 1955.

Miller, M. H. and Daly, J. F. Cerebellar atrophy simulating acoustic neurinoma. *Arch. Otolaryngol.,* 85, 383-386, 1967.

Morales-Garcia, C., and Hood, J. D., Tone decay test in neuro-otological diagnosis. *Arch. Otolaryngol.,* 96, 231-247, 1972.

Naunton, R. F., Proctor, L., and Elpern, B. S., The audiologic signs of ninth nerve neurinoma. *Arch. Otolaryngol.,* 87, 222-227, 1968.

Olsen, W. O., and Noffsinger, D., Comparison of one new and three old tests of auditory adaptation. *Arch. Otolaryngol.,* 99, 94-99, 1974.

Owens, E., Tone decay in eighth nerve and cochlear lesions. *J. Speech Hear. Disord.,* 29, 14-22, 1964.

Owens, E., Bekesy tracings, tone decay and loudness recruitment. *J. Speech Hear. Disord.,* 30, 50-57, 1965.

Owens, E., Personal communication, 1970.

Palva, T., Self recording threshold audiometry and recruitment. *Arch. Otolaryngol.,* 65, 591-602, 1957.

Palva, T., Auditory adaptation. *Acta Otolaryngol.,* 57, 207-216, 1964.

Palva, T., Karja, J., and Palva, A., Auditory adaptation at threshold intensities. *Acta Otolaryngol, Suppl.*, **224**, 195–200, 1967.

Parker, W. P., Personal communication, 1970.

Parker, W. P., Decker, R. L., and Richards, N. G., Auditory function and lesions of the pons. *Arch. Otolaryngol.*, **87**, 228–240, 1968.

Parker, W., and Decker, R. L., Detection of abnormal auditory threshold adaptation. *Arch. Otolaryngol.*, **94**, 1–7, 1971.

Pestalozza, G., and Cioce, C., Measuring auditory adaptation; the value of different clinical tests. *Laryngoscope*, **72**, 240–259, 1962.

Rayleigh, L., Acoustical observations. IV. Phil. Mag. 13, Series 5, 340–347, 1882.

Reger, S. N., and Kos, C. M., Clinical measurements and implications of recruitment. *Ann. Otol. Rhinol. Laryngol.*, **61**, 810–823, 1952.

Reger, S. N., and Kos, C. M., Anatomic localization implications of the functional hearing tests. *Arch. Otolaryngol.*, **67**, 394–402, 1958.

Rosenberg, P. E. Rapid clinical measurement of tone decay. Paper presented at the American Speech and Hearing Association convention, New York, November, 1958.

Rosenberg, P. E., Tone decay. Maico Audiological Library Series, 7, report 6, 1969.

Rosenberg, P. E., Abnormal auditory adaptation (Letter to Editor). *Arch. Otolaryngol.*, **94**, 89, 1971.

Ruben, R. J., Hudson, W., and Chiong, A., Anatomical and physiological effects of chronic section of the eighth nerve in cat. *Acta Otolaryngol.*, **55**, 473, 1962.

Rydell, R., and Pulec, J., Arnold-Chiari malformation. *Arch. Otolaryngol.*, **94**, 8–12, 1971.

Sanders, J. W., Josey, A. F., and Glasscock, M. E., Audiologic evaluation in cochlear and eighth nerve disorders. *Arch. Otolaryngol.*, **100**, 283–289, 1974.

Schubert, K., Horermudung and Hordauer. *Hals-, Nas.-Ohrenheilk.*, **51**, 411, 1944.

Schuknecht, H. F., and Woellner, R., An experimental and clinical study of deafness from lesions of the cochlear nerve. *J. Laryngol.*, **69**, 75–97, 1955.

Sergeant, R. L., and Harris, J. D., The relation of perstimulatory adaptation to other short-term threshold-shifting mechanisms. *J. Speech Hear. Res.*, **6**, 27–39, 1963.

Shimizu, H., Evoked response in eighth nerve lesions. *Trans. Am. Acad. Ophthalmol. Otolaryngol*, **72**, 596–603, 1968.

Shimizu, H., Influence of contralateral noise stimulation on tone decay and SISI tests. *Laryngoscope*, **79**, 2155–2164, 1969.

Sørensen, H., Auditory adaptation in nerve action potentials recorded from the cochlea in guinea pigs. *Acta Otolaryngol*, **50**, 438–450, 1959.

Sorensen, H., Clinical application of continuous threshold recording. *Acta Otolaryngol.*, **54**, 403–422, 1962a.

Sorensen, H., Initial auditory adaptation. I. In normal individuals. *Acta Otolaryngol.*, **55**, 299–308, 1962b.

Sorensen, H., Personal communication, 1970.

Stroud, M. H., and Thalmann, R., Unusual audiological and vestibular problems in the diagnosis of cerebellopontine angle lesions. *Laryngoscope*, **79**, 171–200, 1969.

Sung, S. S., Goetzinger, C. P., and Knox, A. W., A study of the sensitivity and reliability of three tone decay tests. Paper presented at American Speech and Hearing Association convention, Chicago, November 1969.

Tillman, T. Special hearing tests in otoneurological diagnosis. *Arch. Otolaryngol.*, **89**, 25–30, 1969.

Ward, W. D., Auditory Fatigue and Masking. In Jerger, J. (Ed.), *Modern Developments in Audiology*, New York: Academic Press, 1963.

Ward, W. D., Personal communication, 1970.

Yantis, P. A., Clinical applications of the temporary threshold shift. *Arch. Otolaryngol.*, **70**, 779–787, 1959.

chapter 18

BEKESY AUDIOMETRY

Richard L. Hughes, Ph.D.,* and E. W. Johnson, Ph.D.

In 1947 Bekesy introduced a new audiometer that subsequently gained wide acceptance and application in both research and clinical audiology. The instrument was a continuously variable frequency, automatic recording unit. Other automatic audiometers had been introduced by Gardner (1947) and Reger and Newby (1947). The Bekesy instrument placed the variables of test tone intensity and test tone duration under the control of the subject. The new instrument permitted the subject to track his threshold by depressing and releasing a signal key, and allowed measurement of the absolute threshold all along the frequency range instead of at octave and midoctave points. Reger (1952), constructed several clinical versions. Later, the Grason-Stadler Company manufactured production models incorporating many of the design principles devised by Reger.

INSTRUMENTATION

There are a number of Bekesy-type audiometers commercially available. Most of the instruments provide a pure tone signal generated by a continuously variable beat-frequency oscillator. Some audiometers have a frequency range from 100 to 10,000 Hz and others are limited to a 250- to 8,000-Hz range. Either full sweep frequency tracings may be run or specific fixed frequencies may be selected. Frequency presentation may be in an ascending order from low to high frequency or descending from high to low. The test signal may be presented continuously or periodically interrupted at the rate of approximately 2.5 interruptions per second with a 50% duty cycle. An instantly reversible motor-drive controlled by the patient's hand switch is geared to attenuate the signal at the rate of either 2.5 dB/sec or 5 dB/sec (or in one audiometer at 1.25 dB/sec). The total intensity of the audiometers is approximately 120 dB. The instruments utilize broad spectrum white or narrow band noise for masking purposes. A pen, that is coupled to the attenuator, traces a continuous recording of the subject's response on a specially prepared audiogram form placed on a moving table.

*Deceased.

DIAGNOSTIC SIGNIFICANCE

Early Investigations

Many of the early studies with Bekesy audiometry utilized continuous tones at different attenuation rates and steps of intensity change. The main purposes of these investigations were (1) to correlate the sawtooth threshold tracing with conventional audiometric values and (2) to relate tracking behavior with the presence or absence of recruitment.

Correlation to Conventional Audiometry. In conventional pure tone audiometry (see Chapter 9), threshold is usually considered to be a statistical value represented by a point on the audiogram at which the subject responds to 50% of the signals. Bekesy audiometry provides a sawtooth-shaped curve that sweeps across an intensity range. Each ascending arm of the Bekesy trace represents a period of audibility while the descending arm indicates a period of inaudibility. These two arms traverse the same intensity area. The listener continues to hear or not hear within the same area depending on whether it is approached by a signal of increasing or decreasing intensity. In an early investigation of the Bekesy technique, Reger (1952) suggested that threshold is a value at or near the midpoint of the excursions of the recording stylus. Corso (1956, 1957), used the method of adjustment (Hirsh, 1952) instructing his subjects to keep the tone "just barely audible," and found that the peaks representing inaudibility corresponded to thresholds obtained by conventional pure tone audiometry. Burns and Hinchcliffe (1957) used the method of limits (Hirsh, 1952) by instructing their subjects to press the hand switch when the tone was audible and release the switch when the tone was not heard. The instrumentation used in this study had an attenuation rate of 2 dB/sec that changed in 2-dB steps. The midpoint value of the Bekesy trace was found to correlate well with conventional threshold measurements. Later investigators (Harbert and Young, 1966) employed a Grason-Stadler model E-800 audiometer with an almost stepless intensity change (0.25 dB) and found that the peaks of audibility best represented threshold for normal subjects. The difference between 2-dB and 0.25-dB steps is similar to either going up a flight of stairs or walking up an incline. The lower (better) thresholds obtained by Burns and Hinchcliffe were probably generated by an on-effect produced by the relatively large 2-dB intensity steps.

Measurement of Recruitment. Fowler (1928, 1936) first used the term *recruitment* and suggested a method for its measurement. Since then investigators have proposed various other procedures for measuring this phenomenon (see Chapter 15). Bekesy (1947) proposed that, with automatic audiometry, the subject not only traces his absolute threshold through a broad and continuous frequency range, but also records a threshold difference limen for intensity (DLI). It was thought that the DLI determination is an *indirect* measurement of recruitment, equivalent to more direct suprathreshold balance methods. He demonstrated that very narrow tracking behavior was associated with recruitment. Reger (1952) and Liden (1953) supported this observation but later attempts to quantify normal and pathologic excursion widths led to disagreement. Lundborg (1952) proposed the presence of recruitment if the tracking width at 4000 Hz is reduced by one-third to one-half of the excursion size at frequencies below 1000 Hz. Palva (1956) suggested that the normal tracking amplitude is 5 to 15 dB and that recruitment is indicated by excursions of 5 dB or narrower. McLay (1959) judged the tracking envelope to be abnormally small if the width is 3 dB or less. However, normal excursion size is influenced by the variables of the test procedure. Doubling the attenuation rate increases the tracking amplitude by 62% according to Harbert and Young (1966). This relationship seems to exist for pulsed and continuous tones, for normal and pathologic ears and at all frequencies. Epstein (1960) found that the range of normal excursion size for continuous tones increased from 4 to 9 dB, when using a 1 dB/sec attenuation rate, to 10 to 30 dB for a rate of 4 dB/sec. Similar interaction between tracking behavior and attenuation rate was found by Lilly (1965) and Muma and Siegenthaler (1966). Hirsh, Palva and Goodman (1954) in a now classic discussion of the assumptions underlying the use of differential threshold sensitivity, questioned whether loudness recruitment is actually accompanied by an abnormally small DLI. They concluded that Bekesy audiometry does not provide a measure of DLI but rather a variability around absolute threshold. Landis (1958) also contended that the tracking amplitude is not a measurement of DLI at threshold but is dependent on the ear's growth of loudness function. Therefore, the coexistence of recruitment and reduced tracking width should not imply that the restricted amplitude was caused by recruitment nor is it a measurement of DLI.

Attempts to quantify normal and abnormal excursion sizes have been virtually abandoned. However, audiologists continue to inspect the Bekesy tracing for abnormal tracking width from which to draw diagnostic inferences. Although decreased tracking width is considered by many clinicians to be an indication of re-

cruitment, Harbert and Young (1962, a and b) and Suzuki and Kubota (1966) suggested it is an indication of rapid adaptation. They reasoned that reduced amplitude of the trace for continuous tones may be due to the inability of the pathologic ear to hear intensities that are audible to the normal ear. This rapid adaptation, occurring in milliseconds, may indicate lesions at the dendrites or synapse between hair cells and dendrites.

Bases for Current Bekesy Procedure

A study by Dix, Hallpike and Hood (1948) disclosed that patients with hearing impairments of cochlear origin experience recruitment while others with retrocochlear lesions do not. Prior to this study, there was no known measurement to distinguish between the general types of sensory-neural (cochlear and retrocochlear) pathologies. Fowler's alternate binaural loudness balance (ABLB) test was originally considered a clinically useful method of distinguishing only between conductive and sensory-neural impairments. Lundborg (1952) obtained Bekesy audiograms from 50 normal hearing subjects, 51 patients with cochlear lesions (Meniere's disease and acoustic trauma) and from 21 patients with various types of confirmed retrocochlear pathology. Because of the relatively large variation of tracking behavior exhibited by these subjects, the tracings were grouped into four types, based on the criterion of reduced tracking amplitude, which he considered as a corollary phenomenon of loudness recruitment. Type I (not to be confused with Jerger's classification to be discussed later) demonstrated an even, wide trace averaging approximately 6 to 9 dB with extreme limits of 5 to 20 dB throughout the entire tracking range. Such a trace was considered to show a normal DLI and consequently, no recruitment. A Type IV tracing exhibited a pronounced reduction in tracking width, 2 to 3 dB in amplitude, throughout the audiogram and was interpreted as complete recruitment. Types II and III represented intermediate conditions of recruitment to facilitate greater detail of the character of the audiograms. Using this classification system, Lundborg was able to demonstrate the presence of recruitment in cochlear losses by reduced tracking amplitude and the absence of recruitment in retrocochlear lesions by little or no reduction in width.

Hallpike and Hood (1951) and Dix and Hood (1953) also reported the observation of another characteristic of the recruiting ear. They referred to "perstimulatory fatigue" in which the ear fails to maintain a stable threshold as shown by the tracking performance. They reported diminished sensitivity during sustained threshold stimulation amounting to as much as 15 dB and attributed the phenomenon to end organ pathology.

In an attempt to use tracking amplitude as a measure of recruitment, Reger and Kos (1952) made a startling discovery. Patients with presumably cochlear lesions who traced threshold for discrete steady state tones showed a small decrease in threshold sensitivity. The threshold tracing remained relatively stable over a 4-min period. However, the threshold traced by a patient with an acoustic tumor (confirmed by subsequent surgery) grew progressively poorer until it had shifted 30 dB within 2 min before reaching the output limits of the audiometer. These investigators had never before witnessed a threshold shift of such magnitude in which the patient demanded increasingly greater intensity in order to maintain the audibility of the signal. They applied the term "temporary threshold shift" (TTS) to this phenomenon. Subsequent studies (Lierle and Reger, 1955; Kos, 1955) supported the observation that marked and rapid decrease in threshold sensitivity is characteristic of hearing impairments of retrocochlear origin. Despite this evidence, Hood (1955) and Palva (1957, a and b) reiterated that threshold shift (adaptation), regardless of its magnitude, was a manifestation of an end organ abnormality.

These two divergent views concerning the diagnostic significance of threshold adaptation flourished until Jerger, Carhart and Lassman (1958) offered a unifying concept to the phenomenon. Threshold adaptation, they said, could be observed in both cochlear and retrocochlear lesions. However, when marked threshold drift did occur, the underlying pathology related to a cranial nerve VIII defect. Earlier investigations used steady state (continuous) tones as the test signal. Jerger et al. (1958) observed no adaptation in cochlear or retrocochlear lesions for periodically interrupted tones. Comparison of thresholds for interrupted and continuous signals obtained from 8 patients with cochlear pathology yielded an average threshold differential of 8 dB after 3 min of sustained threshold stimulation. The threshold shift in the cochlear group stabilized at a more or less constant level while the threshold reported for a retrocochlear patient showed a rapid and marked shift that never stabilized. Yantis (1959) offered supporting evidence in his observation of extreme threshold shifts in 3 patients with cerebellopontine angle tumor.

One might wonder why dramatic threshold shifts were observed by some investigators and not by others. Surely, Lundborg's (1952) 21 cases of verified acoustic tumors offered ample opportunity to recognize marked threshold adaptation if indeed it did occur. A reasonable explanation for this disagreement may be found in the instruments used by the different investigators. Lundborg, for example, used a Bekesy audiometer in which attenuation changed in 2-dB steps. It is quite likely that each abrupt change of intensity introduced fleeting audible energy that produced a stimulus similar in character to a periodically interrupted signal. Bekesy's original audiometer provided 2-dB steps and the transition from one step to the next was said to generate a "slight click" especially in the high frequency range. On the other hand, observers who noted marked auditory adaptation used Bekesy-type instruments with a virtually stepless change of only 0.25 dB, thus eliminating an apparently critical variable.

Current Bekesy Procedure

Early investigations of Bekesy audiometry attempted to relate tracking behavior to the presence or absence of recruitment. In 1960, Jerger suggested a relationship between Bekesy tracings and the site of lesion. Full range and discrete frequency threshold tracings were obtained for periodically interrupted (I) and continuous (C) tones from 434 subjects. The tracings were obtained with a Grason-Stadler model E-800 audiometer in which the rate of attenuation was 2.5 dB/sec and frequency changed at the speed of one octave per minute. Four basic configurations or types emerged from a qualitative analysis of the tracings.

Type I. An interweaving of I and C thresholds, throughout the audiogram, characterizes this pattern as shown in Figure 18.1. Tracking amplitude usually averages 10 dB although variations as small as 3 dB and as large as 20 dB are sometimes observed. Type I audiograms typify normal hearing and lesions of the middle ear. However, 47% of all Type I audiograms were obtained from subjects with presumably cochlear pathology and sensory-neural loss of unknown etiology.

Type II. The pattern shown in Figure 18.2 represents the Type II configuration that differs from Type I in two aspects. The C threshold separates from I around 1000 Hz and travels parallel to the high frequency end of the audiogram. The separation usually does not exceed 20 dB. In addition, the amplitude of the continuous trace usually narrows considerably to 3 to 5 dB. The fixed frequency Type II tracing (Fig. 18.3) reflects a similar relationship in which separation occurs for mid and high frequencies only. After the C trace stabilizes 5 to 20 dB below I, the two curves travel more or less parallel. Again, the amplitude of the C tracing is reduced in relation to I.

The Type II audiogram is characteristic of cochlear pathology. Not one subject in the normal hearing and acoustic neurinoma groups yielded a Type II tracing. Only 2 out of 69

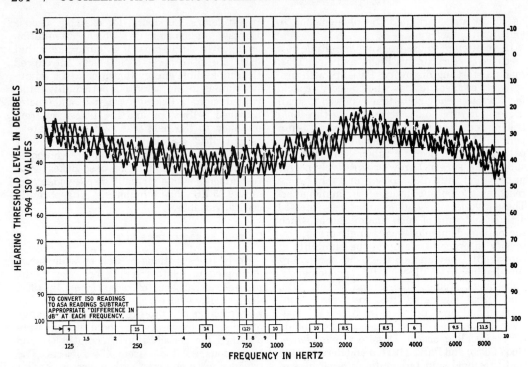

Fig. 18.1. Type I sweep frequency Bekesy audiogram displaying superposition of thresholds for interrupted (*broken lines*) and continuous tones (*unbroken lines*).

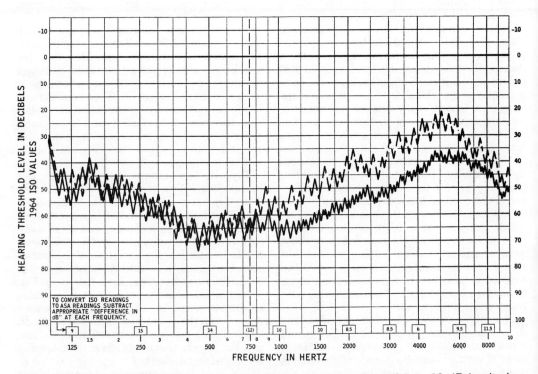

Fig. 18.2. Type II configuration demonstrating curve separation of 5 to 20 dB beginning around 1000 Hz. The amplitude of the C tracing narrows appreciably.

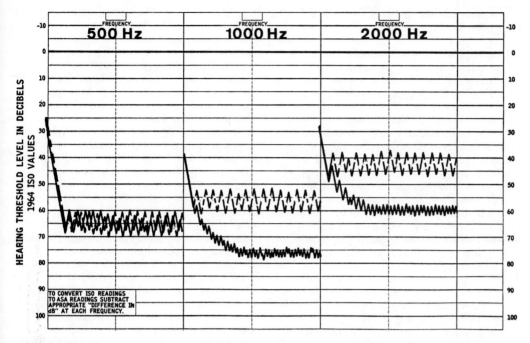

Fig. 18.3. Fixed frequency tracing reflecting Type II characteristics. Curve separation and reduced amplitude of C tracing occur at mid and higher frequencies but not at 500 Hz.

subjects with middle ear pathology traced a Type II pattern.

Type III. The dramatic character of the Type III distinguishes it completely from other configurations (Fig. 18.4 and 18.5). In both the sweep and fixed frequency audiograms, the C trace executes a marked and rapid decline in threshold sensitivity. Deterioration of the C threshold occurs early in the audiogram and continues to the output limits of the audiometer. The amplitude of the continuous tonal tracing is usually undiminished. In discrete frequency measurements, the interrupted threshold takes a horizontal course from which the continuous trace makes a rapid and unaltered decline.

The Type III trace is prevalent in retrocochlear pathology. Six of 10 subjects with acoustic neurinoma yielded Type III audiograms. However, 10 of 16 subjects with sensory-neural loss of sudden onset also generated Type III patterns.

Type IV. The distinguishing feature of the Type IV audiogram (Fig. 18.6) is an early separation of C and I thresholds that occurs below 500 Hz. This separation usually extends into the high frequency area although the two curves may interweave at mid and high frequencies. The tracking envelope of the C trace may or may not be narrowed in relation to the I threshold. The amount of separation inferred from Jerger's text is similar to that observed in

the Type II audiogram (5 to 20 dB). However, one of two illustrative audiograms typifying this configuration demonstrates almost 35 dB of separation at one point. The Type IV audiogram is observed in retrocochlear lesions.

Type V. Shortly after publication of the analysis of Bekesy-type audiograms, Jerger and Herer (1961) added a fifth category. The configuration differs distinctively from the other four types in that the threshold for continuous tones is tracked at significantly less intense levels than threshold for interrupted signals. This threshold relationship is considered suggestive of nonorganic hearing loss. The phenomenon and its relation to children and adults have been studied by other investigators (Rintelmann and Harford, 1963, 1967; Peterson, 1963; Stein, 1963; Hopkinson, 1965; Locke and Richards, 1966) and will be discussed in Chapter 24.

Modifications. Bekesy Types I and III are relatively easy to classify because of their rather distinctive characteristics. Type II and Type IV tracings are occasionally difficult to classify because the two patterns are similar. In an effort to encourage and maintain a standardized classification system, Hopkinson (1966) suggested the continued use of a numerical typing for tracings in addition to a description of the characteristics of an equivocal audiogram in terms of the amount of curve separation and the width of the excursions.

The original description of the Type IV pattern persists despite a subsequent report by Jerger (1962) in which he revised his first definition. The revised description continues to suggest that the two curves begin their separation below 500 Hz. However, Jerger indicated that there is *much greater* separation in the Type IV than in the Type II. Owens (1964) analyzed sweep and discrete frequency tracings obtained from subjects with cochlear lesions and retrocochlear pathology. He found that, in cochlear lesions, the displacement of the C tracing is not confined to any specific frequency area of the audiogram. A new and broader definition of Type II was suggested in which C may separate from I anywhere in the frequency range and remains grossly parallel although it rejoins I in some audiograms. The separation ranged from 4 to 26 dB measured from midpoint to midpoint of the I and C excursions. The Type IV category would thus be eliminated from the classification system. All 13 patients with retrocochlear lesions produced Type III traces. However, 1 of 3 additional subjects diagnosed as having multiple sclerosis who had normal hearing demonstrated an "atypical" tracing in which C shifted more than 30 dB before stabilizing. No reduction was noted in the tracking width of the continuous threshold. Such a tracing would fall under Jerger's revised

Type IV category. The relationship between the Type II and the Type IV tracing as they were initially described was also examined by Hughes, Winegar and Crabtree (1967). Full range Bekesy audiograms of 100 subjects were collected in which half were Type II and half were Type IV. Comparison of the diagnoses demonstrated that almost as many subjects in each group had Meniere's syndrome and a small and equally distributed number had symptoms suggestive of a vascular etiology. One patient in the Type IV group had a nerve VIII tumor while two patients in the Type II group also had confirmed tumors. The investigation concluded that the Type IV (as initially defined by Jerger) is generally produced by the same etiologic factors that produce Type II patterns and that the Type II category should be broadened to include those tracings that demonstrate an early separation not exceeding 20 dB. Hughes (1967) also proposed that the Type IV is one in which the separation of curves is greater than 25 dB regardless of where that separation occurs. Figures 18.7 and 18.8 illustrate the Type IV tracing based on these findings. Confirmed retrocochlear pathology sometimes yields Type III patterns that do not demonstrate curve separation until well along in the audiogram (Jerger and Waller, 1962). Therefore, the classification of Types II,

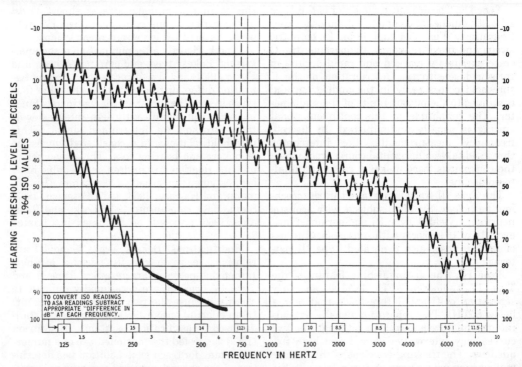

Fig. 18.4. Threshold for C tones undergoes early and rapid decline in sensitivity and typifies the distinctive character of the Type III audiogram.

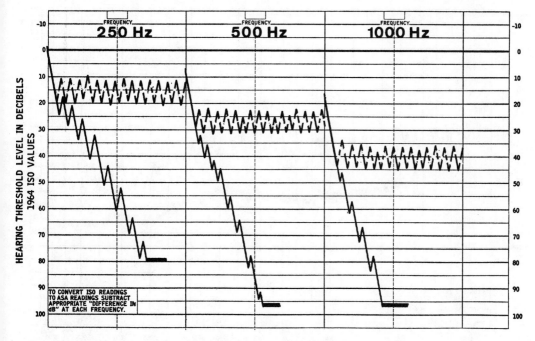

Fig. 18.5. Type III discrete frequency pattern displaying marked drift of the C threshold to the limits of the audiometer. Threshold sensitivity for pulsed tones is unaltered with time as it tracks a horizontal course.

III and IV should be made without regard for frequency.

These revised criteria are more consistent with the concept that cochlear pathology usually produces less auditory adaptation than the retrocochlear lesion. Employing the revised criteria, Johnson (1968, 1970) found that, in 158 cases of confirmed acoustic tumors, 38 patients yielded Type IV audiograms and 53 generated Type II patterns. Fifty-nine patients produced Type III tracings. The 8 remaining patients yielded Type I audiograms. Review of these audiograms discloses that only 11 of the Type II tracings showed curve separation below 500 Hz.

Interpretation of Audiograms

Adults. General agreement with Jerger's findings has been expressed by Harbert and Young (1964, a and b), Owens (1964), Tillman (1966) and Johnson (1968). However, clinical use of Bekesy audiometry requires caution regarding the diagnostic significance of the configurations. Jerger (1962, p. 143) warns, "...we cannot be sure that the absence of a particular pattern necessarily *precludes* the possibility of a disorder at a given site." Johnson (1968) has clearly shown that surgically confirmed acoustic tumors can produce Type I and Type II tracings with striking frequency. Menzel et al. (1964) and Shapiro and Naunton (1967) have

also shown atypical or misleading findings in acoustic neuromas. In this regard, Johnson (1966) suggested that the size of a tumor influences audiologic findings in which small tumors usually yield inconsistent responses. Jerger and Waller (1962) illustrated changes in audiometric responses presumably as a function of tumor growth. They observed the Bekesy audiograms of a patient with a confirmed nerve VIII tumor to shift from Type I to Type II to Type III during a 20-month period. Therefore, an acoustic tumor may generate any one of an assortment of Bekesy patterns contingent on its site and stage of development. Other pathologic conditions may produce findings similar to those of nerve VIII tumor. Robertson (1965) cautions the audiologist to confine his interpretation of audiologic data to an identification of site rather than to the possible etiological factors concerning the suspected lesion. As we have seen, many clinicians have confirmed the value of Bekesy audiometry in demonstrating nerve VIII tumors. However, the following is a list of pathologic conditions that have been reported to produce Type III and Type IV tracings. Acoustic tumor is only one such pathology.

Acoustic tumor (Jerger, 1960)
Cerebellopontine angle tumor (Brand and Rosenberg, 1963)

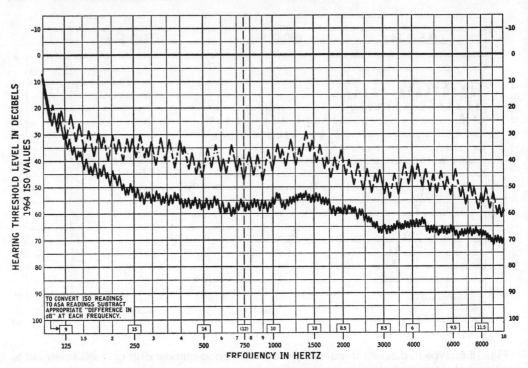

Fig. 18.6. Early and limited curve separation characterize Jerger's initial Type IV pattern. This audiogram would be classified as Type II according to revised criteria.

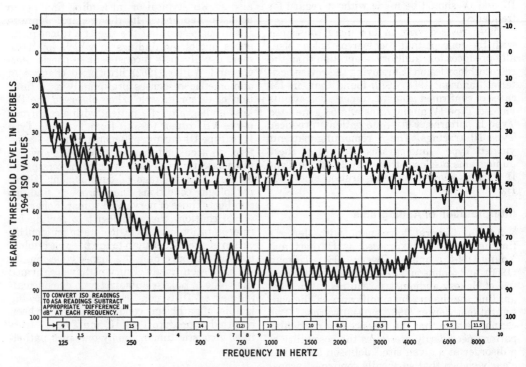

Fig. 18.7. Marked curve separation (without the precipitous drop in audiometer limits seen in Type III audiogram) is the prominent feature of the revised Type IV configuration.

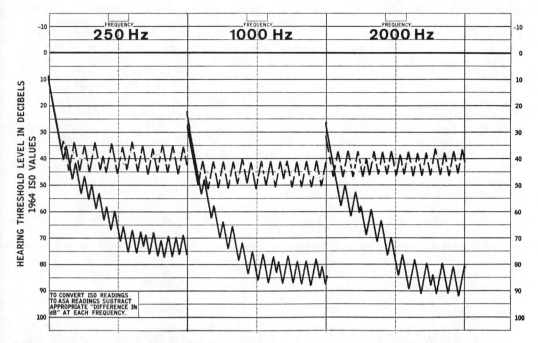

Fig. 18.8. Fixed frequency Type IV (revised) reflects conspicuous threshold drift for C signals that stabilizes with time.

Cerebellar tumor (Jerger et al., 1966)

Cerebral meningioma (Katinsky and Toglia, 1968)

von Recklinghausen's disease (Hitselberger and Hughes, 1968)

Primary cholesteatoma (House and Doyle, 1962)

Ramsay-Hunt syndrome (Harbert and Young, 1967)

Multiple sclerosis (Owens, 1964)

Acromegaly (Menzel, 1966)

Mumps neuritis (Parker, Decker and Richards, 1968)

Head trauma (Suzuki et al., 1964)

Sensory-neural hearing loss of sudden onset (Altshuler and Welsh, 1966)

Sensory-neural hearing loss of unknown origin (Jerger, 1960)

Nerve VIII thermal injury (Harbert and Young, 1964a)

Acquired luetic hearing loss (Robertson, 1965)

Meniere's disease (Jerger, 1960)

Otosclerosis plus sensory-neural hearing loss (Jerger, 1960)

Congenital sensory-neural hearing loss (Hughes, 1970)

Children. Price and Falck (1963) investigated the application of Bekesy audiometry to normal hearing children. The procedure was found clinically useful with children of average intelligence who are at least 7 years of age. Ninety-three percent yielded Type I tracings. Only 5 out of 9 6-year-olds were able to complete the test satisfactorily. The results of a study by Stark (1965) comparing thresholds obtained with conventional and Bekesy audiometry also suggested that the usefulness of automatic audiometry in normal and hearing-impaired children is dependent on age. Almost one-third of 5-year-old subjects did not produce clinically useful tracings while almost all of the 7- to 10-year-old group did.

Hearing-impaired children also generate Bekesy configurations similar to adults. Each pattern except the Type III was observed in children (Stark, 1966; Swisher and Stephens, 1968). A sizable number of hypacusic children yield Type I tracings (Stark, 1966), reflecting, perhaps, pathology similar to the large segment of subjects with sensory-neural losses of unknown etiology in the Jerger (1960) study.

Validity and Reliability. Throughout this chapter we have shown that subject responses are critically dependent not only on pathology but also on the characteristics of the test signal and the test procedure. As in any measurement of psychophysical behavior, a number of other factors influence the validity and reliability of audiometric data (High, Glorig and Nixon, 1961). Not all Bekesy audiograms fit neatly into Jerger's (1960) classification system. Sixteen subjects out of his total population of 434 yielded tracings that could not be classified. These questionable audiograms were rejected mainly because of their apparent lack of validity. Lack of confidence in a particular audiogram is frequently the result of (1) inadequate instructions, (2) confusion of steady state test signals with tinnitus, (3) delays in patient response, (4) inattention or drowsiness and (5) attempts to manipulate test results. Questionable tracings have no common characteristics although classification is obviated, usually, by enormous excursions. Figure 18.9 demonstrates the disruptive influence of tinnitus on the tracking course for steady state signals. Figure 18.10 illustrates how the relationship between I and C is obscured by unusually large excursions produced by a slow responding elderly woman with presbycusis.

The magnitude of a hearing loss may occasionally lead to an unclassifiable audiogram. All we can really say about the classification of the tracing illustrated in Figure 18.11 is that it does not reflect a Type I or Type V configuration. The occasional spiking of the C line does not represent audibility of tone, but rather a response to noise generated by the attenuator mechanism striking against the output stops of the audiometer.

Pollack (1948) has shown that instructions to respond to (1) any sound or (2) only to tone, result in significant threshold differences in conventional audiometry. Bekesy audiograms may be similarly affected. Occasionally during steady state tonal stimulation subjective change of the signal from tone to atonal noise occurs (Sorensen, 1962; Owens, 1965). The signal is usually described by the subject as a "sizzling," "frying" or "buzzing" sound. The change takes place shortly after onset of stimulation and may continue to the limit of the audiometer if the subject is instructed to respond only to tonal quality. The audiogram shown in Figure 18.12 exhibits a curve separation of 20 to 25 dB (Type II) in which both tracings have similar excursion widths. The subject may describe the interrupted tones as "musical" while the continuous signals sound like "buzzing." Instructing the listener to respond only to tonal signals may generate the Type IV pattern of Figure 18.13. Sometimes, a Type III tracing is produced by a subject who hears only a "noisy" (atonal) signal to the limits of the audiometer. Response to atonal sound may produce an audiogram that conceals the underlying pathology.

Effects of Parameter Variations

Stimulus Duration. Temporal auditory summation (Chapter 19) is the process by which threshold for a brief tone increases as the duration of the tone is decreased (Zwislocki, 1960). This temporal integration of acoustic

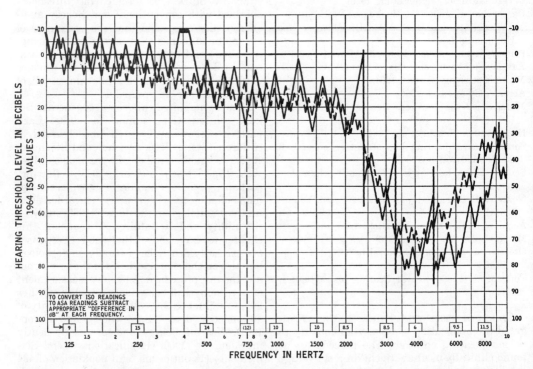

Fig. 18.9. Confusion of tinnitus with steady state signals obscures the relationship between I and C thresholds. *Vertical lines* indicate where control of test tone intensity was assumed by tester to re-establish threshold.

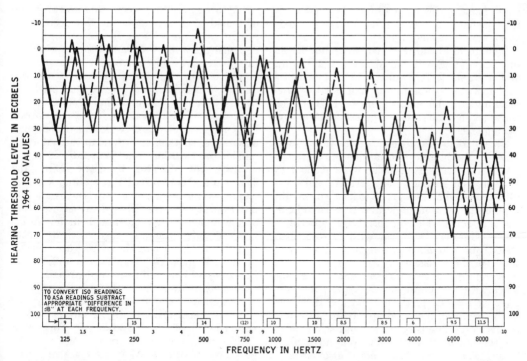

Fig. 18.10. Uncommonly wide excursions prevent accurate classification of this audiogram.

energy is a normal phenomenon. In a series of observations of threshold for tones as a function of their duration, Sanders and Honig (1967) and Wright (1968, a and b; 1969) concluded that threshold duration functions may be more sensitive indicators of cochlear pathology than measures of loudness recruitment. Measurement of temporal auditory summation is feasible clinical procedure if well defined parameters of rise-decay time, duration and repetition rate are employed. Temporal summation is deficient in patients with cochlear lesions in that there is a relatively small improvement in threshold with increased stimulus duration. Cochlear dysfunction may be demonstrated quantitatively by tracking discrete frequency thresholds for each of 500-, 200-, 100-, 50-, 20- and 10-msec tones (employing a 10-msec rise and decay time, a repetition rate of one pulse/sec and an attenuation rate of 2.5 dB/sec). The difference between threshold for the 10-msec signal and each stimulus mode is computed and compared to normative values. Although Wright (1968b) suggests that uncontrolled variables may operate to affect threshold duration functions, the procedure holds promise as an index of temporal processing that can be influenced by cochlear pathology.

Interstimulus Duration. When a patient with sensory-neural hearing impairment tracks threshold for interrupted and continuous tones, he usually requires different sound pres-

sure levels to maintain audibility of the two signals. Threshold, therefore, is intimately related to the temporal characteristics of the test signal.

Systematically varying the interstimulus interval (off-time) of the test signal does not significantly affect threshold values for normal ears (Dallos and Tillman, 1966). Harbert and Young (1962b) found they could generate a family of sweep frequency pulsed-tone curves for a patient with nerve VIII pathology by decreasing the off-time duration. Successive thresholds were elevated with each decrease in off-time until a certain minimal value was reached. The patient's responses then became indistinguishable from those to a steady state signal. Similarly, an ear with retrocochlear pathology maintains a relatively stable fixed frequency threshold but only until the off-time duration is decreased below a certain critical value. Threshold will then deteriorate dramatically (as it does for a steady state pure tone signal) when the interstimulus interval is decreased below the critical off-time (COT) value for that ear (Jerger and Jerger, 1966). COT is subject to individual differences and may be as long as 200 msec or as short as 40 msec. Threshold may be elevated more than 100 dB or as little as 25 dB as the off-time interval is decreased below the subject's critical value. The phenomenon becomes more evident at higher frequencies. Young and Harbert (1968) have found COT for cochlear lesions to be intermediate between values for normal ears and abnormally adapting ears.

Ipsilateral Masking by Noise. A number of investigators (Small and Minifie, 1961; Collins and Menzel, 1965; Young, 1968) have found that ipsilateral broad band and narrow band masking noise have no significant influence on the tracking amplitudes of pulsed and continuous signals.

Sweep frequency thresholds for interrupted tones in the presence of various intensities of ipsilateral broad band noise were studied by Harbert and Young (1965). Broad band noise yields masked thresholds 15 to 20 dB below the level of the noise in subjects with normal hearing and conductive and presumably cochlear losses. However, subjects with retrocochlear lesions generate masked thresholds at or above the level of the masker.

Sweep frequency measurements for pulsed tones with ipsilateral narrow band noise centered at 1000 Hz produce a masked threshold at the center of the band approximately equal to the overall intensity of the masker in normal subjects and those with conductive and cochlear losses. The narrow band noise also elevates thresholds above and below the center of the masking band as would be anticipated from an earlier study by Bilger and Hirsh (1956). Com-

pared to the normal subjects, this lateral spread of masking is less in conductive losses and greater in cochlear losses. Retrocochlear lesions demonstrate a marked lateral spread of masking above and below the center of the narrow band masker yielding a masked sweep frequency threshold approximating that produced by white noise (Harbert and Young, 1965). Therefore, in retrocochlear lesions, a narrow band masker can evoke widespread abnormal adaptation so that an attendant signal (well outside the masking band) is inaudible.

Ipsilateral Masking by Tone. Lilly and Thalmann (1964) tested the assumption that ipsilateral masking of one pure tone by another occurs in the cochlea. They demonstrated that a continuous tone, even though inaudible because of adaptation, masked an interrupted signal in the same ear. Katz (1969) used continuous tone masking (CTM) as a differential index of cochlear and retrocochlear pathology. After determining threshold for a pulsed tone, a continuous tone of identical frequency and phase is added ipsilaterally at successive sensation levels of 10, 20 and 30 dB. Thresholds for the pulsed tone are tracked again in the presence of the continuous masking tone. Lower (better) masked thresholds are observed in patients with cochlear losses while higher thresholds are found in retrocochlear lesions.

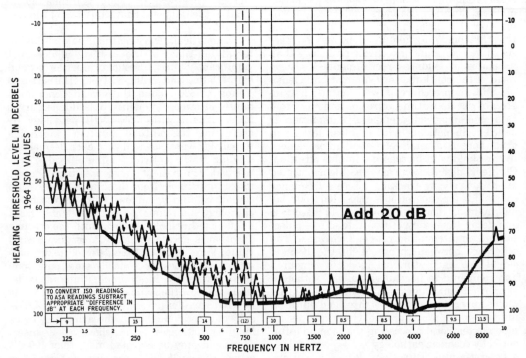

Fig. 18.11. Output limit of Bekesy audiometer restricts threshold measurement of C signals and contributes to an unclassifiable audiogram.

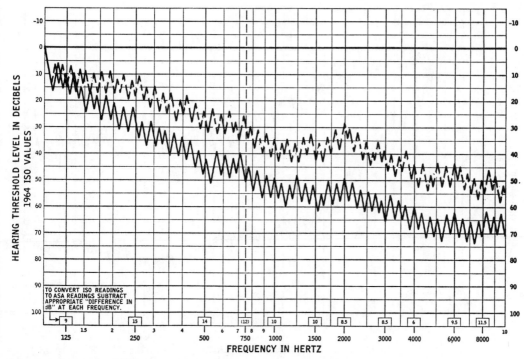

Fig. 18.12. Type II tracing acquired from a subject responding to the atonal quality of C signals.

Contralateral Masking by Noise. The classification of Bekesy tracings is based in large measure on the separation between thresholds for pulsed and steady state tones. In addition, many clinical audiologists inspect the amplitude of the C trace excursions for information regarding recruitment. Bilger (1965) considered the tracking width for continuous tones in fixed frequency audiograms to be the most reliable index of normal and pathologic cochlear function. However, curve separation and tracking width (and consequently, classification of an audiogram) seem to be directly dependent in many instances on the presence or absence of contralateral masking during the test. Dirks and Norris (1966) and Blegvad (1967) have observed that with contralateral masking, fixed frequency audiograms for normal listeners resemble tracings obtained from patients with end organ lesions. They noted curve separation and marked narrowing of the C tracking width at 1000 and 4000 Hz, but not at 250 Hz. The maximum separation between I and C for normal subjects was 20 dB. Grimes and Feldman (1969) utilized frequency-modulated narrow band noise of constant band width. The masker was presented to the contralateral ear and was automatically centered around the test frequency. They found artificial separation between I and C thresholds in nor-

mal subjects. The constant band width was found to be an effective masker of low frequency pure tone signals. However, when the narrow band masker approximates critical band width at higher frequencies the listener encounters difficulty distinguishing between the noise and the continuous signal. False Type II sweep frequency tracings were the result of greater masking of C tones.

Tracking behavior in end organ lesions is similarly affected by contralateral masking. Application of 80 dB SPL broad band noise to the nontest ear occasionally alters Type I tracings to Type II and Type IV while Type II audiograms change to Type IV. Contralateral masking also produces marked reduction in tracking width of the C trace (Blegvad, 1967). Whether these changes are due to interaural interference, distraction of the subject or central masking, the interpretation of Bekesy audiometry may often be influenced even by low level contralateral masking.

Order Effect. Bradford and Goetzinger (1964) have noted that differences in thresholds for C and I tones at 4000 Hz may be produced by the order in which the tones are presented. Wright (1969) found greater threshold differences at all frequencies when C tones preceded presentation of I tones. Although these threshold differences were not statistically significant

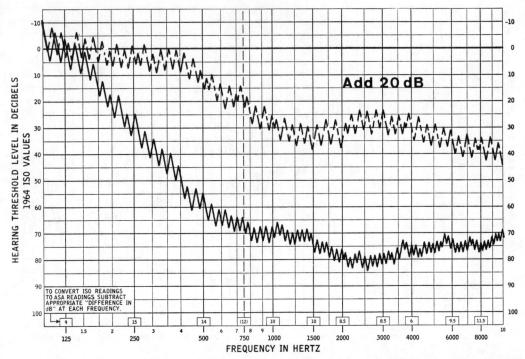

Fig. 18.13. Type IV audiogram obtained from subject instructed to respond only to signals with tonal quality.

in terms of group behavior, it was suggested that they could be of some influence in the interpretation of individual tracings.

Starting Intensity. Rosenblith and Miller (1949) reported a 4-dB better threshold in normal subjects for interrupted signals of decreasing intensity than for similar signals of increasing intensity. They also observed that continuous tones of decreasing intensity generate consistently poorer thresholds than increasing intensity signals. Harbert and Young (1968) investigated the influence of infra- and suprathreshold starting intensities of pulsed and steady state signals on normal and pathologic ears. Various starting intensity levels were employed. Threshold was considered as the point of the first pen reversal for each of the increasing and decreasing intensity modes. They found that thresholds for pulsed tones in subjects with normal hearing and cochlear losses were essentially equal when approached from either intensity direction. Each 20-dB increase in suprathreshold starting intensity for a continuous signal produces a corresponding threshold elevation of 1.5 dB for subjects with normal hearing and 5 dB for patients with cochlear losses. Retrocochlear pathology generates far greater threshold elevations for each 20-dB increase in starting intensity.

Tracking Direction. Rose (1962) compared sweep frequency tracings in which continuous and interrupted tones were each tracked in an ascending mode from 100 to 10,000 Hz and descending from 10,000 to 100 Hz. He observed that pulsed tone thresholds were essentially the same whether tracked from low to high frequencies or the reverse except for abnormally adapting ears. However, the descending mode seems to enhance the tracking behavior for C signals observed in the ascending frequency audiogram. Specifically, separation of I and C thresholds observed in the conventional ascending audiogram is significantly greater in the descending tracking. In addition, the tracking amplitude for continuous tones that narrow in the ascending audiogram is considerably smaller in the descending mode. It should be noted that an attenuation rate of 2.5 dB/sec was employed for I and C tones in ascending audiograms. In descending tracings, I tones were attenuated at the rate of 2.5 dB/sec, while C tones were attenuated by 1.25 dB/sec. We know that reducing the rate of attenuation produces a corresponding reduction of tracking amplitude. Furthermore, Owens (1965) has offered the hypothesis that Type II patterns are the product of an interplay between auditory adaptation and loudness recruitment. He suggested that an attenuation rate of 2.5 dB/sec is often sufficient to overcome an ear's rate of adaptation. Perhaps then, the greater curve separation and reduced amplitude observed in the descending frequency mode were partly the result of the slow attenuation rate (1.25 dB/sec) that was used. Harbert and Young (1968) have observed that ascending and descending frequency audiograms offer an essentially identical relationship between thresholds for pulsed and continuous tones except for ears with abnormal adaptation. Karja and Palva (1970) found differences between ascending and descending continuous tone thresholds in 17 of 221 patients with various sensory-neural losses. When differences occurred, the reverse order sweep frequency tracings always offered poorer thresholds than the forward order audiograms. Young and Harbert (1971), Palva, Karja and Palva (1970), and Jerger et al., (1972) established the fact that poorer reverse frequency tracings were distinguishing characteristics of retrocochlear disorders.

Some frequency areas of an audiogram disclose far more adaptation than others and often, greatest adaptation occurs in the area of greatest loss. We have seen that in a fatigable ear, greater loss will be registered when threshold is approached from high intensity than when it is approached from a subliminal level. Therefore, threshold for a particular frequency area is higher (poorer) in an adapting ear when approached in either direction from a neighboring area of high intensity. Approaching the same area from an adjoining region at lower intensity results in less threshold shift. In addition, approaching a frequency area in any direction from a region of marked adaptation produces far greater threshold elevation than when approaching from a neighboring area of little or no adaptation.

Jerger and Jerger (1974) suggested Bekesy tracings at "comfortable loudness" rather than at threshold. They classified Bekesy comfortable loudness (BCL) audiograms into six different patterns based on the relationships between interrupted and continuous tracings. Three of the patterns showed no unusual adaptation for continuous tracing and were found in patients with cochlear or conductive disorders, or in normal listeners. Three other patterns were found in patients with nerve VIII or extra-axial brain stem disorders. These patterns exhibited marked discrepancies between interrupted and continuous tracings or between continuous forward and continuous backward tracings. Jerger and Jerger concluded that suprathreshold Bekesy tracings are more rewarding than threshold levels in the exploration of nerve VIII and brain stem disorders.

CONCLUSION

For almost a quarter of a century, audiologists have been trying different methods to improve clinical diagnosis with the Bekesy audiometer. Numerous ways have been found to classify responses depending upon whether the signal is continuous or interrupted, the speed of attenuation, the off-time, the tonal duration, the direction of frequency change, the use of masking and comfort level vs. threshold tracings. Almost all of these techniques seem to offer valuable information from the standpoint of differential diagnosis between cochlear and retrocochlear lesions provided the patient is responding to "tone" and that the ear receives a continuous signal or does not get too much rest between pulses. It is obvious that to speak of a patient's responses without identifying the equipment and test parameters is to obscure the significance and reliability of one's findings.

Perhaps in the future audiologists will decide on a few meaningful procedures so that some standardization can be maintained from one audiologist to another. In addition, further research may be able to provide quantitative in addition to qualitative, information presently available from Bekesy audiometry.

REFERENCES

Altshuler, M. W., and Welsh, O. L., Sudden hearing loss with spontaneous recovery. *J. Speech Hear. Disord*, 31, 166–171, 1966.

Bekesy, G. v., A new audiometer. *Acta Otolaryngol.*, 35, 411–422, 1947.

Bilger, R. C., Some parameters of fixed-frequency Békésy audiometry. *J. Speech Hear. Res.*, 8, 85–95, 1965.

Bilger, R., and Hirsh, I., Masking of tones by bands of noise. *J. Acoust. Soc. Am.*, 28, 623–630, 1956.

Blegvad, B., Contralateral masking and Bekesy audiometry in normal listeners. *Acta Otolaryngol.*, 64, 157–165, 1967.

Bradford, L., and Goetzinger, C., A study of the order effects on tracings made with a Bekesy-type audiometer. *Acta Otolaryngol.*, 58, 17–31, 1964.

Brand, S., and Rosenberg, P. E., Problems in auditory evaluation for neuro-surgical diagnosis. *J. Speech Hear. Disord.*, 28, 355–361, 1963.

Burns, W., and Hinchcliffe, R., Comparison of the auditory threshold as measured by individual pure tone and by Bekesy audiometry. *J. Acoust. Soc. Am.*, 29, 1274–1277, 1957.

Collins, J., and Menzel, O. J., The relation between intensity difference limen and Bekesy threshold tracings (Abstract). *ASHA*, 7, 428, 1965.

Corso, J. F., Effects of testing methods on hearing thresholds. *Arch. Otolaryngol.*, 63, 78–91, 1956.

Corso, J. F., Additional variables on the Bekesy-type audiometer. *Arch. Otolaryngol.*, 66, 719–728, 1957.

Dallos, P. J., and Tillman, T. W., The effects of parameter variations in Bekesy audiometry in a patient with acoustic neurinoma. *J. Speech Hear. Res.*, 9, 557–572, 1966.

Dirks, D. D., and Norris, J. D., Shifts in auditory thresholds produced by ipsilateral and contralateral maskers at low-intensity levels. *J.*

Acoust. Soc. Am., **40**, 12–19, 1966.

Dix, M. R., Hallpike, C. S., and Hood, J. D., Observations upon the loudness recruitment phenomenon with especial reference to the differential diagnosis of disorders of the internal ear and VIIIth nerve. *J. Laryngol.*, **62**, 671–686, 1948.

Dix, M. R., and Hood, J. D., Modern developments in pure tone audiometry and their application to the clinical diagnosis of end-organ deafness. *J. Laryngol.*, **67**, 343–357, 1953.

Epstein, A., Variables involved in automatic audiometry. *Ann. Otol. Rhinol. Laryngol.*, **69**, 137–141, 1960.

Fowler, E. P., Marked deafened areas in normal ears. *Arch. Otolaryngol.*, **8**, 151–155, 1928.

Fowler, E. P., A method for the early detection of otosclerosis. *Arch. Otolaryngol.*, **24**, 731–741, 1936.

Gardner, M. B., A pulse-tone clinical audiometer. *J. Acoust. Soc. Am.*, **19**, 592–599, 1947.

Grimes, C. T., and Feldman, A. S., Comparative Bekesy typing with broad and modulated narrow-band noise. *J. Speech Hear. Res.*, **12**, 840–846, 1969.

Hallpike, C. S., and Hood, J. D., Some recent work on auditory adaptation and its relationship to the loudness recruitment phenomenon. *J. Acoust. Soc. Am.*, **23**, 270–274, 1951.

Harbert, F., and Young, I. M., Clinical application of hearing tests. *Arch. Otolaryngol*, **76**, 55–67, 1962a.

Harbert, F., and Young, I. M., Threshold auditory adaptation. *J. Aud. Res.*, **2**, 229–246, 1962b.

Harbert, F., and Young, I. M., Threshold auditory adaptation measured by tone decay test and Bekesy audiometry. *Ann. Otol. Rhinol. Laryngol.*, **73**, 48–60, 1964a.

Harbert, F. and Young, I. M. Audiologic findings in Meniere's syndrome. *Acta Otolaryngol.*, **57**, 145–154, 1964b.

Harbert, F., and Young, I. M., Spread of masking in ears showing abnormal adaptation and conductive deafness. *Acta Otolaryngol.*, **60**, 49–58, 1965.

Harbert, F., and Young, I. M., Amplitude of Bekesy tracings with different attenuation rates. *J. Acoust. Soc. Am.*, **39**, 914–919, 1966.

Harbert, F., and Young, I. M., Audiologic findings in Ramsay-Hunt syndrome. *Arch. Otolaryngol.*, **85**, 632–639, 1967.

Harbert, F., and Young, I. M., Clinical application of Békésy audiometry. *Laryngoscope*, **78**, 487–497, 1968.

High, W. S., Glorig, A., and Nixon, J., Estimating the reliability of auditory threshold measurements. *J. Aud. Res.*, **1**, 247–262, 1961.

Hirsh, I. J., *The Measurement of Hearing*. New York: McGraw-Hill Book Co., 1952.

Hirsh, I. J., Palva, T., and Goodman, A., Difference limen and recruitment. *Arch. Otolaryngol.*, **60**, 525–540, 1954.

Hitselberger, W. E., and Hughes, R. L., Bilateral acoustic tumors and neurofibromatosis. *Arch. Otolaryngol.*, **88**, 700–711, 1968.

Hood, J. D., Auditory fatigue and adaptation in the differential diagnosis of end-organ disease. *Ann. Otol. Rhinol. Laryngol.*, **64**, 507–518, 1955.

Hopkinson, N. T., Type V Bekesy audiograms; spec-
ification and clinical utility. *J. Speech Hear. Disord.*, **30**, 243–251, 1965.

Hopkinson, N. T., Modifications of the four types of Bekesy audiograms. *J. Speech Hear. Disord.*, **31**, 79–82, 1966.

House, W. F., and Doyle, J., Early diagnosis and removal of primary cholesteatoma causing pressure to the VIII nerve. *Laryngoscope*, **72**, 1053–1063, 1962.

Hughes, R. L., Current audiometric practices. *Voice*, **16**, 82–87, 1967.

Hughes, R. L., Unpublished information, 1970.

Hughes, R. L., Winegar, W. J., and Crabtree, J. A., Bekesy audiometry; type 2 versus type 4 patterns. *Arch Otolaryngol.*, **86**, 424–430, 1967.

Jerger, J., Bekesy audiometry in analysis of auditory disorders. *J. Speech Hear. Res.*, **3**, 275–287, 1960.

Jerger, J., Hearing tests in otologic diagnosis. *ASHA*, **4**, 139–145, 1962.

Jerger, J., and Herer, G., Unexpected dividend in Bekesy audiometry. *J. Speech Hear. Disord.*, **26**, 390–391, 1961.

Jerger, J., and Jerger, S., Critical off-time in VIIIth nerve disorders. *J. Speech Hear. Res.*, **9**, 573–583, 1966.

Jerger, J., and Jerger, S., Diagnostic value of Bekesy comfortable loudness tracings. *Arch. Otolaryngol.*, **99**, 351–360, 1974.

Jerger, J., and Waller, J., Some observations on masking and on the progression of auditory signs in acoustic neurinoma. *J. Speech Hear. Disord.*, **27**, 140–143, 1962.

Jerger, J., Carhart, R., and Lassman, J., Clinical observations on excessive threshold adaptation. *Arch. Otolaryngol.*, **68**, 617–623, 1958.

Jerger, J., Jerger, S., Ainsworth, J., and Caram, P., Recovery of auditory function after surgical removal of cerebellar tumor. *J. Speech Hear. Disord.*, **31**, 377–382, 1966.

Jerger, J., Jerger, S., and Mauldin, L., The forward-backward discrepancy in Bekesy audiometry. *Arch. Otolaryngol.*, **72**, 400–406, 1972.

Johnson, E. W., Confirmed retrocochlear lesions. *Arch. Otolaryngol.*, **84**, 247–254, 1966.

Johnson, E. W., Auditory findings in 200 cases of acoustic neuromas. *Arch. Otolaryngol.*, **88**, 598–603, 1968.

Johnson, E. W., Auditory test results in 268 cases of confirmed retrocochlear lesions. *Int. Audiol.*, **9**, 15–19, 1970.

Karja, J., and Palva, A., Reverse frequency-sweep Bekesy audiometry. *Acta Otolaryngol.*, Suppl. **263**, 225–228, 1970.

Katinsky, S. E., and Toglia, J. V., Audiologic and vestibular manifestations of meningiomas of the cerebellopontine angle. *J. Speech Hear. Disord.*, **33**, 351–360, 1968.

Katz, J., The continuous tone masking (CTM) test for identifying site of lesion. *J. Aud. Res.*, **9**, 76–80, 1969.

Kos, C. M., Auditory function as related to the complaint of dizziness. *Laryngoscope*, **65**, 711–721, 1955.

Landis, B., Recruitment measured by automatic audiometry. *Arch. Otolaryngol.*, **68**, 685–696, 1958.

Liden, G., Loss of hearing following treatment with dihydrostreptomycin or streptomycin. *Acta Oto-*

laryngol., **43**, 551–571, 1953.

Lierle, D. M., and Reger, S. N., Experimentally induced temporary threshold shifts in ears with impaired hearing. *Ann. Otol. Rhinol. Laryngol.*, **64**, 263–277, 1955.

Lilly, D. J., The effects of rate of attenuation and mode of signal presentation on the amplitude of the Békésy envelope (Abstract). *ASHA*, **7**, 428, 1965.

Lilly, D. J., and Thalmann, R., The masking of interrupted pure tones by inaudible continuous pure tones in pathologic ears (Abstract). *ASHA*, **6**, 397, 1964.

Locke, J. L., and Richards, A. L., Type V Bekesy audiograms in normal hearers. *J. Aud. Res.*, **6**, 393–395, 1966.

Lundborg, T., Diagnostic problems concerning acoustic tumors. *Acta Otolaryngol.*, Suppl., **99**, 1–110, 1952.

McLay, B., The place of the Békésy audiometer in clinical audiometry. *J. Laryngol.*, **73**, 460–465, 1959.

Menzel, O., Hearing loss secondary to acromegaly; case report. *Eye Ear Nose Throat Mon.*, **45**, 84–85, 1966.

Menzel, O. J., Finney, L. A., David, N. J., and Buermann, A., Atypical audiologic findings in a case of acoustic neurinoma. *Laryngoscope*, **74**, 1391–1400, 1964.

Muma, J. R., and Siegenthaler, B. M., Bekesy excursion size for normal-hearing young adults. *J. Aud. Res.*, **6**, 289–296, 1966.

Owens, E., Bekesy tracings and site of lesion. *J. Speech Hear. Disord.*, **29**, 456–468, 1964.

Owens, E., Bekesy tracings, tone decay, and loudness recruitment. *J. Speech Hear. Disord.*, **30**, 50–57, 1965.

Palva, T., Recruitment tests at low sensation levels. *Laryngoscope*, **66**, 1519–1540, 1956.

Palva, T., Self-recording threshold audiometry and recruitment. *Arch. Otolaryngol.*, **65**, 591–602, 1957a.

Palva, T., Recruitment testing. *Arch. Otolaryngol.*, **66**, 93–98, 1957b.

Palva, T., Karja, J., and Palva, A., Foward vs. reversed Bekesy tracings. *Arch. Otolaryngol.*, **91**, 449–452, 1970.

Parker, W., Decker, R. L., and Richards, N. G., Auditory function and lesions of the pons. *Arch. Otolaryngol.*, **87**, 228–240, 1968.

Peterson, J. L. Nonorganic hearing loss in children and Bekesy audiometry. *J. Speech Hear. Disord.*, **28**, 153–158, 1963.

Pollack, I., The atonal interval. *J. Acoust. Soc. Am.*, **20**, 146–149, 1948.

Price, L. L., and Falck, V. T., Bekesy audiometry with children. *J. Speech Hear. Res.*, **6**, 129–133, 1963.

Reger, S. N., A clinical and research version of the Bekesy audiometer. *Laryngoscope*, **62**, 1333–1351, 1952.

Reger, S. N., and Kos, C. M., Clinical measurements and implications of recruitment. *Ann. Otol. Rhinol. Laryngol.*, **61**, 810–823, 1952.

Reger, S. N. and Newby, H. A., A group pure-tone hearing test. *J. Speech Disord.*, **12**, 61–66, 1947.

Rintelmann, W., and Harford, E., The detection and assessment of pseudo-hypoacusis among school-age children. *J. Speech Hear. Disord.*, **28**, 141–152, 1963.

Rintelmann, W., and Harford, E., Type V Bekesy pattern; Interpretation and clinical utility. *J. Speech Hear. Res.*, **10**, 733–744, 1967.

Robertson, D. G., Use of Bekesy findings in auditory diagnosis. *J. Speech Hear. Disord.*, **30**, 367–369, 1965.

Rose, D. E., Some effects and case histories of reversed frequency sweep in Bekesy audiometry. *J. Aud. Res.*, **2**, 267–278, 1962.

Rosenblith, W. A., and Miller, G. A., The threshold for continuous and interrupted tones. (Abstract). *J. Acoust. Soc. Am.*, **22**, 674, 1949.

Sanders, J. W., and Honig, E. A., Brief tone audiometry. *Arch. Otolaryngol.*, **85**, 640–647, 1967.

Shapiro, I., and Naunton, R. F., Audiologic evaluation of acoustic neurinomas. *J. Speech Hear. Disord.*, **32**, 29–35, 1967.

Small, A. M., Jr., and Minifie, F. A., Intensive differential sensitivity and masked threshold. *J. Speech Hear. Res.*, **4**, 164–171, 1961.

Sorensen, H., Clinical application of continuous threshold recording. *Acta Otolaryngol.*, **54**, 403–422, 1962.

Stark, E. W., Bekesy audiometry with normal-hearing and hearing-impaired children. *J. Aud. Res.*, **5**, 73–83, 1965.

Stark, E. W., Jerger types in fixed-frequency Bekesy audiometry with normal and hypacusic children. *J. Aud. Res.*, **6**, 135–140, 1966.

Stein, L., Some observations on Type V Bekesy tracings. *J. Speech Hear. Res.*, **6**, 339–348, 1963.

Suzuki, T., and Kubota, K., Normal width in tracing on Bekesy audiogram. *J. Aud. Res.*, **6**, 91–96, 1966.

Suzuki, T., Yoshi, N., Sakabe, N., and Igarashi, E., A clinical comparison of two methods for measuring abnormal auditory adaptation by means of the Bekesy audiometer. *J. Aud. Res.*, **4**, 195–205, 1964.

Swisher, L. P., and Stephens, M., Bekesy sweep-frequency and conventional audiometry with hearing-impaired children. *J. Aud. Res.*, **8**, 261–272, 1968.

Tillman, T. Audiologic diagnosis of acoustic tumors. *Arch. Otolaryngol.*, **83**, 574–581, 1966.

Wright, H. N., Clinical measurement of temporal auditory summation. *J. Speech Hear. Res.*, **11**, 109–127, 1968a.

Wright, H. N., The effect of sensori-neural hearing loss on threshold-duration functions. *J. Speech Hear. Res.*, **11**, 842–852, 1968b.

Wright, H. N., Bekesy audiometry and temporal summation. *J. Speech Hear. Res.*, **12**, 865–874, 1969.

Yantis, P. A., Clinical applications of the temporary threshold shift. *Arch. Otolaryngol.*, **70**, 779–787, 1959.

Young, I. M., Effects of ipsilateral masking on Bekesy amplitude. *J. Aud. Res.*, **8**, 357–365, 1968.

Young, I. M., and Harbert, F., Effect of off-time on amplitude and threshold of Bekesy tracings. *J. Aud. Res.*, **8**, 339–343, 1968.

Young, I. M., and Harbert, F., Forward and backward sweep responses in Bekesy audiometry. *Ann. Otol. Rhinol. Laryngol.*, **80**, 612–617, 1971.

Zwislocki, J., Theory of temporal auditory summation. *J. Acoust. Soc. Am.*, **32**, 1046–1060, 1960.

chapter 19

BRIEF TONE AUDIOMETRY

H. N. Wright, Ph.D.

Brief tone audiometry (BTA) is an emerging procedure that may be considered the complement of the more traditional Bekesy audiometry. That is to say, where Bekesy audiometry compares the threshold for pulsed tones at a fixed duration to that obtained for a continuous tone, BTA examines the relative threshold differences among pulsed tones which vary in their duration. As we shall see, comparison of the relative threshold differences among the short tones used in BTA may be utilized to establish a differential among various types of auditory disorders; it is not a procedure which is oriented toward the identification of a single dysfunction of the auditory system. Further, BTA both augments and supplements the findings of Bekesy audiometry and can be incorporated with it to achieve a diagnostic potency which neither alone provides.

CLINICAL PROTOCOL

When the duration of a tone is progressively decreased below 1 sec, the intensity required to maintain its audibility must be continuously increased. Zwislocki (1960, 1969) indicates that this phenomenon is due to the psychophysiologic process of temporal summation. This is in contrast to viewing the auditory system simply as an energy integrator (e.g., Garner and Miller, 1947; Plomp and Bowman, 1959). In substance, the theory of temporal auditory summation, which will not be dealt with in detail here, offers the audiologist a physiologic base for his psychophysical inferences. In any event, the scientific foundation for this theory is substantial (e.g., Irwin and Kemp, 1976).

A number of classical procedures, such as the methods of adjustment, limits, and constant stimuli have been used to establish the functional relation between the threshold and duration for tones. Most of these procedures have been those psychophysical methods of laboratory origin which, by their very nature, do not readily lend themselves to clinical application. One laboratory procedure, however, that does lend itself to clinical application is the tracking method (Stevens, 1958) as provided by a Bekesy

The work reported in this chapter was supported, for the most part, by Grant NS09663 from the National Institute of Neurological Diseases and Stroke of the United States Public Health Services.

audiometer (Bekesy, 1960) functioning in its fixed-frequency mode. This method is consistent with the current conventional wisdom of clinical practice (Jerger, 1960) and is not limited to adult populations (Price and Falck, 1963). Thus, the Bekesy technique is both practical and preferred for BTA. Specifically, if a patient can track his threshold with a Bekesy audiometer where frequency is changing constantly, he certainly should also be able to track his threshold at one frequency for tones which vary only in their duration. Such indeed has been found to be true (Wright, 1968a) and is a relatively easy task for the patient. From the clinician's point of view, however, it is deceptively simple in that a number of criteria must be met to adequately administer BTA.

Criteria

While the tracking method utilizing the conventional Bekesy audiometer is the clinical psychophysical method of choice for BTA, a number of other factors concerned with the manner of tone presentation need careful consideration. Specifically, the parameters of rise-fall time, duration and repetition rate need to be precisely defined for both practical and theoretical reasons. In addition, the parameters of attenuation rate and sampling time need to be considered.

Rise-Fall Time. When tones are turned on and off abruptly, sidebands in the form of transient energy are created. These sidebands can cause as much as a 30-dB error in threshold (Wright, 1967a) as well as cause specious results from BTA for some hearing-impaired patients (Wright, 1967b). No tone is entirely free from the acoustic artifacts associated with switching; their magnitude and extent, however, can be reduced by incorporating a suitable rise-fall time as defined by the time between 10% and 90% of the maximum amplitude of the acoustic waveforms.

In an investigation of the audibility of the acoustic artifacts, 5 normal-hearing listeners tracked their detection of the clicks and thuds associated with 500-msec tones from 125 to 8000 Hz presented once per second and with rise-fall times which varied from virtually instantaneous to 5 msec. Threshold was also obtained for these same tones with rise-fall times of 50 msec. The median results shown in Figure 19.1 for rise-fall times of 1, 3 and 5 msec and for threshold indicate a progressive increase in intensity is required to detect the acoustic artifacts as rise-fall time is increased. The limiting condition for practical purposes is a rise-fall time of 5 msec where, for the most part, the intensity must exceed 100 dB sound pressure level (SPL) before the acoustic artifacts are heard. Similar results were obtained on a hearing-impaired patient as shown in Figure 19.2. These findings indicate that rise-fall times less than 5 msec should not be used in determining thresholds for hearing-impaired listeners. In the present series, the sidebands associated with 10 msec rise-fall time were never heard because the lower limit of intolerance for loud sounds was reached first. The basic conclusion from these studies is that a rise-fall time of 10 msec is more than sufficient to avoid contamination of threshold results by switching artifacts.

Duration. The specification of the duration of the short tones used in BTA is not entirely separate from rise-fall time. Harris (1957) reached the conclusion that duration should be specified somewhere between maximum and mid amplitude of the acoustic wave form. One definition consistent with this conclusion is in terms of effective sound pressure at 0.707 of maximum amplitude. This is achieved technically by adjusting the voltage of the applied tone so that it occupies 1.4 divisions on an oscilloscope graticule and then measure duration where the rise-fall ramps cross at a height of one division.

When rise-fall times are specified between

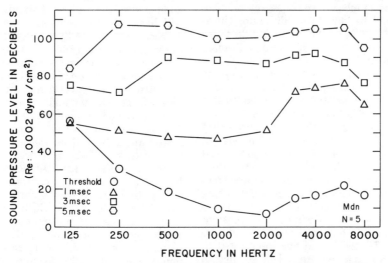

FIG. 19.1. Median sound pressure level (SPL) for 5 normal hearing listeners to detect acoustic transients as a function of frequency. Parameter is rise fall times of 1, 3 and 5 msec.

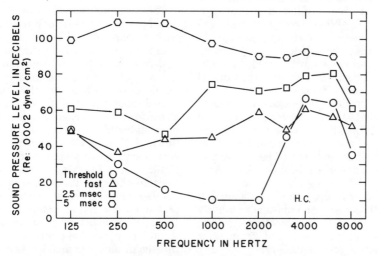

FIG. 19.2. Sound pressure level (SPL) for a hearing impaired listener to detect acoustic transients as a function of frequency. Parameter is rise fall times of virtually instantaneous (fast), 2.5 msec and 5 msec.

10% and 90% of maximum amplitude and duration is in terms of effective sound pressure, the duration of a tone with a 10-msec rise-fall time is essentially the same as that determined by calculating a theoretical equivalent duration (Dallos and Olsen, 1964). That is to say, theory and practice in this instance agree with one another.

A second consideration with respect to duration is to select one which will adequately represent the response of the patient as well as enable the clinician to differentiate among patients. The nature of the complete temporal summation function is such that successive tones should be logarithmically (or geometrically) spaced. Further, in the interest of clinical efficiency the number of tones at any one frequency should be kept to a minimum. Durations that have been found to fulfill these criteria are 500, 200, 100, 50, 20, and 10 msec (Wright, 1968a).

Repetition Rate. The repetition rate at which successive pulsed tones are presented is determined by the longest duration tested and the desired off-time between the end of one tone and the onset of the next. Evidence exists that this critical off-time in the analysis of auditory disorders is 200 msec (Jerger and Jerger, 1966). More exactly, when the silent interval between successive tones is less than 200 msec, the responses of patients presenting with nerve VIII dysfunction are like those to continuous tones. Such findings are consistent with the theory of temporal auditory summation (Zwislocki, 1960), and are interpreted to mean that when a tone is turned off, the neural response of the auditory system does not end abruptly. Instead, the response systematically decays over time. The theory asserts that this rate of decay is exponential with a time constant of 200 msec. When these empirical and theoretical considerations are applied to BTA, they dictate that the silent interval among successive pulsed tones must exceed 200 msec. Neural independence is virtually guaranteed when the off-time is 500 msec.

With an off-time of 500 msec and the longest test tone also of 500 msec, the repetition rate of 1/sec is established. By maintaining this same repetition rate for the all-duration tones, the sampling/unit time and, therefore, the expectations of the listener are held constant. As a consequence, the tracking width for an individual patient should also remain constant. If tracking width is used as an index of reliability for a given patient, then a constant tracking width among all durations and frequencies tested implies the same reliability.

Attenuation Rate. The attenuation rate for Bekesy audiometry (Jerger, 1960) that has found wide use and is generally accepted in the analysis of auditory disorders is 2.5 dB/sec. In BTA, this attenuation rate is maintained so that if the clinician wants to make comparisons among tests, his results will not be compounded by yet another procedural variable.

Sampling Time. In fixed-frequency Bekesy audiometry (Jerger, 1960) the pattern of results among normal and hearing-impaired listeners is reasonably well established during 1 min of test time. In BTA, a 1-min sampling time for each duration tone is also sufficient to establish the threshold for that tone.

Instructions

The instructions for BTA are essentially no different from those for conventional Bekesy audiometry. The patient is simply told that he will hear some tones going "beep-beep-beep." *As soon as* he hears them, he is to push down the response button (demonstrate); *as soon as* they go away, he is to release the response button (demonstrate). In addition, the patient is instructed that every once in a while the tone will get shorter and shorter, but he is to continue to do the same thing; push the button down as soon as he hears the tones (demonstrate) and release it as soon as they go away (demonstrate). These instructions have been found to be effective in the administration of BTA. Occasionally, patients will respond to each pulsed tone as they sometimes do in routine Bekesy audiometry. Such a response pattern on the part of the patient is readily obviated by a clarification of the task to the patient in that he is not to respond to each tone alone, but to the sequence of successive tones.

Interpretation of Results

The interpretation of the BTA results is based on the threshold differences obtained with varying durations at a particular frequency. The threshold for the tones themselves is defined as a visually integrated average of the midpoint of the trackings over the 1-min period during which the thresholds were obtained. Such tracings at 4000 Hz are shown in Figure 19.3 for a normal hearing listener and a hearing-impaired listener with cochlear dysfunction. The first two or three reversals are customarily ignored because they represent an initial search behavior on the part of the patient in the transition from one duration to another and, therefore, should not be interpreted as a reliable index of his threshold. Dean (1974) noted that an actual average of the midpoints and the visual estimates of the threshold, as recommended here, are in good agreement with one another. In addition, pedantic averaging would negate the clinical practicality of BTA.

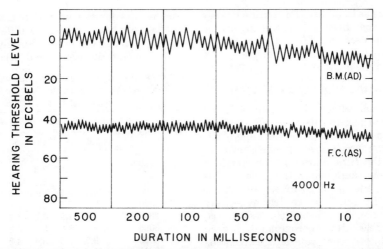

FIG. 19.3. Brief tone audiometry (BTA) results at 4000 Hz for a normal hearing listener (*upper trackings*) and a hearing-impaired listener with cochlear dysfunction (*lower trackings*).

Since the interpretation of results from BTA is based upon relative threshold differences, the threshold for a particular tone at one duration must be selected as the reference threshold against which the other thresholds are compared. In laboratory experiments it has been customary to select the longest duration tested as the reference (e.g., Zwislocki, 1969). For clinical purposes, however, it may be more convenient to select the threshold for a short-duration tone as the reference (Wright, 1968a, 1968b). In either case, the selection of the reference duration is somewhat arbitrary and a matter of convenience. More exactly, when the BTA function is truncated, as is found in cochlear lesions, a short-duration reference facilitates interpretation; whereas, when the function is expanded as is sometimes found in temporal lobe lesions and for the pseudohypoacousic, a long-duration tone reference facilitates interpretation. In any event, the reference duration found to expedite interpretation of the results is either 500 or 20 msec. The theoretical difference between the thresholds for these two tones (Zwislocki, 1960) is approximately 10 dB (9.8 dB, to be exact), a convenient number to use as a base to establish guidelines for the interpretation of clinical findings.

Relation to Bekesy Audiometry

In conventional Bekesy audiometry (Jerger, 1960), the threshold for pulsed tones is compared to the threshold for continuous tones. The pulsed tones used to establish the obtained typings were about 200 msec in duration with rise-fall times of 25 msec, presented at a duty cycle of 50%. In BTA, the longest tone is 500 msec in duration with a rise-fall time of 10 msec and is presented once per second. The thresholds for these two types of pulsed tones among normal hearing listeners are essentially no different from one another (Wright, 1969). Since the sampling/unit time is greater for conventional Bekesy audiometry than for BTA, we might expect that the tracking width would be less; such is indeed the case, but of no practical significance. Specifically, the tracking width for the 500-msec tones used in BTA is 1 dB greater than the width obtained for the 200-msec tones used in Bekesy audiometry. The consequence of these findings, for both thresholds and tracking width, is that the 500-msec tones of BTA are compatible with the pulsed tones of Bekesy audiometry. It should be cautioned, however, that when these thresholds are compared to those for a continuous tone, significant differences are likely to emerge (Wright, 1969).

Summary

The threshold for 500-, 200-, 100-, 50-, 20-and 10-msec tones at a single frequency is tracked at an attenuation rate of 2.5 dB/sec over successive 1-min intervals. All tones are presented at a repetition rate of 1/sec with a rise-fall time of 10 msec as defined between 10% and 90% of maximum amplitude. The durations are specifically defined in terms of the effective sound pressure at the half-power points.

The individual tracking results in BTA are analyzed by visually estimating the threshold for each duration tone from the midpoints of the tracings. The thresholds thus obtained are then referred to those obtained for either the 500- or 20-msec tones to derive relatively complete descriptions of how threshold varies with duration.

The instructions to the listener are essentially the same as those used for routine Bekesy audiometry. The thresholds obtained for the 500-msec tones used in BTA and those for the pulsed tones used in Bekesy audiometry are comparable to one another.

THE NORMAL HEARING LISTENER

Normative values for BTA were obtained from 50 normal hearing listeners with an age range of 17 to 31 years and a mean age of 21. The audiogram for this sample is shown in Figure 19.4; the *bars* represent one standard deviation above and below the mean. This sample was made up of 25 males and 25 females; 25 right ears and 25 left ears were examined at 125, 250, 500, 1000, 2000, 3000, 4000, 6000 and 8000 Hz. Approximately 1 week later, all subjects were retested. Thresholds were obtained for 500- and 20-msec tones alone and compared to the same conditions obtained during the initial determination of the complete function.

Test Condition

The results for the initial administration of BTA are shown in Figure 19.5; the reference duration is 20 msec and the specific values are shown in Table 19.1. The *solid line* represents the theoretical values shown in Table 19.1 at each duration and were derived from the theory of temporal auditory summation (Zwislocki, 1960). The agreement with psychophysiologic expectations is such that we may assume the theoretical values adequately represent the

true results for the normal hearing listener. Further analysis showed no differences with respect to either ear or sex. Finally, the variability among durations and frequencies as

TABLE 19.1. *Brief Tone Audiometry Means and Standard Deviations in Decibels for 50 Normal Hearing Listeners**

Frequency in Hz	Duration in Milliseconds					
	500	200	100	50	20†	10
	MEANS					
125	9.4	8.6	7.3	4.2	0	−3.2
250	9.1	7.9	6.3	3.9	0	−3.6
500	10.1	8.7	6.6	4.0	0	−3.4
1000	9.6	8.1	6.3	3.8	0	−3.2
2000	9.6	7.9	6.0	3.2	0	−3.1
3000	9.7	8.2	5.9	3.3	0	−2.7
4000	9.7	7.5	5.4	3.5	0	−2.9
6000	10.3	8.2	5.7	3.1	0	−2.5
8000	8.9	7.0	5.4	3.1	0	−2.8
Theoretical	9.8	8.2	6.2	3.7		−2.9
	STANDARD DEVIATIONS					
125	3.2	2.9	2.7	2.1		2.3
250	2.2	1.8	1.8	1.4		1.6
500	2.2	2.1	1.5	1.5		1.6
1000	2.4	1.8	1.6	1.5		1.5
2000	2.7	2.0	1.7	1.3		1.5
3000	2.7	2.1	1.5	1.3		1.5
4000	2.8	2.0	1.8	1.4		1.6
6000	2.7	2.5	2.5	2.0		1.4
8000	2.4	2.3	1.8	1.4		1.4

* Comprised of 25 males and 25 females; 25 right ears, 25 left ears.
† Reference duration.

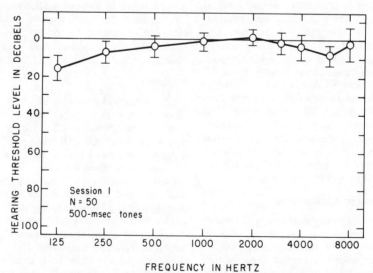

FIG. 19.4. Mean audiogram for a sample of 50 normal hearing listeners to establish normative values for brief tone audiometry (BTA). Sample composed of 25 males and 25 females; 25 right ears, 25 left ears. *Vertical bars* represent one standard deviation above and below the mean.

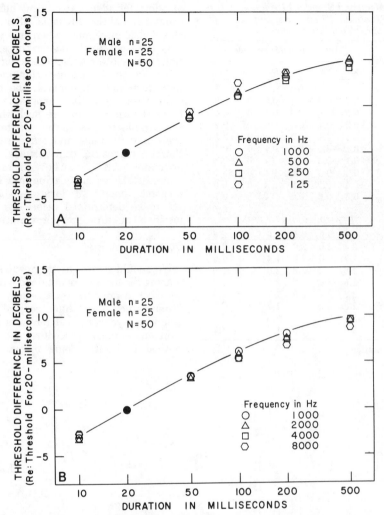

FIG. 19.5. Mean brief tone audiometry (BTA) results, referred to the thresholds for 20-msec tones, at (A) 125, 250, 500, and 1000 Hz; (B) 1000, 2000, 4000, and 8000 Hz. *Solid line* represents the theoretical normal function.

shown by the standard deviations demonstrates that BTA is an extremely stable procedure.

Retest Comparison

Where the normative values show that BTA is extremely stable among listeners, the clinical question remains on how does an individual listener compare to himself when he is retested? To this end, the results for each listener at a particular frequency and duration for the normative condition and the retest session were subtracted from one another in such a way that a higher value on the retest session would be positive, and a lower value, negative. The results from such individual comparisons are shown in Table 19.2. Here we see that the mean differences for all frequencies and durations are always less than 1 dB; the standard

deviations for a comparison of a listener with himself are comparable to those obtained when these same listeners are compared to one another as shown in Table 19.1. It, therefore, is apparent that BTA is not only a stable procedure among listeners, but also for the individual listener as well.

Two-Duration Comparison

During the initial testing, thresholds were obtained first for 500-msec tones, followed immediately by 20-msec tones. It was reasoned that if hearing-impaired listeners respond to BTA in a systematic and relatively continuous way among all six durations, their complete function could be estimated for only two durations; this would shorten the test time for BTA from 6 min to only 2 min, a substantial saving

TABLE 19.2. *Mean and Standard Deviation Values in Decibels of Individual Test-Retest Differences for Brief Tone Audiometry*

Frequency in Hz	Duration in Milliseconds					
	500	200	100	50	20†	10
	MEANS					
125	0.7	0.8	−0.1	−0.8	0	0.8
250	0.5	0.4	0.3	0.1	0	0.4
500	−0.2	−0.1	0.1	0.0	0	−0.2
1000	0.1	0.1	−0.3	0.1	0	−0.1
2000	−0.1	−0.1	−0.3	0.1	0	−0.1
3000	0.1	−0.3	−0.3	−0.1	0	−0.3
4000	0.3	0.5	0.5	0.0	0	0.1
6000	−0.4	−0.2	0.2	0.4	0	−0.5
8000	0.6	0.6	0.2	−0.2	0	−0.1
	STANDARD DEVIATIONS					
125	3.6	3.5	3.5	2.6		2.8
250	2.4	2.0	2.0	1.4		2.0
500	1.7	2.0	2.0	1.4		2.0
1000	2.8	2.6	2.0	2.0		2.0
2000	2.6	2.6	2.0	2.0		2.0
3000	2.2	2.0	2.0	1.7		1.4
4000	2.8	2.2	1.7	1.7		2.0
6000	3.2	3.0	2.8	2.8		2.0
8000	3.0	2.6	2.0	1.4		1.7

† Reference duration.

of effort for identical clinical information. A comparison of the threshold difference between 500- and 20-msec tones when only these thresholds were obtained and for these same durations when the complete function was determined for the 50 listeners combined, is shown in Figure 19.6. In general, the two-duration comparisons and the histograms for each of these determinations are such that they are comparable to one another in terms of both their mean values and standard deviations, thereby suggesting that perhaps two-duration estimates for BTA may be sufficient for clinical purposes. How the hearing-impaired listener responds among all durations, however, has yet to be determined before we are able to justify a two-duration approximation.

Comment

We should note that the results for normal hearing listeners were obtained with the tracking method provided by a Bekesy audiometer. Other values might have been obtained with different psychophysical methods such as the common clinical procedure of a modified method of limits. Some investigators (e.g.,

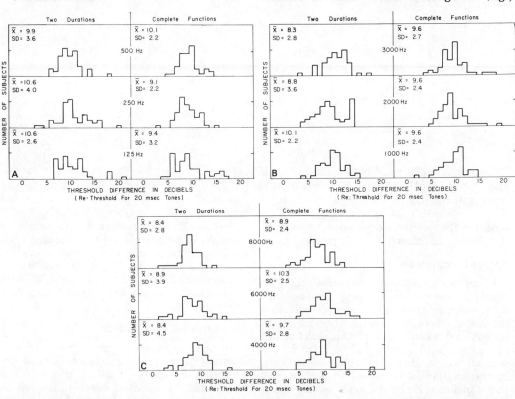

FIG. 19.6. Means, standard deviations, and histograms for the threshold differences between 500- and 20-msec tones when measured directly (two durations) and when extracted from complete functions (six durations) at: (A) 125, 250, 500 Hz; (B) 1000, 2000, 3000 Hz; (C) 4000, 6000, 8000 Hz.

Watson and Gengel, 1969) purport that the threshold difference between long and short tones decreases with an increase in frequency; referred to as a frequency effect. It may be that with the basic adaptive psychophysical procedure of tracking (Levitt, 1971), the listener maintains a constant criterion for "hearing" among all durations and frequencies; whereas in some nonadaptive methods, such as the method of adjustment used by these investigators, the listeners' criterion may vary among durations and frequencies in such a way as to create misleading results. Aside from these methodologic considerations, the frequency effect observed by some may be related to the "normal" listeners investigated. That is to say, BTA is extremely sensitive to cochlear lesions and such lesions commonly manifest themselves in the higher frequencies. Subclinical lesions, not of handicapping significance, therefore, could be the cause for the frequency effect observed by some investigators and not by others.

HEARING-IMPAIRED LISTENERS

Various types of auditory pathology affect the results from BTA in different ways. Each category of hearing impairment will be considered separately, even though it is recognized that they may coexist with one another in any combination within the same patient.

Cochlear Dysfunction

One of the most common impairments seen is the patient with a cochlear hearing loss usually associated with prolonged noise exposure (PTS). A sample of 10 such listeners were tested at octave intervals from 125 through 8000 Hz (Wright, 1968b). The BTA results were then categorized by the threshold difference

between the 500- and 20-msec tones. The results from this analysis are shown in Figure 19.7. Here we see that presumptive cochlear dysfunction will cause a decrease in the difference between the long and short tones. Moreover, this decrease is systematic so that, if the threshold difference between 500- and 20-msec tones is known, the intermediate values for other durations can be estimated. When the relative threshold differences were compared to the amount of hearing loss present, there was a loose correlation on a statistical basis; for the individual listener, however, such a prediction was found to be far too weak for clinical purposes. With a threshold difference between 500- and 20-msec tones of 4 dB, for example, the actual hearing levels varied from 25 to more than 85 dB.

Findings similar to Wright's (1968b) have been obtained in a group of chinchillas with PTS (Hans, Henderson, and Hammernik, 1975). Threshold differences between 500- and 20-msec tones with behavioral audiometry were obtained on the animals both pre-and post-exposure. The threshold differences for the pre-exposure condition were comparable to those found for normal-hearing listeners. Postexposure results, however, showed decreased relative differences between the thresholds for the 500- and 20-msec tones, irrespective of the amount of induced PTS. A clinically significant implication from this investigation was derived from the histopathology on those same animals. Specifically, while the amount of PTS was strongly correlated with a depletion of the inner hair cell population, the brief tone results seemed related to a depletion of the outer hair cell population along the basilar membrane. Such results strongly suggest that cochlear dysfunction will be revealed by BTA in the

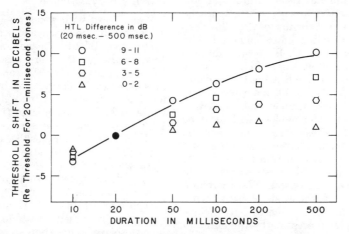

FIG. 19.7. Mean brief tone audiometry (BTA) results from a sample of hearing-impaired listeners presenting with cochlear dysfunction. Parameter is the threshold difference between 500- and 20-msec tones. *Solid line* represents the theoretical normal function.

absence of a hearing loss, thereby explaining away the frequency effect sometimes observed for normal hearing listeners when "normal" is simply defined in terms of hearing levels alone. Similarly, when depressed BTA results are obtained and the hearing levels are within normal limits, the implication is that cochlear dysfunction is present, albeit at a subclinical level. It might be tempting to conclude that loss of outer hair cells will cause depressed BTA results. Such reasoning is just as spurious as concluding that since BTA results are depressed in cochlear dysfunction, the locus for temporal summation is in the cochlea. The present state of scientific knowledge permits us only to conclude that it appears that integrity of the outer hair cells is a necessary condition to obtain normal BTA results.

Patients diagnosed as having Meniere's syndrome have results which are not as clear-cut as those found for listeners whose hearing loss was due, for the most part, to prolonged noise exposure (Olsen, Rose and Noffsinger, 1974). Nevertheless, the relative threshold difference among different-duration tones may serve as an index of cochlear dysfunction. Of course, there are many intervening physiologic processes that need to be accounted for before we can more adequately understand the pathophysiology of cochlear dysfunction. The empirical findings of BTA on patients presenting with cochlear dysfunction are evident and such interpretations can be made with clinical confidence.

Conductive Hearing Loss

The process of temporal auditory summation is neural in nature. Therefore, we should not expect conductive impairments to affect BTA results. This was indeed found to be true (Wright and Cannella, 1969). A group of normal hearing listeners was given a temporarily induced conductive hearing loss by the deep insertion of a Vaseline gauze plug into the external auditory meatus. BTA was administered before and after as well as in the presence of the induced conductive hearing loss of about 40 dB. The BTA results did not vary among the three conditions, thereby substantiating that a conductive hearing loss will have no effect upon BTA. These results were verified in a young patient who presented with a mild conductive hearing loss where the BTA results did not change pre- and post-treatment with the appropriate decongestants. We, therefore, can be confident on the basis of both theory and practice that BTA reflects only neural events in temporal processing by the auditory system.

Mixed Hearing Loss

With the foregoing in mind, it almost seems trivial to consider the compound case of a conductive hearing loss superimposed on a cochlear component. We shall see, however, that, on an individual patient basis, this hearing-loss category deserves attention.

First of all, in an experiment completely analogous to that performed on normal hearing listeners (Wright and Cannella, 1969), a conductive loss was induced over an existing cochlear impairment. When BTA was normal, it remained normal; when the results were consistent with cochlear dysfunction, they remained so. We may then conclude that a conductive overlay on a previously existing cochlear impairment has no effect on BTA; or that deviant BTA results, in the presence of a conductive overlay, reflect the cochlear dysfunction alone.

If we now examine patient material, the implication of this finding will become more apparent. Specifically, consider the audiogram of the patient shown in Figure 19.8 and his BTA results shown in Figure 19.9. This was a patient with a history of noise exposure who presented with the signs and symptoms of clinical otosclerosis, subsequently surgically confirmed. The clinical question is whether the depressed bone conduction results shown in Figure 19.8 reflect true cochlear reserve after the statistical correction for the mechanical depression caused by the Carhart notch. The BTA results shown in Figure 19.9 imply cochlear dysfunction at both 1000 and 4000 Hz prior to the surgical intervention. More exactly, the BTA results for this patient revealed more extensive cochlear involvement than implied by the bone conduction results, thereby lowering treatment expectations. In other words, BTA provided some additional information for this patient which was not otherwise available.

Nerve VIII Dysfunction

When faced with a neural (nerve VIII) involvement in the absence of sensory (cochlear) dysfunction, BTA has been found to distinguish between the two (Sanders, Josey and Kemker, 1971). Sanders et al. (1971) confirmed the findings expected for normal hearing listeners and for those presenting with cochlear dysfunction while extending the diagnostic application of BTA to the patient presenting with a nerve VIII disorder. Their results for these three groups of patients are shown in Figure 19.10. Here we see that nerve VIII involvement is clearly distinguished from cochlear dysfunction, but not from the normal hearing listener. The patient with nerve VIII involvement, however, usually presents with decreased hearing levels, so we know that we are not dealing with normal hearing. On the basis of other procedures, such as tympanometry, we would also be aware of a conductive involvement which would give us the same results. It is,

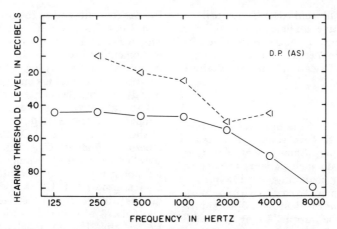

FIG. 19.8. Audiogram of a patient presenting with the signs and symptoms of clinical otosclerosis superimposed upon a history of prolonged noise exposure. *Solid line* represents the results by air conduction; *dashed line*, the results by bone conduction.

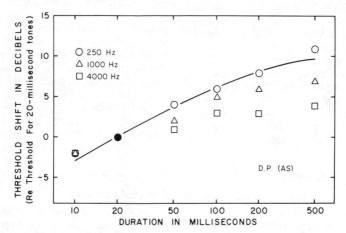

FIG. 19.9. Brief tone audiometry (BTA) results at 250, 1000, and 4000 Hz for the mixed hearing loss shown in Figure 19.8.

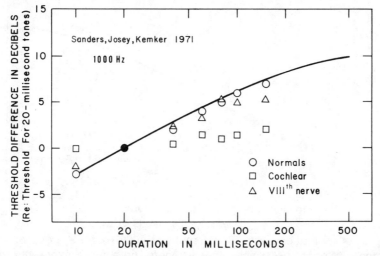

FIG. 19.10. Brief tone audiometry (BTA) results for a group of normal hearing listeners and those presenting with cochlear and nerve VIII dysfunction.

therefore, apparent that BTA alone will not provide a definitive audiologic indication of neural involvement. In the presence of hearing loss and in the absence of a conductive component, however, BTA can indicate retrocochlear dysfunction.

Presbycusis

It is recognized that the presbycusic patient often presents with both sensory and neural signs (Pestalozza and Shore, 1955). The question here is how do such patients respond on BTA and can they be distinguished from those with a history of noise exposure with its consequent presumptive cochlear signs? This question is important because BTA may be capable of sorting out hearing impairment due to presbycusis from a hearing loss due to prolonged noise exposure that would merit compensation. Thus BTA was administered to a group of listeners 51 to 57 years of age, both with and without a previous history of noise exposure (Corso, Wright and Valerio, 1976) and the results compared to those obtained for a group of young noise-exposed listeners (Wright, 1973). These comparisons at 4000 Hz are shown in Figure 19.11. Unfortunately, BTA did not distinguish among the groups. BTA cannot be expected to reveal whether a hearing loss due to aging (at least in the 50-year range) is compounded by one due to excessive noise exposure.

Temporal Lobe Dysfunction

It has been shown in lesions of the temporal lobe, in particular Heschl's gyrus, that the detection of short-duration tones is affected in the ear contralateral to the side of the dysfunction (Gersuni, 1971; Baru and Karaseva, 1972). This was found to be the case with behavioral audiometry in experimentally induced lesions in animals as well as for patient material. In contrast to the findings on patients with cochlear dysfunction, where temporal processing of long-duration tones is affected, the effect of a temporal lobe lesion is to affect the processing of short-duration tones. On the basis of these laboratory findings BTA was administered to some patients with presumptive lesions of the left temporal lobe to determine whether the clinical protocol of BTA would permit this additional differential. Illustrative results from one patient are shown in Figure 19.12. Here we see that the threshold for short-duration tones in the ear contralateral to the side of the lesion was affected, while the threshold for these same tones ipsilateral to the lesion was not. Additional investigations on other patients, and at other frequencies on the same patient, revealed that this effect may occur at some frequencies and not at others within the same patient as well as among patients. Of theoretical importance is that such findings imply tonotopic organization of the auditory cortex in man. Of clinical significance is that when this effect is found there is presumptive evidence of a temporal lobe lesion, probably in Heschl's gyrus. When this effect is not found, it is not possible to rule out other lesions affecting the auditory cortex, at least with BTA (Dean, 1974).

Pseudohypacusic

The last category of patients, not infrequently seen, is the pseudohypacusic. The me-

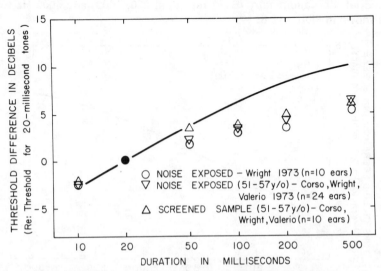

FIG. 19.11. Brief tone audiometry (BTA) results at 4000 Hz for a group of young noise-exposed listeners (Wright, 1973) and older listeners, both noise exposed and non-noise exposed (screened sample).

dian sweep-frequency Bekesy audiogram from 5 such patients is shown in Figure 19.13. Here we see better thresholds for continuous tones (Type V tracings) for the lower frequencies; at 2000 Hz and above the Type V pattern is not seen, probably because of true cochlear involvement (Dean et al. 1976). The BTA results at 250, 1000 and 4000 Hz for this same group of patients are shown in Figure 19.14. Now we see that this group behaves like the patient with a temporal lobe lesion, except that the result is ipsilateral and a "hearing loss" is present. It is also apparent that a cochlear involvement (at 4000 Hz) will interact with the pseudohypacusis to negate the differential of pseudohypacusis and could lead the unsuspecting to the differential of conductive or nerve VIII involvement. Again, it must be emphasized that BTA is only one of many procedures to assist in establishing the audiologic diagnosis. Nevertheless, our clinical experience has shown that the effect observed here for the pseudohypacusic is maximized at 1000 Hz.

Summary

If we rely on BTA results alone as defined by the relative threshold differences among different-duration tones, or more exactly by the threshold difference between 500- and 20-msec tones, and do not take into consideration any other clinical findings (which is, of course, absurd), we arrive at three categorical findings, or guidelines, to interpret our results. First, when the threshold difference is on the order of 10 dB, this is consistent with normal hearing, conductive hearing loss, or nerve VIII dysfunction. Second, when the threshold difference is 5 dB or less, the audiologic differential is cochlear involvement either with or without a conductive component. Finally, when the threshold difference is 15 dB or more, this is audiologic support for temporal lobe dysfunction or pseudohypacusis.

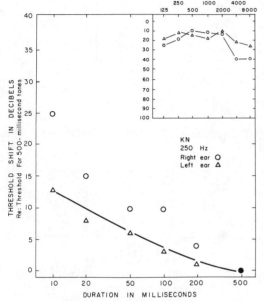

FIG. 19.12. Brief tone audiometry (BTA) results at 250 Hz for a patient presenting with a presumptive lesion in the left temporal lobe. Inset is the audiogram for this patient.

BRIEF TONE BEKESY AUDIOMETRY

Brief tone audiometry, like many other audiologic procedures, has its inherent limitations. However, there are consistent BTA results for normal and hearing-impaired listeners

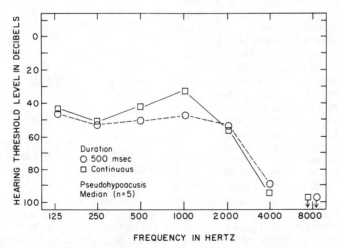

FIG. 19.13. Median sweep-frequency Bekesy audiogram for a sample of five pseudohypacusics. Parameter is the threshold for pulsed and continuous tones.

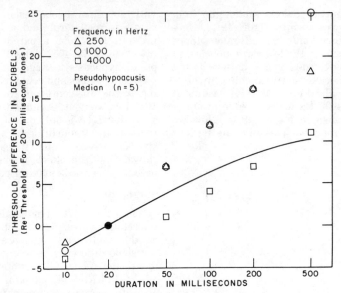

FIG. 19.14. Median brief tone audiometry (BTA) results at 250, 1000, and 4000 Hz for the pseudohypacusic listeners shown in Figure 19.13.

obtained simply by using the threshold difference between 500 and 20-msec tones (Dean, 1974). Therefore, BTA requires only 2 min of testing time per frequency. The equivocation within BTA can be alleviated to establish a more adequate audiologic differential. This is done by combining BTA and traditional Bekesy audiometry. We refer to this as brief tone Bekesy audiometry (BTBA). We compare the threshold for a 500-msec tone to that for a 20-msec tone to obtain the BTA information. If we now compare the threshold for a 500-msec tone to that for a continuous tone, we have Bekesy audiometry. By combining these two procedures into one, the equivocation of each is partially alleviated. In addition, if we take hearing level into account and rule out a conductive component with yet another procedure, such as tympanometry, it is possible to arrive at an unequivocal audiologic differential. Specifically, over three successive 1-min intervals, threshold is determined for a 500-msec tone, a 20-msec tone, and a continuous tone. The threshold patterns you might expect to find for the normal hearing listener, cochlear dysfunction, nerve VIII involvement, temporal lobe dysfunction, and pseudohypacusis are shown in Figure 19.15. Conductive impairment alone would simply be a depression of the normal hearing listener with respect to hearing level. An evaluation of these patterns and the specific procedure of BTBA has been performed and found to be reliable (Dean, 1974). Its advantage lies in its simplicity of interpretation in that we no longer need to measure exactly the differences that we obtained with BTA, but

Category	500 msec	20 msec	Continuous
Normal	-10 / 0 / +10		
Cochlear	50 / 60 / 70		
VIII Nerve	20 / 30 / 40 / 50		
Temporal Lobe	0 / 10 / 20 / 30		
Pseudo-hypoacusis	30 / 40 / 50 / 60 / 70		

FIG. 19.15. Guidelines for the interpretation of brief tone Bekesy audiometry (BTBA) results.

instead base our interpretation on patterns which readily lend themselves to evaluation. Particularly in patients with mixed dysfunctions, flexibility of clinical interpretation comes into play. With a space-occupying lesion in the internal auditory meatus, for example, we would expect to find cochlear as well as retro-cochlear signs and such has indeed been found to be true in some patients. That is to say, we would expect a 5-dB or less difference between the 500- and 20-msec tones and adaptation to the continuous tone. Further, in the pseudohy-pacusic with cochlear involvement, the thresh-old for the continuous tone will begin to approx-imate that for the 500-msec tones, while the threshold difference between 500- and 20-msec tones will remain exaggerated. If the cochlear involvement is more extensive the pseudohy-pacusic aspect will tend to disappear and the results will look like those seen in a severe conductive hearing loss. Other interactions oc-cur, but have not been systematically evalu-ated. When all the limitations and expectations of BTBA are taken into consideration it is apparent that it is a 3-min procedure that materially augments the practicing clinician's confidence in his search to arrive at the most appropriate audiologic diagnosis.

REFERENCES

Baru, A. V., and Karaseva, T. A., *The Brain and Hearing*. New York: Consultants Bureau, 1972.

Bekesy, G. v. *Experiments in Hearing*. New York: McGraw-Hill, Inc., 1960.

Corso, J. F., Wright, H. N., and Valerio, M., Audi-tory temporal summation in presbycusis and noise exposure. *J. Gerontol.*, 31, 58–63, 1976.

Dallos, P. J., and Olsen, W. O., Integration of energy at threshold with gradual rise-fall tone pips. *J. Acoust. Soc. Am.*, 36, 743–751, 1964.

Dean, L. A., Long and Short Tone Diagnostic Audi-ometry. Ph.D. Dissertation, Syracuse Univer-sity, 1974.

Dean, L. A., Wright, H. N., and Valerio, M. W., Brief-tone audiometry in pseudohypacusis. *Arch. Otolaryngol.*, 102, 621–626, 1976.

Garner, W. R., and Miller, G. A., The masked threshold of pure tones as a function of dura-tion. *J. Exp. Psychol.*, 37, 293–303, 1947.

Gersuni, G. V., *Sensory Processes at the Neuronal and Behavioral Levels*. New York: Academic Press, 1971.

Hans, J., Henderson, D., and Hamernik, R. P., The effects of impulse noise on the temporal integra-tion function of the chinchilla. *J. Acoust. Soc. Am.*, 57, 41(A), 1975.

Harris, J. D., Peak vs. total energy in thresholds for very short tones. *Acta Otolaryngol.*, 47, 134–140, 1957.

Irwin, R. J., and Kemp, S., Temporal summation and decay in hearing. *J. Acoust. Soc. Am.*, 59, 920–925, 1976.

Jerger, J. F., Bekesy audiometry in the analysis of auditory disorders. *J. Speech Hear. Res.*, 3, 275–287, 1960.

Jerger, J. F., and Jerger, S., Critical off time in VIII nerve disorders. *J. Speech Hear. Res.*, 9, 573–583, 1966.

Levitt, H., Transformed up-down methods in psy-choacoustics. *J. Acoust. Soc. Am.*, 49, 467–477, 1971.

Olsen, W. O., Rose, D. E., and Noffsinger, D., Brief-tone audiometry with normal, cochlear and eighth nerve tumor patients. *Arch. Otolar-yngol.*, 99, 185–189, 1974.

Pestalozza, G., and Shore, I., Clinical evaluation of presbycusis on the basis of different tests of auditory function. *Laryngoscope*, 65, 1136–1163, 1955.

Plomp, R., and Bowman, M. A., Relation between hearing threshold and duration for tone pulses. *J. Acoust. Soc. Am.*, 31, 749–758, 1959.

Price, L. L., and Falck, V. T., Bekesy audiometry with children. *J. Speech Hear. Res.*, 6, 129–133, 1963.

Sanders, J. W., Josey, A., and Kemker, F. J., Brief-tone audiometry in patients with VIII nerve tumor. *J. Speech Hear. Res.*, 14, 172–178, 1971.

Stevens, S. S., Problems and methods of psycho-physics. *Psychol. Bull.*, 54, 177–196, 1958.

Watson, C. S., and Gengel, R. W., Signal duration and signal frequency in relation to auditory sensitivity. *J. Acoust. Soc. Am.*, 46 (Part 2), 989–997, 1969.

Wright H. N., An artifact in the measurement of temporal summation of the threshold of audibil-ity. *J. Speech Hear. Res.*, 32, 354–359, 1967a.

Wright, H. N., The problem of measuring temporal summation in the hearing-impaired patient. *Int. Audiol.*, 6, 415–422, 1967b.

Wright, H. N., Clinical measurement of temporal auditory summation. *J. Speech Hear Res.*, 11, 109–127, 1968a.

Wright, H. N., The effect of sensori-neural hearing loss on threshold-duration functions. *J. Speech Hear. Res.*, 11, 842–852, 1968b.

Wright, H. N., Bekesy audiometry and temporal summation. *J. Speech Hear. Res.*, 12, 865–974, 1969.

Wright, H. N., and Cannella, F., Differential effect of conductive hearing loss on the threshold-duration function. *J. Speech Hear. Res.*, 12, 607–615, 1969.

Wright, H. N., Unpublished study, 1973.

Zwislocki, J. J., Theory of temporal auditory sum-mation. *J. Acoust. Soc. Am.*, 32, 1046–1060, 1960.

Zwislocki, J. J., Temporal summation of loudness; an analysis. *J. Acoust. Soc. Am.*, 46, 431–441, 1969.

ADDITIONAL READINGS

Barka, K., and Brookler, K. H., Variable on time (V.O.T). *J. Commun. Dis.*, 5, 56–58, 1972.

Barr-Hamilton, R. M., Tempest, W., and Bryan, M. E., The differential monaural test for the locus of hearing disorders. *Sound*, 5, 2–6, 1971.

Bentzen, O., Investigations on short tones with special reference to adaptation of the human ear. *Universitetsforlaget*, 1 Arrhus, 1953.

Dallos, P. J., and Johnson, K. R., Influence of rise-fall time upon short-tone threshold. *J. Acoust. Soc. Am.*, 40, 1160–1163.

Djupesland, G., and Zwislocki, J. J., Effect of tem-poral summation on the human stapedias re-flex. *Acta Otolaryngol.*, 71, 262–265, 1971.

Gamewell, A. D., The temporal integration of en-ergy in noise-fatigued ears. M. A. Thesis, Van-derbilt University School of Medicine, Nashville, Tenn., 1966.

Garner, W. R., The effect of frequency spectrum on temporal integration of energy in the ear. *J. Acoust. Soc. Am.*, 19, 808–815, 1947.

Garner, W. R., Auditory thresholds of short tones as a function of repetition rates. *J. Acoust. Soc. Am.*, 19, 600–608, 1947.

Gengel, R. W., Auditory temporal integration at relatively high masked-threshold. *J. Acoust. Soc. Am.*, 51, 1849–1851, 1972.

Gengel, R. W., and Watson, C. S., Temporal integration; I. Clinical implications of a laboratory study, II. Additional data from hearing-impaired subjects. *J. Speech Hear. Disord.*, 36, 213–224, 1971.

Harris, J. D., Haines, H. L., and Meyers, C. K., Brief-tone audiometry-temporal integration in the hypoacousic. *Arch. Otolaryngol.* 67, 699–713, 1958.

Hempstock, T. I., Bryant, M. E., and Tempest, W., A redetermination of quiet thresholds as a function of stimulus duration. *J. Sound Vib.*, 1, 365–380, 1965.

Henderson, D., Temporal summation of acoustic signals by the chinchilla. *J. Acoust. Soc. Am.*, 46, 474–475, 1969.

Jerger, J. F., Influence of stimulus duration on the pure-tone threshold during recovery from auditory fatigue. *J. Acoust. Soc. Am.*, 27, 121–124, 1955.

Jerger, J., Weikers, N. J., Sharbrough, F. W., and Jerger, S., Bilateral lesions of the temporal lobe. *Acta Otolaryngol.* Suppl. 258, 1969.

Martin, F. E., and Wofford, M., Temporal summation of brief tones in normal and cochlear-impaired ears. *J. Aud. Res.*, 10, 82–86, 1970.

Miskolczy-Fodor, F., Relation between loudness and duration of tonal pulse; I. Response of normal ears to pure tones longer than click-pitch thresholds. *J. Acoust. Soc. Am.*, 31, 1128–1134, 1959.

Miskolczy-Fodor, F., Relation between loudness and duration of tonal pulses; II. Response of normal ears to sounds with noise sensation. *J. Acoust. Soc. Am.*, 32, 482–486, 1960.

Olsen, W. O., and Carhart, R., Integration of acoustic power at threshold by normal hearers. *J. Acoust. Soc. Am.*, 40, 591–599, 1966.

Sanders, J. W., and Honig, E., Brief-tone audiometry; results in normal and impaired ears. *Arch. Otolaryngol.*, 85, 640–647, 1967.

Sheeley, E. C., and Bilger, R. C., Temporal integration as a function of frequency. *J. Acoust. Soc. Am.*, 36, 1850–1857, 1964.

Shoquist, M. L., A comparison of a test of temporal auditory summation with other tests of cochlear function in subjects with Meniere's disease. Ph.D. dissertation, University of Washington, 1971.

Wright, H. N., Switching transients and threshold determination. *J. Speech Hear. Res.*, 1, 52–60, 1958.

Wright, H. N., Temporal summation and backward masking. *J. Acoust. Soc. Am.*, 36, 927–932, 1964.

Zwicker, E., and Wright, H. N., Temporal summation for tones in narrow-band noise. *J. Acoust. Soc. Am.*, 35, 691–699, 1963.

Evaluation of Central Dysfunction

chapter 20

CLINICAL USE OF CENTRAL AUDITORY TESTS

Jack Katz, Ph.D.

In the past few years, since the first edition of the *Handbook,* there has been a dramatic increase in the use of central tests in audiology clinics. The audiologic study of the central auditory nervous system (CANS) has been along two lines. The major activity with CANS disorders has been in site of lesion testing. This approach is typically related to medical diagnosis with the primary focus being the adult patient.

The other aspect of central auditory testing is educationally oriented. It is primarily geared to the study of children to determine whether there is an auditory perception problem. When auditory skills are depressed relative to the child's age and his other abilities, auditory training can be instituted. The discussion of auditory perceptual skills in learning disabled children will be covered in Chapter 34.

The present chapter will provide an overview of the auditory evaluation of brain and brain stem disorders. It will include important concepts and various tests which offer insight into subtle dysfunctions within the central nervous system (CNS). The present status of neuroaudiology will be discussed.

CENTRAL AUDITORY REGION

Audiologists do not agree entirely on what they consider to be the *central auditory system.* This semantic problem seems to retard the clinical application of test procedures for evaluating CANS. For example, after the author worked on a test of brain function with neurologic cases for 3 years, the chairman of his department, an otologist, still thought that the focus of this and other central tests was the patient with cranial nerve VIII tumor. Most otologists limit their work to the conductive mechanism, the cochlea and possibly nerve VIII. Therefore, they might consider nerve VIII as "central."

Among audiologists there is no clear demarcation of the central system. Some audiologists consider their province to be the conductive, cochlear and retrocochlear systems. In fact, many audiologists consider the retrocochlear system to be composed solely of nerve VIII. Consequently, their interest in auditory brain and brain stem disorders has been thwarted.

The auditory system appears to be continually refining auditory information from the time a signal enters the ear canal until it is processed in the brain. Therefore, setting up very specific criteria for peripheral and central function (or narrower distinctions) are difficult to make with precision. On the other hand, to ignore distinctive trends would limit the unusual capabilities of audiology to detect and locate auditory dysfunction.

One can speculate about the proper division of the auditory system between peripheral and central portions. Depending on the orientation and specific criteria different landmarks could be arrived at. This chapter will refer to the system up to and including cranial nerve VIII as the peripheral system and the brain stem and brain as the central system. This agrees with the division used by neurologists and anatomists (Elliott, 1969) and therefore is a convenient demarcation. Thus, the nerve VIII-brain stem junction will serve as the boundary between the peripheral and central systems.

The audiologist is capable of making distinctions within the peripheral system and there is ample evidence that he can make distinctions in the central portion as well. Auditory tests can divide pathologic responses into at least four groups: conductive, cochlear, retrocochlear (nerve VIII and brain stem) and cerebral (Katz, 1970). Based on our present knowledge, the cerebellum is difficult to group. In many respects cerebellar cases appear retrocochlear

(Miller and Daly, 1967), in other ways their responses are similar to cases with cerebral dysfunction and in still other ways they are unique.

Figure 20.1, *row A,* shows nine paired anatomical subdivisions of the auditory system. The auditory mechanism is shown to begin with the outer ear and to end in the cerebrum. The auditory reception (AR) center refers to Heschl's gyrus (the middle, posterior portion of the superior temporal gyrus in each cerebral hemisphere). The nonauditory reception (NAR) portion includes the entire cerebrum excluding the AR centers. Another division which may not be familiar is the high and low brain stem. The high brain stem region refers to the upper portion of the brain stem (no doubt including at least the inferior colliculus) and the low brain stem refers to the inferior portion (most probably including the cochlear nuclei and the superior olivary complex). It is not clear how the thalamic level (medial geniculate body) relates to the areas in Figure 20.1.

Although *row A* shows nine basic subdivisions, finer distinctions may be made in both the peripheral and central systems; however, they are beyond the scope of this chapter. The right and left members are represented to help keep in mind that one or both sides can be involved. The cerebellum is shown with *dashed lines* to indicate uncertainty about its exact status.

Row B simply designates the overall classification of the auditory system. Obviously, there are portions of the CNS which do not handle direct or indirect auditory information and therefore are not included in this classification. For example, the occipital poles are not part of the auditory system. However, they are represented as part of the nonauditory reception region.

Row C shows the two-division breakdown, peripheral and central, as previously discussed (which divides at nerve VIII and low brain stem). *Row D* is a narrower breakdown. Here we see that *neural* problems (as in the term sensory-neural can include not only nerve VIII and the entire brain stem but also may include the cerebellum. The other dashed line indicates that the cerebellum is classified as part of the brain as well. *Row E* shows the simple division of the brain into cerebral and cerebellar sections.

A number of the subdivisions are particularly difficult to discriminate. This includes nerve VIII from lower brain stem pathology; upper brain stem from cerebellar lesions and a right-sided AR disorder from one in the transhemispheric tracts. It will be noted that the corpus callosum and anterior commissure have not been included in Figure 20.1 because of our limited clinical knowledge at this time.

AUDITORY FINDINGS IN CENTRAL CASES

In order to get some information about the comparative performance of various groups of patients with auditory dysfunction, 67 cases from the author's files were studied. The peripheral and central lesions in these cases were

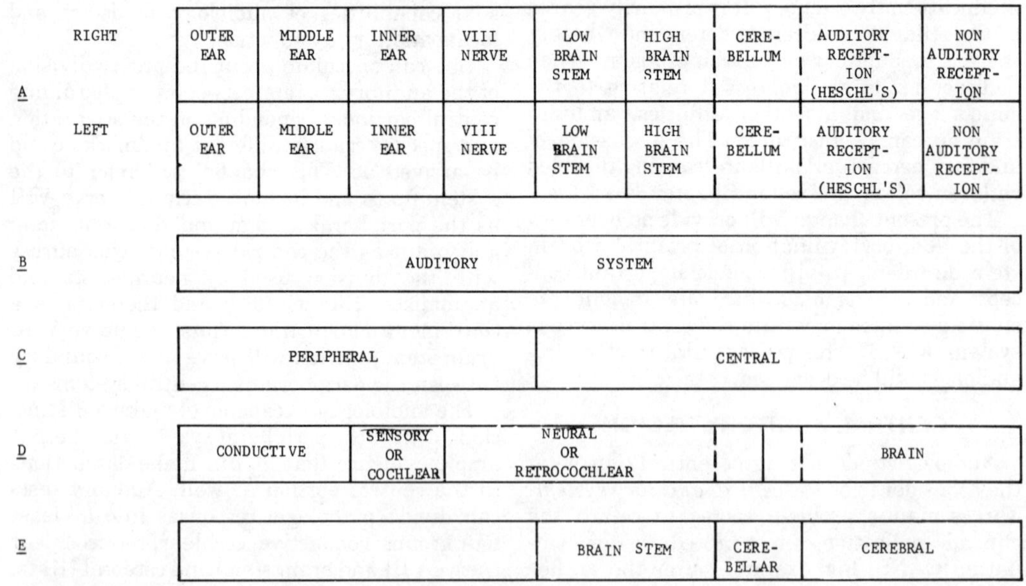

Fig. 20.1. Schematic diagram of the sections of the auditory system (*row A*) and the terms used to classify them (*rows B–E*).

well documented by medical and audiologic tests. Diagnosis of patients with brain and brain stem lesions was made by neurologists or neurosurgeons using surgical, autopsy, radiologic and other methods for locating the disorders.

There was a sample of cochlear ($N=22$), retrocochlear ($N=10$) and cerebral ($N=35$) cases. Patients with mixed cerebral and brain stem disorders were excluded from the study although some of the cerebral and retrocochlear cases had conductive or cochlear problems which were incidental to their primary disorders. The records of patients with cerebral lesions were primarily drawn from the subjects in two previous studies (Katz and Pack, 1975; Katz, Kushner and Pack, 1975). The results of this investigation will be referred to in various sections that follow.

There is no disagreement on the peripheral end that damage to the system can produce a hearing loss in the ipsilateral ear. There is not much disagreement that cerebral lesions produce little if any hearing loss but that the results of difficult speech tests show up in the contralateral ear. However, two important misconceptions have hindered the accuracy of audiologic diagnosis in central cases, especially with lesions at the level of the brain stem and cerebellum.

Hearing Loss and Side of Lesion. Comparatively little clinical emphasis has been placed on the auditory system between nerve VIII

and the cerebrum. This is unfortunate because lesions in the posterior fossa (which includes the brain stem and cerebellum) are often difficult to detect radiologically and by other medical tests. It should be emphasized that (1) *brain stem and cerebellar lesions frequently produce hearing loss and have other effects on auditory functioning* (these abnormalities can be readily noted on various audiologic procedures) and (2) *lesions to the brain stem produce primarily ipsilateral auditory dysfunction.* Because the audiologic response behavior which typifies cerebellar lesions is vague at present, discussion of such lesions will be omitted here.

The groups of cases (previously described) were studied to determine which ear was primarily affected by the auditory lesions. Figure 20.2 shows the pure tone and word discrimination (WDS) results for the 10 retrocochlear cases. These data show that there is a definite effect on the *ipsilateral* ear in retrocochlear cases for both pure tone thresholds and WDS. Since there is no quarrel about nerve VIII lesion cases having hearing loss in the ipsilateral ear, the data for the brain stem and nerve VIII cases are shown separately as well. All of the nerve VIII ($N=3$) and brain stem ($N=7$) cases were depressed in the ipsilateral ear, although there appear to be differences in the respective audiometric configurations. The results for the contralateral ear were much better than the ipsilateral ear and the contralateral thresholds can be classified as relatively nor-

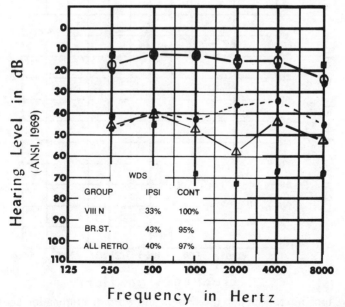

Fig. 20.2. Pure tone air-conduction thresholds and word discrimination scores (WDS) for a group of nerve VIII tumor cases (■) and brain stem lesion cases (●) as well as combined information for all retrocochlear cases for the ipsilateral (△) and contralateral ears (○).

mal. The mean difference of 30 dB between the ears ($t=13.8$) was significant at the 0.001 level of confidence. WDS was also studied. The ipsilateral ear was severely depressed for both nerve VIII and brain stem patients (40%) while the contralateral ear was essentially normal (97%).

Since there are many similarities in the test results for nerve VIII and brain stem lesion cases, the audiologist must not jump to the conclusion that there is a nerve VIII lesion simply because the disorder is of a retrocochlear nature. More properly he should seek other information which might help in differentiating a lesion which primarily involves nerve VIII from a disorder of the brain stem (or cerebellum). One clue which we have noted is a tendency toward low frequency hearing losses in the ipsilateral ear in early brain stem lesion cases. There is often some evidence of a low frequency deviation which shows up in the contralateral ear as well. The relationship between the thresholds for nerve VIII and brain stem cases can be seen in Figure 20.2. For brain stem cases threshold in the ipsilateral ear improves from 47 dB at 250 Hz to 34 dB at 4000 Hz. For nerve VIII cases threshold drops from 42 dB at 250 Hz to 73 dB at 2000 Hz.

Nerve VIII cases are more likely to have middle or high frequency losses. Caloric responses are nil in nerve VIII tumor patients but this is not usually the case in brain stem

cases. Other approaches in differentiating some retrocochlear disorders might be through the use of acoustic reflex measurement.

The confusion about brain stem and cerebellar hearing losses and the ipsilateral and contralateral effects is not the only source of conflict. Another misconception among audiologists is the notion that there is no hearing loss or simple discrimination problem with cerebral defects. Karp, Belmont and Birch (1969) have noted pure tone hearing losses among hemiplegic patients in the ear contralateral to the brain lesion. The present sample of 35 cerebral lesion cases (14 AR, 21 NAR subjects) was used to gather the same type of information on another population. Pure tone thresholds (for octave frequencies between 250 and 8000 Hz) were averaged for each ear and WDS (W-22 lists, typically in the recorded mode and presented at 40 dB sensation level (SL)) was calculated. The information was summed for the ears ipsilateral and contralateral to the involved hemisphere. Pure tone data were not available for four of the AR cases.

Figure 20.3 shows the audiometric curves for the ipsilateral and contralateral ears for the AR and the combined ear curve for the NAR subjects. The WDSs are also presented. The mean age for the AR cases was 51 years and for the NAR cases 39 years. The age difference may account in part for the poorer performance in the AR cases but other factors appear to be

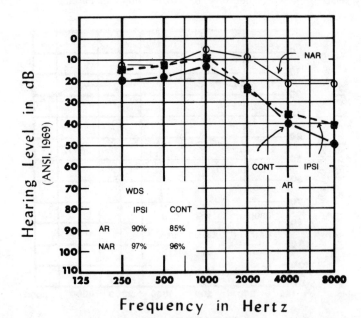

Fig. 20.3. Pure tone air-conduction thresholds and word discrimination scores (WDS) for a group of nonauditory reception (NAR) cases (○) and auditory reception (AR) cases. The ipsilateral (■) and contralateral (●) pure tone thresholds are shown separately for the AR group.

operating as well. In both groups there was a tendency toward poorer hearing in the contralateral ear.

A t-test was computed between the ipsilateral and contralateral ears for each group based on the pure tone average (6 frequencies). The difference of almost 4 dB for the AR cases was significant at the 0.01 level of confidence ($t=4.4$) but the mean difference of about 1 dB for the NAR group was not significant at the 0.05 level ($t=1.11$). Thus, there appears to be a small but consistent difference between the pure tone thresholds for AR cases favoring the ipsilateral ear. With cerebral lesions outside of Heschl's gyrus there is a slight but nonsignificant tendency toward better hearing ipsilaterally.

For the WDSs for the two cerebral groups, t-test comparisons were computed between the ears. The 5% difference for the AR group was statistically significant ($t=5.59$) at the 0.01 level, however, the 1% difference for the NAR cases was not significant. The pure tone and WDS comparisons for the cerebral cases show that there is a slight contralateral effect as a result of brain impairment when the region around Heschl's gyrus is involved. With lesions in other parts of the brain there appears to be no consistent effect on either pure tone thresholds or WDS.

This section provides information about pure tone air conduction loss and standard discrimination (W-22) problems in patients with central lesions. The ipsilateral ear is depressed for pure tone thresholds and WDSs in brain stem cases. The contralateral ear is depressed in cases with cerebral lesions involving the AR centers. The magnitude of difficulty on these so-called peripheral tests is much less in cerebral cases than in cases with brain stem lesions.

SENSITIVITY OF CENTRAL TESTS

Pure tone hearing loss is no doubt greater in sensory-neural disorders than conductive disorders. The maximum conductive loss is perhaps 60 to 65 dB (ANSI-1969) whereas the maximum sensory-neural loss exceeds the limits of the audiometer. Cochlear hearing loss especially in the high frequencies is typically more depressed than nerve VIII hearing losses. The latter can have severely depressed WDS with very little effect on pure tone thresholds. With lesions higher in the CANS (more central) hearing loss per se continues to decrease (Figs. 20.2 and 20.3).

It seems rather clear that there is a progression of pure tone threshold sensitivity from the conductive outer ear to the cerebrum, with the peak of sensitivity in the vicinity of the cochlea. The sensitivity curve of other tests may be quite different. For example, WDS is only mildly affected in conductive hearing loss cases, more so in cochlear cases, but maximally sensitive in nerve VIII or low brain stem cases. Higher brain stem lesions are less effective in reducing WDS than low stem dysfunction, even less so for AR disorders and WDS is essentially nonaffected in cases with NAR problems.

We have measured tone decay in so many ways, at different frequencies and only with certain patients that it was difficult to follow the sensitivity curve with our present data. However, nerve VIII and low brain stem lesion cases have greater amounts of tone decay than those with cochlear or high brain stem disorders. Those with cerebral lesions have less tone decay than high brain stem cases.

Figure 20.4 is a schematic representation of test performance for various lesion groups on pure tone air conduction, WDS, tone decay and staggered spondaic word (SSW) tests. Nerve VIII and low brain stem lesion categories were combined because of their audiometric similarity. The ordinate shows the sensitivity of responses. Scores falling below the normal line are supranormal or overcorrected.

The SSW test can be used to illustrate the selective sensitivity of central auditory procedures. The most sensitive pathologic regions which can be demonstrated by the corrected staggered spondaic word (C-SSW) score (moderate or severely depressed) are the AR centers and high brain stem. With low brain stem lesions there is a sharp drop in errors into the overcorrected category (significantly negative) as opposed to high brain stem and AR cases (highly positive).

The C-SSW score is an excellent discriminator between high and low brain stem lesions (Katz, 1970). Because the brain stem is so differentially sensitive, care must be taken not to combine high and low brain stem results when studying the SSW test. Otherwise there will be a wide range of scores for brain stem cases (Jerger and Jerger, 1975). Combining C-SSW scores for high and low brain stem cases is like mixing apples and elephants.

The 67 pathologic subjects, previously mentioned, were subdivided into six subgroups to compare their performance on various tests. The six subgroups are cochlear ($N=22$), nerve VIII ($N=3$), low brain stem ($N=3$), high brain stem ($N=4$), AR ($N=14$) and NAR ($N=21$) cases. The tests were pure tone air conduction (ANSI-1969), WDS and the SSW. Tone decay tests were not administered routinely at specific frequencies, using specific methods nor to all of the test subgroups. Therefore, tone decay information is not included.

Figure 20.5A shows the mean results in the ipsilateral ear on the three tests for the six

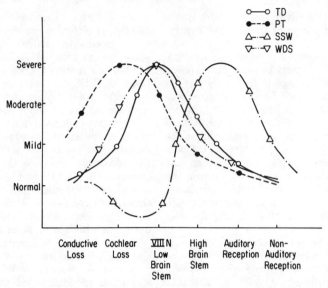

Fig. 20.4. Author's conception of the specificity of test response for various procedures when there has been dysfunction from the conductive mechanism to the nonauditory reception areas of the brain. The relative test performance is shown on the ordinate. Because of the great similarity of performance for nerve VIII and low brain stem groups they are represented together. This conception was drawn prior to the actual data compilation for the 67 subjects shown in Figures 20.5 and 20.6. The actual data differ in a number of ways from the original conception; however, each test seems maximally sensitive in certain regions. The tests are pure tone air-conduction (*PT*), word discrimination score (*WDS*), tone decay (*TD*) and the staggered spondaic word test (*SSW*).

pathologic groups. Because of the small sample size the figure should be taken as representing general tendencies rather than as specific means. (Since these data were compiled, other nerve VIII and brain stem patients have been studied without changing these interpretations in any important way.) As expected, the figure shows that the peripheral groups (cochlear and nerve VIII) have the greatest deficit for pure tone hearing. The ipsilateral ear also shows deficits in WDS peripherally and in the brain stem group. The central test (SSW) is quite variable from group to group in the ipsilateral ear, peaking at the high brain stem level and dropping sharply when the lesion is slightly more central or more peripheral. In the ipsilateral ear the cerebral lesion cases have relatively little deficit on any of the tests.

Figure 20.5*B* shows the same parameters for the contralateral ear. In this case the results are relatively flat except for the C-SSW score for the AR group. The NAR performance is indistinguishable from the cochlear and the retrocochlear results when dealing with group data. The primary method of differentiation and localization of NAR disorders is the use of response bias and not the C-SSW score (Katz and Pack, 1975).

Figure 20.6 shows the mean performance in the *more abnormal ear* (ipsilateral and contralateral) based on the data in Figures 20.5*A* and *B*. The ipsilateral ear was the more deviant in the cochlear and the three retrocochlear groups for each of the three tests. The contralateral ear was the more abnormal on the three tests for the cerebral groups (AR and NAR).

Unilateral lesions at specific levels in the auditory system are noted primarily in one ear, if at all, regardless of the type of test. This consistency may not hold up in the cerebellar cases. Just by using three clinical tests we are able to demonstrate important differences in these six pathologic groups. This should not be interpreted as advocating such a limited test battery when dealing with these serious problems. One should keep in mind that these subjects in this study are not average, typical cases. Rather they are individuals with relatively "pure" problems.

CLINICAL USE OF CENTRAL TESTS

Chapter 3 shows some clinical application of central auditory tests. Chapters 21 through 23 provide information about specific tests with clinical utility.

Some audiologists feel that central testing is

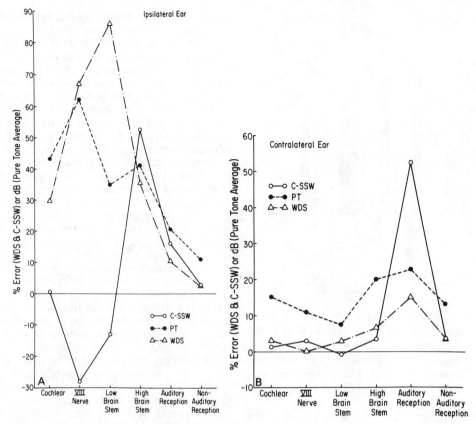

Fig. 20.5. Performance of patients with unilateral disorders from the cochlea to nonauditory reception regions of the brain on three tests: pure tone air-conduction thresholds (*PT*); word discrimination scores (*WDS*) and the corrected staggered spondaic word test scores (C-SSW). The data are shown separately for the ipsilateral ear (*A*) and for the ear contralateral to the dysfunction (*B*). The ordinate shows the pure tone thresholds in dB and the WDS and C-SSW in the percentage of error.

unimportant in their setting because there is no call to evaluate brain and brain stem patients. There are, no doubt, a number of cases with central problems seen in every audiology clinic. Brain stem lesions frequently masquerade as cochlear and nerve VIII abnormalities while brain pathology may be noted in patients with a wide variety of communication disorders. At times a brain lesion will be demonstrated which is incidental to the reason for the person's hearing evaluation. Recently, a patient was being evaluated audiometrically because of a hearing loss. Abnormal central findings bore out the presence of a brain lesion. It turned out that the patient was in the hospital for a suspected seizure disorder. Medical tests neither confirmed the audiologic results nor even the presence of seizures until the patient was readmitted to the hospital several months later. Newer radiologic techniques confirmed the presence of a large tumor which

was then successfully removed from the patient's brain.

Many clinical procedures are used for testing the integrity of the CANS. These tests tend to be less challenging than the procedures used to differentiate normal subjects in the laboratory setting. Central tests are usually monaural or dichotic procedures since they offer more information about the site of the lesion.

Lynn, Gilroy and their associates (1972a, 1972b; 1974; 1975a, 1975b) have been particularly successful in demonstrating the clinical value of CANS tests. They have demonstrated systematic performance on central auditory tests in patients with lesions in the brain and brain stem. Lynn and his associates use low-pass filtering, the SSW test, Willeford's competing sentences and rapidly alternating speech discrimination test. They find the last named test useful in locating lower brain stem lesions and the other three tests helpful in

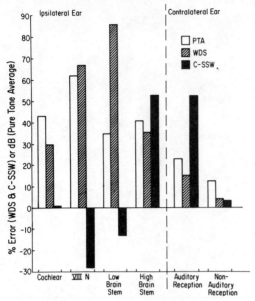

Fig. 20.6. Data derived from Figure 20.5. The poorer ear for each test is shown for each locus of lesion. For each test the poorer ear changed from the ipsilateral to contralateral between the high brain stem and the auditory reception center of the brain.

identifying superficial and deep lesions in the cerebrum.

Lynn does not use the correction for discrimination of the SSW test (Lynn, 1975b) as prescribed (Katz, Basil and Smith, 1963; Katz, 1968; Brunt, 1972), neither does he use specific norms nor response bias. While the present author considers this unfortunate, Lynn does provide the information to make the appropriate correction for WDS. The elimination of reversals and other forms of response bias is also regrettable. Lynn (1973) points out that his use of many tests makes this exploitation of just one test unnecessary. A further discussion of Lynn's work will be found in Chapters 21 to 23.

Jerger and Jerger (1975) investigated the clinical validity of central auditory tests. They found the SSW test to be the best of the procedures used in identifying cerebral lesions, and the synthetic sentence index in the ipsilateral competing mode to be the best for locating brain stem lesions. They indicated the SSW test to be quite variable in brain stem cases. However, since they combined all brain stem patients they were no doubt including both low brain stem cases (our mean C-SSW score ipsilaterally was −13) with high brain stem cases (our mean C-SSW score was +52). Obviously, the results would appear quite variable but in

reality the test is probably more specific than the experimental design permitted.

Smith and Resnick (1972) used the dichotic binaural fusion test for identification of brain stem lesions. The technique which is based on Matzker's (1959) test was successful in differentiating patients with brain stem lesions from normals, cochlear impaired, and brain pathology cases. Performance was depressed in the dichotic conditions as opposed to the diotic when there was brain stem involvement.

Many clinicians use the Rush Hughes recording of the PB-50 words as a convenient test of central auditory function (Goldstein, Goodman and King, 1956). Another approach to the problem of CANS testing is the use of accelerated speech. Quiros (1964) evaluated patients with various pathologies and noted useful diagnostic information with brain lesions.

One of the difficult diagnostic problems associated with clinical auditory tests of brain function is the interhemispheric tracts. Sparks and Geschwind (1968) point out that the nondominant ear is depressed when the corpus callosum (or possibly the anterior commissure) is involved. Lesions in the interhemispheric tracts make auditory tests appear to be positive for the right hemisphere (nondominant for speech). That is, performance is depressed in the left ear. Katz, Kushner and Pack (1975) have reported on a competing environmental sound (CES) test to aid in identifying the abnormal hemisphere and to help determine if the corpus callosum is involved.

Katz and Pack (1975) suggested another approach to the study of the interhemispheric tracts. Since the corpus callosum and anterior commissure are deep structures not involving the auditory reception center, they suggest that standard word discrimination scores should be essentially normal bilaterally as opposed to the true AR case who would have depressed WDS in the contralateral ear or bilaterally. Both right AR and interhemispheric lesions would show depressed scores in the left ear on a dichotic competing procedure like the SSW test. The data of Lynn (1975b) and Lynn and Gilroy (1976) seem to support this notion. Lynn (1975b) uses the filtered speech score as an indicator. If filtered speech scores are good this is reasonable evidence that the AR center is not impaired. This would lend support to the presence of an interhemispheric lesion. Other monaural tests such as the Rush Hughes test could be used in a like manner.

REPORTING CANS TEST RESULTS

Many audiologists have not had intensive practicum experience in central test report writing. Therefore, they may have some reticence in explaining their findings. Especially because of the potential seriousness of CNS lesions it is important that the audiologist neither overstates nor understates the results.

The results of the entire audiologic battery should be consolidated and harmonized. It would be most unfortunate to ignore the peripheral condition in central cases and vice versa. Peripheral and central designations are arbitrary and lesions to them are by no means mutually exclusive.

Since audiologic jargon may be strange to the referral source just as his jargon may be strange to the audiologist, it is vital that both understand each other (see Chapter 3). When reporting important data it is well to do this in person or over the phone and follow up by a written report to avoid misunderstandings. When a patient is referred to rule out a peripheral disorder but the results show it to be a CANS problem the physician's focus must be brought from the periphery to the CNS. For example, "Dr. Jones, I'm calling about Mrs. Brown. I know that she was referred because of possible Meniere's disease, but is there some information to suggest that the disorder might be more central? How does this relate to your findings? Our test results suggest that it might be at the brain stem or cerebellar level. If it was a cochlear problem like Meniere's we would have expected a greater loss for pure tone and less difficulty with discrimination. In addition there were other retrocochlear signs that made it look more like a brain stem or cerebellar problem on the left side. It seems to resemble more of a low brain stem problem than one involving the entire brain stem or cerebellum but neither of the latter conditions can be ruled out on the basis of our data. Is there any way to check out our results?"

Professional jargon, semantic problems, lack of time and other interferences cause breakdown in important communications. One means of increasing the accuracy of communication is the use of graphics to reinforce or summarize the written report. Figure 20.7 would be a useful diagram to be printed on an audiologic report form. Some large "Xs" and "?s" appropriately placed on the figure could summarize a complex report and give the essence to the physician instantly. By the use of four "Xs" and one "?" the audiologist can summarize—a conductive hearing loss on the right side, a cochlear hearing loss bilaterally, high brain stem involvement on the left side and possibly an auditory reception problem, also on the left side. Of course, if there are specific indications of other sites of brain lesions these should be detailed beyond the simple "X" in the nonauditory region.

SURVEY OF NEURO-AUDIOLOGY

There is considerable amount of variation in central testing from one audiology clinic to another. Many audiologists use no tests of central auditory function while others have extensive neuro-audiologic test batteries. Among the centers which concentrate on central problems there is considerable variation in the percentage of patients who are actually subjected to these tests.

In order to get a glimpse of the work going on in various centers a survey was taken of various contributors to the *Handbook*. Of the 20 audiologists who were queried, 15 responses were obtained in time to be included. In some ways they represent a very sophisticated group and in other ways they may be typical of U. S. audiologists in general. It is difficult to know if the sample is biased in favor of the SSW test because of the author's association with it.

The audiologists were asked whether they used CANS tests. Eighty percent indicated that they were using tests of central auditory function. Some had been using these tests for many years but an equal number of the respondents had just begun this testing within the past 5 years or were just ready to begin their use of central tests. The average length of time that central tests had been used (for those who were already administering CANS tests) was 6 years. They ranged from 2 to more than 10

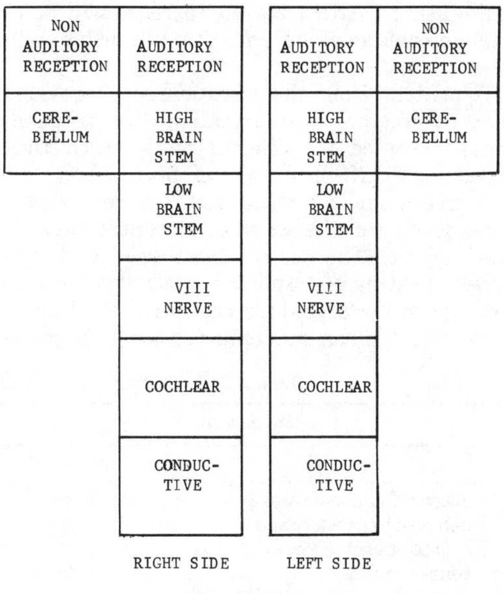

NON AUDITORY RECEPTION	AUDITORY RECEPTION		AUDITORY RECEPTION	NON AUDITORY RECEPTION
CERE-BELLUM	HIGH BRAIN STEM		HIGH BRAIN STEM	CERE-BELLUM
	LOW BRAIN STEM		LOW BRAIN STEM	
	VIII NERVE		VIII NERVE	
	COCHLEAR		COCHLEAR	
	CONDUC-TIVE		CONDUC-TIVE	

RIGHT SIDE   LEFT SIDE

AUDITORY SYSTEM

Fig. 20.7. A graphic system for summarizing the results of auditory test information. A bold "X" or "?" can be noted in the appropriate boxes.

years. Three centers were not testing for CNS disorders.

For the 15 years after Bocca, Calearo and Cassinari (1954) reported the use of a test for brain function, 6 of the 15 audiologists began their work with central tests (an average increase of 1 audiologist every 2½ years). In the next 5 years, 5 audiologists began using these tests (1 audiologist per year). Three audiologists indicated plans for central testing in the near future. This seems to reflect the interest among audiology centers in this country with perhaps even more dramatic interest in the past few years. One might speculate that the 5 audiologists who did not respond to the questionnaire were neither using CANS tests nor perhaps considering its use in the near future.

Eighty percent of the respondents who deal with adults use central tests. This is higher than we would expect to find in the general clinical practice of audiology. On the average about 7.5% of adults who are seen in these clinics are administered central tests.

Two thirds of the clinics which deal with children provide CANS testing. However, only 5% of the children who are seen in the clinics are given such tests. If the small percentage of patients given central tests is representative of audiology clinics at large it is most likely that this percentage will increase in the future. For audiologists at large one can expect the greatest change to be an increase in the percentage using central tests. For those who are successfully using CANS tests the increase will be in the percentage of patients who are tested with them.

The data from the questionnaire provided two other types of information. The respondents indicated the clinical tests which they used for CANS testing and from whom the referrals came for these tests. A rating of 5 was given for the most used central test in each clinic. The second most used test was given a rating of 4 and so on. A rating of zero was given if a procedure was not used at all at a center. A mean was obtained for each procedure and then multiplied by 20. Therefore, a rating of 100 was given if the same procedure was used as the primary one for each of the clinics. Table 20.1 shows the ratings. Thirteen different tests were used to test adults and nine different procedures were used with children.

Table 20.1 shows that the SSW test was the most commonly used procedure for evaluating either adults or children. With adults the Rush Hughes difference test was the next most used, followed by filtered speech procedures. For children filtered speech was the second most commonly used. Acoustic reflex testing was frequently used with children and adults, presumably as a measure of brain stem function.

Among centers which deal with adult populations the greatest percentage of referrals for central tests were from otologists (44%) followed by neurologists (37%). The remaining 19% were made up of referrals from speech pathologists, other physicians and various other professionals.

In the centers dealing with children the referrals were more distributed. The primary referral source was from neurologists (32%), otologists (22%), various other sources combined (15%) followed by pediatricians and schools (each with over 10%). Speech pathologists and other physicians made up the remainder of the referrals.

One healthy sign is that the audiologists receive their referrals from a wide variety of sources. The testing is carried out in many settings by a growing number of audiologists and there is a growing armamentarium of procedures to suit the evaluation of children and adults for various test situations. Elliott (1969), in the following quotation, described the growing interest of the CNS for the medical student and physician. He could just as easily have been discussing the CANS for the audiology student and audiologist.

The central nervous system is only today beginning to yield its mysteries to research, so that

TABLE 20.1. *Ratings of Central Tests Used in Audiology Clinics**

For Adults		For Children	
Test	Mean rating	Test	Mean rating
Staggered spondaic word	56	Staggered spondaic word	58
Rush Hughes difference	34	Filtered speech (Bocca)	36
Filtered speech (Bocca)	28	Acoustic reflex	28
Acoustic reflex	20	Competing message (S/N)	20
Competing message (S/N)	16	Binaural integration (Matzker)	16
Binaural integration (Matzker)	12	Synthetic sentence index	10
Synthetic sentence index	10	3 other tests	<10
Sentence integration	10		
5 other tests	7		

* If all 15 clinics had used the *same* test as their primary procedure it would have received a mean rating of 100. If each center had used the same procedure second most often it would receive a mean rating of 80. If a center did not use a test at all, a 0 was averaged into the mean rating.

almost yearly the practitioner finds new resources where his predecessors found only meaningless complexities; yet so vast are the complexities of the system that the prospects of further discoveries, some of them dramatic, seem inexhaustible. The scientifically curious student and the . . . practitioner may, therefore, approach the subject with a lively quickening of interest.

SUMMARY

In increasing numbers, audiologists are becoming involved in central auditory testing which may be referred to as neuro-audiology. Some concepts were presented to aid the audiologist in identifying central auditory problems and specifying their locations. Lesions to the brain stem show up in the ipsilateral ear and those to the brain show up in the contralateral ear when the auditory reception center is involved. Intrahemispheric localization is also within the province of the audiologist.

It is critical that audiologists communicate their findings effectively. This may be aided by graphic representation of the diagnosis. In the years following we are likely to witness a dramatic increase in the number of audiologists who are testing for auditory symptoms of brain and brain stem pathology. Similarly we can expect growth in the percentage of audiology patients who are given CANS tests.

REFERENCES

Bocca, E., Calearo, C., and Cassinari, V., A new method for testing hearing in temporal lobe tumors; preliminary report. *Acta Otolaryngol.,* **44,** 219–221, 1954.

Brunt, M. A., The Staggered Spondaic Word Test. In Katz, J. (Ed.), *Handbook of Clinical Audiology* pp. 334–356. Baltimore: Williams & Wilkins Co., 1972.

Elliott, H. C., *Textbook of Neuroanatomy,* Ed. 2. p. 357. Philadelphia: J. B. Lippincott Co., 1969.

Gilroy, J., and Lynn, G. E., Reversibility of abnormal auditory findings in cerebral hemisphere lesions. *J. Neurol. Sci.,* **21,** 117–131, 1974.

Goldstein, R., Goodman, A., and King, R., Hearing and speech in infantile hemiplegia before and after left hemispherectomy. *Neurology,* **6,** 869–875, 1956.

Jerger, J., and Jerger, S., Clinical validity of central auditory tests. *Scand. Audiol,* **4,** 147–163, 1975.

Karp, E., Belmont, I., and Birch, J., Unilateral hearing loss in hemiplegic patients. *J. Nerv. Ment. Dis.,* **148,** 83–86, 1969.

Katz, J., The SSW test, an interim report. *J. Speech Hear. Disord.,* **33,** 132–146, 1968.

Katz, J., Audiologic diagnosis, cochlea to cortex. *Menorah Med. J.,* **1,** 25–38, 1970.

Katz J., Basil, R., and Smith, J., A staggered spondaic word test for detecting central auditory lesions. *Ann. Otol. Rhinol. Laryngol.,* **72,** 908–918, 1963.

Katz, J., Kushner, D., and Pack, G., The use of competing speech (SSW) and environmental sound (CES) tests for localizing brain lesions. Presented at *American Speech and Hearing Association Meeting,* Washington, D.C., November 1975.

Katz, J., and Pack, G., New Developments in Differential Diagnosis Using the SSW Test. In Sullivan, M. (Ed), *Central Auditory Processing Disorders,* pp. 84–107. Omaha: University of Nebraska Press, 1975.

Kimura, D., Left-right differences in the perception of melodies. *Q. J. Exp. Psychol.,* **16,** 355–358, 1964.

Lynn, G. E., Personal communication, 1973.

Lynn, G. E., Perception of rapidly alternating speech in patients with brain stem and cerebral hemisphere lesions. Presented at the 9th Colorado Medical Audiology Workshop, Vail, Colorado, March 1975a.

Lynn, G. E., Dichotic speech discrimination in patients with deep cerebral hemisphere lesions. Presented at the 9th Colorado Medical Audiology Workshop, Vail, Colorado, March 1975b.

Lynn, G. E., Benitez, J. T., Eisenbrey, A. B., Gilroy, J. and Wilner, H. I., Neuro-audiological correlates in cerebral hemisphere lesions; temporal and parietal lobe tumors. *Audiology,* **11,** 115–134, 1972a.

Lynn, G. E. and Gilroy, J., Neuro-audiological abnormalities in patients with temporal lobe tumors. *J. Neurol. Sci.,* **17,** 167–184, 1972b.

Lynn, G. E. and Gilroy, J., Central Aspects of Audition. In Northern, J. L. (Ed.), *Communicative Disorders Related to Hearing Loss,* pp. 102–118. Boston: Little, Brown & Co., 1976.

Matzker, J., Two new methods for the assessment of central auditory functions in cases of brain disease. *Ann. Otol. Rhinol. Laryngol.,* **68,** 1185–1197, 1959.

Miller, M., and Daly, J., Cerebellar atrophy simulating acoustic neurinoma. *Arch Otolaryngol.,* **85,** 383–386, 1967.

Quiros, J., Accelerated speech audiometry: An examination of test results. *Translations of the Beltone Institute for Hearing Research,* 1964, #17. (Translated from Interpretacion de los resultados obtenidos con logoaudometria accelerado. *Revista Fonoaudiologica,* **17,** 128–164, 1961.

Smith, B. B., and Resnick, D. M., An auditory test for assessing brain stem integrity; preliminary report. *Laryngoscope,* **82,** 414–424, 1972.

Sparks, R., and Geschwind, N., Dichotic listening in man after section of neocortical commissures. *Cortex,* **4,** 3–16, 1968.

chapter 21

MONOSYLLABIC SPEECH TESTS*

James H. Stevens, Ph.D.

The traditional audiometric techniques provide site of lesion information in hearing loss cases. However, these techniques are much less useful in locating disorders of the central auditory nervous system (CANS). The neural fibers from each cochlea are represented bilaterally in the system central to the cochlear nuclei. There are numerous commissural connections at various levels in the auditory neuroanatomy. This arrangement provides for duplicate information in various parts of the system and is referred to as internal redundancy (Korsan-Bengtsen, 1973) or intrinsic redundancy (Bocca and Calearo, 1963).

Extrinsic redundancy refers to the wealth of information inherent in the speech message. Specifically, extrinsic redundancy refers to those aspects of normal speech such as frequency range, tempo, rhythm, duration and length. Included in extrinsic redundancy is an individual's knowledge that a verbal message is going to follow, or at least should follow, certain phonologic and syntactical rules. As long as the message follows these dictates there should be no difficulty in understanding it.

Assuming that the peripheral and central auditory nervous systems are intact, considerable reduction in the extrinsic redundancy of the message should not interfere with its comprehension. Similarly, patients with lesions of the central auditory nervous system but with a normal peripheral hearing mechanism should not show a loss of understanding for an extrinsically redundant message. The implication is that the loss of intrinsic redundancy is compensated for by the full extrinsic redundancy of the message. However, if the extrinsic redundancy of the message is purposely reduced as well as the patient having a loss of intrinsic redundancy due to a central auditory lesion, the result would be a breakdown in comprehension.

The purpose of this chapter is to review the results of filtered and distorted monosyllabic word tests with patients having CANS lesions. Filtered speech reduces the extrinsic redundancy of the speech signal by selectively attenuating portions of its frequency spectrum. Distorted speech tests, such as the Rush Hughes discrimination recording, provide reduced extrinsic redundancy because of various alterations.

The first portion of this chapter will deal with the monosyllabic word tests which have been used to study brain function, and the second with tests of brain stem pathology.

MONOSYLLABIC WORD TESTS FOR CORTICAL PATHOLOGY

Early investigators attempted to study the effects of central auditory lesions by means of conventional auditory testing. In most cases, no systematic defect could be determined which related to the central lesion.

Filtered Speech Tests

Bocca, Calearo and Cassinari (1954) were pioneers in the field of central auditory assessment. They noted that patients with temporal lobe tumors complained of the lack of clarity for speech presented to the ear contralateral to the tumor, even though conventional audiometry failed to demonstrate any loss of sensitivity or speech discrimination. In view of the patients' complaints, it was decided to increase the difficulty of the speech discrimination task by routing the speech signal through a low-pass filter. It was reasoned that distorting the speech in this manner would place greater demands on the integrative function of the auditory cortex, and would thus be more likely to demonstrate cortical dysfunction.

Bocca et al. showed that a patient with a right-sided temporal lobe tumor achieved normal discrimination scores bilaterally for disyllabic meaningful phonetically balanced (PB)-words. However, with the same speech material routed through a low-pass filter with a cut-off frequency of 800 Hz, the patient achieved a lower score for the ear contralateral to the lesion. The score for the contralateral ear was reduced by 20 to 25% compared with that of the ipsilateral ear (Fig. 21.1).

In a follow-up investigation, Bocca, Calearo, Cassinari and Migliavacca (1955) showed the general validity of their filtered speech test in 18 patients with unilateral temporal lobe disorders. In those instances where the test results were equal for both ears, surgery confirmed that the tumor had not destroyed the auditory cortex. Bocca and his co-workers thus showed the potential utility for filtered speech as a means of exploring cortical auditory function.

In 1958, Bocca published normative data for his low-pass filtered speech test. At a 50-dB

---

* This chapter is based, in part, on the previous chapters of Hodgson (1972) and Goetzinger (1972).

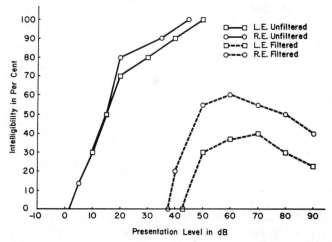

Fig. 21.1. Discrimination scores for unfiltered and filtered speech for a subject with right temporal lobe tumor. (From E. Bocca, C. Calearo, and V. Cassinari: *Acta Otolaryngologica,* **44,** 219–221, 1954.)

sensation level (SL), normals received scores of 70 to 80% for each ear when the test material was presented monaurally. Individuals with temporal lobe tumors obtained scores of approximately 50% with contralateral ear stimulation, and 65 to 75% with ipsilateral ear stimulation.

Jerger (1960a) corroborated Bocca's filtered speech findings by routing English PB-50 lists through a 500 Hz low-pass filter. Two patients with temporal lobe lesions served as subjects for his study. Both subjects showed no significant loss of hearing or speech discrimination problems when tested by conventional audiometric means. However, the subjects scored approximately 30% lower in the ear contralateral to the temporal lobe tumor when filtered speech was used.

Antonelli and Calearo (1968) studied the significance of filtered speech testing with 11 patients having right-sided temporal lobe epilepsy both before and after surgery. They invariably found reduced performance with filtered speech on the left (contralateral) ear whether Heschl's gyrus (the "primary auditory area") had been removed or not. They attributed this reduction to the disease or surgery with secondary defects in auditory functioning in spite of the absence of anatomical changes in Heschl's gyrus.

Hodgson (1967) reported pre- and postoperative audiologic findings on an individual with extensive congenital left hemisphere damage. A left hemispherectomy was performed to alleviate seizures and destructive behavior. Postoperative testing was done 3 weeks and 3 months following the surgery. Pure tone sensitivity, speech reception thresholds and word discrimination scores (WDS) for unfiltered speech were similar both before and after the operation (Fig. 21.2). Hodgson also reported the patient's WDS resulting from routing PB-50 lists through a 500-Hz low-pass filter for each ear on each evaluation. Results were reported as WDSs for an unfiltered and filtered condition, as well as a score that represented the difference between the unfiltered and filtered presentations for each ear. The filtered speech discrimination scores were consistently lower when presented to the right ear (contralateral to the damaged hemisphere). In addition, the unfiltered/filtered speech difference scores were always greater for the right than for the left ear. However, the left ear superiority for the final postoperative assessment amounted to only 2%, and was too small to be considered significant.

The following section will describe the clinical application of a central monaural distorted speech test based upon two readily available phonograph recordings.

The Rush Hughes/W-22 Difference Score

Silverman and Hirsh (1955) investigated the relationship between the relatively easy CID W-22* PB word recording and the more difficult Rush Hughes* recording of the Harvard PB words. A subject population consisting of 218 patients from various hearing clinics individually listened to two lists of the Rush Hughes recordings, three lists of the CID W-22 record-

---

* Manufactured and distributed by Technisonic Studios, 1201 South Brentwood Blvd., St. Louis, Mo., 63117.

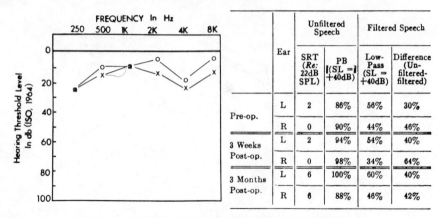

Fig. 21.2. Auditory test results in a case of left hemispherectomy. Pure tone thresholds are re ISO-1964 norms. (From W. Hodgson: *Journal of Speech and Hearing Disorders*, **32**, 39–45, 1967.)

ings, and three additional lists recorded by a female speaker. Statistical analysis of the results indicated that the CID W-22 recording (recorded by Ira Hirsh) and the recording made by the female speaker were: (1) more alike in their intelligibility than was either speaker paired with Hughes, and (2) were significantly more intelligible than was Hughes. Based upon their data, the authors concluded that the difference between the CID W-22 and Rush Hughes (PB-50) lay not in the restriction of vocabulary but in the person who served as the speaker.

Goldstein, Goodman and King (1956) compared speech discrimination results utilizing the Rush Hughes and W-22 recordings presented to four individuals with right infantile hemiplegia both before and after surgical removal of the diseased (left) cerebral hemispheres. Pre- and postoperative assessment indicated that the patients' hearing sensitivity for speech and pure tones was generally within normal limits. The patients' WDS for the Rush Hughes and W-22 recordings indicated a poorer performance when the speech signal was presented to the ear which was contralateral to the diseased or removed hemisphere. Although not stated per se, the data also showed a larger average Rush Hughes/W-22 difference score for the ear contralateral to the lesion (32%) as compared to the ear ipsilateral to the lesion (16%).

In an investigation concerning hearing problems of the elderly, Goetzinger and Rousey (1959) discovered that the Rush Hughes and CID W-22 recordings provided diagnostic information concerning central auditory processing. It was postulated that a large difference score (D/S) reflected a weakness in an individual's ability to cortically integrate the more difficult

speech signal. Table 21.1 represents WDSs from the W-22 and Rush Hughes recordings, as well as D/Ss for normal hearing subjects as a function of age. The same information is also reported for a group of subjects exhibiting sensory-neural hearing loss. As can be seen, the D/S remains relatively constant up to a mean chronologic age of 74 years. The increased D/S in the most elderly group reflects a difficulty in processing the more difficult speech material in old age. This conclusion was supported in a later study (Goetzinger, Proud, Dirks, and Embrey, 1961) which showed a larger bilateral D/S with advancing age. It was concluded that there is an inability to integrate difficult speech material in the aged due to senile changes in the auditory system.

Goetzinger (1972) emphasized that the D/S was generally greater for patients exhibiting peripheral hearing losses than for normal hearing patients (Table 21.1). However, this greater D/S with sensory-neural losses is generally less than in patients having temporal lobe lesions. It has been estimated that a D/S of 30% or greater in one ear is suggestive of a lesion in the contralateral auditory cortex (Goetzinger and Angell, 1965). Clinical experience with the procedure has also shown it to be sensitive to subcortical pathology (Goetzinger, 1972, 1976). In most instances, confirmed brain stem lesions have been demonstrated by either ipsilateral or bilaterally significant D/Ss.

Lilly and Franzen (1968) reported that the 1953 American Standards Specifications for Speech Audiometers (ASA Z24.13-1953) recommended the utilization of a recording stylus with a bottom radius of 2.5 mil (1 mil = $^1/_{100}$ inch). This recommendation was made in accordance with the standards for recording transcriptions at that time. However, between 1956

TABLE 21.1. *Means and Standard Deviations for Recorded W-22 and Rush Hughes (RH) Tests as well as for Difference Scores (D/S) of Normal Hearing Subjects with Reference to Age** Data are shown also for subjects with sensory-neural hearing loss.

N (Ears)	C.A. Mean	SRT Mean	W-22 Mean	W-22 S.D.	RH Mean	RH S.D.	D/S	D/S S.D.
	yr							
30	11½	Normal	94.3	1.8	75.1	5.2	19.2	4.7
40	27	5.0	97.0	2.1	81.0	4.6	16.0	4.5
10	46	1.2	97.8	1.7	81.6	4.4	16.2	4.8
64	66	12.8	88.0	10.2	67.8	12.0	20.2	7.0
64	74	15.9	81.2	12.7	58.0	14.9	23.2	9.3
64	84	26.5	78.1	8.5	43.8	14.5	34.3	10.8
			Sensory-neurals					
18	56	39.9	86.7	10.8	62.6	16.1	24.1	8.5

Adapted from C. P. Goetzinger (1972).

and 1958, the manufacturers of the CID W-22 and Rush Hughes PB-50 speech material changed the groove shape of their recordings to a "universal micro-groove" appropriate for a 1-mil stylus. The new groove size was considered necessary for improved fidelity in reproduction. Until recent years, the change in the transcription characteristics of the recordings failed to become common knowledge to manufacturers of most commercially available speech audiometers. As a result, many clinics with older model speech audiometers continue to play the W-22 and Rush Hughes PB-50 recordings with styli which are inappropriately large. Such a recording groove-stylus mismatch serves to create additional harmonic distortion (Lilly and Franzen, 1968).

The W-22/Rush Hughes PB-50 D/S norms (Goetzinger and Rousey, 1959; Goetzinger et al., 1961) were generated using a 2.5-mil stylus with "universal micro-groove" recordings (Goetzinger, 1976). Accordingly, the 30% D/S deemed as significant for central auditory nervous system pathology (Goetzinger and Angell, 1965) may be a conservative estimate if the recordings are played back with an appropriate 1-mil stylus.

Hall (1970) conducted a normative study investigating articulation functions for the W-22 and Rush Hughes PB-50 "universal micro-groove" recordings utilizing a 1-mil stylus. Normals obtained a mean D/S of only 6% when the recordings were presented at 92 dB sound pressure level (SPL). Such findings were not in agreement with previous indications (Goetzinger and co-workers, 1959, 1961, 1965) that D/Ss of approximately 20% are manifested in both normal and sensory-neural ears. In light of the reduced D/S utilizing "universal micro-groove" recordings in conjunction with a 1-mil stylus, a D/S of less than 30% may be indicative of central auditory nervous system pathology,

particularly in light of normal pure tone sensitivity and slightly suspicious symptomatology.

Clinical Procedure

Goetzinger (1972) advocated certain procedures in the clinical administration of the W-22 and Rush Hughes PB-50 recordings for purposes of obtaining a diagnostic D/S.

The recommended presentation level of the W-22 recording is 40 dB above the patient's speech reception threshold. In the event that the patient demonstrates a tolerance problem at this level, the intensity is gradually reduced until the patient indicates that the signal is comfortably loud. The appropriate loudness level is determined by playing a different list of W-22 monosyllabic words as a practice session prior to test administration. In addition to setting a comfortable loudness level, the practice session also allows the patient to experience listening to recorded words over earphones.

During the practice period, the patient should be trained to enunciate the test words clearly, and to ignore the carrier phrase ("You will say___") preceding the test word. The patient should be seated in such a manner that he is clearly visible to the examiner. In the event of uncertainty concerning whether the stimulus word was correctly repeated, the patient should be urged to quickly spell the word (assuming he has this skill). A prearranged visual gesture between the examiner and patient may be used as a means of informing the patient that he is requested to spell the test word. As soon as (1) the most comfortable listening level has been established, and (2) the patient is aware of what is expected of him, a full 50-word W-22 recording is presented for purposes of assessing his word discrimination score for the D/S.

The test procedure for the administration of the Rush Hughes PB-50 recording is essentially the same as that of the W-22 recording. The only difference is that the recommended presentation level is at least 50 dB above the patient's speech reception threshold. In the event that the patient demonstrates a tolerance problem, the presentation level may be reduced to a comfort level in a similar manner as previously described for the W-22 recording.

The D/S is computed by subtracting the score obtained on the Rush Hughes recording from that obtained on the W-22 recording. Patients with large D/Ss are generally retested for purposes of verifying the results.

Tests Combining Faint and Filtered Speech

Bocca (1955) provided evidence that two low-redundant messages could be centrally summated or integrated by normal hearing listeners. Speech was presented at a very low intensity to one ear, and the same speech, sufficiently intense (45 dB SL) but routed through a 500-Hz low-pass filter, was simultaneously presented to the other ear. The intensity level of the unfiltered speech signal was determined by progressively attenuating it for each subject until a point was reached at which the average score from three presentations did not exceed 30%. The low-pass filtered speech performance did not exceed 50% for any subject. Results of the experiment indicated that, when the speech was delivered simultaneously to both ears, the binaural discrimination score was approximately equal to the sum of the individual monaural scores.

Calearo (1957) used this binaural test in patients with temporal lobe disorders. He found there was no summation if the low-intensity speech was presented to the ear contralateral to the lesion. By reversing the presentation, the patients received a satisfactory binaural summation. The author concluded that the test method could thus be utilized as a means of assessing central hearing disorders.

Jerger (1960b) used the same testing technique in patients with lesions of the auditory cortex. He demonstrated that the speech discrimination score was decreased when either type of signal was presented to the ear contralateral to the lesion. The binaural summation under either combination of signal delivery was little better than the score for the ipsilateral ear alone.

In summary, several investigators have documented that reducing the extrinsic redundancy of the speech signal by filtering causes a breakdown in intelligibility to the ear contralateral to the temporal lobe lesion. Other methods of reducing extrinsic redundancy are described elsewhere in this book, and are similarly effective in the diagnosis of cortical pathology. Perhaps the greatest advantage in the utilization of frequency distorted speech materials is that they may be easily prepared and presented with a minimum investment in equipment and clinical time.

TESTS FOR BRAIN STEM PATHOLOGY

General Discussion

Lesions of the auditory cortex are relatively specific in their auditory effects. Lesions involving the subcortical pathways, on the other hand, manifest themselves in a variety of ways. In light of our present knowledge concerning the neuroanatomy and physiology of the central auditory nervous system, one might expect a lesion specific to the cochlear nuclei to show ipsilateral effects (Matzke and Foltz, 1972). If the lesion is superior to the major decussation of fibers occurring at the level of the trapezoid body, contralateral effects might be expected. However, clinical research has failed to demonstrate such specific effects from confirmed tumors of the brain stem. One possible explanation might be the relatively small anatomical dimensions of the brain stem as compared to that of the neocortex. For example, a left brain stem lesion could conceivably exert sufficient pressure upon the right ascending fibers to result in bilateral effects.

Jerger and Jerger (1975) have presented evidence that auditory symptoms vary as a function of whether the brain stem is affected by an extra- or intra-axial tumor. Extra-axial tumors (tumors located on the outside of the brain stem) gave ipsilateral central auditory symptoms, whereas intra-axial tumors (tumors located within the brain stem) gave either bilateral or contralateral symptoms. Extra- and intra-axial tumor cases were dichotomized further in terms of their audiologic manifestations. For example, individuals with extra-axial brain stem tumors exhibited a greater loss of pure tone sensitivity (50 to 60 dB for 500, 1000, and 2000 Hz, and 80 dB for 4000 Hz) as compared to those with intra-axial tumors (approximately 10 to 15 dB at all frequencies).

Other researchers have reported similar variable findings in tumors involving the auditory pathways. Parker, Decker and Richards (1968) investigated the auditory findings of 20 cases afflicted with pontine lesions. They reported pure tone sensitivity ranging from normal to a severe loss of sensitivity, with a high frequency loss being the most predominant configuration. WDS varied between 0 and 100%, and loudness recruitment varied from absent to complete.

Carhart (1967) felt that lesions specific to the cochlear nucleus may result in high frequency sensory-neural hearing losses which show similar symptomatology to that of cochlear disorders. Experimental evidence has indicated that Rh incompatibility at birth can cause damage to the cochlear nuclei (Haymaker et al., 1961; Malamud, 1961). There has also been less conclusive evidence indicating that the cochlea remains intact in such cases (Crabtree and Gerrard, 1950; Hall, 1964). Typically, individuals with hearing losses resulting from Rh incompatibility demonstrate bilateral high frequency sensory-neural losses with indications of loudness recruitment (e.g., high short increment sensitivity index (SISI) scores in conjunction with Type II Bekesy tracings) with speech discrimination scores suggestive of cochlear pathology.

Other confirmed brain stem lesion cases have shown more subtle audiologic indications. Jerger (1960b) discussed a case of a right-sided brain stem lesion with bilaterally normal pure tone sensitivity, but with a considerably reduced unfiltered speech discrimination score for the left (contralateral) ear. This individual received a score of 100% for the right ear, and only 24% for the left ear when the speech was presented at 40 dB SL.

As may be gleaned from the evidence cited above, subcortical lesions involving the auditory pathways show a wide variety of auditory symptoms. Small differences in the size and location of a brain stem tumor may result in markedly different test results.

Filtered Speech Tests for Brain Stem Pathology

Arnold (cited by Fletcher, 1953) was the first to demonstrate that the brain is capable of combining or synthesizing incomplete speech sounds from the two ears into an intelligible message. He presented low-pass filtered speech to one ear, and the same test words, but high-pass filtered, to the other ear. The cut-off frequency for both the high and low pass filters was 1000 Hz. Monaural discrimination scores were very low, while binaural listening permitted good discrimination.

Matzker (1959) was the first to apply the binaural resynthesis of two bands of filtered speech as an index to brain stem pathology. A list of 41 two-syllable German phonetically balanced words were simultaneously passed through a low-pass band (500 to 800 Hz) and high-pass band (1815 to 2500 Hz) filter at intensities which were preset for maximum intelligibility for each pass band. Initially, the binaural signal was presented so that the right ear received only the low frequency band, and the left ear received only the high frequency band. This was followed by a second presenta-

tion of 41 words in which both frequency bands were presented to both ears in a diotic manner. The final presentation involved a repetition of the initial test procedure. Normal test results were reflected by relatively fewer errors in the third presentation than in the first. The author's examples implied that the number of errors in the diotic (second presentation) and second binaural presentation (third presentation) were approximately the same. In contrast, pathologic results were reflected by a high number of errors in the two binaural presentations, and an improvement under diotic stimulation.

Matzker felt that his test procedure was sensitive to lesions of the brain stem affecting the auditory pathways, and to the generalized atrophy of the central auditory nervous system due to aging (presbycusis). Unilateral cortical auditory pathology should not result in abnormal test results due to the normal auditory cortex's ability to receive sufficient synthesis from the intact brain stem.

Linden (1964) utilized a similar test of binaural fusion with a low-pass band of 560 to 715 Hz and a high-pass band of 1800 to 2200 Hz. When the binaural resynthesis test was presented to subjects with various central pathologies, the ability to resynthesize speech was reduced to the same percentage value as the intelligibility of filtered speech presented monaurally. Linden failed to replicate Matzker's findings and concluded that his version of the test was not sensitive to central auditory lesions.

Hayashi, Ohta and Morimoto (1966) and Ohta, Hayashi and Morimoto (1967) studied Matzker's test principle utilizing bands of 300 to 600 Hz and 1200 to 2400 Hz with nonsense syllables serving as the signals. These researchers reported that individuals afflicted with sensory-neural hearing loss could successfully resynthesize the binaurally presented material. It was therefore concluded that the test could be used in the assessment of both brain stem and cortical pathology in the presence of peripheral hearing loss.

Smith and Resnick (1972) published preliminary results from the so-called "dichotic binaural fusion (DBF) test." The DBF test was based upon Matzker's original test procedure, and was primarily designed to differentiate brain stem from temporal lobe pathologies. The authors were also interested in being able to differentiate brain stem from cochlear pathology. The DBF test materials consisted of three 50-word consonant-nucleus-consonant type (CNC) lists presented over bands of 360 to 890 Hz and 1750 to 2220 Hz. The test was presented under three conditions. The first condition (dichotic A) consisted of a dichotic presentation of the low band signal to one ear and the high band to the other. The second condition consisted of a diotic presentation where both bands were presented to both ears simultaneously. The third condition (dichotic B) consisted of another dichotic presentation similar to the first condition, except that the low band was presented to the ear which originally received the high band signal, and vice versa. It was reported that subjects with normal hearing, bilateral sensory-neural hearing losses, and those with confirmed temporal lobe lesions scored similarly under all three conditions. However, in the case of confirmed brain stem pathology, there was a significant enhancement in the diotic condition over at least one of the dichotic conditions.

Palva and Jokinen (1975) reported the results of over 2000 patients tested with a resynthesis of filtered speech procedure based upon Matzker's (1959) original principle. The test involved the presentation of two bands of filtered words. The band widths were 480 to 720 Hz and 1800 to 2400 Hz. Each separate band yielded a discrimination score of approximately 15 to 20%. However, when the bands were presented simultaneously in either a binaural or monaural mode, the discrimination score typically increased to about 80% in normal hearing young subjects. The test words were presented at 50 dB SL.

The test was designed to yield three discrimination scores. The first score was obtained by presenting both bands to the right ear. The second score resulted from the same two bands being presented to the left ear. The third score resulted from the dichotic presentation of the filtered speech bands (the low frequency band presented to the right ear, and the high frequency band presented to the left ear). The scores were reported in the following manner:

$$\frac{\text{Right Ear}}{\text{Left Ear}} \text{Binaural}$$

Results of the study indicated that peripheral hearing losses often showed binaural discrimination reduced to the same level as that of the poorer ear. In central lesions involving the auditory cortex, the most typical finding was asymmetry in the monaural test in the ear contralateral to the lesion combined with relatively good binaural discrimination. In cases of brain stem pathology, asymmetry in the monaural test was found in either the contralateral or ipsilateral ear combined with poor binaural discrimination, or poor discrimination scores under all three modes of presentation. It was reasoned that the binaural score should be a significant factor in distinguishing a cortical

from a brain stem central auditory disorder. If brain stem lesions occur in areas peripheral to those regions responsible for binaural hearing, the binaural score should be reduced to the same level as that of the poorer ear. However, the binaural discrimination score should be relatively high in lesions involving the auditory cortex because normal fusion occurs in the intact brain stem and may be successfully integrated by the nondiseased hemisphere.

CONCLUSION

The use of filtered or distorted monosyllabic word materials has proven to be useful as an aid in the diagnosis of central auditory disorders. It should be re-emphasized that the results of any central test should be interpreted in light of additional auditory test information and a complete and accurate case history.

REFERENCES

Antonelli, A., and Calearo, C., Further investigations on cortical deafness. *Acta Otolaryngol.*, **66**, 97–100, 1968.

Bocca, E., Binaural hearing; another approach. *Laryngoscope*, **65**,1164–1171, 1955.

Bocca, E., Clinical aspects of cortical deafness. *Laryngoscope*, **68**, 301–309, 1958.

Bocca, E., and Calearo, C., Central Hearing Processes. In Jerger, J. (Ed.), *Modern Developments in Audiology*, pp. 337–370, Ch. 9. New York: Academic Press, 1963.

Bocca, E., Calearo, C., and Cassinari, V., A new method for testing hearing in temporal lobe tumors; preliminary report. *Acta Otolaryngol.*, **44**, 219–221, 1954.

Bocca, E., Calearo, C., Cassinari, V., and Migliavacca, F., Testing "cortical" hearing in temporal lobe tumors. *Acta Otolaryngol.*, **45**, 289–304, 1955.

Calearo, C., Binaural summation in lesions of the temporal lobe. *Acta Otolaryngol.*, **47**, 392–395, 1957.

Carhart, R., Probable mechanisms underlying kernicteric hearing loss. *Acta Otolaryngol.*, Suppl. 221, 1967.

Crabtree, N., and Gerrard, J., Perceptive deafness associated with severe neonatal jaundice. *J. Laryngol.*, **64**, 482–506, 1950.

Fletcher, H., *Speech and Hearing in Communication*. New York: D. van Nostrand Co., Inc., 1953.

Goetzinger, C. P., The Rush Hughes Test in Auditory Diagnosis. In Katz, J. (Ed.), *Handbook of Clinical Audiology*, pp. 325–333, Ch. 17. Baltimore: Williams & Wilkins Co., 1972.

Goetzinger, C. P., Personal communication, 1976.

Goetzinger, C. P., and Angell, S., Audiological assessment in acoustic tumors and cortical lesions. *Eye Ear Nose Throat Mon.*, **44**, 39–49, 1965.

Goetzinger, C. P., Proud, G. O., Dirks, D., and Embrey, J., A study of hearing in advanced age. *Arch. Otolaryngol.*, **73**, 662–674, 1961.

Goetzinger, C. P., and Rousey, C. L., Hearing problems in later life. *Med. Times*, 87, 771-780, 1959.

Goldstein, R., Goodman, A., and King, R., Hearing and speech in infantile hemiplegia before and after left hemispherectomy. *Neurology*, 6, 869-875, 1956.

Hall, J., Cochlea and the cochlear nuclei in asphyxia. *Acta Otolaryngol.*, Suppl. 194, 1964.

Hall, L. W., A study of the speech discrimination ability for normal hearing and sensori-neural subjects on three tests employing a 1 mil stylus. Unpublished master's thesis, University of Kansas, 1970.

Hayashi, R., Ohta, F., and Morimoto, M., Binaural fusion test; a diagnostic approach to the central auditory disorders. *Int. Audiol.*, 5, 133-135, 1966.

Haymaker, W., Margoles, C., Penschen, A., Jacob, H., Lindenberg, R., Arroyo, L., Stockdorph, O., and Stowens, D., Pathology of Kernicterus and Posticteric Encephalopathy. In American Academy for Cerebral Palsy, *Kernicterus and Its Importance in Cerebral Palsy*, pp. 21-228. Springfield, Ill.: Charles C Thomas, 1961.

Hodgson, W. R., Audiological report of a patient with left hemispherectomy. *J. Speech Hear. Disord.*, 32, 39-45, 1967.

Hodgson, W. R., Filtered Speech Tests. In Katz, J. (Ed.), *Handbook of Clinical Audiology*, pp. 313-324, Ch. 16. Baltimore: Williams & Wilkins Co., 1972.

Jerger, J., Observations on auditory behavior in lesions of the central auditory pathways. *Arch. Otolaryngol.*, 71, 797-806, 1960a.

Jerger, J., Audiological manifestations of lesions in the auditory nervous system. *Laryngoscope*, 70, 417-425, 1960b.

Jerger, S., and Jerger, J., Extra- and intra-axial brain stem auditory disorders. *Audiology*, 14, 93-117, 1975.

Korsan-Bengsten, M., Distorted speech audiometry. *Acta Otolaryngol.*, Suppl. 310, 1973.

Lilly, D., and Franzen, R., Reproducing styli for speech audiometry. *J. Speech Hear. Res.*, 11, 817-824, 1968.

Linden, A., Distorted speech and binaural speech resynthesis tests. *Acta Otolaryngol.*, 58, 32-48, 1964.

Malamud, N., Pathogenesis of Kernicterus in the Light of Its Sequelae. In American Academy for Cerebral Palsy, *Kernicterus and Its Importance in Cerebral Palsy*, pp. 230-244. Springfield, Ill.: Charles C Thomas, 1961.

Matzke, H. A., and Foltz, F. M., *Synopsis of Neuroanatomy*. New York: Oxford University Press, 1972.

Matzker, J., Two new methods for the assessment of central auditory functions in cases of brain disease. *Ann. Otol. Rhinol. Laryngol.*, 68, 1185-1197, 1959.

Ohta, F., Hayashi, R., and Morimoto, M., Differential diagnosis of retrocochlear deafness; binaural fusion test and binaural separation test. *Int. Audiol.*, 6, 58-62, 1967.

Palva, A., and Jokinen, K., The role of the binaural test in filtered speech audiometry. *Acta Otolaryngol.*, 79, 310-314, 1975.

Parker, W., Decker, R., and Richards, N., Auditory function and lesions of the pons. *Arch. Otolaryngol.*, 87, 228-240, 1968.

Silverman, S., and Hirsh, I., Problems related to the use of speech in clinical audiometry. *Ann. Otol. Rhinol. Laryngol.*, 64, 1234-1243, 1955.

Smith, B. B., and Resnick, D. M., An auditory test for assessing brain stem integrity; preliminary report. *Laryngoscope*, 82, 414-424, 1972.

chapter 22

SENTENCE TESTS OF CENTRAL AUDITORY DYSFUNCTION

Jack A. Willeford, Ph.D.

Sentence-type stimuli have been employed clinically in a variety of ways for the purpose of identifying the site-of-lesion in adult patients who have sustained damage to areas of the brain. Sentence materials have also been used to confirm the presence and nature of central auditory processing difficulties in children with learning disabilities. It is the purpose of this chapter to review the major types of sentence tests, their application to adults and children, and their clinical and theoretical relationships to other types of central auditory measures.

TYPES OF SENTENCE TESTS

Synthetic Speech Sentences

Sentences which are purposely and systematically diverted from the standard rules of grammar and syntax were developed as an adjunct to standard speech audiometry by Speaks and Jerger in 1965. Later, they were utilized in competing message paradigms for measuring functions in the central auditory system (Jerger and Jerger, 1974; Speaks, 1975; Jerger and Jerger, 1975). Their rationale for developing this technique was to avoid the use of single words, and single-syllable words in particular. They felt that such short signals impose limitations in evaluating the capacity to manipulate the changing of pattern with time, which they considered a crucial parameter. They used a closed message set to minimize the subject's reliance on previous linguistic history. Thus, the subject could simply identify the stimulus sentence from among a group of sentences which had controlled lengths and informational content (Speaks and Jerger, 1965; and Jerger, Speaks, and Trammell, 1968). The details and additional rationale are discussed in the reference articles. A particular group of synthetically determined sentences, employed in two major studies (Jerger and Jerger, 1974, 1975), was selected from among various word-order approximations and sentence lengths. Several random orders of a list having 10 sentences of 7 words each were made. All were third-order approximations of actual sentences as shown in Table 22.1. One additional study by Speaks in 1975 refers to the use of synthetic sentences as a clinical tool for diagnosing central lesions. However, no details were provided about which sentence set was used nor were specifics offered about procedure except that it was employed as a dichotic listening test with a passage of connected discourse as the competition. For this reason, the present discussion will focus on the two explicit studies by Jerger and Jerger.

In the first of these studies synthetic sentence identification (SSI) materials were administered to a series of patients with carefully defined intra-axial brain stem lesions. That is, great care was taken to eliminate all patients in whom there was evidence of coexisting eighth nerve involvement or lesions not arising from within the brain stem. This study was unique, in the writer's judgment, from that standpoint alone, but was also of special interest from another aspect. The latter involved an unusual combination of test-mode presentations of competing messages. In the first mode, tape recorded synthetic sentences were presented by melodious male voice to one ear while the other simultaneously received a narrative by the same speaker about events in the life of Davy Crockett. Following this technique the ears receiving the message and competition, respectively, were reversed. The second test mode combined the sentences and the competition of connected discourse for presentation to first one ear and then the other. In both the opposite side, or contralateral competing message (CCM), and the ipsilateral competing message (ICM), or same side procedures, performance was measured at various message-to-competition ratios (MCRs). With the competition narrative generally fixed at 50 dB sound pressure level (SPL), the MCRs were varied in 20-dB steps from 0 dB to −40 dB for the CCM condition, and in 10-dB steps from +10 dB to −20 dB for the ICM condition. Results on both measures were plotted as the averages of the scores of the various MCRs. Normal performance was 100% correct at all MCRs for CCMs, and ranged from nearly 100% to about 20% on the ICMs with increasing competition intensities. The latter is illustrated in Figure 22.1.

The results on 11 patients with carefully defined intra-axial brain stem lesions, who were given both the CCM and ICM tasks, were strikingly dissimilar for the two tests. All 11 patients exhibited very poor performance on the ICM test, 6 of them on both ears and 5 of them just on the contralateral ear (CE). No patient performed poorly on the ipsilateral ear (IE) alone. Performance scores on these patients averaged 37% on both IE and CE when averaged across MCRs of 0, −10, and −20 dB, whereas normals average 76%. The ICM results are summarized in Figure 22.2, together with those for the CCM test which shows that 8 of the 11 patients, by sharp contrast, had normal scores even at the most difficult MCR of −40 dB.

A typical result for one of the patients receiving SSI materials is shown in Figure 22.3. This is the performance of a 17-year-old girl with a

TABLE 22.1. *Synthetic Sentence Identification (SSI)**

1. Small boat with a picture has become
2. Built the government with the force almost
3. Go change your car color is red
4. Forward march said the boy had a
5. March around without a care in your
6. That neighbor who said business is better
7. Battle cry and be better than ever
8. Down by the time is real enough
9. Agree with him only to find out
10. Women view men with green paper should

* Supplied by J. Jerger in a personal communication; also in J. Jerger, C. Speaks, and J. A. Trammell: *Journal of Speech and Hearing Disorders*, 33, 318–328, 1968.

left-side pontine glioma who had normal pure tone sensitivity. CCM performance was normal, bilaterally, whereas ICM performance was normal on the IE and showed a marked deficit on the CE.

The major finding in this study was that ICM performance, though variable, was consistently poor in all cases having intra-axial brain stem lesions. CCM performance, on the other hand, remained normal in all except three cases with mildly abnormal results. An intriguing aspect of these results is the fact that they show ICM to be a measure of brain stem dysfunction. This finding has pertinence since two other tests in current use involve ipsilateral competing stimuli. Those tests are the Flowers-Costello test of central auditory abilities (Flowers, Costello and Small, 1970), and the composite auditory perception test (CAPT) developed by Butler, Hedrick and Manning (1972), for the Alameda County Schools, Hayward, California. However, the descriptive literature with both of these tests fails to identify the nature of the test protocol except to describe them as "competing message" measures. Moreover, no mention is made of what these tests are presumed to measure in terms of neurophysiologic processes or levels. They are simply ascribed the function of identifying central auditory disorders in children with learning disabilities, specifically in those children who have difficulty with auditory closure or auditory figure-ground events.

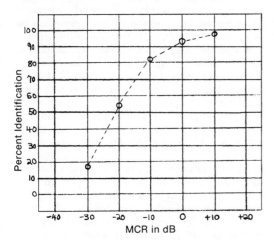

Fig. 22.1. SSI-ICM norms. (Adapted from data in a personal communication from J. Jerger, 1975.)

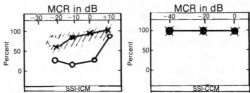

Fig. 22.3. SSI-ICM and SSI-CCM test results for a 17-year-old girl with an intra-axial brain stem lesion on the left side. (Adapted from Jerger and Jerger, 1974.)

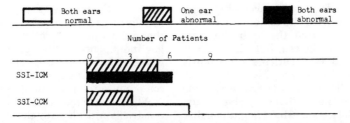

Fig. 22.2. Pattern of SSI-ICM and SSI-CCM test results on 11 patients with intra-axial brain stem lesions. The number of normal results, and abnormal findings on one or both ears, is shown. (Adapted from Jerger and Jerger, 1974.)

The second investigation (Jerger and Jerger, 1975) was one in which, as part of a larger study, the SSI as well as the staggered spondaic word (SSW) test (Katz, 1962; see Chapter 23) were administered to two groups of patients with medically diagnosed disorders of the central auditory system. One group consisted of 10 patients with intra-axial brain stem lesions, and the other group was comprised of 10 patients with temporal lobe lesions.

The results of this investigation were in general agreement with the earlier study. Specifically, on the ICM test, the brain stem group had an impairment of about 40% on the CE only. In the temporal lobe group, mean ICM performance was depressed about 30% on the IE and 40% on the CE. CCM results, on the other hand, were in the normal range for the brain stem group, and the temporal lobe group had a deficit of approximately 20% on the CE. The Jergers summarized as follows:

For brainstem patients, the SSI procedure shows poor performance for ICM and relatively good performance for CCM. The ICM deficits are observed on the C ear only and CCM performance is within normal limits on both ears . . . For temporal lobe patients, the SSI procedure yields poor performance on both ICM and CCM. The ICM deficits are observed on both ears and the CCM deficit is observed on the C ear only (p. 20).

A few differences may be noted between the results of this and the previous study. However, changes in the later study are largely accounted for by the authors' acknowledgment that some exceptional findings did occur. They stated that their major observation was one which recognizes that brain stem patients have "relatively more" difficulty on ICM tasks than on CCM tasks, and that the reverse is true for temporal lobe subjects.

The Jergers' comparison of SSI and SSW results is of considerable interest, especially since the SSW results are also compared with other sentence material in a subsequent discussion. The SSW was found to show significantly reduced scores for the temporal lobe group, but not for the brain stem group. These findings led them to conclude . . . "The overriding principle that characterized the combination of the two procedures was that the brain stem patients consistently showed SSI-ICM deficits whereas temporal lobe patients consistently showed SSW deficits" (p. 20).

A possible limitation of the SSI test, using the Jergers' technique, is that it involves visual as well as auditory tasks which might penalize or have limited application for a small population of illiterate or retarded adults who cannot read, and those with visual handicaps. Its use would also preclude younger children with undeveloped reading skills, or those in whom the central visual and auditory processes are not mutually facilitating events. The latter appears to be the case, in the writer's experience, for certain children with learning disabilities. This possibility might be circumvented in some cases by simply having the subject repeat the stimulus as Speaks (1975) has suggested as an optional response method.

Natural Speech Sentences

Willeford developed a competing sentence test (CST) in 1968 for the specific purpose of evaluating central auditory function. Unlike the SSI, the CST is composed of simple, natural English sentences. Inspiration for the test evolved partly from a consideration of some early tests designed by Jerger (1964) and a test which Frager (1968) employed in a thesis study under Willeford's direction. Each of these measures involved a variety of techniques utilizing sentences. Additional motivation was for one of the same reasons the SSI was developed — to avoid dependence on identification of highly transient single words, particularly monosyllabic words. Such words place a premium on one's concentration and attention. Another reason was the desire to simulate language constructions one might encounter in everyday life. It was hoped that the test might provide insight into a subject's ability to process standard forms of spoken language. Thus, factors of temporal patterns, the acoustic spectra, linguistic features, and syntactical characteristics were considered as important attributes of the signal.

Identification of the target sentences through key word recognition was not a great concern as it was stated to be in construction of the SSI materials where only "identification" of a given sentence is involved in a closed set (Speaks and Jerger, 1965). The "real" sentences involve "message perception" and were designed so as to minimize that perception by key words alone. The sentences were employed in an open-set paradigm which brings language performance and skill somewhat to bear on the success of the message to be decoded. However, an effort was made to select a level of language that did not penalize children, the person with low intelligence or literacy levels, or patients whose reduced physical well-being as a result of central nervous system (CNS) lesions might compromise their maximum test performance.

While one major consideration in the test construction dealt with the nature of the test stimuli, an equally important factor was the nature of the competing message. In many dichotic tests (Katz' SSW and Berlin's CVs (consonant-vowel) are notable exceptions), and in *all* tests where the primary messages are sentences, the competition takes some other form. Continuous discourse, by a single speaker as in the SSI procedure, a babble of several voices, environmental noise, white noise, accelerated speech, and backward speech have been used. The point at issue is that the competition "differs" from the test stimulus. Influenced by the work of Treisman (1964), competition signals were sought that were similar in character to the test items. She showed that selective attention to a desired message during a dichotic sentence task is influenced by the transitional probabilities between words. Her evidence suggested that irrelevant (competing) words are discarded during their identification rather than before or after. She found that an irrelevant message, delivered by the same voice (talker) and involving similar content material, was a more difficult task than that presented by two different voices, different languages, and reversed speech. Speaks (1975), Berlin et al. (1972) and Berlin and McNeill (1976) have shown similar results. The latter is a comprehensive review of the variables in dichotic listening tasks, and should be read by anyone seeking to develop such measures.

A sample of the competing sentences (CSs) is presented in Table 22.2. It may be observed that the content of these pairs concerns time, weather, or some common theme. One sentence of each set is presented simultaneously to opposite ears. The sentences are of similar length and content. No attempt was made to time-match the onsets of the paired stimuli precisely, a factor Berlin et al. (1973) have since shown to be critical with dichotic CVs where brief signals differ by only a single consonant. However, the two sentences do begin and end very nearly at the same time. Precise time matching was not considered essential since it was believed that correct responses would be dependent on a combination of the several ongoing factors mentioned earlier.

Wingfield (1975) has recently suggested that the perceptual act, when listening to sentences,

is not a passive handling of the speech on a word-by-word basis. He maintains that, so long as there is some minimal intelligibility, a person actively reconstructs the heard fragments so as to produce responses that are meaningful, fully grammatical, and that match the syntactic form of the heard speech when it can be detected. He concluded that speech perception on the sentence level is an active process based on analysis with larger than individual word components which probably correspond to higher syntactic constituents. Thus, the CST would seem to challenge a subject's skill for a task that occurs continuously in everyday living.

Both sentences in each pair of CSs were recorded on a magnetic stereo tape by the same male talker with general American dialect. Attempt was made to avoid emphasizing important words, pauses, and intonation patterns that would aid the perception process.

Three lists, each with 25 pairs of sentences were recorded. Each list also had slightly different construction paradigms. To date, however, only one list has had major use. Thus, discussion will be restricted to that list. On the basis of pilot experiments, 35 dB SL (*re* the pure tone average (PTA)) was established as the test level of the primary message. The competition sentence was set for a level of 50 dB SL (*re* the PTA). Thus, a signal-to-competition ratio (SCR) of −15 dB was adopted.

Using all 25 pairs of sentences, Ivey (1969) standardized the test on 20 subjects between the ages of 19 and 33 years, all of whom had negative otologic and neurologic histories. Instructions to Ivey's subjects were based on Kimura's (1963) statement that hemispheric dominance must be controlled in the dichotic mode by commanding subjects to listen to the material in one ear and to ignore the material presented to the other ear. Thus, the sentence-test protocol has been to instruct subjects to listen to and repeat the "primary" message (35 dB SL) and ignore the "competing" message (50 dB SL) in their other ear. To control for ear and sentence list differences, half of the subjects received the "A" sentences in their right ear and the "B" sentences in their left ear. The remaining half of the subjects received the sentences in the reverse order. The results, shown in Table 22.3, revealed that: (1) the two lists were approximately equal in difficulty and (2) differences between the ears of normal subjects slightly favor the right ear (994 total correct responses out of 1000 items for right ears as compared to 980 total correct left ear responses out of the 1000 sentences presented to left ears). Twelve of the 20 subjects had slightly better performance in the right ear. Nine of those 12 missed only 1 more item in

TABLE 22.2. *Selected Examples of Willeford's Competing Sentences*

(weather)	a.	I think we'll have rain today.
	b.	There was frost on the ground.
(time)	a.	This watch keeps good time.
	b.	I was late to work today.
(family)	a.	My mother is a good cook.
	b.	Your brother is a tall boy.
(food)	a.	Please pass the salt and pepper.
	b.	The roast beef is very good.
(safety)	a.	Fasten your seat belt.
	b.	Get ready for take-off.

TABLE 22.3. *Response Performance for 20 Normal Adult Subjects on Dichotic Competing Sentence Test*

Ear	No. of Sentences Presented	Test List A	Test List B	Total
		Correct – Incorrect	Correct – Incorrect	Correct – Incorrect
Right	500	497 – 3	497 – 3	994 – 6
Left	500	494 – 6	486 – 14	980 – 20
Total	1000	991 – 9	983 – 17	1974 – 26

Adapted from Ivey (1969).

the left ear and 3 subjects missed 2 more items in the left ear. Identical scores for both ears were obtained in 7 subjects, 6 of whom scored 100% in each ear and 1 subject missed 1 item in each ear. Just 1 person had superior performance in the left ear and he missed only 1 of the 25 items in his right ear. These data established that young adult normals find the CS task very easy, and show little differences in skill between ears.

Clinical Use of Natural Sentences with Adults

Since 1968, the CST has been used rather extensively on adult subjects with carefully defined neurologic lesions. Lynn and Gilroy (1972, 1975), Lynn et al. (1972), Lynn (1973), and Gilroy and Lynn (1974), have consistently reported results showing that the CST, as one of a battery of central auditory measures, is useful in detecting the presence of structural lesions in the brain. Moreover, they have found it helpful for monitoring changes in a patient's neurologic status with time, or as the result of treatment or surgery. The recent report by Lynn and Gilroy (1975) summarizes the present state of knowledge reported in the series of other reports by Lynn and his colleagues at the Wayne State University School of Medicine where they have access to a large clinical population for study. Table 22.4 presents the mean scores on a series of tests for 10 patients with tumors in the posterior region of the temporal lobe. These patients ranged in age from 23 to 66 years. Five patients had involvement representing the left hemisphere and 5 had right hemisphere lesions. The mean undistorted speech discrimination (UD PB) score was slightly poorer on the contralateral ear (CE), but was thought to be influenced by significant sensory-neural hearing loss and its accompanying inner ear distortion combined with the temporal lobe tumor. Low-pass filtered speech (LPFS) and each of the other tests show unilateral asymmetries with poorer scores in the CE. The alternate binaural and simultaneous binaural scores refer to part of Lynn's modification of Katz' SSW procedure. The simultaneous binaural represents the overlapping (right-competing and left-competing) por-

TABLE 22.4. *Subjects with Tumors in Posterior Region of Temporal Lobe**

Test	Ear	Mean	Range
UD PB	IE	95.8	88–100
	CE	84.0	48–100
LPFS	IE	45.1	2–92
	CE	35.5	0–68
Alt Bin	IE	93.7	82–100
	CE	70.5	25–95
Sim Bin	IE	77.4	38–100
	CE	42.9	0–88
Comp Sent	IE	84.0	0–100
	CE	33.0	0–100

* Mean scores in percentage correct; $N = 10$. UD PB, undistorted speech discrimination; LPFS, low-pass filtered speech; Alt Bin, alternating speech, binaural; Sim Bin, simultaneous speech, binaural; Comp Sent, competing sentence; IE, ipsilateral ear; CE, contralateral ear. (After Lynn and Gilroy, 1975.)

tions of the SSWs spondaic words, and the alternate binaural represents the nonoverlapping (right-noncompeting and left-noncompeting) portions. The CST constituted a second dichotic measure, and permitted a comparison of test results between the sentences and the SSW. It is now generally known that persons with unilateral temporal lobe lesions commonly exhibit abnormally poor test performance on the ear which is contralateral to the damaged hemisphere. This was illustrated in the studies cited earlier (Jerger and Jerger, 1974, 1975). This is true for either dichotically competing speech or for monotic degraded-speech. The mean data in Table 22.4 confirm this standard of behavior. It may be observed that there is a corresponding pattern of scores between the SSW and the CST. Dr. Lynn related, in a personal communication early in his experience with the CST, that 10 pairs of sentences were entirely adequate to test one ear. In fact, he stated that 5 test items were all that he needed to make a determination about a given patient. Since that time, the use of 10 sentences has become the standard test length. Thus, the 25 pairs of sentences provide enough items to test both ears (10 to each ear). The last 5 may be ignored, used for rechecking either ear in competition, for evaluating sentence discrimination without competition, or for assessing patients' skill at repeating both messages, which normals can also easily do. In the latter case, both ears receive a stimulus at 50 dB SL (SCR = 0 dB).

The range of scores for the sentences in Table 22.4 illustrates the commonly observed result of a 100% score in the ipsilateral ear (IE) and complete failure (0%) in the CE. Group data are misleading, however, since exceptions may be observed to the CE effect in some patients. Moreover, the ear-difference scores may range from 100% to slight on some patients. It seems that variations in performance are dependent on factors such as lesion size and location. For example, most patients with temporal lobe lesions show dramatic CE effects for CSs. Table 22.5 presents data for such a case and the dramatic result of the CST and the SSW may be noted. The difference in scores between the two ears is extreme for both tasks and the CE is down. Table 22.6, on the other hand, shows results on a subject where CS and SSW scores are normal, bilaterally, and only monotic distorted speech provided a clue to abnormality by virtue of a weak CE performance. Note that the lesion in this case is in the inferior region of the temporal lobe. Lynn and his colleagues have noted a trend which suggests that both the CST and the SSW are highly sensitive to lesions in the posterior regions of the temporal lobe, the SSW to posterior and slightly anterior areas of the lobe, and distorted monotic speech to lower and broader (more anterior) aspects of the temporal lobe. These factors are evident in the group data in Table 22.7 and the specific

TABLE 22.5. *Auditory Findings (in Percent) in Patient (Male: age 66) with Left Temporal Lobe Astrocytoma and Evidence of Upper Brain Stem Involvement**

Ear	UD PB	LPFS	Alt Bin	Sim Bin	Comp Sent	Binaural Fusion
Right	100	32	70	0	0	10
Left	100	46	100	98	100	0
Binaural	–	–	–	–	–	10

* Abbreviations as in Table 22.4. (After Lynn and Gilroy, 1975.)

TABLE 22.6. *Auditory Findings (in Percent) in Patient (Female: age 23) with Left Temporal Lobe Astrocytoma, Inferior Region**

Ear	UD PB	LPFS	Alt Bin	Sim Bin	Comp Sent
Right	100	32	100	98	100
Left	100	56	100	98	100

* Abbreviations as in Table 22.4. (After Lynn and Gilroy, 1975.)

TABLE 22.7. *Subjects with Temporal Lobe Tumors in Anterior-Inferior Regions**

Test	Ear	Mean	Range
UD PB	IE	98.0	96–100
	CE	99.0	96–100
LPFS	IE	47.7	28–72
	CE	32.7	20–56
Alt Bin	IE	95.8	85–100
	CE	91.5	73–100
Sim Bin	IE	90.8	73–98
	CE	75.8	28–98
Comp Sent	IE	100.0	100–100
	CE	96.7	90–100

* Mean scores in percentage correct; $N = 6$. Abbreviations as in Table 22.4. (After Lynn and Gilroy, 1975.)

case cited in Table 22.5. Such results lead one to wonder whether these differences are a matter of the relative sensitivity of the various tests for identifying deficiencies in the higher auditory system, or whether it is simply that each test is looking at the critical neural processing areas for the nature of the stimuli involved in these three diverse auditory tasks. Perusal of the literature indicates some investigators have assumed that all speech processing takes place in the same fashion regardless of the nature of the stimulus used, and that it is simply a matter of whether the test material has sufficient sensitivity to expose a processing breakdown. It seems more likely to the writer, on the contrary, that different test materials and strategies challenge the integrity of the auditory processors in different ways. Thus, each test appears to have relative strengths and weaknesses. Although they concern themselves only with CVs and digits as signals, Porter and Berlin (1975) have presented an excellent theoretical discussion of this topic and arrive at a similar conclusion, at least as far as how language processing may function developmentally with increasing age.

Lynn and Gilroy (1975) report further on the use of CSs with extratemporal lobe tumors in which they have observed the following pattern of results:

Parietal Lobe Tumors. When the parietal lobe tumor was deeply situated (and involved the corpus callosum), no difference between ears is noted on monotic distorted-speech tests. For dichotic speech material, on the other hand, performance seems to be routinely poorer in the IE regardless of the hemisphere in which the tumor resided. Such results have also been reported by Sparks, Goodglass and Nickel (1970), and Speaks (1975) for dichotic tests. Lynn and Gilroy (1975) had earlier stated that patients with parietal tumors which invade only the superficial tissues perform normally on all of the tests discussed. It seems apparent from such reports that we still have a great deal to learn about relating auditory test results to specific anatomic sites of damage in the CNS.

Frontal Lobe Tumors. The presence of frontal lobe tumors in 11 patients produced widely varying results on the central auditory tests discussed, ranging from normal results on all tests for 5 subjects, to abnormal findings on the other 6. Four cases had abnormal results for the dichotic CS and SSW tests on the IE, offering further testimony to the limitations of our knowledge regarding central auditory disorders.

Other Types of Brain Lesions. Lynn and Gilroy (1975) reported data on selected cases of intracranial damage other than tumors. These involved vascular and degenerative-type lesions. In each instance the results of the CST were highly significant. Thus, CSs would appear to be an important addition to a central auditory test battery. Experience suggests that they have the added advantage of being applicable to subjects within a wide age range, and that they are minimally influenced by the coexistence of peripheral hearing impairment in many instances.

Clinical Use of Natural Sentences with Children Having Learning Disabilities

For the past 3 years, the writer and his staff colleagues at Colorado State University have been using the CST as part of a four-test battery for children with learning disabilities (LD). All of the children seen to date were were referred because they were known to have, or else suspected of having, some kind of an "auditory problem."

The test battery consisted of the CST, a monotic test of low-pass filtered speech (FS) which utilized selected CNC words as stimuli, a modified binaural-fusion (BF) task which Ivey (1969) adapted from the technique by Matzker (1959, 1962), and an alternating speech (AS) test similar to one suggested by Lynn and Gilroy (1975). The CS and BF tests were used by Lynn and his colleagues, together with different versions of the FS and AS tasks. This fact has permitted continuing comparisons between the data on adults with well-documented lesions, and those of children with bizarre academic and social histories. In the case of adults, the tests served to detect the presence of central auditory lesions, and to monitor changes in a patient's neurologic condition following surgery or therapy. In the case of children, they are used to help identify subtle dysfunctions in auditory behavior and to follow changes in performance with maturation, training, counseling and environmental controls. Attention in this section will again necessarily focus on CSs. It should be mentioned at this point that the AS tests used by both Lynn and the writer involve sentences. However, they are not stressed in this chapter because data is still limited and, with LD children at least, the test seldom results in an abnormal performance.

CS scores for a group of presumed normal children are shown in Table 22.8. These data show a consistently strong competition performance for the right ear on which nearly all children score 100%. Left ear scores, however, reflect very poor performance for 5-year-olds (not shown here is the fact that children who are only 4 do essentially as well as those who are 5) but show progressive improvement through the 9-year level. By the time most children are 10 they can perform at the 100% level in both ears. Thus, skill on the CST would appear to be related to maturation. Moreover, evidence from three youngsters of 11 years of age revealed that once bilateral skill is achieved, primary signal levels in either ear can be reduced from 35 dB SL to as low as 10 dB SL before their performance begins to deteriorate. Stated differently, selective attention to the primary sentence remains undiverted by the 50 dB SL competing sentence even when the SL of the primary sentence is made very faint.

Table 22.9 presents an analysis of these youngsters in terms of ear strength. One can follow the progression of dominance by the right ear in most of the younger children to the converging symmetry of ear performance by the age of 9. It can be observed, however, that a few children show no ear differences at the lower age levels, and that an occasional child achieves better scores in the left ear. This result is achieved much less often as a child reaches the age of 9 according to these data. This trend is even more evident in Table 22.10 where comparison is drawn between children in the 5 to 9 age group, and a group comprising various ages from 10 to 31.

TABLE 22.8. *Competing Sentences Scores on Right-Handed Children with Presumed Normal Central Auditory Function**

Age	N	Mean Scores LE – RE	Range
5	12	30 – 94	0–100
6	19	55 – 92	0–100
7	18	71 – 92	0–100
8	14	88 – 97	60–100
9	14	91 – 98	80–100

* Each child scored 100% in both ears in the absence of dichotic competition. LE and RE, left and right ear, respectively.

Considerable variability in skill has been noted in children. We have seen one individual at age 5 and two at age 6 who perform normally in both ears, while others may still be scoring poorly in one ear (usually the left) at ages 10, 11, or in one case even 12. The 12-year-old youngster, incidentally, was doing very poorly in school and had obvious problems with auditory processing, even to the lay observer. Examined 2 years later, her strong ear score improved from 80% to 100% and her weak ear score jumped from 10% to 80%. This case appeared to have been one of delayed maturation. Interpretation of a processing problem on the basis of poor performance on one ear is somewhat hazardous. However, it seems reasonable to assume that a child in whom dichotic listening skills have not yet developed is as functionally handicapped in auditory processing as the adult who fails to perform as the result of a cortical lesion.

It should be mentioned that scoring is liberalized for younger children. That is, their responses are counted as correct if they paraphrase the sentence to a lower level of language as long as they do not alter the essential content or meaning of the sentence, and do not interchange the language of the two competing sentences. The task requires the examiner to make only simple judgments. The job is frequently made easier by the fact that there are

often all-or-none type responses. The child responds easily and correctly, or fails to respond at all. Reasons for failing to respond include such statements as "I couldn't hear it, I don't know, I couldn't understand, this ear (pointing) won't let the other ear listen." An example of acceptable language level transitions would be as follows:

Test Pair	Correct Responses
Primary message (35 dB SL)	I like the roast.
	The meat is good.
The roast beef is very good.	The roast is good to eat.
	Roast beef is good.
Competition Message (50 dB SL)	*Incorrect responses*
	I don't know.
Please pass the salt and pepper.	Put salt on the beef.
	The salt and pepper are very good.
	The roast has too much pepper.

Referring to young children, Menyuk (1969, p. 32) indicates "We can definitely state that the child does not simply repeat what he hears, although there are instances in which he will . . . the child is using the items in his lexicon generatively to create new utterances."

Data for the four-test battery on 75 subjects referred for suspected auditory perceptual difficulties are presented in Table 22.11. These subjects ranged in age from 5 to 18 years. Each was having academic difficulties and social-adjustment problems for reasons undetermined since most also had normal intelligence, normal peripheral hearing skills (pure tone and speech sensitivity and speech discrimination), and average performance on most tests of speech-language-auditory behavior administered in the schools. A study of these relationships is presently in process, and portend some very interesting results. One tentative finding at the moment is the frequent observance of a slightly reduced verbal IQ, on the Wechsler Intelligence Scale for Children in comparison to the performance scale of that measure. (Subsequent data, obtained as this chapter was

TABLE 22.9. *Competing Sentence Performance for Normal Right-Handed Children* *

Age	Strong Ear		No Ear Difference	Total
	Right	Left		
5	9	2	1	12
6	10	3	6	19
7	10	2	6	18
8	7	2	5	14
9	4	0	10	14
Total	40	9	28	77

* Values indicate number of children who had better scores in left and right ears. Each child scored 100% in both ears in the absence of competition.

TABLE 22.10. *Ear Strength on Competing Sentences for Two Age Groups of Normal Subjects* *

Age	N	Strong Ear		No Ear Difference	Percent
		Right	Left		
5–9	77	40	9	28	36
Over 9	38†	4	1	33	87
Total	115	44	10	61	

* Values indicate number of subjects who had better scores in left and right ears.
† Twenty-nine subjects were 10 to 15 years old, 8 were 16 to 25 years old, and 1 subject was 31 years of age.

TABLE 22.11. *Distribution of Abnormal Test Results on Four Measures of Central Auditory Function* *

C	F	B	A – 3	F	B	A – 2
C	F	B – 15			F	B – 16
C	B	A – 3			F	A – 0
	C	F – 4			F	– 7
	C	B – 3			B	A – 3
	C	A – 4			B	– 15
	C	– 0			A	– 0

* Subjects, age 5 to 18 years, all had learning disabilities; N = 75. C, competing sentences; F, low-pass filtered CNC words; B, binaural fusion; A, alternating speech.

about to go to press, failed to confirm this observation. In fact, the reverse has often since been observed in several children.) The test distribution shows that FS and BF tests were the ones most often found abnormal, either alone or in combination. Poor performance on the combination of CS, FS, and BF tests ranked third. It seems noteworthy that the CST and the AS task were never the only tests failed. In fact, the AS measure was seldom failed in any combination of test results. CST results, however, though they were never judged abnormal in isolation, were below normal performance levels in some inter-test pattern for 32 of the 75 subjects.

Table 22.12 presents the results obtained on four selected 6-year-olds who were within 2 months of each other in chronologic age. Each child was righthanded and had normal intelligence and normal hearing by traditional audiometric standards. Each had also been labeled as a LD child even though a multitude of tests by public-school diagnostic teams failed to identify abnormal behaviors on diagnostic tests. All were referred because their academic performances were well below the levels expected of them. The highlight of these results is the tremendous variability in performance among these youngsters on the CST as well as on each of the other measures. These results can best be described as astonishingly diverse. And, while these cases were chosen to show the extremes of test performance we have observed, they are unique only in terms of the magnitude of score differences. Results in many children are readily judged as abnormal, but most are not this dramatic. Identification of unique auditory behavior in these children together with counseling has, in most cases, remarkably altered the child's self-image as well as the opinion in which the child is held by parents and teachers.

Table 22.13 illustrates similar results in a group of older children, each of whom were also righthanded, had normal IQs, and normal peripheral hearing. It is almost superfluous to add that these youngsters lack self-confidence, avoid social events, are noted for misunderstanding instructions at home and assignments at school. Typically, such children and their perplexed parents have spent many hours with school teachers, counselors, in mental health centers, juvenile courts, etc. Thus, evaluation of central auditory function in LD children would seem to hold great promise for literally legions of public school children, and CSs appear to be capable of contributing importantly to that evaluation process.

Other Sentence Applications

Sentences have been used in other applications of central auditory evaluation by Jerger (1964), Frager (1968), Marston and Goetzinger (1972), and by Masterson (1975). The reader is referred to these references for details, or to Berlin and McNeill's (1976) comprehensive review of literature. The references by Frager and by Marston and Goetzinger deal with aging and may be of particular interest. In general, these studies utilized sentence material which was employed as competing messages for monosyllabic test words, asked simple questions which required a yes-no answer against contin-

TABLE 22.12. *Central Auditory Test Results (in Percent) on Selected 6-Year-Olds with Learning Disabilities*

| Subject | Sex | Age | Test Scores by Ear* | | | | | | | |
| | | | CS | | FS | | BF | | AS | |
			L	R	L	R	L	R	L	R
SR	F	6.4	70	30	58	38	60	70	100	100
AM	M	6.5	0	0	70	72	0	10	80	60
CI	M	6.5	0	100	54	48	0	20	100	100
SP	M	6.6	100	100	0	0	5	15	10	20

* CS, competing sentence; FS, filtered speech; BF, binaural fusion; AS, alternating speech.

TABLE 22.13. *Central Auditory Test Results (in Percent) on Selected Older Children with Learning Disabilities*

| Subject | Sex | Age | Test Scores by Ear* | | | | | | | |
| | | | CS | | FS | | BF | | AS | |
			L	R	L	R	L	R	L	R
RW	M	13	100	100	86	76	5	10	100	100
MB	M	14	90	100	48	74	100	90	100	100
LH	F	13	80	10	56	52	50	40	100	100

* Abbreviations as in Table 22.12.

uous discourse competition, etc. However, the SSI and CS materials reviewed in this chapter presently constitute the major use of sentences in the clinical evaluation of central auditory disorders.

REFERENCES

Berlin, C. I., Lowe-Bell, S. S., Cullen, J. K., Thompson, C., and Stafford, M., Is speech "special?" Perhaps the temporal lobectomy patient can tell us. *J. Acoust. Soc. Am.*, 52, 702–705, 1972.

Berlin, C. I., Lowe-Bell, S. S., Cullen, J. K., Thompson, C. L., and Loovis, C. F., Dichotic speech perception; an interpretation of right-ear advantage and temporal offset effects. *J. Acoust. Soc. Am.*, 53, 699–709, 1973.

Berlin, C. I., and McNeill, M. R., Dichotic Listening. In Lass, N.J. (Ed.) *Contemporary Issues in Experimental Phonetics*. New York: Academic Press, 1976.

Butler, K., Hedrick, D., and Manning, C., *Composite Auditory Perceptual Test*. Hayward, Calif.: Alameda County School Department, Revised, 1972.

Flowers, A., Costello, M., and Small, V., *Tests of Central Auditory Abilities*. Dearborn, Mich.: Perceptual Learning Systems, 1970.

Frager, C., Auditory integration in geriatrics. Unpublished master's thesis, Colorado State University, Fort Collins, Col., 1968.

Gilroy, J., and Lynn, G. E., Reversibility of abnormal auditory findings in cerebral hemisphere lesions. *J. Neurol. Sci.*, 21, 117–131, 1974.

Ivey, R. G., Tests of CNS auditory function. Unpublished master's thesis, Colorado State University, Fort Collins, Col., 1969.

Jerger, J., Auditory Tests for Disorders of the Central Auditory Mechanism. In Fields, W. S., and Alford, B. R. (Eds.): *Neurological Aspects of Auditory and Vestibular Disorders*, pp. 77–93. Springfield, Ill.: Charles C Thomas, 1964.

Jerger, J., Speaks, C., and Trammell, J. A., A new approach to speech audiometry, *J. Speech Hear. Disord.*, 33, 318–328, 1968.

Jerger, J., and Jerger, S., Auditory findings in brainstem disorders. *Arch. Otolaryngol.*, 99, 342–349, 1974.

Jerger, J., and Jerger, S., Clinical validity of central auditory tests. *Scand. Audiol.*, 4, 147–163, 1975.

Katz, J., The use of staggered spondaic words for assessing the integrity of the central auditory nervous system., *J. Aud. Res.*, 2, 327–337, 1962.

Kimura, D., A note on cerebral dominance in hearing. *Acta Otolaryngol.*, 56, 617–618, 1963.

Lynn, G. E., and Gilroy, J., Neuro-audiological abnormalities in patients with temporal lobe tumors. *J. Neurol. Sci.*, 17, 167–184, 1972.

Lynn, G. E., Benitez, J. T., Eisenbrey, A. B., Gilroy, J., and Wilner, H. I., Neuro-audiological correlates in cerebral hemisphere lesions; temporal and parietal lobe tumors. *Audiology*, 11, 115–134, 1972.

Lynn, G. E., Auditory Correlates of Neurological Insult. Address delivered as part of "Guest Lecturers in Science" series, Colorado State University, Fort Collins, June 15, 1973.

Lynn, G. E., and Gilroy, J., Effects of Brain Lesions on the Perception of Monotic and Dichotic Speech Stimuli. In Sullivan, M. (Ed.), *Central Auditory Processing Disorders*. Omaha: University of Nebraska Press, 1975.

Marston, L. E., and Goetzinger, C. P., A comparison of sensitized words and sentences for distinguishing nonperipheral auditory changes as a function of aging. *Cortex*, 8, 213–223, 1972.

Masterson, P., Psychoacoustic processing of dichotic sentences by preschool children. *J. Aud. Res.*, 15, 130–139, 1975.

Matzker, J., The binaural test. *J. Int. Audiol.*, 1, 209–211, 1962.

Matzker, J., Two new methods for the assessment of central auditory functions in cases of brain disease. *Ann. Otol. Rhinol. Laryngol.*, 68, 1185–1197, 1959.

Menyuk, P., Sentences children use. M.I.T. Research Monograph No. 52, Cambridge, Mass., 1969.

Porter, R., and Berlin, I., On interpreting developmental changes in the dichotic right-ear advantage. *Brain Lang.*, 2, 186–200, 1975.

Sparks, R., Goodglass, H., and Nickel, B., Ipsilateral vs. contralateral extinction in dichotic listening resulting from hemisphere lesions. *Cortex*, 6, 249–260, 1970.

Speaks, C., Dichotic Listening; A Clinical or Research Tool? In Sullivan, M. (Ed.), *Central Auditory Processing Disorders*. Omaha: University of Nebraska Press, 1975.

Speaks, C., and Jerger, J., Method for measurement of speech identification. *J. Speech Hear. Res.*, 8, 185–194, 1965.

Treisman, A. M., The effect of irrelevant material on the efficiency of selective listening. *Am. J. Psychol.*, 77, 533–546, 1964.

Wingfield, A., Acoustic redundancy and the perception of time-compressed speech. *J. Speech Hear. Res.*, 18, 96–104, 1975.

Willeford, J., Competing sentences for diagnostic purposes, Unpublished material, Colorado State University, Fort Collins, Col., 1968.

chapter 23

THE STAGGERED SPONDAIC WORD TEST

Michael Brunt, Ph.D.

The other chapters in this section provide the reader with a wealth of information about the central auditory process as it relates to differential diagnosis. Speech audiometry seems to be the most useful approach to the evaluation of the central auditory nervous system (CANS). The present chapter is devoted to the staggered spondaic word (SSW) test, a speech procedure which is used as a measure of central auditory dysfunction. The SSW test is a dichotic procedure (i.e., different signals are presented to each ear). The subject is expected to repeat both messages. Unlike most of the available tests of CANS, the SSW test has been standardized on a rather large sample of normal subjects as well as on patients with a variety of peripheral and central problems.

CONSIDERATIONS IN DEVELOPING THE TEST

In devising the SSW test, Katz (1962, 1968) sought a task free of contamination from peripheral hearing disorders which would require very little patient sophistication, but still would be sensitive to central auditory disorders. Spondaic words were chosen to reduce test errors due to peripheral hearing problems. Spondaic words are relatively familiar to most patients and are essentially 100% intelligible over a wider range of intensities than monosyllabic words. In order to capitalize as much as possible on the advantages of spondees and yet sensitize them to central problems they were given in the dichotic mode.

TECHNIQUE AND EQUIPMENT

General Comments

Each test item is composed of two spondees recorded in a partially overlapped fashion. One spondee is sent to each ear. Figure 23.1 illustrates that each ear receives stimulation in isolation as well as in competition with the other. For example, "up" is heard as a right noncompeting (R-NC) condition while "stairs" and "down" are heard as right competing (R-C) and left competing (L-C) conditions, respectively. Finally, "town" is heard as the left noncompeting (L-NC) condition. As shown, the ear stimulated first changes from item to item.

Equipment and Presentation

The standard SSW test (List EC*), consisting of 4 practice and 40 test items is available as a 2-channel tape. Total test time is about 10 min. Test administration requires independent control of presentation level for each ear. A high fidelity stereo tape recorder routed through a 2-channel speech audiometer is most appropriate.

The SSW test was standardized at a presentation level of 50 dB re speech reception threshold (SRT) to eliminate the influence of intensity on word accuracy. This presentation level of 50 dB sensation level (SL) should be used when at all possible although Balas and Simon (1964) found near 100% accuracy with normal subjects at 30 dB SL. Obviously, 50 dB SL would be contraindicated for patients with severe hearing loss or tolerance problems.

Explanation and Example of Scoring Procedure

Figure 23.2 illustrates the final page of the SSW test form. In this example the hypothetical patient received the odd numbered items first in the right ear (right ear first or right ear leading) and the even numbered items first in the left ear. For example, Column A is for the right-noncompeting (R-NC) condition, Columns B and C for the right competing (R-C) and left competing (L-C) conditions with Column D for the left noncompeting (L-NC) condition. In scoring, an error is counted for each monosyllable or half-spondee incorrect. Account is taken of all errors whether they are word substitutions (Item 29), nonlinguistic substitutions (Item 28) or omissions (Item 34).

Other patterns of response also are given on the SSW test by some patients. These responses have been termed "reversals," "ear effect" and "order effect." These factors will be mentioned after the basic scoring is discussed.

Raw SSW (R-SSW) Score

1. **Number of Errors.** Initially, errors for each condition (R-C, R-NC, L-C and L-NC) are individually summed. Individual ear performance is the average of the competing and noncompeting errors for the ear in question. From our example (Fig. 23.2) for the right ear there were 22 errors; i.e., (R-NC + R-C)/2 or, (17 errors + 27 errors)/2. Accordingly, the total SSW score is the average of the two ear scores.

* Test as well as test manual and score sheets available from AUDITEC of St. Louis, 402 Pasadena Avenue, St. Louis, MO 63119.

TIME SEQUENCE

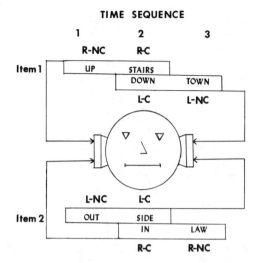

Fig. 23.1. Example of two SSW test items illustrating temporal sequence of word presentation and reversal of the leading ear.

From our example the raw errors would be classified as:

R-NC	R-C	L-C	L-NC
17	27	10	5
Right ear		Left ear	
22		8	
	Total SSW		
	15		

2. Percent of Error. These errors are then converted to percentage error by the appropriate multiplier. For the usual test presentation of 40 items the multiplier is 2.5 ($2.5 \times 40 = 100\%$). Multipliers are listed on the test form for a 20-, 25- or 30-item test. As with the raw number of errors, the percent of error is computed for each condition (R-NC, R-C, L-C and L-NC). Ear scores are the average percent error of the competing and noncompeting conditions for the ear in question while the total SSW percent error score is the average of the two ear scores.

To elucidate this we may turn to the number of errors for our patient above. There was a total of 17 R-NC and 27 R-C errors. Multiplying each by 2.5 results in 42% error for the R-NC and 68% for the R-C conditions. For the right ear, then, the average percent error is 55%. Summarizing all raw SSW scores in percentage of error we have:

R-NC	R-C	L-C	L-NC
42%	68%	25%	12%
Right ear		Left ear	
55%		18%	
	Total SSW		
	36%		

Corrected SSW (C-SSW) Score

Katz originally chose spondaic words as the signals to avoid contamination by peripheral hearing disorders. However, Katz, Basil and Smith (1963) noted a high, positive correlation ($r = 0.92$) between SSW performance and word discrimination for W-22s in subjects with conductive and sensory-neural losses. Katz (1968) replicated this finding ($r = 0.93$) in a study of patients with cochlear losses. Therefore, raw SSW scores are corrected to reduce the effects of word discrimination errors. The percentage of word discrimination error is subtracted from the SSW error score for the same ear.

Let us assume our patient's discrimination score was 92% for the right ear and 82% for the left leaving 8 and 18% error for the right and left ears, respectively. For the R-NC condition the corrected SSW (C-SSW) score would now be 34% (42% − 8%). The average word discrimination error for the two ears would be subtracted from the total SSW error leaving an error of 23% (36% − 13%). The corrected (C-SSW) error scores are then:

R-NC	R-C	L-C	L-NC
34%	60%	7%	−6%
Right ear		Left ear	
47%		0%	
	Total SSW		
	23%		

Using the C-SSW score widens the application of the SSW to patients with peripheral hearing loss. Valuable information then may be derived from patients as to their central auditory system even if they do evidence peripheral loss.

Other Patterns of Response on the SSW

Three patterns of response sometimes encountered on the SSW are the reversal, the ear effect and the order effect. Reference to Figure 23.2 will provide a useful guide for the following discussion of these responses.

For each test item most patients report the leading spondee first. However, some will give word reversals which are noted on the answer sheet but are not included in the basic scoring. The two most common classes of reversals are the *true reversal* and the *probable reversal*. Item 23 in Figure 23.2 illustrates a true reversal in which the second spondee is given first. A *probable* (formerly called *partial*) reversal is similar with the exception that an error on one monosyllable is either a substitution or a distortion (Item 35). The sum of these reversals is termed *total reversals*. In our example there were 11 reversals, 6 true and 5 probable.

Recently Katz and Pack (1975) also have included the category of *questionable reversal*.

PAGE 3

	(A)	(B)	(C)	(D)	Rev	WRONG		(E)	(F)	(G)	(H)	Rev	WRONG
21.	hair 3	clip (net) 4	tooth 1	brush 2	T Ⓟ Q	1	22.	pro (fruit)	team (juice)	— (cup)	steak (cake)	T P Q	4
23.	ash 3	tray 4	tin 1	can 2	Ⓣ P Q	•	24.	nite	light	guard (yard)	— (stick)	T P Q	2
25.	key 3	note (chain) 4	tooth (suit) 1	paste (case) 2	T P Q	3	26.	play	ground	bat	— (boy)	T P Q	1
27.	corn	starch	— soap —	— flakes —	T P Q	2	28.	birth	day	[z3] (first)	place	T P Q	1
29.	day	light (break)	lamp	light	T P Q	1	30.	door 2	knob 3	— (low)	bell 1	T P Ⓠ	1
31.	bird 3	cage 4	crow's 1	nest 2	Ⓣ P Q	•	32.	week	— (end)	— (work)	day	T P Q	2
33.	— book —	— shelf —	— drug —	— store —	T P Q	4	34.	wood	work	— (beach)	craft	T P Q	1
35.	hand 3	shake (butt) 4	milk 1	shake 2	T Ⓟ Q	1	36.	fish	net	sky	line	T P Q	•
37.	— for —	— give —	milk	man	T P Q	2	38.	sheep	skin	— (bull)	rug (dog)	T P Q	2
39.	lace (rose)	[ʃɜ] (horse)	street	car	T P Q	2	40.	green	house	— (string)	bean	T P Q	1
SUM Page 3	3	7	3	3		16	SUM Page 3	1	2	8	4		15
SUM Page 2	3	6	1	0		10	SUM Page 2	1	4	6	7		18
TOTAL	6	13	4	3		26	TOTAL	2	6	14	11		33
Left First	L-NC	L-C	R-C	R-NC				R-NC	R-C	L-C	L-NC		
	(A)	(B)	(C)	(D)				(E)	(F)	(G)	(H)		
Right First	R-NC	R-C	L-C	L-NC				L-NC	L-C	R-C	R-NC		

EAR EFFECT	RE First	LE First
Total Errors		
☑ Sig. ☐ N. Sig.	26	33

REVERSALS		
True	Prob.	Quest.
6	5	1

Maximum Rev's = 12

ORDER EFFECT			
1	2	3	4
8	19	18	14

FIRST SPONDEE 27   SECOND SPONDEE 32

☑ Sig   ☐ N. Sig

COMBINED TOTALS	RNC	RC	LC	LNC
(A) - (D) or (E) - (H)	6	13	4	3
(H) - (E) or (D) - (A)	11	14	6	2
	17	27	10	5

Enter these figures on Page 1.

Fig. 23.2. Final page of an SSW test form.

A questionable reversal (Item 30) is where one of the four half-spondees is omitted while the other three are given out of order. The sum of true, probable and questionable reversals is termed *maximum reversals*. Reversal responses have been useful in providing qualitative information on patients with lesions in the cortex but outside the primary auditory reception area.*

Since test items are presented so each ear serves as the leading ear for half the test items and the trailing ear for the other half the SSW scores should not be contaminated by various response biases. In spite of item counterbalancing an ear effect and/or an order effect is evident in some patients.

The ear and order effects, if significant, call for an adjustment in the SSW score; also correction for discrimination errors is made. If both effects are significant, adjustment is made only for the one showing the most difference between the halves of the test (i.e., either between right ear first and left ear first (ear effect) or between the first spondee and the second spondee (order effect). Such an adjustment provides a "cleaner" representation of auditory reception function with regard to the SSW test findings (Katz and Pack, 1975).

* The "primary auditory reception area" or center is Heschl's gyrus or Brodmann's area 41 — the anatomical site being the area of the superior temporal gyrus posterior and inferior to the fissure of Rolando.

Examination for an ear effect is done by summing the errors for Columns A through D and comparing them to the summed errors for Columns E through H. These sums are placed in the appropriate spaces on the answer sheet (Fig. 23.2) under "ear effect." A difference of 5 or more is considered significant.

Analysis of the SSW results considers the corrected and the adjusted (A-SSW) scores. The A-SSW score is based on the half of the test least in error. In our example, this comprises Columns A through D (26 errors versus 33 errors for Columns E through H). Since only half of the test items are used in the analysis the multipliers to determine raw percent error are double those for the whole test. Let us examine this scoring considering only the condition scores. The errors would be:

R-NC	R-C	L-C	L-NC
6	13	4	3

For the usual 40-item test to find raw percent error per condition we would multiply by 2.5. For the A-SSW conditions we would multiply by 5. For the R-NC condition the raw percent error adjusted for the ear effect would be 30% (6 errors times 5). Our raw percent errors are then:

R-NC	R-C	L-C	L-NC
30%	65%	20%	15%

Following that we merely correct these scores for discrimination errors giving results adjusted for the ear effect and corrected for word discrimination score (WDS) errors. Previously we assumed 8% WDS error for the right ear and 18% error for the left. Subtracting these errors appropriately we find the A-SSW scores of:

R-NC	R-C	L-C	L-NC
22%	57%	2%	−3%

For the order effect the errors for the first spondee (Columns A, B, E and F) are summed and compared to the errors for the second spondee (Columns C, D, G and H). As with the ear effect, these sums are entered on the test form. A difference of 5 or more is considered significant. Adjusting for an order effect is similar to that for the ear effect. For the order effect one also scores the half of the SSW test least in error; i.e., either all the first spondees or all the second.

NORMAL PERFORMANCE ON THE SSW TEST

A series of studies have dealt with normal hearing subjects on the SSW test, List EC and its forerunners. In all instances the format of test presentation has been identical. The lists differed in the number of test items and there was some variation in the equipment used for the test preparation and presentation. These variations were shown to have had very little effect on the results.

Table 23.1 summarizes normative studies on the SSW test. Overall findings suggest that normal individuals from 11 to 60 years of age will make few errors on the SSW test. Furthermore, the small standard deviations for all studies indicate little variability among normal listeners. It may be noted that some total corrected SSW scores are listed as negative. This means that there was a greater percent error on the routine speech discrimination test than on the SSW. Therefore, when the R-SSW was corrected for discrimination errors the C-SSW was overcorrected. This overcorrection is usually minor and most commonly seen in patients with sensory-neural losses. A more detailed discussion of these normative studies may be found in Brunt (1972).

SSW STANDARD BASED ON CORRECTED SCORES

The SSW standard (Table 23.2) for corrected scores was offered by Katz in 1968 as an interim one. This standard was based on a portion of

TABLE 23.1. *Means and Standard Deviations for Total Raw and Corrected Staggered Spondaic Word (SSW) Scores for Various Age Groups and Lists*

Study	N	List	Age	Age Range	Total Raw SSW	Total Corrected SSW	S.D. Corrected SSW
Katz, Basil, and Smith (1963)	20	1A	20	14–28	98.8	−0.4	1.5
Katz and Fishman (1964)	10	1B	22	20–29	98.3	0.8	1.9
	10	1B	35	31–39	97.7	1.4	1.9
	10	1B	44	40–48	97.7	1.3	1.9
Burgess (1964)	10	1B	55	51–59	97.0	3.0	2.6
Goldman and Katz (1966)	24	1B	24	18–39	98.3	−0.3	2.2
Katz and Myrick (1965)	10	C-EC	23	19–29	97.8	−1.3	2.2
Brunt (1969) (40 diabetics and 40 non-diabetics)	80	EC	45	16–61	97.1	−4.6*	4.97

* This lower mean is attributed to poorer word discrimination than the other groups.

TABLE 23.2. *Upper and Lower Limits for 5 Corrected Staggered Spondaic Word Score (C-SSW) Categories*

	Overcorrected	Normal	Mildly Abnormal	Moderately Abnormal	Severely Abnormal
Total score	− −5	−4–5	6–15	16–35	36–100
Ear score	− −7	−6–10	11–20	21–40	41–100
Condition score	− −10	−9–15	16–25	26–45	46–100

(Adapted from Katz, 1973.)

the normal hearing subjects from studies cited in Table 23.1 as well as on 17 patients with surgically confirmed or medically diagnosed brain lesions. Ten of these patients had unilateral auditory reception lesions while the other 7 had lesions sparing the middle, and posterior superior temporal gyri. In an attempt to avoid bias by comparing only normals to those with central nervous systm (CNS) lesions, results from patients with conductive and sensory-neural losses were included as well. Experience with the test by Katz and associates (1970a, 1970b, 1973, 1975) and others has shown that the interim standard can be accepted as the standard with only minor modification.

As would be expected, individuals with normal hearing, conductive and sensory-neural losses generally perform in the "normal" range. The "overcorrected" category, which was added to the standard, includes patients with sensory-neural losses. Patients with moderate or severe scores can be suspected of having disorder of the auditory reception center. We are left with the mildly abnormal category.

Patients with mildly abnormal scores may or may not have a CANS lesion. Some patients have been called, for want of more definitive information, "abnormal listeners." More commonly this category includes individuals with conductive or sensory-neural losses or patients with CNS lesions lying outside the primary auditory reception area.

In clinical application one compares the most extreme corrected SSW scores, either positive or negative, for condition, ear and total SSW score to the standard. Katz and associates (1973, 1975) note that, among the three score categories, the ear score often is the most sensitive to the presence or absence of a CANS problem. Adjustment of SSW scores is appropriate in cases of significant ear or order effects. Even with such adjustment the SSW standard above (Table 23.2) still is advocated.

SSW AND CENTRAL AUDITORY NERVOUS SYSTEM DYSFUNCTION

General Comments

Thus far we have discussed the results found in normal subjects and patients with peripheral hearing loss. More detail may be found elsewhere (Brunt, 1972). The following sections will describe the results, value and limitations of the SSW test. Discussion of the SSW generally will follow an historical pattern. Remarks will center on new as well as previous information stressing results on patients with medically or surgically confirmed CNS disorder. A brief mention will be made of early findings, the details of which are in Brunt (1972) or the original sources. Where reference is made to C-SSW scores as "normal," "mildly abnormal," etc., these will refer to the standards of Table 23.2.

Early Findings on the SSW Test

Tests such as the SSW, which are sensitive to cerebral auditory dysfunction show reduced performance in the ear opposite the involved hemisphere. The C-SSW score is moderately to severely reduced when there is dysfunction in the auditory reception center. Figure 23.3 illustrates raw and corrected SSW findings on one such case as well as SSW results in a patient with a central nonauditory reception lesion.

Preliminary findings on the SSW were reported in 1962 (Katz) on three cases of suspected CANS involvement. One, a 24-year-old male patient, as the result of an automobile accident at 5 years of age had residual scars on the temporal, parietal and occipital regions of the right side of the skull. Another was an 11-year-old cerebral palsied female patient with primarily left-sided involvement while the third was a 60-year-old man. All had normal hearing sensitivity and very good WDS for both ears. However, the man with a history of skull trauma had a moderately abnormal (L-C = 38%) score and the girl with cerebral palsy had a severely abnormal (R-C = 70%) C-SSW score. In both cases the reduced performance was for the competing condition in the ear opposite the supposed lesion. The 60-year-old man evidenced moderate to severely abnormal (R-C = 48%, L-C = 30%) C-SSW scores for the competing conditions. Further discussion of older cases will be found in the section on the elderly.

Katz, Basil and Smith (1963) reported on six cases of unilateral head trauma as evidenced by head scars, unilateral paralysis or both. For all six, hearing sensitivity was normal with excellent speech discrimination scores for both ears. The mean C-SSW score for the competing

SSW TEST

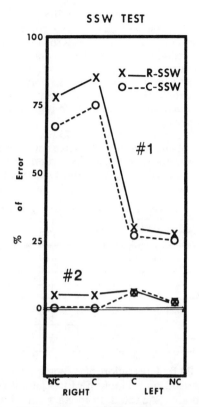

Fig. 23.3. Raw (R-SSW) and corrected (C-SSW) test results on two cases with central nervous system lesions. *Case 1:* 26-year-old male patient with left temporoparietal vascular accident; *Case 2:* 20-year-old male patient with right parietal vascular accident.

they could be classified in the moderately abnormal category (R-C = 34.5%, L-C = 34.8%). Figure 23.4 presents the findings for all cerebral palsied subjects as well as for the "older" and "younger" CP groups.

The above studies lend support to the SSW as a measure of CANS function although there was no direct evidence specifically concerning central auditory areas. However, in 1965 Berlin, Chase, Dill and Hagepanos reported on a series of patients with right ($N = 17$) and left ($N = 12$) temporal lobe lesions as compared to normals ($N = 11$). All were given seven verbal test procedures, including the SSW test. On the SSW the patients did significantly poorer for the ear opposite the lesion. Their performance placed them in the mildly abnormal category. It is interesting that of the seven procedures evaluated, only on the SSW (a) did both the right and left temporal lobe subjects exhibit a significant difference between ears (more depressed in the ear contralateral to the lesion) and (b) did patients in *both* groups perform significantly poorer than normals. Berlin et al. stated that the SSW was a promising clinical measure for assessing CANS function.

In determining the norms as well as the validity of the SSW test Katz (1968) administered the SSW test to 17 patients with medically diagnosed or surgically confirmed cerebral problems. At the time of testing the site of lesion was not known but determined independently by a neurologist. Neurologic judgments were made on a six-point scale ranging from "definitely nonauditory" reception to "definitely auditory" reception lesions of the brain.

condition for the ear contralateral to the suspected lesion was moderately abnormal (27%) indicating a central auditory reception problem.

In another study the SSW was administered to 26 cerebral palsied individuals and matched controls (Katz, Myrick and Winn, 1966). The total mean C-SSW was normal for the controls. However, the C-SSW results for the cerebral palsied group on competing items (R-C = 20.9, L-C = 22.5) placed them in the mildly abnormal category. Katz, Myrick and Winn noted better C-SSW performance by the older cerebral palsied subjects than the younger. Therefore, both control and cerebral palsied subjects were each divided into two groups of "older" and "younger"; younger defined as 13 years (the median) of age or below.

For each group competing conditions were pooled and an analysis of variance was carried out. Results showed that the younger cerebral palsied group differed significantly from the other three groups. On the competing items

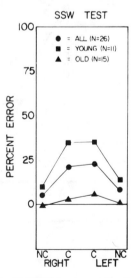

Fig. 23.4. C-SSW test results for all cerebral palsied subjects, "older" and "younger" cerebral palsied subjects. See text.

Figure 23.5 presents the SSW results on these patients as related to neurologic judgments.

The close correspondence of the total C-SSW scores with neurologic judgments is apparent. Note, too, that the scores adjusted for either ear or order effect still approximate the original C-SSW scores for those patients judged as having "definitely" or "very likely" auditory reception lesions. This close correspondence is the usual case for patients with damage in or very close to the primary cortical auditory reception area. On the other hand, when scores are adjusted for ear or order effects and adjusted results tend to be normal or mild, CNS damage is not near the primary auditory reception area.

Recent Findings on the SSW for Patients with Known CNS Lesions

Katz and Pack. Katz and Pack (1975) assumed that a more precise relationship could be established between SSW results and CANS problems if patients with carefully localized lesions were studied. They surmised that a three-dimensional representation of the lesion would be most accurate in correlating the SSW findings. To this end they obtained and cut an average sized human brain into 12 1-cm sagittal sections. A grid pattern consisting of 1-cm sides was placed over a drawing of the brain. Figure 23.6 illustrates this grid pattern in re-

lation to the sagittal view of the brain. By comparing these sections and the grid pattern to medical and surgical findings the extent and depth of cerebral lesions of patients could be more accurately estimated than without such aids. For example, in Figure 23.6 Area E-9 corresponds to the primary auditory reception area, commonly known as Brodmann's area 41 or Heschl's gyrus.

After the preliminary work 75 patients with CNS problems were evaluated in a double-blind procedure. For each patient the extent of CNS lesion was localized from autopsy, surgical re-

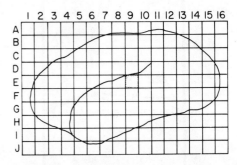

Fig. 23.6. Illustration of a labeled grid superimposed on a diagram of the lateral view of a brain. (Adapted from Katz and Pack, 1975.)

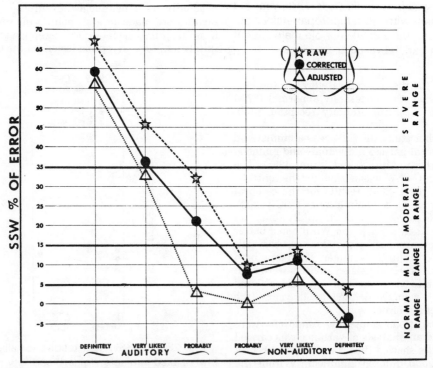

Fig. 23.5. Total SSW scores versus neurologic categorization of cortical lesions.

port, radiologic data or neurologic evaluation and plotted relative to the brain sections and grid pattern.

Independent of these judgments all patients were evaluated on various audiologic tests including the SSW. From these 75 patients 30 were selected for study based on the neurologist's information. Sixteen had tumors, 9 had vascular disease, 3 had damage from trauma and 2 from surgery.

The 30 subjects retained were those with clear-cut lesions confined and clearly localized to one hemisphere, those excluded were patients with lesions outside the cerebrum. Thirteen of the cases were considered by the neurologist to have lesions affecting grid area E-9 or the primary auditory reception area. These were termed the *auditory reception* (AR) group. The other 17 had lesions outside grid area E-9 and were called the *nonauditory reception* (NAR) group.

The mean age of the 30 subjects was 48 years. There were 14 female and 16 male patients. No subjects were excluded because of hearing loss. The mean SRT was 3 dB hearing threshold level (HTL) in each ear and ranged from −10 to 48 dB HTL. Word discrimination means were 92% and 91% for the right and left

ears, respectively, with a range from 68% to 100%.

Figure 23.7, *A* and *B,* presents mean C-SSW results with standard deviations for the AR and NAR cases. Findings are given relative to performance for the ear contralateral versus the ear ipsilateral to the lesion. The 13 AR cases mean C-SSW ear error for the ear contralateral to the lesion was 53% (severely abnormal) with individual results ranging from 34 to 77% error. In short, on these patients there was 100% correct diagnosis of hemisphere and site of lesion.

In contrast the mean C-SSW ear error for the 17 NAR cases was 5 (normal) for the ear contralateral to the damaged hemisphere. The NAR contralateral C-SSW ear score ranged from −4 to 18% (normal to mildly abnormal). Table 23.3 presents results for the NAR group relative to the damaged hemisphere and the ear with the poorer competing condition. These data show that of the 17 NAR cases the peak errors occurred for the ear contralateral to the lesion in 12 cases, peaked in the ipsilateral ear in three cases and showed equivalent errors bilaterally in two patients.

If one only examines the peak errors as indicating which hemisphere is damaged, the SSW test was successful in picking out 71% of these NAR patients. However, the NAR patients as a group and individually performed within normal limits in most cases. Extreme caution should be used in identifying the side of lesion in NAR cases based on the peak SSW error. Even when the SSW test is normal or mild some qualitative information about intrahemispheric lesions may be obtained from "reversals."

In previous work Katz (1970a) had noted that patients who had reversals on test items had lesions which tended to involve especially the pre- and post-central gyri (frontoparietal region) as well as the anterior temporal lobe. He had tentatively identified this area as the "reversal strip." This reversal strip in general corresponds to Columns 6 and 7 on the grid pattern (Fig. 23.6), especially squares C-6 and

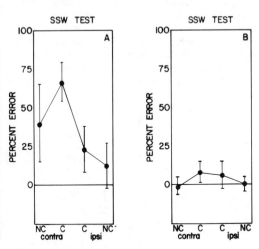

Fig. 23.7. (A) Means and standard deviations for the four competing and noncompeting C-SSW conditions for the thirteen AR patients of Katz and Pack (1975). Data presented relative to ear contralateral and ipsilateral to the damaged hemisphere. (B) Means and standard deviations for the four competing and noncompeting C-SSW conditions for the 17 NAR subjects of Katz and Pack (1975). Data presented relative to ear contralateral and ipsilateral to the damaged hemisphere.

TABLE 23.3. *Distribution of 17 Nonauditory Reception (NAR) Subjects Relative to Damaged Hemisphere and Ear with Poorer Competing Condition*

Damaged Hemisphere	C-SSW* Competing Condition			
	Right poorer	Left poorer	Right equal left	Total
Left	5	2	1	8
Right	1	7	1	9
Total	6	9	2	17

* C-SSW, corrected staggered spondaic word score.
(Adapted from Katz and Pack, 1975.)

C-7. Katz and Pack (1975) indicated some similar findings by Luria (1970) and Efron (1965, as cited by Masland, 1969) with aphasics who evidenced trouble in auditory sequencing.

Among the 17 NAR cases who had damage anterior to Area E-9, 9 had shown reversals ranging from 1 to 28 with a mean of 11. Therefore, Katz and Pack correlated the reversal data to the areas of damage in the NAR cases. The sagittal sections used in this comparison were the two most lateral 1-cm sections for each hemisphere as well as the two sections per hemisphere medial to these. The data were combined for both right and left hemisphere cases as there was no difference in performance between them.

The presence or absence of reversals for the 17 NAR patients was considered with regard to site of lesion. Overall, the relationship of site of lesion and reversals was most predictable for Columns 6 and 7. For example, of the 13 patients who had damage to Column 6, 9 showed reversals. Four of the 13 with Column 6 damage showed no reversals. Out of 17 NAR patients 13 would have been correctly diagnosed as to site of lesion. Four patients fell into the false negative category; i.e., damage to Column 6 but no reversals. The overall data suggest that reversals strongly imply damage to Column 6 but their absence, because of false negative findings, does not rule out Column 6 damage.

For the nine NAR patients who evidenced reversals the majority of the reversals occurred when there was damage to cortical areas corresponding to Row C (Fig. 23.6). The trend was for reversals to decrease from Row C down to Row I. Overall, the data suggest that the reversals or lack of them more closely correspond to the condition of Columns 6 and 7 than to any other.

In summary, the present findings suggest that if there is damage to the motor and sensory strips along the fissure of Rolando and, to some degree in the anterior temporal lobe, there will tend to be reversals. Pending additional cases the "reversal strip" would appear to comprise the motor and sensory strip (Columns 6 and 7) as well as the anterior temporal lobe.

SSW Findings of Other Researchers. Lynn, Benitez, Eisenbrey, Gilroy and Wilner (1972), Lynn and Gilroy (1972) and Gilroy and Lynn (1974) present data on the SSW and other CANS procedures relative to CNS tumors affecting the temporal or parietal lobes. The following discussion will show the importance of comparing the SSW results to other audiologic data. All SSW results are given here as C-SSW scores as opposed to raw scores in the original articles. Tests other than the SSW which Lynn, Gilroy and their associates have

employed were a version of Matzker's (1959) binaural resynthesis test, low-pass filtered (LPF) speech (Hodgson, 1972) and Willeford's (1968, 1974; see also chapter 22) competing sentence (CS) test.

Lynn et al. (1972) presented results on a 56-year-old man initially diagnosed and later surgically confirmed as having a right parietal lobe tumor with no direct effect on the right temporal lobe. Figure 23.8 presents pre- and postoperative results on the SSW, LPF speech and on the CS test. As would be expected, none of the preoperative tests suggested a temporal lobe problem. Six months later the patient returned because of recurrent seizures. The postoperative findings from Figure 23.8 illustrate a significant change on the SSW, LPF speech and on the CS test. Together they are suggestive of a right temporal lobe problem. (Note, however, that the L-C condition falls in the mildly abnormal range, not a strong indicator of auditory reception involvement. The authors did note that in their experience such SSW performance may be taken as abnormal but not what would be expected in cases of "primary temporal lobe tumor.") The binaural resynthesis test also suggested a brain stem problem in the CANS. Interestingly, medical information at that time gave no indication of temporal lobe or brain stem pathology. However, 2 months later medical examination did suggest temporal lobe pathology while autopsy showed tumor invasion of the temporal lobe as well as significant brain stem involvement.

In 1972 Lynn and Gilroy reported on 11 patients with temporal lobe lesions of whom 10

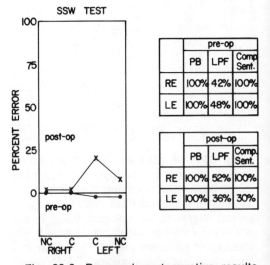

Fig. 23.8. Pre- and postoperative results on a 56-year-old male patient with a recurrent tumor of the right parietal lobe. (Adapted from Lynn et al., 1972.)

were administered the SSW. These 10 were divided into one group of 5 with "posterior" temporal lobe tumors and 5 with "anterior-inferior" temporal lobe tumors. Figure 23.9A presents C-SSW results on 4 of the posterior tumor group while Figure 23.9B illustrates findings on the 5 anterior-inferior lesion patients. All results are given relative to the ear contralateral and ipsilateral to the tumor.

Of the four posterior temporal lobe patients illustrated all evidenced three or more C-SSW scores (i.e., total, ear or condition scores) which

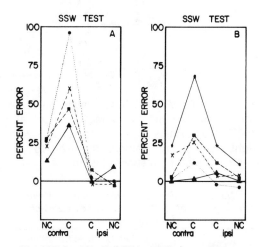

Fig. 23.9. (A) C-SSW results on four patients with posterior temporal lobe tumors. Results given relative to ear contralateral and ipsilateral to the damaged hemisphere. (Adapted from Lynn and Gilroy, 1972.) (●-----●, OW-M; ×-·-×, MB; ■---■, RH; △——△, OW-F). (B) C-SSW results on five patients with anterior-inferior temporal lobe tumors. Results given relative to ear contralateral and ipsilateral to the damaged hemisphere. (Adapted from Lynn and Gilroy, 1972.) (*——*, SS; ■---■, GL; ×-·-×, HR; ●-----●, FA; ▲——▲, CL.)

placed them in the moderately to severely abnormal range suggesting a lesion in the region of the primary auditory reception area. None showed abnormal scores for the ear ipsilateral to the lesion. Thus, these four were correctly identified by the SSW test, alone, as having an auditory reception lesion without recourse to the rest of the battery. It was enlightening to see that results for three of the posterior temporal lobe patients could be correctly diagnosed despite cochlear hearing loss, abnormal discrimination and exceeding of the 60-year-old limit for normal performance.

The fifth patient performed abnormally on the SSW according to Lynn and Gilroy although the C-SSW results fell within the normal range. Overall findings on this patient as summarized in Table 23.4 point out the value of inter-test relationships. In this particular case, all information taken together suggested a unilateral temporal lobe lesion for the left hemisphere.

The five patients with anterior-inferior temporal lobe tumors (Figure 23.9B) had fewer errors than the patients with posterior tumors. On the SSW test two patients showed severely and moderately abnormal scores, one evidenced mildly abnormal results while two had quantitatively normal scores. Without response bias the SSW test would not have identified the latter two CNS lesions. (On these same five cases only one did poorly on the competing sentence test.) Such findings would suggest that, in general, these patients had temporal lobe disruption away from or minimally affecting the primary auditory reception area as based on the Katz and Pack data. Such is the supposition given by Lynn and Gilroy. Overall, the Lynn and Gilroy data provide independent support for Katz' SSW findings.

Finally, Gilroy and Lynn (1974) provide pre- and postoperative data on three cases with CNS damage indicating CANS test value in following the course of the disorder. One case is given as illustration.

TABLE 23.4. *Audiologic Findings on Patient (BH-53-F) with Posterior Left Temporoparietal Tumor*[*]

Ear	PTA	PB	LPF	Comp Sent	Ear	Binaural Resynthesis	
		%	%	%		R-LB	R-HB
						L-HB	L-LB
Right ear	32	48	0	0			
Left ear	30	100	2	100		%	%
					Right ear	0	45
		C-SSW			Left ear	40	20
	R-NC	R-C	L-C	L-NC	Binaural	75	85
	−20	13	10	2			

* PTA, pure tone average; PB, phonetically balanced; LPF, low-pass filtered; Comp Sent, competing sentences; C-SSW, corrected staggered spondaic word score; R-NC and R-C, right noncompeting and competing; L-C and L-NC, left competing and noncompeting; R-LB: right low pass band, L-LB: left low pass band, R-HB: right high pass band, L-HB: left high pass band.

(Adapted from Lynn and Gilroy, 1972, and Lynn et al., 1972.)

A 24-year-old normal hearing woman was found to have a right parietal lobe tumor. Initial preoperative findings showed mildly abnormal SSW findings for the contralateral (left) ear but normal results on routine and LPF speech discrimination. Postoperative results were normal on all three tests and on the CS test.

Subsequent tumor regrowth occasioned a second preoperative audiologic examination. Among the four measures mentioned above the SSW was mildly abnormal; the others suggesting no problem. A third operation also followed with two postoperative evaluations before the patient succumbed. On these latter two, results for the SSW were moderately abnormal and competing sentence test findings were abnormal while no problem was suggested by routine and LPF speech discrimination.

The SSW results at first glance appear atypical as the tumor was in the parietal lobe. However, surgical and autopsy findings confirmed that there was interference with corpus callosal auditory pathways deep in the parietal lobe. These medical-surgical results confirmed Gilroy and Lynn's contention that the SSW can pick up auditory pathway interference at the corpus callosum which would go undetected with LPF speech. Johnson and Katz (1971) had noted such results on patients with lesions affecting the corpus callosal structures but not the primary auditory reception area.

The SSW test was given to 15 normals and two groups of patients with left (N = 15) and right (N = 15) hemisphere lesions by McClellan, Wertz and Collins (1973). Among the three groups there was no significant difference with respect to age, education, pure tone thresholds, SRTs or speech discrimination.

Both pathologic groups performed abnormally on the SSW and significantly different from the normals. Figure 23.10 presents mean results for all three groups as a function of condition (R-NC, R-C, etc.). The right hemisphere lesion group performed poorly in the left ear as would be expected. The left hemisphere lesion patients showed abnormal results for both ears but somewhat poorer for the right ear.

Table 23.5 summarizes data for the two pathologic groups relative to normal and abnormal performance. Twenty-four of the 30 CNS patients evidenced abnormal performance. The four who performed normally may not have had damage to primary auditory reception areas. Of more interest are the patients who showed significant errors for both ears, especially the left hemisphere group. An obvious suggestion is that those with bilateral errors had damage to both hemispheres except for the

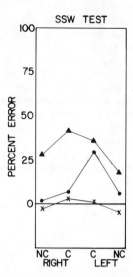

Fig. 23.10. Mean C-SSW results on three groups of patients (from McClellan et al., 1973). (15 normals, ×——×; 15 patients with right hemisphere lesions, ●——●; 15 patients with left hemisphere lesions, ▲——▲.)

TABLE 23.5. *Frequency Distribution of Error Performance of 15 Right and 15 Left Hemisphere Damaged Patients*

Damage	Normal	Left Errors	Right Errors	Bilateral Errors
Right hemisphere	4	8	0	3
Left hemisphere	2	2	0	11

(Adapted from McClellan et al., 1973.)

preponderance of left as opposed to right hemisphere patients with bilaterally poor scores.

Other authors have commented on such findings. Johnson and Katz (1971) noted bilateral deficits on the SSW with left hemisphere patients who had concomitant corpus callosal lesions. Corpus callosal influence would not show up in McClellan et al.'s right hemisphere patients since the left ear is already depressed. Another explanation may be two-fold. The language deficit from aphasia per se may have interfered with test response. For example, Hutchinson (1973) reported that aphasics given a dichotic listening task showed a right ear preference although performance for both ears was poorer than for her normal controls. Speaks, Gray, Miller and Rubens (1975) compared performance on monaurally versus dichotically presented consonant-vowel (CV) syllables in patients with unilateral damage of *either* the right *or* the left hemisphere. Results suggested that even with damage confined to one hemisphere there will be some effect evident for both ears on a dichotic listening task.

Summary of SSW Results in Patients with Brain Lesions

Clinical findings as reported by Katz and others suggest that the SSW test is most useful in detecting cortical auditory problems especially in patients with primary auditory reception disorders. Damage outside of this area may result in normal or mildly abnormal performance except perhaps in cases with corpus callosum disorder. Patients who have reversals may be suspected of having a CNS problem affecting the area of the sensory and motor strip around the fissure of Rolando or perhaps the anterior temporal lobe.

OTHER CONSIDERATIONS OF THE SSW TEST

SSW Test and Ear Laterality

Dirks (1964) has suggested that if verbal dichotic tests were employed to detect CANS problems ear laterality might confound results. Studies with normals on dichotic listening tasks have clearly shown an ear laterality effect favoring the right ear for both semantic and nonsemantic verbal items (Kimura, 1961a; Dirks, 1964; Curry, 1967; Berlin and Lowe, 1972). The same has been shown with patients with temporal lobe lesions (Kimura, 1961b; Hutchinson, 1973; Speaks et al., 1975).

Small ear differences sometimes are evident on the SSW test when testing normal subjects. These usually are seen between the R-C and L-C items and favor the right ear but are considered clinically nonsignificant. For example, Katz and Fishman (1964) noted a R-C/L-C ear difference of only 1.7%. Brunt and Goetzinger (1968) found a mean of 0.3 errors for the right ear as opposed to 1.0 errors for the left. Generally, all studies of the SSW test conventionally presented have shown no readily apparent laterality effect for individuals between 11 and 60 years of age.

Apparently significant ear laterality on the SSW test is demonstrable only when drastic changes are made in method of presentation. Goldman and Katz (1966) noted a significant right ear superiority when the entire test item (both competing and noncompeting monosyllables) were sent to one ear. Chapnick and Brunt (1970) found the right ear to be superior when a 900 Hz low pass filtered version of the test was given dichotically and subjects were required to respond by free recall or to first repeat the signals in the right ear and then the stimuli heard in the left.

The resistance of the SSW test to ear laterality effects when conventionally presented may be for two main reasons. For each test item one ear is leading in time relative to stimulation. This may allow the listener to better separate both spondaic words as opposed to a condition where all portions of a test item are temporally overlapped.

Aside from item formation, correct responses are facilitated by word association as the two monosyllables of each spondaic word are highly associated. Emmerich, Goldenbaum, Hayden, Hoffman and Treffts (1965) and Bryden (1964) noted fewer errors on dichotic tasks designed with high associative value among the test words. In a similar vein, in Curry's (1967) investigation fewer errors were evident for familiar, dichotically presented words than for nonsense syllables.

SSW Test Results for Children Under 11 and Adults Over 60

Children and the SSW Test. At present there are some limitations to the use of the SSW with children under 11 years of age. In comparison to the norms presented in Table 23.2, there is more variability in performance for children younger than 11. In an attempt to reduce this variability Katz and Myrick (1965) selected 20 of the most familiar items from the standard 40-item test (List EC) to form a children's list (List C-EC). With the shortened version errors and variability decreased from 7 to 11 years of age with the 11-year-olds performing like normal adults. The general error pattern for the younger children was a significant ear laterality effect favoring the right ear. Brunt (1965) also had noted a similar laterality effect on an early 50-item version of the SSW test on 60 children aged 8 to 10 years of age with functional articulation disorders.

The Elderly and the SSW Test. Reports by Balas (1962) and Katz (1962) had shown that individuals over 60 years of age, had more errors and variability than those from 11 to 60 years of age. These findings suggested that frequently individuals over 60 will not perform within the limits of the normative standard (Table 23.2). The SSW may prove useful in studying CANS changes with age.

Results on 5 patients ranging in age from 61 to 91 years of age to illustrate the variability encountered in the elderly are shown in Figure 23.11 (Brunt, 1975). Table 23.6 summarizes pure tone and speech audiometric results. All five had sensory-neural losses. SSW performance ranged from normal to severely abnormal while ear and order effects ranged from none to both an ear and an order effect. Curiously enough, there were no reversals. Figure 23.11A

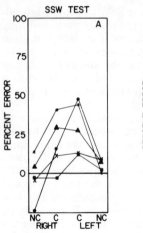
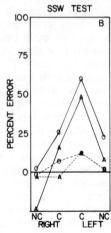

Fig. 23.11. (*A*) C-SSW results for five elderly patients. (*——*, GG-61; ×——×, FB-67; ▲——▲, EB-68; ■——■, FW-76; ●——●, JR-91.) (*B*) Corrected (*O*) and adjusted (*A*) SSW results for two elderly patients. (——, JR-91; -----, FW-76).

TABLE 23.6. *Summary of Pure Tone and Speech Audiometric Results on 5 Elderly Patients (See Text)**

Patient	PTA		SRT		WDS	
	RE	LE	RE	LE	RE	LE
					%	%
GG-61-M	45	37	45	45	86	88
FB-67-F	33	35	25	25	86	98
EB-68-M	27	30	20	15	84	92
FW-76-F	33	35	30	30	92	92
JR-91-M	38	43	35	35	76	78

* PTA, pure tone average; SRT, speech reception threshold; WDS, word discrimination score; RE and LE, right and left ear, respectively.

illustrates the variability in results in terms of C-SSW scores which, in some cases, were adjusted for ear or order effects. Figure 23.11*B* presents C-SSW and A-SSW data on two of these patients. These findings were like two of the others where adjustment for ear or order effects was made; i.e., adjusted scores were somewhat "better" but closely paralleled scores just corrected for WDS errors.

The absence of reversals for all 5 patients and the abnormal scores for some do suggest that the SSW may pick out CANS changes in the elderly. The question still remains whether the SSW test would be able to separate CANS age changes from a centrally located auditory lesion. However, some work is in progress by Deptula (1977) and others which may provide a more definitive picture of SSW performance in the elderly.

Summary. At the present time SSW results on children younger than 11 and adults over 60 should be interpreted with caution. It would seem appropriate to stress, again, the importance of inter-test audiologic findings, especially when considering these two populations. It may be that the variability seen in the above two groups is related partially to the language process. For the youngsters variability may reflect various degrees of developing language competence in all its aspects while for the elderly, just the opposite; the gradual breakdown of CANS connections related to normal linguistic processing.

CONCLUSION

This chapter was designed to give the reader an overview of the development, normalization and clinical utility of the SSW test. A discussion of scoring procedures was given pointing out factors to take cognizance of in test interpretations such as speech discrimination errors, reversals and ear and order effects. As presented above, sufficient data has been collected by Katz as well as others on individual patients to suggest that the SSW is a strong clinical instrument in examining for central auditory nervous system disorders.

REFERENCES

Balas, R. F., Results of the staggered spondaic word test with an old age population. Unpublished master's thesis, Northern Illinois University, 1962.

Balas, R. F., and Simon, G. R., The articulation function of a staggered spondaic word list for a normal hearing population. *J. Aud. Res.,* **4,** 285–289, 1964.

Berlin, C., Chase, R. A., Dill, A., and Hagepanos, T., Auditory findings in patients with temporal lobectomies. Paper presented at American Speech and Hearing Association Convention, Chicago, 1965.

Berlin, C., and Lowe, S., Temporal and Dichotic Factors in Central Auditory Testing. In Katz, J. (Ed.), *Handbook of Clinical Audiology,* Ch. 15. Baltimore: Williams & Wilkins Co., 1972.

Brunt, M. A., Performance on three auditory tests by children with functional articulation disorders. Unpublished master's thesis, University of Pittsburgh, 1965.

Brunt, M., Auditory sequelae of diabetes. Doctoral dissertation, University of Kansas, 1969.

Brunt, M., The Staggered Spondaic Word Test. In Katz, J. (Ed.), *Handbook of Clinical Audiology,* Ch. 18. Baltimore: Williams & Wilkins Co., 1972.

Brunt, M., Unpublished research, 1975.

Brunt, M., and Goetzinger, C. P., A study of three tests of central function with normal hearing subjects. *Cortex,* **4,** 288–297, 1968.

Bryden, M. P., Manipulation of strategies of report in dichotic listening. *Can. J. Psychol.,* **18,** 126–137, 1964.

Burgess, C., Unpublished study, 1964.

Chapnick, B., and Brunt, M., Ear laterality as a function of method of recall on a filtered version of the staggered spondaic word test. Unpublished master's thesis, Ohio State University, 1970.

Curry, F. K. W., A comparison of left-handed and right-handed subjects on verbal and nonverbal dichotic listening tasks. Cortex, 3, 343–352, 1967.

Deptula, P., Personal communication, 1977.

Dirks, D., Perception of dichotic and monaural verbal material and cerebral dominance for speech. Acta Otolaryngol., 58, 73–80, 1964.

Efron, R., Temporal Perception, Aphasia, Deja Vu. In Mischelevich, D., and Chase, R. (Eds.), Interdisciplinary Seminar Program Temporal Lobe Function in Man, II. Language and Speech, Part 2, Neurocommunications Laboratory, Department of Psychiatry. Baltimore: The Johns Hopkins University School of Medicine, 1965.

Emmerich, D. S., Goldenbaum, D. M., Hayden, D. L., Hoffman, L. S., and Treffts, J. L., Meaningfulness as a variable in dichotic hearing. J. Exp. Psychol., 69, 433–436, 1965.

Gilroy, J., and Lynn, G. E., Reversibility of abnormal auditory findings in cerebral hemisphere lesions. J. Neurol. Sci., 21, 117–131, 1974.

Goldman, S., and Katz, J., A comparison of the performance of normal hearing subjects on the staggered spondaic word test given under four conditions – dichotic, diotic, monaural (dominant ear) and monaural (nondominant ear). Paper presented at American Speech and Hearing Association Convention, Chicago, 1966.

Hodgson, W. R., Filtered Speech Tests. In Katz, J. (Ed.), Handbook of Clinical Audiology, Ch. 16. Baltimore: Williams & Wilkins Co., 1972.

Hutchinson, B. B., Performance of aphasics on a dichotic listening task. J. Aud. Res., 13, 64–70, 1973.

Johnson, M., and Katz, J., Relationships between dichotic listening and language abilities of aphasic subjects. Paper presented at First Annual Conference on Clinical Aphasiology, Albuquerque, N. M., 1971.

Katz, J., The use of staggered spondaic words for assessing the integrity of the central auditory nervous system. J. Aud. Res., 2, 327–337, 1962.

Katz, J., The SSW test – an interim report. J. Speech Hear. Disord., 33, 132–146, 1968.

Katz, J., Differential Diagnosis of Auditory Impairments. In Fulton, R. T., and Lloyd, L. L. (Ed.), Audiometry for the Retarded: With Implications for the Difficult-to-Test. Baltimore: Williams & Wilkins Co., 1970a.

Katz, J., Audiologic diagnosis; cochlea to cortex. Menorah Med. J., 1, 25–38, 1970b.

Katz, J., The SSW test manual. Auditec of St. Louis, Brentwood, Mo., 1973.

Katz, J., Basil, R. A., and Smith, J. M., A staggered spondaic word test for detecting central auditory lesions. Ann. Otol. Rhinol. Laryngol., 72, 908–918, 1963.

Katz, J., and Fishman, P., The use of the staggered spondaic word test as a means of detecting differences between age groups. Unpublished study, 1964.

Katz, J., and Myrick, D. K., A normative study to assess performance of a group of children, aged seven through eleven, on the staggered spondaic word (SSW) test. Unpublished study, 1965.

Katz, J., Myrick, D. K., and Winn, B., Central auditory dysfunction in cerebral palsy. Paper presented at American Speech and Hearing Association Convention, Washington, D. C., 1966.

Katz, J., and Pack, G., New Developments in Differential Diagnosis using the SSW Test. In Sullivan, M. (Ed.), Central Auditory Processing Disorders. Omaha: University of Nebraska Press, 1975.

Kimura, D., Cerebral dominance and the perception of verbal stimuli. Can. J. Psychol., 15, 166–171, 1961a.

Kimura, D., Some effects of temporal lobe damage on auditory perception. Can. J. Psychol., 15, 156–165, 1961b.

Luria, A. R., Traumatic Aphasia, pp. 104–141, 267–268. The Hague: Mouton Co., 1970.

Lynn, G. E., Benitez, J. T., Eisenbrey, A. B., Gilroy, J., and Wilner, H. I., Neuro-audiological correlates in cerebral hemisphere lesions. Audiology, 11, 115–134, 1972.

Lynn, G. E., and Gilroy, J., Neuro-audiological abnormalities in patients with temporal lobe tumors. J. Neurol. Sci., 17, 167–184, 1972.

Masland, R. L., Paper presented to the Orton Society, "Brain Mechanisms Underlying the Language Function." Reprinted in Human Communication and Its Disorders: An Overall View. National Advisory Neurological Diseases and Stroke Council, pp. 85–109, 1969.

Matzker, J., Two new methods for the assessment of central auditory functions in cases of brain disease. Ann. Otol. Rhinol. Laryngol. 68, 1185–1197, 1959.

McClellan, M., Wertz, R. T., and Collins, M. J., The effects of interhemispheric lesions on central auditory behavior. Paper presented at American Speech and Hearing Association Convention, Detroit, Michigan, 1973.

Speaks, C., Gray, T., Miller, J., and Rubens, A. B., Central auditory deficits and temporal lobe lesions. J. Speech Hear. Disord., 40, 192–205, 1975.

Willeford, J., Competing Sentences for Diagnostic Purposes. Unpublished material, Colorado State University, Fort Collins, Co., 1968.

Willeford, J., Central auditory function in children with learning disabilities. Paper presented at American Speech and Hearing Association Convention, Las Vegas, Nevada, 1974.

Evaluation of Pseudohy-pacusis

chapter 24

PSEUDOHYPACUSIS PERSPECTIVES AND PURE TONE TESTS

Frederick N. Martin, Ph.D.

Not every patient seen in the audiology clinic is fully cooperative during the hearing evaluation. This lack of cooperation may be because the patient (1) does not understand the test procedure, (2) is poorly motivated, (3) is physically or emotionally incapable of appropriate responses, (4) wishes to conceal a handicap, (5) is deliberately feigning or exaggerating a hearing loss for personal gain or exemption or (6) fails to respond accurately due to unconscious motivation. This chapter will describe some of the concepts underlying false or exaggerated hearing test results. It will also present some pure tone test procedures which aid in the detection of inaccuracies and in the determination of a patient's true hearing thresholds.

Many terms have been used to describe a hearing loss which appears greater than can be explained on the basis of pathology in the auditory system. The most popularly used terms in the literature today are "nonorganic hearing loss," "pseudohypacusis," "psychogenic hearing loss," and "malingering." Williamson (1974) cautions that such terms do not necessarily describe the same phenomenon. Since clinicians typically do not know whether an inflated auditory threshold is the result of conscious or unconscious motivation, it seems appropriate to use generic terms. Because of its specific reference to hearing loss the term "pseudohypacusis," which was proposed by Carhart (1961), appears most descriptive. Both "pseudohypacusis" and "nonorganic hearing loss" will be used interchangeably in this chapter to describe responses obtained on hearing exami-

nation which are above the patient's true organic thresholds.

Over the years a number of related terms have been proposed. Chaiklin and Ventry (1963) prefer the term "functional" to describe hearing disorders with either no organic pathology or with pathology insufficient to explain the extent of a hearing loss. Other terms used for this purpose include: "pseudo deafmuteness" (Fromm, 1946), "pseudo organic deafness" (Getz, 1954), "pseudodeafness" (Hefferman, 1955), "pseudo neural hypacusis" (Brockman and Hoversten, 1960) and "pseudohypacusis" (Carhart, 1961). The term "auditory malingering" refers to those persons who deliberately falsify their responses on hearing tests for some personal gain (Guttman, 1938; Doerfler and Stewart, 1946; Fournier, 1958).

Many terms have been used to describe exaggerated performance on hearing tests which are unconsciously motivated. The literature reveals such labels as "psychic deafness" (Froeschels, 1944; Myklebust, 1954), "hysterical deafness" (Rosenberger and Moore, 1946) and "psychogenic deafness" (Martin, 1946; Doerfler, 1951; Truex, 1946). The term "hysterical deafness" was popular several years ago but is used little today. This term implies a form of conversion neurosis wherein the patient loses his ability to hear due to some unconscious emotional conflict. "Psychogenesis" literally means beginning (genesis) in the mind (psyche). Even such exotic labels as "sinistrosis" (Fournier, 1958) appear in the literature.

If one thinks of a hearing loss which is due to physical impairment in the auditory system as being "organic" then the term nonorganic is immediately clear. Many individuals with pseudohypacusis have nonorganic aspects superimposed on an organic hearing loss (Johnson, Work and McCoy, 1956). The audiologist must remember that his function is to determine the extent of the organic component rather than to determine the precise reason for the nonorganic results.

PSEUDOHYPACUSIS IN ADULTS

A number of factors may encourage some persons to either feign a hearing loss which does not exist or to exaggerate an existing hearing loss. One of these factors is financial gain, based upon the increasing number of awards made by the courts for incurred disability or pensions paid by the Veterans Administration for service-connected hearing loss. Other factors are psychosocial, based on the desire to avoid situations which are regarded as undesirable. There may be many other "gains" which the individual may feel are afforded to hearing-handicapped persons. There are many rationalizations for nonorganic behavior.

The number of persons with pseudohypacusis may be increasing since the implementation of the Walsh-Healey Act of 1969 (Alberti, 1970). More recently the Occupational Safety and Health Act of 1970 has passed. Some state laws regarding noise in industry are even more stringent than federal legislation. The promise of financial reward is bound to be a factor precipitating pseudohypacusis in workers who are in danger of incurring noise-induced hearing loss. Barelli and Ruder (1970) gathered data on 162 medicolegal patients and found that 24% of the 116 workers applying for compensation proved to have a nonorganic hearing loss. Gaynor (1974) also predicts an increasing number of cases applying for compensation, citing the $52 million paid in 1970 by the Veterans Administration for service-connected hearing loss.

Studying social and psychological characteristics of adult males with pseudohypacusis, Trier and Levy (1965) reported psychological and psychiatric evaluations of patients with and without hearing complaints. The nonorganic group achieved lower scores on all measures of current socioeconomic status and scored significantly lower on measures of verbal intelligence. They showed a greater degree of clinically significant emotional disturbance. Trends of hypochondriasis were also noted, including many complaints of tinnitus. These findings are similar to other reports which state that adults with nonorganic hearing loss also manifest a reliance on denial mechanisms. Such patients appear to have a diminished sense of confidence in their ability to meet the needs of everyday life and may feel a sense of some gain by appearing to be hearing-impaired.

There is disagreement over whether a nonorganic hearing loss may be psychogenic at all, or whether all exaggerated hearing thresholds are deliberately and consciously manifested with an eye toward personal gain. Beagley and Knight (1968) stated that, while psychogenic deafness is rare, it does occur and

can be diagnosed if careful attention is paid to the diagnostic criteria. They summarized 21 cases of nonorganic hearing loss and specified one case as fulfilling all the criteria for a psychiatric or "hysterical" background. Goldstein (1966) does not believe that psychogenic hearing loss exists as a clinical entity. He feels that criteria for this etiology would have to include the discovery of lower hearing thresholds on electrophysiologic tests or under hypnosis, and that consistency should exist between everyday auditory behavior and results on voluntary hearing tests. In addition, hearing improvement should be evident on tests subsequent to resolution of the psychological difficulty. In short, Goldstein believes that all nonorganic hearing losses are consciously simulated (malingered).

Disagreeing with Goldstein's criteria for psychogenicity, Ventry (1968) presented a case report of a patient diagnosed as having a unilateral psychogenic hearing loss. According to Ventry and Chaiklin (1962) the term psychogenesis does not separate conscious from unconscious behavior and so if there is some psychological origin in a nonorganic hearing loss it is by definition psychogenic.

Two groups of servicemen were compared by Cohen et al. (1963). One group was consistent on auditory tests and the other was not. The inconsistent group manifested deviant neurosensory signs and psychological abnormalities, gave reports of head injuries out of proportion to the actual extent of the injury, but showed no difference from the control subjects in predisposing factors. Cohen et al. concluded that individuals who present inconsistent results on hearing tests may be influenced by psychodynamic factors.

In a study of military personnel with pseudohypacusis Gleason (1958) found that the patient who is inconsistent on audiologic tests is likely to be deviant psychologically but not necessarily psychiatrically ill. Fifty-five percent of the population studied were judged to be emotionally immature and 30% neurotic. Of 278 consecutive cases, 30% showed inconsistencies and exaggerated hearing losses and 86% of this subgroup had medically confirmed losses. The inconsistent group had many psychosomatic complaints, deviant social behavior and in general made poor adjustments to their hearing losses. Most of these men had done poorly in school. The conclusion of this study was that in many cases of pseudohypacusis the problem is on an unconscious level in order to gain a favored goal, or to explain to society that the patient is blameless for inadequate social behavior. From this point of view, exaggerated hearing loss may be one symptom of a personality disturbance.

It does not seem likely that the near future

will bring resolution to the dispute over the etiologies of pseudohypacusis. Everyone would agree that there are some patients who deliberately lie and attempt to convey the impression of a greater hearing loss than they actually have, or who pretend to have a hearing difficulty when their hearing is perfectly normal. Regardless of how they deviate psychologically these people are malingerers. The argument for conversion neurosis is supported by the documentation of other psychogenic disorders such as hysterical blindness, aphonia or paralysis. Although this question remains moot the function of the audiologist is the same regardless of his orientation toward this question.

PSEUDOHYPACUSIS IN CHIDREN

A number of case reports of pseudohypacusis in children appear in the literature. Dixon and Newby (1959) reported on 40 children between the ages of 6 and 18 years with pseudohypacusis. Despite claimed hearing losses, 39 of these children were able to follow normal conversational speech with little difficulty. Most experienced audiologists can report similar experiences with marked exaggeration of hearing thresholds for pure tones in the presence of normal speech reception thresholds.

There are also cases of apparent malingering with psychological undertones. For example, Bailey and Martin (1961) reported on a boy with normal hearing sensitivity who manifested a great many nonorganic symptoms. Following the audiometric examination he admitted a deliberate attempt to create the impression that he had a hearing loss. He claimed he did this so that he could be admitted to the state residential school for the deaf where his parents taught and his sister and girl friend were students. Investigation into this boy's background revealed that he was a poor student in a high school for normal hearing students which he attended. Hallewell et al. (1966) described a 13-year-old boy with a severe bilateral hearing loss who revealed essentially normal hearing sensitivity under hypnosis.

Cases of presumed psychogenic hearing loss have also been reported. Lumio, Jauhiainen and Gelhar (1969) reported on three sisters whose hearing losses all appeared to develop over a period of a few months. Two of the three girls also had complaints of visual problems and were fitted with eyeglasses. All three apparently had their hearing return to normal in one day during a visit with their aunt. When the hearing returned the visual disorders also disappeared. These authors reported that the pseudohypacusis was due to family conflicts. They felt that it was probable that the hearing loss of the youngest child was entirely unconscious, but the other two may have been partly simulated.

Thirty-two cases diagnosed as psychogenic hearing loss are reported by Barr (1963). While pure tone audiograms showed levels in the 60- to 80-dB range, hearing for speech was considerably better than would be anticipated based on both formal and informal tests. Overall, these children were of normal intelligence but did not perform well in school. Since they were from homes where high scholastic performance was considered important their parents willingly accepted the idea of hearing loss (based on failure of a school hearing test) as explanation of poor academic achievement. It was felt that the attention paid to the children encouraged them to consciously or unconsciously feign a hearing loss on subsequent examinations. Barr stresses that the nonorganic difficulty must be detected as early as possible before the child realizes that there are secondary gains to be enjoyed from a hearing disorder.

Sometimes children who fail school screening tests become the object of a great deal of attention. This may cause the children to continue to feign a hearing loss. A number of such school children are discussed by Campanelli (1963). These children behaved on formal tests as if they had a hearing loss but behaved normally in other situations. This study further emphasized the need for caution against preferential seating, special classes, hearing therapy and hearing aids until the extent of the hearing problem is defined by proper audiologic diagnosis. In a study evaluating one hearing conservation program (Leshin, 1960), a number of cases of nonorganic hearing loss were discovered. A team including otologists, audiologists, medical social consultants and local health department staff worked to: (1) reconcile medical, audiologic and psychosocial data to arrive at a diagnosis; (2) determine familial and environmental factors contributing to nonorganic loss and (3) outline and implement courses of action to relieve the child's need to use pseudohypacusis as a personality mechanism.

Identification audiometry is a significant step in discovering school children with hearing disorders. There is some reason to fear that a child may fail a school test in spite of his normal hearing due to such factors as noisy acoustic environment, improper testing technique, insufficient motivation or poorly calibrated equipment. If attention is attracted to this incorrect failure the child may get the notion that a hearing loss provides a variety of secondary gains, such as an excuse for poor school performance. The end result may be referral to an otologic or audiologic clinic for further evaluation of hearing. Several authors (Miller, Fox and Chan, 1968; Ross, 1964) have stressed the need to uncover nonorganic hearing losses before referrals are made. Ross cited four cases which illustrate the problems of such referrals and the commitment to simulated hearing loss this may bring to the child.

Pseudohypacusis in children appears to occur with sufficient frequency to cause concern. Whether the notion of simulating a hearing loss comes out of a school screening failure or from some conscious or unconscious need, it must be recognized as early as possible by the audiologist in order to avoid a variety of unfortunate circumstances. Performance or supervision of hearing tests on young children by an audiologist may serve to avert what may later develop into serious psychological or educational difficulties.

INDICATIONS OF PSEUDOHYPACUSIS
The Nontest Situation

Frequently the source of referral will suggest the possibility of pseudohypacusis. When an individual is referred by an attorney following an accident that has resulted in his client's sudden loss of hearing, it is only natural to suspect that nonorganicity may play a role in test results. This is also true of veterans referred for hearing tests, the results of which decide the amount of monthly pension to be paid for perhaps an indefinite period. It must be emphasized that the majority of patients referred for such examinations are cooperative and well meaning; however, the VA population consists of a higher risk group for nonorganicity than self-referred or physician-referred patients. Pseudohypacusis must be on the mind of the clinical audiologist or he may miss some of the symptoms which indicate its presence.

A case history is always of value, but it is particularly valuable in compensation cases. It is obviously beneficial for the examining audiologist to take the history statement himself so that he can observe not only the responses given to questions, but also the manner in which these responses are offered. The patient may claim an over-reliance on lip reading, may ask for inappropriate repetitions of words, and may constantly readjust a hearing aid. It is usual for hard-of-hearing patients to be relatively taciturn about their hearing problems, whereas exaggerated or contradictory statements of difficulty or discomfort, vague descriptions of hearing difficulties and the volunteering of unasked-for supplementary information may be symptomatic of pseudohypacusis.

We sometimes see in patients with nonorganic loss exaggerated actions and maneuvers to watch every movement of the speaker's lips, or the turning away with hand cupped over the ear, ostensibly to amplify sound. As a rule, hard-of-hearing adults face the speaker with whom they are conversing, but their watching postures are not nearly so tortuous as described above. Not all patients who intend to exaggerate their hearing thresholds create such caricatures, and even patients who do should not be condemned as having a nonorganic hearing loss on the basis of such evidence alone.

The Test Situation

During the hearing examination the pseudohypacusic patient is frequently inconsistent in his test responses. A certain amount of variability is to be expected of any individual, however, when the magnitude of this variability exceeds 10 dB for any threshold measurement one must consider the possibility of nonorganicity. With the exception of some unusual conditions it can be expected that the cooperative patient will give consistent audiometric readings.

Two types of patient error are frequently seen in the clinical testing of pure tone thresholds. These are false positive and false negative responses. When the subject does not respond at levels at, or slightly above, his threshold he is giving a false negative response. False negative responses are characteristic of nonorganic hearing loss. Frequently the highly responsive patient will give false positive responses, signaling that he has heard a tone when none was introduced or when the tone was below his threshold. False positive responses, although sometimes annoying, are characteristic of true hearing loss. Feldman (1962) points out that the patient with pseudohypacusis does not offer false positive responses during silent periods on pure tone tests. Chaiklin and Ventry (1965a) found that only 22% of their group of adult subjects with nonorganic hearing loss gave a "false alarm" while 86% of those with organic loss gave such false responses. Thus one simple check for nonorganicity is to allow silent intervals of a minute or so from time to time. A false alarm is more likely to indicate that the patient is trying to cooperate and believes he has heard a tone. Extremely slow and deliberate responses may be indicative of a nonorganic problem since most patients with organic hearing losses respond relatively quickly to the signal, particularly at levels above threshold.

The Audiometric Configuration

A number of authors have suggested that an audiometric pattern emerges which is consistent with pseudohypacusis. Some have described this pattern as a relatively flat audiogram showing an equal amount of hearing loss across frequencies (Semenov, 1947; Fournier, 1958). Others have suggested that the "saucer-shaped audiogram" similar to a supra-liminal equal loudness contour is the typical curve illustrating nonorganicity (Doerfler, 1951; Carhart, 1958; Goetzinger and Proud, 1958). On the other hand, Chaiklin et al. (1959) observed that saucer-shaped audiograms can also occur in true organic hearing losses and that these curves are seen infrequently in non-organic hearing loss. They conclude that there is no typical pure tone configuration associated with nonorganic hearing loss. Since the patient with nonorganic hearing loss may attempt to give responses that are of equal loudness at all frequencies, ignorance of the manner in which loudness grows with respect to intensity at different frequencies does suggest that the result should be a saucer-shaped audiogram. The logic of this is apparently not borne out in fact.

In a study of 64 men with nonorganic hearing loss and 36 men with true organic loss, Ventry and Chaiklin (1965) asked a panel of three experienced audiologists to judge the configurations of the audiograms. Saucer-shaped curves appeared in only 8% of the nonorganic cases and were also seen in true organic losses. This research indicates, as many experienced audiologists have observed, that the saucer audiogram has limited utility in identifying nonorganicity.

Test-Retest Reliability

One indication of nonorganicity is lack of consistency on repeated measures. Counseling the patient about his inaccuracies may encourage more accurate responses; however, it should seem obvious that if this counseling is done in a belligerent way it can hardly be expected to increase cooperation if pseudohypacusis is being attempted. Sometimes a brief explanation of the test discrepancies encourages improved patient cooperation. By withholding any allegations of guilt on the part of the patient the audiologist can superficially assume responsibility for not having conveyed instructions properly. This provides a graceful way out for many patients even if they are highly committed to nonorganic loss. Berger (1965) found that some children can be coaxed into "listening harder," thereby improving results on pure tone tests.

The Shadow Curve

It is generally agreed that a patient with a severe hearing loss in one ear will hear a test tone in the opposite ear if the signal is raised to a sufficient level during a pure tone test. The sound travels to the nontest ear by bone conduction. For an air-conduction signal the levels required for contralateralization range from 40 to 70 dB, depending on frequency (Zwislocki, 1953). The interaural attenuation,

the loss of energy of the sound due to contralateralization, is much less for bone conduction than for air conduction. With the vibrator placed on the mastoid process there is almost no interaural attenuation although it can be as much as 20 dB for the higher frequencies in some cases. If a person has no hearing for air conduction or bone conduction in one ear, the audiogram taken from the bad ear would suggest a moderate conductive loss. Unless clinical masking is applied to the better ear a "shadow curve" of the better ear should be expected. A complete discussion of interaural attenuation, the shadow curve and masking are presented in Chapter 11.

It may seem advantageous to a patient feigning a hearing loss to claim that loss in only one ear. Appearing to have one normal ear is convenient since the individual need not worry about being "tripped up" in conversation by responding to a sound which is below his admitted threshold. In this way all hearing can occur in the "good ear" and the claim can be made that hearing is poor in the "bad ear." Normal activities can be carried on for the unilaterally hearing-impaired individual without any special abilities at speechreading.

The naive pseudohypacusic patient may give responses indicating no hearing in one ear and very good hearing in the other ear. The lack of contralateral response, especially by bone conduction, is a very clear symptom of unilateral nonorganic hearing loss and offers a good reason why all patients should be tested initially without masking, even if it appears obvious at the outset of testing that masking will be required later in the examination.

SRT and Pure Tone Average Disagreement

The speech reception threshold (SRT) is generally expected to compare favorably with the average of the best two of the three thresholds obtained at 500, 1000 and 2000 Hz (Siegenthaler and Strand, 1964). Lack of agreement between the pure tone average (PTA) and the SRT, in the absence of explanations such as slope of the audiogram or poor word discrimination (Noble, 1973) is symptomatic of nonorganic hearing loss. Carhart (1952) was probably the first to report that in confirmed cases of nonorganic hearing loss the SRT is *lower* (better) than the pure tone average. Ventry and Chaiklin (1965) reported that the SRT-PTA discrepancy identified 70% of their patients with confirmed pseudohypacusis, in each case the SRT proving to be at least 12 dB lower than the PTA. The lack of SRT-PTA agreement is often the first major symptom of pseudohypacusis.

The person exaggerating his thresholds undoubtedly uses some kind of a loudness judgment to maintain consistency throughout testing. In attempting to remember the loudness of a suprathreshold signal at which he previously responded he might easily become confused between pure tones and spondaic words. Very little research has been carried out to explain why the discrepancy generally occurs favoring the SRT, but a possible explanation may refer to the fact that the loudness of speech occurs primarily in the low frequencies. According to the equal loudness contours, the low frequencies grow more rapidly than tones in the speech-frequency range. This speculation is supported by the work of McLennan and Martin (1976) who concluded that when pure tones of different frequency are compared in loudness against a speech signal, the difference between the loudness of speech and pure tones is a function of the flattening equal loudness contours. Hirsh (1952, p. 212) likens the phon lines to loudness recruitment in that these low frequency sounds increase in loudness more quickly per decibel than the mid-frequencies. More will be said about speech audiometry and nonorganic hearing loss in the next chapter.

PURE TONE TESTS FOR PSEUDOHYPACUSIS

The function of the audiologist is to determine the organic hearing thresholds for all his patients, including those with pseudohypacusis. In many cases the audiologist simply gathers evidence against the nonorganic patient to prove a case. This is sometimes necessary but unfortunately too common, for the unmasking of nonorganic cases should not be an end in itself. While it is easier to make a diagnosis on a cooperative patient in terms of his hearing thresholds, any lack of cooperation in no way justifies a disinterest on the part of the audiologist, whatever the hearing problem might be.

There are pure tone tests which prove the presence of pseudohypacusis, those which approximate the true threshold and those which actually quantify the patient's threshold without his voluntary cooperation. Discussion of some pure tone tests for pseudohypacusis will follow.

PURE TONE TESTS FOR DETECTION OF PSEUDOHYPACUSIS

Automatic Audiometry

The use of the Bekesy automatic audiometer has increased dramatically since Jerger's (1960) report in which he described the usefulness of Bekesy audiometry for determination of the locus of auditory lesion by comparison of the threshold tracings obtained with continuous and periodically interrupted tones. Patients with nonorganic hearing loss sometimes manifest a distinct Bekesy pattern (Jerger and

Herer, 1961) with the tracings for interrupted tones showing poorer hearing than for continuous tones. Following Jerger's (1960) four organic diagnostic types this nonorganic type of tracing was called Type V. The same kind of tracing in patients with pseudohypacusis was also reported by Resnick and Burke (1962). Since these original reports Type V patterns have been reported for pseudohypacusic adults (Stein, 1963) and children (Peterson, 1963).

While the Type V tracing has not been completely explained the work of Rintelmann and Carhart (1964) suggests that it is related to a patient's own internal standard for most comfortable loudness or to his recalled loudness for a sustained tone. Hattler (1968) indicated that the Type V tracing may be attributed to differential effects of memory upon the loudness of sustained and interrupted pure tones. In any case, normal hearing subjects require greater intensity for interrupted tones to match the loudness of continuous tones.

Hattler (1970) altered the normal pulsed-tone duty cycle (200 msec on, 200 msec off) to 200 msec on, 800 msec off. He called this the lengthened off-time (LOT) test. The LOT test has the effect of increasing the tracing level of the interrupted tones for nonorganic patients but has no effect on the tracings of normal listeners or organic hypacusics. LOT identified 95% of a series of nonorganic cases while Type V tracings using the standard 50% duty cycle identified only 40%.

Rintelmann and Harford (1967) feel that the Type V Bekesy classification should be based on sweep frequency rather than fixed-frequency tracings. They define the Type V as a separation of pulsed and continuous tracings for at least two octaves with a minimum of a 10 -dB separation between midpoints. Using these criteria they found Type V tracings in none of their series of normal hearing subjects, 2% of their patients with conductive hearing loss, 3% of their sensory-neural group and 76% of their nonorganic group. These figures, although they betray a small number of false positives on Type V classification, speak well of the procedure for identification of pseudohypacusis using strict criteria for classification. The criteria described above have been validated by others (Ventry, 1971).

The effects of sophistication and practice on Type V tracings were recently studied (Martin and Monro, 1975). In three groups of normal hearing subjects simulating a hearing loss the LOT procedure was consistently superior to standard off-time (SOT) in the elicitation of Type V patterns. Subjects who were familiarized with the principle of the Type V pattern did better than those who were not informed. A third group was allowed practice with the procedure while observing the action of the pen of the Bekesy audiometer and did consistently better in producing organic types of Bekesy tracings than either of the other two groups. A recommendation was made that in cases of suspected pseudohypacusis the continuous tones should be compared to both the SOT and LOT tones, and the two pulsed-tone tracings should be compared to each other to increase the efficiency of this test. The conclusion was inescapable that practice and sophistication do assist the motivated subject to avoid the Type V pattern when a hearing loss is simulated.

To add greater difficulty in Bekesy tracings for pseudohypacusic patients Hood, Campbell and Hutton (1964) developed a technique called BADGE (Bekesy ascending descending gap evaluation). The patient tracks his threshold for a fixed frequency over a 1-min period for a continuous tone. The level is set at 0 dB and the tone is automatically increased in intensity until the subject presses the key, indicating that he has heard the tones. This is called the continuous ascending (CA) test. After 1 min of tracing, the pen is replaced to the 0-dB hearing threshold level (HTL) position and the audiometer is set in the automatic pulse mode. One minute of tracing is then obtained in the pulsed ascending (PA) condition. Following these tracings the tone is switched off and the pen is set in a position so that the tone is at a level 30 to 40 dB above the pulsed ascending tracing or at the maximum output of the audiometer, whichever is lower. The tone is then switched on in the pulse mode and the patient tracks his threshold for 1 min. This is called the pulsed descending (PD) test. Hood et al. found that using a combination of pulsed and continuous, ascending and descending modes of tracing apparently destroys the pseudohypacusic patient's yardstick for the level he attempts to simulate as his threshold. Using this method a number of subjects gave positive BADGE results, but did not show a Type V tracing. The test is obviously confusing to the patient and therefore useful in identification of exaggerated hearing thresholds.

A high incidence of Type V tracings reported among otherwise cooperative listeners unaccustomed to Bekesy audiometry suggests that this type of tracing may not be a good indicator of pseudohypacusis (Stark, 1966; Hopkinson, 1965). It has been suggested (Price, Shepherd and Goldstein, 1965) that a psychological, but not necessarily psychopathologic explanation may be offered for the Type V tracing. Although very wide pen excursions during Bekesy audiometry may be seen in hypacusic patients, Istre and Burton (1969) reported on a

patient with nonorganic hearing loss with swings up to 45 dB. They felt that the wide Bekesy swings are diagnostic since the normal swing is usually 6 to 16 dB (assuming an attenuation rate of 2.5 dB/second). It seems unwarranted to assume pseudohypacusis on the basis of swing width alone since this can be caused by factors other than nonorganicity, such as reaction time (Suzuki and Kubota, 1966) and personality (Shepherd and Goldstein, 1968).

Arguments over the usefulness of Bekesy audiometry techniques for diagnosis of pseudohypacusis are bound to continue. It can be said at this point, however, that the LOT and BADGE tests are certainly of value although it must be recognized that they do not indicate the true threshold. While a Type V tracing may suggest nonorganicity and the need for further tests, it is not evidence in and of itself.

Pure Tone Tests with Ipsilateral Masking

Most subjects find it difficult to maintain consistent suprathreshold responses to auditory signals in the presence of several levels of noise in the same ear. This known difficulty was the principle of the Doerfler-Stewart test (1946) which utilizes spondaic words in the presence of sawtooth noise. Martin and Hawkins (1963) modified the Doerfler-Stewart test for use with pure tones, finding it useful in discovering nonorganic hearing disorders. For the procedure to be of value the clinician must know the precise effect of his audiometer's noise generator on pure tone thresholds for tones of different frequencies so that he can compare the masking levels which shift the threshold of a tone on normal ears. Martin and Hawkins' research indicated that the effective masking levels are similar for subjects with normal hearing as well as those with conductive and sensory-neural losses. Pang-Ching (1970) also found that the introduction of noise to the test ear confuses the patient with a nonorganic hearing loss, causing him to lose his loudness yardstick.

While the sensory-neural acuity level (SAL) test (Jerger and Tillman, 1960) was designed to be used in lieu of bone-conduction audiometry in determining sensory-neural sensitivity, Rintelmann and Harford (1963) found that it also proves helpful in identifying nonorganic hearing loss. They studied 10 children with suspected pseudohypacusis and reported that, in addition to other test findings suggesting nonorganicity, air-SAL gaps appeared without other evidence of conductive hearing loss.

The introduction of a noise to the test ear, either by air conduction or bone conduction, may cause elevations in auditory threshold which suggest nonorganic hearing disorders because of their inconsistencies with predicted findings on patients with true hypacusis. While such methods identify the probable presence of some nonorganic hearing disorder they fail to provide evidence regarding the true thresholds of hearing.

Miscellaneous Tests for Detection of Pseudohypacusis

Tests continue to be developed for the detection of pseudohypacusis. Most of these tests are based on confusing the patient so that he cannot recall a previously established level at which he responded to an acoustic signal. Some of these procedures will be described briefly in the following paragraphs.

The use of both an ascending and descending approach to pure tone threshold measurements was recommended a number of years ago as a rapid and simple procedure (Harris, 1958). A greater than 10-dB difference between these two measurements suggests a nonorganic problem since the two thresholds should be identical. Personal use of this procedure indicates that this difference is often as large as 30 dB for pseudohypacusic patients. For patients with nonorganic loss the ascending method generally reveals lower (better) thresholds than the descending approach. The Harris test is quick and easy to perform with the simplest clinical audiometer and is the basis for the BADGE test described earlier. Recently Kerr, Gillespie and Easton (1975) modified Harris' original procedure and suggested that the test is improved slightly by performing the descending portion in 10-dB rather than 5-dB steps.

Some tests may be carried out by presenting a number of pure tone pulses in rapid succession and asking the patient to count and recall the numbers of pulses he has heard. The intensity of the tones may be varied above and below the admitted threshold of the tone in one ear (Ross, 1964) or above the threshold in one ear and below the threshold in the other ear (Nagel, 1964). If the originally obtained thresholds are valid the patient should have no difficulty in counting the pulses. Inconsistency should occur only if all the tone pulses are above threshold and the patient has to sort out the number of louder ones from the number of softer ones. This can be very difficult to do.

One procedure has been suggested (Gaynor, 1974) which requires that the patient be tested for pure tone thresholds in the normal fashion, and while humming both audibly and inaudibly. The humming produces masking and elevation of threshold in subjects with normal hearing. The practical value of such procedures in dealing with the larger problems of pseudohypacusis is yet to be determined.

PURE TONE TESTS WHICH SUGGEST THRESHOLDS OF PSEUDOHYPACUSIC PATIENTS

The Stenger Test

As stated earlier, some patients manifest unilateral nonorganic hearing complaints. One of the best ways to test for this is by use of the Stenger test. The Stenger principle states that when two tones of the same frequency are introduced simultaneously into both ears, only the louder tone will be perceived. This principle has been used in a variety of ways through the years in detecting unilateral pseudohypacusis and has gone through a number of modifications, one of which will follow.

Since its introduction as a tuning fork test more than 75 years ago the Stenger test has been modified many times. If unilateral nonorganic hearing loss is suspected the Stenger test may be performed quickly as a screening procedure. This is most easily done by introducing a tone of a desired frequency into the better ear at a level 10 dB above the threshold and into the poorer ear at a level 10 dB below the (admitted) threshold. If the loss in the poor ear is genuine, the patient will be unaware of any signal in his poor ear and will respond to the tone in his good ear readily, since at 10 dB above threshold it should be easily heard. Such a response is termed a negative Stenger, indicating that the poorer ear threshold is probably correct. If the patient does not respond, this is a positive Stenger which proves that the postulated threshold for the "poorer" ear is incorrect. A positive Stenger results because the tone is above the true threshold in the "bad" ear and precludes hearing the tone in the good ear. Since the patient does not want to admit hearing in the bad ear and is unaware of the tone in the good ear, he simply does not respond.

The screening procedure described above rapidly identifies the presence or absence of unilateral nonorganic hearing loss if there is a difference in admitted threshold between the ears of at least 20 dB. The test is most likely to be positive in nonorganic cases with large interaural differences (exceeding 40 dB) or large nonorganic components in the "poorer" ear (Chaiklin and Ventry, 1965b).

A positive result on the Stenger test does not identify the true organic hearing threshold. To obtain threshold information the Stenger test can also be performed by seeking the *minimum contralateral interference levels*. The procedure is as follows: The tone is presented to the good ear at 10 dB sensation level (SL). There should be a response from the patient. A tone is presented to the bad ear at 0 dB HTL, simultaneously with the tone at 10 dB SL in the good ear. If a response is obtained the level is raised 5 dB in the *bad ear,* keeping the level the same in the good ear. The level is continuously raised in 5-dB steps until the subject fails to respond. Since the tone is still above threshold in the good ear the lack of response must mean that the tone has been heard loudly enough in the bad ear so that the patient experiences the Stenger effect and is no longer aware of a tone in the good ear. Being unwilling to respond to tones in the bad ear, he simply stops responding. The lowest hearing level of the tone in the bad ear producing this effect is the minimum contralateral interference level, and should be within 20 dB of the true threshold.

In one study (Peck and Ross, 1970) the Stenger test was performed on 35 normal hearing subjects feigning a total hearing loss in one ear. Ascending and descending methods of tone presentation were used. No differences in the interference levels were observed between the two methods. The interference levels were found to be within 14 dB of the true thresholds, resulting in the general conclusion that the Stenger test can identify the general hearing threshold of the poor ear in a unilateral nonorganic hearing loss. This conclusion was supported by Kintsler, Phelan and Lavender (1970) who found that the Stenger test correctly identified 25 out of 31 cases of nonorganic hearing loss.

Since their results were better than suggested by the study of Chaiklin and Ventry (1965b), Kintsler, Phelan and Lavender (1972) replicated the Chaiklin and Ventry study, which found the Stenger not to be a good identifier of nonorganic hearing loss. They found very high correlations between positive findings on the Stenger test and pseudohypacusis. In conflict with this Hattler and Schuchman (1971) found that of 225 patients with nonorganic hearing loss the Stenger test was applicable only in 57% of the cases and had the poorest efficiency of all the tests tried even when applicable, correctly labeling only one-half of the patients with pseudohypacusis.

The studies cited above illustrate that the accuracy and efficiency of the Stenger test continue to be contested. While the Stenger, like most tests, has certain shortcomings I personally regard it as an efficient test for quick identification of unilateral nonorganic hearing loss. Equipment for the test requires only a pure tone audiometer with separate hearing level dials for the right and left ears. To be sure, if the test is performed by an inexperienced clinician a series of patterns and rhythms of tone introductions may betray the intentions of the test to an alert patient.

Acoustic Impedance Measurements

No procedure in recent years has had such a profound effect upon diagnostic audiology as impedance measurements (Chapters 29 and 30). Among the valuable contributions which impedance testing makes to our field is the detection of pseudohypacusis. This section is devoted to the use of tympanic membrane impedance measurements and ways in which they may help in the identification of nonorganic hearing loss.

Concerning pseudohypacusis the greatest value of acoustic impedance measurements is through determination of the middle ear muscle reflex threshold. Since it is generally agreed that this reflex is produced by the *loudness* of an acoustic signal rather than its physical intensity, the elicitation of this reflex at a low SL has been construed to suggest the presence of a cochlear lesion. If the SL (the difference between the reflex threshold and the voluntary pure tone threshold) is extremely low (5 dB or less) it is difficult to accept even an explanation of quick loudness recruitment as an explanation for this sudden increase in loudness (Lamb and Peterson, 1967). As an example of this, Feldman (1963) cited a case with a unilateral nonorganic hearing loss, with acoustic reflexes observed with the test tone in the "poor ear" at levels below the patient's voluntary threshold. If the audiologist is certain that no artifact contaminates the readings, the suggestion that the acoustic reflex may be achieved by a tone which cannot be heard must be rejected and a diagnosis of pseudohypacusis may be made.

More than merely identifying pseudohypacusis, acoustic reflex measurements may be useful in actual estimation of thresholds. Jerger et al. (1974) describe a procedure based on the work of Niemeyer and Sesterhenn (1972) in which the middle ear muscle reflex thresholds for pure tones are compared to those for wideband noise and low and high frequency filtered wide-band noise. In this manner the approximate degree of hearing loss (if any) can be determined, as well as the general audiometric configuration. Details of this procedure may be found elsewhere but it certainly appears that this method may have utility in estimating thresholds of patients with pseudohypacusis. Jerger (1975) is now calling this procedure SPAR, an acronym for sensitivity prediction from the acoustic reflex.

There is no way to know how many patients with pseudohypacusis appear to have a conductive hearing loss. Of course the middle ear muscle reflex measurement cannot be used in cases with nonorganic components overlying even the mildest of conductive problems (Alberti, 1970) since reflexes are absent in both ears when even one ear has a conductive disorder. While the present state of the art does not allow determination of a middle ear problem on the basis of absolute impedance (or otoadmittance) alone, tympanometry, with its various types suggesting different kinds of middle ear disorders is very useful in such cases.

The elaborateness of middle ear measurements, including the cautions to the patient that he be quiet and immobile, may have the effect of discouraging nonorganic behavior if this test is performed early in the battery of diagnostic procedures. It is often good practice to perform middle ear measurements as the first test on adults and cooperative children. They are asked to sit quietly and are told that the measurements made will reveal a great deal about their hearing. I have no hesitancy in recommending this approach in general and believe it is a useful deterrent to pseudohypacusis.

PURE TONE TESTS WHICH IDENTIFY THRESHOLDS OF PSEUDOHYPACUSIC PATIENTS

Electrodermal Audiometry

The subject of electrodermal audiometry (EDA) is covered comprehensively in Chapter 26. This procedure lends itself nicely to threshold exploration on subjects with pseudohypacusis (Grove, 1966; Stride, 1966). While EDA was once used with great frequency on patients unwilling or unable to cooperate on voluntary tests, including babies and small children, the test is used much less often today. Its primary function is to determine pure tone thresholds on patients with suspected pseudohypacusis.

EDA is used in Veterans Administration audiology clinics, where a constant vigil for nonorganic hearing loss must be kept in view of the large amounts of compensation which may be given to veterans with service-connected hearing loss. Since 1955 EDA has been listed as a required test for patients seeking pensions for hearing loss. Its routine use has diminished since 1967 owing to the fact that the percentage of veterans evidencing nonorganic hearing loss has decreased over the years. It is now felt that less than 5% of the VA hearing-impaired population shows some degree of nonorganic hearing loss (Causey, 1975). At the present time EDA is carried out only if there are seemingly uncorrectable indications of nonorganicity among veterans. Administration of this test is left up to the discretion of the individual audiologist.

It is possible for the patient who is knowledgeable about EDA to confound the test in several ways. For example, moving about, squirming or coughing will increase the activity of the stylus on the psychogalvanometer, requiring that the sensitivity be decreased, causing the actual changes in skin resistance to be more difficult to discern. While the examiner may suspect that this activity is deliberately undertaken there is little more that can be done to eliminate it than merely making the request.

While EDA may be useful in revealing true thresholds in pseudohypacusic patients, it is fraught with difficulties. Not the least among these is the potential legal hazard in presenting electric shocks which, while mild in degree, may be claimed to be painful or harmful. The audiologist must approach the use of this technique with care and consideration.

Evoked Response Audiometry

Since many audiologists have become disappointed in EDA as a method of objective audiometry, recent attention has been focused on other electrophysiologic methods. Prominent among these is the cortical evoked response (Chapter 27). Since this procedure involves no electric shocks or other annoying stimuli it appears as a useful tool in determining pure tone thresholds for noncooperative patients (Beagley, 1973; Beagley and Knight, 1968; McCandless and Lentz, 1968). It has been recommended that evoked response audiometry (ERA) be used as an objective test for *all* patients complaining of noise-induced hearing loss (Heron, 1968) and has even been called the "crucial test" in diagnosis of pseudohypacusis (Knight and Beagley, 1970).

As an example of the enthusiasm generated for ERA, Alberti (1970) called the cortical audiometer the most important instrument in the detection of pseudohypacusis. He finds that results obtained from this technique and from voluntary pure tone testing agree within 10 dB, and recommends that ERA be used not only for uncooperative patients but also for patients who cannot speak English.

The evoked response procedure just described allows the use of pure tones because it looks, via an electroencephalograph (EEG) and averaging computer, at the later components of the evoked response (50 to 300 msec). Examination of the earlier components, probably arising from the brain stem, constitutes the procedure called brain stem evoked response (BSER).

BSER has the advantage of the easy application of surface electrodes plus the fact that the response is stable and repeatable (Schulman-Galambos and Galambos, 1975). Disadvantages include the necessity of using clicks or transients as stimuli and the fact that the cochlear portion of the responses are rarely elicited below about 60 dB HTL. Berlin (1978) feels that BSER, in combination with electrocochleography, tympanometry and acoustic reflexes, forms a powerful test battery for noncooperative patients (such as small children). It seems logical to extend this conclusion to pseudohypacusic patients.

The development of modern techniques for digital averaging allows the recording of synchronous firings in response to low frequency tones, minimizing the disadvantages to BSER and electrocochleography that clicks or transients be used as stimuli. This procedure has been called the frequency following response (FFR) (Marsh and Worden, 1968) and may have potential as one of the procedures to be used in diagnosis of pseudohypacusis.

ERA may have the effect of eliminating or determining the presence of nonorganic overlays on true organic hearing losses. The mere elaborateness of the procedure along with the suggestion that hearing can be measured without patient cooperation might have a deterring effect on the would-be malingerer.

Not all audiology centers are equipped with the expensive equipment required to perform ERA and not all audiologists are skilled in its use. Even in the hands of experienced clinicians high correlations between evoked response and voluntary thresholds are not always found (Rose et al., 1972) and so caution should be used in interpreting ERA data. Obviously further research and clinical reports will determine the value of ERA as a diagnostic tool for pseudohypacusis.

Electrocochleography

A procedure which has drawn considerable attention in recent years is electrocochleography (Chapter 28), the recording of cranial nerve VIII action potentials. Although measurements of this kind have been made since the 1930s it is only within the last decade that this procedure has offered feasibility as a diagnostic tool. The obvious advantage of electrocochleography in dealing with pseudohypacusis is that actual measurements can be determined with fewer contaminating artifacts than are seen with either ERA or EDR procedures.

Like EDA and ERA, electrocochleography may be categorized as "objective" since determinations of hearing may be made without the conscious cooperation of the patient. Until recent years the procedure was naturally limited to those patients who could be anesthetized so that the tympanic membrane could be surgically reflected, exposing the round window. More recently the intratympanic needle electrode has been used to obviate the need for surgery. It is obvious that either procedure could rationally be refused by a patient suspected of pseudohypacusis as being painful or dangerous. A recent procedure utilizing saline impregnated cotton with a meatal disc electrode (Cullen et al., 1972) eliminates the above objections and requires only that the patient remain quiet during the test.

The extent to which electrocochleography is and will be used as a method of determining hearing in pseudohypacusic patients is as yet unknown. In addition to the fact that responses during electrocochleography lack frequency information because clicks or brief transients are the necessary acoustic stimuli, limitations are placed by the cost of equipment, the time required to obtain results and, of greatest importance, the skill and training needed by the examiner. Not all audiologists can or should engage in electrophysiologic hearing tests. To some extent the cost of the equipment itself deters proliferation of the use of this procedure.

Delayed Feedback Audiometry

General dissatisfaction has been expressed with delayed speech feedback audiometry (DFA) since it does not reveal the true threshold of the patient with nonorganic hearing loss. A procedure has been described which uses the delayed feedback notion with pure tones, and which can be used on patients who appear unwilling or unable to give accurate readings on threshold audiometry (Ruhm and Cooper, 1964).

Pure tone DFA requires the use of a special apparatus, some variations of which are now commercially available. The patient is asked to tap out a continuous pattern such as four taps, pause, two taps, pause, etc. (----□--□----). The electromagnetic key on which the patient taps is shielded from the visual field of the patient. After the patient has demonstrated that he can maintain the tapping pattern and rhythm, an audiometer circuit is added so that for each tap a tone pulse is introduced into an earphone worn by the patient. The tone has a duration of 50 msec at maximum amplitude but is delayed by 200 msec from the time the key is tapped. If the tone is audible its presence causes the subject to vary his tapping behavior in several ways, such as a loss of tapping rhythm, a change in the number of taps or an increase of finger pressure on the key.

It has been demonstrated (Ruhm and Cooper, 1962) that changes occur in tapping performance at sensation levels as low as 5 dB and are independent of test tone frequency and manual fatigue (Ruhm and Cooper, 1963). Once a subject has demonstrated key-tapping ability any alterations seen after introduction of a delayed pure tone must be interpreted as meaning that the tone was heard.

Not all researchers have found the 5-dB SL change in tapping performance using pure tone delayed auditory feedback. Alberti (1970) found that tapping rhythms were disturbed in general at 5 to 15 dB above threshold, but has observed variations as great as 40 dB. He reported that some subjects are difficult to test with this procedure because they either cannot or will not establish a tapping rhythm, a phenomenon which I have also observed. At times the patients appear to fail to understand the instructions and at other times complain that their fingers are too stiff to tap the key.

We are presently investigating the effects of sophistication on key-tapping performance at the University of Texas. Experience apparently does play a role at suprathreshold levels with unpracticed subjects showing many more time and pattern errors than practiced subjects (Cooper and Stokinger, 1977). Practice notwithstanding, the pure tone DFA procedure is considerably less time consuming than many of the electrophysiologic methods and does not necessitate the use of an unpleasant electric shock, as does EDA. This test has been found to be accurate, reliable and simple (Robinson and Kasden, 1973), and it seems safe to predict that the future will see wider use of pure tone DFA in threshold identification of patients with pseudohypacusis. It will very likely prove to be one of the best tests for this purpose.

It is difficult to assess the degree of sophistication the would-be pseudohypacusic patient takes to the audiologic examination. Martin and Monro (1975) showed that the patient desiring to deceive the audiologist on Bekesy audiometric procedures improves his chances of avoiding the Type V classification if he becomes more knowledgeable about, or has the opportunity to practice the procedure. In a later study we (Monro and Martin, 1977) found some tests easier to "beat" than others; the Stenger test is most difficult to defeat, patients taking the pure tone DAF test were helped only slightly by sophistication, but the confusion of ascending vs. descending approaches to "threshold" or the old reliable SRT-PTA discrepancy were compensated for to a considerable degree by subject preknowledge. Effects of sophistication on other tests for pseudohypacusis are yet to be determined.

DISCUSSION

In the vast majority of cases the detection of pseudohypacusis is not a difficult task for the alert clinician. The more challenging responsibility of the audiologist is to determine his patient's organic thresholds of hearing. The difficulty of this task increases as the coopera-tion of the patient decreases. Some pseudohypacusic patients are overtly hostile and unwilling to modify their test behavior even after counseling (Ventry, Trier and Chaiklin, 1965).

It is not likely that a single approach to diagnosis and resolution of pseudohypacusis is forthcoming. It seems important to say at this juncture that there are certain points upon which we should all agree. For example, it is far better to discourage exaggeration of hearing thresholds at the outset of testing than to detect these exaggerations later. Once nonorganicity is observed the audiologist is faced with the responsibility of determining the true organic thresholds. Tests which may aid in deterring pseudothreshold responses include all the electrophysiologic and electroacoustic procedures. In my own opinion, acoustic impedance measurements should be accomplished initially in all routine audiologic assessments, thereby discouraging some pseudohypacusis. Pure tone DFA and the Stenger tests are quick and easy to perform and allow the patient to realize that the examiner has methods of determining pure tone thresholds even without patient cooperation.

There are times when the audiologist feels his patient with pseudohypacusis should be referred for psychological or psychiatric guidance. Such decisions should not be made recklessly or arbitrarily, but rather after considerable thought. Suggestions of this nature to an individual or to his family must be made carefully because of the unfortunate stigma that may be associated with psychological referrals.

Great care must be taken in writing reports about patients with suspected pseudohypacusis. It must be borne in mind that once an individual has been diagnosed as a "malingerer," "uncooperative" or "functional" his reputation and prestige may be damaged. To label a patient in such ways is a grave matter since it implies deliberate falsification. Such labels are difficult to expunge and may be tragically unjust. The only way an audiologist can be absolutely certain that his nonorganic patient is truly a malingerer is for the patient himself to admit to the intent and most experienced audiologists would probably agree with Hopkinson (1967) that such admissions are rare indeed. Value judgments are not within the purview of the audiologist and should be avoided.

Counseling sessions should be carried out following all audiologic evaluations. Counseling the pseudohypacusic individual is naturally more difficult than counseling patients with organic hearing disorders. If the patient is a child he may be told only that his hearing appears to be normal (if this is felt to be the case) despite audiometric findings to the contrary. Parents should be warned not to discuss the child's difficulties in his presence or to provide any secondary rewards which may be accrued to a hearing loss. Pseudohypacusic adults may simply have to be told that a diagnosis of the extent of the hearing disorder cannot be made because inconsistencies in response preclude accurate diagnosis. If a referral for psychological evaluation or guidance is indicated the clinician must choose his words extremely carefully lest the patient be offended. It is at this point of the examination when audiology must be practiced as more of an art than a science.

REFERENCES

Alberti, P., New tools for old tricks. *Ann. Otol. Rhinol. Laryngol.*, 79, 900–907, 1970.

Bailey, H. A. T., Jr. and Martin, F. N., Nonorganic hearing loss—case report. *Laryngoscope*, 71, 209–210, 1961.

Barelli, P. A., and Ruder, L., Medico-legal evaluation of hearing problems. *Eye Ear Nose Throat Mon.*, 49, 398–405, 1970.

Barr, B., Psychogenic deafness in school children. *Int. Audiol.*, 2, 125–128, 1963.

Beagley, H. A., The role of electro-physiological tests in the diagnosis of non-organic hearing loss. *Audiology*, 12, 470–480, 1973.

Beagley, H. A., and Knight, J. J., The evaluation of suspected nonorganic hearing loss. *J. Laryngol. Otol.*, 82, 693–705, 1968.

Berger, K., Nonorganic hearing loss in children. *Laryngoscope*, 75, 447–457, 1965.

Berlin, C. I., Electrophysiological indices of auditory function. In Martin, F. N. (Ed.), *Pediatric Audiology*. Englewood Cliffs, N. J.: Prentice-Hall, 1978 (in press).

Brockman, S. J., and Hoversten, G. H., Pseudo neural hypacusis in children. *Laryngoscope*, 70, 825–839, 1960.

Carhart, R., Speech audiometry in clinical evaluation. *Acta Otolaryngol.*, 41, 18–42, 1952.

Carhart, R., Audiometry in diagnosis. *Laryngoscope*, 68, 253–279, 1958.

Carhart, R., Tests for malingering. *Trans. Am. Acad. Ophthalmol. Otolaryngol.*, 65, 437, 1961.

Campanelli, P.A., Simulated hearing losses in school children following identification audiometry. *J. Aud. Res.*, 3, 91–108, 1963.

Causey, G. D., Personal communication, 1975.

Chaiklin, J. B., and Ventry, I. M., Functional Hearing Loss. In Jerger, J. (Ed.), *Modern Developments in Audiology*, pp. 76–125, New York: Academic Press, 1963.

Chaiklin, J. B., and Ventry, I. M., Patient errors during spondee and pure-tone threshold measurement. *J. Aud., Res.*, 5, 219–230, 1965a.

Chaiklin, J. B., and Ventry, I. M., The efficiency of audiometric measures used to identify functional hearing loss. *J. Aud. Res.*, 5, 196–211, 1965b.

Chaiklin, J. B., Ventry, I. M., Barrett, L. S., and Skalbeck, G. S., Pure-tone threshold patterns observed in functional hearing loss. *Laryngoscope*, 69, 1165–1179, 1959.

Cohen, M., Cohen, S. M., Levine, M., Maisel, R., Ruhm, H., and Wolfe, R. M., Interdisciplinary pilot study of non-organic hearing loss. *Ann. Otol. Rhinol. Laryngol.*, 72, 67–82, 1963.

Cooper, W. A., and Stokinger, T. E., Pure tone delayed auditory feedback; effect of prior experience. *J. Aud. Res.*, 1977 (in press).

Cullen, J. K., Ellis, M. S., Berlin, C. I., and Lousteau, R. J., Human acoustic nerve action potential recordings from the tympanic membrane without anesthesia. *Acta Otolaryngol.*, 74, 15–22, 1972.

Dixon, R. F., and Newby, H. A., Children with non-organic hearing problems. *Arch. Otolaryngol.*, 70, 619–623, 1959.

Doerfler, L. G., Psychogenic deafness and its detection. *Ann. Otol. Rhinol. Laryngol.*, 60, 1045–1048, 1951.

Doerfler, L. G., and Stewart, K., Malingering and psychogenic deafness. *J. Speech Disord.*, 11, 181–186, 1946.

Feldman, A. S., Functional hearing loss. *Maico Audiological Library Series*, 1, 119–121, 1962.

Feldman, A. S., Impedance measurements at the ear-drum as an aid to diagnosis. *J. Speech Hear. Res.*, 6, 315–327, 1963.

Fournier, J. E., The detection of auditory malingering. *Translation Beltone Inst. Hear. Res.*, 8, 1958.

Froeschels, E., Psychic deafness in children. *Arch. Neurol. Psychiatry*, 51, 544–549, 1944.

Fromm, E. O., Study of a case of pseudo deafmuteness (psychic deafness). *J. Nerv. Ment. Dis.*, 103, 37–59, 1946.

Gaynor, E. B., Humming and nonorganic hearing loss. *Arch. Otolaryngol.*, 100, 199–200, 1974.

Getz, S. B., Note on pseudo-organic deafness. *Arch. Otolaryngol.*, 60, 718–719, 1954.

Gleason, W. J., Psychological characteristics of the audiologically inconsistent patient. *Arch. Otolaryngol.*, 68, 42–46, 1958.

Goetzinger, C. P., and Proud, G. O., Deafness; examination techniques for evaluating malingering and psychogenic disabilities. *J. Kans. Med. Soc.*, 59, 95–101, 1958.

Goldstein, R., Pseudohypoacusis. *J. Speech Hear. Disord.*, 31, 341–352, 1966.

Grove, T. G., Performance of naive and role-playing pseudo-malingerers on an unconditioned EDR audiometric test. *J. Aud. Res.*, 6, 337–350, 1966.

Guttman, J., A new method of determining unilateral deafness and malingering. *Laryngoscope*, 38, 686–687, 1938.

Hallewell, J. D., Goetzinger, C. P., Allen, M. L., and Proud, G. O., The use of hypnosis in audiologic assessment *Acta Otolaryngol.*, 61, 205–208, 1966.

Harris, D. A., A rapid and simple technique for the detection of non-organic hearing loss. *Arch. Otolaryngol.*, 68, 758–760, 1958.

Hattler, K. W., The Type V Bekesy pattern; the effects of loudness memory. *J. Speech Hear. Res.*, 11, 567–575, 1968.

Hattler, K. W., Lengthened off-time; a self-recording screening device for nonorganicity. *J. Speech Hear. Disord.*, 35, 113–122, 1970.

Hattler, K. W., and Schuchman, G. I., Efficiency of the Stenger, Doerfler-Stewart and lengthened off-time Bekesy tests. *Acta Otolaryngol.*, 72, 262–267, 1971.

Hefferman, A., A Psychiatric Study of Fifty Pre-school Children Referred to Hospital for Suspected Deafness. In Caplan, G. (Ed.), *Emotional Problems of Early Childhood.* New York: Basic Books, 1955.

Heron, T. G., Industrial deafness and the summed evoked potential. *S. Afr. Med. J.*, 42, 1176–1177, 1968.

Hirsh, I., *The Measurement of Hearing*, p. 212. New York: McGraw-Hill, 1952.

Hood, W. H., Campbell, R. A., and Hutton, C. L., An evaluation of the Bekesy ascending descending gap. *J. Speech Hear. Res.*, 7, 123–132, 1964.

Hopkinson, N. T., Type V Bekesy audiograms; specification and clinical utility. *J. Speech Hear. Disord*, 30, 243–251, 1965.

Hopkinson, N. T., Comment on Pseudohypoacusis. *J. Speech Hear. Disord*, 32, 293–294, 1967.

Istre, C. O., and Burton, M., Automatic audiometry for detecting malingering. *Arch. Otolaryngol.* 90, 326–332, 1969.

Jerger, J., Bekesy audiometry in analysis of auditory disorders. *J. Speech Hear. Res.*, 3, 275–287, 1960.

Jerger, J., Personal communication, 1975.

Jerger, J., Burney, L., Mauldin, L., and Crump, B., Predicting hearing loss from the acoustic reflex. *J. Speech Hear. Disord.*, 39, 11–22, 1974.

Jerger, J., and Herer, G., An unexpected dividend in Bekesy audiometry. *J. Speech Hear. Disord.*, 26, 390–391, 1961.

Jerger, J., and Tillman, T., A new method for the clinical determination of sensorineural acuity level (SAL). *Arch. Otolaryngol.*, 71, 948–955, 1960.

Johnson, K. O., Work, W. P., and McCoy, G., Functional deafness. *Ann. Otol. Rhinol. Laryngol.*, 65, 154–170, 1956.

Kerr, A. G., Gillespie, W. J., and Easton, J. M. Deafness; a simple test for malingering. *Br. J. Audiol.*, 9, 24–26, 1975.

Kintsler, D. P., Phelan, J. G., and Lavender, R. B., Efficiency of the Stenger tests in identification of functional hearing loss. *J. Aud. Res.*, 10, 118–123, 1970.

Kintsler, D. P., Phelan, J. G., and Lavender, R. B., The Stenger and speech Stenger tests in functional hearing loss. *Audiology* 11, 187–193, 1972.

Knight, J., and Beagley, H., Nonorganic hearing loss in children. *Int. Audiol.*, 9, 142–143, 1970.

Lamb, L. E., and Peterson, J. L., Middle ear reflex measurements in pseudohypacusis. *J. Speech Hear. Disord.*, 32, 46–51, 1967.

Leshin, G. J., Childhood non-organic hearing loss. *J. Speech Hear. Disord.*, 25, 290–292, 1960.

Lumio, J. S., Jauhiainen, T., and Gelhar, K., Three cases of functional deafness in the same family. *J. Laryngol.*, 83, 299–304, 1969.

Marsh, J. T., and Worden, F. G., Sound evoked frequency-following responses in the central auditory pathway. *Laryngoscope*, 78, 1149–1163, 1968.

Martin, F. N., and Hawkins, R. R., A modification of the Doerfler-Stewart test for the detection of non-organic hearing loss. *J. Aud. Res.*, 3, 147–150, 1963.

Martin, F. N., and Monro, D. A., The effects of sophistication on Type V Bekesy patterns in simulated hearing loss. *J. Speech Hear. Disord.*, 40, 508–513, 1975.

Martin, N. A., Psychogenic deafness. *Ann. Otol. Rhinol. Laryngol.*, 55, 81–89, 1946.

McCandless, G. A., and Lentz, W. E., Evoked response (EEG) audiometry in non-organic hearing loss. *Arch. Otolaryngol.*, 87, 123–128, 1968.

McLennan, R. O. and Martin, F. N., On the discrepancy between the speech reception threshold and the pure-tone average in nonorganic hearing loss. Poster Session at the annual convention of the American Speech and Hearing Assoc., Houston, 1976.

Miller, A. L., Fox, M. S., and Chan, G., Pure tone assessments as an aid in detecting suspected non-organic hearing disorders in children. *Laryngoscope*, 78, 2170–2176, 1968.

Monro, D. A., and Martin, F. N., Effects of sophistication on four tests for nonorganic hearing loss. *J. Speech Hear. Disord.*, 42, 528–534, 1977.

Myklebust, H. R., *Auditory Disorders in Children.* New York: Grune & Stratton, 1954.

Nagel, R. F., RRLJ – A new technique for the non-cooperative patient. *J. Speech Hear. Disord.*, 29, 492–493, 1964.

Niemeyer, W., and Sesterhenn, G., Calculating the hearing threshold from the stapedius reflex threshold for different sound stimuli. Paper presented at the 11th International Congress of Audiology, Budapest, Hungary, 1972.

Noble, W. G., Pure-tone acuity, speech-hearing ability and deafness in acoustic trauma; a review of the literature. *Audiology*, 12, 291–315, 1973.

Pang-Ching, G., The tone-in-noise test: a preliminary report. *J. Aud. Res.*, 10, 322–327, 1970.

Peck, J. E., and Ross, M., A comparison of the ascending and the descending modes for administration of the pure-tone Stenger test. *J. Aud. Res.*, 10, 218–220, 1970.

Peterson, J. L., Non-organic hearing loss in children and Bekesy audiometry. *J. Speech Hear. Disord.*, 28, 153–158, 1963.

Price, L. L., Shepherd, D. C., and Goldstein, R., Abnormal Bekesy tracings in normal ears. *J. Speech Hear. Disord.*, 30, 139–144, 1965.

Resnick, D. M., and Burke, K. S., Bekesy audiometry in non-organic auditory problems. *Arch. Otolaryngol.*, 76, 38–41, 1962.

Rintelmann, W. F., and Carhart, R., Loudness tracking by normal hearers via Bekesy audiometer. *J. Speech Hear. Res.*, 7, 79–93, 1964.

Rintelmann, W., and Harford, E., The detection and assessment of pseudohypoacusis among school-age children. *J. Speech Hear. Disord.*, 28, 141–152, 1963.

Rintelmann, W., and Harford, E., Type V Bekesy pattern; interpretation and clinical utility. *J. Speech Hear. Res.*, 10, 733–744, 1967.

Robinson, M., and Kasden, S. D., Clinical application of pure tone delayed auditory feedback in pseudohypacusis. *Eye Ear Nose Throat Mon.*, 52, 91–93, 1973.

Rose, D. E., Keating, L. W., Hedgecock, L. D., Miller, K. E., and Schneurs, K. K., A comparison of evoked response audiometry and routine clinical audiometry. *Audiology,* 11, 238–243, 1972.

Rosenberger, A. I., and Moore, J. H., The treatment of hysterical deafness at Hoff General Hospital. *Am. Psychiatry,* 102, 666–669, 1946.

Ross, M., The variable intensity pulse count method (VIPCM) for the detection and measurement of the pure tone threshold of children with functional hearing losses. *J. Speech Hear. Disord.,* 29, 477–482, 1964.

Ruhm, H. B., and Cooper, W. A., Jr., Low sensation level effects of pure tone delayed auditory feedback. *J. Speech Hear. Res.,* 5, 185–193, 1962.

Ruhm, H. B., and Cooper, W. A., Jr., Some factors that influence pure-tone delayed auditory feedback. *J. Speech Hear. Res.,* 6, 223–237, 1963.

Ruhm, H. B., and Cooper, W. A., Jr., Delayed feedback audiometry. *J. Speech Hear. Disord.,* 29, 448–455, 1964.

Schulman-Galambos, C., and Galambos, R., Brain stem auditory evoked responses in premature infants. *J. Speech Hear. Res.,* 18, 456–465, 1975.

Semenov, H., Deafness of psychic origin and its response to narcosynthesis. *Trans. Am. Acad. Ophthalmol. Otolaryngol.,* 51, 326–348, 1947.

Shepherd, D. C., and Goldstein, R., Intrasubject variability in amplitude of Bekesy tracings and its relation to measures of personality. *J. Speech Hear. Res.,* 11, 523–535, 1968.

Siegenthaler, B. M., and Strand, R., Audiogram — average methods and SRT scores. *J. Acoust. Soc. Am.,* 36, 589–593, 1964.

Stark, E. W., Jerger types in fixed-frequency Bekesy audiometry with normal and hypacusic children. *J. Aud. Res.,* 6, 135–140, 1966.

Stein, L., Some observations on Type V Bekesy tracings. *J. Speech Hear. Res.,* 6, 339–348, 1963.

Stride, R. D., Psychogalvanic audiometry without conditioning. *Int. Audiol.,* 5, 226–229, 1966.

Suzuki, T., and Kubota, K., Normal width in tracing on Bekesy audiogram. *J. Aud. Res.,* 6, 91–96, 1966.

Trier, T., and Levy, R., Social and psychological characteristics of veterans with functional hearing loss. *J. Aud., Res.,* 5, 241–255, 1965.

Truex, E. H., Psychogenic deafness. *Conn. State Med. J.,* 10, 907–915, 1946.

Ventry, I., A case for psychogenic hearing loss. *J. Speech Hear. Disord.,* 33, 89–92, 1968.

Ventry, I. M., Bekesy audiometry in functional hearing loss; a case study. *J. Speech Hear. Disord.,* 36, 125–141, 1971.

Ventry, I. M., and Chaiklin, J. B., Functional hearing loss; a problem in terminology. *ASHA,* 4, 251–254, 1962.

Ventry, I. M., and Chaiklin, J. B., Evaluation of pure tone audiogram configurations used in identifying adults with functional hearing loss. *J. Aud. Res.,* 5, 212–218, 1965.

Ventry, I., Trier, T., and Chaiklin, J., Factors related to persistence and resolution of functional hearing loss. *J. Aud. Res.,* 5, 231–240, 1965.

Williamson, D., Functional hearing loss; a review. *Maico Audiol. Lib. Ser.,* 12, 33–34, 1974.

Zwislocki, J., Acoustic attenuation between the ears. *J. Acoust. Soc. Am.,* 25, 752–759, 1953.

chapter 25

SPEECH TESTS FOR PSEUDOHYPACUSIS*

Norma T. Hopkinson, Ph.D.

This chapter will deal with those speech audiometry tests which are used in the evaluation of pseudohypacusis. Many audiologists have ambivalent feelings about nonorganicity, suspecting it, evaluating it and reporting it. The same audiologists or others view pseudohypacusis as a relic of the past and not a part of the new morality.

It is easy to see why an audiologist might prefer to look the other way and make believe the problem does not exist. The audiologist does not want to be the person who would deny another his rights of privacy, just compensation, or to assume some dishonesty or psychopathology without a court appearance or the word of a psychiatric panel. We are inclined to grant maximum freedom to the individual and to accept his behavior at face value.

It is indeed a simple solution to suggest that he is just another variety of patient with an organic problem or that his understanding of English causes him to be too lax in his criteria for responding. While this approach ensures some of the patient's rights it also does him and our society a disservice. It could prove to the malingerer that a society so naive deserves what it gets; it keeps the psychiatric patient from the therapy he needs; and as for society it takes from the more deserving recipient and gives to the less deserving.

It seems that the audiologist's job is clear. He must take precautions that he is not stating evidence of a 60-dB loss when it is actually 10 dB. It is not his job to determine guilt or innocence or who needs the money and who does not. He must ascertain to the best of his ability what the patient can and cannot hear and indicate on the basis of his background and experience the conditions under which the data were obtained.

Hopkinson (1975) points out that even a small degree of nonorganicity is still quite dangerous in terms of rehabilitation for the patient. She reported on an example of a recent variety of nonorganic hearing loss with its

* The work reported in this chapter was supported in part by grants NS 04105 and NS 12501 CDR from the National Institutes of Neurological Diseases and Stroke of the United States Public Health Services.

concomitants in which the motivations were not apparent. The patient described symptoms that were compatible with an eighth nerve tumor and revealed some test behavior that was consistent with the interpretation. Sophisticated testing of both auditory and visual senses was necessary in order to learn the nonorganic component.

Nowadays it seems as if the pseudohypacusic component is 20 to 25 dB as opposed to the claims in the past. Also, the motivation for the problem seems less clear-cut. Despite the reduced extent of the loss and the subtle dynamics of the problem the audiologist must obtain the facts (although, he must be more clever than in the past) and should refer the patient in the direction of rehabilitation. Philosophically, these tests are presented on the basis of a continuum of nonorganicity, ranging from the one extreme of psychiatric aberrancy, through the gray area in which the patient finds himself believing that he has a problem, through the area of malingering which is identified as pure and simple knowledge of the act, through to the other end of the continuum which would be criterial listening problems, defined by the patient's inability to listen critically and to make appropriate responses.

RESPONSES TO TRADITIONAL SPEECH AUDIOMETRY

The alert audiologist can pick up important clues regarding the patient's responsiveness on the standard test procedures. For example, the patient who repeats only the first or second half of the spondaic words on the speech reception threshold (SRT) test is very likely to be uncooperative. Since spondaic words have equal emphasis on each syllable if he hears one monosyllable he should hear both. While this unusual test behavior does not indicate the patient's true threshold it serves as a warning to the audiologist about the quality of responses he can expect. A patient with poor hearing in one ear may have convinced himself that he is "deaf." Therefore, he may not respond to speech or other signals in that ear regardless of the level. However, when the unmasked signal to the poorer ear exceeds 50 or 60 dB above the threshold in the better ear the audiologist has an indication of a problem because the signal was not referred to the better ear (Bekesy, 1960). This lack of response shows some uncooperativeness but not the true threshold.

Since spondaic words are identified as part of the hearing test, a pseudohypacusic patient might not respond to them, even when they are well above threshold; however, he might engage in normal conversation at lower levels. Additional clues that help to identify the patient with nonorganic hearing loss are as follows:

1. SRTs vary significantly from responses to pure tone signals in the speech range. Pure tone thresholds are usually higher because the loudness level for a pure tone is easier to set to sensitive difference limens (DLs) in the low frequencies (Martin, 1972).

2. Certain spondees are missed at every level even though the words are homogeneous with respect to intelligibility (Egan, 1948; O'Neill and Oyer, 1966). This presumes that the patient has seen or been told the words.

3. Retests for SRTs differ by 10 dB or greater from the original thresholds (Chaiklin and Ventry, 1963). Among cooperative subjects, test-retest agreement has been shown to be ±5 dB (Menzel, 1960). False speech thresholds are believed to be difficult to duplicate because of the transient nature of speech and the temporal pattern of the speech signal (Chaiklin and Ventry, 1963). However, obtaining inconsistent SRTs is not a guarantee that the problem is not organic (Glorig, 1965).

In Chapter 12 a method for obtaining SRT was proposed that controls for the patient's listening criteria. When the poorer ear is approached, the patient is not made conscious of which ear is being tested. If he does not respond when spondees are presented, a contralateral noise is used. At increasing intensity levels, he is asked if he hears the noise until he responds to the question. The response to the question tells the audiologist that he hears in the poorer ear. Consequently, the response guides the audiologist to know where to begin the presentation of spondees in descending mode. This method leads to a threshold quantity. The speech tests for nonorganic hearing loss that will be described may be used so that threshold can be quantified.

SPECIAL TESTS

Doerfler-Stewart Test

History and introduction. The Doerfler-Stewart test was developed during World War II to detect binaural pseudohypacusis. The test compares responses to speech versus noise. Most listeners will continue to respond even when noise is presented at a level 10 to 15 dB more intense than the speech. The nonorganic patient tends to stop responding even when the noise is less intense than speech (Doerfler and Stewart, 1946).

The Doerfler-Stewart test was first standardized on 100 patients with organic and nonorganic hearing problems (Muth, 1952). In 1956 Epstein and Hopkinson reported a set of norms that had been established in a study of patients with both organic and nonorganic hearing problems. Doerfler and Epstein (1956) reported this test procedure and norms in a monograph prepared for the Veteran's Administration.

Procedure. The test procedure is based on instructions from a variety of contributors.[†] The results can be recorded efficiently on the form shown in Figure 25.1. The speech audiometer must have the same binaural output for speech and noise with independent control over attenuation for each of the signals. Both the speech and noise signals should be calibrated separately in terms of 0 dB hearing level. The SRT for spondaic words is used as the reference level for speech. A sawtooth noise was recommended originally (Doerfler and Stewart, 1946) because the spectrum with base frequency of approximately 125 Hz was believed to be psychologically more noisy than a white noise at the same sensation level. A "complex noise" was substituted by Ventry and Chaiklin (1965). "Speech noise" (Grason-Stadler speech audiometers, models 162,1701 and 1704) has been as effective as sawtooth noise. Although there is not a great deal of formal evidence, it appears that the real strength of the Doerfler-Stewart test does not depend specifically on the kind of noise, as long as it has strong energy components between 125 and 500 Hz.

Instructions. The patient is instructed:

"I am going to say words to you, words like airplane, cowboy, baseball, outside, etc. My voice will be very faint when you first hear me. Just say the words after me, as soon as you begin to hear them."

It is important not to mention the noise signal. Earphones are placed on the patient and the clinician begins the test immediately. The self-assurance with which he administers this test is of significant value in uncovering a pseudohypacusic problem. Each step of the test should be continuous with the next. The equipment should be set for binaural input of both speech and noise signals. The audiologist presents the spondees by live voice, monitoring the volume unit (VU) meter to 0, with equal emphasis on each syllable.

Speech Reception Threshold One (SRT$_1$ and SRT$_1$ + 5). SRT$_1$ is accomplished using an ascending technique. The test begins at 0 dB hearing level (HL) and the intensity is increased in 5-dB steps for each presentation of three spondees. If there has been no response

---

† Test procedures based on the following: (a) instructions for university students by Francis L. Sonday, Indiana University Medical Center; (b) Doerfler and Epstein (1956); (c) instruction manual for Grason-Stadler Speech audiometer, model 162.

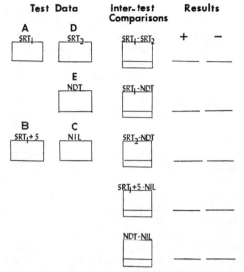

FIG. 25.1. Form used to record responses on the Doerfler-Stewart test. Columns labeled positive and negative on the right are a convenient check system for the normative calculations.

after two or three increments, a few of the words should be repeated, using a tone of voice that suggests the patient might have heard faintly but did not respond. If there is no response, the intensity may be increased in successive 5-dB steps until the patient responds correctly to two out of three spondees. The intensity is then increased another 5 dB. If the patient repeats three out of three words correctly, the previous level is recorded as his speech threshold one (SRT$_1$), and the latter increment is recorded as SRT$_1$ + 5.

Noise Interference Level (NIL). NIL is established by raising the noise level from 0 dB HL, as the clinician continues to present spondees at the SRT$_1$ + 5 dB level. The noise is brought up in 10-dB steps until a level 20 dB below the SRT$_1$ + 5 is reached. Then the increments may be in steps of 5 dB/spondee until the patient no longer repeats spondees. The point at which he does not repeat any of four spondees is the NIL. If the patient reports the presence of the noise, it is important that the clinician say nothing about it, except perhaps to nod so the patient can see that he knows the noise is present. Otherwise the patient may become very distracted, thinking that the equipment is defective. The patient should not be told that the noise is part of the test. The level at which the noise was first mentioned should be recorded separately for future reference.

When the NIL is obtained the intensity level of the speech signal should not be changed. The clinician continues to increase the noise in 5-dB steps giving one spondee at each level until the noise is 15 to 20 dB above NIL. Under the cover of this noise level, the intensity of speech should be lowered in 5-dB steps, presenting one spondee at each decrease. If no words have been repeated by the time the reading is 15 dB below SRT$_1$, the speech setting need not be reduced further. Rather the noise level can be reduced. The decrease should be in 10-dB steps/spondee until the previously obtained NIL is reached. The noise level then can be reduced in 5-dB steps/spondee until 0 dB HL or less.

Sometimes the pseudohypacusic listener will become confused and will begin repeating these fainter spondees during the decrease in the noise. This now represents the SRT$_1$ and a new NIL should be obtained. A record should be kept of the "bonus response." The results can be kept separately or, if one is able to continue to manipulate the speech and noise while responses continue, then the final set of results may not be positive but may represent the organic level of speech.

Speech Reception Threshold Two (SRT$_2$). A second SRT is obtained if no spondees were repeated when the levels of speech and noise signals were reduced. The level is raised 5 dB/three spondaic words until the patient repeats two out of three words. The level is recorded on the form in Figure 25.1 as SRT$_2$.

Noise Detection Threshold (NDT). NDT is determined following simple instructions to the patient. The intensity of the speech should be only as high as necessary (10 dB above the lower SRT). The clinician should allow the patient to see his face. An example of the instructions is as follows: "I am going to put a noise in your ears again. Please raise your hand as soon as you hear the noise, even if it is very faint. Put your hand down when the noise goes away."

The noise should be rechecked for calibration in this part of the test. While the noise is increased from −10 dB HL in 5-dB steps, the clinician should continue to look at the patient. The noise should be interrupted before each increase. After obtaining an ascending, descending and ascending threshold for the noise, the reading is recorded as NDT.

Interpretation. The norms as they were first reported (Epstein and Hopkinson, 1956; Doerfler and Epstein, 1956) are as follows:

SRT$_1$–SRT$_2$	−4 to +5 dB
SRT$_1$–NDT	−7 to +15 dB
SRT$_2$–NDT	−7 to +15 dB
SRT$_1$ + 5-NIL	−18 to +3 dB
NDT-NIL	−31 to −2 dB

Using the original set of norms in a study of the efficiency of the Doerfler-Stewart test, Ventry and Chaiklin (1965) considered the absence of positive (suspicious) difference scores as a negative result; one positive difference score equivocal, and two or more were considered a positive result. Based on their findings, they presented a revised set of norms. By taking this approach, they suggest that the only value of the measures is an overall classification of positive or negative outcome. For the clinician who is seeking insight into the response of the patient, the normative results are only the beginning. If the one positive result on the Doerfler-Stewart test is the NDT-NIL, the clinician may very well have a very important result. However, one positive result must be evaluated against the responses to the remainder of the measures, just as two or three positive results must be evaluated. The clinician may have learned that the patient tends to exaggerate certain measures, or he may have learned that the speech reception score is no doubt considerably lower than either SRT_1 or SRT_2. The clinician will now use these guidelines in presenting other test materials.

An interrelationship exists among the five measures either because they have measured the same signals, in the same or related context, or they have measured different signals in a threshold context. The first and second speech reception thresholds should relate closely. SRT_1 and SRT_2 have a close association with the detection of noise. Noise interference and speech reception above threshold are relevant to one another. Noise detection and noise interference should correlate.

Menzel (1960) described the efficiency of the Doerfler-Stewart test as a detector of nonorganic hearing loss when it is used early in the battery of tests. He concluded from his work that it was a common occurrence for the first speech reception score in the Doerfler-Stewart test to be inflated, but not the monaural SRT that followed the Doerfler-Stewart test. He concluded that the test served as "an important motivational device in discouraging the would be malingerer" (Menzel, 1960).

In Figure 25.2 representative results for a patient with organic hearing loss are shown. These scores would show a negative result.

Examination of the two SRTs shows that they are consistent. The relationship of noise detection with noise interference is reasonable. NIL is higher (15 dB) when compared with the noise detection score.

To show that pseudohypacusis is still with us the results for a patient who was tested on two recent occasions are shown in Figure 25.3. Doerfler-Stewart norms gave evidence of positive (nonorganic) results on the first visit. Regardless of the norms, the clinical data themselves show significant inconsistencies. Analy-

sis of the individual scores shows that the binaural sensitivity was 30 dB or better (note interrelationship among SRT_1, SRT_2, and NIL). The relationship between SRT_2 and NDT was not logical, and showed a degree of exaggeration for the noise signal. The noise was subjectively loud enough to interfere with speech at a level of 40 dB, yet the patient did not admit to detecting the noise until the noise reached 46 dB. On the second visit, three of the calculations continued to show significant results. The sensitivity level for the better ear now was essentially normal. Again, the noise interfered at a level lower than that which the patient admitted hearing. Retests of the better ear using standard pure tone audiometry showed an average of 10 dB.

The audiologist had manipulated the speech and noise signals to get two valuable interpretations. One was an overall qualitative evaluation, obtained through the use of the norms. The other was a quantitative evaluation, obtained through the analysis of each measure. One could say that the listener in this case had poor listening criteria. Needless to say, we did not recommend a hearing aid for this patient.

The Doerfler-Stewart test has universality because of the norms. Within the clinic, normative data make possible classifications of patients according to their performances on tests. Outside the clinic, normative data make possible a communication with the referral source and other sources concerned with the patient. The referring neurologist is not interested in the details of how the NIL is less than the NDT. He is interested in the patient's performance on tests, whether positive or negative, and in the audiologist's interpretation.

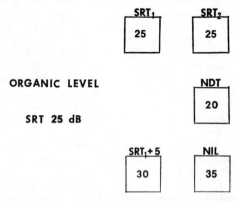

FIG. 25.2. Results that represent the responses of a patient with organic loss of hearing to the Doerfler-Stewart test. Persons with normal hearing will show lower scores with the same relationships among the scores.

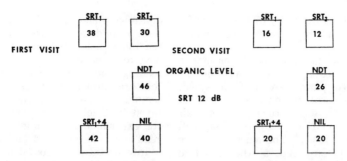

FIG. 25.3. Responses to the Doerfler-Stewart test by a patient who was tested on two separate occasions. The results show the kinds of responses that characterize nonorganic hearing loss.

Delayed Auditory Feedback Test (DAF)

Defensive audiology can be played very well with DAF because a lawsuit is unlikely over hearing one's own pleasant voice. In fact the effects of delayed speech feedback were studied before it became evident that it was appropriate for investigating hearing thresholds (Lee, 1950).

At $1/8$-sec delay between the time of reading aloud and hearing the playback, the effects of side tone on the speaker-reader were quite marked; at $1/4$ sec, the effects were still present, but at $1/15$ of a sec delay, little or no effect was noted. These effects on the listener's speech were studied by Black (1951). He described them as changes in vocal rate and intensity as a result of the subject's hearing his own voice delayed in time.

A tape recorder-reproducer is necessary to give the test. The spacing of the recording and playback heads makes it possible to insert a delay between what the speaker monitors from his kinesthetic movements during oral reading and what he monitors from his speech through earphones. In order to serve as a test of hearing levels, a means of controlling intensity level must also be available in the equipment. A variety of delay times makes the instrument more versatile. A monitor meter for observing changes in the reader's vocal intensity, and a stop watch to time his reading rate provide the clinician with a good objective measure of speech disruption.

College students with normal hearing who "feigned malingering" were subjects in one of the early attempts to use DAF as a test of hearing levels (Tiffany and Hanley, 1952). The effect on reading rate was significant when the signal was at 75 dB HL. In auditory procedures, most writers choose a delay between 0.1 and 0.2 sec. They have suggested that the test is effective at high levels of the feedback signal (Tiffany and Hanley, 1952; Chaiklin and Ventry, 1963). For the most part, studies have been reported on subjects with normal hearing or on persons who are pretending to have nonorganic hearing losses (Chaiklin and Ventry, 1963). Investigators reporting on DAF have stressed that a great deal of individual variation has been shown in response to feedback, and that in general the test is not helpful in obtaining a quantifiable threshold. Thresholds are inferred as 20 dB or more below the lowest level of positive effect. The test can be used either as a binaural or as a monaural test with equal effectiveness (Gibbons and Winchester, 1957). If the monaural procedure is used, appropriate contralateral masking is necessary.

The earliest investigators suggested starting the test at high feedback levels, and then decreasing the intensity for successive readings until the effect (a change in reading rate) no longer occurred (Hanley and Tiffany, 1954). Others have suggested starting without feedback for a baseline measure and then increasing the hearing threshold levels until a change in reading rate occurs (McGranahan, Causey and Studebaker, 1960). A speech time analyzer may be used for precision of measurement (McGranahan et al., 1960); however, a stopwatch is sufficient in lieu of special equipment.

Suggested Procedure. Hanley and Tiffany (1954) reported that a 0.18-sec delay time was a critical setting in a study of five patients who demonstrated questionable motivation for listening and one who was a classical malingerer. The procedure which follows uses a 0.18-sec time delay. The procedure begins with several readings while there is no feedback, followed by 10-dB increments. The use of decreasing intensity was discontinued because patients tended to adapt to the feedback, especially at low levels.

A stopwatch is recommended for the procedure. The reading passage should be chosen to conform to the patient's general level of intelligence and ability to read. Prior to the use of the equipment for testing for pseudohypacusis the threshold of intelligibility (50% correct) for running speech should be established for normal ears.

The microphone is adjusted on the patient so that he cannot readily move away from it. Instructions to the patient are brief. He is told, "When I put the earphones on you, please read this passage aloud. Read it through, then wait until I ask you to read it again. That will happen several times." The earphones are placed on the patient and, at the signal to begin reading, the watch is triggered to time the reading. Feedback is not yet part of the procedure. At the end of the passage, the reading time is written down as the first reading without feedback. A second baseline reading is obtained in a similar manner; however, the recording apparatus is turned on so that the patient can see it operating. There is still no feedback or intensity increment. If a VU meter is available a gross measurement of volume peaks may provide a useful basis for comparison. At the end of the second reading the time is recorded along with the gross measurement of volume. The results of a third pretest reading are obtained the same way as the first reading.

The next time the patient reads the passage the equipment is set 10 dB above the normal 0 dB intelligibility level with a feedback delay of 0.18 sec. Again the reading time is written down. The level is raised another 10 dB and the procedure continues until levels have been reached that cause the patient obvious difficulty in reading. During the readings, each time, a VU meter level should be written down for comparison purposes.

If the instrumentation is sufficiently flexible, two additional features may be beneficial. The first of these is the change of delay times. The second is the facility to switch to a simultaneous feedback rather than a delay. Some listeners who may know what to expect during the test may be able to control reading rate at low levels of feedback. When the clinician notices any tendency to control reading rate, he should repeat the test at the same level. At the same time he should vary the delay time from 0.15 to 0.5 sec and in reverse. If the reading rates are consistent with those obtained at 0.18-sec delay, the patient probably has not heard at that level.

Simultaneous feedback may be used to substantiate a change of a few seconds in reading rate at a certain level. At the same level, the patient's reading is fed back to the earphones without delay, but with amplification. The reading rate obtained in this manner may be compared with the first reading obtained at the same level with 0.18 sec delay.

When all of the readings that are necessary with delay have been completed, the earphones and microphone are left in place, and the patient is told to read the passage again. The reading is not taped. Delay and feedback are now removed as part of the procedure. The reading time is recorded for comparison against the three pretest readings. The basis for this comparison comes from the early study of delayed feedback which showed that following the experimental readings subjects seemed to read faster (Hanley and Tiffany, 1954).

Interpretation. A good deal has been written about individual differences in the response to delayed feedback, although it may be that these differences are no greater than for any other auditory test. The differences noted may be more related to the lack of procedural controls than to individual differences. Although most readers will slow their rate of reading at low levels, some readers will increase their rate. Using the above procedure a change in reading rate of 3 sec or greater is considered a significant effect of the delay when the base time for comparison is an average of the three pretest readings. Others have reported a change of 3.5 sec as significant for a threshold measure when a speech time analyzer is used (McGranahan et al., 1960).

If the reader did not show facility with the reading passage at the beginning of the test and the clinician believes the post-test reading without delay is a more accurate indicator of his reading ability, the final reading may be used as the basis for comparison. The reading rate is usually slower under a delayed condition than under the base condition.

To use a 3-sec critical difference the passage should take the average reader about 30 sec to read. Time differences on a briefer passage will be difficult to measure. One that is too long will tire the patient and provide no additional information.

For the procedure described, a level within 10 dB of speech reception threshold has been obtained when a 3-sec change in reading rate occurs. This measure is considered clinically useful as quantifiable support for threshold measures, except in those instances where the pure tones are more sensitive at either the 250- to 8000-Hz end of the scale. At high levels of feedback, distortion products may be generated in the electronic system. These distortion products may be amplified and cause the patient to show reading differences that do not reflect his thresholds within the speech range. Under the circumstances, a spuriously low threshold could be inferred from the results of the delayed feedback test.

A word about the choice of pseudohypacusic tests is appropriate here. The major emphasis should be on tests which yield results within 10 dB of the organic level of hearing. Rather than using nonquantifiable procedures the audiologist would be better off getting subjective impressions and influencing the patient by simply "chatting" with him.

Speech Stenger Test

Development. A test using speech signals to verify a monaural loss of hearing has been based on the classical pure tone Stenger Test (Taylor, 1949; Johnson, Work and McCoy, 1956; Watson and Tolan, 1967). Spondaic words are most frequently used as the speech signal. Both ears are stimulated as in the pure tone Stenger with differing sensation levels in each ear. The patient with normal hearing or a binaural hearing loss is conscious of hearing the speech in only one ear, the louder one. A two-channel speech audiometer is necessary, so that the speech signal can be presented to both ears simultaneously with intensity levels in each ear controlled independently (Newby, 1972).

Advantages of Speech Stenger. The results of the speech Stenger provide quantitative information to compare with the cross-hearing levels from traditional air conduction and speech reception tests. The speech Stenger has a decided advantage over the pure tone Stenger. Beats cannot be heard in speech signals as they are heard in the pure tone Stenger when the frequency presented to the opposite ear is a few cycles disparate from the test frequency (Zwislocki, 1963). Diplacusis can interfere with accurate administration of the pure tone Stenger, but not the speech Stenger.

Suggested Procedure. Instructions for the test are delivered over earphones to the better ear. An example of the instructions is as follows:

"Please continue to say words after me. Most of the words will be heard in your right (better) ear. Sometimes I will ask you a question. If I do, please answer the question; do not repeat it. At the same time as you repeat and answer, please raise the hand of the ear you hear me in. For example, if I say 'airplane' in your right (better) ear, put your (right) hand up and repeat 'airplane,' and then put your hand down."

The instructions are purposely complicated in order to ensure the patient's close attention to the test response (Johnson et al., 1956). The speech signals are then delivered only to the better ear of the patient at a level 15 or 16 dB sensation level (SL). Several spondees should be presented until the patient feels comfortable repeating spondees and raising his hand. If the patient forgets to raise his hand at any time, he should be reminded immediately and never be allowed to skip this part of the response.

Interrupt the presentation after each word, because, as the levels increase, the malingerer with good hearing in the "poorer" ear will be able to hear the increase and be aware of when the "poorer" ear has become part of the test. If there is an interruption, he will not be as aware that levels in the "poorer" ear are increasing.

The first binaural presentation is a simple question with the poorer ear receiving a level 20 dB above the dial reading in the better ear. A few questions are interspersed in a list of spondees. The intensity levels of the two ears should be varied dependent upon the kind of response the patient gives to successive signals. If the patient continues to respond, the level for the poorer ear should be increased until there is some indication that he hears speech in the poorer ear. At whatever level the patient stops responding, the level for the poorer ear then should be decreased until he begins to respond again (Table 25.1).

The level in the better ear should be reduced only after the audiologist has gained insight about the relationship of the two ears. Then she/he should seek to elicit a descending speech reception threshold by gradually removing the signal from the better ear. Then the signal to the poorer ear may be reduced until the patient is no longer able to repeat words, or answer questions, and does not raise his hand.

Interpretation. An interpretation of the responses can be divided into three categories: (1) crossover levels, (2) admitted interference levels and (3) interference levels.

1. Crossover levels are consistent with conventional hearing levels obtained when masking is *not* used. Usually these levels indicate that hearing for speech in the poorer ear is at least a 35-dB greater loss than in the better ear. The patient traditionally continues to respond at high levels when the signal to the better ear has been removed. As the signal in the poorer ear is reduced, the patient stops responding at a level that agrees relatively closely (±10 dB) with the unmasked levels on pure tone and speech measures. Ordinarily the level of the last response would be called responses from the better ear or "crossover" responses.

2. When the patient admits that he hears a speech signal in his poorer ear and raises his hand to designate the level, this constitutes a kind of interference, and the lowest level of that interference is called "admitted interference." It should show a relatively close relationship to other pure tone and speech test results that have been obtained voluntarily for the poorer ear. Admitted interference levels can be checked just as crossover levels were by reducing the intensity of the speech signal to the

TABLE 25.1. *Sample of Response to Speech Stenger by Organic and Nonorganic Patient*

A. Patient with Organic Loss

Organic HL .... Better ear = 30 db; Poorer ear = 70 dB
Volunteered HL .... Better ear = 30 dB; Poorer ear = 70 dB

	Ear				Response
Presentation	Better	Poorer	Verbal	Hand to	Interpretation of response
1.	46*	0	Yes	Better ear	Agrees with standard test results
2.	46	86	Yes	Poorer	Agrees with standard test results

B. Patient with Nonorganic Overlay

Organic HL .... Better ear = 30 dB; Poorer ear = 30 dB
Volunteered HL .... Better ear = 30 dB; Poorer ear = 50 dB

	Ear				Response
Presentation	Better	Poorer	Verbal	Hand to	Interpretation of response
1.	46*	0	Yes	Better ear	Agrees with standard test results
2.	46	66	No	No	Should still hear in better ear
3.	46	56	No	No	Obviously hears sound in "poorer" ear
4.	46	46	No	No	"Poorer" ear no doubt as good as "better" ear
5.	46	36		Confusion	Aware of sound in "poorer" ear – not lateralized to either ear
6.	46	26	Yes	Better ear	Not aware of sound in "poorer" ear
7.	46	30	Yes	Better ear	Not aware of sound in "poorer" ear
8.	46	34	No	No	Aware of sound in "poorer" ear Therefore, HL = 30 dB ± 4 dB

* Presentation level to better ear 16 dB above threshold.

better ear until only the poorer ear is being stimulated.

3. Finally, interference levels infer that the patient no longer responded to speech in his better ear, when the signal was presented simultaneously at a higher intensity to his poorer ear. This response is the classical response to Stenger procedures. In order to check a threshold level for the poorer ear, the intensity level to the poorer ear should be reduced until the response occurs again for the better ear. A final check can be made then, by gradually removing the signal from the better ear, to determine whether the patient will continue to respond to stimulation of the poorer ear, although he may not identify correctly the ear in which he hears the signal (Table 25.1).

After the clinician has become experienced with the speech Stenger, he may improvise methods of manipulating the levels to each ear, so that the reliability of response can be checked carefully. Threshold levels for the poorer ear can be supported with this test unless the patient (like many nonorganics) has not been cooperative during traditional speech procedures. If that is so, the results of the Stenger may be used to identify the levels at which to proceed with other tests of speech or with retests. The degree of disparity in level between the ears also can be supported when using the procedure as described.

The Story Tests

Introduction. Although story tests are no longer considered part of the stylish repertoire of nonorganic tests, they still may be used to verify a monaural loss of hearing, and quantitative results can be obtained if the technique is controlled for that purpose. A two-channel speech audiometer is necessary with the facility for switching from one ear to the other and to a binaural position. One of these kinds of tests will be described here. In Table 25.2, a sample of a story test is shown.

A number value can be obtained from this test to support the organic level of a unilateral loss. The patient is advised that he will hear a story over the earphones. He should listen to all of it, then repeat as many parts of the story as he remembers. The choice of level for presenting the test signals is very important. The level will be the same for both ears; however, it should be chosen so that it is slightly above the admitted threshold in the better ear. The clinician should be aware that cross-hearing will interfere with the validity of the test if the level for the poorer ear is more than 30 to 35 dB greater than the level for the better ear (Newby, 1972).

Parts of the story are delivered to the better ear, parts to the poorer ear, and parts to both ears. If the level has been chosen effectively at

TABLE 25.2. *Sample of a Story Test*
Swinging Story

Better Ear	Poorer Ear	Both Ears
(1) A bootblack	(2) A tailor	(3) and two cabdrivers won
	(4) 400 and	(5) 75 dollars
(6) shooting dice	(7) in the alley.	(8) They
(9) went on a spree		(10) and spent
	(11) 33 dollars of	
(12) it on	(13) wine	(14) women
(15) and song.		(16) Before they
(17) started they	(18) met three bums to whom they	(19) lost every cent
(20) in a game of	(21) draw	(22) poker.
(23) The moral of this story is it never		(24) pays to gamble
	(25) especially with bums.	

the outset, and if the patient repeats parts of the story delivered to the poorer ear, then the hearing can be said to be at least at that level. The story should be designed so that it is wholly integrated and makes sense, in the event that the patient has an organic monaural loss and hears only those parts delivered to the better ear or both ears.

Suggested Procedure. The procedure for the test is that the clinician reads through the whole story, switching parts of it to either ear without interruption. At the end of the story, a simple "OK" from the clinician with intonation suggesting that it is all right to repeat the story now, should be sufficient to start a cooperative patient repeating parts of the story. If the patient remains silent or repeats only a few words, a longer silence should be maintained to allow the patient time to think about his responses. It is important not to rush him or push him into stating that he heard nothing. If he continues to remain silent, he should be permitted to see the clinician's face. He should be asked if he did not hear the story. If the patient says he did not, he should be advised that the story is loud enough to be heard, that he should try again and that the whole thing will be repeated for him.

To be successful, this test must provide the listener with the feeling of continuity so that he is not sharply aware that the story is being switched from ear to ear. Levels are not changed in this procedure because the differing levels may cue the patient that the poorer ear is louder than the other. He could then respond only to the ear receiving less intense signals. Using equal levels in each ear the malingerer cannot make this evaluation if the actual hearing levels in each ear are similar.

Interpretation. At the end of the story, the patient should repeat only those parts that were delivered to the good ear or both ears.

Many times, parts of the story, or at least words delivered to the poorer ear, will be mixed in with better ear responses. This gives the clinician some idea that the poorer ear is at least as sensitive as the level at which the test was presented. Often these levels relate within 10 dB of the SRT for the poorer ear.

The technique may be changed a little to investigate thresholds for speech lower than the admitted levels. A level is chosen that is approximately 10 dB below the admitted thresholds for each ear. The patient is given instructions face-to-face before earphones are placed, and the whole story is delivered at the selected intensity level. At the end of the story, the long silence is used to await any response. If a response is forthcoming, the audiologist is encouraged to seek better SRTs. If a response does not occur, one may choose to accept the initially admitted thresholds.

Speech Measures by Electrodermal Audiometry (EDR)

Introduction. In a few years or less, the clinical audiologist will see the passing of EDR from the nonorganic battery of tests, largely because of legal implications. As one who has never viewed the test as a method of torture, but rather as a boon to the listener because he cannot help himself and to the audiologist in the resolution of many difficult nonorganic losses, the writer sees this passing as a misfortune, and as another contributor to the "defensive" approach to audiology. In the meantime, so that clinical audiologists should not be unaware that these tests had some value in the history of clinical audiology, speech measures by EDR will be described.

Classical Conditioning of Speech Signals. Successful use of EDR or galvanic skin response (GSR) techniques in pure tone audiometry led to attempts to condition similar responses to speech signals. A validation study using normally hearing subjects and conductively impaired subjects was reported (Ruhm and Carhart, 1958). A followup study indicated the value of the test on 30 patients who had pseudohypacusis (Ruhm and Menzel, 1959).

The following procedure and interpretation are suggested for classically conditioned speech signals. The patient was instructed to listen to the words and not to repeat them. He was made aware that a shock would be part of the test. The procedure reported by Ruhm and Carhart (1958) involved conditioning the skin response to a spondaic word that was presented in a group of spondees by monitored live voice. The unconditioned stimulus (shock) was always used when the key word was presented during the conditioning schedule. All of the words were presented at a level that could be heard easily during conditioning. The threshold for intelligibility was established, by omitting the shock and presenting words at supposed subthreshold levels. In the brief series of words, the key word or conditioned stimulus was always one of the spondees. Other words may have shown minimal inkwriter movement, but not of sufficient amplitude to be identified as the conditioned word.

Conventional EDR equipment was used in conjunction with a speech audiometer. The test was conducted monaurally. Classical conditioning was used to elicit skin responses and was successful if a rigid conditioning procedure was carried out prior to the investigation of thresholds. Chaiklin (1959) found GSR speech thresholds (for the tape recorded message, "Now you hear me") to be equivalent to the standard SRT in normal listeners. Interpretation of the responses was *objective* in that the patient did not make overt responses to the signals, even though the clinician still decided whether the criteria for a skin response were met.

Instrumental Avoidance Conditioning. A test was described that used instrumental avoidance conditioning to obtain verbal responses to speech signals (Hopkinson, Katz and Schill, 1960). The test took two practical measurements of SRT at the same time, the GSR recording to the conditioned speech signals as well as the actual verbal response.

The following procedure was suggested. The patient was instructed to listen for words. Several spondees were identified for the patient. He was told that if the correct word were spoken *just as soon as it was heard*, he could avoid a shock. If the correct word were not spoken or if it were said too late, the shock would *not* be avoided. Electrodes were affixed and earphones were put in place as for conventional EDR audiometry. A spondee was presented to the better ear at an intensity level 15 dB less intense than the professed threshold. If a response was obtained, a second spondee was presented 10 to 20 dB lower. If no response was obtained, the intensity was increased in 5-dB steps until a response was obtained. After the first response, another but less familar spondee, such as "hedgehog" was presented at the threshold level and a moderate shock was administered within 1 sec. It is assumed that the patient would not make a correct response in the allotted time because of the faintness of the signal and the unfamiliarity of the word. The unconditioned stimulus (the shock) served as reinforcement for the preconditioning carried out in the verbal instructions. At a level 5 dB less intense, a spondee which was used in the instructions to the patient was presented with the shock reinforcement (a second shock). If there was a response at this level, the reinforcing sequence would be used again. This type of procedure was followed until there was sufficient evidence to support a voluntary threshold from verbal response and a GSR threshold from skin resistance changes.

A comparison of two conditioning techniques in a study of GSR speech audiometry with normals showed that the instrumental avoidance technique was superior in the following: (1) more rapid acquisition of conditioning, (2) greater resistance to extinction, (3) wider intensity generalization and (4) less stimulus intensity dynamism (Katz and Connelly, 1964). Some of these same findings were noted in a study of instrumental versus classical conditioning using pure tones (Shepherd, 1964). In view of these findings, the accomplishment of voluntary verbal responses along with objective skin responses was a major advantage to the audiologist.

LESS DEFINITIVE SPEECH TESTS

Although quantitative levels are less likely to be obtained using certain speech tests, their results might verify the suspicion of lower quantitative thresholds. They may also lead the less cooperative patient to perform more reliably in a retest using a quantitative test. When they are used, successive retests or additional threshold measures are necessary to ascertain organic levels of hearing.

Lombard Test

The Lombard test is well known as a screening procedure in otologists' offices (Chaiklin and Ventry, 1963). The principle of the test is that the listener-speaker's own vocal intensity is regulated by him to accommodate to the noise in his environment. Unless one does not hear the noise in his surroundings, he will raise his vocal intensity to compensate for the level of noise.

Description. The audiologist uses the Lombard effect by having a patient read a paragraph aloud, and gradually increasing masking noise through the patient's earphones to determine whether vocal output changes. If the patient raises his reading volume while the noise is being increased and lowers it while the noise is being decreased, the patient is assumed to be hearing the intensity changes. The results of this method are gross evidence that the patient hears (Simonton, 1965). If the vocal reflex occurs at levels of intensity less than the patient's admitted threshold, the audiologist knows that the threshold is in error, but he does not know the magnitude of the error (Newby, 1972).

A modification of the Lombard has been described that recommends that the patient read aloud into the microphone input of a live voice speech audiometer. The talkback and attenuator dial are left at one position so that the VU meter peaks at zero. Masking noise is then introduced into both ears and is slowly increased until the VU meter is observed to increase peak value. Reducing the level brings the VU meter back to zero (Harris, 1965).

Modifications such as the one described represent attempts to obtain quantitative levels; however, neither normative data nor pathologic data have been circulated. There appear to be wide variations in response among individuals. A person who has disciplined himself to listen in noisy conditions can control the intensity of his own voice in spite of intense masking levels.

Modifications of Conventional Speech Tests

Modifications of conventional speech tests may be used to encourage a patient who is reticent to respond. These should be noted, although they are limited as methods of measurement in and of themselves. Used in conjunction with a threshold measure, they may serve a purpose.

Three Spondaic Words. The patient is instructed that two-syllabled words will be said in groups of three, after which the clinician will wait for all three to be repeated. Emphasis should be placed on remembering and repeating all three of the words. The method is begun at approximately 4 dB above admitted threshold. The cooperative patient will repeat all three spondees at each level until he is not able to hear them. The less cooperative patient responds in a variety of ways. The most frequent response is to say one spondee of the three. At the beginning of the method, the clinician should take some time to ask the patient if he could not remember all three words, so that stress is laid to three words. Under these conditions, the clinician may become aware of the range below the previously admitted threshold, in which the patient continues to find speech intelligible. He may then initiate a retest of SRT beginning at a lower level.

Monosyllables at Low Sensation Level. When the SRTs are discrepant from other threshold measures, phonetically balanced monosyllables may be presented by live voice at 5 or 10 dB above admitted thresholds. The reliability of the admitted threshold may be checked in a general way by evaluating the percentage of correct score against the articulation curves shown in the studies of social adequacy index (Davis, 1948). The articulation curves are available in a more recent text (Harris, 1965). Theoretically, a listener with 0 dB HL will score approximately 25% on phonetically balanced (PB) words at 5 dB SL, 50% correct at 10 dB SL, 75% correct at 20 dB SL, 88% at 28 dB SL, 92% at 32 dB SL and 100% at 40 dB SL. Of course, many factors can vary the scores such as the monosyllabic materials used, the fact that live voice rather than recorded voice has been used, and true distortions in the hearing mechanism.

If a patient has admitted to hearing speech at a level of 40 dB, but on other tests in the audiologic battery of tests he has shown evidence of hearing levels lower than 40 dB, a repeat test of discrimination for speech using live voice may be attempted. Snyder (1977) has shown an extreme example of this kind of nonorganic response in which an unusually high percentage word recognition score was obtained by a patient. The level of presentation of PB words could be chosen as 20 dB HL. If the patient obtains a score of 80% correct, the repeat of speech reception testing may begin at the level of the first speech reception score. A score of 80% correct suggests that the threshold for speech may be near normal. If no response is obtained at 20 dB, the level should be raised to 40 dB HL. A score close to 100% suggests essentially normal hearing, although a lower percentage does not preclude normal hearing.

Repeat Discrimination Measures. If the clinician suspects that recorded discrimination scores have been exaggerated, checks on consistency of cooperation are available. Unlike retests of discrimination lists to check the consistency of the score, these tests are given to find out the consistency of response. The former purpose might require the use of a different scrambling of the list of words; but the latter purpose requires the use of the same recording. The method allows the clinician to observe whether the same words are identified incorrectly in the same way or in similar ways. The percentage correct score might be the same, but an entirely different set of words might be missed. Initial consonants might be substituted rather than final consonants. This is not meant to infer that all legitimate errors will be repeated in exactly the same way; however, a certain consistency of error should be apparent.

This method only provides clinical evidence that the speech discrimination scores sometimes reflect a lack of patient cooperation. Other methods of checking hearing levels for speech may be improvised as the clinician works with the patient. The clinician may learn how the patient responds and what might motivate him to respond. In any event, the clinician's ultimate purpose is to identify the magnitude of the patient's problem.

One last word about the study of nonorganic hearing loss. Several researchers believe that persons who are simulating hearing loss or pretending to have hearing difficulty are appropriate subjects for the study of nonorganicity. If it were true that these persons were good subjects we could learn a great deal about the problem; however it might not be any more appropriate to substitute any other kind of person for the nonorganic patient than it would be to substitute a person who pretends to have an acoustic tumor. The investment of the pretender who is a subject in a study of nonorganicity is like that of the financial investment one makes in playing Monopoly. The use of pretenders is fraught potentially with misleading assumptions. Unfortunately, many misunderstandings about nonorganicity probably have developed because we have taught students of clinical audiology that nonorganicity is only someone pretending not to hear. Surely we must know that pretending for kicks will never be like having a personal, emotional investment in the behavior.

REFERENCES

Bekesy, G. von, *Experiments in Hearing*. New York: McGraw-Hill, Inc., 1960.

Black, J. W., The effect of delayed side-tone upon vocal rate and intensity. *J. Speech Hear. Disord.*, 16, 56-60, 1951.

Chaiklin, J. B., The conditioned GSR auditory speech threshold. *J. Speech Hear. Res.*, 2, 229-236, 1959.

Chaiklin, J. B., and Ventry, I. M., Functional Hearing Loss. In Jerger, J. (Ed.), *Modern Developments in Audiology*, Ch. 3, pp. 76-125. New York: Academic Press, 1963.

Davis, H., The articulation area and the social adequacy index for hearing. *Laryngoscope*, 58, 761-778, 1948.

Doerfler, L. G., and Epstein, A., The Doerfler-Stewart test for functional hearing loss. *Monogr. Vet. Adm.*, 1956.

Doerfler, L. G., and Stewart, K., Malingering and psychogenic deafness. *J. Speech Disord.*, 11, 181-186, 1946.

Egan, J. P., Articulation testing methods. *Laryngoscope*, 58, 955-991, 1948.

Epstein, A., and Hopkinson, N. T., An investigation into the clinical validity of the Doerfler-Stewart test in the determination of non-organic hearing loss. Paper presented at the Convention of the American Speech and Hearing Association, Chicago, November 1956.

Gibbons, E. W., and Winchester, R. A., A delayed side tone test for detecting uniaural functional deafness. *Arch. Otolaryngol.*, 66, 70-78, 1957.

Glorig, A. (Ed.), Evaluation of Non-organic Hearing Loss. In *Audiometry: Principles and Practices*, Ch. 12, pp. 235-242. Baltimore: Williams & Wilkins Co., 1965.

Hanley, C. N., and Tiffany, W. R., An investigation into the use of electromechanically delayed side tone in auditory testing. *J. Speech Hear. Disord.*, 19, 367-374, 1954.

Harris, J. D., Speech Audiometry. In Glorig, A. (Ed.), *Audiometry: Principles and Practices*, Ch. 7, pp. 151-169. Baltimore: Williams & Wilkins Co., 1965.

Hopkinson, N. T., Katz, J., and Schill, H. A., Instrumental avoidance galvanic skin response audiometry. *J. Speech Hear. Disord.*, 25, 349-357, 1960.

Hopkinson, N. T., Iatrogenic nonorganic hearing loss. *Trans. Pa. Acad. Ophthalmol. Otolaryngol.*, 28, 51-55, 1975.

Johnson, K. O., Work, W. P., and McCoy, G., Functional deafness. *Ann. Otol. Rhinol. Laryngol.*, 65, 154-170, 1956.

Katz, J., and Connelly, R., Instrumental avoidance vs. classical conditioning in GSR speech audiometry. *J. Aud. Res.*, 4, 171-179, 1964.

Lee, B. S., Some effects of side-tone delay. *J. Acoust. Soc. Am.*, 22, 639-640, 1950.

Martin, F. N., Nonorganic Hearing Loss: An Overview and Pure Tone Tests. In Katz, J. (Ed.), *Handbook of Clinical Audiology*, Ch. 19, pp. 357-373. Baltimore: Williams & Wilkins Co., 1972.

McGranahan, L. M., Causey, D., and Studebaker, G. A., Delayed side tone audiometry (abstract). *ASHA*, 2, 357, 1960.

Menzel, O. J., Clinical efficiency in compensation audiometry. *J. Speech Hear. Disord.*, 25, 49-54, 1960.

Muth, E. B., An attempt to standardize the Doerfler-Stewart test for malingering and psychogenic deafness. Masters thesis, University of Maryland, 1952.

Newby, H. A., *Audiology*, Ed. 3. New York: Appleton-Century-Crofts, 1972.

O'Neill, J. J., and Oyer, H. J., *Applied Audiometry*. New York: Dodd, Mead & Co., 1966.

Ruhm, H. B., and Carhart, R., Objective speech audiometry; a new method based on electrodermal response. *J. Speech Hear. Res.*, 1, 169-178, 1958.

Ruhm, H. B., and Menzel, O. J., Objective speech audiometry in cases of nonorganic hearing loss. *Arch. Otolaryngol.*, 69, 212-219, 1959.

Shepherd, D. C., Instrumental avoidance conditioning versus classical conditioning in electrodermal audiometry. *J. Speech Hear. Res.*, 7, 55–70, 1964.

Simonton, K. M. Audiometry and Diagnosis. In Glorig, A. (Ed.), *Audiometry: Principles and Practices*, Ch. 9, pp. 185–206. Baltimore: Williams & Wilkins Co., 1965.

Snyder, J. M., Characteristic patterns of etiologic significance from routine audiometric tests and case history. *Maico Audiol. Lib. Ser.*, 15, Report 5, 1977.

Taylor, G. J., An experimental study of tests for the detection of auditory malingering. *J. Speech Hear. Disord.*, 14, 119–130, 1949.

Tiffany, W. R., and Hanley, C. N., Delayed speech feedback as a test for auditory malingering. *Science*, 115, 59–60, 1952.

Ventry, I. M., and Chaiklin, J. B., Efficiency of five audiometric measures. *J. Aud. Res.*, 5, 201–211, 1965.

Watson, L. A., and Tolan, T., *Hearing Tests and Hearing Instruments* ("Facsimile of the 1949 Edition"). New York: Hafner Publishing Co., 1967.

Zwislocki, J. (Ed.), Critical evaluation of methods of testing and measurement of nonorganic hearing impairment. Report of Working Group 36, NAS-NRC Committee on Hearing, Bioacoustics and Biomechanics, 1963.

Physiological Tests of Auditory and Vestibular Function

chapter 26

ELECTRODERMAL AUDIOMETRY

Albert W. Knox, Ph.D.

The purpose of this chapter is to familiarize the reader with the bases, history, development, rationale, applications and the future of galvanic skin response (GSR) audiology. Students and clinicians who are interested in the techniques of administering and interpreting the GSR test will find very thorough step by step coverage in Engelberg (1970).

The practice of compensating people financially for losses to the auditory system has created unique problems in the field of audiology. The usual protocol of testing requires the clinician to present a signal to the patient and then depend upon the willingness of the patient to respond to it. If this response is at threshold and can be repeated the test is valid. This ideal behavior has not always been obtainable in cases where large sums of money are concerned. Workmen's compensation, disability retirement, veterans compensation or criteria of acceptability into the military services are some of the circumstances wherein people have been known to take liberties with their voluntary reporting of true organic threshold. Some normal subjects have even made it appear as though a stimulus of 120 dB (ANSI-1969) was insufficiently intense to activate their auditory system. While there are a number of tests the audiologist can use to determine that the thresholds had been exaggerated, as long as the patient has the option of voluntary response, the tester cannot be certain of the true organic threshold. Shrewd individuals, well informed in audiometric procedures, were capable of defeating the purposes of the tests and benefiting by many hundreds of thousands of

dollars. Some means are necessary of ascertaining auditory sensitivity without involving voluntary responses by the patient.

Physiologic foundations for objective audiometry were well known and in practice in physiologic and psychological research. Recording reflexes elicited by sound signals were reported by Johannes Mueller in 1838 using the cochleopalpebral reflex (a quick blinking of the eyelids). Bechterew (1905), who is famous for his work with vestibular nuclei, suggested that this reflex could be employed when testing patients who may be malingering total deafness. Gault (1920) employed this reflex in 1916 in medicolegal cases arising from military service in the German Army in the First World War.

The psychogalvanic reflex (PGSR) was the next phenomenon to be tried. Observed by Féré (1888) and named by Veraguth (1909) the PGSR was reportedly used to measure hearing sensitivity by Albrecht (1918). However, because the change in resistance was small and quickly extinguished, the method was considered unreliable and the use of the test was discontinued.

Two basic methods of assessing the PGSR were developed. The exosomatic (Lindsley, 1963) system of Féré, which involves application of electric current with a low voltage potential between the electrodes and measuring the change of resistance directly from the electrodes, is the one in clinical and experimental use because of the ease of measurement. A second method, sometimes called endosomatic, was developed by Tarchanoff (Lindsley, 1963). The Tarchanoff method measures the difference in electric potential arising from currents in the skin. The currents and their electric potential, or voltage pressure, are of extremely low magnitude and require DC amplifiers of high stability and great sensitivity. Such instruments have not yet been developed.

It was World War II which precipitated the

next development. The return of nearly twelve million American service men to civilian life, following its conclusion, gave impetus to the search.

Bordley, Hardy and Richter (1948) utilizing modern audiometric equipment applied the technique of classical Pavlovian conditioning by pairing pure tone stimuli with mild electric shock. They found that after several paired presentations the tone alone was capable of eliciting the desired PGSR.

It appeared that the conditioned PGSR met the severest tests of objectivity. The utilization of the conditioned electrodermal response (EDR) eliminated the need for any judgmental or decisive response by the subject about the presence of signals near or at threshold levels. Doerfler and McClure (1954) established the efficiency of this technique in threshold measurement. After the problems of equipment calibration were solved and the schedules of presentation were determined and substantiated by experimental data, the EDR test became clinically practical. The test data were graphic in nature and required interpretation by the examining audiologist. This had the effect of taking the subjectivity from the patient but giving it to the audiologist.

THE PSYCHOGALVANIC REFLEX

The human skin has properties of electrical conductance as well as electrical resistance. If electrodes are placed on a subject's skin, for example one on the index finger and one on the ring finger of one hand, the resistance of the skin to current flow between the electrodes can be measured. This measurement is made by determining the voltage pressure of one electrode and comparing it to the voltage at the other electrode. The drop in voltage between these electrodes is converted to resistance measurement by the application of Ohm's law. Usually this resistance is of the order of 5,000 to 20,000 ohms. This is the static resistance or resistance level of the skin and not the GSR. This static resistance can be measured with almost any kind of voltmeter and recorded with simple galvanometers. When some stimulus causes the skin resistance to change, such as a loud noise or change in emotional state as a result of an unexpected event, the resistance across the electrodes decreases; it undergoes a slow change to a lower level and then gradually builds up to its static level. It is this change which is the PGR (or sometimes called GSR, PGSR, PGΔSR or EDR).

The source of the reflex is clouded in controversy. Almost certainly it arises from some activity that parallels or precedes sweating. There are also those who believe that the reflex source is the result of dilation or contraction of the blood vessels in the vicinity of the electrodes. Others believe it results from muscle activity because of a correlation approaching unity with visceral muscle activity.

McCleary (1950) identified the central mechanism of the GSR as starting in the premotor area (Brodmann's area 6) of the cortex. Electric stimulation of the premotor cortex elicits the reflex and severing the premotor area causes the reflex to disappear.

A word should be said about the conditioning process. PGSR testing is not an operant process; it is a reflex or respondent process. As the noxious stimulus is paired with the tone there is no operant behavior elicited. An operant response would change the environment; a reflex changes the physiologic state of the individual only. The subject, short of ripping off the electrodes and aborting the test, is unable to avoid the shock. The subject is instructed to remain as quiet as possible, to relax and not move any more than is necessary. When his cooperation is obtained and adequate conditioning is possible, transient changes in skin resistance can provide a valid measure of auditory threshold.

Equipment necessary for the EDR audiometric test includes an adequate sound-isolated environment for both the individual to be tested and the audiologist and his instruments. Adequate wiring is necessary between the rooms for pure tone signals, masking, patient monitor circuits, shock and resistance electrodes, as well as the ground or indifferent electrode, if the equipment requires it.

An audiometer serves as the signal source generating the auditory (conditioned) stimulus and controlling its frequency and intensity. The onset and duration of the tone are controlled by a psychogalvanometer, as well as the onset, intensity and duration of the electric shock (unconditioned stimulus).

ELECTRODERMAL AUDIOMETRY

Electrodermal audiometry (EDA) is an exacting procedure. Every step must be carefully controlled if errors are to be avoided and valid results obtained. The approaches to it are many; however, the procedure for adult application established by Chaiklin, Ventry and Barrett (1961) has probably gained the widest acceptance. For use with children the routine suggested by Hardy and Pauls (1952) has been recommended by most writers, but its reported use has been limited to hospital clinics. The following considerations epitomize the thinking and research of audiologists who regularly employ EDA.

Pretest Considerations

The candidacy of a patient for taking the GSR test must be established in three areas.

First he must be able to tolerate the shock (unconditioned stimulus, UCS). This eliminates people who have a medical history of heart trouble or seizures; they should not be tested by EDA. Second, he must be responsive to conditioning. Patients on tranquilizers or analgesic medication or those habituated to alcohol or narcotics either psychedelic or opiate, are almost impossible to condition. In some instances the procedure of having the patient remain in the hospital overnight and attempting to test in the morning after a drug- or medicine-free night is sufficient to obtain adequate conditioning. Subjects who have earned their living as farmers or laborers, however cooperative, may be poor candidates for EDA because of difficulty in conditioning. These subjects have usually developed callouses on their hands which are as hard and impervious as bone and either do not experience the shock or do not demonstrate GSR. Electricians frequently have experienced so many shocks they are not affected by them.

For those interested in the effect of drugs on behavior with respect to GSR, Uhr and Miller (1960) have reported a series of studies which utilize the GSR to measure the effects of drugs on the autonomic system. Their findings in brief are that skin conductivity was reduced by depressants and at least one stimulant was capable of improving conditioning.

Third, the patient must be emotionally capable of conditioning. Certain psychiatric patients are incapable of responding and avenues other than noxious electric shock may provide the preferred method of examination. This is particularly true of catatonic patients but should not be generalized to all psychiatric patients.

Although EDA has been advocated as useful with children (O'Neill and Oyer, 1966), the uninhibited nature of children almost precludes them from candidacy. It is mandatory that the subject hold still and not vocalize, two conditions almost unknown in a population of children, particularly after receiving a noxious stimulus. Irwin and his colleagues (Hind, Aronson and Irwin, 1958) working with mentally retarded children advocated further research with depressants to find dosage levels wherein a child would be tractable and still be responsive to conditioning. Spradlin, Locke and Fulton (1969) reviewed the state of the art of EDA with mentally retarded children and found it to be essentially ineffective.

Preparation of the Patient

Most clinicians agree that EDA testing should be done after the patient has had adequate rest and that electrodes should not be attached to adjacent fingers. Those two points

seem to be the only areas of agreement. The instructions given to the patient, the methods of attaching electrodes, the type and properties of electrodes to use, the use of cleaning agents for the fingers, the electrode paste and other considerations vary greatly with the audiologists, most of whom stoutly maintain the supremacy of their systems over all others. What is probably true is that the mechanical aspects of preparation vary greatly with the clinical skill and manner of each audiologist, and those differences do not reflect the critically important aspects of patient preparation.

After adequate rest and use of the rest room facilities, the usual steps of patient preparation are as follows:

1. Seat the patient comfortably in the chair in the testing suite.

2. Examine his hands and fingers for signs of signal interferences: (a) grease should be cleaned off with alcohol or surgical soap; (b) callouses and blisters should be avoided as nonreactionary; (c) burns, insect bites, cuts, sore areas should be avoided because of contamination of the patient's wound.

3. Fasten the electrodes to the surface you have selected. Common sense has dictated the policy of separating the shock electrodes to one hand and response electrodes to the other for ease of application. The use of alternate fingers to prevent the accidental shorting of the signal to ground is generally accepted when conditions allow. What is important is that the electrodes be adequately fastened and sufficiently separated to ensure signal validity.

Lykken (1959), studying the effect of physical properties and dimensions in electrodermal measurement, found that the size and area of electrodes did not seem to be critical factors. The optimal site for the response electrode was the undersurface of the tip of the index finger. He recommended that electrodes should be (a) of negligible resistance, (b) not a source of current flow themselves (battery effect), (c) stable in chemical property in the presence of electrode paste, (d) nondehydrating, (e) constant in skin pressure, (f) clean and (g) reasonably comfortable.

4. Instructions can be given to the patient throughout his preparation. The goals of the instructions are that he is to sit quietly, not to move, not to speak, but stay awake and as alert as possible. Some clinicians tell the patient he will receive a shock (Engelberg, 1970), others do not (O'Neill and Oyer, 1966).

5. It is advisable to start the test with the ear and frequency for which clinical information is more important. It is very possible for conditioning to extinguish and be ineffective for the second ear test. Therefore, select the ear and place the earphones with this in mind.

Calibration of equipment, individually by components should be undertaken prior to the test in all other audiologic activities, in order to assure the clinician that the components are performing at least at factory specifications. Then the components must be calibrated as a single system. Here the patient becomes part of the composite instrumentation. His static resistance must be calibrated into the resistance bridge of the response circuits so that *changes* in resistance can be measured and provide the basis for decision. It is therefore the ΔR, or change in resistance, that is recorded on the strip chart recorder. (The Grason-Stadler Company uses the symbol ΔR to refer to measurement of resistance from an arbitrary base rather than the static resistance.) On the chart paper the *ordinate* represents the magnitude of response and base resistance level; the *abscissa* provides an accurate representation of time, usually at the rate of 1 mm/sec.

Perception of movement by visual and auditory monitoring method is necessary. It is important that the clinician observe the patient without being seen himself. A window in the sound suite is adequate if the patient is seated facing away from it. The patient's movement will interfere with the base resistance; the clinician's movement, if observed by the subject, could elicit an EDR. In addition to visual monitoring, a sensitive microphone and auditory monitor system can be set up to detect patient behavior as slight as changes in respiration or the noise of clothing in slight movement.

The variables to be set to the personal preference of the clinician are (a) stylus heat if the recorder paper is thermosensitive, (b) the sensitivity to change in resistance, (c) the intensity of shock, (d) the duration of the shock, (e) the intensity of the signal, (f) the delay between the tone (condition stimulus, CS) and the shock (UCS) and (g) the interval between events.

Taking each of these points in order, the stylus heat must be adjusted so that the response tracing is clear and in sharp contrast to the graphic grid on the paper. The sensitivity adjustment is necessary to obtain a clear differentiation between the excursion of the writing stylus in response to shock and random fluctuations. Shock should cause a visible deflection; the spontaneous or random fluctuations should only displace the stylus to a small, nonobjectionable deflection. Shock adjustment should be adequate to obtain conditioning. Chaiklin et al. (1961) presented half-seconds of shock in increasing intensity until the subject reported it to be "distinctly unpleasant" and then increased the shock until the subject reported he could not tolerate a shock of higher intensity. The range of distinct unpleasantness was 0.58

ma to 4.10 ma with a mean of 1.78 ma. The maximum tolerable shock ranged from 0.58 ma to 4.3 ma with a mean of 1.94.

The 0.5-sec duration of the shock has had wide acceptance, primarily because that was what was reported in the Chaiklin, Ventry and Barrett study. Shock duration longer than this appears to be necessary only with extremely lethargic patients. As in all of these variables, the guideline is "what is necessary to obtain and maintain conditioning?" This question poses two discrete problems for the clinical audiologist. The intensity of tonal signal must be sufficient to make the conditioned stimulus (CS)-UCS pairing a physiologically significant event until conditioning is obtained. Subsequent to conditioning, the reduction or increase of the intensity of the CS with its corresponding GSR constitutes the test. The final two points, the delay between the tone and shock (CS-UCS) and the interval between events provide for reliability and validity. Research indicates that a 0.5 sec interval between the tone and shock provides the best conditioning (Bitterman, Reed and Krauskopf, 1952). By varying the interval between events and following an appropriate reinforcement schedule, such as the 40% schedule advocated by Chaiklin et al. (1961) the clinician can accomplish his goals. These goals are (a) to condition the patient to the auditory stimuli, (b) to provide adequate and systematic reinforcement of the conditioning, (c) to test the reliability and validity of the subject's responses and the clinical decisions of the audiologist and (d) to obtain valid measurement of the patient's true organic threshold.

APPLICATIONS

The major clinical application of EDA is the compensation examination of demobilized servicemen by the audiology service of the Veterans Administration. Under the guidelines in contemporary use, any voluntary threshold which is of a compensable level must be verified by EDA unless the patient's health contraindicates use of the test. It is possible, that even though it is a valid and reliable test, its greatest value may be as a deterrent to exaggerating. Those who have considered exaggerating, or attempted it, quickly abandon the idea when confronted with the test.

One of the most important aspects of its administration is that of providing an avenue of voluntary response in the presence of EDA confirmed exaggerated thresholds. It is poor practice to confront the patient in an accusatory manner which he is almost certain to consider threatening or which deprives him of his dignity. The method many audiologists have found to be very acceptable, without embarrassment to the patient, is that of telling him that we have test scores that do not agree, or do not support each other, and that it is possible that he did not understand the directions for the voluntary pure tone test. Then the directions for pure tone test are repeated with emphasis on threshold responses. A sample statement is "we have reason to believe that you are waiting too long before you respond. Please do not wait until you are absolutely certain that you heard the tone, if you hear the tone, or think you hear the tone, please respond; we will verify your response with the test." Then repeat the pure tone thresholds with the GSR electrodes in place. Malingerers will usually get the message, while those who are confused will have the issue clarified, and the incidence of hostile patients may be reduced.

RESEARCH

Research in conditioned GSR audiology has taken two avenues: first, its application to clinical audiology for adults; second, the use of EDA to measure other phenomena of auditory behavior. In the first instance there has been a very thorough experimental documentation of the validity and reliability of EDA. As mentioned earlier, Doerfler and McClure (1954) established the thresholds with hard of hearing adults. Burk (1958), using a planned sampling procedure, a conditioning schedule, and a prior commitment to response criteria reported validity for subjects with normal hearing. Chaiklin (1959) and Ruhm and Carhart (1958) extended the validity data to speech audiometry, but at the time of this writing it has never achieved widespread use. Experimental verification of procedures and levels with children has not been published.

An example of the application of EDA or the conditioned GSR to provide objectivity in audiologic or psychophysiologic research is the study of Epstein and Eldot (1966). They used conditioned GSR as an objective measure of the recruitment of loudness.

FUTURE

Recently, the Occupational Health and Safety Act has become the law of the land. Safety standards have been advocated which audiologic instrument producers have been hard pressed to achieve. First, these standards primarily represent the safety thinking of American National Standards Institute (ANSI), National Laboratory Standards Institute (NLSI), and Underwriters Laboratories (UL). Recent among their recommendations is that no electric current be administered to the body in excess of 5 microamperes. Because this is

actually less than the polarization current in the skin, this proposal, if adopted, would preclude the use of shock as the aversive stimulus. That would not constitute an insurmountable problem as other stimuli could be provided. Puffs of air to the eye or ice to the skin has been used but are difficult to calibrate and even more objectionable to some people than the mild electric shock.

Second, the Underwriters Laboratories has also recommended that any instrument connected to the patient must be able to provide isolation to a surge of 2500 volts (Medical and Dental Equipment Standard, 1974). Because most of the audiometers manufactured today cannot meet that specification, certainly not with the metal disc magnetic transducer used in the headphones, it may be a while before this recommendation for audiologic equipment becomes operational and applicable if it is enacted into law.

Finally, the techniques of signal averaging (electroencephalic response audiometry and electrocochleography) may provide the solution to the amplification of the DC signal necessary for the Tarchanoff method of measuring the EDA if the test survives at all. Certainly, if the antagonists of electric current prevail the very least they would accept would be an unconditioned stimulus other than electric shock.

REFERENCES

Albrecht, W., Die Trennung der nicht organischen von der organischen Horstorung mite Hilfe des psychogalvanischen Reflexes. *Arch. Ohr.-Nas.-Kehlk.-heilk.*, 101, 1–19, 1918.

Bechterew, W., Obosrenji psichiatrii neurolgii i experimentalnoj psichologii. Heft, 1905.

Bitterman, M. E., Reed, P. C., and Krauskopf, J., The effect of the duration of the unconditioned stimulus upon conditioning and extinction. *Am. J. Psychol.*, 65, 256–262, 1952.

Bordley, J. E., Hardy, W. G., and Richter, C. P., Audiometry with the use of galvanic skin-resistance response. *Bull. Johns Hopkins Hosp.*, 82, 569, 1948.

Burk, K. W., Traditional and psychogalvanic skin response audiometry. *J. Speech Hear. Res.*, 1, 275–278, 1958.

Chaiklin, J. B., The conditioned GSR auditory speech threshold. *J. Speech Hear. Res.*, 2, 229–236, 1959.

Chaiklin, J. B., Ventry, I. M., and Barrett, L. S., Reliability of conditioned GSR pure-tone audiometry with adult males. *J. Speech Hear. Res.*, 4, 269–280, 1961.

Doerfler, L. G., and McClure, C. T., The measurement of hearing loss in adults by measurement of galvanic skin response. *J. Speech Hear. Dis.*, 19, 184–189, 1954.

Engelberg, M., *Audiological Evaluation for Exaggerated Hearing Level*. Springfield, Ill.: Charles C Thomas, 1970.

Epstein, A., and Eldot, H., An objective measure of the recruitment of loudness phenomenon. Final Report No. NB 03952, NINDB, Public Health Services, Bethesda, Md., January 1966.

Féré, C., Note sur des modifications de la resistance electrique sans l'influence des exitations sensorilles et des emotions. *C. R. Soc. Biol.*, 5, 217, 1888.

Gault, H., Presse med. 1916, 15. *Zit. nach A. J. Cemach Passow-Schaeters Beitr. Hals-Nas-Ohrenheilk.*, 14, 1-81, 1920.

Hardy, W. G., and Pauls, M. D., The test situation of PGSR audiometry. *J. Speech Hear. Disord.*, 17, 13-24, 1952.

Hind, J. E., Aronson, A. E., and Irwin, J. V., GSR auditory threshold mechanisms: instrumentation, spontaneous response and threshold definition. *J. Speech Hear. Res.*, 1, 220-226, 1958.

Lindsley, D. B., Emotion. In Stevens, S. S. (Ed.), *Handbook of Experimental Psychology*. New York: J. Wiley & Sons, 1963.

Lykken, D. T., Properties of electrodes used in electrodermal measurement. *J. Comp. Physiol. Psychol.*, 52, 629-634, 1959.

McCleary, R. A., The nature of the galvanic skin response. *Psychol. Bull.*, 47, 97-117, 1950.

Medical and Dental Equipment Standard, UL 544, effective September 30, 1974. Underwriters Laboratories Inc., Melvill, New York, 1974.

O'Neill, J., and Oyer, H., *Applied Audiometry*. New York: Dodd & Mead, 1966.

Ruhm, H. B., and Carhart, R., Objective speech audiometry: A new method based on electrodermal response. *J. Speech Hear. Res.*, 1, 169-178, 1958.

Spradlin, J., Locke, B., and Fulton, R., Conditioning and audiological assessment. In Fulton, R. T. and Lloyd, L. L. (Eds.), *Audiometry for the Retarded*. Baltimore: Williams & Wilkins Co., 1969.

Uhr, L., and Miller, J. G. (Eds.), *Drugs and Human Behavior*. New York: John Wiley & Son, 1960.

Veraguth, I., *Das psychogalvanische Reflexphanomen*. Berlin: Karger, 1909.

BIBLIOGRAPHY

Barr, B., Pure-tone audiometry for pre-school children. A clinical study with particular reference to children with severely impaired hearing. *Acta Otolaryngol. Suppl.*, 121, 1-84, 1955.

Baumeister, A. A., Beedle, R., and Urguhart, D., GSR conditioning in normals and retardates. *Am. J. Ment. Defic.*, 69, 114-120, 1964.

Bechterew, W., Uber cinen besonderen Gehors-ober den akustiko-palpebralen Reflex. *Z. Ohrenheilk*, 52, 367-368, 1906.

Blank, I., and Finsinger, J. E., Electrical resistance of the skin. *Arch. Neurol. Psychiatry*, 56, 544-557, 1946.

Bordley, J. E., and Hardy, W. G., A study in objective audiometry with use of the psychogalvanic response. *Ann. Otol. Rhinol. Laryngol.*, 58, 751-760, 1949.

Bordley, J. E., and Haskins, H. L., The role of the cerebrum in hearing. *Ann. Otol. Rhinol. Laryngol.*, 64, 370-382, 1955.

Conklin, J. E., Three factors affecting the general level of electrical skin resistance. *Am. J. Psychol.*, 64, 78-86, 1951.

Cook, S. W., and Harris, R. E., The verbal conditioning of the galvanic skin reflex. *J. Exp. Psychol.*, 21, 202-210, 1937.

Coombs, C. H., Adaptation of the galvanic response to auditory stimuli. *J. Exp. Psychol.*, 22, 244-268, 1938.

Davis, R., Factors affecting the galvanic reflex. *Arch. Psychol.*, 18, 1-64, 1930.

Davis, R. C., Buchwald, A. M., and Frankmann, R. W., Autonomic and muscular responses in relation to simple stimuli. *Psychol. Monogr.*, 69, No. 20, Whole No. 405, 1-71, 1955.

Doerfler, L. G., and Kramer, J. C., Unconditioned stimulus strength and the galvanic skin response. *J. Speech Hear. Res.*, 2, 184-192, 1959.

Duffy, E., and Lacey, O. L., Adaptation of energy mobilization; changes in general level of palmar skin conductance. *J. Exp. Psychol.*, 36, 437-452, 1946.

Feldman, H., A history of audiology. *Translations Beltone Inst. Hear. Res.*, No. 22, January 1970.

Fulton, R. T., and Lloyd, L. L. (Eds.), *Audiometry for the Retarded*. Baltimore: Williams & Wilkins Co., 1969.

Furer, M., and Hardy, J. D., The reaction to pain as determined by the galvanic skin response. *Res. Publ. Assoc. Res. Nerv. Ment. Dis.*, 29, 72-89, 1950.

Giolas, M. H., and Epstein, A., Intensity generalization in EDR audiometry. *J. Speech Hear. Res.*, 7, 47-53, 1964.

Girden, E., The galvanic skin response "set," and the acoustic threshold. *Am. J. Psychol.*, 65, 233-243, 1952.

Goldstein, R., Detection and assessment of auditory disorders in children less than three years old; a critical review. *Volta Rev.*, 57, 215-219, 1955.

Goldstein, R., Effectiveness of conditioned electrodermal responses (EDR) in measuring pure-tone thresholds in cases of non-organic hearing loss. *Laryngoscope*, 66, 119-130, 1956.

Goldstein, R., Electrophysiologic Audiometry. In Jerger, J. (Ed.), *Modern Developments in Audiometry*. New York: Academic Press, 1963.

Goldstein, R., and Derbyshire, A., Suggestions for terms applied to electrophysiologic tests of hearing. *J. Speech Hear. Disord.*, 22, 696-697, 1957.

Goldstein, R., Ludwig, H., and Naunton, R. F., Difficulties in conditioning galvanic skin response: its possible significance in clinical audiometry. *Acta Otolaryngol.*, 44, 67-77, 1954.

Goldstein, R., Polito-Castro, S. B., and Daniels, J. T., Difficulty in conditioning electrodermal responses to tone in normally hearing children. *J. Speech Hear. Disord.*, 30, 26-34, 1955.

Goodhill, V., Rehman, I., and Brockman, S., Objective skin resistance audiometry. *Ann Otol. Rhinol. Laryngol.*, 63, 22-39, 1954.

Grant, D. A., Meyer, D. R., and Hake, H. W., Proportional reinforcement and extinction of the conditioned GSR. *J. Gen. Psychol.*, 42, 97-101, 1950.

Grant, D. A., and Schneider, D. E., Intensity of the

conditioned stimulus and strength of conditioning; II. The conditioned galvanic skin response to an auditory stimulus. *J. Exp. Psychol.*, 39, 35–40, 1949.

Grings, W. W., Methodological considerations underlying electrodermal measurements. *J. Psychol.*, 35, 271–282, 1953.

Grings, W. W., Lowell, E. L., and Honard, R. R., Electrodermal responses of deaf children. *J. Speech Hear. Res.*, 3, 120–129, 1960.

Grings, W. W., Lowell, E. L., and Rushford, G. M., Role of conditioning in GSR audiometry with children. *J. Speech Hear. Disord.*, 24, 380–390, 1959.

Hardy, W. G., and Bordley, J. E., Special techniques in testing the hearing of children. *J. Speech Hear. Disord.*, 16, 122–131, 1951.

Hovland, C. I., The generalization of conditioned responses; I. The sensory generalization of condition-responses with varying frequencies of tone. *J. Gen. Psychol.*, 17, 125–148, 1937.

Hovland, C. I., The generalization of conditioned responses; II. The sensory generalization of conditioned responses with varying intensities of tone. *J. Genet. Psychol.*, 51, 279–291, 1937.

Hovland, C. I., and Riesen, A. H., Magnitude of galvanic and vasomotor response as a function of stimulus intensity. *J. Gen. Psychol.*, 23, 103–121, 1940.

Hull, C. L., Stimulus intensity dynamism (V) and stimulus generalization. *Psychol. Rev.*, 56, 67–76, 1949.

Humphreys, L. G., Extinction of conditioned psychogalvanic responses following two conditions of reinforcement. J. Exp. Psychol., 27, 71–75, 1940.

Jenkins, W. O., and Stanley, J. C., Partial reinforcement; a review and critique. *Psychol. Bull.*, 47, 193–234, 1950.

Kimble, G. A., Conditioning as a function of the time between conditioned and unconditioned stimuli. *J. Exp. Psychol.*, 37, 1–15, 1947.

Kimble, G. A., *Hilgard and Marquis' Conditioning and Learning*. Ed. 2. New York: Appleton-Century-Crofts, 1961.

Knapp, P. H., and Gold, B. H., Magnitude of galvanic and vasomotor response as a function of stimulus intensity. *J. Gen. Psychol.*, 23, 103–121, 1940.

Lacey, O. L., and Siegel, P. S., An improved potentiometric circuit for measuring the galvanic skin response. *Am. J. Psychol.*, 61, 272–274, 1948.

Lacey, O. L., and Siegel, P. S., An analysis of the unit of measurement of the galvanic skin response. *J. Exp. Psychol.*, 39, 122–127, 1949.

Littman, R. A., Conditioned generalization of the galvanic skin reaction to tones. *J. Exp. Psychol.*, 39, 868–882, 1949.

McCurdy, H. G., Consciousness and the galvanometer. *Psychol. Rev.*, 57, 322–327, 1950.

Meritser, C. L., and Doerfler, L. G., The conditioned galvanic skin response under two modes of reinforcement. *J. Speech Hear. Disord.*, 19, 350–359, 1954.

Michels, M. W., and Randt, C. T., Galvanic skin response in the differential diagnosis of deafness. *Arch. Otolaryngol.*, 45, 302–311, 1947.

Moeller, G., The CS-UCS interval in GSR conditioning. *J. Exp. Psychol.*, 48, 162–166, 1954.

Newby, H. A., *Audiology*, Ed. 3. New York: Appleton-Century-Crofts, 1972.

Nober, E. H., GSR magnitudes for different intensities of shock, conditioned tone and extinction tone. *J. Speech Hear. Res.*, 1, 316–324, 1958.

Rosen, J., The place of GSR audiometry in work with young children. *Volta Rev.*, 58, 387–391, 1957.

Schlosberg, H., and White, C. T., Degree of conditioning of the GSR as a function of the period of delay. *J. Exp. Psychol.*, 43, 357–362, 1952.

Shimuzu, H., Sugano, T., Segawa, Y., and Nakamura, F. A., A study in psychogalvanic skin resistance audiometry. *Arch. Otolaryngol.*, 65, 499–508, 1957.

Sortini, A. J., Skin resistance audiometry with young children. *Hearing Dealer,* May 1955.

Statten, P., and Wisehart, D. E. S., Pure-tone audiometry in young children; psychogalvanic-skin-resistance and peep-show. *Ann. Otol. Rhinol. Laryngol.*, 65, 511–534, 1956.

Stewart, K. C., A new instrument for detecting the galvanic skin response. *J. Speech Hear. Disord.*, 19, 169–173, 1954a.

Stewart, K. C., Some basic considerations in applying the GSR technique to the measurement of auditory sensitivity. *J. Speech Hear. Disord.*, 19, 174–183, 1954b.

Strauss, R. B., Premedication in clinical audiometry. *Arch. Otolaryngol.*, 67, 354–363, 1958.

White, C. T., and Schlosberg, H., Degree of conditioning of the GSR as a function of the period of delay. *J. Exp. Psychol.*, 43, 357–362, 1952.

Wilcott, R. C., A search for subthreshold conditioning at four different auditory frequencies. *J. Exp. Psychol.*, 46, 271–277, 1953.

chapter 27

ELECTROENCEPHALIC RESPONSE AUDIOMETRY

Paul H. Skinner, Ph.D.

The discovery of the perpetual fluctuation of electrical potentials in the animal cortex was made in 1875 by Caton who described them as "feeble currents of the brain." The discovery of these potentials was quite remarkable in that the amplitude is in the order of microvolts and Caton's discovery preceded the availability of electronic amplifiers for biologic research. The first recordings from the human brain were made in 1924 by Hans Berger (1929). The publication of his work, represented the first use of the term electroencephalogram (EEG) to describe these potentials. Berger established that these potentials originated in neuronal tissue and that the potentials changed with sensory stimulation (Brazier, 1958).

THE K COMPLEX OR VERTEX POTENTIAL

Study of the EEG was undertaken in laboratories throughout the world and information was rapidly obtained. Loomis, Harvey and Hobart (1938) studied the effects of sensory stimulation on the EEG in sleeping subjects and described a special pattern which they designated the "K complex." Briefly, this was described as a nonspecific triphasic response which appeared after signal onset (Fig. 27.1).

Attention was given to the effects of sound stimulation on the EEG in awake subjects by Davis (1939), and in sleeping subjects by Davis et al. (1939). Changes in the EEG (K complex) which occurred in response to sound stimulation, while not always observable, were reported to be most prominent from the vertex of the scalp, and therefore have been referred to as "V potentials."

EXTRICATING THE RESPONSE FROM THE BACKGROUND EEG

An accurate and detailed description of the V potential awaited the development of the special purpose summing computer. In the initial EEG work of Caton (1875) with experimental animals, the recording electrodes were placed directly on the sensory cortex. The EEG described by Berger (1929) was recorded from the intact scalp of man. The decrease in the electrical potentials of the cortex when recorded from the intact scalp is significantly reduced by a factor of 10 to 20 as compared to direct measurement at the cortex (Lindsey, 1961; Domino et al., 1964). Also, the evoked potentials produced by sensory stimulation are relatively low voltage and are often masked out by the greater voltage of the on-going, spontaneous cortical activity. The responses to sensory stimuli are consequently very difficult to detect and extricate from the background EEG.

Many techniques were applied to reveal the relatively small V potential from the on-going EEG potentials. The problem was at least conceptually overcome by Dawson (1954) who utilized a photographic superimposition technique to reveal changes in the EEG to sound.

The consummation of this technique was achieved by Clark (1958) and Clark et al. (1961) with the development of the average response computer. They reported a computer which converted analogue data (EEG voltages) into digital form from which averages (amplitude and time histograms) could be computed. The principle of averaging to extricate consistent changes from a background of random noise is straightforward. If a given stimulus produces a consistent change (positive or negative) in the cortical potentials at a fixed time delay after stimulus onset; and, this information is stored or preserved by a computer, the algebraic sum of these changes or responses should result in increased amplitude as the number of responses is increased. In order for the response to be extricated from the on-going EEG, this background activity must have essentially random polarities (positive and negative) and amplitudes so that they would sum to zero. This is somewhat analogous to the theoretical proof that the sum of positive and negative deviations about a mean or null point will sum to zero. Since in this case reliance is placed upon an assumption of randomness of the EEG, in general the larger the number of samples or sensory stimuli, the greater the reduction in background EEG, and the greater the summation of response amplitude. The goal in the study of auditory potentials is to present a sufficient number of stimuli so that the signal to noise ratio will permit detection of the auditory electroencepahalic response.

NATURE OF THE AUDITORY ELECTROENCEPHALIC RESPONSE

The auditory electroencephalic response (AER) can be divided somewhat arbitrarily into four classes of responses on the bases of latency, different properties and presumably different anatomical sources. They have been identified by their latencies from the onset of the signal as "early," 4 to 8 msec, "middle," 8 to 50 msec, "late," 50 to 300 msec, and "very late," 300 msec to several seconds (DC shift). As might be expected, there is some overlap in the latency of the various responses.

The early response is comprised of a series of "very fast waves" (100 to 2000 Hz) which presumably arise from the brain stem (Jewett and Williston, 1971; Lev and Sohmer, 1972). The middle response is comprised of a series of "fast waves" (5 to 100 Hz) (Goldstein, 1969) which presumably arise from the primary cortical projection areas. The late AER is comprised essentially of "slow waves" (2 to 10 Hz) (Appleby, 1964; Scott, 1965) which presumably arise from the primary cortical projection and secondary association areas. The "very late" responses have been described as the expectancy wave which is the last peak in the late response and the contingent negative variation which is a long latency negative potential (DC shift). This response presumably arises from the frontal cortex (Walter, 1964). These responses are displayed schematically in Figure 27.2. It should be clear, however, that each response must be recorded separately under different stimulus and recording conditions.

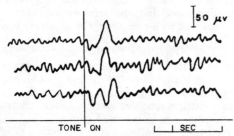

Fig. 27.1. K complexes evoked from an adult male in stage II of sleep in response to 1000 Hz stimuli at 50 dB SL.

The AER classifications are summarized in Table 27.1.

The Early or Brainstem Response

It is important to distinguish between the early and middle responses. Prior to the detection of the "brain stem" responses in electroencephalic response audiometry (ERA), the responses within the 8 to 50 msec latency range were referred to as the early response. Since the brain stem responses have an earlier latency from about 4 to 8 msec, they now are referred to as the early latency response, and the 8 to 50 msec latency responses currently are referred to as the middle response. One must note this change to avoid confusion in the identification of early versus middle responses in the literature.

The early response typically includes peaks from 1 to 4 msec which presumably arise from the auditory nerve. Since these responses are considered in electrocochleography, they will not be included among electroencephalic responses.

The early or brain stem responses can be observed as a series of fast waves described by Jewett (1970), Jewett and Williston (1971) and Sohmer and Feinmesser (1970), and also by the so-called "frequency following response" described by Worden and Marsh (1969).

Seven peaks can be observed numbered in order of latency of occurrence, which comprise the early, fast wave response. Inferences have been made regarding the origin of the various peaks based upon comparisons of the amplitudes and latencies of the responses in humans to those recorded in cats from electrodes placed in specific regions of the brain (Jewett, 1970; Lev and Sohmer, 1972; Picton et al., 1974). Presumably the first peak typically shown in configurations of the early response arises from

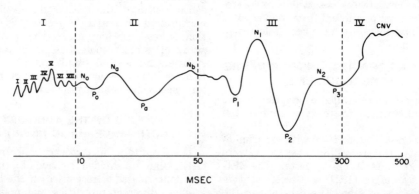

Fig. 27.2. Schematic representation of the four classes of auditory evoked responses. The amplitude and latency of the first three responses are not linearly related but rather approximate more nearly logarithmic relationships. Responses III and IV approximate a linear relationship.

TABLE 27.1. *Classes of Auditory Evoked Neural Responses*

Classification	Origin	Wave Form	Latency	Amplitude
Early	Brain stem	Fast (100–2000 Hz)	4–8 msec	50 nanovolts-1 μv
Middle	Primary cortical projection area	Fast (5–100 Hz)	8–50 msec	0.7–3 μv
Late	Primary cortical projection and secondary association areas	Slow (2–10 Hz)	50–300 msec	8–20 μv
Very late:				
Expectancy wave	Secondary association areas	Slow	230–360 msec	10–20 μv
CNV	Prefrontal cortex and secondary association areas	DC	300 + msec	10–30 μv

CNV = contingent negative variation.

the cochlear nerve (N_1) response with a latency of 0 to 4 msec, prior to the brain stem potentials. The second peak may be confounded with the second response of the cochlear nerve (N_2), but presumably arises from the brain stem. There is speculation that various waves may be associated with different brain stem nuclei or associated tracts; e.g., the largest and most stable peaks are wave II, associated with the primary cochlear nuclei, and wave V, associated with the inferior colliculus. As indicated previously, the early or brain stem response must be distinguished from the middle responses associated with the primary projection area. Actually, there may be overlap between the late peaks of the early response and the early peaks of the middle response as indicated.

The wave form of the early response is shown in Figure 27.3 as described by Jewett (1970), Hecox and Galambos (1974), Skinner and Glattke (1977). It is a fast wave, polyphasic response with a latency from about 4 to 10 msec and a peak to peak amplitude from about 50 nanovolts to over 1 microvolt. Largest amplitude occurs at peak V which also is the most stable of the various peaks.

The frequency following response described by Worden and Marsh (1969) is a microphonic-like response. As its title would indicate, this neural response follows the driving frequency of the stimulus. While it has not been investigated adequately for clinical utility, it may provide some valuable insight (Davis, 1976; Stillman, Moushegian, and Rupert, 1976).

The Middle Response

The middle response was revealed by the work of Geisler, Frishkopf and Rosenblith (1958), which was among the earliest studies in which the summing computer was used to study the AER. They concluded that the response was of neurogenic origin. Suspicion was cast upon the origin by Bickford, Jacobson and Cody (1964) who indicated it to be myogenic. They reported that recordings at the inion to

high intensity clicks had increased response amplitude with tense neck muscles and reduced amplitude with relaxed muscles. In response to the work of Bickford et al. (1964), Geisler (1964) suggested that the middle response represented cortical potentials with the amplitude dependent on muscular tension.

The origin of the middle response when recorded postauricularly was evaluated by Kiang et al. (1963) and by Cody et al. (1964) and they concluded that the response recorded from that location was myogenic. The origin of the middle response was evaluated further by Mast (1963; 1965) who studied this short latency response recorded with parietal and vertex electrode placement rather than the inion or postauricular response. He concluded that the response recorded from the vertex was consistent in the presence of muscle contraction and indicated that the response was probably comprised of both neurogenic and myogenic components. Other investigators have supported essentially a neurogenic origin of the middle response when recorded from the vertex (Borsanyi and Blanchard, 1964; Lowell, 1965; Goldstein, 1965). A compelling study was reported by Ruhm, Walker and Flanigin (1967) which supports a neurogenic origin of the middle response. They compared the middle response in two normal hearing subjects before surgery (scalp recordings) and during cortical ablation (cortex recordings). In one subject, it was possible to record simultaneously from the scalp and the cortical surface near the vertex. The response components under these conditions were similar in latency. They were also similar to the vertex recordings of normal subjects. In the second subject, pre- and persurgical recordings taken from the same area (scalp versus cortex) were also quite similar. As expected, the amplitude was greater in the cortical record. A study by Picton et al. (1974) also provided important insight in the origin of the middle and other AER components.

The middle response has been compared to responses from the primary sensory cortex. As

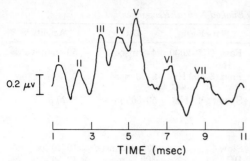

Fig. 27.3. Typical configuration of the brainstem response showing peak designation.

described by Walter (1964), evoked potentials from the primary sensory cortex are stable (stereotyped) responses that persist over thousands of repetitions. There is little change in the wave form of the primary response within the records of the same subject. The latency of the primary response is consistent with the latency throughout the specific sensory pathway and is relatively short. If the middle components of the cortical potentials do arise from the primary sensory areas, they would likely be modified by the relatively large surrounding tracts of nonspecific parietal and temporal cortex. Later discussion on the middle AER will reveal that it demonstrates many of the characteristics that Walter associates with a primary response.

The wave form of the middle response has been described by Lowell (1965), Ruhm et al. (1967), Goldstein (1969) and others. It is a polyphasic wave form with a vertex negative peak at about 8 msec (No), positive at 12 msec (Po), negative at about 18 msec (Na) and the major peaks, positive at 32 msec (Pa) and negative at about 52 msec (Nb) (Fig. 27.4). Peak to peak amplitude of these responses varied from about 0.7 to about 3μvolts with the greatest voltage occurring at the major peaks at about 32 to 52 msec.

The Late Response

The late response was described by McCandless and Best (1964), Derbyshire and McCandless (1964), Walter (1964) and Davis et al. (1964). This response is generally accepted as a neurogenic response and in sleeping subjects probably gives rise to the familiar K complex described in the classical studies of Loomis et al. (1938) and Davis et al. (1939).

Considerable insight has been gained on the nature of the late potential in the early work of Loomis et al. (1938), Davis et al. (1939), Forbes and Morison (1938), and more recently by Walter (1964), Vaughan (1969) and Picton et al. (1974). While late responses can be evoked

by auditory, visual and tactile signals, and recorded from many areas on the cortex or intact scalp, the wave forms differ among sensory modalities. The largest amplitude occurs to auditory stimuli (Walter, 1964).

The late response appears to be a secondary discharge. This response was first described by Forbes and Morison (1938) as a nonspecific on effect with relatively long latency, variable components and subject to habituation (reduced by repetitive stimuli). They noted the long delay between the primary and secondary responses and the synchronism of appearance in various regions of the cortex. They suggested that the afferent discharge acted upon the thalamus and other subcortical centers and that the charge was then distributed throughout the cortex.

The wave form of the late response has been described as polyphasic with vertex positive peaks at about 75 and 200 msec and vertex negative peaks at about 150 and 275 msec. A typical wave form of the late response is presented in Figure 27.5. The primary peaks of the late response in fully conscious subjects are the first negative and second positive peaks which range in amplitude from about 8 to 20 μvolts.

Very Late Responses: The Expectancy Wave and Contingent Negative Variation

The effects of conditioning in man and animals have been investigated by electrophysiologic methods, and under certain conditions, EEG modifications have been observed. Two very late responses have been discovered to be conditioned responses.

The first of these responses is revealed as a particularly large and reliable increase in amplitude of the P_{300} peak. This peak is a component of the late response described before as arising from the primary projection and secondary association areas. It is termed the expectancy wave (Davis, 1973). The second response is a very slow negative potential which actually is a DC shift. It is called the contingent negative variation (CNV) (Walter, 1964). These two responses are independently variable cortical events, yet both are evoked by similar experimental techniques (Donald and Goff, 1971). Both types of responses can be related to specific conditioning stimuli to test certain cognitive or psychological operations in children as well as in adults. In this regard, they hold unique potential among the various classes of electrophysiologic responses, in addition to simple threshold estimation.

The CNV is a protracted, widespread, negative potential which emanates from the frontal cortex and generally sweeps back from prefrontal to motor cortex following the response (Wal-

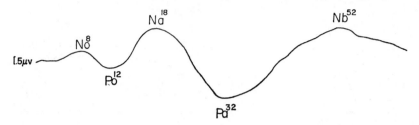

Fig. 27.4. Typical configuration of the middle response showing peak designation.

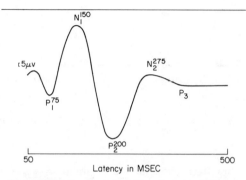

Fig. 27.5. Typical configuration of the late auditory electroencephalic response showing peak designation.

ter, 1964). The CNV can be observed in response to a stimulus only when the stimulus is conditional, i.e., associated with a second, "imperative" stimulus (one which requires a mental decision or motoric action). The conditional stimulus evokes a primary response in the nonspecific frontal cortex which is followed by a CNV leading up to the response (mental decision or motor task) to the imperative stimulus. This negative potential persists until the subject responds by some action to the second or imperative stimulus. The CNV reflects the expectancy of signal association by the subject and is independent of the intensity of the conditional stimulus. Its amplitude and consistency are related to the semantic content of the imperative stimuli if they are meaningful to the subject and require some decision or action (Walter, 1964). The CNV apparently reflects cognition and in this respect is a very important finding.

The CNV is recordable from all parts of the scalp with maximum amplitude recorded by anterior electrodes. It occurs at the completion of the late or slow wave V potential with a latency beyond 300 msec and an amplitude of about 20 μvolts (Fig. 27.6). About 10 to 12 stimulus pairs are sufficient to observe the CNV. The amplitude of the CNV is related to the probability of occurrence of the imperative stimuli. The CNV disappears if the imperative

stimuli are omitted for about 30 trials and in about 6 to 12 trials if the subject is told that no imperative stimulus will be presented. It is restored if the imperative stimulus is reinstated with 100% conditioning (Walter et al., 1964; Low et al., 1966).

The CNV lacks stability when recorded from very young children, and subjects with learning and emotional problems. Davis, Hirsh and Lauter (1975) report, however, that children as well as adults give reliable CNVs. It may prove to be a very helpful measure in differential diagnosis (Cohen and Offner, 1967; Walter, 1964). Primary attention for clinical utility of the expectancy wave and the CNV has been focused upon their unique potential to gain information about psychological functions (Reneau and Hnatiow, 1975). The CNV, at least, also holds potential to estimate threshold and in this regard offers the advantage of independence from stimulus intensity. Both aspects warrant consideration; neither has been adequately explored.

METHODOLOGY

The audiologist interested in recording AERs may use a commercial system preassembled as a unit or obtain the individual components and assemble them for standard or special capabilities. A commercial self-contained system would be more convenient for clinical use and the assemblage of special components preferable for experimental versatility.

Instrumentation

Either system must be able to produce a signal and electronically switch, time and shape it so the signals can be presented with variable but controlled parameters in appropriate time sequences. Attention will be given to the subject of signal parameters in a later section. The timing device which controls signal presentation must also control the computer triggering (sweep time) so the computer's scan following the signal is synchronized with signal onset. The signal must be led from the generation and switching networks

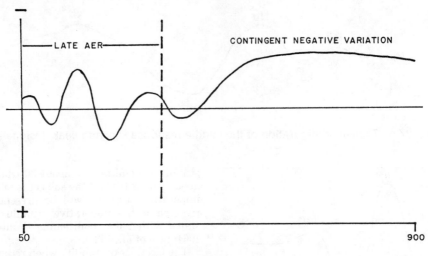

Fig. 27.6. Schematic of the contingent negative variation in relation to the late auditory evoked response.

through impedance matching and attenuation devices to subject earphones.

The low voltage (microvolt range) potentials which radiate from the scalp are picked up by surface electrodes and amplified to within the sensitivity required by the associated instruments. The key instrument for the analysis of the recorded potentials is the summing computer or averaging computer. A response display or recording system (X-Y plotter) is also required. EEG equipment or an oscilloscope, if not a necessity, is indeed useful to monitor the on-going electrophysiologic activity from the scalp. A schematic demonstrating the necessary components for the study of the AER is presented in Figure 27.7

Procedure

Electrode Placement. Recording or pick-up electrodes most commonly used are the disc type attached to the surface of the intact scalp. It is critical that the surface of the scalp be carefully cleaned chemically (e.g., by acetone) in the areas where electrodes are to be attached. Electrode paste, such as bentonite mixture or commercially available electrode pastes, are used to serve as an electrolyte to conduct the potentials between the scalp and the electrode. The electrodes must be securely attached to the scalp by tape or glue to prevent artifacts from physical displacement.

A monopolar technique is most commonly used to record the auditory evoked potential. This simply indicates that a "pick-up" electrode is used in conjunction with a reference electrode. The voltage potential between these two electrodes demonstrates on-going as well as consistent changes due to auditory excitation of the brain. The "active electrode" usually is placed on the vertex of the scalp or slightly forward of the vertex. This placement is most effective for the very early components of the brain stem response as well as for the recording of the middle and late responses (Martin and Moore, 1974). The reference electrode should be placed on a relatively inactive area, i.e., an area which is minimally affected by bioelectrical activity of the brain. The earlobes or mastoids are convenient for reference electrode placement. The voltage or the potential changes between these electrodes provide the input for the amplifiers and are the first stage in the input. A third electrode is used to ground the subject to reduce the effect of the body as an antenna.

Sweep Time. With the onset of each signal the summing computer must be triggered so that its sweep will be time-locked to the stimulus. Changes in the brain waves following the signal will be sampled, stored and summed by the computer. The sweep time that is set on the computer depends on the latency (time between the signal presentation and response) of the AER. The early and middle responses occur at about 4 to 8 and 8 to 50 msec, respectively. Subject state does not affect the latency of these responses, Hecox and Galambos (1974) and Mendel and Goldstein (1969b). The primary peaks of the late response are usually complete 200 to 300 msec after the onset of the signal. Latency is primarily dependent on subject state and maturity. Ordinarily a 500 msec sweep time is sufficient to ascertain the primary peaks of the late response. In sedated or natural

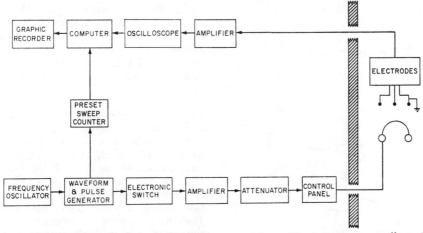

Fig. 27.7. Schematic of the instrumentation used for evoked response audiometry.

sleep conditions or in very young children, the primary peak latency may shift to 900 to 1000 msec at culmination(Skinner and Antinoro, 1969a, 1969b).

Signal Paradigm. The number and rate of auditory signals necessary to evoke the AER differ for the various components described. Rosenblith (1957) has explained that the signal to noise ratio is improved by the square root of the number of responses.

The early response (4 to 8 msec) may be obtained with very high stimulus repetition rates but optimally with 5 to 10 per second and requires 1000 or more stimulus samples (Glattke, 1975). The middle response may be obtained with stimulus repetition rates of 8 to 10 per second and requires 500 or more stimulus samples, Karlovich and Goldstein (1969). Apparently the early and middle responses do not habituate or adapt as a function of signal number or rate. Several studies (Keidel and Spreng, 1965; Davis et al., 1966; Nelson and Lassman, 1968) demonstrated increased AER amplitude of the late response with decreased rate of signal presentation. One signal per 10 sec yielded the largest potentials, but such slow rates are too time-consuming for clinical use. McCandless and Best (1966) investigated click rates, either random or fixed intervals, from 3 per sec to 1 per 2 sec. With more than 1 click per 2 sec, certain components of the response wave form were reduced in amplitude.

Leibman and Graham (1967) and Rose and Ruhm (1966) indicated that 100 or more signals may be used without risk of inhibition. The least number of runs which have been reported as adequate for AER resolution are from 32 (Davis et al., 1966) to about 50 (Cody and Bickford, 1965; Leibman and Graham, 1967; McCandless and Best, 1964; Price and Goldstein, 1966).

Testing Environment. A sound-treated room with electrical shielding and provision for visual and auditory monitoring is an ideal testing environment. Electrical shielding may not be necessary in some settings if the amount of electrical interference is negligible. The subject should be placed in a comfortable reclining chair or cot to reduce neck and shoulder tension which may introduce myogenic potentials.

Threshold Determination

The determination of threshold is a special problem in ERA. As signal intensity decreases, the amplitude of the AER also decreases. This makes it difficult to determine the AER near psychophysical threshold levels since it is hard to distinguish from the background cortical activity. Under these circumstances, ERA lacks the objectivity implicit in the procedure.

Threshold can be estimated by comparing the silent control (baseline) condition with conditions in which audible signals were used. The determination of threshold by these comparisons is a difficult task and requires a knowledge of the wave form characteristics and the factors which modify the wave form. There is considerable individual variability among AER wave forms due to subject state (awake or asleep), age, signal parameters and auditory pathology.

A preliminary step is to present moderate to high intensity signals which are of sufficient intensity to evoke a clear averaged response. A descending or ascending procedure may then be used to establish a dB-AER trend based upon three or four AERs. The trend can be used for mathematical or intuitive extrapolation to estimate threshold (Skinner, Antinoro, and Shimoto, 1972). Figure 27.8 shows that often a small response can be determined only in relation to other responses in a trend.

A

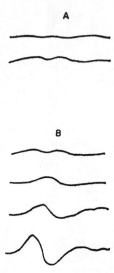

B

Fig. 27.8. (A) Comparison of a control condition (no audible signal presented) with an auditory electroencephalic response threshold recording, and (B) comparison of the same threshold response with AERs obtained with successively more intense signals.

With appropriate signal characteristics and recording techniques, wave V of the early response may be apparent within 10 dB of the individual's psychophysical threshold for the stimulus used. The other peaks or wavelets of the early response usually are detectable at levels of 30 to 40 dB sensation level (SL) (Hecox and Galambos, 1974; Glattke, 1975; Sohmer and Feinmesser, 1970; Wolfe, Skinner and Burns, 1976). These brain stem responses are of very low amplitude and have a similar latency to myogenic responses. Thus, the early response may be obscured or ablated by the background activity. Skinner and Glattke (1977) indicated that an analysis of the various ERA responses led to the conclusion that the brain stem responses appear to be the most promising for threshold determination in children.

Adequate attention has not been given to threshold determination by the middle response. Goldstein and Rodman (1967) established objective criteria based upon peak latency of the middle response. They were able to judge threshold within 5 dB in at least half of the subjects. About 10% of their silent control conditions resulted in averaged patterns that could have been mistaken for responses.

Several studies have pointed up remarkably good agreement between ERA thresholds based upon the late response and psychophysical thresholds at 500, 1000 and 2000 Hz in normal hearing adults. These ERA thresholds were within 10 dB of psychophysical thresholds for all but a small percentage of subjects (McCandless and Best, 1964; Price et al. 1966). Davis (1965) noted that some adult subjects with normal hearing did not yield discernible responses until 20 to 25 dB above psychophysical threshold.

Cody, Klass and Bickford (1967) reported similar thresholds by ERA and conventional audiometry in subjects with normal hearing and subjects with sensory-neural hearing losses. Davis et al. (1967) estimated psychophysical thresholds from ERA data for 162 hearing-impaired children from 4 to 10 years of age, and reported only a 2.2-dB difference between these data and the clinical audiograms. They also reported an average deviation for estimates at a single frequency to be only 8 dB.

Threshold determination in ERA has not received adequate attention as yet in subjects who demonstrate differing kinds of hearing loss. A comparison between ERA thresholds and psychophysical thresholds will no doubt be more complicated and erratic in these subjects. In children below about age 7, the determination of thresholds remains nebulous and comparisons between psychophysical and ERA thresholds have not been very reliable. Reportedly, the early response may offer special value in this problem, Hecox and Galambos (1974).

Effects of Signal Parameters on AER

Intensity. Several investigators have studied the effect of signal intensity on the AER. All unconditioned response components are influenced by this parameter.

The relationship between signal intensity and amplitude of early and middle components is not definitive. In general, response amplitude increases monotonically at least at low intensity levels, but components may vary in amplitude with increased intensity at moderate and higher intensity levels. The relationship is confounded among the early components by the relative influence of the emergence and growth of the various wavelets. Conflicting reports exist regarding the relationship between stimulus intensity and response amplitude for the most consistent peak, wavelet V. Glattke (1975) and Starr and Achor (1975) indicate no consistent relationship, however, Wolfe et al. (1976) found at least a monotonic relationship. Latency of the various peaks of the early response consistently diminishes with increased signal intensity and provides the most stable, stereotyped characteristic (Hecox and Galambos, 1974; Glattke, 1975; Wolfe et al., 1976).

Conflicting reports also exist regarding the relationship between stimulus intensity and response amplitude for the middle components. Latency of the middle response diminishes consistently with increased stimulus intensity.

The relationship between the amplitude of the late response and signal intensity has been studied by Suzuki and Taguchi (1965), Keidel and Spreng (1965), Rose and Ruhm (1966), Davis and Zerlin (1966), Davis, Bowers and Hirsh (1968) and Antinoro, Skinner and Jones (1969). It has been clearly demonstrated that an increase in intensity produces an increase in peak amplitude and a decrease in latency. Skinner and Antinoro (1969b) and Antinoro et al. (1969), have shown that the relationship between signal intensity in dB and AER amplitude in microvolts is linear for low and middle frequencies.

Rise Time. It is well known that early, brain stem responses can be elicited only by signals with a very fast rise time. Tone pips or bursts with rise times slower than 2.5 msec do not elicit the early response (Cobb, Skinner and Burns, 1977).

There is a significant effect of rise time on the middle response. Lane and Kupperman (1969) reported that the AER to pure tones is not as clear as the AER to clicks. Some subjects yielded no response to tones. Skinner and Antinoro (1970b) also studied the effects of signal rise time on the middle response using fast (about 10 μsec), 0.5, 2.5, 5, 10 and 25 msec, rise times. The responses were consistently elicited with a stable wave form at the fast rise time, but both factors diminished with increased rise time. A middle response was not obtained at the 25-msec rise time for any of the 20 subjects, and the high stability of the wave form maintained only with the fast rise time (10 μsec).

These data indicate that one must rely on the use of very fast signal rise times in order to elicit clear and stable early and middle response wave forms in ERA. This, of course, would require the use of filtered clicks or tone pips to gain frequency information.

Skinner and Jones (1968) and Onishi and Davis (1968) reported similar results in studying the effects of signal rise time on the late AER. Onishi and Davis indicated that AER amplitude of the primary peaks fell off very gradually with increased rise time up to 30 msec, where a more distinctive amplitude reduction occurred. With rise times from 5 msec to 50 msec, Skinner and Jones found a more distinctive drop in AER amplitude at about 25-msec rise time. No interaction between sensation level and rise time was observed from 30 to 90 dB SL. Thus, a rise time of 25 to 30 msec is optimal, since it is gradual enough to produce a pure tone and sufficiently abrupt to evoke a clear AER.

Stimulus Duration. It is well known that stimulus duration is related to perceived loudness of an auditory signal. Zwislocki (1960) has shown that threshold at 1000 Hz improves 10 dB for a 10-fold increase in duration up to about 200 msec. Temporal summation revealed by increased perceived loudness is essentially complete after durations of about 200 msec at 1000 Hz. Shorter durations at this frequency will result in decreased loudness or poorer threshold values.

The early and middle responses apparently are "on effect" responses produced by onset of the signal and unrelated to signal duration. The effects of signal duration on the middle AER were studied by Lane and Kupperman (1969) and Skinner and Antinoro (1970b). In the latter study, no consistent changes in the middle response were observed with acoustic durations from about 1.5 to 40 msec.

The effects of signal duration on the late AER components have been investigated by Skinner and Jones (1968) and Onishi and Davis (1968). Skinner and Jones used a fast rise signal (10 μsec) and observed a slight tendency for the AER amplitude to increase with signal durations up to 25 to 50 msec. No increase in AER amplitude was observed with further increases in signal duration up to 150 msec. In general, they reported no consistent increase in AER amplitude with increased signal duration.

Onishi and Davis studied the effect of signal duration with two rise times. They indicated with the shorter rise time (3 msec) that the amplitude of the primary AER peak increased significantly when the duration of the plateau was increased from 0 to 30 msec. They reported with the slower rise time (30 msec) that no effect was observed in the AER with increased signal duration.

Onishi and Davis recommended a rise time of 25 to 30 msec as optimal in producing a sinusoidal signal which is sufficiently abrupt to elicit the late AER without significant decrease in AER amplitude. Onishi and Davis reported further that with such a rise time, any effect of signal duration was negated.

Both studies indicated that the amplitude of the AER was fully determined within approximately 30 msec after signal onset. To ensure optimal signal presentation, a signal duration with a 25- to 50-msec plateau should be used in conjunction with a 25- to 30-msec rise time.

Actually, any signal duration might be used, but it would appear superfluous to duplicate signal durations that are required for conventional audiometry. The primary peaks of the late auditory evoked response are of course completed in awake subjects by about 200 to 300 msec after signal onset.

Frequency. The abrupt signal rise times

which are required to elicit the brainstem evoked response (BSER) produce wide energy dispersion across frequency. Thus it is necessary to use tone pips or filtered clicks to limit energy dispersion and gain information on the frequency response or "audiometric curve" of the hearing mechanism. The problem is confounded further since evidence exists that the BSER, like the action potential (N_1), arises from stimulation of the basal end of the cochlea coincident with the traveling wave regardless of stimulus frequency. Moreover, information obtained by the frequency following response may be limited in the same manner (Davis, 1976). Other investigators have studied this problem by using high pass band masking and indicate in contradiction that characteristic BSERs do reflect changes in stimulus frequency and thus place of stimulation along the basilar membrane (Terkildsen, Osterhammel, and Huis in't Veld, 1975). This matter requires further study for clarification. Whereas, the middle response may also require the use of tone pips for audiometric purposes, presumably different band limited signals do reflect the responses from different areas of the cochlea.

Antinoro and Skinner (1968), Antinoro et al. (1969), and Rothman (1970) reported that a significant interaction occurred between amplitude of the late AER and signal frequency, particularly at the high frequencies. Antinoro and Skinner reported a continued decline in AER amplitude from 250 to 8000 Hz at 30 and 60 dB SL. They reported further that this decline in amplitude was not the result of loudness differences at different frequencies, since similar results were obtained at 30 and 60 dB equal loudness levels. The decline in AER amplitude was more dramatic at equal SLs and was consistently 20% per octave from 1000 to 8000 Hz. There was relatively little difference in amplitude of the AER at 250, 500, 1000 and 2000 Hz.

Energy Dispersion. The effect of energy spread of complex auditory signals on the auditory electroencephalic response has been given little attention. Keidel and Spreng (1965) reported a relationship between critical band theory and the late AER. They reported that when two sinusoids were separated symmetrically about a narrow Gaussian noise band of 50 dB SPL, changes occurred in the AER when the frequency of the sinusoids was extended beyond the width of the critical band. Skinner and Antinoro (1970a) performed two experiments in which pure tones and noise bursts were employed to stimulate regions inside and outside of the critical band at several frequencies. Neither experiment revealed any change in the late AER amplitude or latency with changes in stimulus bandwidth.

SPECIAL CONSIDERATIONS IN ERA

ERA with Children

While the determination of hearing levels by ERA has proven to be very successful with more mature subjects, the most urgent need is for the very young. Compelling evidence has revealed detrimental effects of sensory deprivation during the early and formative stages (Barnet, 1964). In order to cope with the effects of sensory deprivation, auditory function must be assessed as soon as possible to permit appropriate educational and medical habilitation. It is clear that such assessment requires the development of an objective audiometric procedure such as ERA. The determination of hearing levels in very young children by the ERA technique is a very difficult task indeed, and lacks the objectivity implicit in the procedure. Serious problems are inherent in this procedure with young children which require recognition and discussion.

Maturation. Apparently subject maturation is the most important variable in ERA since it is well known that response stability and detectability are excellent in mature subjects. Davis et al. (1967) reported the strong impression that response wave forms tend to stabilize and resemble adult patterns in subjects who are about 7 years of age.

It is known that progressive myelinization occurs in the auditory nervous systems of infants (Langworthy, 1933). Moreover, even in the orderly development of behavioral auditory response mechanisms and morphologic maturation of the nervous system, wide variation exists. This process often is postulated as the basis for variability in AER latency and thus poor "time locking" between signal and response in very young subjects.

High Voltage Background EEG Activity. As was reported by Davis et al. (1967), the records of very young children are difficult to evaluate because the spontaneous background EEG activity is of high voltage, which intensifies the problem of extricating the response from the "biologic noise." Improvement of the signal to noise ratio does not necessarily improve by an increase in the number of signal presentations, since as reported by Shimizu (1966), the AER amplitude from young subjects does not always increase linearly by the number of samples, as a result of wave form instability.

Subject Cooperation. Young children are commonly apprehensive about ERA and many refuse to cooperate sufficiently to permit the procedure. Even the most cooperative children present problems. Their abrupt movements introduce muscle potentials which may obliterate a neural response and displace electrodes, which introduces artifacts. Few children are patient enough to tolerate adequate study time, since more than 1 hr is commonly required. Handicapped children are in general even more difficult to control, presumably in part because of greater anxiety from poor communication ability.

Subject State. The early BSER and middle components are remarkably stable responses and appear to be relatively unaffected by subject state; i.e., waking or sleeping states. The early response, however, can be recorded more reliably in relaxed or sleeping subjects since these potentials are of very low voltage and may be obscured easily by myogenic potentials. Dramatic changes are known to occur in the wave form of the late response from waking to sleeping states in subjects.

Threshold Determination. The determination of a response in very young children is a special problem in ERA. While the subject of threshold determination was discussed from a more general point of view in an earlier section, additional comments are warranted in this section. The use of a template can be justified to evaluate the response of sufficiently mature subjects. The nature of the atypical response of young subjects limits and frequently precludes this method. In the absence of repeatable responses, in view of the marked variability of the response of the young subject, a valid criterion often is lacking to judge presence or absence of response.

ERA is not an objective audiometric technique for young children, and must be interpreted with caution in the absence of corroborative data.

Encouraging results were obtained in young subjects by ERA as reported by Hecox and Galambos (1974). They studied the early responses of 35 infants aged 3 weeks to about 3 years. Their report focused primarily on wave V since it is known to be the most stable and reliable component of the early response. They indicated that the early response was obtained for young subjects, and that these responses were remarkably consistent with adult responses. It was indicated further that a reasonably accurate estimate of threshold can be obtained in young subjects by the early response. This report certainly warrants further research on the clinical utility of ERA with the early response.

Mixed reports exist regarding the value of the middle response to estimate hearing levels of very young children. Discouraging results have been experienced by Skinner (1973) and Davis et al. (1974). Davis et al. reported that of 18 very young children tested by middle response ERA, only a 6-year-old child yielded clear recordings at about 70 dB hearing level

(HL). In 10 cases with apparently normal hearing (by late response criteria) the middle responses were too inconsistent to allow any estimate of threshold. Lowell (1965) reported some findings using the middle response with children, but indicated that better results were obtained with the late response. Conversely, McRandle, Smith and Goldstein (1974) reported that middle responses were obtained from 10 newborns during sleep with clicks at 55 dB HL. A clear middle component was evident from each neonate. Moreover, several case studies of preschool children were cited in which middle response data were consistent with varying levels of hearing as tested by behavioral methods. In view of conflicting and inadequate research reports, the effectiveness of the middle response in ERA with very young children remains controversial. It is an important area for more extensive research.

Several studies have been conducted on large numbers of very young children in which ERA was focused on the late response. Appleby (1964) studied auditory sensitivity as measured by ERA in 40 presumably normal neonates using tone pips equated in loudness to pure tones. He reported that 85% of these infants yielded detectable responses to 50-dB tone pips; only 40% to 40-dB tone pips; and that responses could not be reliably detected for signal levels below 40 dB.

Barnet and Goodwin (1965) studied the AER of normal, sleeping infants using clicks presented at a rate of 1 per sec. They reported that the late response was discernible in all subjects at about 45 dB above normal threshold, and in 11 of 15 subjects at 35 dB. They suggested that depth of sleep influenced the response latency.

The preceding studies were conducted with presumably normal children. McCandless (1967) used ERA to assess the hearing of 128 clinical patients who were unable or unwilling to respond to conventional audiometry. One hundred and two of these children were 10 years of age or younger, and, of this group, definable responses at some signal level were obtained in 90. Most of the subjects who did not yield clearly distinguishable responses were under the age of 2 years. McCandless suggested that the most frequent cause of unsatisfactory results was myogenic artifact or intermittent electrode contact resulting from movement. Changes in the level of consciousness also were indicated as a problem, since subject state altered late AER wave form. Test-retest reliability in ERA was determined. In cooperative children, when the test was technically good, test-retest agreement was within 10 dB. With children under age 2, the retest thresholds often varied as much as 30 dB.

ERA in Diagnosis

Origins of the various classes of AERs can be attributed to only general areas of the auditory nervous system; e.g., brain stem, primary projection, secondary association areas. Also, these potentials are recorded in ERA by distant or far field recording techniques which result in very diffuse responses. The multiplicity of pathways in these diffuse responses confounds inferences on the origin of the responses. Moreover, considerable variability is found in the responses within and among subjects, which is compounded in the responses from very young or pathologic auditory systems.

The primary objective in ERA is the estimation of hearing levels in very young subjects. Since this objective remains problematic, attention to diagnosis in ERA has been secondary. While several different rationale have been formulated, Best and Tabor (1968), Shimizu (1968), Shepherd and McClaren (1969), Goldstein (1969), and Starr and Achor (1975); these strategies for ERA in diagnosis lack adequate validation. The relationship of auditory pathology to the various classes of responses perhaps lends more information to understanding factors that affect the responses than inferences about pathology. For example, as would be expected, conductive loss results in ERA threshold elevation; i.e., lower peak response amplitude and increased peak latency. Loudness recruitment, of course, results in unusual increase in peak response amplitude and decrease in peak latency. The CNV, a unique response, has been used successfully to gain information on a patient's ability to understand speech, Burian et al. (1972).

ERA is concerned with four classes of responses which involve brain stem, primary projection area, cortical and surrounding association areas, frontal cortical areas, and related functions. Indeed, pathology in these areas may likely affect the associated AERs. As techniques are refined and extended, ERA may contribute uniquely to diagnosis in auditory disorders. Diagnostic implications of ERA are sufficiently stimulating that the topic is a compelling area for future research.

Effects of Arousal and Sedation on AER

The level of arousal reportedly has no significant effect on the early or middle components, and these responses are remarkably stable in awake and sleeping subjects, Hecox and Galambos (1974) and Mendel and Goldstein (1969a). Since both of these responses are vulnerable to myogenic effects, responses can be recorded with greater clarity if the subject is able to relax the scalp musculature.

This can be accomplished more successfully through sleep than voluntary relaxation, Picton et al. (1974). Thus, both BSER and middle components recording may be enhanced by sleep.

A dramatic difference is apparent in the wave form of the late AER obtained from awake subjects versus subjects in sleep (Williams, Tepas and Morlock, 1962; Weitzman and Kremen, 1965; Cody, Klass and Bickford, 1967; Skinner and Antinoro, 1969a). Typical AER wave forms for awake and asleep subjects were compared by Skinner and Antinoro. The most prominent peak in the late AER of awake subjects was N_1-P_2; and N_2-P_3 was commonly obscure or absent in the response. In sleeping subjects, however, a reversal occurred in which N_2-P_3 became the prominent peak and N_1-P_2 was considerably diminished. (The prominent N_2 peak is probably the familiar K-complex seen in the unaveraged EEG of sleeping subjects.) Moreover, the amplitude of N_2-P_3 obtained in sleeping subjects exceeded the amplitude of N_1-P_2 in the awake condition. For this reason, the late AER was observed more readily in the records of sleeping subjects. The changes in the wave complexes obtained under two conditions, awake and sedated sleep (chloral hydrate), are apparent in the late AER curves based upon the average amplitude and latency of eight subjects as shown in Figure 27.9. While these curves are based on averages, they depict quite well the typical wave complexes observed under the two conditions. The largest peak, N_1-P_2, in the awake condition never exceeded 10 μvolts, whereas the largest peak, N_2-P_3, in the asleep condition was as great as 19 μvolts. A significant latency shift was also apparent in subjects under sedation. While the N_2-P_3 peak was usually apparent in the half-second sweep time, occasionally a full second sweep time was necessary to include the N_2-P_3 peak.

Skinner and Antinoro also studied the late response in 20 children in awake versus asleep conditions. Such a comparison is of course more difficult in children than in adults because of the problems in controlling awake preschoolers and the great variability in the late AERs of very young subjects.

In the AERs of awake children, the wave complex was highly variable among subjects and could not be typified by a single wave form. As has been reported by others, peak latencies were considerably greater than those of the adult responses. In the same subjects, however, the late responses obtained under sedation frequently assumed a more typical wave complex as compared to the responses of adult subjects in sleep. Again, however, the latency of the prominent peaks was considerably greater in children. Occasionally the la-

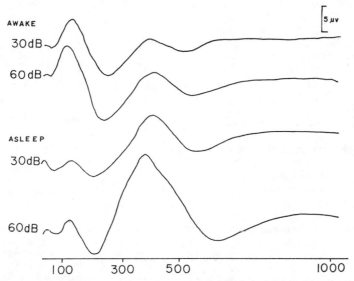

AWAKE
30dB
60dB

ASLEEP
30dB
60dB

5 µv

100   300   500   1000

Fig. 27.9. Evoked response wave complexes derived from the average amplitude and latency of the late auditory electroencephalic responses of eight adult subjects under awake and asleep conditions. These constructed wave forms are quite typical of individual adult responses.

tency of the prominent peaks observed during sleep was surprisingly great, and in one subject N_2-P_3 was completed at about 930 msec. It was routinely necessary to maintain a full second sweep time on the computer to observe responses in sedated children.

Without exception, in the late AERs obtained from children, as well as adults, the amplitude of N_2-P_3 obtained during sleep exceeded the amplitude of any of the major peaks obtained from awake subjects. Response variability was so great among the children, however, that average amplitude and latency data are not meaningful. Much clearer responses were obtained from sedated children than from awake children.

Attention has been given to the effects of sleep stage on the late response. Different stages of sleep have been described as they relate to cyclic variations in EEG and their relation to eye movements, body motility and dreaming (Dement and Kleitman, 1957). Several investigators have indicated that sleep stages affect certain aspects of the late AER. Derbyshire et al. (1956) and Toriyama, Matsuzaki and Hayaski (1966) reported that the detectability of the late AER is related to sleep stage. Williams et al. (1964) reported that response detection at threshold was greater during deeper stages (third and fourth) of sleep. Similarly, Davis and Onishi (1969) and Skinner and Shimota (1975) reported that deeper sleep (stage 3) seemed to be optimal for eliciting the late AER. The characteristics of the late AER

have been found by a number of investigators to change with stage of sleep. Williams et al. (1964) indicated that in deeper stages of sleep an increase was apparent in the amplitude of the late peaks in the response. Weitzman and Kremen (1965) also reported increased peak latency for the later peaks.

Effects of Sedatives

The use of sedation in ERA with very young children has been reported to be advantageous and often imperative. The obvious purpose of sedation is to permit evaluation of otherwise uncooperative or uncontrollable patients. Sedation usually reduces the confounding effects of movement and myogenic artifacts. In addition, sleep may enhance AER potentials as well as the recording process. Some sedatives, however, ablate or obscure the AER. The benefits to be derived depend in part on the sedatives used and, more importantly, on the class of components under study in that the effects of sedatives vary accordingly.

It would appear that the use of sedatives might prove to be very advantageous in studying the early AER. It has been reported by Picton et al. (1974). Wolfe et al. (1976) and Davis (1976) that the early response can be recorded more clearly in sleeping subjects since sleep may reduce myogenic artifacts by reduction of tension of the scalp musculature. In addition, it has been reported that the BSER components are quite stable in sleeping subjects. Although no systematic studies have been reported on the effects of sedatives on human brain stem potentials, there is encouraging evidence. It has been documented that sedatives apparently have no effect on the brain stem potentials of animals. Also, Galambos (1976) reported that the early response was recorded successfully in preschool subjects under sedation. If this response is stable in young children and unaffected by sedatives, ERA with the early AER may prove to be of great value.

The middle AER components, like the early components, are known to be very stable and reportedly clearer in sleeping subjects as a result of reduced muscle tension (Mendel and Goldstein, 1969b; Picton et al., 1974). The effects of sedatives on the middle AER have not been investigated extensively, however, at least two such investigations have led to somewhat different conclusions. Skinner and Shimota (1975) studied the middle response under a variety of sedatives, using adult subjects as their own control, and found that response detectability at 40 dB SL was reduced under all the sedatives used, but particularly by barbiturates. In contrast, Kupperman and Mendel (1974) reported that ERA thresholds were obtained (which closely approximated behavioral thresholds) for adult subjects sedated with a barbiturate (secobarbital). While testing was done under different sleep stages in the two studies, it is questionable that the difference in results could be attributable primarily to that factor. Sufficient data are not available to permit inferences about the successful use of the middle AER in young children under sedation. Further research is needed in this area.

Considerable attention has been given to the effects of sedatives on the late AER, however, few studies have provided adequate control conditions, if any. It is not certain that the late response can be observed satisfactorily in sedated subjects. Although the response amplitude is enhanced significantly in sleep; the late response wave form is more variable and, in fact, changes dramatically with varying levels of arousal. The late response can be observed with rather good reliability in adult subjects with certain sedatives; however, sedation by barbiturates markedly reduced the detectability of the late response, Skinner and Shimota (1975). These problems are intensified in ERA with young children.

REFERENCES

Antinoro, F., and Skinner, P., The effects of frequency on the auditory evoked response. J. Aud. Res., 8, 119–123, 1968.

Antinoro, F., Skinner, P., and Jones, J., Relation between sound intensity and amplitude of the auditory evoked response at different stimulus frequencies. J. Acoust. Soc. Am., 46, 1433–1436, 1969.

Appleby, S., The slow vertex maximal sound evoked responses in infants. Proceedings of a conference held in Toronto, Canada, October 8–9, 1964. Acta Otolaryngol. Suppl. 206, 146–152, 1964.

Barnet, A. B., Average evoked electroencephalographic response to clicks in infants. Proceedings of a conference held in Toronto, Canada, October 8–9, 1964. Acta Otolaryngol. Suppl. 206, 134–146, 1964.

Barnet, A. B., and Goodwin, R. S., Averaged evoked electroencephalographic responses to clicks in the newborn. Electroenceph. Clin. Neurophysiol., 18, 445–450, 1965.

Berger, H., Uber das Elektrenkephalogramm des Menschen. Arch. Psychiat. Nervenkr., 87, 527–570, 1929.

Best, L., and Tabor, J., Cortical audiometry as an otologic procedure. Trans. Am. Acad. Ophthalmol. Otolaryngol., March-April, 142–152, 1968.

Bickford, R. G., Jacobson, J. L., and Cody, D. T. R., Nature of average evoked potential to sound and other stimuli in man. Ann. N. Y. Acad. Sci., 112, 204–223, 1964.

Borsanyi, S. J., and Blanchard, C. L., Auditory evoked brain responses in man. Arch. Otolaryngol., 80, 149–154, 1964.

Brazier, M. A. B., The Electrical Activity of the Nervous System. New York: Macmillan, 1958.

Burian, K., Gestring, G., Gloning, K., and Haider, M., Objective examination of verbal discrimination and comprehension in aphasia using the contingent negative variation. Audiology, 11, 310–316, 1972.

Caton, R., The electric currents of the brain. Br. Med. J., 2, 278, 1875.

Clark, W. A., Jr., Average response computer (ARC-1). Q. Rep. Electronics (MIT), 114–117, 1958.

Clark, W. A., Goldstein, M. H., Brown, R. M., Molnar, C. E., O'Brien, D. F., and Zieman, H. E., The average response computer (ARC); a digital device for computing averages and amplitudes and time histograms of electrophysiological responses. Trans. Int. Radio Engineers, 8(1), 46–51, 1961.

Cobb, J., Skinner, P., and Burns, I., The effect of signal rise time and frequency on the BSER. Presented to the American Speech and Hearing Association convention, Chicago, 1977.

Cody, D. T. R., and Bickford, R. G., Cortical audiometry: an objective method of evaluating auditory acuity in man. Mayo Clin. Proc., 40, 273–287, 1965.

Cody, D. T. R., Jacobson, J. L., Walker, J. C., and Bickford, R. G., Averaged evoked myogenic and cortical potentials to sound in man. Ann. Otol. Rhinol. Laryngol., 73, 763–777, 1964.

Cody, D. T. R., Klass, D. W., and Bickford, R. G., Cortical audiometry; an objective method of evaluating auditory acuity in awake and sleeping man. Trans. Am. Acad. Ophthalmol. Otolaryngol., 71, 81–91, 1967.

Cohen, J., and Offner, F., Some clinical applications of the CNV and evoked potentials. Electroenceph. Clin. Neurophysiol., 22, 190, 1967.

Davis, H., Slow cortical responses evoked by acoustic stimuli. Proceedings of a conference on the Young Deaf Child held in Toronto, Canada, October 8-9, 1964. *Acta Otolaryngol. Suppl.* 206, 128-134, 1965.

Davis, H., Classes of auditory evoked responses. *Audiology,* 12, 464-469, 1973.

Davis, H., Principles of electric response audiometry. *Ann. Otol. Rhinol. Laryngol.,* 85 (Suppl. 28): No. 3, part 3, May-June 1976.

Davis, H., and Onishi, S., Maturation of auditory evoked potentials. *Int. Audiol.,* 8(1), 24-33, 1969.

Davis, H., and Zerlin, S., Acoustic relations of the human vertex potentials. *J. Acoust. Soc. Am.,* 39, 109-116, 1966.

Davis, H., Davis, P. A., Loomis, A. L., Harvey, P. N., and Hobart, G., Electrical responses of the human brain to auditory stimulation during sleep. *J. Neurophysiol.,* 2, 500-514, 1939.

Davis, H., Engebretson, M., Lowell, E. L., Mast, T., Satterfield, J., and Yoshie, N., Evoked responses to clicks recorded from the human scalp. *Ann. N. Y. Acad. Sci.,* 112, 224-225, 1964.

Davis, H., Mast, T., Yoshie, N., and Zerlin, S., The slow response of the human cortex to auditory stimuli: recovery process. *Electroenceph. Clin. Neurophysiol.,* 21, 105-113, 1966.

Davis, H., Hirsh, S., Shelnutt, J., and Bowers, C., Further validation of evoked response audiometry (ERA). *J. Speech Hear. Res.,* 10, 717-732, 1967.

Davis, H., Bowers, C., and Hirsh, S., Relations of the human vertex potential to acoustic input: loudness and masking. *J. Acoust. Soc. Am.,* 43, 431-438, 1968.

Davis, H., Hirsh, S. K., Shelnutt, J., and Dinges, D. F., Validation of clinical ERA at Central Institute for the Deaf. *Rev. Laryngol.,* 95, 475-480, 1974.

Davis, H., Hirsh, S. K., and Lauter, J., The contingent negative variation (CNV) as an indicator of discrimination or of concept formation. *Central Institute for the Deaf Progress Report,* 18, 4, July, 1974-June, 1975.

Davis, P. A., Effects of acoustic stimuli on the waking human brain. *J. Neurophysiol.,* 2, 494-499, 1939.

Dawson, G., A summation technique for the detection of small evoked potentials. *Electroenceph. Clin. Neurophysiol.,* 6, 65-84, 1954.

Dement, W., and Kleitman, L., Cyclic variations in EEG during sleep and their relations to eye movements, body motility, and dreaming. *Electroenceph. Clin. Neurophysiol.,* 9, 673-690, 1957.

Derbyshire, A. J., and McCandless, G. A., Template for the EEG response to sound. *J. Speech Hear. Res.,* 7, 96-102, 1964.

Derbyshire, A. J., Fraser, A. R., McDermott, M., and Bridge, A., Audiometric measurements by electroencephalography. *Electroenceph. Clin. Neurophysiol.,* 8, 467-478, 1956.

Domino, E., Matsuoka, S., Waltz, J., and Cooper, I., Simultaneous recordings of scalp and epidural somatosensory-evoked responses in man. *Science,* 145, 1199-1200, 1964.

Donald, M., Jr., and Goff, W., Attention-related

increases in cortical responsivity dissociated from the contingent negative variation. *Science,* 172, 1163-1166, 1971.

Forbes, A., and Morison, B. R., Cortical responses to sensory stimulation under deep barbiturate narcosis. *J. Neurophysiol.,* 2, 112-128, 1938.

Galambos, R., Personal communication, 1976.

Galambos, R., and Hecox, K., Brainstem evoked response audiometry in man. Paper presented at annual convention of the American Speech and Hearing Association, Detroit, 1974.

Geisler, C. D., Discussion of C. D. Geisler. Average responses to clicks in man recorded by scalp electrodes (Technical Report 380, Research Laboratory of Electronics, MIT, Nov. 4, 1960). *Ann. N. Y. Acad. Sci.,* 112, 218-219, 1964.

Geisler, C. D., Frishkopf, L. S., and Rosenblith, W. A., Extracranial responses to acoustic clicks in man. *Science,* 128, 1210-1211, 1958.

Glattke, T., Personal communication, 1975.

Goldstein, R., Early components of the AER. Proceedings of a conference on the Young Deaf Child in Toronto, Canada, October 8-9, 1964. *Acta Otolaryng. Suppl.* 206, 127-128, 1965.

Goldstein, R., Use of averaged electroencephalic response (AER) in evaluating central auditory function. Paper presented to Annual Convention of the American Speech and Hearing Association, Chicago, November 12, 1969.

Goldstein, R., and Rodman, L. B., Early components of averaged evoked responses to rapidly repeated auditory stimuli. *J. Speech Hear. Res.,* 12, 697-705, 1967.

Hecox, K., and Galambos, R., Brain stem auditory evoked responses in human infants and adults. *Arch. Otolaryngol.,* 99, 30-33, 1974.

Jewett, D., Volume-conducted potentials in response to auditory stimuli as detected by averaging in the cat. *Electroencephalogr. Clin. Neurophysiol.,* 28, 609-618, 1970.

Jewett, D., and Williston, J., Auditory-evoked far fields averaged from the scalp of humans. *Brain,* 94, 681-696, 1971.

Karlovich, R., and Goldstein, R., The amplitude of the AER as a function of stimulus rate and number. Reviewed in a paper presented to the Annual Convention of the American Speech and Hearing Association, Chicago, November 14, 1969.

Keidel, W. D., and Spreng, M., Neurophysiological evidence for the Stevens power function in man. *J. Acoust. Soc. Am.,* 38, 191-195, 1965.

Kiang, N. Y.-S., Crist, A. H., French, M. A., and Edwards, A. G., Post-auricular electric response to acoustic stimuli in humans. *Q. Progr. Report (MIT),* 2, 218-225, 1963.

Kupperman, G. L., and Mendel, M. I., Threshold of the early components of the averaged electroencephalic response determined with tone pips and clicks during drug-induced sleep. *Audiology,* 13, 379-390, 1974.

Lane, R., and Kupperman, G., The effects of rise time and duration of pure tones on the amplitude, latency and general identifiability of the early components of the AER. Reviewed in a paper presented by R. Goldstein to the Annual Convention of the American Speech and Hearing Association, Chicago, November 14, 1969.

Langworthy, O., Development of behavior patterns and myelination in the nervous system in the human fetus and infant. *Contrib. Embryol. Carnegie Inst.*, **139**, 3–57, 1933.

Leibman, J., and Graham, J. T., Changes in parameters of averaged auditory evoked potentials related to number of data samples analyzed. *J. Speech Hear. Res.*, **10**, 782–785, 1967.

Lev, A., and Sohmer, H., Sources of averaged neural responses recorded in animal and human subjects during cochlear audiometry (Electro-Cochleogram). *Arch. Klin. Exp. Ohren. Nasen. Kehlkopfheilkd.*, **201**, 79–90, 1972.

Lindsey, D., The Reticular Activation System and Perceptual Integration. In Sheer, D. (Ed.), *Electrical Stimulation of the Brain*. Austin, Tex.: University of Texas Press, 1961.

Loomis, A. L., Harvey, P. N., and Hobart, G., Distribution of disturbance patterns in the human electroencephalogram, with special reference to sleep. *J. Neurophysiol.*, **1**, 413–430, 1938.

Low, M. D., Frost, J. D., Borda, R. P., and Kellaway, P., Surface negative slow potential shift associated with conditioning in man and subhuman primates. *Electroencephalogr. Clin. Neurophysiol.*, **21**, 413, 1966.

Lowell, E., Early components of the AER in the hearing of young children. Proceedings of a conference on the Young Deaf Child in Toronto, Canada, October 8–9, 1964. *Acta Otolaryngol. Suppl.* **206**, 124–126, 1965.

Martin, M. E., and Moore, E. J., Spatial distribution of eighth nerve and brain-stem responses to clicks in man using surface electrodes. Paper presented at annual convention of the American Speech and Hearing Association, 1974.

Mast, T., Muscular versus cerebral sources for the short latency human evoked responses to clicks. *Physiologist*, **6**, 229, 1963.

Mast, T., Short latency human evoked responses to clicks. *J. Appl. Physiol.*, **20**, 725–730, 1965.

McCandless, G. A., Clinical application of evoked response audiometry. *J. Speech Hear. Res.*, **10**, 468–478, 1967.

McCandless, G. A., and Best, L., Evoked responses to auditory stimuli in man using a summing computer. *J. Speech Hear. Res.*, **7**, 193–202, 1964.

McCandless, G. A., and Best, L., Summed evoked responses using pure tone stimuli. *J. Speech Hear. Res.*, **9**, 266–272, 1966.

McRandle, C., Smith, M., and Goldstein, R., Early averaged EER to clicks in neonates. *Ann. Otol. Rhinol. Laryngol.*, **83**, 695–701, 1974.

Mendel, M., and Goldstein, R., The effect of test conditions on the early components of the averaged electroencephalographic response. *J. Speech Hear. Res.*, **12**, 344–350, 1969a.

Mendel, M., and Goldstein, R., Stability of the early components of the averaged electroencephalographic response. *J. Speech Hear. Res.*, **12**, 351–361, 1969b.

Nelson, D. A., and Lassman, F. M., Effects of intersignal interval on the human auditory evoked response. *J. Acoust. Soc. Am.*, **44**, 1529–1532, 1968.

Onishi, S., and Davis, H., Effects of duration and rise time of tone bursts on evoked potentials. *J.*

Acoust. Soc. Am., **44**, 582–591, 1968.

Picton, T., Hillyard, S., Krausz, H., and Galambos, R., Human auditory evoked potentials; I. Evaluation of components. *Electroencephalogr. Clin. Neurophysiol.*, **36**, 179–190, 1974.

Price, L. L., and Goldstein, R., Averaged evoked responses for measuring auditory sensitivity in children. *J. Speech Hear. Res.*, **31**, 248–256, 1966.

Price, L. L., Rosenblut, B., Goldstein, R., and Shepherd, D. C., The averaged evoked response to auditory stimulation. *J. Speech Hear. Res.*, **9**, 361–370, 1966.

Reneau, J., and Hnatiow, G., *Evoked Response Audiometry; A Topical and Historical Review*, pp. 119–137. Baltimore: University Park Press, 1975.

Rose, D. E., and Ruhm, H. B., Some characteristics of the peak latency and amplitude of the acoustically evoked response. *J. Speech Hear. Res.*, **9**, 412–422, 1966.

Rosenblith, W., Some quantifiable aspects of the electrical activity of the nervous system. *Rev. Mod. Phys.*, **31**, 532–545, 1957.

Rothman, H. H., Effects of high frequencies and intersubject variability on the auditory evoked cortical response. *J. Acoust. Soc. Am.*, **47**, 569–573, 1970.

Ruhm, H., Walker, E., and Flanigin, H., Acoustically evoked potentials in man; mediation of early components. *Laryngoscope*, **77**, 806–822, 1967.

Scott, J., Simplified instrumentation for AER. Proceedings of a conference on the Young Deaf Child, held in Toronto, Canada, October 8–9, 1964. *Acta Otolaryngol. Suppl.* **206**, 155, 1965.

Shepherd, D., and McClaren, K., Diagnostic aspects of AER. *Excerpta Medica*, No. 189, 44, 1969.

Shimizu, H., Variation of electroencephalic auditory response with maturation. Paper presented to American Association for the Advancement of Science, Baltimore, December 29, 1966.

Shimizu, H., Evoked response in VIII nerve lesions. *Trans. Am. Acad. Ophthalmol. Otolaryngol.*, **72**, 596–603, 1968.

Skinner, P., Unpublished data, 1973.

Skinner, P., and Antinoro, F., Auditory evoked responses in normal hearing adults and children before and during sedation. *J. Speech Hear. Res.*, **12**, 394–401, 1969a.

Skinner, P., and Antinoro, F., The effects of signal parameters on the auditory evoked response. Paper presented to 1969 Congress of Oto-Rhino-Laryngology, Mexico Federal District. *Excerpta Medica*, **189**, 43–44, 1969b.

Skinner, P., and Antinoro, F., Critical band theory and the auditory evoked slow wave V potential. *J. Acoust. Soc. Am.*, **48**, 557–560, 1970a.

Skinner, P., and Antinoro, F., The effects of rise time and signal duration on the early components of the auditory evoked cortical response. Submitted for publication, 1970b.

Skinner, P., and Glattke, T., Electrophysiologic response audiometry; state of the art. *J. Speech Hear. Disord.*, **42**, 179–198, 1977.

Skinner, P., and Jones, H., Effects of signal duration and rise time on the auditory evoked potential. *J. Speech Hear. Res.*, **11**, 301–306, 1968.

Skinner, P., and Shimota, J., A comparison of the effects of sedatives on the auditory evoked cortical response. *J. Am. Audiol. Soc.*, 1, 71–78, 1975.

Skinner, P., Antinoro, F., and Shimota, J., An evaluation of linear extrapolation to threshold in electroencephalic response audiometry. *J. Aud. Res.*, 12, 26–31, 1972.

Sohmer, H., and Feinmesser, M., Cochlear and cortical audiometry. *Israel J. Med. Sci.*, 6, 219–223, 1970.

Starr, A., and Achor, L. J., Auditory brain stem responses in neurological disease. *Arch. Neurol.*, 32, 761–768, 1975.

Stillman, R. D., Moushegian, G., and Rupert, A. L., Early tone-evoked responses in normal and hearing-impaired subjects. *Audiology*, 15, 10–22, 1976.

Suzuki, T., and Taguchi, K., Cerebral evoked response to auditory stimuli in waking man. *Ann. Otol. Rhinol. Laryngol.*, 74, 128–139, 1965.

Terkildsen, K., Osterhammel, P., and Huis in't Veld, F., Far field electrocochleography. Frequency specificity of the response. *Scand. Audiol.*, 4, 167–172, 1975.

Toriyama, M., Matsuzaki, T., and Hayaski, H., Some observations on auditory average response in man. *Int. Audiol.*, 5, 234–237, 1966.

Vaughan, H., The relationship of brain activity to scalp recordings of event related potentials (Monograph). Albert Einstein College of Medicine, 1969.

Walter, H., The convergence and interaction of visual, auditory, and tactile responses in human nonspecific-cortex. *Ann. N. Y. Acad. Sci.*, 112, 320–361, 1964.

Walter, W., Cooper, R., McCallum, C., and Cohen, J., The origin and significance of the contingent negative variation or "expectancy wave." *Electroencephalogr. Clin. Neurophysiol.*, 18, 720, 1964.

Weitzman, E., and Kremen, H., Auditory evoked responses during different stages of sleep in man. *Electroencephalogr. Clin. Neurophysiol.*, 18, 65–70, 1965.

Williams, H., Hammack, J., Daly, R., Dement, W., and Rubin, A., Responses to auditory stimulation, sleep loss and the EEG stages of sleep. *Electroencephalogr. Clin. Neurophysiol.*, 16, 269–279, 1964.

Williams, H., Tepas, D., and Morlock, H., Evoked responses to clicks and electroencephalographic stages of sleep in man. *Science*, 138, 685–686, 1962.

Wolfe, J., Skinner, P., and Burns, J., The relationship of brain stem response amplitude to stimulus intensity. Presented at the American Speech and Hearing Association Convention, Houston, Texas, 1976.

Worden, F., and Marsh, J., Frequency-following (microphonic-like) neural responses evoked by sound. *Electroencephalogr. Clin. Neurophysiol.*, 25, 42–52, 1969.

Zwislocki, J., Theory of temporal auditory summation. *J. Acoust. Soc. Am.*, 32, 1046–1060, 1960.

chapter 28

ELECTRO-COCHLEOGRAPHY

Theodore J. Glattke, Ph.D.

Electrocochleography (ECoG) is an electrophysiologic approach to the study of hearing. In ECoG, electrical activity that originates within the cochlea or the auditory nerve is recorded and evaluated. Unlike measures of ongoing electrical activity, ECoG represents an evoked or stimulus dependent measure.

There are three classes of electrical potentials which could be analyzed in ECoG. These are the compound action potential (AP) of the auditory nerve, the summating potential (SP), and the cochlear potential (CP), also known as the cochlear microphonic (Wever, 1966). The AP has proven to be the most sensitive indicator of the functional state of the peripheral auditory system, yielding information about both the threshold and suprathreshold characteristics of the cochlea and auditory nerve. Therefore, analysis of the AP forms the basis for the majority of ECoG examinations.

Auditory nerve APs were first observed in 1910, and many of the essential features of both CPs and APs had been described by various investigators by 1935 (Derbyshire and Davis, 1935). Among the early studies, that of Wever and Bray (1930) ushered in an era of careful evaluation of AP and CP characteristics based upon recordings obtained from the vicinity of the cochlea. Derbyshire and Davis (1935) compared CP and AP recordings obtained from two sites: the auditory nerve and the round window of the cochlea. Their stimulus techniques enabled them to segment the responses into CPs *or* APs, and these same techniques are in use today in modern ECoG.

The early animal laboratory studies were soon followed by attempts to record electrical activity from the cochlea of man (Fromm, Nylen and Zotterman, 1935; Andreev, Arapova and Gersuni, 1939; Perlman and Case, 1941; Lempert, Weaver and Lawrence, 1947; Lempert et al., 1950). In these studies, the recording electrodes were placed on or near the round window of individuals undergoing ear surgery. The initial results were discouraging because the recordings were contaminated with unwanted noise, and the surgical procedures produced a significant conductive hearing loss. Responses were observed only for high intensity stimulation, and the responses were dominated by CP activity. Lempert and his co-workers contributed two important concepts, the "cochleogram" as an indicator of the integrity of the ear, and the suggestion that recordings should be made without disruption of the normal air-conduction route to the ear.

During the 1950s, studies using laboratory animals advanced the understanding of the stimulus dependent cochlear potentials. Davis identified the SP in 1950, and with his co-workers summarized the early studies of this response (Davis et al., 1958). Tasaki, Davis and Legouix (1952) demonstrated that the CP is intimately related to the mechanical events in the cochlea, and Bekesy (1960) showed that the CP amplitude was dependent upon specific hair cell displacement patterns. Goldstein and Kiang (1958) described the APs dependence upon the rise-time or abruptness of the stimulus.

Ruben and his co-workers (1960) studied recordings obtained from man at the time of surgery. Their recordings were of CP activity, and they were unable to obtain specific information about the amount or the frequency characteristics of hearing loss (Ruben, 1967).

The use of an averaging computer (Clark et al., 1961) was extended to human cochlear recordings by Ronis (1966). This event opened the current era of ECoG, in which the existence of a hearing loss of peripheral origin can be established or ruled out unequivocally. All ECoG techniques use averaging procedures. Averaging is used in order to extract the desired response from unwanted background noise and other stimulus dependent responses. The differences among the various techniques are concerned with recording site and signal selection. The details of these techniques, and the relative advantage of each, will be described in the sections which follow.

RECORDING AND STIMULATION TECHNIQUES

When recordings of the AP, CP, or SP are obtained from locations near the generators of these potentials, the evoked responses associated with them are quite large. For example, APs recorded directly from the auditory nerve have been in the range of 1000 to 2000 μvolts (Peake and Kiang, 1962). CPs also range to more than 1000 μvolts, and SPs with amplitudes in the 100-μvolt range have been observed when intracochlear recording sites are used (Dallos, 1973). Intracochlear, direct nerve, or round window recording sites are impractical and potentially dangerous for humans, and these are not used for clinical cochleography. As the recording electrode is moved away from the generator site, the amplitude of the response decreases dramatically, and practical ECoG techniques represent a compromise between ideal recordings and those which may be obtained wih minimal risk.

Electrodes and recording sites used in ECoG fall into three groups. These are the *transtympanic membrane* needle electrodes, which make contact with the promontory of the cochlea; *intrameatal* surface electrodes; and surface electrodes which are attached *outside* of the ear canal. The transtympanic membrane technique was developed by Portman, LeBert and Aran (1967) and by Yoshie, Ohashi and Suzuki (1967). Transtympanic membrane electrodes are made from no. 22 or smaller hypodermic needles which are 3 to 6 inches in length, and which are insulated except at the point and outer ends. The point of the electrode contacts the promontory after the needle is passed through the posterior/inferior quadrant of the tympanic membrane. Yoshie (1973) fixes the electrode in place with medical grade cement applied to the tragus. Others support the electrode with elastic bands which, in turn, are attached to a circumaural ring (Portmann and Aran, 1971; Eggermont and Odenthal, 1974b; Naunton and Zerlin, 1976b). The circumaural ring is held on the patient's head by a large elastic band placed around the head. A small metal cup attached to the preamplifier lead provides a cap for the outer end of the electrode. This type of electrode is illustrated in Figure 28.1*A*. These electrodes are used with a reference electrode attached to the earlobe on the same side, and a ground electrode placed on the forehead.

The transtympanic membrane electrodes can be placed after administration of a local anesthetic to the ear canal of a cooperative patient. In the case of young children or fearful individuals, a general anesthetic is used to permit electrode placement and subsequent recording (Eggermont and Odenthal, 1974b; Naunton and Zerlin, 1976a). Yoshie (1973) reports good success by simply sedating the patient, rather than using a general anesthetic.

One alternative to the transtympanic membrane approach has involved the use of electrodes placed within the external meatus near the tympanic membrane (Yoshie and Ohashi, 1969; Cullen et al., 1972; Coats, 1974). The electrode developed by Coats is illustrated in Figure 28.1*B*. It consists of a small insulated wire which has a balled end (Vernon and Meikle, 1974) and which is fitted to an 0.005-inch thick piece of acetate that has been formed into an open spring. The electrode/spring combination is passed into the external meatus with the aid of an otoscope and middle ear forceps until the electrode is approximately 2

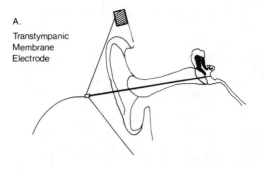

A.
Transtympanic Membrane Electrode

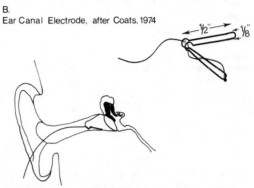

B.
Ear Canal Electrode, after Coats, 1974

½" ⅛"

Fig. 28.1. Examples of electrode placement for electrocochleography (ECoG). (*A*) Electrode arrangement for obtaining recordings from the promontory of the cochlea. (*B*) Electrode developed by Coats (1974) for obtaining recordings from the external auditory meatus.

to 4 mm from the tympanic membrane. When released, the acetate expands to contact the walls of the external meatus, thereby holding the electrode against the skin surface. The electrode may be placed without any anesthesia or sedation in a cooperative patient. In clinical use, it is placed after sedation of the patient. This electrode is used with a reference electrode placed on the earlobe, and a ground electrode attached to the forehead.

Surface electrodes outside of the ear include those which are clipped to the earlobe (Sohmer and Feinmesser, 1967) or fitted to a device which holds them in contact with the hard palate (Keidel, 1971).

Recordings from the promontory reveal evoked response amplitudes that are larger than those obtained at any of the other commonly used recording sites. AP amplitudes of 10 to 20 μvolts are obtained from normal ears when signals of 80 to 90 dB sensation level (SL) are presented. For signals near 0 dB SL the AP responses range between 0.1 and 1 μvolt. These response amplitudes constitute the chief advantage associated with the use of the transtympanic membrane electrodes. The amplitudes are adequate to provide reliable records at or within 10 dB of an individual's voluntary threshold for the same auditory signal. Furthermore, the large response amplitude helps to preserve the response wave form, thereby providing additional diagnostic information. (See "Clinical Findings.")

The advantages of the transtympanic membrane procedure must be weighed against the disadvantages associated with it. When the transtympanic membrane procedure is used, there is greater risk to the patient. This increased risk is related to the use of the general anesthetic, and the possibility of damage due to placement of the electrode. A survey based upon 3696 cases has suggested that the risk due to general anesthesia is less than 1.0%, and the risk of undesirable effects due to electrode placement is less than 0.1% (Crowley, Davis and Beagley, 1975). Although the risk to the patient is quite low, this consideration must not be taken lightly.

The costs of personnel and hospital space required for the transtympanic membrane approach are considerable. An anesthesiologist monitors and controls the levels of anesthesia. An otolaryngologist places the electrode and is responsible for the pre- and postrecording medical care of the patient, and an audiologist carries out the test procedure. An operating room, or similarly equipped facility, must be used to provide the life-support equipment dictated by the use of the general anesthesia. Hospital inpatient time may be required for postanesthesia recovery.

The principal advantage of the intrameatal and other surface recording techniques is that they are less dangerous and less costly than the promontory-based techniques. While sedation may be required for the intrameatal procedure, local or general anesthesia is not necessary (Coats, 1974). The likelihood of complications due to electrode placement is very slight.

The disadvantages of the intrameatal or surface techniques arise from the fact that they yield relatively small evoked responses. The response amplitudes for moderate to high signal levels are 0.1 to 2 μvolts (Sohmer et al., 1972; Cullen et al., 1972; Coats, 1974). Small response amplitudes could contribute to erroneous threshold estimates. For example, Cullen et al. (1972) report AP response thresholds corresponding to signal levels of 40 dB SL in their normal hearing subjects. Sohmer et al. (1972) show responses down to levels of 35 dB SL. Only Coats (1974) has reported AP thresholds to be in the range of 0 to 10 dB SL.

If the AP threshold elevation were always due to a given recording technique, an appropriate extrapolation could be made for estimating hearing threshold. Unfortunately, AP response characteristics for cases of sensory-neural hearing loss do not permit such extrapolation. The technique suggested by Cullen et al. (1972), which is based upon latency measures of the observed responses, is not capable of differentiating patients with moderate sensory-neural hearing loss from normal hearing patients. Extremely noisy recordings, or those with moderate to severe AP threshold elevations must be viewed very cautiously when the intrameatal or surface techniques are used.

When the intrameatal and surface techniques are compared with the transtympanic membrane technique, it seems that the intrameatal and surface records might be obtained as a *screening* procedure, only. If AP response thresholds can be obtained in the range of 0 to 20 dB for a given patient, one might safely assume that no hearing impairment exists. The promontory recording techniques, on the other hand, are appropriate when conventional behavioral and other forms of objective audiometric technqiues have produced equivocal results (Schmidt and Spoor, 1974; Montandon et al., 1975a, 1975b).

Acoustic signal selection for ECoG adheres to the tenet that was described by Goldstein and Kiang (1958). The appropriate signal is one which is sufficiently abrupt as to cause a great number of auditory nerve fibers to discharge nearly simultaneously. Acoustic signals which have a rise-time of more than 5 to 10 msec will fail to produce an AP response at normal threshold levels, and may cause a threshold *overestimation* (poorer) of as much as 20 dB (Eggermont, 1974).

Acoustic "click" signals are satisfactory for the purpose of providing abruptness, and have been used extensively (Portmann and Aran, 1971; Yoshie, 1968, 1973). Acoustic clicks are produced by passing a 0.1-msec pulse to a conventional earphone or a high frequency emphasis loudspeaker. This type of signal is characterized by a broad distribution of energy through the audible spectrum. The actual spectrum produced by this technique is dependent upon the transducer characteristics and the outer and middle ear characteristics of the patient. Studies of the spread of excitation resulting from the use of such clicks with humans have suggested that low intensity signals cause maximal excitation in the 2000 to 4000 Hz region, and high intensities extend this range from 2000 to 8000 Hz or more (Glattke, 1972; Simmons and Glattke, 1975).

Attempts to control for the spectrum include the use of high-pass filters with the clicks (Aran et al., 1971) or the use of tone-bursts formed by switching brief sinusoids to a transducer (Yoshie, 1971). A particularly useful technique was suggested by Davis, Silverman and McAuliffe (1951). According to this technique, a tone "pip" is produced by passing a pulse through a 1/3rd octave filter. The output of the filter is a brief series of sinusoidal waves that rises to maximum amplitude in two or three cycles, and decays in four to six cycles after passing through the maximum. The major frequency component to the tone pip is located in the center of the 1/3rd-octave passband determined by the filter setting. Since the rise-time is over a fixed number of cycles, the rise-time also varies with the filter setting. A 500-Hz tone pip will rise to its maximum in 4 to 6 msec. A 2000-Hz tone pip will rise in 1 to 1.5 msec, and an 8000-Hz tone pip will rise in 0.25 to 0.375 msec (Zerlin and Naunton, 1975). Tone pips have been used in human ECoG evaluations by Eggermont (1974), Eggermont and Odenthal (1974b) and by Naunton and Zerlin (1976b).

A second advantage associated with the use of clicks or tone pips is that the phase of each signal can be held constant or inverted 180° during the course of gathering responses without the use of additional complex equipment. This is useful, because the CP portion of the observed responses will mimic the phase of the click or tone pip, and the CP portion can be eliminated from the mean evoked response by presentation of equal numbers of signals in opposite phase (Peake and Kiang, 1962; Dallos, 1973). Electrical, and possibly mechanical, artifacts associated with the stimulus may also be eliminated from the mean response by this same signal-inversion technique.

Sound pressure levels (SPLs) of the acoustic signals for ECoG must be variable. The range should extend from perceptual thresholds of normal hearing individuals to 80 or 100 dB SL. The AP response is easily influenced by the effects of immediate prior stimulation, and because of this, it is advisable to use either an ascending or random sound pressure series for ECoG, rather than beginning the evaluation with high intensity signals and using a descending series.

Measurement of the SPL for clicks and tone pips cannot be accomplished with conventional sound-level meters because the signals are too brief to be read accurately by the metering equipment. Rather, the method of determining peak equivalent SPL advocated by Teas, Eldredge and Davis (1962) typically is used. In this technique the output of the transducer is monitored while clicks or tone pips are being produced. The repetition rate of the acoustic signals should be the same as that used for the ECoG evaluations. The monitoring is accomplished with a conventional calibration microphone. The transducer is placed in the testing environment at its usual position for ECoG, and the microphone is placed in a position corresponding to the location of the patient's pinna.

The output of the monitoring microphone is observed on an oscilloscope while the clicks or tone pips are generated by the transducer. This output will consist of a brief series of sinusoidal waves reflecting the *ringing* action of the transducer for clicks, or the tone pip characteristics. The peak amplitude and the principal frequency of the transducer output are noted. The click or tone pip is then replaced with a continuous sinusoid which is matched to the amplitude and frequency observed previously. The sound pressure level is measured for this substitute signal, and it is called the "peak equivalent SPL."

The peak equivalent SPL corresponding to perceptual threshold for acoustic click signals is typically in the range of 30 to 35 dB SPL for normal hearing individuals (Eggermont and Odenthal, 1974c). The peak equivalent SPL for tone pip voluntary thresholds in normal hearing individuals varies with the tone pip frequency, as in the case of conventional audiometric signals. In general, the peak equivalent SPL for thresholds obtained using tone pips is approximately 10 dB greater than the ANSI-1969 reference SPL for the corresponding audiometric frequency (Zerlin and Naunton, 1975).

In clinical practice, it has become common to express signal levels in dB relative to the voluntary thresholds for normal listeners, rather than using the peak equivalent SPL measures. In this way, results can be reported with a measure that is similar to the audiometric hearing threshold level (HTL).

Rate of presentation of the acoustic signals used in ECoG is in the range of 5 to 10 clicks or tone pips per second. Selection of these rates is based upon the finding that the auditory nerve AP response exhibits a reduction in amplitude for higher stimulation rates. This reduction probably results from neural refractory characteristics, and the 50% reduction point is reached with rates of approximately 30 per second (Eggermont and Odenthal, 1974a). Parenthetically, it may be noted that the 50% point is reached in laboratory animals (cat) when the repetition rate is greater than 100 per second (Peake, Goldstein and Kiang, 1962).

The number of samples required for ECoG response means is dependent upon the response amplitude, and, hence, the recording site. Intrameatal and surface recordings require more than 500 samples, and recordings obtained from the promontory require between 50 and 500 samples.

Recording amplifiers for ECoG should be of

a low-noise differential-input type. The differential-input amplifier cancels the electrical noise which is common to the active and reference electrodes and thereby enhances the readability of the AP responses. The amplifier filters should pass frequencies between 100 Hz and at least 3000 Hz in order to study the fastest components of the AP response without phase distortion. The amount of amplification will depend upon the anticipated size of the AP response and the input sensitivity of the computer. It has been common to use the maximum amount of gain possible without saturating the computer input. Amplification is typically in the range of 1000 to 100,000 times the recorded potential. See Goff (1974) for a thorough review of these principles.

Computer selection is likely to be determined by financial limitations and programming skills available to the facility that would undertake ECoG. The so-called "dedicated" averaging computers are suitable for analysis of the AP response, and require no programming skills.The flexibility of small general-purpose computers makes them more desirable to facilities which have computer programming skills available. Among additional considerations related to computer selection is the computer speed. The device must be able to sample the ongoing or evoked activity from the recording amplifier, store that brief sample, and return to get the next brief sample at a very high rate. This rate must be at least twice the highest frequency passed by the recording amplifier, and will be four or more times that frequency under ideal conditions. Sampling rates that are too low will cause a decrease in the signal-to-noise ratio of the entire recording/averaging system (Vaughan, 1974).

Additional equipment that may be required, together with the basic computer and signal generator, is schematized in Figure 28.2. It should be noted that the signal generator, recording amplifier, and tape recorder may be used separately from the computer to record the evoked responses. The averaging process may then be conducted from the prerecorded potentials and the results of the averaging may be plotted at a later time.

Environmental considerations are very important for successful ECoG measures. The AP evoked response is very susceptible to ambient acoustic noise (Teas et al., 1962), and a sound-treated test room is essential if reliable measures are to be obtained for signal levels corresponding to normal hearing thresholds. If the ECoG procedure must be carried out in an operating room or other nontreated area, careful noise surveys should be conducted prior to testing. Ambient background noise should be maintained at a constant level during the ECoG recording. Failure to do this could result in an elevation of the apparent threshold of the response, distortion of the response wave form, or modification of the response growth pattern with changes in signal intensity. All of these factors are critical in the evaluation of ECoG responses, and their modification by extraneous factors could lead to erroneous interpretation of the results of an ECoG evaluation.

Specific principles of the averaging process, and additional considerations related to the extraction of the AP response from other background or evoked activity will not be presented here. Thorough reviews of this material may be found in Goff (1974), Vaughan (1974), Eggermont (1974), Eggermont and Odenthal (1974b), and Dallos (1972, 1973).

ACTION POTENTIAL CHARACTERISTICS

The APs of the auditory nerve in humans have been studied by a number of investigators for a variety of auditory signals. Prior to consideration of clinical findings, normal response characteristics will be reviewed for the click and tone pip signals.

Acoustic clicks result in AP responses characterized by one or more negative peaks. The first peak usually dominates the response wave form, and is called the N_1 component. Subsequent peaks are called N_2, etc., in the order of their appearance. A normal AP response labeled according to this convention is illustrated in Figure 28.3.

AP amplitudes are measured from the baseline of the tracing preceding the response to the peak value of the N_1 component. The latency of the N_1 peak is usually measured from the estimated or actual signal arrival at the ear. The CP response, if present, may be used to estimate the actual time-of-arrival of the signal because the CP will mirror the signal wave form and will have no significant latency itself. The CP may not be present at low or moderate levels of stimulation, or for record-

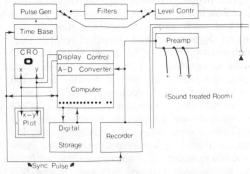

Fig. 28.2. Typical apparatus used for electrocochleography (ECoG) procedures.

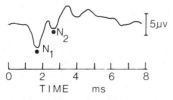

Fig. 28.3. Action potential (AP) response showing multiple negative-going peaks.

ings obtained from intrameatal or surface sites. When the CP is not present, the signal arrival time must be estimated by considering the distance between the transducer and the patient's ear.

The characteristics of the normal AP response with changes in click intensity may be observed in Figure 28.4. Within 10 dB of the individual's perceptual threshold, the AP can be identified as a shallow negative wave with a response latency of 4 to 5 msec. As the intensity of the click is increased, the latency of the N_1 component decreases until it reaches 1 to 1.5 msec at levels of 80 dB or more. The amplitude of the N_1 component grows slowly with intensity increments near threshold, and then grows more rapidly with increments above about 60 dB SL. The transition point, at about 60 dB SL, is also the point at which the response develops into clear multiple components (N_1, N_2, etc.). Figure 28.5 shows the amplitude and latency characteristics of the AP response for a group of 8 normal-hearing subjects. In order to arrive at a standard scale against which all response amplitudes could be plotted, the N_1 amplitude was first measured for the response of greatest magnitude. All other response amplitudes were then expressed as a percentage of the amplitude of the largest response. The resulting graphical representation is the "growth function" for the amplitude of the N_1 component. The shaded area of Figure 28.5A shows the range of the individual growth functions for the 8 normal hearing individuals. The normal growth rate for the AP response is between 0.5 and 1.0% per dB up to the 60 dB SL point, and 1.5 to 3.0% per dB above that point.

The latency changes in the N_1 component associated with changes in the click intensity are shown in Figure 28.5B. The data points show the mean N_1 latency for all subjects at a specific intensity. The vertical bars intersecting the data points show the group standard deviation. As is apparent, the latency changes from about 4.4 msec at threshold to about 1.2 msec for clicks at 80 dB SL. Standard deviations range from about 200 to 500 μsec, and are greatest in the transition range for amplitude, near 60 dB SL.

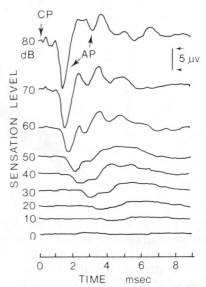

Fig. 28.4. Action potential (AP) for acoustic clicks at several sensation levels. These tracings are the mean responses for 64 presentations of a click at a rate of 5 clicks per second. Note the very early cochlear potential (CP) components present in the responses to clicks at 70 and 80 dB sensation level (SL). These data were collected with the assistance of Dr. F. Blair Simmons, and they are reproduced with his permission.

The latency and amplitude curves become asymptotic in the 90- to 100-dB SL region. Within the 0- to 80-dB range, any serious departure from the growth and latency functions as suggested by Figure 28.5 should alert the clinician to the possibility of impaired cochlear or auditory nerve function.

Tone pip signals result in AP responses with amplitude and latency characteristics which are related to the frequency region and temporal features of the individual signal. Examples of this interdependence are illustrated in Figures 28.6 and 28.7. Figure 28.6 shows AP responses obtained for tone pips at 500, 2000, and 8000 Hz, and the amplitude and latency characteristics of those responses are summarized in Figure 28.7.

The 2000 Hz tone pip results in responses which are very similar to those observed for clicks (Fig. 28.4). The response to low-level signals is a shallow negative-going wave. It develops into a clear AP having multiple negative-going components when high intensities are used. Responses associated with the 8000 Hz tone pip tend to be more succinct than those observed for clicks or the lower frequency tone pips.

The responses to the 500 Hz tone pips reveal

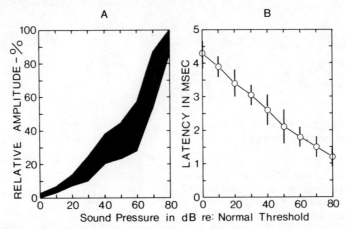

Fig. 28.5. Normal action potential (AP) growth and latency for acoustic clicks. (*A*) Range of AP amplitudes as a function of click intensity for 8 normal hearing subjects; (*B*) mean latency measures for the same subjects. The *vertical bars* intersecting the data points in *B* reflect the standard deviations for the latency measures. These data were collected with the assistance of Dr. F. Blair Simmons, and they are reproduced with his permission.

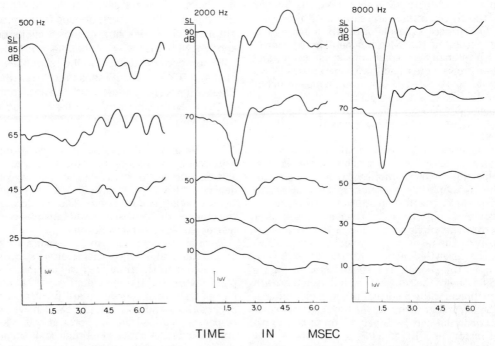

Fig. 28.6. Action potential responses for tone pips at various frequencies. These tracings are the mean responses for 500 presentations of the tone pips, at a rate of 10 per second. (From R. F. Naunton and S. Zerlin: *Audiology,* **15,** 1–9, 1976a. Provided through the courtesy of Dr. Zerlin.)

an abrupt N_1 component only at high intensities, and they show a cyclical pattern over time. This cyclical pattern reflects the fact that the AP will "follow" low frequency stimulation with individual negative peaks that are synchronized with the "rarefaction" phase of the individual cycles of the tone pip (Peake et al., 1962). Careful observation of the responses to the 500 Hz tone pips will show that the frequency-following behavior appears to occur at a rate of 1000 Hz, rather than 500 Hz. This occurs because the tone pip phase was alter-

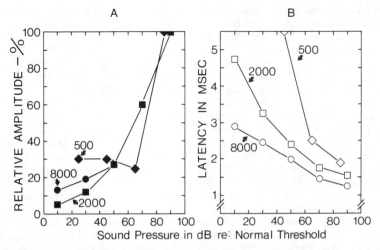

Fig. 28.7. Amplitude and latency measures for the action potential (AP) responses shown in Figure 28.6. (A) Growth functions for the AP responses; (B) the latency measures. The *diamond shaped symbols* represent the data for 500 Hz; *squares*, 2000 Hz; and *circles*, 8000 Hz.

nated between sequential presentations of the signal in order to eliminate the CP response from the mean tracings. The CP was eliminated because it followed the signal wave form when the phase was alternated. The AP wave form was not eliminated, but it did change in latency according to the phase change of the tone pips. The resulting evoked response, therefore, is a series of negative waves that occur at points in time corresponding to half-period intervals for the 500-Hz stimulus, or 1-msec intervals.

The growth functions in Figure 28.7A show a shallow portion for signal intensities near threshold. The functions become steeper as the intensity of the tone pip increases above 50 to 60 dB SL. As was the case for the gross wave forms of the responses, the growth function for 2000 Hz is most similar to that obtained for clicks.

The latency functions shown in Figure 28.7B help to clearly differentiate among the three tone pip frequencies. The AP latencies are inversely related to the tone pip frequency (at equal sensation levels). Therefore, the delay between the onset of the 8000 Hz tone pip and the N_1 response is consistently shorter than the delay for 2000 Hz or 500 Hz (Zerlin and Naunton, 1976b).

Thresholds for the APs produced by tone pip signals appear to be closely related to perceptual threshold for the same sounds when the tone pips are above 1000 Hz. Data from Eggermont and Odenthal (1974c) and Naunton and Zerlin (1976a) suggest that ECoG thresholds may be greater than 10 dB above (poorer than) perceptual thresholds for 500 and 1000 Hz tone

pips, but that they are likely to be within 10 dB of perceptual thresholds for 2000, 4000 and 8000 Hz.

CLINICAL FINDINGS

The individual who must interpret ECoG findings should consider four features of the evoked responses: (a) response threshold, (b) response wave form, (c) rate of change of the response amplitude and (d) rate of changes of the response latency (Aran et al., 1972). This section will be concerned with how these response characteristics may vary with certain audiometric configurations.

Regardless of the type of signal (click or tone pip) used, conductive hearing loss with a flat audiometric configuration produces AP responses with an elevated threshold. Once the threshold is reached, the AP response appears normal in terms of wave form and amplitude/latency characteristics (Aran et al., 1971; Odenthal and Eggermont, 1974). The cochleogram associated with a conductive hearing loss will show amplitude and latency results that are parallel to those associated with a normal ear, but the amplitude/latency curves will be shifted on the intensity axis.

Sensory-neural hearing loss resulting in deafness or audiometric thresholds at profound levels will result in an absence of AP responses. When this occurs, there is no doubt that the patient has no functional hearing.

In cases of mild and moderate sensory-neural hearing loss, a variety of response patterns has been described. The most common of these is the "recruiting" response (Portmann, Aran and Lagourgue, 1973) which is based on the use of clicks. Figure 28.8 illustrates this type of finding. The audiometric configuration may be sloping (as indicated in the figure) or flat. The apparent threshold of the AP will approximate the mid-frequency thresholds shown on the audiogram. The "recruiting" aspect of the response is that it will grow in amplitude very rapidly, and it will not show the gradual increase in amplitude with near-threshold signal levels as seen in the normal hearing or conductive hearing loss patient. The latency of the "recruiting" AP response will be very short, and will fail to show the progression seen in the normal cochleograms. The recruiting cochleogram, in essence, is similar to the high intensity portion of the normal cochleogram.

The response wave form associated with the "recruiting" cochleogram appears to be grossly normal. However, the transition between a broad, shallow AP response near threshold and the abrupt N_1 component of the response for higher intensities is much more rapid than in the case of the normal ear. Rather than extending over a 30- to 40-dB range (as in Fig. 28.4) it occurs within a 10-dB step. Similar findings regarding the growth and latency of AP responses to tone pips at 2000, 4000 and 8000 Hz have been reported by Odenthal and Eggermont (1974).

Another response classification associated with sensory-neural hearing loss is the result of an aberration in the response wave form. It is called the "dissociated" response, after Aran et al. (1971). The dissociated response is obtained when clicks are used, and when there is an audiometric configuration similar to that shown in Figure 28.9. The audiogram reveals normal hearing through 2000 Hz, a precipitous "notch" to 60 dB at 6000 Hz, and a near normal threshold at 8000 Hz.

The AP response threshold for the dissociated response is only slightly elevated, corresponding with the mid-frequency audiometric thresholds for the patient. Once the AP threshold is reached, the response grows normally until the mid-intensity region is reached. At about 60 dB, a "new" N_1 component appears in the response, and this earlier component dominates the response at higher click intensities.

The cochleogram reflects this change in response wave form by the abrupt disjuncture of the amplitude and latency curves at 60 dB. The low intensity portion of the amplitude curve appears grossly normal, changing at a rate of approximately 0.5% per dB, and the high intensity protion is also within normal limits. The latency curve behaves in a similar fashion. Near threshold response latency is approximately normal, and the latency changes at a normal rate until the break in the AP response at 60 dB. The dominance of the early N_1 component in the AP then determines that the latency drops to less than 2 msec, and the progression of latency beyond that point is very slight. It is clear that the two portions of the amplitude and latency curves are reflecting

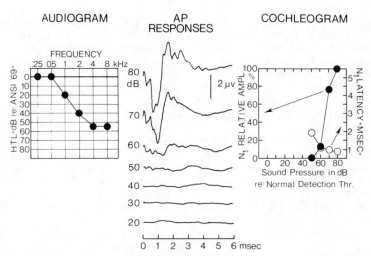

Fig. 28.8. Example of a "recruiting" cochleogram, together with action potential (AP) responses and audiogram. The responses are means of 64 samples based upon clicks presented at a rate of 5 per second. The cochleogram portion of the figure shows the amplitude (*solid data points*) and latency (*open data points*) on the same coordinates. The solid data points refer to the left ordinate, and the open data points refer to the right ordinate. These data were collected with the assistance of Dr. F. Blair Simmons, and are reproduced with his permission.

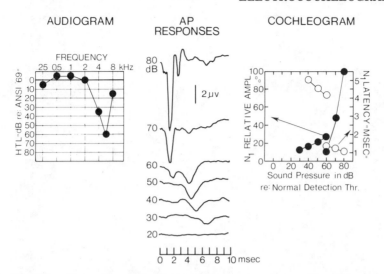

AUDIOGRAM AP RESPONSES COCHLEOGRAM

Fig. 28.9. Example of a dissociated cochleogram, together with action potential (AP) responses and audiogram. The responses are means of 64 samples based upon clicks presented at a rate of 5 per second. The cochleogram portion of the figure shows the amplitude (*solid data points*) and latency (*open data points*) on the same coordinates. The solid data points refer to the left ordinate, and the open data points refer to the right ordinate. These data were collected with the assistance of Dr. F. Blair Simmons, and are reproduced with his permission.

the characteristics of two discrete components of the AP response. The dissociated ECoG response category has not been reported for tone-pips (Odenthal and Eggermont, 1974).

Hearing loss due to retrocochlear lesions may also produce variations of the response wave form. In particular, the evoked responses for high intensity signals fail to develop into the succinct N_1 that is characteristic of all other classes for click stimuli. These "larges" (Portmann and Aran, 1972) responses are characterized by broadened wave forms, and have been observed for patients with a variety of central nervous system disorders.

Sensory-neural hearing loss confined to the low frequency region may not fit neatly into the above categories when clicks are used. Figure 28.10 shows an example of a cochleogram associated with this type of hearing loss. The audiogram shows a 35-dB loss at 500 Hz, and normal hearing above and below that frequency. The AP responses appear to be within normal limits, showing the two-part growth function that is characteristic of responses obtained from normal ears. In addition, the response wave form develops normally from a broad to a sharp AP. The latency of the AP response is also within normal limits, although it is somewhat shorter than the normal finding in the 40- to 60-dB range. Failure to detect hearing loss with click signals when the loss is confined to the low frequency region has led

others to the use of tone pips with encouraging results.

Two such examples are shown in Figure 28.11. The estimated ECoG thresholds are good indicators (±10 dB) of the extent and slope of the hearing loss in the mid and high frequency region. Such correspondence between audiometric configuration and ECoG threshold has been observed by Eggermont and Odenthal (1974b) and Naunton and Zerlin (1976b) for a variety of audiometric configurations. The use of tone pips seems superior to clicks because some of the speculation regarding audiometric contour is removed when tone pips are used. In addition, analysis of the growth and latency of the wave form of the tone pip responses provides useful information in the case of sensory-neural hearing loss, as does the "recruiting" cochleogram in the case of click signals (Odenthal and Eggermont, 1974).

RATIONALE FOR INTERPRETATION

It is much easier to compare known audiometric information with ECoG responses than to estimate audiometric threshold for ECoG information for a patient who has defied every other evaluation technique. The ECoG results are easy to interpret in cases of normal hearing, significant conductive hearing loss, or complete deafness. In other cases, associated with various degrees and types of sensory-neural hear-

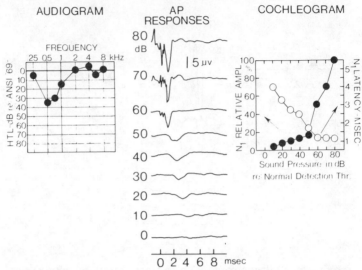

Fig. 28.10. Low frequency hearing loss, and associated action potential (AP) responses and cochleogram. The responses are means of 64 samples based upon clicks presented at a rate of 5 per second. The first positive-going component in the response at 70 and 80 dB is the electrical signal artifact. The smaller components preceding the AP response at 60, 70, and 80 dB are cochlear potentials (CPs). The cochleogram shows both the amplitude (*solid data points*) and latency (*open data points*) on the same coordinates. The solid data points refer to the left ordinate, and the open data points refer to the right ordinate. These data were collected with the assistance of Dr. F. Blair Simmons, and are reproduced with his permission.

ing loss, interpretation of the ECoG findings requires consideration of a number of elements that contribute to the normal AP response. The intent of this section is to provide information that will aid the reader in understanding *why* the clinical results look the way they do.

At the outset, it should be noted that the AP response measured from the recording sites used in ECoG represents the complex sum of the electrical potentials related to the discharge of a number of individual neurons located in the modiolus. In addition, the presence of a succinct AP response with a well-defined N_1 component is dependent upon the use of a signal which causes the responding neurons to discharge nearly simultaneously. Finally, the mechanical events in the cochlea which precede neural excitation strongly influence the latency and the cadence of the discharge of individual neurons.

It should be obvious that a large number of discharging neurons is needed in order to observe an AP. The discharge of a single neuron is too small to be seen at a great distance from that neuron. More subtly, the electrical filtering effects caused by the tissue, fluid, bone, and electrode itself cause a reduction in the observable amplitude of the "spikes" produced by single neurons.

Neural synchrony is also needed, for if the neurons contributing to the response were not time-locked to some stimulus-related point, no distinct evoked response could be seen. This requirement was illustrated best by Goldstein and Kiang (1958). They studied AP responses using white noise that was switched on with variable rise times. Regardless of the rise time, white noise would cause a great number of neurons to discharge, but the cadence of those discharges would be unstable because of the randomness of the stimulation caused by the noise. When slow rise times were used, no AP responses were seen at near threshold levels of stimulation. When brief rise times were used, the AP responses appeared normally, as with acoustic clicks.

When a brief signal is used, the temporal characteristics of this signal provide the necessary prerequisite for neural synchrony. However, brief signals necessarily have broad spectral representations. This broad spectrum contributes to excitation along a considerable length of the basilar membrane, with the high frequency components providing maximal stimulation in the basal region, and the lower frequencies extending this toward the apex. The time course of this spread of excitation will be determined by the mechanical characteristics of the basilar membrane. The latency to excitation for neurons innervating the basal

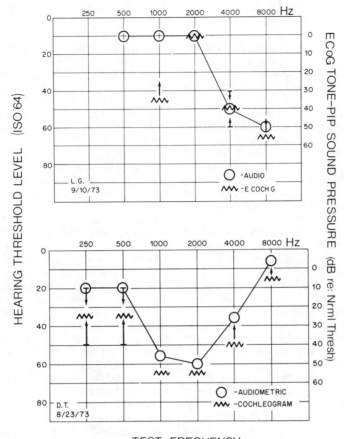

Fig. 28.11. Audiometric and electrocochleogram (ECoG) thresholds for two patients. The *open circles* show the audiometric thresholds. The ECoG thresholds are shown as actual (*jagged lines*) or estimated (*arrows*). When an arrow shows an estimated threshold, it means that the action potential (AP) response was seen at the intensity indicated by the ECoG symbol, and that testing was not done at intensities below that point. When the ECoG symbol is between two arrows, it means that the AP response was seen at the greater intensity (indicated by the lower arrow) and not seen at the lesser intensity (indicated by the arrow above the symbol). Note that the ordinate for the ECoG signal intensities is shifted 10 dB relative to the hearing threshold level ordinate. (From R. F. Naunton and S. Zerlin: *Laryngoscope*, **86**, 475–482, 1976b. Provided through the courtesy of Dr. Zerlin.)

end will be much briefer than the latency to excitation in the more apical regions. Consequently, neurons which are normally responsive to high frequency stimulation will tend to respond sooner than neurons innervating the lower frequency regions of the cochlea (Kiang, 1965).

Linked to the time delay associated with the spread of excitation from base to apex is the fact that a given neuron is likely to respond only during the period of time that the basilar membrane is displaced toward the scala vestibuli. This occurs during the rarefaction phase of the acoustic signal (Peake and Kiang, 1962). For a single point on the basilar membrane,

this period of time is equivalent to one-half of the period of the frequency to which that point is responding. Thus, neurons innervating the cochlea in the region which responds maximally to 8000 Hz energy that is present in a brief click have only 0.0625 msec in which to initiate a discharge. On the other hand, neurons innervating the cochlear region normally responsive to 1000 Hz have a 0.5 msec time "window" within which to discharge. It should follow from this that neurons innervating the region of the cochlea which is responsive to higher frequencies therefore have a higher probability of discharging within a brief time period, and with a cadence that is more stable.

All of this reasoning leads to the conclusion that the short latency, succinct, N_1 component represents neural activity which is dominated by neurons innervating the basal region of the cochlea (the high frequency region).

The normal latency progression of the AP response (Figure 28.5) extends from more than 4 msec to approximately 1 msec as the click intensity is increased from threshold to 80 dB SL. The AP responses to low intensities do not have a succinct N_1 component, but the well-defined N_1 appears at levels 50 to 60 dB above threshold. This suggests that the low intensity clicks cause maximal excitation in the low mid-frequency range of the cochlea, and that the basal dominance occurs for high intensity stimulation.

The response latency progression and the AP wave form changes associated with the use of tone pips also support this general line of reasoning. Responses to low frequency tone pips are less abrupt and have a longer latency than responses to high frequency tone pips. This finding supports the concept that the low to mid-frequency region of the cochlea contributes to long latency broad AP responses, and that the high frequency region yields short latency abrupt AP responses.

When considering the tone pip responses as support for this reasoning, one caution should be borne in mind. It should be recalled that the lower frequency tone pips have rise times that are inherently longer than the rise times associated with high frequency tone pips. The change in rise time could contribute to the change in response latency. In addition, the longer period of the low frequency tone pips could result in greater temporal dispersion of the neural discharges associated with them. This temporal feature could contribute to broadened AP response wave forms. The implication here is that the temporal features of the acoustic signals, rather than the place of excitation in the cochlea, influence the latency and waveform of the AP response. If this is true, it could be argued that the AP response associated with low frequency tone pips might not originate from the appropriate region of the cochlea. In other words, low frequency tone pips fail to test the low frequency region of the cochlea.

Evidence that the tone pips do provide effective stimulation for restricted regions of the cochlea comes from two sources. The first is the general agreement between audiometric configurations and ECoG threshold configurations (Odenthal and Eggermont, 1974; Naunton and Zerlin, 1976b). The second type of support is obtained from studies using masking over selected frequency regions where tone pips or clicks are used. The frequency selective properties of such bands of masking noise are well known. With restricted cochlear regions removed from participation in the AP response as a result of the masking, the resulting click and tone pip AP thresholds, latencies, and wave forms are consistent with the rationale that those features are a reflection of the region of the cochlea experiencing maximum stimulation (Glattke, 1972; Simmons and Glattke, 1975; Zerlin and Naunton, 1976a; Özdamar and Dallos, 1976).

Considering that the latency and shape of the AP response may be a reflection of the region of the cochlea responding to the stimulus, the dissociated responses in Figure 28.9 should be reexamined. The low intensity responses are broad, and develop into a succinct AP at approximately 60 dB. This intensity is the same at which the "new" AP response emerges, some 2 msec earlier than the later "old" N_1 component. Recalling that these response patterns are associated with a notched audiometric configuration, it seems reasonable to suggest that the "hole" in the latency function relates to the region of the cochlea corresponding to the 4- to 6-kHz notch in the audiogram. Instead of excitation progressing from the mid to high frequency region of the cochlea in a normal fashion, the abrupt jump relates to the loss of sensory cells (or nerve fibers) in the 4- to 6-kHz region.

In the case of sloping sensory-neural hearing loss (Fig. 28.8) one might continue the same reasoning. Low intensity stimulation is not effective because there is a hearing loss which extends to the mid-frequency region of the cochlea. Long latency broad AP responses are not seen. When the AP response does appear, it is succinct and has a short latency. This suggests that the sensory elements and nerve fibers remaining in the more basal regions of the cochlea are determining the character of the response.

The broad responses that have short latencies, fitting into the "larges" category of Portmann and Aran (1972) are also consistent with the concept that high intensity clicks provide maximal stimulation in the basal region of the cochlea. The short latency is most suggestive of the basal excitation, and the aberration of the response wave form corresponds with the finding that these responses are associated with a variety of pathologies that may contribute to abnormalities of the metabolic properties of the auditory nerve or cochlea. In such instances, the failure of the AP response to be dominated by a succinct N_1 could be the result of the inability of the available neurons to discharge with a normal cadence. This, in turn, could result from abnormal patterns of neural refraction, or abnormal mechanical excitation in the cochlea due to structural deviations secondary to vascular or metabolic disturbances.

The rate of growth and latency changes with increments in click or tone pip intensity may also be affected by a complementary mechanism, namely the presence of two distinct groups of receptors in the cochlea. It is well known that approximately 75% of the receptor cells in the cochlea are outer hair cells, and the remaining 25% are inner hair cells. The exact role of each type of hair cell is not understood completely, but it is known that selective destruction of the outer hair cells in laboratory animals results in a 50- to 60-dB elevation of the AP response threshold (Wang and Dallos, 1972). The AP response growth and latency characteristics after selective outer hair cell destruction are similar to the "recruiting" responses seen in ECoG or the high intensity responses for normal ears (Wang and Dallos, 1972). This type of finding leads to the conclusion that the neurons innervating the outer hair cells contribute to the low intensity portion of the response growth and latency curves, and that the high intensity portion of the curves may be dominated by the neurons innervating the inner hair cells (Yoshie, 1973; Eggermont and Odenthal, 1974a). Additional support for this two-population theory stems from the fact that more than 90% of the sensory neurons of the ear innervate the small group of inner hair cells, and that the remaining 10% of the sensory neurons innervate the much larger group of outer hair cells (Spoendlin, 1973). Proponents of the two-population theory have suggested that this innervation pattern is reflected in the slow growth of the responses near threshold (because there are relatively few neurons available), and the rapid growth of the response at high intensities (where inner hair cells and their associated neurons dominate the response) (Eggermont and Odenthal, 1974c).

CONCLUSIONS

Analysis of the AP response to transient signals is an inexact art at present. Nonetheless, it is clear that the AP response is an extremely sensitive indicator of cochlear and auditory nerve integrity. It is likely that the place of maximal stimulation in the cochlea, the status of the auditory nerve, and the relative contribution of neurons innervating the inner and outer hair cells all contribute to the configuration of an AP response. It is difficult to parcel out each attribute of the response, and then trace that attribute to a single factor. However, all of the characteristics of the response can contribute to the clinician's impression about the status of a patient's cochlea or auditory nerve.

If the clinician is to use all of the features of the AP response, it seems imperative that recordings be obtained from the promontory of the cochlea. The role of recordings obtained from other sites seems to be limited to screening.

Cochleography methods are geared to documenting hearing impairment or normal hearing unequivocally. Audiometric configurations based upon ECoG remain incomplete at present, but it appears that the high frequency portion of a conventional audiogram may be described adequately by ECoG thresholds for tone pips.

Finally, consideration of the other stimulus-dependent potentials, the CP and the SP, may provide great assistance in splitting "sensory-neural" hearing loss into "sensory" and "neural" components. The first steps toward this goal have already been taken (Odenthal and Eggermont, 1974; Naunton and Zerlin, 1976b). While it appears that recordings of the CP and SP from locations used in ECoG will not produce results that are interpretable in terms of audiometric configuration (Simmons and Beatty, 1962), such measures may become useful in estimating site-of-lesion where hearing loss has been demonstrated by other means.

REFERENCES

Andreev, A. M., Arapova, A. A., and Gersuni, S. V., On electrical potentials in the human cochlea. *J. Physiol. USSR*, 26, 205–212, 1939.

Aran, J.-M., Charlet de Sauvage, R., and Pelerin, J., Comparison des seuiles electrocochleographiques et de l'audiogramme. Etude statistique. *Rev. Laryngol. Otol. Rhinol.*, 92, 477–491, 1971.

Aran, J.-M., Portmann, M., Portmann, C., and Pelerin, J., Electrocochleogramme chez l'adulte et chez l'enfant. *Audiology*, 11, 77–89, 1972.

Bekesy, G., *Experiments in Hearing*. New York: McGraw-Hill Book Co., 1960.

Clark, W. A., Brown, R. N., Goldstein, M. H., Jr., Molnar, C. E., O'Brien, D. F., and Zieman, H. E., The average response computer (ARC); a digital device for computing averages and amplitude and time histograms of electrophysiological response. *IRE Trans. Bio-Med. Electronics BME-8*, 46–51, 1961.

Coats, A. C., On electrocochleographic electrode design. *J. Acoust. Soc. Am.*, 56, 708–711, 1974

Crowley, D. E., Davis, H., and Beagley, H. A., A survey of the clinical use of electrocochleography. *Ann. Otol. Rhinol. Laryngol.*, 84, 297–307, 1975.

Cullen, J. K., Jr., Ellis, M. S., Berlin, C. I., and Lousteau, R. J., Human acoustic nerve action potential recordings from the tympanic membrane without anesthesia. *Acta Otolaryngol.*, 74, 15–22, 1972.

Dallos, P., Cochlear potentials; status report. *Audiology*, 11, 29–41, 1972.

Dallos, P., *The Auditory Periphery*. New York: Academic Press, 1973.

Davis, H., Deatherage, B. H., Eldredge, D. H., and Smith, C. A., Summation potentials of the cochlea. *Am. J. Physiol.*, 195, 251-261, 1958.

Davis, H., Silverman, S. R., and McAuliffe, D. R., Some observations on pitch and frequency. *J. Acoust. Soc. Am.*, 23, 40-42, 1951.

Derbyshire, A. J., and Davis, H., The action potentials of the auditory nerve. *Am. J. Physiol.*, 113, 476-504, 1935.

Eggermont, J. J., Basic principles for electrocochleography. *Acta Otolaryngol. Suppl. 316.* 7-16, 1974.

Eggermont, J. J., and Odenthal, D. W., Electrophysiological investigation of the human cochlea. *Audiology*, 13, 17-24, 1974a.

Eggermont, J. J., and Odenthal, D. W., Methods in electrocochleography. *Acta Otolaryngol. Suppl. 316*, 17-24, 1974b.

Eggermont, J. J., and Odenthal, D. W., Action potentials and summating potentials in the normal human cochlea. *Acta Otolaryngol. Suppl. 316*, 39-61, 1974c.

Fromm, B., Nylen, C. O., and Zotterman, Y., Studies in the mechanisms of the Wever and Bray effect. *Acta Otolaryngol.*, 22, 477-483, 1935.

Glattke, T., J., Human auditory nerve responses obtained in the presence of band-limited noise. Presented at the meeting of the American Speech and Hearing Association, San Francisco, Calif., 1972.

Goff, W. R., Human Averaged Evoked Potentials; Procedures for Stimulating and Recording. In Thompson, R. F., and Patterson, M. M. (Eds.), *Bioelectric Recording Techniques,* Part B, pp. 102-157. New York: Academic Press, 1974.

Goldstein, M. H., Jr., and Kiang, N. Y.-S., Synchrony of neural activity in electric responses evoked by transient acoustic stimuli. *J. Acoust. Soc. Am.*, 30, 107-114, 1958.

Keidel, W. D., The use of quick correlators in electrocochleography. *Rev. Laryngol. Otol. Rhinol.*, 92 (Suppl.), 709-721, 1971.

Kiang, N. Y.-S., *Discharge Patterns of Single Fibers in the Cat's Auditory Nerve,* Research Monograph 35. Cambridge, Mass.; MIT Press, 1965.

Lempert, J., Wever, E. G., and Lawrence, M., The cochleogram and its clinical applications; a preliminary report. *Arch. Otolaryngol.*, 45, 61-67, 1947.

Lempert, J., Meltzer, P. E., Wever, E. G., and Lawrence, M., The cochleogram and its clinical applications; concluding observations. *Arch. Otolaryngol.*, 51, 307-311, 1950.

Montandon, P., Megill, N., Kahn, A., Peake, W., and Kiang, N., Recording auditory-nerve-potentials as an office procedure. *Ann. Otol. Rhinol. Laryngol.*, 84, 2-10, 1975a.

Montandon, P., Shepard, N., Marr, E., Peake, W., and Kiang, N., Auditory-nerve potentials from ear canals of patients with otologic problems. *Ann. Otol. Rhinol. Laryngol.*, 84, 164-173, 1975b.

Naunton, R. F., and Zerlin, S., Human whole-nerve response to clicks of various frequency. *Audiology*, 15, 1-9, 1976a.

Naunton, R. F., and Zerlin, S., Basis and some diagnostic implications of electrocochleography.

Laryngoscope, 86, 475-482, 1976b.

Odenthal, D. W., and Eggermont, J. J., Clinical electrocochleography. *Acta Otolaryngol. Suppl 316*, 62-74, 1974.

Özdamar, O., and Dallos, P., Input output functions of whole nerve action potentials. Interpretation in terms of one population of neurons. *J. Acoust. Soc. Am.*, 59, 143-147, 1976.

Peake, W. T., and Kiang, N. Y.-S., Cochlear responses to condensation and rarefaction clicks. *Biophys. J.*, 2, 23-34, 1962.

Peake, W. T., Goldstein, M. H., Jr., and Kiang, N. Y.-S., Responses of the auditory nerve to repetitive acoustic stimuli. *J. Acoust. Soc. Am.*, 34, 562-570, 1962.

Perlman, M. B., and Case, T. J., Electrical phenomena of the cochlea in man. *Arch. Otolaryngol.*, 34, 710-718, 1941.

Portmann, M., and Aran, J.-M., Electrocochleography. *Laryngoscope*, 81, 899-901, 1971.

Portmann, M., and Aran, J.-M., Relations entre "pattern" electrocochleographique et pathologie retro-labyrinthique. *Acta Otolaryngol.*, 73, 190-196, 1972.

Portmann, M., Aran, J.-M., and Lagourgue, P., Testing for "recruitment" by electrocochleography, preliminary results. *Ann. Otol. Rhinol. Laryngol.*, 82, 36-43, 1973.

Portmann, M., LeBert, G., and Aran, J.-M., Potentials cochlearies obtenus chez l'homme en dehors de toute intervention chirurgicale. Note preliminaire. *Rev. Laryngol Otol. Rhinol.*, 88, 157-164, 1967.

Ronis, B. J., Cochlear potentials in otosclerosis. *Laryngoscope*, 76, 212-231, 1966.

Ruben, R. J., Cochlear Potentials as a Diagnostic Test in Deafness. In Graham, A. B. (Ed.), *Sensorineural Hearing Processes and Disorders,* pp. 313-337. Boston: Little Brown & Co., 1967.

Ruben, R. J., Sekula, J., Bordley, J. E., Knickerbocker, G. G., Nager, G. T., and Fisch, U., Human cochlear responses to sound stimuli. *Ann. Otol. Rhinol. Laryngol.*, 69, 459-479, 1960.

Schmidt, P. H., and Spoor, A., The place of electrocochleography in clinical audiometry. *Acta Otolaryngol. Suppl. 316*, 5-6, 1974.

Simmons, F. B., and Beatty, D. L., The significance of round window recorded cochlear potentials in hearing. *Ann Otolaryngol.*, 71, 767-801, 1962.

Simmons, F. B., and Glattke, T. J., Electrocochleography. In Bradford, L. (Ed.), *Physiological Measures of the Audio-Vestibular System.* New York: Academic Press, 1975.

Sohmer, H., and Feinmesser, L., Cochlear action potentials recorded from the external ear in man. *Ann Otol. Rhinol. Laryngol.* 76, 427-435, 1967.

Sohmer, H., Feinmesser, M., Bauberger-Tell, L., Lev, A., and David, S., Routine use of cochlear audiometry in infants with uncertain diagnosis. *Ann. Otol. Rhinol. Laryngol.*, 81, 72-75, 1972.

Spoendlin, H., The Innervation of the Cochlear Receptor. In Møller, A. (Ed.), *Basic Mechanisms in Hearing,* pp. 185-234. New York: Academic Press, 1973.

Tasaki, I., Davis, H., and Legouix, J. P., The space time pattern of the cochlear microphonics (guinea pig) as recorded by differential electrodes. *J. Acoust. Soc. Am.*, **34**, 502–519, 1952.

Teas, D. C., Eldredge, D., and Davis, H. Cochlear responses to acoustic transients; an interpretation of whole-nerve action potentials. *J. Acoust. Soc. Am.*, **34**, 1438–1459, 1962.

Vaughan, H. G., Jr., The Analysis of Scalp-Recorded Brain Potentials. In Thompson, R. F., and Patterson, M. M. (Eds.), *Bioelectric Recording Techniques,* Part B, pp. 158–209. New York: Academic Press, 1974.

Vernon, J., and Meikle, M., Electrophysiology of the Cochlea. In Thompson, R. F., and Patterson, M. M. (Eds.), *Bioelectric Recording Techniques,* Part C, pp. 4–63. New York: Academic Press, 1974.

Wang, C. Y., and Dallos, P., Latency of whole-nerve action potentials; influence of hair-cell normalcy. *J. Acoust. Soc. Am.*, **52**, 1678–1686, 1972.

Wever, E. G., Electrical potentials of the cochlea. *Physiol. Rev.*, **46**, 102–127, 1966.

Wever, E. G., and Bray, C., Action currents in the auditory nerve in response to acoustic stimulation. *Proc. Natl. Acad. Sci. U.S.*, **16**, 344–350, 1930.

Yoshie, N., Auditory nerve action potential responses to clicks in man. *Laryngoscope,* **78**, 198–215, 1968.

Yoshie, N., Clinical cochlear response audiometry by means of an average response computer. *Rev. Laryngol. Otol. Rhinol.*, **92** (Suppl.), 646–672, 1971.

Yoshie, N., Diagnostic significance of the electrocochleogram in clinical audiometry. *Audiology,* **12**, 504–519, 1973.

Yoshie, N., and Ohashi, T., Clinical use of cochlear nerve action potential responses in man for differential diagnosis of hearing losses. *Acta Otolaryngol. Suppl. 252,* 71–87, 1969.

Yoshie, N., Ohashi, T., and Suzuki, T., Non-surgical recording of auditory nerve action potentials in man. *Laryngoscope,* **77**, 76–85, 1967.

Zerlin, S., and Naunton, R. F., Physical and auditory specifications of third-octave clicks. *Audiology,* **14**, 135–143, 1975.

Zerlin, S., and Naunton, R. F., Effects of high-pass masking on the whole-nerve response to third-octave audiometric clicks. In Rubin, R., and Salomon, G. (Eds.), *Proceedings of an International Conference on Electrocochleography.* Springfield: Charles C Thomas pp. 207–214, 1976a.

Zerlin, S., and Naunton, R. F., Whole Nerve Response to Third-Octave audiometric clicks at Moderate Sensation Level. In Rubin, R., and Salomon, G. (Eds.), *Proceedings of an International Conference on Electrocochleography.* Springfield: Charles C Thomas, pp. 199–206, 1976b.

chapter 29

INTRODUCTION TO ACOUSTIC IMPEDANCE

Jerry L. Northern, Ph.D., and Alison M. Grimes, M.A.

The determination of acoustic impedance is an important aspect of the clinical audiologic test battery. Acoustic impedance measurements are particularly useful to audiologists because the objective results often substantiate or clarify behavioral audiometric findings. Some audiologists use impedance audiometry initially with each patient to predict audiometric results, thereby increasing efficiency and accuracy in the clinic routine; other audiologists use impedance measures to confirm behavioral audiometric observations with difficult-to-test patients. In the past few years acoustic impedance test procedures have had an important part in every type of hearing evaluation.

The study of impedance enhances the audiologist's understanding of auditory physiology, anatomy and pathologic manifestations. It also helps to elucidate principles underlying the complex relationship among factors of acoustic impedance. The technical manipulations of operating acoustic impedance equipment are easily mastered. However, the relationships and interpretations of impedance audiometry require in-depth study and considerable clinical experience. Initially impedance audiometry was used only for identifying and evaluating conductive hearing impairment, but now these procedures have many clinical applications. Impedance measurements contribute to the evaluation of the site of auditory pathology, the nature of hearing loss, identification of retrocochlear and brain stem disorders, and study of Eustachian tube and facial motor nerve function. Many clinical uses of impedance procedures may be found in Chapter 30, in Jerger (1973, 1975b), or in Northern (1976a, 1977). In the hands of an experienced audiologist, impedance audiometry is especially valuable in the clinical evaluation of young children, the mentally retarded, the multiply handicapped and other difficult-to-test patients (Northern and Downs, 1974).

Currently, there is a basic battery of three impedance procedures: tympanometry, static compliance (or acoustic impedance) and the acoustic reflex threshold. Some clinicians use the Eustachian tube evaluation as part of the basic impedance battery. Although each test provides some information about the function and integrity of the auditory system, the information becomes most meaningful when relationships among the tests are considered.

HISTORICAL PERSPECTIVE

The measurement of acoustic impedance is by no means a new technique. Otto Metz of Denmark, in 1946, using an early mechanical impedance bridge, reported many of the applications of impedance audiometry currently in use today. The Scandinavians were quick to appreciate the clinical use of impedance measurements for testing the acoustic reflex and Eustachian tube function (Jepsen, 1963; Kristensen and Jepsen, 1952; Thomsen, 1955a, 1955b). The Scandinavians developed tympanometry and a wide variety of clinical uses for acoustic reflex measures, but have paid little attention to static compliance (absolute impedance) of the middle ear system.

In the late 1950s and early 1960s impedance interests in the United States were directed toward a mechanical device developed by Zwislocki (1963) which was designed to measure the absolute impedance at the tympanic membrane. The Zwislocki acoustic impedance bridge received an initial warm welcome from audiologists who were intrigued by its clinical potential. Investigators described various clinical applications of the Zwislocki acoustic impedance bridge (Feldman, 1963, 1967, 1969; Nilges, Northern and Burke, 1969; Zwislocki and Feldman, 1970). The Zwislocki bridge was never widely accepted because of difficulties in its routine use and clinical limitations of the absolute impedance measurement, however, the device brought attention to the potential use of impedance measurements in auditory assessment.

While audiologists in the United States abandoned acoustic impedance measurement, activity in Scandinavia developed at a rapid rate. An impedance audiometer was developed in Denmark by Terkildsen and Scott-Nielsen (1960). These authors described their new instrument as an "exact electronic counterpart of the bridge employed by Metz." During this period of time, Onchi (1963), a respected Japanese physician-scientist working independently in the Far East, developed a similar electroacoustic impedance device which he called an "aural reflex indicator." Onchi reported that his meter was not totally accurate in measuring acoustic impedance of the tympanic membrane, but he felt that its use in measuring the acoustic reflex was of clinical value. Scandinavians, led by Jepsen (1963), Ewertsen et al. (1958), Moller (1958) and Klockhoff (1961), studied normal and pathologic parameters of the acoustic reflex.

The origins of tympanometry were reported in 1959 by Terkildsen and Thomsen of Copenhagen. A paper by Thomsen a year earlier (1958) contains the first tympanograms ever published. Thomsen demonstrated the principle that middle ear pressure could be determined by changing air pressure in the auditory meatus until minimal impedance was obtained. At that time the mechanical impedance bridge in use could not be sealed airtight in the ear canal so his experiments were conducted in a pressure chamber. Terkildsen is credited with the initial use of the word "tympanometry" to describe the pressure-compliance function of the tympanic membrane (Northern, 1976b).

In 1970 there was a resurgence of interest in impedance in the United States. Two important articles appeared in American journals advocating the routine use of impedance measurements in audiologic and otologic clinics. Alberti and Kristensen (1970) described the use of impedance measurements in the routine evaluation of otologic patients. They stressed the broad spectrum of information provided through impedance which supplemented the otologic diagnosis. Jerger (1970) reported impedance findings from a series of 400 consecutive patients seen for evaluation at the Audiology Service of Baylor Medical Center. Jerger's lucid description and utilization of impedance results were to serve as the basis for a new era in hearing evaluation which stresses the acoustic impedance test battery as a routine procedure with every patient.

Recent applications of impedance audiometry continue to emphasize its broad impact on the field of hearing evaluation. Brooks (1971) of England has long advocated the use of impedance in mass screening programs. In the United States, the importance of the impedance contribution to school hearing screening is being recognized (McCandless and Thomas, 1974; Cooper et al., 1975). An objective technique for estimating sensory-neural hearing loss from acoustic reflex thresholds was developed in Germany by Niemeyer and Sesterhenn (1974) and improved into a clinical procedure by Jerger and associates (1974). In addition to standard contralateral acoustic reflex measurements, instrument developments have made ipsilateral acoustic reflex elicitation possible, and clinicians have been alerted to the applications of "contra" and "ipsi" acoustic reflex comparisons (Greisen and Rassmussen, 1970; Jerger, Neely and Jerger, 1975). Djupesland (1975) has published a comprehensive treatise concerning non-acoustic stimulation of acoustic reflex activity. Pediatric specialists are showing keen interest in the possible use of impedance measurements to evaluate otologic problems in children. (Keith, 1973; Bluestone and Shurin, 1974; Northern, Rock and Frye, 1975).

PHYSICAL PRINCIPLES OF ACOUSTIC IMPEDANCE

Definitions and Terminology

Students of impedance audiometry are confronted with a vast number of terms. Jerger (1972, 1975a, 1975c) has attempted to elucidate this terminologic strife. Feldman (1976) has recommended simplification and standardization of the currently used impedance nomenclature. Academicians and manufacturers tend to make much more of the terminology chaos than is clinically necessary. Audiologists need to understand physical principles of impedance measures in largely a conceptual fashion, rather than through advanced mathematical operations. The technically inclined audiologist is referred to the excellent material published by Zwislocki (1963), Lilly (1972) or Berlin and Cullen (1975).

Some authors suggest a dichotomy of impedance measures based on "dynamic" versus "static" tests (Lilly, 1972; Eliachar and Northern, 1974; Jacobson, Kimmel and Fausti, 1975). Dynamic refers to measures of impedance when the eardrum is under varying amounts of pressure. Static measurement refers to the impedance assessment when the eardrum is at a normal resting position. The various authors seem to have little agreement about the definition and classification of which measurements are "dynamic" or "static." The "dynamic" measures consisting of tympanometry and acoustic reflex evaluation are reported to be more clinically valuable than the "static" measurement of impedance (Dempsey, 1975).

On a conceptual basis *impedance* may be defined as resistance to motion. It is an objective measure of the degree of immobility of a mechanical system set into motion. Mechanical impedance (Zm) is technically a ratio of force acting on an object and the resulting velocity of motion generated by this force:

$$Zm = \frac{\text{Force}}{\text{Velocity}} \tag{1}$$

Impedance is therefore a ratio of two measureable phenomena: energy and motion. When the force is in the form of a sound pressure wave, the special case of mechanical impedance, known as *acoustic impedance,* is operational.

Impedance audiometers measure the acoustic

impedance by "looking into" the outer canal. This is done on a noncontact basis, with an air space in front of the impedance probe, for the purpose of measuring characteristics of the mechanical system of the entire middle ear mechanism. The acoustic impedance measured in this way is directly analogous to the ratio shown in formula (1),

$$Za = \frac{\text{Pressure}}{\text{Volume velocity}} \qquad (2)$$

except that an area factor is involved. Force is considered to be applied in terms of pressure (force/unit area) and the result of the applied sound pressure is manifested in the volume velocity of the air into which the sound pressure is applied. Conceptually then, acoustic impedance is an ordered way of noting a physical result. The unit of measure is the acoustic ohm. For example, if a sound pressure of one dyne produces a volume velocity of air of one cubic centimeter per second, this is arbitrarily defined as one acoustic ohm. (ANSI Acoustic Terminology, 51.1, 1960).

An alternate way to express the characteristics of a mechanical system is in terms of compliance (mobility) and stiffness (immobility). A system that is highly compliant will have low impedance and vice versa. The choice of term is no different than the proverbial problem of whether to describe a glass of water as "half-full" or "half-empty." Compliance (rather than impedance) is the term most often used in contemporary clinical literature. Use of this term is based on the fact that compliance (or its reciprocal, stiffness) is the dominant factor in the total impedance of the middle ear with low frequency probe tones.

Some mechanical systems move easily; other mechanical systems move only with difficulty. Three inherent characteristics of impedance interact in a complex manner to determine the mobility of a mechanical system: *mass, resistance* and *stiffness* (or its reciprocal compliance) as shown in Figure 29.1. All moving systems include various proportions of the three impedance factors (Wever and Lawrence, 1954).

Mass is related to the weight and density of the elements within a moving system. Mass causes the system to obey the laws of inertia, i.e., bodies at rest tend to remain at rest while bodies in motion tend to remain in motion. In the middle ear, mass is composed of the weight of the three ossicles and tympanic membrane.

Resistance comes from the change of the applied energy in a moving system, to an alternate form of energy and may be known as *friction*. This alternate form of energy is usually released as heat in moving systems. The resistance factor in the middle ear system is slight, due primarily to suspension of the ossicles by ligaments and muscles.

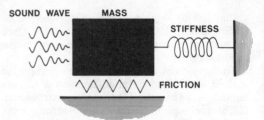

Fig. 29.1. Impedance is a ratio of energy and motion. In acoustic impedance, the energy is due to sound pressure, while motion is a function of the complex relationship among the mass, friction and stiffness of the moving system.

Stiffness is the reciprocal of compliance or elasticity. It is the tendency for the moving system to retain its original shape and position. Stiffness in the middle ear is generally attributed to the motion of the stapes footplate and the resistance of the inner capsule fluids.

The operational relationship of mass, friction and stiffness determines the total, or complex, impedance of a mechanical system. The effect of mass and stiffness on the resultant motion is known as *reactance* (see Fig. 29.2 for impedance/admittance terminology). The formula shown previously (1) is a conceptual operation in which the three innate physical characteristics dictate the resulting impedance of the system. The working impedance formula is presented below:

Zm (mechanical impedance)

$$= \sqrt{\underbrace{R^2}_{\text{(resistance)}} + \left(\underbrace{2\pi f \cdot M}_{\substack{\text{(reactance} \\ \text{due to mass)}}} - \underbrace{\frac{S}{2\pi f}}_{\substack{\text{(reactance} \\ \text{due to} \\ \text{stiffness)}}}\right)^2} \qquad (3)$$

where Zm = mechanical impedance, R = resistance, M = mass, S = stiffness, f = frequency, and π = 3.14.

A mathematical description of total impedance is incomplete without also expressing an additional parameter—*time*. The ratios previously expressed do not indicate whether the applied energy and the resultant velocity of motion are synchronous in time. It is convenient to express time in angular fractions of one wavelength of the applied energy (i.e., 360° may represent one cycle of a 1000-Hz tone with a volume velocity lag of 45°). This is a more convenient means of expression than indicating a lag of 125 μsec. Thus, total impedance at a "phase angle of 45°" describes not only the amplitude of impedance but also the time phase relationship involved. These phase relationships are determined by the mass and compliance factors in the system. In a pure resistance system without reactance factors, the applied energy and resultant velocity of motion would be "in-time synchronism," or be represented by a 0-phase angle.

Whereas phase angle is of interest in research, clinical applications have not been rewarding. By use of phase angle one can calculate and display resistance or conductance. Most impedance instruments display compliance. One instrument displays resistance. No commercially available impedance audiometers directly measure *mass,* probably because of technical difficulties. Most clinicians accept impedance measurements in terms of compliance since this physical characteristic dictates the resultant motion of the middle ear when low frequency sound pressure is applied to the tympanic membrane.

Mathematical descriptors of physical phenomena which involve both magnitude and phase are called vector quantities. Vectors lend themselves to graphic representation and are combined geometrically. The operational formula expressed above (3) is shown in vector diagrams in Figure 29.3. Impedance is the *vector sum* of resistance and reactance (Lilly, 1972; Jerger, 1975c). Friction (resistance) operates in the impedance formula at an orthogonal direction to the total reactance (difference between reactance due to mass and reactance due to stiffness). This diagram represents each impedance component separately; all lines shown are vectors. Total impedance, according to Figure 29.3, is the geometric combination of reactance and resistance vectors. Resistance and reactance are right-angle vectors with impedance equal to the hypotenuse to either right triangle. Students of geometry will recall the Pythagorean theorem which states that "the hypotenuse of a right triangle is equal to the square root of the sum of the square of the two sides." Review of formula (3) will show that Zm equals the "square root of the sum of two squares," i.e., the square root of resistance squared plus reactance squared. The resultant total impedance vector as graphically portrayed shows both its magnitude and phase angle.

In the working formula for mechanical impedance (3), friction (resistance) is frequency independent. However, the same frequency component (f) influences both the mass reactance and stiffness reactance in a reciprocal fashion. While the total mass reactance is calculated through a multiplication process, the stiffness reactance is calculated by division. Thus, any change in frequency will cause an increase in one term with a concomitant decrease in the other term. The total reactance can be described as the *quotient* of stiffness taken away from the *product* of mass. It is apparent that there is a certain frequency where mass and stiffness effects cancel each other out, making the total reactance nearly equal to zero. At that point, the only factor that creates impedance for the mechanical system is the small component of resistance (or friction). In the middle ear as with all mechanical systems, there is a certain frequency at which the ear has very little acoustical imped-

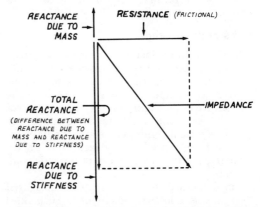

Fig. 29.3. Impedance can be demonstrated geometrically as the hypotenuse of a right triangle in which resistance and reactance are the sides of a right triangle.

	IMPEDANCE		PHYSICAL CHARACTERISTICS	ADMITTANCE		
Units of measure	Associated terms			Associated terms		Units of measure
Ohms	Resistance (R)		Friction (Resistance)	Conductance (G)		Mhos
Ohms	Positive (X_A)	Reactance	Mass	Susceptance (B)	Negative $(-B_A)$	Mhos
Ohms or cc	Negative $(-X_A)$		Stiffness		Positive (B_A)	Mhos or cc

Fig. 29.2. Impedance terminology.

ance. At this frequency sound is transmitted very easily and the reactance term equals zero. The *resonant frequency* of the middle ear is 1200 to 1800 Hz. Resonance occurs when a body undergoing forced vibration oscillates with greatest amplitude for applied frequencies near its own natural frequency, resulting in an increase in amplitude with no increase in driving energy. It is at middle ear resonance where acoustic energy is transmitted most effectively. At low frequencies well below resonance the system operates in a compliance dominated mode and the measurement of compliance is made with clinical accuracy and repeatability.

An alternative device, known as an otoadmittance meter, for measuring middle ear function has been introduced. The otoadmittance system measures the element of *admittance* (defined as the reciprocal of impedance) (Jacobson et al., 1975; Greenberg, 1975). The two components of admittance, *conductance* and *susceptance,* are reciprocally related to the impedance components of resistance and reactance. The advent of the otoadmittance technique, accompanied by terms less familiar, has added to the terminology confusion that now exists.

Units of Compliance

The impedance factors of mass and friction are independent of the compliance of the auditory system. Using a low frequency probe tone these two elements are negligible in the middle ear which is predominantly a compliance (or stiffness) controlled mechanical system. Let us examine possible units of measure of a mechanical spring as a preliminary exercise to understanding the unit of measure of acoustic compliance.

Springiness or elasticity may be measured by hanging a known weight on a suspended spring and noting the distance of extension per unit of weight. A "tight" spring does not extend much; a "loose" spring may extend a great amount. Units of measure, for example, can be inches per pound or centimeters per dyne.

Another way to measure springiness is through equivalent volumes of trapped air. Entrapped air acts as a spring, as anyone who has ever pumped up a flat tire with a manual air pump can verify. As the tire fills with air the pump handle "bounces" back. A small volume of air acts like a stiff spring; a larger volume of air acts like a looser spring. Volumes of air are measured in cubic centimeters. The equivalent volume of air concept expresses *compliance* as if one had that amount of air trapped in a container. The cubic centimeters unit of measure may have no bearing on the actual physical volume—only the springiness of trapped air. Thus 0.2-cc equivalent volume

describes a "tight" spring, while 5.0-cc equivalent volume might be considered a loose spring. Thus, compliance may be measured in cubic centimeters of equivalent volumes of air.

The absolute measure of impedance is an acoustic ohm defined as the ratio of a sound pressure of one dyne per square centimeter (to a volume velocity of air which displaces one cubic centimeter of air per second). The ohm is the traditional measure of acoustic impedance or resistance. High ohm values represent increased resistance while low ohm values represent mobile systems. Since the admittance system is the reciprocal of impedance, and the terminology is also reciprocal, the admittance unit of measure is the mho (ohm spelled backwards). A composite summary of impedance/admittance terminology relating physical characteristics to common units of measure is presented in Figure 29.2.

PRINCIPLES OF OPERATION

The electroacoustic impedance meter is actually a specially designed sound level meter. The theory of operation of the electroacoustic impedance audiometer is relatively simple, and the technical manipulations of the equipment to perform the test procedures can be learned in a few hours. Interpretating test results, however, requires the knowledge of a skilled clinician who understands and appreciates the subtle diagnostic patterns and acoustic impedance test battery relationships.

The electroacoustic impedance technique relies on the principle that sound intensity is a function of cavity size. There are standard couplers for calibrating audiometer earphones (6-cc cavity) and performing electroacoustic measurements with hearing aids (2-cc cavity). A signal of fixed intensity introduced into a large cavity and a small cavity will produce two different sound pressure levels in the two cavities. The larger cavity will have a lower sound pressure level; a higher sound pressure level will exist in the smaller cavity (Fig. 29.4).

The schematic diagram of the impedance meter (Fig. 29.5) illustrates the closed cavity between the impedance meter probe tip in the external auditory canal and the tympanic membrane. The electroacoustic impedance meter simply measures the sound pressure level in this closed cavity by emitting a probe signal through one probe tip hole and measuring its intensity with a pick-up microphone from another one of the probe tip holes. The third hole in the probe tip is connected to an air manometer capable of varying the air pressure conditions within the closed cavity.

As indicated previously, the electroacoustic impedance audiometer is a miniature sound pressure level measurement device. The sound pressure level of the probe tone in the ear canal cavity is determined by the compliance of the tympanic membrane and middle ear system. The pick-up microphone quantifies the sound pressure level (or intensity) of acoustic energy that is reflected back into the external auditory canal. A high amount of reflected energy is measured when the middle ear system is stiff as in ossicular fixation or otitis media. In contrast, discontinuity of the middle ear system creates a flaccid tympanic membrane that absorbs much of the probe tone

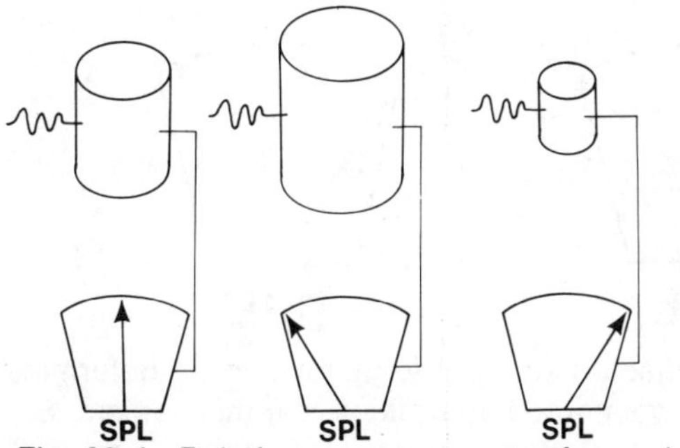

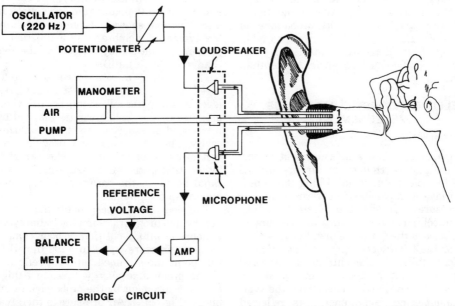

Fig. 29.4. Relative measurements of sound pressure level from various sized volumes, related to a fixed-intensity stimulus, indicate volume size. Therefore, relationships between sound pressure level (SPL) and volume (cubic centimeters) can be established.

sound energy and reflects very little back into the external auditory canal. The impedance meter measures the reflected sound energy for clinical determinations regarding the compliance of the tympanic membrane and the middle ear mechanism (Fig. 29.6).

With a hermetically sealed auditory meatus, an artificial "hard-walled" cavity can be created with the application of +200 mm H_2O pressure. Within the external auditory canal, the tympanic membrane is the only structure that is susceptible to changes in air pressure. The degree of sound energy absorption by the tympanic membrane and/or reflection of sound from the tympanic membrane, has a direct relationship to the impedance (or compliance) of the middle ear conductive mechanism. Obviously, any pathologic conditions that exist in the middle ear will influence the stiffness and compliance of the tympanic membrane, and accordingly, the reflection of probe sound energy.

The middle ear is a stiffness-dominated mechanical system; and, as noted in "stiffness"-type audiograms, the stiffness factors are sensitive to low frequency pure tones. Thus, most impedance audiometers use a low frequency probe tone of approximately 220 Hz. Low frequency probe tones are less likely to be influenced by the resonant properties of the ear canal. The long wave length property of low frequency probe tones contributes to a uniform

Fig. 29.5. Schematic diagram of an electroacoustic impedance meter with the probe tip sealed in the external auditory meatus. The probe tip has three holes: (1) probe tone, (2) cavity air pressure control, and (3) pick-up microphone to compare sound pressure level (SPL) in ear canal cavity with reference to SPL in impedance meter.

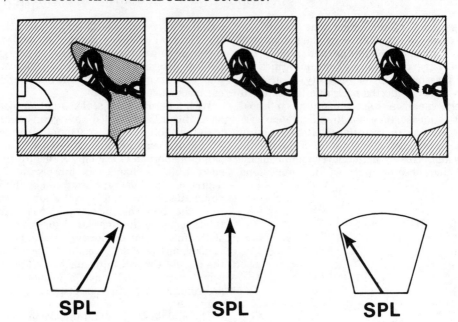

Fig. 29.6. The impedance meter measures reflected sound energy for clinical determinations regarding the compliance of the tympanic membrane and middle ear mechanism. SPL = sound pressure level.

sound pressure reference level in the external ear canal. Some researchers advocate the use of higher frequency probe tones such as 660 and 800 Hz in addition to the 220-Hz signal (Liden, Peterson and Bjorkman, 1970; Feldman, 1974; Harford and Liden, 1972; Liden, Harford and Hallen, 1974). Alberti and Jerger (1974) evaluated 1143 ears with probe tones of 220 and 800 Hz and concluded that no additional significant diagnostic information is obtained with probe-tone frequencies higher than 220 Hz.

ELECTROACOUSTIC IMPEDANCE MEASUREMENT

Tympanometry

Tympanometry is the measurement of eardrum compliance change as air pressure is varied in the external canal. Using the impedance bridge it is possible to determine middle ear pressure and quantitate Eustachian tube function behind an intact tympanic membrane. Compliance of the tympanic membrane is measured as the *relative change in the sound pressure level* (SPL) in the entrapped ear canal cavity as the air pressure is increased and decreased. When sound waves strike the tympanic membrane, some energy is reflected back, identical in frequency to the probe tone frequency, but differing in phase and amplitude. The amount of difference in phase and amplitude between the probe frequency and

the reflected wave depends upon the impedance characteristics of the tympanic membrane and the middle ear system. Acoustic impedance purists worry about measurements of the phase difference, but knowledge of the phase offers little, if any, clinical information. The resultant graph or tympanogram (pressure-compliance function) shows the compliance change of the tympanic membrane as a function of air pressure variations by measuring the relative change in the SPL (dB).

The point of maximum compliance (measured as the point of lowest sound pressure level in the external cavity) occurs when the pressure in the middle ear is balanced by the introduced pressure in the closed external ear cavity. Thus, tympanometry provides an indirect measure of existing middle ear pressure by identifying the air pressure in the external canal at which the eardrum shows a peak of maximum compliance.

The mechanical aspects of tympanometry begin by pushing or "clamping" the tympanic membrane into a position of poor compliance with air pressure equal to +200 mm H_2O. At this point the stiffened eardrum reflects most of the probe tone energy creating a high dB SPL measurement by the probe pick-up microphone (Fig. 29.7). Air pressure is then reduced in the ear canal cavity, permitting the compliance of the tympanic membrane to increase; the impedance meter now measures a decrease in reflected SPL (dB). The lowest SPL is achieved at the maximum compliance of the tympanic membrane, and as negative air pressures are created in the external auditory canal, compliance decreases and is noted by an increase in the SPL meter. Clinicians tend to conceptualize the tympanogram as "the way the eardrum moves." Actually, the tympanogram is a graphic recording of changes in *SPL* in the external ear canal as air pressure is varied by the clinician.

By displaying the tympanograms in terms of the relative change in compliance from a standard arbitrary reference compliance at +200 mm H₂O, the amplitude of the tympanogram is independent of the size of the ear canal. In this way a "standard range" of normal tympanograms is available for most impedance meters independent of patient, age and individual variance in anatomy. Utilization of the tympanogram "norm" pattern is an important guide for clinical interpretation.

Pathologic conditions which render the tympanic membrane nonmobile simply show no SPL change as a function of varied air pressure. Tympanograms from ears with perforations (it is possible in some cases to obtain tympanograms from ears with perforated tympanic membranes or with ventilation tubes in place) have a constant SPL in the external auditory canal and middle ear cavity. Alteration of air pressure has no influence on the entrapped SPL. Tympanic membranes retracted from serous otitis media may not be influenced by pressure equal to ±200 mm H₂O. Ear canals occluded with cerumen demonstrate a constant small volume size with no change in "compliance" as air pressure is varied.

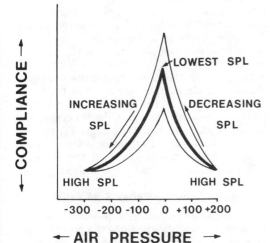

Fig. 29.7. The tympanogram is a graphic record of change in sound pressure level (SPL) in the external ear canal as air pressure is varied.

Static Compliance

Static compliance is also a measure of middle ear mobility. The factors of compliance include mass, friction, and stiffness, which work together in a complex manner to facilitate or impede motion of the middle ear system. Historically, this test procedure is referred to as *acoustic impedance*. Currently, however, *compliance* seems to be a more appropriate term than *impedance*. Considerable controversy exists in the United States concerning the clinical contribution of static compliance to otologic and audiologic diagnosis. Unfortunately, because a wide range of compliance values exist for various otologic pathologies that overlap with normal middle ear mechanisms, diagnosis of ear pathology based only on the static compliance measure must be considered with extreme caution.

Static compliance is measured in terms of equivalent volume in cubic centimeters based on two volume measurements. The first volume measurement (C_1) is made with the tympanic membrane clamped in a position of poor compliance with +200 mm H₂O air pressure in the external ear canal. The second volume measurement (C_2) is made with the tympanic membrane at the maximum compliance pressure. Since sound is more easily transmitted by the tympanic membrane during the second volume measurement (C_2), the probe-sound pressure in the enclosed cavity of the external canal is lower than noted in the first volume measurement (C_1), and a larger "equivalent volume" will be indicated (Fig. 29.8).

The static compliance measure is contaminated by the compliance of the air in the external canal itself. Static compliance is calculated by subtracting C_1 from C_2, which cancels out the external ear canal compliance and leaves a final compliance value that is the amount of compliance of the middle ear mechanism. Thus, $C_2 - C_1$ equals the static compliance of the ear in units of equivalent air volume in cubic centimeters. In general clinical use, static compliance is abnormally low when the value is smaller than 0.28 cc and abnormally high when the value is larger than 2.5 cc. The major clinical contribution of the static compliance measurement is to differentiate between the fixated middle ear and the middle ear with an ossicular discontinuity. Only static compliance values that clearly exceed the 0.28 or 2.5 cc norms should be considered diagnostically significant.

Middle ear compliance is influenced by many variables including patient age, sex, and pathologic state. The static compliance measure is corroborative information following tympanometry since both these tests measure "compliance." The static compliance measure is consid-

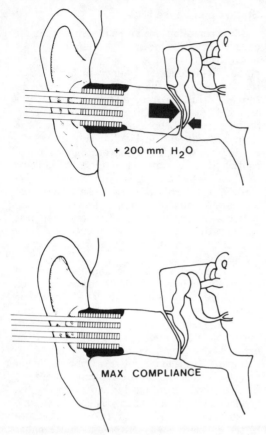

+ 200 mm H₂O

MAX COMPLIANCE

Fig. 29.8. Static compliance is based on two volume measurements. The first measurement represents the near-absolute volume between the probe-tip and the "clamped" tympanic membrane; the second measurement is made with the tympanic membrane in a position of maximum compliance.

ered by many to be the least valuable test in the impedance battery, and many clinicians omit it in routine clinical assessment. Indeed, Feldman (1974) indicates that the static compliance measure is appropriate only when the patient's tympanic membrane is devoid of any abnormalities. Dempsey (1975) summarizes the current status of static compliance by pointing out the irony that this "impedance" measure — for which the meter is named — is of questionable usefulness.

An interesting application of the C_1 measure has been suggested to identify a perforation of the eardrum (Northern and Downs, 1974). If the tympanic membrane is not intact and has a hole due to a perforation or a ventilating tube, the probe tone circulates sound into the entire middle ear space, and the C_1 volume measure will be quite large, often exceeding

4.0 cc or 5.0 cc in an adult patient. The C_1 measure in an average sized adult with an intact eardrum should be 1.0 to 1.5 cc; in a child the C_1 measure may be 0.6 cc to 0.8 cc. Thus, the static compliance C_1 measurement can be used to identify nonobservable perforations of the tympanic membrane or for the evaluation of patency of ventilating tubes in the eardrum. This technique is known as the physical volume test, or PVT (Rock, 1974; Northern, 1976a, 1977).

Acoustic Reflex Threshold

The stapedial muscle contracts reflexively when the ear is stimulated with a sufficiently loud sound. This contraction occurs bilaterally, even when only one ear is stimulated. Researchers have consistently documented that the necessary loudness range is 70 dB to 100 dB hearing threshold level (HTL). The median threshold value for the stapedial reflex to pure tone signals is approximately 85 dB HTL and approximately 65 dB HTL for white noise (Metz, 1952; Jepsen, 1963).

In the demonstration of the acoustic reflex, the electroacoustic impedance technique measures the sudden change in sound pressure caused by the change in compliance of the middle ear system as the muscles contract. The acoustic signal is introduced through an earphone attached to the impedance audiometer headset. If the signal is sufficiently loud to the earphone ear to elicit the bilateral acoustic reflex, the contraction of the stapedius muscle in the ear containing the probe tip will suddenly decrease the compliance of that eardrum (creating a sudden increase in the cavity sound pressure level) synchronously with the presentation of the stimulating earphone signal. The contralateral technique of eliciting the stapedial reflex is shown in Figure 29.9. The lowest signal intensity capable of eliciting the acoustic reflex is recorded as the acoustic reflex threshold for the stimulated ear. Under some circumstances the clinician is interested in the presence or absence of the acoustic reflex in the probe ear; on other occasions, the ear of interest is the earphone or stimulated ear. Regardless of which ear is under examination, it is standard clinical practice to record the acoustic reflex for the stimulated ear (Northern, 1975).

Ipsilateral Acoustic Reflex Stimulation

Recent developments in impedance audiometer design have made possible the presentation of stimulating signals through the probe tip itself to elicit stapedial reflex contraction. Ipsilateral stimulation eliminates the need to delineate the "earphone ear" and the "probe ear." Ipsilateral acoustic reflex measurement has

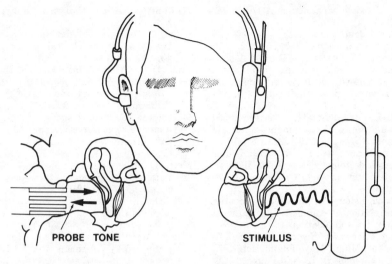

PROBE TONE   STIMULUS

Fig. 29.9. Diagrammatic representation of the physical principles underlying the measurement of the acoustic reflex. When the earphone stimulus is loud enough to stimulate stapedial muscle contraction, the compliance of the middle ear system is decreased, and the increase in cavity sound pressure level of the probe tone is monitored by the impedance meter.

generally taken two forms: real time and shared time measurement. In the real time technique, the equipment permits reflex identification while the probe tone and stimulus signal occur simultaneously; in the shared time technique, the equipment compares the prestimulus SPL with the poststimulus SPL. If an acoustic reflex has occurred, the relatively slow latency of the acoustic reflex will cause the poststimulus SPL to be greater (because contraction of the stapedius muscle decreases the compliance of the tympanic membrane) than the prestimulus level.

Experience at the time of this writing shows the real time (stimulus and probe tone together) ipsilateral reflex testing to contain artifacts. Caution must be exercised in interpreting these data until there is further investigation.

Research reports which compare acoustic reflex threshold sensitivity between contralateral and ipsilateral stimuli have been published indicating that ipsilateral thresholds are 3 to 6 dB more sensitive than contralateral thresholds (Moller, 1962; Fria et al., 1975).

REFERENCES

Alberti, P. W., and Jerger, J. F., Probe-tone frequency and the diagnostic value of tympanometry. *Arch. Otolaryngol.*, 99, 206–210, 1974.

Alberti, P. W., and Kristensen, R., The clinical application of impedance audiometry. *Laryngoscope*, 80, 735–746, 1970.

Berlin, C., and Cullen, J. K., The Physical Basis of Impedance Measurement. In Jerger, J. (Ed.),

Handbook of Clinical Impedance Audiometry, pp. 1–20. New York: American Electromedics Corp., 1975.

Bluestone, C. D., and Shurin, P. A., Middle ear disease in children. *Pediatr. Clin. North Am.*, 2, 379–400, 1974.

Brooks, D. N., A new approach to identification audiometry. *Audiology*, 10, 334–339, 1971.

Cooper, J. C., Jr., Gates, G. A., Owen, J. H., and Dickson, H. D., An abbreviated impedance bridge technique for school screening. *J. Speech Hear. Disord.*, 40, 260–269, 1975.

Dempsey, C., Static Compliance. In Jerger, J. (Ed.), *Handbook of Clinical Impedance Audiometry*, pp. 71–84. New York: American Electromedics Corp., 1975.

Djupesland, G., Advanced Reflex Considerations. In Jerger, J. (Ed.), *Handbook of Clinical Impedance Audiometry*, pp. 85–126. New York: American Electromedics Corp., 1975.

Eliachar, I., and Northern, J., Studies in tympanometry; validation of the present technique for determining intra-tympanic pressures through the intact eardrum. *Laryngoscope*, 84, 247–255, 1974.

Ewertsen, H., Filling, S., Terkildsen, K., and Thomsen, K. A., Comparative recruitment testing. *Acta Otolargyngol. Suppl. 140*, 116–122, 1958.

Feldman, A., Impedance measurements at the eardrum as an aid to diagnosis. *J. Speech Hear. Res.*, 6, 315–327, 1963.

Feldman, A., A report of further impedance studies of the acoustic reflex. *J. Speech Hear. Res.*, 10, 616–622, 1967.

Feldman, A., Acoustic impedance measurement of post-stapedectomized ears. *Laryngoscope*, 79, 1132–1155, 1969.

Feldman, A., Eardrum abnormality and the measurement of middle ear function. *Arch. Otolaryngol.*, **99**, 211–217, 1974.

Feldman, A., Impedance terminology — letter to the Editor. *Arch. Otolaryngol.*, **102**, 251–252, 1976.

Fria, T., LeBlanc, J., Kristensen, R., and Alberti, P. W., Ipsilateral acoustic reflex stimulation in normal and sensorineual impaired ears; a preliminary report. *Can. J. Otolaryngol.*, **4**, 695–703, 1975.

Greenberg, H. J., Fundamentals of acoustic impedance or admittance measurement — a tutorial presentation. *ASHA*, **17**, 729–732, 1975.

Greisen, O., and Rasmussen, P. E., Stapedius muscle reflexes and oto-neurological examinations in brain-stem tumors. *Acta Otolargyngol.*, **70**, 366–370, 1970.

Harford, E., and Liden, G., Clinical Application and Interpretation of Automatic Tympanometry. In Rose, D., and Keating, L. (Eds.), *Mayo Foundation Impedance Symposium*, pp. 127–138. Rochester, Minn., Mayo Foundation, 1972.

Jacobson, J. T., Kimmel, B. L., and Fausti, S. A., Clinical application of the Grason-Stadler otoadmittance meter. *ASHA*, **17**, 11–16, 1975.

Jepsen, O., The threshold of the reflexes of the intra-tympanic muscles in a normal material examined by means of the impedance method. *Acta Otolaryngol.*, **39**, 406–408, 1951.

Jepsen, O., Middle Ear Muscle Reflexes in Man. In Jerger, J. (Ed.), *Modern Developments in Audiology.* pp. 193–239. New York: Academic Press, 1963.

Jerger, J., Clinical experience with impedance audiometry. *Arch. Otolaryngol.*, **92**, 311–324, 1970.

Jerger, J., Suggested nomenclature for impedance audiometry. *Arch. Otolaryngol.*, **96**, 1–3, 1972.

Jerger, J., Diagnostic Audiometry. In Jerger, J. (Ed.), *Modern Developments in Audiology*, pp. 75–115. New York: Academic Press, 1973.

Jerger, J., Impedance terminology. *Arch Otolaryngol.*, **101**, 589–590, 1975a.

Jerger, J., Diagnostic Use of Impedance Measures. In Jerger, J. (Ed.), *Handbook of Clinical Impedance Audiometry*, pp. 149–174. New York: American Electromedics Corp., 1975b.

Jerger J., A Word about Terminology. In Jerger, J. (Ed.), *Handbook of Clinical Impedance Audiometry*, pp. xii–xiii. New York: American Electromedics Corp., 1975c.

Jerger, J., Burney, P., Mauldin, L., and Crump, B., Predicting hearing loss from the acoustic reflex. *J. Speech Hear. Disord.*, **39**, 11–22, 1974.

Jerger, S., Neely, G., and Jerger, J., Recovery of crossed acoustic reflexes in brain stem auditory disorders. *Arch Otolaryngol.*, **101**, 329–332, 1975.

Keith, R. W., Impedance audiometry witn neonates. *Arch. Otolaryngol.*, **97**, 465–467, 1973.

Klockhoff, I., Middle ear reflexes in man; a clinical and experimental study with special references to diagnostic problems in hearing impairment. *Acta Otolaryngol. Suppl. 164*, 1–91, 1961.

Kristensen, H., and Jepsen, O., Recruitment in otoneurological diagnostics. *Acta Otolaryngol.*, **42**, 553–560, 1952.

Liden, G., Peterson, J. L., and Bjorkman, G., Tympanometry; a method for analysis of middle ear function. *Acta Otolaryngol. Suppl. 263*, 218–224, 1970.

Liden, G., Harford, E., and Hallen, O., Automatic tympanometry in clinical practice. *Audiology*, **13**, 126–139, 1974.

Lilly, D. J., Acoustic Impedance at the Tympanic Membrane. In Katz, J. (Ed.), *Handbook of Clinical Audiology*, pp. 434–469. Baltimore: Williams & Wilkins Co., 1972.

McCandless, G. A., and Thomas, G. K., Impedance audiometry as a screening procedure for middle ear disease. *Trans. Am. Acad. Ophthalmol. Otolaryngol.*, **78**, ORL 98–102, 1974.

Metz, O., The acoustic impedance measured on normal and pathological ears. *Acta Otolaryngol. Suppl. 63*, 1–254, 1946.

Metz, O., Threshold of reflex contractions of muscles of middle ear and recruitment of loudness. *Arch. Otolaryngol.*, **55**, 536–543, 1952.

Moller, A., Intra-aural muscle contraction in man, examined by measuring acoustic impedance of the ear. *Laryngoscope*, **68**, 48–62, 1958.

Moller, A., The sensitivity of the contraction of the tympanic muscles in man. *Ann. Otolaryngol.*, **71**, 86–95, 1962.

Niemeyer, W., and Sesterhenn, G., Calculating the hearing threshold from the stapedius reflex threshold for different sound stimuli. *Audiology*, **13**, 421–427, 1974.

Nilges, T. C., Northern, J., and Burke, K., Zwislocki acoustic bridge; clinical correlations. *Arch. Otolaryngol.*, **89**, 69–86, 1969.

Northern, J., Clinical Measurement Procedures. In Jerger, J. (Ed.), *Handbook of Clinical Impedance Audiometry*, pp. 21–46. New York: American Electromedics Corp., 1975.

Northern, J., Clinical Applications of Impedance Audiometry. In Northern, J. (Ed.), *Hearing Disorders*, pp. 20–32. Boston: Little, Brown & Co., 1976a.

Northern, J., *Selected Readings in Impedance Audiometry.* New York: American Electromedics Corp., 1976b.

Northern, J., *Impedance Audiometry for Otologic Diagnosis.* Presented at Shambaugh Fifth International Workshop on Middle Ear Microsurgery and Fluctuant Hearing Loss, Chicago, March, 1976. Shambaugh, G. and Shea, J. (Eds.), Huntsville, Ala: Strode Publications, Inc., 1977.

Northern, J., and Downs, M., *Hearing in Children*, pp. 174–191. Baltimore: Williams & Wilkins Co., 1974.

Northern, J., Rock, E., and Frye, D., Tympanometry; a technique for identifying ear disease in children. *Pediatric Nursing*, April 1975.

Onchi, Y., Aural reflex indicator. *Trans. Am. Acad. Ophthalmol. Otolaryngol.*, **67**, 785–789, 1963.

Rock, E. H., Practical otologic applications and considerations in impedance audiometry. *Impedance Newsletter*, **3**, 10, New York: American Electromedics Corp., 1974.

Terkildsen, K., and Scott-Nielsen, S., An electroacoustic impedance measuring bridge for clinical use. *Arch. Otolaryngol.*, **72**, 339–346, 1960.

Terkildsen, K., and Thomsen, K. A., The influence of pressure variations on the impedance of the human ear drum. *J. Laryngol. Otol.*, **73**, 409–418, 1959.

Thomsen, K. A., Employment of impedance measurement in otologic and otoneurologic disorders. *Acta Otolaryngol.*, **45**, 159–167, 1955a.

Thomsen, K. A., Eustachian tube function tested by employment of impedance measuring. *Acta Otolaryngol.*, **45**, 252–267, 1955b.

Thomsen, K. A., Investigations on the tubal function and measurement of the middle ear pressure in pressure chamber. *Acta Otolaryngol., Suppl. 140*, 269–278, 1958.

Wever, E. G., and Lawrence, M., *Physiological Acoustics*. Princeton, N. J.: Princeton University Press, 1954.

Zwislocki, J., An acoustic method for clinical examination of the ear. *J. Speech Hear. Res.*, **6**, 303–314, 1963.

Zwislocki, J., and Feldman, A., Acoustic impedance of pathological ears. *ASHA, Monogr. 15*, 1970.

chapter 30

ACOUSTIC IMPEDANCE-ADMITTANCE BATTERY

Alan S. Feldman, Ph.D.

The impedance-admittance battery using electroacoustic instrumentation has evolved in recent years into three basic segments. These are tympanometry, intra-aural muscle reflex testing, and Eustachian tube evaluation. Each aspect of the battery with its subtests contributes certain information to the diagnostic capabilities of the entire battery. The weaknesses which any one test may have as an independent contributor are greatly outweighed by the strength of the information to be derived from the combined results. At the same time, it is important to stress that this battery of middle ear measurements will rarely supplant other diagnostic audiologic procedures. With the exception of the reduced reliance on traditional bone conduction audiometry (Feldman, 1972, 1975; Jerger, 1975) the astute clinician will still rely strongly on a thorough case history and a comprehensive audiologic evaluation before arriving at an audiologic diagnosis.

Certain aspects of the test battery should be considered more routine than others, and the order in which these measures are given is worth considering. It is suggested that the clinical battery begin with the middle ear measurements. The results of these measurements will often dictate the directions the clinician should follow. For example, some aspects of the battery may provide objective indications of normal hearing. This kind of a priori knowledge is helpful in dealing with a patient who may be difficult in a subjective audiometric test situation.

Middle ear measurements need not always come first. For example, children between the ages of 6 months to 24 months might be more suitably tested first in the sound field which is physically less restricting and less likely to induce fear and crying. This can be followed by objective middle ear measurements.

The battery of acoustic impedance-admittance measurements helps to evaluate (a) the air pressure status in the middle ear space, (b) the static impedance of the middle ear, (c) the integrity and mobility of the tympanic membrane, (d) the integrity and mobility of the ossicular chain, (e) the function of the intra-aural muscles, and (f) the patency and function of the Eustachian tube. In addition, the measurement battery can differentiate between different types of pathology within the middle ear and can provide some indication of the sensory-neural hearing level and locus of pathology in the sensory-neural system. In this chapter we will examine the specific tests within the battery and the interpretation of the results as they relate to possible pathologic entities.

The middle ear normally functions as a mediator which facilitates the flow of acoustic energy from the environment to the cochlea. The mechanical system of the middle ear behaves as an impedance matching device minimizing the difference between the low impedance of air in the environment and high impedance of fluid in the cochlea. A signal presented into the ear canal is "looking" at a certain impedance at the eardrum. Electroacoustic measurements of middle ear function simply assess certain aspects of this middle ear impedance. Pathology alters the impedance matching function of the middle ear by either increasing or decreasing it.

One problem the clinician must cope with is the current lack of standardization in this area of measurement. There is no standard form of notation or measurement unit or parameter. While it is true that all instruments presently measure either complex acoustic admittance (Y_A) or its components acoustic susceptance (B_A) and acoustic conductance (G_A), the lack of a standard for measurement notation has resulted in different instruments utilizing different but related display parameters. For example, these may be in terms of pure acoustic susceptance in acoustic millimhos or in a unit of volume having an equivalent value—cubic centimeters or microliters. At the same time, some instruments convert the acoustic admittance to acoustic impedance and provide an expression of the magnitude of the impedance vector.

Despite the differences in approach, there is a marked similarity among low frequency probe tone measurements. Differences in approach become important when dealing with higher frequency probe tones. Static measurements of high frequency signals are generally invalid unless they are performed with a system that either evaluates components of the acoustic admittance or establishes the phase angle of the acoustic admittance vector magnitude (Lilly, 1972).

There are certain basic similarities in all commercial clinical instruments used for tympanometry:

1. They depend on the measurement being performed in an hermetically sealed ear canal;

2. They are designed to generate a probe tone into the sealed ear canal and operate on

the basis that the probe tone will be maintained at a constant sound pressure level (SPL);

3. They contain a variable air pressure system in order to compare (a) the probe tone reflected off the eardrum under a condition of ear canal air pressure stress with (b) the probe tone reflected off the eardrum when air pressure is equal on both sides of it;

4. They are calibrated so that the driving current into the probe-tone transducer is known for specified acoustic volumes (i.e. compliance);

5. The measurement of the change in current required to maintain the probe tone at a constant SPL, as the air pressure is varied in the ear canal, provides the information for calculating static acoustic impedance of the middle ear;

6. They provide a display of the changes in acoustic energy that occur in the ear canal as air pressure is varied from positive to ambient and finally negative atmospheric pressure;

7. They employ a low frequency probe tone, although some also feature a higher frequency.

One distinction between instruments is the method by which the probe tone level in the ear canal is controlled. Instruments fall into two groups in this regard: bridges and meters. The former instruments require a manual manipulation of a balance or compliance control (attenuator) to measure static values while the latter automatically adjust and maintain the probe tone at a predetermined level. Examples of the bridge type of instrument are the Madsen Z070, Peters AP61 and American Electromedics 83.

Two steps are necessary in tympanometry with the bridge type instrument, whereas the meter type provides directly calibrated static values derived from the tympanogram. The Grason Stadler 1720B, Teledyne TA2C and Madsen ZS75 are examples of meters. This distinction is the basis for the two different shapes of tympanograms seen with bridges and meters (Fig. 30.1). Even these distinctions, however, apply to only one aspect of the entire middle ear measurement battery, the slope of the tympanogram. The derived information is identical with all instruments for middle ear pressure, static acoustic impedance (or compliance, or admittance, or susceptance) measured with low frequency probe tones, intra-aural muscle reflexes and Eustachian tube evaluation.

TYMPANOMETRY

Tympanometry may be best understood as a measurement of the ease with which sound flows at the plane of the tympanic membrane as air pressure is varied in the ear canal (Terkildsen, 1962). The specific acoustic parameter being measured (whether it is admittance or impedance or a component of either one) is not a restricing factor. When a probe tone is introduced into the sealed ear canal some of the acoustic energy is reflected off the eardrum and the rest flows into or through the middle ear into the cochlea. This energy transfer is optimal when the pressure in the ear canal is the same as the pressure in the tympanic cavity. In the normal ear sound energy flows best at ambient atmospheric pressure. When the eardrum and middle ear are stiffened, either by pathology or externally induced air pressure in the ear canal, there is a greater amount of acoustic energy reflected off the eardrum. The difference between the minimal and maximal reflected acoustic energy is attrib-

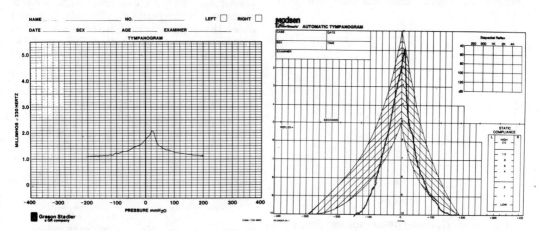

Fig. 30.1. Tympanograms of the same ear obtained with an electroacoustic meter (AVC) instrument, the Grason Stadler Otoadmittance Meter, Model 1720B (*left*) and an electroacoustic bridge, the Madsen Z070 impedance bridge (*right*). The tympanogram on the left is on a calibrated scale, while the right is on an arbitrary scale.

uted to the impedance properties of the middle ear.

Tympanometry Subtests

Tympanometry is the general term for measuring the flow of acoustic energy with an electroacoustic instrument. The procedure evolved from studies of impedance of the ear and pressure chamber studies of middle ear ventilation (Terkildsen and Thomsen, 1959; Terkildsen and Scott Nielsen, 1960; Thomsen, 1958). There are two fundamental subtests that are an integral part of basic tympanometry and a third which is a by-product.

1. *Middle ear pressure determination* is the most dependable test in this portion of the middle ear battery. Because energy flows best through the middle ear when the pressure on either side of the eardrum is the same, and both positive and negative pressure exert an extreme stiffening of the eardrum, it is possible to identify that pressure in the ear canal which corresponds to the pressure in the tympanic cavity by determining the point of peak energy flow (Fig. 30.2). This is the point of lowest impedance in the middle ear system. Early studies of acoustic impedance were directed toward a measurement of the static acoustic impedance but this focus was changed because of the unreliability of that measurement (Metz, 1946). As a result, the interest then shifted to studies of middle ear pressure and the procedure of tympanometry as we know it today was developed (Thomsen, 1958; Terkildsen and Thomsen, 1959; Terkildsen, 1961; Brooks, 1968; Liden, Peterson and Bjorkman, 1970). The accuracy of electroacoustic instruments in following pressure changes is quite high (Peterson and Liden, 1970; Eliachar and Northern, 1974)

with only a slight overestimation in ears with negative pressure because of volume changes in the middle ear that develop when a negative air pressure is established in the ear canal (Holmquist, 1976).

The determination of middle ear pressure simply involves finding the ear canal pressure corresponding to the peak of a tympanogram. When the tympanogram is flat with no obvious peak, even when sensitivity of the measuring system is increased, it would imply an infinite negative pressure or a negligible air space in the middle ear. Negative pressure should correspond to visible retraction of the eardrum. However, this measuring system is more sensitive than the human eye, even with the aid of magnification and pneumatic massage (Bluestone, Beery and Paradise, 1974). As a consequence, it is not uncommon for negative pressure readings to be unconfirmed by visual examination of the ear.

2. *Static acoustic impedance determination* is the second subtest within the tympanometry battery. With the advent of the Zwislocki mechanical acoustic bridge (Zwislocki, 1963; Feldman, 1963), interest increased in the assessment of the absolute magnitude of the acoustic impedance of the middle ear. Although the mechanical acoustic bridge has not become a clinical instrument, the principle of measurement of the actual acoustic impedance magnitude has been incorporated into current electroacoustic instruments. In tympanometry the *amplitude* of a tympanogram relates to the magnitude of the acoustic impedance in that the greater amplitude indicates a low impedance and a shallow amplitude a high impedance. Depending upon how the instruments are calibrated this information will be displayed in terms of acoustic compliance, acoustic ohms or acoustic millimhos. Table 30.1 compares the popularly used notations according to their respective parameters. The results for all instruments are directly comparable with

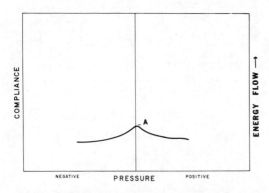

Fig. 30.2. Normal tympanogram. Point (A) represents the point of peak energy flow (maximum compliance or admittance) and occurs at a point when ear canal and middle ear pressure are equal.

TABLE 30.1. *Parameters of Measurement and Their Respective Notations*

Acoustic Impedance (Z_A) acoustic ohm	Acoustic Admittance (Y_A) acoustic millimho
Acoustic Reactance (X_A) acoustic ohm	Acoustic Susceptance (B_A) acoustic millimho Acoustic Compliance cubic centimeters
Acoustic Resistance (R_A) acoustic ohm	Acoustic Conductance (G_A) acoustic millimho

low frequency probe tones where the compliance of the ear is the fundamental contributor to the admittance. The mass and resistance contribute very little to the magnitude of impedance in the low frequencies. For clinical purposes the actual magnitude of the static acoustic impedance is not as great a concern as is the relationship to a normal range. Consequently, static acoustic impedance or admittance need be viewed only in terms of *whether a particular ear is stiffer than normal or more flaccid than normal and what may be contributing to these findings*. Certain pathologies or abnormalities result in the former, while others result in the latter.

3. *Shape aberration of tympanograms* is a by-product of automatic tympanometry. Normal tympanograms present typically smooth and symmetrical shapes. The specific forms they will take are, in part, instrument dependent, but certain features are a consequence of pathologic conditions or eardrum abnormalities (Liden, Harford and Hallen, 1974; Feldman, 1974). There is a distinct relationship between static acoustic impedance and many shape aberrations. It is due to the sudden change in flow of acoustic energy through the middle ear system that develops as eardrum stiffness induced by air pressure in the ear canal is removed and then reintroduced in automatic tympanometry (Feldman, 1976a). This stiffness change is proportionally much greater in abnormal conditions than it is in normal ears and results in peaking, notching and "W" patterns of tympanograms. This is particularly true with higher frequency probe tones which approximate the resonant point of the eardrum or middle ear. Shape aberrations assist in the identification of certain clinical entities and also contribute to the validation of static impedance measures obtained with low frequency probe tones (Feldman, 1974, 1976b).

PROCEDURES IN TYMPANOMETRY

Each instrument manufacturer provides instructions for the operation and maintenance of his specific instrument as well as instructions in its use. In clinical practice some common procedures and problems seem to occur often enough that they deserve mention here. It is important to remember that while this is an objective measurement, it does require at least passive cooperation of the patient. Instructions to the patient should include an explanation that extraneous head and mouth movement, as well as speaking, should be avoided during the test. Swallowing should also be avoided after an initial several swallows before the test begins. The patient should be advised that the small probe must be sealed tightly in the entrance to the ear canal and

that the initial discomfort which may be felt will pass as soon as the test begins. Most commonly the procedure will involve some discomfort but no pain. With very young children it will be important to work rapidly and provide assurance that the test will take a very short time. As with any clinical activity with children, cooperation increases as the child develops confidence in the clinician and the clinician develops self-confidence. There may be times when the test will not be possible, but if the clinician is willing to sacrifice some precision in the measurement it is even possible to obtain valuable measurements with infants while they are crying or sucking a bottle or pacifier. Figure 30.3 shows very interpretable tympanograms obtained in a crying 3-month-old infant. One ear falls within the normal pressure range although somewhat low in amplitude and the other shows both negative pressure and low amplitude. This suggested serous otitis media which was surgically confirmed.

Inspection of the ear with an otoscope is a necessary preliminary activity prior to the actual measurement. There are several reasons for this. First, it is essential to establish that cerumen is not impacted in the ear and obstructing the canal thus preventing the measurement at the eardrum. Secondly, cerumen in the canal which is not obstructive, but which may plug the probe tube, destroys the calibration of the instrument. Even flakes of cerumen can be pulled on to the front of the probe and act like a valve as pressure is varied in the ear canal. Many bizarre tympanometric patterns are attributable to innocuous looking particles of cerumen (Feldman, 1976a). As a consequence, potentially complicating cerumen should be removed prior to the measurement. A third reason for the visual inspection of the ear is the need to determine the size and shape of the ear canal. It is important to establish the size of the probe tip and the angle at which to insert the probe.

Achieving an airtight seal is perhaps the greatest problem the novice encounters in middle ear measurements. This problem disappears with experience. Difficulties in obtaining a seal should be drastically reduced if one is resourceful and has available a wide variety of probe tips. The most successful method of sealing the ear canal is to have the patient relax the jaw while the clinician lifts the pinna up and back with one hand and inserts the probe with the other hand. The probe should be rotated about 90° as it is pushed into the lumen of the ear canal. In those rare cases when it is not possible to seal the ear it can often be done by hand holding the probe, fit with a large tip, in the concha at the canal orifice. This is a more common occurrence among the elderly

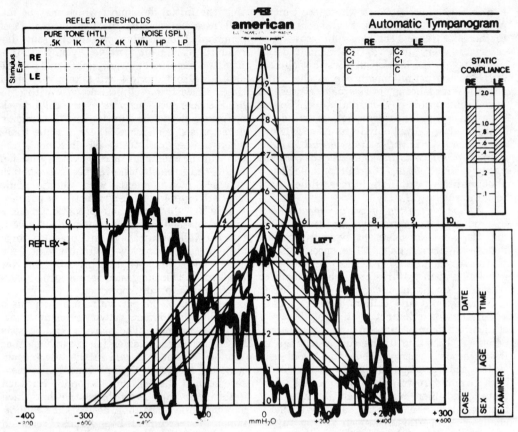

Fig. 30.3. Tympanograms obtained on a crying infant. Middle ear pressure on the left ear is within normal limits and amplitude is somewhat restricted. The right ear exhibits negative pressure and a similar borderline low amplitude. Irregular spiking is due to physical and vocal interference with the measurement but it does not inhibit effective interpretation.

populations whose canals tend to be collapsed or slit shaped. Some tips may never quite do the job and as a last resort the clinician may resort to the use of a silicone putty which can be pushed around the probe tip. Care must be taken not to allow this material to obstruct the probe.

Obtaining the measurement is rarely a problem once the ear is sealed. Validating a seal is best accomplished by adjusting the pressure in the ear canal and observing the pressure meter. If the positive or negative air pressure cannot be maintained then there is a leak, either in the seal or in the test system. A leak which occurs only when high positive pressure is introduced implies an open tympanic membrane with the increased pressure being evacuated through the Eustachian tube. Once the ear is sealed, tympanometry is performed according to the instructions provided by the manufacturer.

The actual measurement in tympanometry

may be performed either manually or automatically or, as with most instruments, in a combination of automatic and manual operation.

Manual tympanometry refers to the determination of the two points of minimum and maximum flow by measuring with the ear canal air pressure at either a high positive or high negative setting and then varying the pressure until a maximum deflection of the balance or component meter is observed. The minimum flow setting is usually ± 200 mm H_2O and in normal ears the maximum will be around ± 25 mm H_2O. In pathologic ears the peak will occur at the pressure setting that corresponds to the pressure in the tympanic cavity. The first measurement, often called C_1, is intended to be made with the eardrum in a rigid state resulting in maximum reflection of the signal. A low frequency probe tone will permit an accurate measurement of the volume of the ear canal. The second measurement, often called C_2, combines information about ear canal volume with properties of the middle ear. This set of measurements is frequently referred to as acoustic compliance, implying that the measurement is reported in terms of a volume of air having a compliance equivalent to the ear canal (C_1) or the combined ear canal and middle ear (C_2). While this is not technically correct (Lilly, 1972; Jerger, 1975, p. xii), it is a sufficiently close approximation to be permissible in most clinical measurements. The determination of the static acoustic compliance or admittance properties of the middle ear in manual tympanometry is achieved by subtracting the measurement performed with the eardrum under induced pressure (C_1) from the measurement at peak flow (C_2). In most clinical instruments (bridges) the static measurement must be obtained in this two point manual manipulation. In those instruments (meters) which automatically adjust the probe tone SPL, no balancing is necessary and the reading is made directly from the meter or the tympanogram at these two pressure levels. If desired, a series of discrete measurements can be made and a complete manual tympanogram may be plotted. This is not usually necessary in the clinical setting.

Automatic tympanometry refers to the automatic recording, usually on an XY plotter, of changing acoustic admittance as the air pressure is continuously varied in the ear canal over the same range (± 200) as in manual tympanometry. With the electroacoustic bridge,

which is not calibrated for tympanometry, the amplitude of the tympanogram is in arbitrary units while the meter type instruments yield calibrated values which relate directly to the parameter being measured. Typical tympanograms of a normal ear measured with each type of instrument were shown in Figure 30.1. As was noted, there is a different shape in each instance as well as amplitude, but in both cases the tympanogram falls within the normal range for that instrument and the pressure peak is identical. The elevation of the tympanogram on the electroacoustic meters is equivalent to the C_1 manual measurement. For example in Figure 30.1 the elevation at + 200 mm H_2O is 1.1 cc, and is an index of ear canal volume. Thus, despite the differences in certain features, the basic information yielded by each instrument is the same with low frequency probe tones. In Figure 30.4, the four separate tympanograms of a normal ear are displayed for a component measuring admittance system. The B220 (susceptance at 220 Hz) tympanogram is essentially equivalent to the single curve measured with complex admittance (impedance) bridges or meters.

INTERPRETATION OF TYMPANOGRAMS

There have been two approaches to tympanogram interpretation that have been advocated. Jerger (1970) has used a coding system which types various patterns of tympanograms. This classification system is shown in Figure

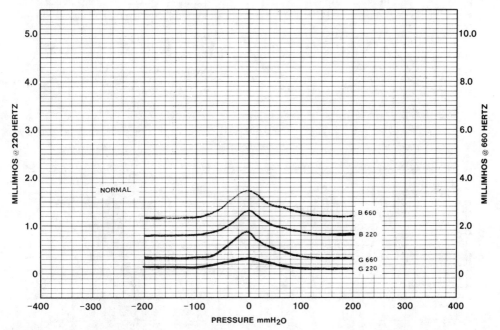

Fig. 30.4. Normal tympanograms obtained for high and low frequency probe tones with a component measurement system (Grason Stadler Otoadmittance Meter Model 1720B).

30.5. His approach tends to oversimplify interpretation and becomes somewhat limited when combined pathologies exist. Also there tends to be a proliferation of subcategories and classifications which ends up in a myriad of confusion. Its limitations are further compounded with the use of high frequency tympanometry. This classification system is generally confined to one type of instrument. Another approach that has been suggested is a descriptive analysis of tympanograms (Feldman, 1975, 1976a). Rather than the use of a code which needs translation in the end, this approach describes the three features that are displayed by the tympanogram: pressure, amplitude and shape.

It will be recalled that every tympanogram tells us something about (a) the *pressure* status of the middle ear. It is either normal, positive or negative (or absent) and can be specified in actual mm H_2O. (b) The *amplitude* of the tympanogram is an indication of the static acoustic impedance or compliance at the eardrum. It is either within normal limits, stiff or flaccid, i.e., normal impedance, high impedance or low impedance. (c) The *shape* of the tympanogram is a source of information about the resonant point at the eardrum, the integrity of the eardrum and other abnormalities in the system. The shape reflects modifications of slope and smoothness. It follows that the interpretation of tympanometry by descriptive analysis involves a consideration of (a) pressure peak, (b) amplitude and (c) shape. Within this framework one may now view pathologies as pressure related, amplitude related and/or shape related. The effects of pathology on these tympanogram characteristics are as follows:

A. *Pressure peak*. Pressure related pathologies may be categorized as follows:
  1. Pathologies with negative pressure
    a) Blocked Eustachian tube
    b) Serous otitis media
  2. Pathologies with normal pressure
    a) Ossicular bony fixation
    b) Adhesive fixation
    c) Ossicular discontinuity
    d) Middle ear tumor
    e) Eardrum abnormality
  3. Pathologies with positive pressure
    a) Early acute otitis media
  4. Absence of pressure peak
    a) Middle ear effusion
    b) Open tympanic membrane
    c) Artifact.

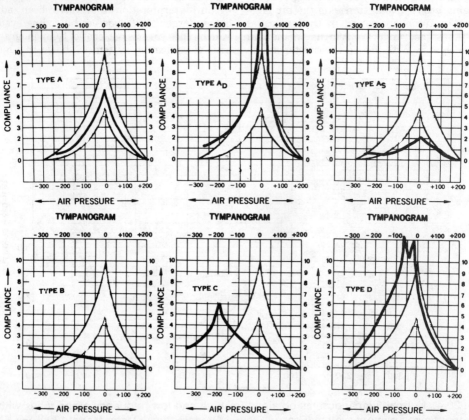

Fig. 30.5. Tympanogram typing system after that advanced by Jerger (1970);.

It is important to note that any of the pathologies in (2) above may be combined with a blocked Eustachian tube. Most commonly adhesive fixation, cholesteatoma type tumor and eardrum abnormality would fit this combined category.

B. *Amplitude*. Pathologies as they influence amplitude may be categorized as follows:
1. Pathologies with increased tympanogram amplitude
   a) Eardrum abnormality
   b) Ossicular discontinuity
2. Pathologies with decreased tympanogram amplitude
   a) Ossicular fixation bony or adhesive
   b) Serous otitis media
   c) Cholesteatoma, polyps, granuloma
   d) Glomus tumors
3. Pathologies not influencing tympanogram amplitude
   a) Blocked Eustachian tube
   b) Early acute otitis media.

As with pressure related pathologies, the possibility of combined effects is always a consideration. In this instance, it is fair to say that in the case of combined pathologies, the amplitude will be most influenced by that pathology that is closest to the eardrum, and eardrum abnormality will obscure accurate measurement of static properties of the middle ear itself (Feldman, 1974, 1976b; Møller, 1965). Any time there is a condition which would result in increased tympanogram amplitude it will overshadow an "in series" stiffening pathology. Similarly, a condition such as a fixed malleus will be revealed as stiff even though an interruption may exist medially.

C. *Shape*. Pathologies altering tympanogram shape may be categorized as follows:
1. Slope
   a) Pathologies which flatten or decrease tympanogram slope
      1) Serous otitis
      2) Ossicular fixation
      3) Tumors of the middle ear
   b) Pathologies which increase slope
      1) Eardrum abnormality
      2) Ossicular discontinuity
2. Smoothness
   a) Pathologies altering tympanogram smoothness
      1) Eardrum abnormality
      2) Ossicular discontinuity
      2) Vascular tumors
      4) Patulous Eustachian tube.

The interpretation of tympanograms based on a descriptive analysis is not solely an over-simplified coding of a pressure compliance function. Instead, it recognizes that some of the more subtle influences of pathology on tympanograms will become apparent when the interpretation process considers the features of pressure, amplitude and shape and relates each of these to potential pathological entities.

Discussed below are the interpretations of the tympanograms shown in Figure 30.6 which are compared according to classification by typing (Jerger, 1970 and Liden et al., 1974) and by descriptive analysis. It is apparent that some tympanograms (especially with high frequency probe tones) cannot fit a simple classification system:
1. Normal ear.
2. Flaccid ear with a peaking tympanogram suggests possible pathology that is undefineable without additional information from a high frequency probe tone and the acoustic reflex. It could be eardrum abnormality or ossicular discontinuity if this is a low frequency probe tone.
3. An otosclerotic ear. This would appear similar with all probe tones and analysis systems.
4. These converging tympanograms are found with high (4A in Fig. 30.6) and low (4B in Fig. 30.6) frequency tympanograms and are quite typical of fluid (or mass) filled middle ears.
5. Typical low compliant middle ear system commonly observed in serous otitis media.
6. The positive pressure peak with any frequency probe tone and normal compliance would be consistent with an overinflated middle ear (post Valsalva) or acute otitis media.
7. This mild notching and peaking is typical of a scarred eardrum usually more discernible to tympanometry than to otoscopic inspection.
8. High frequency probe tone. Tympanograms with broad, deep and often multiple (not shown) notching are characteristic of ossicular discontinuity.
9. and 10. Flaccid systems revealed by the large value for a low frequency probe tone (9) and deep broad notching are consistent with ossicular discontinuity. The negative pressure in these ears also suggests retraction and poor Eustachian tube function. The ear has a natural myringostapediopexy (in the case of ossicular degeneration the eardrum is displaced and rests on the head of the stapes).
11. The systematic pulsing aberration of the smoothness of the tympanogram and low amplitude disclose a glomus tumor.

SPECIAL CONSIDERATIONS WITH TYMPANOMETRY

The effectiveness of this procedure in the identification of middle ear disease has led to a growing interest in its application to screening

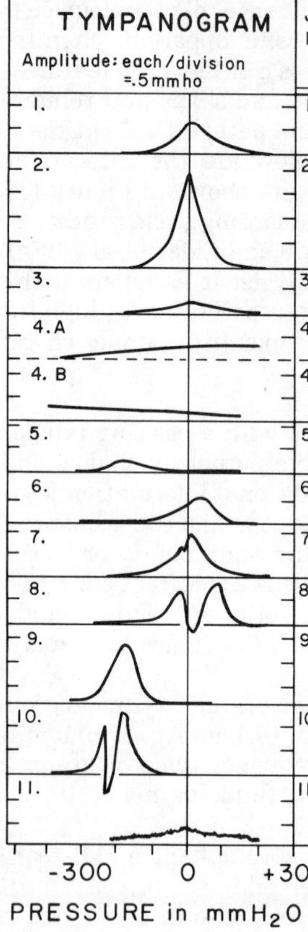

TYMPANOGRAM	CLASSIFICATION			
	JERGER (1970) LIDEN et al (1974)	FELDMAN (1975)		
Amplitude: each / division =.5 mmho	TYPE	PRESSURE	AMPLITUDE	SHAPE
1.	1. A	NORMAL	NORMAL	NORMAL
2.	2. A$_D$	NORMAL	FLACCID	PEAKED
3.	3. A$_S$	NORMAL	STIFF	NORMAL
4.A	4.A ? B	ABSENT-NEG.	STIFF	FLAT
4. B	4.B ? B	ABSENT-NEG.	STIFF	FLAT A+B CONVERGE
5.	5. C	−125 mm	STIFF	NORMAL
6.	6. ?	+ 90 mm	NORMAL	NORMAL
7.	7. D	NORMAL	FLACCID	NOTCHED
8.	8. E	NORMAL	FLACCID	DEEP, BROAD NOTCHING
9.	9. C	−200mm	FLACCID	NORMAL
10.	10. ? C/E	−200 mm	FLACCID	DEEP, BROAD NOTCHING
11.	11. A$_S$	NORMAL	STIFF	VASCULAR PERTURBATION

−300   0   +300

PRESSURE in mmH$_2$O

Fig. 30.6. Series of different tympanograms classified according to typing and descriptive analysis. (See text for discussion.) (From A. S. Feldman: *Annals of Otology, Rhinology and Laryngology (Supp. 25)*, **85**, No. 2, 1976c.

programs, both in the pre-school and school-age population (Brooks, 1968, 1969, 1971, 1973, 1974; Keith, 1973; McCandless and Thomas, 1974; Walton, 1975; Cooper et al., 1975; Lewis et al., 1975). The use of audiometry as a screening technique is a limited measure of middle ear disorders in these populations.

If the goal of a screening program is to identify hearing loss, then audiometry is the method of choice. If, however, the identification of ear disease is the goal, then impedance measurement is the preferred route. The basic techniques in testing are no different than they are in the clinical situation. What is necessary is instrumentation which permits rapid and valid assessment of the middle ear. It should be easy to operate and criteria for referral should be set so that over-referral is at a minimum and under-referral is close to nonexistent. Such instrumentation is beginning to be commercially available (Fig. 30.7).

Criteria for referral continue to be a problem (Lewis et al., 1975; Walton, 1975). In large part

this is because many middle ear problems in children are self-resolving or transient. They may be detected in screening tympanometry and resolved by the time examination by the physician takes place. Furthermore, the sensitivity of tympanometric measurement is such that it may not be corroborated by visual inspection of the ears. These findings would be classified as subclinical. It will take some time before definitive criteria can be agreed upon. At this point the consensus appears to be to monitor children who are possibly "at risk" as a means of minimizing too high an over-referral rate (Lewis et al., 1975). Figure 30.8 provides such criteria. It establishes a greater than −150 mm H$_2$0 as the pressure referral point and less than 0.25 mmho (or cc if calibrated for altitude) as the amplitude referral criterion. It also incorporates the concept of verifying results that are outside the normal range with the acoustic reflex. The additional finding of the absence of an acoustic reflex strengthens the need for referral.

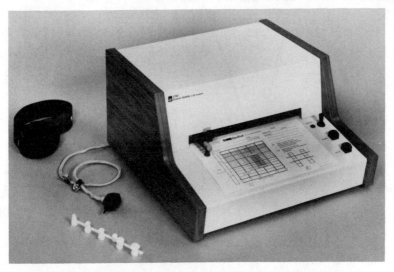

Fig. 30.7. Instrument for automatic tympanometry and acoustic reflex for use in identification programs. (Courtesy Enviromedics Division, GenRad, Bolton, Mass.)

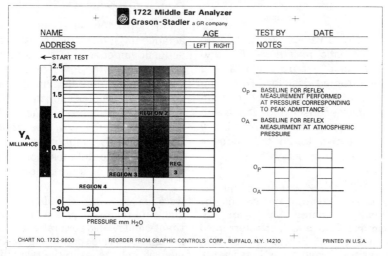

Fig. 30.8. Referral criteria for automatic tympanometry and acoustic reflex for use in identification programs. *Region 1*, pass; *Region 2*, pass if acoustic reflex present; *Region 3*, monitor; *region 4*, refer.

PROBE TONE FREQUENCY

All electroacoustic admittance (impedance) instruments use a low frequency probe tone (220 Hz to 275 Hz). Some use a higher frequency as well. The low frequency probe tone is particularly versatile because the transmission in the ear changes with frequency. The influence of stiffness predominates for low frequencies but diminishes with increasing frequency. The influence of the mass of the system increases in conjunction with increasing frequency. When the two have an equal effect the system is said to be in resonance. By confining measurements to low frequency probe tones one

can generally ignore both mass and resistance in the ear and measurements of either complex acoustic admittance or its stiffness influenced component of susceptance are essentially identical. This is the reason the measurements made with the Madsen type of instrument, which measures the absolute admittance vector magnitude, and the Grason Stadler Otoadmittance meter (Model 1720B, 1721), which measures the admittance components, correlate very highly when using the 220-Hz probe tone.

Figure 30.9 shows that the complex acoustic impedance of both a normal ear and one with an ossicular interruption are made up of primarily the stiffness component (negative acous-

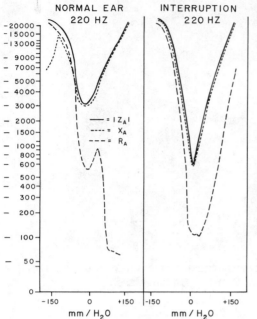

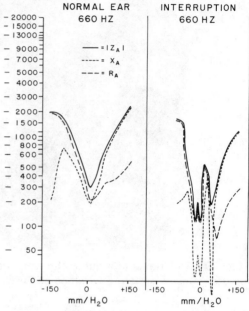

Fig. 30.9. Absolute values of acoustic reactance (X_A), acoustic resistance (R_A) and acoustic impedance (Z_A) in a normal ear and an ear with interrupted ossicles. This demonstrates the contribution of each component to the complex acoustic impedance with a low frequency probe tone. The primary contribution is shown to be the acoustic reactance in both middle ear systems.

Fig. 30.10. Absolute values of acoustic reactance (X_A), acoustic resistance (R_A) and acoustic impedance (Z_A) in a normal ear and an ear with interrupted ossicles. This demonstrates the contribution of each component to the complex acoustic impedance with a high frequency probe tone. At the point of maximum energy flow the contribution of both X_A and R_A is about equal in the normal ear while R_A contributes most to energy flow in the ear with an interruption.

tic reactance). With the 660-Hz probe tone the relationship between the components and the complex acoustic impedance changes in both the normal ear and the one with an interrupted ossicular chain. Figure 30.10 demonstrates that the acoustic resistance and acoustic reactance are equally important in the contribution to the complex acoustic impedance in the normal ear, while the interrupted ear impedance is primarily a consequence of the resistance, and the reactance is actually slightly mass controlled. This shifting relationship between the stiffness and mass control occurs when stiffening air pressure is introduced into the ear canal and varied across the plane of the eardrum. The changing characteristics result in the measured reactance becoming lower than the resistance. This in turn shifts the phase angle of the absolute impedance vector magnitude and is displayed as a notch on a tympanogram (Vanhuyse, Creten and Van Camp, 1975).

Many people have minimized the value of high frequency tympanometry because of an inability to categorize the "W" or notching patterns in some meaningful manner. These

were first described by Liden et al. (1970, 1974) and were related to ears with ossicular discontinuity and healed perforations of the tympanic membrane. This patterning with high frequency probe tones in the two different conditions makes a distinction difficult. At the same time it should also be pointed out that this patterning of high frequency probe tone tympanometry is not the only effect of healed perforations (Feldman, 1974, 1975). The absence of notching does not mean that an abnormal eardrum is not influencing the tympanogram. It is as much a complicating factor with low frequency probe tone tympanograms as it is with high frequencies. As seen in Figure 30.11 the range of acoustic susceptance (or compliance) with a 220-Hz probe tone is completely different in normal ears when compared to ears with healed perforation (Feldman, 1974). This is the reason for much of the frustration experienced by the clinician, such as for example when other audiologic tests are at odds with static compliance values in a patient with presumed otosclerosis. The usual com-

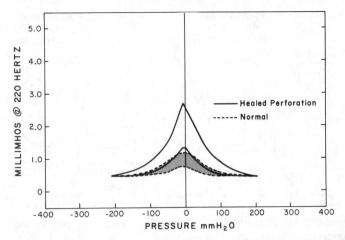

Fig. 30.11. Range of acoustic susceptance (compliance) with a 220 Hz probe tone for normal eardrums (*shaded*) and abnormal eardrums (*open area*).

ment is that there is too much overlap with normal ears and that less reliance must be placed on static compliance values. When one is working in the semi-vacuum generated by restricting the measurement to only low frequency probe tones such reasoning is completely justifiable. A unique feature of high frequency probe tones is the patterning effect of healed perforations. One needs to bear in mind that when the impedance of the eardrum is lower than the impedance of the rest of the middle ear it prevents the measurement of the middle ear itself (Møller, 1965; Feldman, 1976b; Williams, 1976). Consequently, the high frequency probe tone serves an important function of validating the measurement of static impedance made with any probe tone frequency. The clinical importance of eardrum abnormality is minimal. The value of its identification exists only to establish the validity of static measurements. The presence of eardrum abnormality is best established with high frequency probe tones and explains the 10 to 20% overlap between pathologic and normal populations. Furthermore, most notching due to eardrum abnormality is sharp and peaking while tympanogram notching due to ossicular discontinuity is usually multiple, broad, deep and undulating. Differentiation between eardrum and middle ear generated notching is possible in most instances (Fig. 30.6).

INTRA-AURAL MUSCLE REFLEX BATTERY

The measurement of the acoustic reflex has been actively pursued in clinical settings for a longer period than any other aspect of the middle ear measurement battery (Metz, 1946; Klockhoff, 1961; Jepsen, 1963). This was the most applicable feature of Metz's pioneering efforts to measure the impedance of the ear in a clinical population. Based on the fact that loud signals presented to one ear elicit a bilateral contraction of the stapedius muscle, it became common practice to monitor the impedance change which occurs as a consequence of the muscle contraction. This monitoring has traditionally been performed in the contralateral ear (crossed reflex). In recent years, instrumentation has become available which permits both the eliciting signal and the impedance monitoring to take place in the same ear. This is referred to as ipsilateral (uncrossed) reflex testing. The contralateral acoustic reflex can be expected to occur at 70 to 95 dB sensation level (SL) in normal ears (Jepsen, 1951; Deutsch, 1972; Peterson and Liden, 1972) and about 3 to 12 dB lower SL for ipsilateral (Møller, 1962; Fria et al., 1975).

In addition to acoustic reflex measurement, considerable work has been carried on in the area of nonacoustic elicitation of either or both the stapedius and tensor tympani muscles (Klockhoff, 1961; Djupesland, 1964, 1975, 1976). Nonacoustic stimulation of the intra-aural muscles is helpful when hearing loss precludes the presentation of loud acoustic reflex eliciting stimuli. Nonacoustic testing confines the reflex studies to the middle ear and cranial nerves V and VII, whereas acoustic reflex testing also contributes to the accumulation of information about the sensory-neural and central auditory systems as well as the middle ear.

ACOUSTIC REFLEX

In order to obtain an acoustic reflex the monitoring probe and the transducer presenting the eliciting stimulus are coupled to the patient as indicated in Figure 30.12. As illustrated the test ear varies in the contralateral test setup. If the middle ear function is being

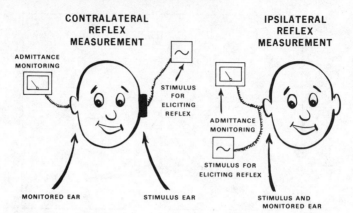

Fig. 30.12. Acoustic reflex eliciting stimulus and impedance monitoring setup for contralateral and ipsilateral testing modes.

evaluated, then the test ear is the one in which the monitoring probe sits (probe ear). If the threshold or other dynamic characteristics of the reflex are being studied, then the ear being stimulated (stimulus ear) is the test ear. Obviously the probe ear and stimulus ear are the same in ipsilateral testing.

In the acoustic reflex test itself the reflex stimulus (tone or noise) is introduced and varied at either ascending or descending levels and the response is monitored, either on the meter of the measuring instrument or through some form of automatically written display (Woodford, Feldman and Wright, 1975). In clinical practice it is rarely necessary to go beyond a visual detection level on the instrument panel meter.

For an acoustic reflex to be present, certain conditions must be met. They are:

1. There must be sufficient residual hearing to induce a reflex.
2. Cranial nerve VII must be functional on the monitored ear.
3. The stapedial tendon must be intact and properly attached to the head of the stapes.
4. The ossicular chain must be continuous through the point of stapedial tendon insertion and sufficiently mobile to allow for stapedial contractions to change the impedance characteristics at the tympanic membrane.

In clinical testing the acoustic reflex battery can be used to help in the detection of:

1. Middle ear pathology.
2. Sensory pathology.
3. Neural pathology.
4. Central pathology.
5. Hearing threshold level.
6. Nonorganic hearing loss.

Detection of Middle Ear Pathology

The broadest application of the acoustic reflex has been as an aid in the detection of middle ear pathology. When contraction of the stapedius muscle cannot be effective in stiffening the ossicular chain and the tympanic membrane, no measurable change in acoustic impedance will be discernible. Not all middle ear pathologies inhibit the acoustic reflex, although most do. For example crural interruption still permits a stapedial contraction to be transmitted to the eardrum through the still continuous link of the stapedial tendon attachment to the neck of the stapes. Some ears with minimal serous otitis media will exhibit a reflex although it will usually be obliterated at the later stages. A conductive loss may elevate the threshold for the acoustic reflex, but care should be taken not to attribute all reflex threshold elevation to a conductive loss.

Detection of Sensory Pathology

One of the earliest applications of acoustic reflex testing was in the study of abnormal loudness growth. The Metz recruitment test (Metz, 1952) demonstrated that the normal 70 to 95 dB SL required for elicitation of the acoustic reflex is markedly reduced in ears with cochlear pathology. This has been repeatedly observed in routine clinical practice. It has the unique advantage over other tests of loudness growth of being both objective and independent of the hearing sensitivity in either ear. Jerger, Jerger and Mauldin (1972) have pointed out that the probability of eliciting a reflex diminishes with increasing sensory hearing loss. However, the probability is as high as 95% with as much as a 65-dB loss and does not drop to a 20% probability until a 95-dB HL is reached.

In clinical practice the presence of an acoustic reflex at reduced SLs has been used to infer a reduction of the dynamic range of comfortable listening (McCandless and Miller, 1972). In this regard it may have application in helping to establish the maximum power output (MPO) of hearing aids, particularly in children when subjective tests of loudness discomfort are tenuous. In our own application of this finding we tend to limit the MPO of a hearing aid to no more than 20 dB above the threshold for the acoustic reflex.

Detection of Neural Pathology

The basic acoustic reflex battery focuses on the presence or absence of an acoustic reflex and the threshold at which it occurs. An extension of this testing can provide helpful diagnostic information about the function of the facial and cochlear nerves. Abnormal adaptation of the acoustic reflex has been observed in patients with nerve VIII tumors (Anderson, Barr and Wedenberg, 1970). An even more common finding than abnormal adaptation in neural pathology is either an elevation of acoustic reflex threshold or its complete obliteration (Jerger et al., 1974; Jerger and Jerger, 1974; Olsen, Noffsinger and Kurdziel, 1975). Any of these three observations, abnormal decay of greater than 50% amplitude to 10 dB reflex SL stimulus within 10 sec (for pure tones 1000 Hz and below), abnormal elevation of the reflex threshold, i.e., greater than 95 dB SL or absence of the reflex in the presence of good auditory threshold should raise the index of suspicion about possible nerve VIII pathology. The acoustic reflex also has application in the testing of nerve VII function. For example, it is common for the acoustic reflex to be absent in early stages of Bell's palsy. It is also one of the earlier signs of return of function. The monitoring of the stapedius reflex is a helpful addition to the tests which otolaryngologists use for this difficult to treat pathology.

Detection of Central Pathology

Some reports have dealt with abnormalities in the acoustic reflex response in the presence of brain stem disorders (Greisen and Rasmussen, 1970; Jerger and Jerger, 1975). These abnormalities are presumed to be a consequence of pathology in the area of crossed brain stem pathways. In the presence of normal hearing one may observe an absence of contralateral reflexes. Ipsilateral reflexes are unimpaired in these instances.

Detection of Hearing Threshold Level

This application has received much attention since it was first advanced by Niemeyer and Sesterhenn (1974). This technique is based on the broadened critical bands for loudness summation of broadband signals that occurs with increasing sensory-neural hearing loss. The test is variously referred to as SPAR, temporal summation audiometry or threshold estimation. The current clinical procedure was described in detail by Jerger et al. (1974) and involves a comparison of the reflex threshold for pure tones (500, 1000 and 2000 Hz) with the reflex threshold for a broad band noise. The reflex is more sensitive to broad band noise. The normal difference in reflex threshold for these signals is 20 to 30 dB. Reduction in this normal difference serves as the basis for prediction of the amount of hearing loss. The criteria developed by Jerger et al. (1974) are shown in Table 30.2.

Detection of Nonorganic Hearing Loss

We have noted that the greater the hearing loss the less the likelihood there is of obtaining an acoustic reflex. The lower the SL of the reflex the more question there is about the validity of the pure tone threshold. For example, it would be an impossible situation for an acoustic reflex to be present at a lower hearing level (HL) than the pure tone threshold. Such a finding would clearly establish the presence of a nonorganic hearing loss. It would not establish the actual hearing threshold level but would suggest that it is no greater than 30 dB more sensitive than the acoustic reflex threshold, and could conceivably be normal.

This battery of acoustic reflex tests provides the examiner with a variety of measures of integrity and mobility of the middle ear system as well as a considerable amount of information about the rest of the auditory system. The

TABLE 30.2. *Criteria for Prediction of Sensitivity Loss (A) and Criteria for Categorizing Audiograms According to Pure Tone Average (PTA) (B)**

(A) Difference (in dB)	Broadband Noise Reflex (in SPL)	Prediction
20 or larger	Any level	Normal
15–19	80 dB or less	Normal
15–19	81 dB or more	Mild-moderate
10–14	Any level	Mild-moderate
Less than 10	89 dB or less	Mild-moderate
Less than 10	90 dB or more	Severe
Reflexes not observed		Profound

(B) Category	Criteria
Normal	PTA less than 20 dB HL
Mild-moderate	PTA 20 to 49 dB HL inclusive
Severe	PTA 50 to 84 dB HL inclusive
Profound	PTA 85 dB HL or more

* From Jerger et al. (1974). SPL = sound pressure level.

entire battery is not routine, but portions may be selected as particular diagnostic questions are raised. Figure 30.13 presents a matrix for comparing the expected results of acoustic reflex testing with contralateral and ipsilateral stimulation in some selected pathologies.

NONACOUSTIC REFLEX

Nonacoustic reflex testing has not received as broad acceptance as has the acoustic reflex.

There are times when the clinician might resort to this method of evaluation of the middle ear, although with the advent of ipsilateral reflex measurement it becomes less pertinent in the routine clinical battery. One problem complicating nonacoustic stimulation is the possibility of artifact as a consequence of head movement in relation to the probe. Both artifact and valid responses appear similar on a meter and are somewhat difficult to distin-

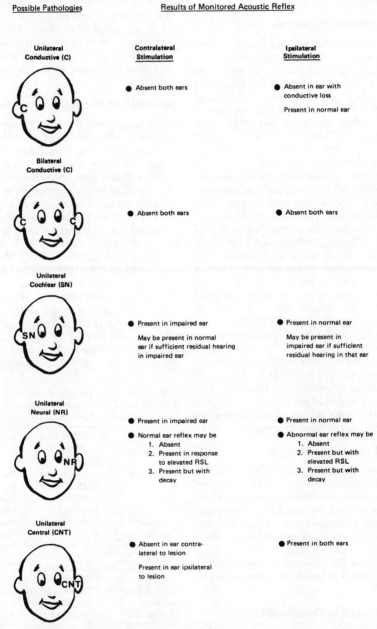

Fig. 30.13. Probable results of a monitored acoustic reflex for contralateral and ipsilateral stimulation in a variety of hearing losses due to different pathologic conditions. The responses are reported relative to the monitored ear.

guish. However, the true nonacoustic response extinguishes rapidly (Djupesland, 1976) and the artifact does not. This could be used to validate the response. Another problem is to ascertain exactly which of the intra-aural muscles is responding.

Electrical stimulation of the ear canal has been reported by Klockhoff (1961) but it has not gained acceptance. Perhaps the most accepted method is a light touch of the facial area around and in front of the auricles. Djupesland (1975, 1976) has discussed the nonacoustic reflex and its contribution to diagnosis. He advocates stroking this facial area with a piece of cotton wool. Fee, Dirks and Morgan (1975) found no more than 60% response to this type of nonacoustic stimulation in the cheek area between the eye and the lower jaw. This is presumed to elicit a stapedius muscle response. Clinically one observes increasing incidence of response the closer the stimulation is to the ear canal. However, this area is also innervated by cranial nerve V which supplies the tensor tympani muscle, and it becomes difficult to distinguish which muscle is controlling the response or whether both are responding.

The use of an air jet to the orbital region and to the contralateral ear has also been reported (Djupesland, 1975, 1976). Both probably elicit the tensor response but are difficult to control for artifact because of head movement associated with a startle response.

In general, the absence of response to nonacoustic stimulation may be viewed as supportive of middle ear pathology. The presence of a response may be ambiguously viewed depending upon the confidence of the examiner that an artifact was not present.

Flottorp and Djupesland (1970) have described a diphasic impedance change (on/off response), which suggests a lowering of impedance, in some instances of middle ear pathology. They observed this with acoustic as well as nonacoustic stimulation and associated this phenomenon with an early stage of otosclerosis. Similar observations have been reported by Terkildsen (1976). An on/off lowering of impedance has also been noted by Feldman and Williams (1976) with acoustic stimulation in many normal ears but this has been accompanied by an intervening period of increased impedance. It has been attributed to a mechanical decoupling of the incudostapedial joint at the onset and end of the stapedius muscle contraction.

EUSTACHIAN TUBE BATTERY

Tympanometry has also been advocated as a technique for the evaluation of Eustachian tube function (Bluestone, Paradise and Beery, 1972; Holmquist, 1969; Holmquist and Miller, 1972;

Bluestone, 1975; Holmquist, 1976). One of the functions of the Eustachian tube is the ventilation of the middle ear space. Information about the middle ear pressure from the tympanogram provides insight about this function. The peak of the tympanogram is an indication of the pressure status in the tympanic cavity. Normal pressure in the middle ear should be ± 25 mm H_2O (Holmquist and Miller, 1972; Feldman, 1975). When the tympanogram peak deviates much beyond that range Eustachian tube malfunction is indicated. It is, however, only an indication of status at one point in time and may not be a true indication of basic tubal function. Deviations in the positive pressure direction will be rare as gases are constantly being absorbed through the middle ear mucosa. This occurs at a rate of about 50 mm H_2O per hour. However, the periodic opening of the normal Eustachian tube with swallowing maintains the pressure within the normal range.

The distinction should be made between patency and function of the Eustachian tube. The former refers to the ability to open the tube under any conditions whereas the latter refers to its ability to open and perform a proper ventilation function. Another function of the tube, of course, is to permit drainage of exudate from the middle ear.

Testing of the Eustachian tube can be performed in the presence of both open and closed tympanic membranes. Testing protocols have not been rigidly developed and this is an area where interpretation of the test results is somewhat controversial. The testing involves observation of (a) deviations in tympanogram peak pressure point, (b) changes in tympanogram peak pressure point associated with swallowing or (c) in the case of an open tympanic membrane, the ability to sustain or evacuate induced pressure in the middle ear without and with swallowing (Bluestone, 1975; Williams, 1975; Holmquist, 1976).

Testing with an Intact Tympanic Membrane

In the presence of an intact, tympanic membrane it is necessary to induce some change in pressure in the middle ear space and, with tympanometry, to record shifts in pressure peak that occur with swallowing. Pressure within the middle ear space can be modified by a Valsalva or Toynbee maneuver or Politzerization. Positive pressure will be generated in the middle ear with all of these if the tube is patent, except for the Toynbee which may induce either negative or positive pressure. Pressure shifts can be recorded by tympanometry which, when compared to the original tympanogram, should show a pressure peak displacement. Following this, the patient is instructed to swallow some water, and after several swallows the tympanogram is rerun. A poorly functioning tube will not result in a peak shift back toward normal pressure.

Because most pathologic conditions involve negative pressure, testing for a shift with positive pressure in the middle ear may not provide appropriate information about tubal function under conditions mimicking stress. Another procedure has been described by Williams (1975) which compares the tubal function for both positive and negatively induced pressure. This test, called the pressure-swallow (PSW) test involves the following six steps:

1. Obtain a tympanometric tracing in the usual manner.
2. Increase the air pressure to a positive value of $+$ 400 mm H_2O and ask the patient to swallow (one swallow will usually suffice, but up to five may be required).
3. Retrace the tympanometric curve. The peak should be displaced 15 to 20 mm negative.
4. Return the air pressure to the peak pressure point of the original tracing (Step 1) and ask the patient to swallow a few times. This will equalize the pressure to the original peak pressure point.
5. Decrease the air pressure to a negative value of -400 mm H_2O and have the patient swallow.
6. Retrace the tympanometric curve. The peak should be displaced 15 to 20 mm positive.

Failure to displace the tympanogram peak suggests poor Eustachian tube function. It is important that all tracings be administered in the same direction of air pressure change to preclude confusion created by possible hysteresis effects.

In all of the above tests an abnormally patent Eustachian tube will not permit a pressure build up in the middle ear to be sustained. Consequently no pressure peak shifts will be measurable. In these patients the best clue is the instrument meter (admittance or balance meter), which will fluctuate synchronously with respiration.

Open Perforation of the Tympanic Membrane

For this test (Bluestone et al., 1972) only the pressure meter is observed.

1. After the probe is sealed in the ear a positive pressure is introduced gradually toward 400 mm H_2O. If the Eustachian tube opens the pressure will drop. The maximum pressure introduced should be noted. If the pressure drops, record this point as opening pressure.
2. Record the point at which the pressure meter stops dropping to indicate the closing pressure.
3. Ask the patient to swallow. Note the point to which pressure meter indication drops after each swallow until no further drop in pressure occurs.
4. Introduce negative pressure to -200 mm H_2O and record point of maximum stable pressure.
5. Ask the patient to swallow and record the point of each residual pressure. If no drop occurs at -200 mm pressure reduce it to -100 and repeat the swallow.

The inability to sustain positive pressure buildup to 300 mm H_2O is associated with abnormal Eustachian tube function and the inability to evacuate positive pressure is highly suspect. Negative pressure equalization is a more difficult task and some patients with normal ears will not be able to equalize to ambient pressure. Figure 30.14 illustrates a data form for use in recording Eustachian tube function test results.

SUMMARY

The battery of middle ear measurement tests involving tympanometry, the intra-aural muscle reflex testing, and Eustachian tube function is an extensive one. The basic procedure in a clinical testing situation usually involves obtaining a tympanogram and testing for the acoustic reflex threshold at several frequencies. This involves about 5 to 10 min of clinical time. Obviously, it is unnecessary, as with diagnostic audiometry, to perform the whole test battery on each patient. However, basic tympanometry and the acoustic reflex rapidly answer the question "Is the middle ear normal?" This can be the starting point for the selection of other appropriate tests in the complete audiologic battery as well as within the middle ear battery itself.

It is important to stress that the value of both tympanometry and intra-aural muscle reflex testing increases when they are done to-

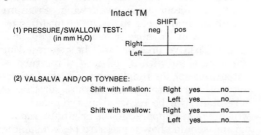

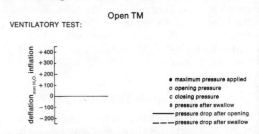

Fig. 30.14. Form for recording different tests of Eustachian tube function.

gether. Discrepancies between them should not be ignored but should be explored until they are explained.

REFERENCES

Anderson, H., Barr, B. and Wedenberg, E., Early diagnosis of VIII nerve tumors by acoustic reflex tests. *Acta Otolaryngol. Suppl. 263,* 232–237, 1970.

Bluestone, C. D., Assessment of Eustachian Tube Function. In Jerger, J. (Ed.), *Handbook of Clinical Impedance Audiometry,* Ch. 6. New York: American Electromedics Corp., 1975.

Bluestone, C. D., Paradise, J. L., and Beery, Q. C., Physiology of the Eustachian tube in the pathogenesis and management of middle ear effusions. *Laryngoscope,* 82, 1654–1670, 1972.

Bluestone, C. D., Beery, Q. C., and Paradise, J. L., Audiometry and tympanometry in relation to middle ear effusions in children. *Laryngoscope,* 83, 594–603, 1974.

Brooks, D. N., An objective method of detecting fluid in the middle ear. *Int. Audiol.,* 7, 280–286, 1968.

Brooks, D. N., The use of the electroacoustic impedance bridge in the assessment of middle ear function. *Int. Audiol.,* 8, 563–569, 1969.

Brooks, D. N., A new approach to identification audiometry. *Audiology,* 10, 334–339, 1971.

Brooks, D. N., Hearing screening, a comparative study of an impedance method and pure tone screening. *Scand. Audiol.,* 2, 67–76, 1973.

Brooks, D. N., The role of the acoustic impedance bridge in pediatric screening. *Scand. Audiol.,* 3, 99–104, 1974.

Cooper, J. C., Jr., Gates, G. A., Owen, J. H., and Dickson, H. D., An abbreviated impedance bridge for school screening. *J. Speech Hear. Disord.,* 40, 260–269, 1975.

Deutsch, L., The threshold of the stapedius reflex for pure tone and noise stimuli. *Acta Otolaryngol.,* 74, 248–251, 1972.

Djupesland, G., Middle ear muscle reflexes elicited by acoustic and nonacoustic stimulation. *Acta Otolaryngol. Suppl. 188,* 287–292, 1964.

Djupesland, G., Advanced Reflex Considerations. In Jerger, J. (Ed.), *Handbook of Clinical Impedance Audiometry,* Ch. 5. New York: (Ed.), American Electromedics Corp., 1975.

Djupesland, G., Non-acoustic Reflex Measurement: Procedures, Interpretations and Variables. In Feldman, A. S., and Wilber, L. A. (Eds.), *Acoustic Impedance and Admittance – The Measurement of Middle Ear Function,* Ch. 10. Baltimore: Williams & Wilkins Co., 1976.

Eliachar, I., and Northern, J., Studies in tympanometry; validation of the present technique for determining intra-tympanic pressures through the intact eardrum. *Laryngoscope,* 84, 247–255, 1974.

Fee, W. E., Dirks, D. D., and Morgan, D. E., Nonacoustic stimulation of the middle ear muscle reflex. *Ann. Otol. Rhinol. Laryngol.,* 84, 80–87, 1975.

Feldman, A. S., Impedance measurements at the eardrum as an aid to diagnosis. *J. Speech Hear. Res.,* 6, 315–327, 1963.

Feldman, A. S., An Historic Review and Current Status of the Acoustic Measurement of Middle Ear Function. In *Mayo Foundation Impedance Symposium,* p. 40–49, June 1972. Rochester, Minn., Mayo Foundation, 1972.

Feldman, A. S., Eardrum abnormality and the measurement of middle ear function. *Arch. Otolaryngol.,* 99, 211–217, 1974.

Feldman, A. S., Acoustic Impedance-Admittance Measurements. Chapter 4 In Bradford, L. J. (Ed.), *Physiological Measures of the Audio-Vestibular System,* New York: Academic Press, 1975.

Feldman, A. S.: Tympanometry. In Feldman, A. S., and Wilber, L. A. (Eds.), *Acoustic Impedance and Admittance – The Measurement of Middle Ear Function,* Ch. 6. Baltimore: Williams & Wilkins Co., 1976a.

Feldman, A. S., Instrumentation and probe tone frequency in tympanometry. *The Reflex, Grason Stadler,* 2, 1, 1976b.

Feldman, A. S., Tympanometry; application and interpretation. *Ann. Otol. Rhinol. Laryngol.* (Supp. 25) 85, No. 2, 1976c.

Feldman, A. S., and Williams, P. S., Tympanometric measurement of the transmission characteristics of the ear with and without the acoustic reflex. *Scand. Audiol.* 5, 43–47, 1976.

Flottorp, G., and Djupesland, G., Diphasic impedance change and its applicability in clinical work. *Acta Otolarynol. Suppl. 263,* 200–204, 1970.

Fria, T., LeBlanc, J., Kristensen, R., and Alberti, P. W., Ipsilateral acoustic reflex stimulation in normal and sensori-neural impaired ears; a preliminary report. *Can. J. Otolaryngol.,* 4, 695–703, 1975.

Greisen, O., and Rasmussen, P. E., Stapedius muscle reflexes and oto-neurological examinations in brain stem tumors. *Acta Otolaryngol.,* 70, 366–370, 1970.

Homlquist, J., Eustachian tube function assessed with tympanometry. *Acta Otolaryngol.,* 68, 501–508, 1969.

Holmquist, J., Eustachian Tube Function. In Feldman, A. S., and Wilber, L. A. (Eds.), *Acoustic Impedance and Admittance – The Measurement of Middle Ear Function,* Ch. 7. Baltimore: Williams & Wilkins Co., 1976.

Holmquist, J., and Miller, J., Eustachian Tube Evaluation Using the Impedance Bridge. *Mayo Foundation Impedance Symposium* pp. 297–307, June 1972. Rochester, Minn.: Mayo Foundation, 1972.

Jepsen, O., The threshold of the reflexes of the intra-tympanic muscles in a normal material examined by means of the impedance method. *Acta Otolaryngol.,* 39, 406–408, 1951.

Jepsen, O., Middle Ear Muscle Reflexes in Man. In Jerger, J. (Ed.), *Modern Developments in Audiology,* Ed. 1, Ch. 6. New York: Academic Press, 1963.

Jerger, J., Clinical experience with impedance audiometry. *Arch. Otolaryngol.,* 92, 311–324, 1970.

Jerger, J., Diagnostic Use of Impedance Measures. In Jerger, J. (Ed.), *Handbook of Clinical Impedance Audiometry,* Ch. 7. New York: American

Electromedics Corp., 1975.

Jerger, J., Jerger, S., and Mauldin, L., Studies in impedance audiometry; I. Normal and sensorineural ears. *Arch. Otolaryngol.*, **96**, 513–523, 1972.

Jerger, J., and Jerger, S., Audiological comparison of cochlear and eighth nerve disorders. *Ann. Otol. Rhinol. Laryngol.*, **83**, 275–286, 1974.

Jerger, S., and Jerger, J., Extra- and intra-axial brain stem auditory disorders. *Audiology*, **14**, 93–117, 1975.

Jerger, J., Burney, P., Mauldin, L., and Crump, B., Predicting hearing loss from the acoustic reflex. *J. Speech Hear. Disord.*, **39**, 11–22, 1974.

Keith, R. W., Impedance audiometry with neonates. *Arch. Otolaryngol.*, **97**, 465–467, 1973.

Klockhoff, I., Middle ear reflexes in man. *Acta Otolaryngol. Suppl. 164*, 1–91, 1961.

Lewis, N., Dugdale, A., Canty, A., and Jerger, J., Open-ended tympanometric screening; a new concept. *Arch Otolaryngol.*, **101**, 722–725, 1975.

Liden, G., Peterson, J., and Bjorkman, G., Tympanometry. *Arch. Otolaryngol.*, **92**, 248–257, 1970.

Liden, G., Harford, E., and Hallen, O., Tympanometry for the diagnosis of ossicular disruption. *Arch Otolaryngol.*, **99**, 23–29, 1974.

Lilly, D. J., Acoustic Impedance at the Tympanic Membrane. In Katz, J. (Ed.), *Handbook of Clinical Audiology*, Ch. 23. Baltimore: Williams & Wilkins Co., 1972.

McCandless, G. A., and Miller, D. L., Loudness discomfort in hearing aids. *Natl. Hear. Aid. J.*, **25**, 7, 1972.

McCandless, G. A., and Thomas, G. K., Impedance audiometry as a screening procedure for middle ear disease. *Trans. Am. Acad. Ophthalmol. Otolaryngol.*, **78**, ORL 98–102, 1974.

Metz, O., The acoustic impedance measured on normal and pathological ears. *Acta Otolaryngol. Suppl. 63*, 1–254, 1946.

Metz, O., Threshold of reflex contractions of muscles of middle ear and recruitment of loudness. *Arch. Otolaryngol.*, **55**, 536–543, 1952.

Møller, A. R., The sensitivity of contraction of the tympanic muscles in man. *Ann. Otol. Rhinol. Laryngol.*, **71**, 86–95, 1962.

Møller, A. R., An experimental study of the acoustic impedance of the middle ear and its transmission properties. *Acta Otolaryngol.*, **60**, 129–149, 1965.

Niemeyer, W., and Sesterhenn, G., Calculating the hearing threshold from the stapedius reflex threshold for different sound stimuli. *Audiol-*

ogy, **13**, 421–427, 1974.

Olsen, W. O., Noffsinger, D., and Kurdziel, S., Acoustic reflex and reflex decay. *Arch. Otolaryngol.*, **101**, 622–625, 1975.

Peterson, J., and Liden, G., Tympanometry in human temporal bones. *Arch. Otolaryngol.*, **92**, 258–266, 1970.

Peterson, J., and Liden, G., Some static characteristics of the stapedial muscle reflex. *Audiology*, **11**, 97–114, 1972.

Terkildsen, K., Conduction of sound in the human middle ear. *Arch. Otolaryngol.*, **73**, 69–79, 1961.

Terkildsen, K., Akustiske impedansmalingu og mellemørets funktion. Thesis Københavns Universitet, Denmark, 1962.

Terkildsen, K., Pathologies and Their Effect on Middle Ear Function. In Feldman, A. S., and Wilber, L. A. (Eds.), *Acoustic Impedance and Admittance – The Measurement of Middle Ear Function*, Ch. 5. Baltimore: Williams & Wilkins Co., 1976.

Terkildsen, K., and Scott Nielsen, S., An electroacoustic impedance measuring bridge for clinical use. *Arch. Otolaryngol.*, **72**, 339–346, 1960.

Terkildsen, K., and Thomsen, K. A., The influence of pressure variations on the impedance of the human eardrum. *J. Laryngol. Otol.*, **73**, 409–418, 1959.

Thomsen, K. A., Investigations on the tubal function and measurement of the middle ear pressure in pressure chamber. *Acta Otolaryngol. Suppl. 140*, 269–278, 1958.

Vanhuyse, V. J., Creten, W. L., and Van Camp, K. J., On the W-notching of tympanograms. *Scand. Audiol.*, **4**, 45–50, 1975.

Walton, W. K., A tympanometry – ASHA model for identification of the hearing impaired child. Capital Region Education Council, Windsor, Conn., May 1975.

Williams, P. S., A tympanometry pressure swallow test for assessment of Eustachian tube function. *Ann. Otol. Rhinol. Laryngol.*, **84**, 339–343, 1975.

Williams, P. S., Effects of rate and direction of air pressure changes on tympanometry. Unpublished doctoral dissertation, University of Washington, 1976.

Woodford, C. M., Feldman, A. S., and Wright, H. N.: Stimulus parameters, the acoustic reflex and clinical implications. *N.Y.S. Speech Hear. Rev.*, **7**, 29–37, 1975.

Zwislocki, J., An acoustic method for clinical examination of the ear. *J. Speech Hear. Res.*, **6**, 303–314, 1963.

chapter 31

ELECTRONYSTAGMOG-
RAPHY

Theodore J. Glattke, Ph.D.

Electronystagmography (ENG) is a clinical tool which involves the acquisition of a permanent, quantifiable record of eye motion. When ENG records are obtained during a clinical evaluation they may be interpreted with consideration of a growing body of information regarding normal and abnormal patterns of eye motion associated with the function of the oculomotor and vestibular systems. The assessment of ENG recordings has become an important element in the complete neuro-oto-audiologic diagnostic procedure, particularly for individuals with unilateral hearing loss, tinnitus, dizziness or vertigo. This chapter will review the principles and practices related to the acquisition of ENG recordings, the more common tests with which they are used and guidelines for determining if a specific set of recordings falls within the normal range.

VESTIBULO-OCULAR INTERACTION

The peripheral vestibular system consists of five sensory receptors that are contained within each membranous labyrinth. These receptors are (1) the macula of the *saccule,* (2) the macula of the *utricle* and (3–5), the *crista-cupula apparatus* in each of the three semicircular canals. Each of these receptors contains sensory cells having cilia that are in intimate contact with an overlying membrane in a fashion similar to that of the cochlear hair cells and tectorial membrane. The spiral cochlea is phylogenetically newer than the vestibular apparatus, and represents a refinement of the vestibular sensory system.

The sensory nerve fibers from each of the five vestibular receptors join together to form the vestibular branch of the auditory nerve and they project into the brain stem to form synaptic connections in the vestibular nucleus. An example of the innervation scheme for a portion of the vestibulo-ocular system is shown in Figure 31.1. The vestibular nucleus consists of four discrete divisions from which neurons emerge to supply information to the visual and somatosensory systems. The medial division of the nucleus receives a portion of its input from the semicircular canals, and sends projections to the oculomotor, trochlear and abducens nuclei. The abducens nerve (cranial nerve VI) emerges from its nucleus and innervates the

lateral rectus muscle, which pulls the eye outward. The trochlear (cranial nerve IV) innervates the superior oblique muscle, which pulls the eye downward. The oculomotor (cranial nerve III) supplies the medial rectus, which rotates the eye inward. The oculomotor nerve also supplies the inferior oblique and inferior rectus muscles.

While the overall organization of the vestibulo-ocular system is very complex, the innervation pattern just described allows each of the semicircular canal receptors to influence eye motion *in the plane of the canal in which the receptor resides.* Of particular importance to the ENG evaluation is the fact that the horizontal canal receptors have a substantial effect upon the motion of the eye in the horizontal plane, or "to and fro" from the individual's right to left side. In the normal case, this influence results from motion of the head. Specifically, the vestibular labyrinth contains endolymph which lags behind the motion of the head itself whenever the head is *accelerated* or *decelerated.* The fluid lag is due to inertia, and it results in a brief relative motion within the membranous labyrinth. The fluid motion, in turn, results in a displacement of the crista-cupula apparatus housed within each canal, in a manner that would occur with any pliable object placed in the path of a flowing liquid.

The diagrams in Figure 31.2 illustrate these effects. *Part A* of the figure is a schematic of the horizontal semicircular canal in the resting position. The crista-cupula apparatus is shown to be contained within an enlargement of the canal which is called the ampulla. The ampulla is located in the rostral portion of the canal (the portion closest to the front of the head). When the head is rotated toward the left side, as shown in *part B,* the endolymph which is present in the canal lags briefly and undergoes a relative motion toward the ampulla. The direction of this motion is called *ampullo-petal.* The crista-cupula apparatus will be displaced in the direction of the momentary flow of the endolymph. When experiencing rotation of this type, the normal individual will produce compensatory eye motion toward the right side, *which is opposite to the direction of rotation.* The eyes will move slowly to the right until a maximum deviation is reached and they will return quickly before repeating the slow compensatory motion to the right. It is the left horizontal canal which has promoted this compensatory eye motion, acting, of course, in concert with the canal on the right side of the head.

Part C of the figure illustrates the effects of head rotation to the right. Rotation to the right

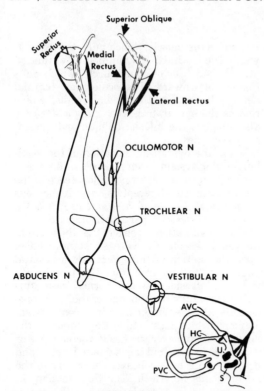

Fig. 31.1. Simplified innervation scheme for a horizontal semicircular canal. *PVC,* posterior vertical canal; *HC,* horizontal canal; *AVC,* anterior vertical canal; *U,* utricle; *S,* saccule. The brain stem nuclei involved in control of the extrinsic eye muscles are shown in schematic form with their possible connections via the vestibular nucleus to the sensory receptors in the horizontal canal. In the case of a right labyrinth, note that principal connections are made to the medial rectus of the right eye and the lateral rectus of the left eye.

results in a relative motion of the endolymph away from the ampulla, or in an *ampullo-fugal* direction. The crista-cupula displacement corresponds to this fluid motion, and the resulting slow compensatory eye motion is toward the left side, with rapid recovery to the right.

The "to and fro" motion of the eyes, with slow travel in one direction and rapid travel in the other, is *true vestibular nystagmus.* When true vestibular nystagmus is present, *its direction is named by the direction of the fast phase* of eye motion. The *magnitude of the nystagmus is measured in terms of rate of eye motion,* in degrees of rotation per second, *during the slow phase of the motion.* The fast-phase direction and the slow-phase velocity (SPV) of nystagmus are two of its features that are used in clinical descriptions.

A. AT REST

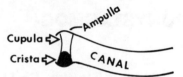

B. FLOW TOWARD AMPULLA (Petal)

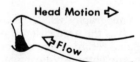

C. FLOW AWAY FROM AMPULLA (Fugal)

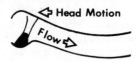

Fig. 31.2. Effects of head acceleration or deceleration on fluid flow in the horizontal semicircular canal. (*A*) The canal at rest, with its sensory apparatus, the cupula and crista located within the ampulla of the canal. This is a schematic of the left canal, and when the head is accelerated to the left, as in *B,* the resulting lag in fluid motion causes a net displacement toward the ampulla with associated displacement of the crista-cupula. Acceleration in the opposite direction, as shown in *C,* will result in flow and displacement in the opposite direction, away from the ampulla.

CALORIC STIMULATION

In the normal case, both the left and right vestibular systems function to influence eye motion. A major portion of the complete ENG examination consists of observing and measuring eye motion under normal conditions of stimulation, for example, under conditions of changes in head or body position. A portion of the examination requires that each vestibular labyrinth be stimulated singly, without known stimulation of the opposite labyrinth. This cannot be accomplished by spinning or otherwise moving the individual, since both labyrinths would receive stimulation when motion was introduced. The usual method of single-labyrinth stimulation involves the use of a *caloric stimulus.*

When caloric stimuli are used, the individual reclines, and the head is brought to an elevation of 30° above a true horizontal plane. The head position appropriate for caloric stimuli is illustrated in *part A* of Figure 31.3. As suggested by the figure, the 30° elevation results in a nearly vertical orientation of the horizontal

A. Head & Canal Position

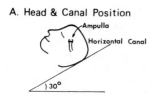

B. Ampullo-petal Flow

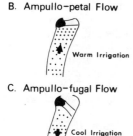

C. Ampullo-fugal Flow

Fig. 31.3. Effects of caloric irrigation on fluid flow in the horizontal canal. When the head is brought to the position indicated by A, warm irrigation will cause the fluid motion suggested in B, and cool irrigation will result in the motion indicated in C.

canals. The ampulla of the canal is placed in a position above the canal itself, when the appropriate position is assumed. The caloric stimulus consists of liquid (water or air) which is different than normal body temperature and which is introduced into the external auditory meatus. The meatus, tympanic membrane and middle ear all undergo a temperature change. Since the horizontal canal passes very close to the middle ear space, the fluid in the horizontal canal also undergoes a change in temperature. When a warm stimulus is used, as shown in part B of Figure 31.3, the fluid nearest the middle ear space becomes warmer and less dense than normal. Because of the change in density, the warmed fluid effectively "rises" toward the ampulla of the horizontal canal. This ampullo-petal motion corresponds to that which would result from head rotation to the left, which was illustrated in part B of Figure 31.2. Left rotation and warm irrigation of the left ear both produce a nystagmus with a slow compensatory motion to the right side, and a fast phase to the left side.

When a cool irrigation is used, the fluid nearest the middle ear becomes more dense than normal, as illustrated in part C of Figure 31.3. The fluid "falls" toward the dorsal part of the canal due to its density and the effects of gravity. The resulting ampullo-fugal flow of endolymph corresponds to head rotation to the right. The nystagmus which is evoked by this form of stimulation will have a slow phase

toward the left side and a fast phase toward the right side.

In summary, caloric stimulation provided to either labyrinth may produce nystagmus effects which correspond to rotation. Warm stimulation of a labyrinth results in nystagmus effects which would follow from rotation toward the irrigated side. Cool stimulation produces effects which would normally result from rotation away from the irrigated side. The slow and fast phases of the nystagmus complement this form of stimulation. Cool irrigation produces nystagmus with a fast phase away from the irrigated side. Warm irrigation results in a fast phase toward the irrigated side. The specific applications of this form of stimulation in clinical testing will be described in a later section of this chapter.

PHYSICAL BASIS FOR ENG

The ENG recording is made possible because the eyeball behaves as an electrical *dipole*. In this sense, the eye might be thought of as a battery which is constantly maintained and renewed by the metabolic processes associated with it. The dipole characteristic of the eye results in a *corneal-retinal potential* (CRP), or voltage, with a relatively positive (+) value at the cornea and a negative (−) value at the retina. Although the CRP is quite small, it may be detected at some distance from the eye.

A typical ENG recording situation is illustrated in Figure 31.4. Disc-shaped electrodes are placed over each outer canthus, as close to the eye as is possible without interference with eye or eyelid motion. A third electrode is placed between the eyes on the lower forehead. The lead from the electrode nearest the right eye is connected to the active or "+" input of a "differ-

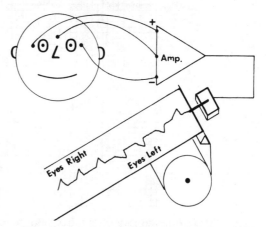

Fig. 31.4. Electronystagmography (ENG) recording apparatus. The corneal-retinal potential is recorded from sites close to the eyes, and after amplification, is displayed on a conventional strip-chart recorder.

ential" amplifier. The lead from the left side is attached to the reference or "−" input of the amplifier, and the third lead is attached to the grounded terminal of the amplifier. The amplifier is called "differential" because it functions to detect the difference in the voltages appearing at the active and reference inputs relative to the grounded point. In amplifying only the differences, the amplifier excludes noise which is common to the active and reference electrodes, such as 60 Hz line-frequency interference.

Eye rotation toward the right side of the skull results in the development of a positive voltage at the active input of the amplifier, and rotation toward the left side of the skull results in a negative voltage at the active input. When the amplifier is attached to a strip chart recorder, eye rotation toward either direction will result in a pen deflection having a magnitude and direction proportional to the magnitude and direction of the eye motion. In Figure 31.4, rotation to the right results in a pen motion toward the upper part of the recording paper, and left rotation results in pen motion in the opposite direction. If recordings of vertical motion of the eyes are desired, the active and reference electrodes are placed above and below the eye, and the same recording principles obtain.

CALIBRATION AND MEASUREMENT OF NYSTAGMUS

In order to obtain an accurate measurement of the magnitude of eye motion, the electrodes are applied and the individual is instructed to look at a spot or a light source which has been placed at some distance to the right or left of the center point of his field of vision. The distance should be sufficient to cause eye rotation in the amount of 10° to the right of center and 10° to the left of center. The recorder is activated and the amount of pen deflection, in millimeters (mm), corresponding to the 10° eye rotation is noted. The tracing in *part A* of Figure 31.5 shows an example of a calibration tracing where the individual was instructed to look at a center line target and then one to the right of center. Examination of the tracing reveals that 10° of eye rotation corresponds to 8 mm of pen deflection. This means that 1 mm of pen deflection is equivalent to 1.25° of eye rotation.

Part B of Figure 31.5 illustrates how the calibration information would be used to measure the SPV of a nystagmus beat. The nystagmus illustrated in *part B* has a slow component reflected in gradual pen motion toward the top of the tracing and a fast phase toward the bottom. According to our convention, the slow phase corresponds to right rotation of the eye, and the fast phase corresponds to left rotation of the eye. The paper speed has been set to 10 mm/sec. If the distance between the start of one nystagmus beat and the next is measured, then the time course of a beat may be computed by dividing the distance by 10 mm/sec. In the example shown in Figure 31.5, the distance covered by the slow phase portion of each beat is 14 mm. Therefore, the duration of the slow

A. Calibration

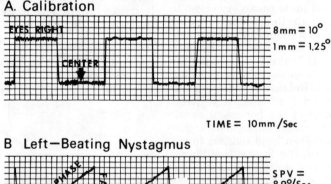

TIME = 10mm/Sec

B Left−Beating Nystagmus

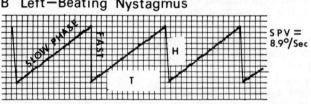

Fig. 31.5. An example of electronystagmography (ENG) calibration and subsequent measurement. The calibration tracing in *A* shows that 8 mm of pen displacement corresponds to 10° of eye rotation. Therefore, the slow phase velocity shown in *B* may be taken as the total slow phase height (*H*) divided by time (*T*). In the example in *B*, *H* = 10 mm (or 12.5° of eye displacement), and the time for one beat is 14 mm (1.4 sec at 10 mm/sec), giving a slow phase velocity of 8.9°/sec.

phase component is 1.4 sec. This is symbolized by the T inset in the graph. The height of the nystagmus beat, symbolized by H in the figure, is 10 mm, corresponding to a total eye rotation of 12.5°. If total eye rotation (H) is divided by the time course (T) of the slow phase component, the resulting number will be the rate or velocity of eye motion. For the example in Figure 31.5, the computation would be:

$$\frac{\text{Magnitude of slow phase}}{\text{Duration of slow phase}}$$

$$= \frac{12.5° \text{ (10 mm)}}{1.4 \text{ sec (14 mm)}} = 8.9°/\text{sec}$$

A complete description of the nystagmus shown in Figure 31.5, *part B*, would state that *it is a left-beating nystagmus with an SPV of 8.9°/ sec.*

Another approach to the calibration and measurement of nystagmus is to require that the individual look at points which are 10° off center and then to *adjust the recorder sensitivity* until the 10° of eye rotation results in exactly 10 mm of pen deflection. Then, 1 mm of pen deflection will correspond to 1° of eye motion, and the examiner need only measure the height of the pen deflection (in mm) to arrive at eye rotation directly. The CRP may be too small in some individuals to permit this, however.

CALIBRATION VARIABILITY

The CRP is highly variable over time. It varies with the dark adaptation of the eye, in particular. Since dark adaptation will be affected by room illumination, calibration procedures should be accomplished with illumination which is approximately equal to that which will be used during the various phases of the ENG examination. Many portions of the examination are accomplished with the individual's eyes closed, and, therefore, subdued illumination is the best condition to use in the examining room.

The CRP will vary over time, even with constant illumination in the test facility. Since the magnitude of the CRP will influence the amount of pen deflection, the true calibration of the recording will vary over time, as well. *It is imperative to recalibrate the recorder sensitivity for eye displacement several times during the course of a complete evaluation.* Failure to do so may invalidate recordings taken as few as 5 min subsequent to a calibration procedure.

THE ENG EXAMINATION

The complete ENG examination includes at least the 11 steps shown in the outline below. The steps numbered 3 through 11 require between 60 and 90 min for completion. Each of the steps, and the specific tests associated with them, will be described in the sections which follow.

ENG Examination Sequence

1. Preevaluation instruction
2. History (dizziness questionnaire)
3. Nondiagnostic otoscopy
4. Electrode application
5. Calibration
6. Gaze nystagmus
7. Optokinetic nystagmus
8. Visual tracking
9. Spontaneous nystagmus
10. Positional nystagmus
11. Caloric testing

Preevaluation Instruction

Several forms of medication, and alcohol, may affect the vestibular system. In order to obtain valid ENG recordings, it is imperative that the patient who is to be evaluated be instructed to abstain from sedatives, tranquilizers, antihistamines and pain medication for 72 hours prior to the evaluation. Additionally, no alcoholic beverages should be consumed by the patient within 24 hours prior to the evaluation. It is advisable that, upon making the appointment for the evaluation, instructions regarding medications be provided to the patient in written form to minimize the possibility of misunderstanding.

Occasionally, a patient who will not or cannot abstain from medications will be encountered. Therefore, even though instructions have been provided to them, the examiner should ask all patients about their medications, and should report the results of that inquiry along with the examination findings.

History

The ENG evaluation, like a hearing evaluation, is only a portion of a complete oto-neurologic examination. The patient's history with respect to vertigo, dizziness, medications and hearing may all be of value to the physician who must ultimately arrive at a medical diagnosis. In most instances, the history may be gathered by using a questionnaire which is sent to the patient prior to his arrival at the clinic. Among the items which might be included on such a questionnaire, the following topics may be most helpful:

Tinnitus — whether unilateral or bilateral, episodic or constant, long standing or of recent onset.
Vertigo — (True spinning sensation), whether long standing or recent, episodic or constant, associated with tinnitus, sudden motion, hearing loss, etc.
Dizziness — whether long standing or recent, episodic or constant, motion induced, etc.

Hearing Loss — extent of loss, duration of loss, medical or surgical history related to the loss, unilateral or bilateral.

General Physical Condition — including cardiovascular, neurologic, and surgical history.

Medications and Drugs — use of sedatives, stimulants, tobacco, alcohol, antihistamines, pain relievers.

Nondiagnostic Otoscopy

Referrals for ENG evaluations will usually originate with a physician who has determined that the patient's ears are normal otoscopically. However, it is prudent to examine the patient's ears at the time of the evaluation to be certain that there are no conditions which would preclude the successful or safe administration of caloric stimulation. If such a condition exists, the noncaloric portions of the examination may be completed, and the basis for refusal to obtain caloric-induced responses may be noted in the report.

Electrode Application

Misapplication of the electrodes is a common problem encountered in ENG evaluations. Proper application requires that the skin at the electrode sites be cleansed thoroughly with alcohol or some other solvent. A small amount of electrode paste or jelly is rubbed onto the recording sites. Additional amounts are applied to the electrodes, and the electrodes are placed on the sites and fixed there with suitable adhesive tape or collars.

The electrode paste application and the cleansing of the skin help to improve the electrical conductivity of the skin. Several problems may result from a failure to apply the electrodes properly. The most serious of these is that unwanted electrical signals which should appear to be identical at the active and reference electrode sites will actually appear to be different. The unwanted signal will be amplified by the differential amplifier and obscure the desired CRP recording. Loose electrodes may produce small voltage changes due to their motion at the electrode recording site. The small voltages may result in an impression of erratic eye motion, even though eye motion may be normal. Finally, failure to clean the recording site or apply the electrode paste properly may result in a significant reduction in the apparent amplitude of the CRP with a subsequent failure to detect ocular motion. Practically, difficulties encountered with electrodes may result from a combination of all three factors, and reapplication of *all* electrodes is the most prudent course of action if erratic recordings are encountered.

Calibration

The steps for calibration have been described previously, and will not be repeated here. It should be noted that the patient must be able to see the calibration target, and glasses or contact lenses should be left in place if the patient requires them for calibration and the other visual tracking tasks. Clinically useful data may be obtained from the calibration procedures, and normal and abnormal findings are described below.

Normal Findings. The calibration procedure should result in tracings which are essentially rectangular, and which resulted from accurate and repeatable deviation of the patient's eyes to the right or left. Figure 31.6 shows an example of a normal calibration tracing as well as an abnormal result.

Abnormal Findings. Some individuals cannot move their eyes accurately or precisely in the manner required by the calibration procedure. When instructed to look toward an illuminated point or spot and then change to a new spot or point without moving their heads, the patients' eyes may move beyond the target and then retreat back toward it. This phenomenon is known as *ocular dysmetria*. It is manifested in ENG recordings as overshoots in the tracings corresponding to the calibration procedure. An example of overshoot is shown in the lower tracing in Figure 31.6.

Some individuals may blink their eyes during the calibration procedure, with each eye blink corresponding to a change in eye position. If the presence of overshoot is suspected, the examiner should ensure that eye blinks are not occurring coincident with the required eye motion.

Gaze Nystagmus

During the test for gaze nystagmus, a target is held about 15 to 20 inches from the patient's

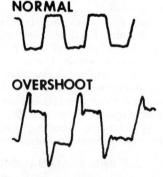

Fig. 31.6. Example of a normal and overshoot calibration finding.

eyes and the patient is instructed to fix his gaze on the target without changing head position. The target is placed and held so that approximately 20-sec recordings are obtained for (1) eyes center, (2) eyes right-of-center 30° and (3) eyes left-of-center 30°. It should be noted that 30° deviation from center is not the maximum possible deviation, and the examiner should use a protractor or other device to move the target accurately.

Normal Findings. Deviation of the eyes to 30° left or right of center should not induce nystagmus in normal individuals (though deviations to the end-point of ocular rotation may do so).

Abnormal Findings. Gaze nystagmus appears similar to true vestibular nystagmus, with distinct slow and fast phases. The fast phase will be in the direction of the deviation of the eyes from center. In order to be considered true gaze nystagmus, it must occur *only* upon the deviation of the eyes from center.

Optokinetic Nystagmus

Optokinetic (OPK) nystagmus occurs in normal individuals when a significant portion of their visual field moves by them, but they remain stationary. A common example of this effect occurs with individuals seated in an automobile at a railroad crossing while a fast-moving train is passing by. The eyes will follow a specific target across the visual field, and then return rapidly to fix on the next available target.

The eye motion resembles true vestibular nystagmus, with a "slow" phase corresponding to the tracking of the target and a "fast" phase associated with the return of the eyes to pick up the new target. During an ENG evaluation, the target may be established by holding a small rotating drum, upon which stripes have been placed, about 2 feet from the patient's eyes. Alternatively, a large striped drum may be lowered over the patient's head, so that the entire visual field is dominated by the moving targets. A third technique involves projecting moving targets along the walls of the examination room with a filmstrip projector.

Normal Findings. Normal individuals will experience an OPK nystagmus which is equivalent for both directions of target motion. Equivalence, in this case, refers to the speed of the induced nystagmus and the pattern of eye motion resulting from the stimulus. Examples of a normal tracing are shown in the upper portion of Figure 31.7.

Abnormal Findings. An example of abnormal OPK findings is also shown in Figure 31.7. The departure from normal may take the form of unequal amplitudes or poor formation of the induced nystagmus. The abnormal patterns may be characterized by erratic breakup of the following-activity of the eyes, or even become rectangular, as if a calibration stimulus had been used.

Visual Tracking

OPK nystagmus is a normal compensatory eye motion, but visual tracking requires pursuit of the eyes after a target which oscillates from side to side. The target may be a spot placed on a metronome, a hanging pendulum, or a moving source of illumination.

Normal Findings. Normal individuals are able to pursue an oscillating target which causes eye deviation as much as 20° to either side of center at rates of deviation from 10° to 20° per second. An example of a normal finding is shown in Figure 31.8.

Abnormal Findings. The principal feature of abnormal findings is a disruption of the smooth sinusoidal tracking pattern which characterizes the normal result. This breakup may be characterized by a few random eye movements superimposed upon the sinusoidal pattern, or, at an extreme, reflect an inability to track the target successfully over any portion of its range of motion. The poor tracking example in Figure 31.8 reveals an inability to follow the change of direction of the target successfully, with a consequent disruption of the sinusoidal pattern.

RIGHT   OPK   LEFT   OPK

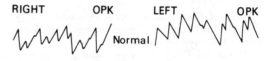
Normal

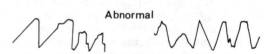
Abnormal

Fig. 31.7. Example of a normal and abnormal optokinetic (OPK) tracing. The *top tracings* show normal results, and the lower tracings show abnormal results for an OPK stimulus. The column labeled *right* shows the results for the stimulus moving to the patient's right, and the *left* column shows the results for the stimulus moving to the patient's left. Note the clear differentiation of slow and fast phases in the normal tracings, reflecting the patient's OPK-induced nystagmus.

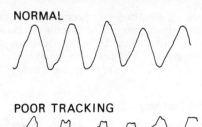

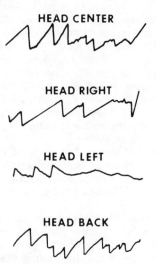

Fig. 31.8. Examples of normal and abnormal visual tracking for a target in pendular motion. The *upper tracing* shows a sinusoidal pattern which mimics the pendular motion of the target, whereas the abnormal tracing reflects poor pursuit of the eyes.

Spontaneous Nystagmus

True spontaneous nystagmus is present without any known stimulus. When testing for spontaneous nystagmus, the patient should be placed in a neutral position and not be provided with any visual target. This may be accomplished by placing the patient in a comfortable seated or supine position, by lowering the illumination of the test room, and by requesting that the patient's eyes be closed.

Additionally, it is important that the *patient be alert and not attending to eye motion*. Therefore, it is common to assign the patient a mental arithmetic task while testing for spontaneous nystagmus. ENG recordings are obtained for approximately 30 sec.

Normal Findings. Normal individuals may demonstrate irregular eye motion and occasional true nystagmus beats.

Abnormal Findings. Examples of abnormal findings are shown in Figure 31.9. In general, spontaneous nystagmus which is of vestibular origin will be characterized by the presence of distinct fast and slow phases, and will have a SPV of more than about 5° per sec. In the examples shown in Figure 31.9, tracings show the presence of nystagmus in the neutral position (head center, patient supine), and that nystagmus is considered to be spontaneous. (The other tracings will be discussed in the next section of this chapter.)

Spontaneous nystagmus of vestibular origin may be abolished by visual fixation. Therefore, if its presence is suspected, the examiner should provide a stationary target upon which the patient can fixate visually. In the normal course of testing, this condition would have already been met by the "eyes center" portion of the test for gaze nystagmus.

There are several forms of nonvestibular nystagmus which may be present in the neutral position and are, hence, spontaneous. These

Fig. 31.9. Example of spontaneous nystagmus which changes with head position. The *top tracing* shows a left-beating spontaneous nystagmus. The spontaneous nystagmus changes to a right-beating type with the body in the supine position, but head turn to the left side.

forms may occur congenitally with normal vision, with blindness, or after long periods of exposure to poorly illuminated surroundings. Nonvestibular nystagmus may or may not include specific slow and fast phases and will fail to be suppressed upon visual fixation.

Positional Nystagmus

Following the test for spontaneous nystagmus in a neutral position, recordings of approximately 30-sec duration are obtained with the patient in each of the positions listed below. No visual targets are provided, and peak alertness is required. The positions are:

1. Supine (if not already used for spontaneous nystagmus).
2. Supine with head turned to the right.
3. Supine with head turned to the left.
4. Supine, with head and neck extended over the edge of the examining table.
5. Body and head turned to the right side with neck supported.
6. Body and head turned to the left side, with neck supported.

Normal Findings. As with spontaneous nystagmus, normal individuals may show occasional true nystagmus beats, often immediately after assuming a new head or body position. These beats will not be sustained.

Abnormal Findings. Nystagmus which is not present in the "neutral" position, but which appears upon the assumption of one or more of the other positions is *position-induced*. Position-induced nystagmus will have specific fast and slow phases and will be sustained for a major portion of the time period over which the recording is obtained. It may occur with delayed onset, and the recording time should not be shortened to less than 30 sec.

If spontaneous nystagmus is present, it may change its direction or other characteristics during head and body position changes. Examples in Figure 31.9 show changes in both direction and speed of the nystagmus as different head positions are assumed. Taken together, all of the tracings in Figure 31.9 reflect a *spontaneous nystagmus which changes magnitude and direction with changes in head position*.

A true position-induced nystagmus would not appear until the nonneutral positions were assumed, and like the examples shown in Figure 31.9, it could change direction or magnitude with changes in body or head position.

Caloric Tests

The caloric tests are performed with the patient in the supine position and with the patient's head elevated 30° in order to bring the horizontal canals into the proper position for irrigation. Air caloric stimulation is now increasing in popularity, but the most effective forms of this stimulus remain to be described completely. Stimulation with water irrigation has been the most popular method for more than 3 decades, and that technique will be described here.

Each irrigation requires sufficient time to permit the flow of approximately 250 ml of water, or approximately 40 sec. The recordings are obtained with the patient's eyes closed, except as noted below. Recordings of the responses evoked by the stimulus should be made

for at least 3 min following the onset of irrigation. *The patient should be brought to peak alertness* during the recording. At the end of each recording period, a 5-min rest period should be allowed in order to permit complete recovery from prior stimulation. The ENG recorder should be *recalibrated* just prior to or subsequent to a recording period.

The irrigation sequence usually followed is:

1. Right cool (RC) (water at 30°C).
2. Left cool (LC) (water at 30°C).
3. Left warm (LW) (water at 44°C).
4. Right warm (RW) (water at 44°C).

Between 60 and 90 sec following the onset of irrigation, during the time of maximal response, the patient should be instructed to open his eyes briefly and should be provided with a visual target. After approximately 10 sec, the eyes-closed conditions should be restored. This step is analogous to testing for *fixation suppression* in the case of spontaneous nystagmus.

Normal Results. Caloric stimulation results in transient vertigo and nystagmus with direction properties that are predictable on the basis of the temperature and side of stimulation. Cool stimulation produces a nystagmus with a fast phase to the opposite side, and warm stimulation produces nystagmus with a fast phase toward the stimulated labyrinth.

The magnitude of the effects produced by caloric stimulation can be measured by examining the slow-phase velocity, according to the techniques described earlier. The measurements are obtained as an average of 5 or more consecutive nystagmus beats at selected intervals during the response, and may be graphically portrayed as shown in Figure 31.10. Responses protrayed in that figure show maximum SPV in the range between 22 and 28° per sec with a gradual reduction in response velocity until a cessation of nystagmus at approxi-

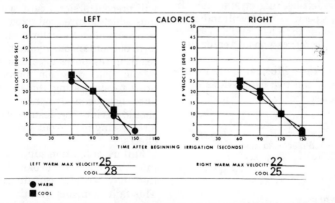

Fig. 31.10. Example of bilaterally symmetrical normal caloric-induced responses. See text for computation of the vestibular asymmetry and direction preponderance values for these responses.

mately 2½ min following the onset of irrigation.

Once the nystagmus has been measured, the recordings are evaluated according to two aspects: (1) the relative sensitivity of each labyrinth and (2) the preponderance of the direction of the evoked nystagmus. Responses obtained from normal individuals vary widely, and the establishment of norms in terms of the absolute magnitude of a response has not been possible. Therefore, impressions regarding the normalcy of a response are based upon comparisons of the effects of the four stimulus conditions on an individual. This is done by determining the maximum SPV for each stimulus, and then comparing the velocity measures by using the expressions shown below:

For vestibular asymmetry:

$$\frac{(RC + RW) - (LC + LW)}{(RC + RW + LC + LW)} \times 100 = \%$$

For direction preponderance:

$$\frac{(RW + LC) - (LW + RC)}{(RC + RW + LC + LW)} \times 100 = \%$$

where:

RC = maximum slow-phase velocity for right cool stimulation

RW = maximum slow-phase velocity for right warm stimulation

LC = maximum slow-phase velocity for left cool stimulation

LW = maximum slow-phase velocity for left warm stimulation.

Inspection of the expressions shown above will reveal that the estimate of vestibular asymmetry is based upon a comparison of the magnitude of the right response versus the left response. The direction preponderance expression compares the stimuli which should cause a right-beating nystagmus with those which should produce a left-bearing nystagmus. In both expressions, a positive (+) result indicates *right* response greater than left, and a negative (−) result indicates a *left* response greater than right.

For the normal case illustrated in Figure 31.10, evaluation of the two expressions gives the following results:

Vestibular asymmetry:

$$\frac{(25°/\text{sec} + 22°/\text{sec}) - (28°/\text{sec} + 25°/\text{sec})}{25°/\text{sec} + 22°/\text{sec} + 28°/\text{sec} + 25°/\text{sec}}$$
$$\times 100 = -6\%$$

Direction preponderance:

$$\frac{(22°/\text{sec} + 28°/\text{sec}) - (25°/\text{sec} + 25°/\text{sec})}{25°/\text{sec} + 22°/\text{sec} + 28°/\text{sec} + 25°/\text{sec}} \times 100 = 0\%$$

Abnormal Results. There are four possible outcomes of the caloric evaluation in the case of abnormal responses. These are (1) bilateral weakness, (2) unilateral weakness, (3) direction preponderance and (4) failure of fixation suppression.

Impressions of bilateral weakness may be based on widely varying criteria. At an obvious extreme, failure to evoke any caloric-induced nystagmus is a certain indicator of bilateral weakness. Normative data in the literature suggest that normal maximal responses should exceed 20°/sec, and that normal standard deviations may be greater than 10°/sec. Therefore, a conservative interpretation of responses as abnormal due to bilateral weakness would require that they not exceed a range of 5° to 10°/sec. Results suggestive of bilateral weakness should alert the examiner to review the entire test procedure and patient history to be certain that the examination was not affected by patient medications and patient alertness during the course of the ENG procedure.

Unilateral weakness is determined by a comparison of the patient's responses due to right irrigation with those due to left irrigation. Differences as much as 10% may be encountered in 66% of the normal population, and a conservative interpretation would require that the observed difference be at least 20%. A clear example of unilateral weakness is shown in Figure 31.11, *part A*, where the computation for vestibular asymmetry gives a result of −72.7%.

Direction preponderance is susceptible to the same interpretation variability as is associated with unilateral weakness. Requiring a 20% difference would seem to be the minimum acceptable rule of thumb, on the basis of normal standard deviations. Figure 31.11, *part B*, shows results suggestive of direction preponderance with a computed value of −56.98%. It should be noted here that some individuals will present a significant spontaneous nystagmus which is direction fixed, and which cannot be overridden by caloric stimulation. If that form of spontaneous nystagmus exists, it would result in responses to caloric stimulation which mimic true direction preponderance. Thus, prior to suggesting that direction preponderance has been demonstrated, the examiner should review the results which preceded caloric testing to rule out spontaneous nystagmus effects.

Failure of fixation suppression of the nystagmus that has been evoked by caloric stimulation may occur in certain classes of patients. This failure means that the individuals cannot suppress the nystagmus beats, even with eyes open. Normal individuals may not be able to suppress nystagmus completely, but should be

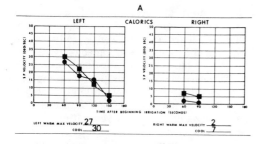

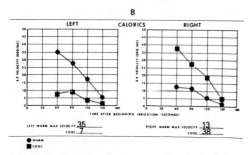

Fig. 31.11. Examples of responses showing unilateral weakness (*A*) or direction preponderance (*B*). The computations for the results shown in the figure are as follows:

A. Vestibular Asymmetry

$$\frac{(7°/\text{sec} + 2°/\text{sec}) - (30°/\text{sec} + 27°/\text{sec})}{(7 + 2 + 30 + 27)}$$
$$\times\ 100 = -72.7\%$$

Direction Preponderance

$$\frac{(2°/\text{sec} + 30°/\text{sec}) - (27°/\text{sec} + 7°/\text{sec})}{(7 + 2 + 30 + 27)}$$
$$\times\ 100 = -3\%$$

B. Vestibular Asymmetry

$$\frac{(38°/\text{sec} + 13°/\text{sec}) - (7°/\text{sec} + 35°/\text{sec})}{(38 + 13 + 7 + 35)}$$
$$\times\ 100 = 9.6\%$$

Direction Preponderance

$$\frac{(13°/\text{sec} + 7°/\text{sec}) - (35°/\text{sec} + 38°/\text{sec})}{(38 + 13 + 7 + 35)}$$
$$\times\ 100 = -56.98\%$$

The results in *A* suggest right unilateral weakness. The results in *B* show left direction preponderance.

able to reduce the nystagmus magnitude by at least 25% when their eyes are open. Therefore, failure to reduce the nystagmus by 25% might be considered as evidence for failure of fixation suppression.

THE ENG REPORT

The report of the results of an ENG evaluation would, ideally, contain as much of the data gathered on the patient as is possible. With a strip-chart recorder paper speed of 10 mm/sec, and a total actual recording time of about 20 min, the record obtained on a patient could exceed 35 feet in length! A practical solution to reducing the size of the permanent record without loss of significant information would be to prepare a report which contains three parts: (1) a narrative description of the patient's responses in all phases of the examination, together with comments regarding any unusual events and a statement regarding the normalcy of the overall results; (2) an abstraction of the ENG recordings during each of the test procedures obtained by actually cutting out samples of the record and pasting them on forms which are labeled for that purpose and (3) a graphical representation of the slow phase velocity measures obtained after caloric stimulation. Taken together, all of this information will enable the referring physician to fully integrate the examination results into the oto-neurologic evaluation. Further, a report following this format serves as a competent and complete record of the patient's visit which will be useful to other interested parties and in studies which involve review of patient records.

DIAGNOSTIC SIGNIFICANCE OF ENG TESTS

The ENG techniques described in this chapter unquestionably provide for a means of documentation of patients' ocular behavior with great sensitivity and precision. However, just as an accurate diagnosis cannot be obtained from the results of a single hearing test without consideration of other factors, neither can an ENG evaluation produce all of the information required for a complete oto-neurologic picture. It would be irresponsible to overinterpret ENG findings, which, like the tip of an iceberg, represent only a small peek at the interaction of the vestibular, ocular, proprioceptive and other neurologic systems. Such interpretation should be undertaken only by an individual whose training and experience regarding these phenomena, as well as specific knowledge about the patient, enable him to do so.

Nonetheless, in order to apply the tests comprising an ENG evaluation in an intelligent manner, and to modify a test situation as conditions may dictate, the audiologist or other individual who is responsible for the administration of the evaluation must be aware of some general considerations regarding diagnosis.

At the outset, it must be remembered that the normal stimulation of the vestibular system is based in the acceleration or deceleration of the head or of the head and body, and the resulting ocular behavior results from a combination of labyrinthine and proprioceptive or exteroceptive cues. Attempting to segment these facets of the overall response into individual components is tenuous. This is particularly so for the forms of vestibular stimulation which comprise the ENG evaluation. The normal situation requires the interaction of both labyrinths, yet testing both labyrinths simultaneously may fail to detect unilateral problems. Such testing is analogous to the evaluation of hearing in a sound field situation, which, while more "normal" than conditions involving earphones, may also be less specific in terms of result interpretation.

In spite of these limitations, there is a growing body of evidence to suggest that abnormalities encountered in a clinical ENG examination may point to three general types of interpretation regarding lesions of the vestibular or nervous system. The first of these categories is "central." Central lesions, as viewed in the context of ENG results, refer to those which involve central nervous system control over *ocular motion*. Lesions of the labyrinth or vestibular branch of the auditory nerve are not considered to be "central." Central lesions are manifested in abnormal findings for those tests which involve visual, rather than vestibular, stimulation. These tests include (1) calibration, (2) gaze, (3) optokinetic, and (4) tracking tasks along with (5) fixation suppression of evoked or spontaneous nystagmus. Abnormal findings for these five tests may not pinpoint the exact focus of a lesion, but they do point to aberrations of the visual, oculomotor, cerebellar, or other systems which serve to coordinate oculomotor behavior.

An impression of peripheral involvement may be obtained from the caloric findings. *After central signs have been ruled out,* the finding of bilateral weakness or unilateral weakness after caloric stimulation appears to be a clear indicator of end-organ or vestibular nerve involvement. Direction preponderance abnormalities, on the other hand, do not appear to be of localizing value. In the simplest sense, direction preponderance may represent a subtle manifestation of oculomotor coordination difficulties which are not apparent when visual cues or fixed targets are provided to the patient. Alternatively, the finding of direction preponderance may also represent a subtle labyrinthine imbalance which provides some constant error in its input to the combined vestibulo-ocular system.

The presence of spontaneous nystagmus may also be a manifestation of one of several types of peripheral or central problems. After central or ocular signs have been ruled out, it is tempting to interpret direction-fixed spontaneous nystagmus in terms of the absence of input from one labyrinth. However, equally compelling interpretations of spontaneous nystagmus can also be based on the presumption that the central nervous system can produce compensatory control in the case of unilateral labyrinthine dysfunction, and the exact cause of spontaneous nystagmus in a given patient may be elusive.

Taken as a whole, the ENG evaluation has great power in detecting pathology. The interpretation of the findings must be made very cautiously, and only in the context of the patient's history, audiologic, vestibular, neurologic and other signs. Clear findings of unilateral or bilateral weakness in response to caloric stimulation are helpful in localizing lesions in the periphery, and the central tests involving visual targets are useful in ruling out central involvement. Electronystagmography has had a rich and controversial history extending over a period of some 40 years. As more patient records are examined systematically and reported in the literature, this form of evaluation will clearly move from an anecdotal base to one that is more substantial.

REFERENCES

I. Overviews on Test Techniques and Interpretation

Aschan, G., Bergstedt, M., and Stahle, J., Nystagmography; recordings of nystagmus in clinical neuro-otological examinations. *Acta Otolaryngol.,* Suppl. 129, 1956.

Coats, A. C., Electronystagmography. In Bradford, L. (Ed.), *Physiological Measures of the Audio-Vestibular System.* New York: Academic Press, 1975.

Jung, R., and Kornhuber, H., Results of Electronystagmography in Man. In Bender, M. (Ed.), *The Oculomotor System.* New York: Harper & Row, 1964.

Jongkees, L., and Philipszoon, A., Electronystagmography. *Acta Otolaryngol.,* Suppl. 189, 1964.

Naunton, R., *The Vestibular System.* New York: Academic Press, 1975.

Spector, M., *Dizziness and Vertigo.* New York: Grune & Stratton, 1967.

Wolfson, R. J., *The Vestibular System and its Diseases.* Philadelphia: University of Pennsylvania Press, 1966.

II. Anatomy of the Vestibulo-Ocular System

Engstrom, H., Bergstrom, B., and Ades, H., Macula utriculi and macula sacculi in the squirrel monkey. *Acta Otolaryngol.,* Suppl. 301, 1972.

Flock, Å., Sensory Transduction in Hair Cells. In Lowenstein, W. R. (Ed.), *Handbook of Sensory Physiology, Vol. I.* New York: Springer Verlag, 1971.

Gacek, R. R., Anatomical studies of the vestibulo-ocular pathways in the cat. *Adv. Otorhinolaryngol.,* **19,** 66–75, 1973.

Lindeman, H. H., Anatomy of the otolith organs. *Adv. Otorhinolaryngol.,* **20,** 405–433, 1973.

Wersall, J., and Bagger-Sjoback, D., Morphology of the Vestibular Sense Organs. In Kornhuber, H. H., (Ed.), *Handbook of Sensory Physiology, Vol. VI, Part 1.* New York: Springer Verlag, 1974.

III. Calibration, Optokinetic, and Tracking Abnormalities

Benitez, J., Eyetracking and OPK tests. *Laryngoscope,* 80, 834–848, 1970.

Coats, A., Central and peripheral OPK asymmetry. *Ann. Otol. Rhinol. Laryngol.,* 77, 938–948, 1968

Eviator, A., Interpretation of electronystagmographic results. *Laryngoscope,* 82, 1059–1067, 1972.

Haring, R., and Simmons, F. B., Cerebellar defects detectable by electronystagmography calibration. *Arch. Otolaryngol.,* 98, 14–17, 1973.

Hetter, G. P., Corneal-retinal potential behind closed eyelids. *Arch. Otolaryngol.,* 92, 433–436, 1970.

IV. Position Testing

Barber, H. O., Clinical manifestations of otolith dysfunction. *Adv. Otorhinolaryngol.,* 20, 396–404, 1973.

Coats, A. C., The diagnostic significance of spontaneous nystagmus as observed in the electronystagmographic examination. *Acta Otolaryngol.,* 67, 33–43, 1969.

Harrison, M. S., Positional vertigo. *Brain,* 95, 369–372, 1972.

Nylen, C., The posture test. *Acta Otolaryngol.,* Suppl. 109, 1953.

V. Caloric Interpretation

Brookler, K., Directional preponderance in clinical electronystagmography. *Laryngoscope,* 80, 747–754, 1970.

Fitzgerald, G., and Hallpike, C., Studies in human vestibular function. *Brain,* 65, 115–180, 1942.

Coats, A., Directional preponderance and unilateral weakness. *Ann. Otol. Rhinol. Laryngol.,* 74, 655–662, 1965.

Coats, A., Directional preponderance and spontaneous nystagmus. *Ann. Otol. Rhinol. Laryngol.,* 75, 1135–1144, 1966.

Coats, A., Central electronystagmographic abnormalities. *Arch. Otolaryngol.,* 92, 43–53, 1970.

Eviatar, A., and Wassertheil, S., The clinical significance of directional preponderance concluded by electronystagmography. *J. Laryngol. Otol.,* 85, 355–368, 1971.

Henricksson, N., Speed of slow component and duration in caloric nystagmus. *Acta Otolaryngol.* Suppl. 125, 1956.

Jongkees, L. Electronystagmography, use and usefulness. *Ann. Otol. Rhinol. Laryngol.,* 77, 732–739, 1968.

Koch, H., Henriksson, N., Lundgren, A. and Andren, G., Directional preponderance and spontaneous nystagmus in eye-speed recording. *Acta Otolaryngol.,* 50, 517–525, 1959.

Rubin, W., and Smith, T., Electronystagmography in patients with vestibular disorders. *Arch. Otolaryngol.,* 86, 38–43, 1967.

Simmons, F. B., Patients with bilateral loss of caloric response. *Ann. Otol. Rhinol. Laryngol.,* 82, 175–178, 1973.

Evaluation of Young Children and the Elderly

chapter **32**

A CASE HISTORY FOR CHILDREN

Carol H. Ehrlich, Ph.D.

A child is very special. He has special charm, special needs, special skills and special problems. We who serve him must find special ways to do so, and we must do it in the time he will allow.

A case history has been described by Rosenberg (see Chapter 7) as "the first test." The beauty of this first test for pediatric audiology is that it does not deplete the child's time, yet it offers a potential wealth of information. Such an achievement is known in common parlance as money in the bank.

The value of a case history for children grows out of a conceptual framework of the role of the audiologist. If that role is seen as being a hearing measurer and site of lesion tester, there is obviously no need for a case history. One can do those things with no information as long as there is a responding body under the earphones. Fortunately audiology has matured beyond that position. Our present role which is described in policy papers of the American Speech and Hearing Association and the Academy of Rehabilitation Audiology charges the audiologist to address the needs of the *human being* who presents possible, real or potential hearing loss. We must view the child and not just his ears. Knowledge of his background and behaviors and of his parents' attitudes and concerns is absolutely essential if we are to evaluate problems and assist him and his family in a way that will make a difference in their lives.

Pediatric referrals to the audiologist are made for a number of reasons. Middle ear pathology and known impairment of hearing may cause the child's physician to refer for purposes of gaining diagnostic information and determining rehabilitation needs. Most other referrals are made to identify the cause of speech and language delay, for of the several possible causes, hearing loss is the simplest and most straightforward. Some referrals are made seeking information about the peripheral and central auditory (and in some clinics, vestibular) systems because of other medical or behavioral problems. The audiologist can supply information about the hearing loss, recommend steps (medical, rehabilitative and supportive) to be taken to meet the needs of the hearing impaired child, and direct families appropriately for other help if hearing is found to be normal.

A good case history serves at least three important purposes for the audiologist, and in the case of children whose response repertoire and test capacity may be limited, it is particularly helpful. First, it involves the parents actively in the evaluation. By this means parents can be made to feel they are an essential part of the team. They will contribute their insights to the total picture, and their coping with the findings and cooperation with the recommendations may thereby be facilitated. Second, it will specify the presenting concerns and give direction to the testing. Case history information should suggest appropriate test techniques and levels. It may point to middle ear problems, congenital deafness, language disorders, functional hearing loss, disease of some other bodily system, and parental needs for counseling—to mention just a few. Third, it provides information which can support or challenge the test results. This inherent value alone is sufficient to warrant the time it takes to obtain the case history.

The techniques and timing of history taking are decisions which vary legitimately according to the needs of the clinic and the experience and opinion of the audiologist. There is no single right or best way. Northern and Downs (1974) advise against the audiologist taking a history because the information may introduce a tester bias, and they do not wish to duplicate the work of the physician, social worker or geneticist. Others, including Katz and Struck-mann (1972) and Hannah and Sheeley (1975), favor history taking as the first step of the evaluation in order to plan testing appropriately. While unnecessary duplication is to be avoided, our experience leads us to believe that a basic history is necessary to all professionals involved with the child. Then each discipline must plumb its own concerns in greater depth. Less than this amount of attention to the child and his background leads to audiologic care which is superficial and mechanical, and is very apt to sacrifice desired quality of care.

Time constraints have led us to mail a case history form to parents prior to the evaluation with a request to mail or bring the completed form back to us. Essential information the parent has provided, much of which may be routine, can be reviewed quickly by the audiologist in the sound room as the evaluation begins. Valuable clinic time can be used efficiently, exploring in more depth only those matters which appear to be important. The quiet moments this allows at the beginning of the test session will serve to put the child at ease as he becomes accustomed to the strange surroundings.

Obtaining and using parents' reports effectively require all the skills the audiologist can muster—as a human being and as a scientist. He must strike a balance between sympathetic warmth and clinical objectivity in his interaction with the parent, and he must regard the bits of information as clues or pieces of the puzzle without drawing premature conclusions from them. Bias is clearly a risk. I accept this risk because the potential value of the information makes it eminently worthwhile. (Precautions are in order, however, and frequent self-conscious questioning of assumptions during the testing helps to avoid error.) Eliciting important information without opening the sluice for a stream of extraneous or redundant material, and finally closing off the interview gracefully are the marks of an able, seasoned clinician.

Information germane to the audiologist's care of a child should include presenting concerns, genetic and pregnancy/birth/medical history, developmental history, social and educational history, and in some detail a description of his hearing, speech and language.

PRESENTING CONCERNS

The parents' expression of their concerns should help us if we listen, for our evaluation and recommendations must respond to those concerns. The importance of real communication cannot be overstressed. Some parents are able to state their real concerns directly. Oth-ers, and we all have seen them, say one thing while their real message is quite different and can only be heard in their voice quality, their posture, or in the questions they evade. Considerable skill and sensitivity are needed to complete this portion of the case history. To fail to do so accurately results in isolation of the evaluation from its true objective, so no matter how legitimate the evaluation and valid the results, the process is of little value. Parents must know that their concern is recognized, and at least to some degree answered when they leave.

GENETIC AND PREGNANCY/BIRTH/MEDICAL HISTORY

Genetic and pregnancy/birth/medical history provide the data which trigger red flags—red flags for problems in hearing, vision, intelligence, perception, language and motor function.

A joint committee of the American Academy of Pediatrics, the American Academy of Ophthalmology and Otolaryngology and the American Speech and Hearing Association in October 1973 listed five high risk perinatal conditions associated with hearing impairment: (1) history of genetically determined childhood hearing impairment; (2) rubella or other nonbacterial intrauterine fetal infection (e.g., cytomegalovirus infections, herpes infection); (3) defects of ear, nose, or throat: malformed, low-set or absent pinnae, cleft lip or palate (including submucous cleft), a residual abnormality of the otorhinolaryngeal system; (4) birthweight less than 1500 g; (5) any indirect or free bilirubin concentration that is potentially toxic (toxic level differs in each baby). Feinmesser and Bauberger-Tell (1971) found a 0.5% incidence rate of hearing loss in a broad prospective study of high risk babies. Lubchenco et al. (1972) found 18% of very low birth weight babies were hearing impaired. The incidence rate of hearing loss in the Johnson et al. (1972) study of respiratory distress babies who were treated with positive pressure ventilation was 11.5%. Our study found hearing loss in 2.5% of a sample of 5-year-old children who had been premature, respiratory distressed or hyperbilirubinemic babies in The Newborn Center intensive care unit of The Children's Hospital, Denver (Ehrlich et al., 1973).

The role of respiratory distress during the neonatal period in the child's ultimate problems (hearing, vision, motor, learning, etc.) has been controversial. Lubchenco (1973) regards it simply as a concomitant of the primary offender, prematurity. The support for a causal relationship is found in studies reported by Fisch et al. (1968), Robertson (1969), Windle (1966) and Johnson et al. (1972).

In addition to the loss of hearing experienced

by the infants in our Newborn Center study, a significant number of them presented handicapping disorders of auditory/verbal processing and visual/perceptual/motor function at 5 years of age. Auditory/verbal difficulties (in various combinations of tasks including auditory memory, auditory discrimination in noise, expressive vocabulary, word retrieval, articulation and sound blending) occurred in 34.5% of the 81 children studied. Visual/perceptual/motor disorders (in visual memory, figure/ground discrimination, block design, maze tracking, and geometric design reproduction) occurred in 36% of the children. One third of each of these groups overlapped, presenting problems in both auditory/verbal and visual/perceptual/motor areas.

While only 2.5% of the children studied had hearing loss, 54% of them presented these other problems which can be expected to impede learning. (Post-study data from 24% of the children support this notion, for the schools they now attend have sought information from us to help in dealing with their learning problems). Another 30% of the children in the study had mild or discrete difficulties for which it was felt they could compensate. Only 15% were functioning normally.

An interesting clinical note is that 51% of the children in the significantly impaired group were undetected by physician's examination, while only 7% were missed by examination of the audiologist, speech pathologist and psychologist. The findings point up the need for every consultant down the line to be alert to the possibility of these communication/learning disorders. The audiologist will often be the first person; it is his responsibility to recognize the risk and symptoms. To send the child on his way with the narrow assurance that his hearing is normal is to renege on one's commitment as a health-care professional. He should receive the other services he needs, whether they are available in a speech and hearing clinic or must be delivered elsewhere. Our job is to direct him appropriately. The genetic and pregnancy/birth/medical history should assist the audiologist greatly in detecting the problems so he can respond to the needs they present.

DEVELOPMENTAL HISTORY

Developmental history including gross and fine motor, adaptive and language functions, provides an essential framework for evaluating a child's current performance. The audiologist is alerted by these data to irregularities of development, and can plan test techniques and assess response behavior as they relate to the child's maturational levels.

Audiometric test techniques must obviously be geared to the child's developmental level rather than his chronologic age, with some modifications for physical handicaps. In a practical sense, we have categorized five levels of response behavior which testing should utilize:

Level 1. Basic bodily reactions, including arousal, startle, twitch, temporary cessation or alteration of a regular breathing pattern, heart rate change, or electroencephalograph (EEG) change. We are largely dependent on these reactions in assessing hearing during the first 3 months of life in the normally developing baby.

Level 2. Specific and spontaneous body response behaviors, including eye shifts, eye widening, head turns, quieting/listening postures. The normally developing baby between 4 and 7 to 8 months demonstrates these behaviors in response to attractive and novel sound signals at a distraction, suprathreshold level.

Level 3. Learned simple response behaviors, such as turning to see a blinking light when an associated sound is presented (Conditioned Orientation Reflex), or clapping each time a signal is heard, or laughing, or rocking, or mimicking the sound, or a variety of other behaviors which can be stimulated with the help of the audiologist. Most babies between 8 or 9 and 24 months can be tested for these target behaviors, with measured levels sometimes representing listening (threshold) and sometimes distraction (suprathreshold).

Level 4. Learned elaborate behaviors, such as placing pegs in holes or rings on a stake, etc. (play audiometry, light boards, puppet in the window illuminated (PIWI), etc.). The typical 2- to 5-year old handles this task well, yielding quite accurate and reliable threshold response curves.

Level 5. Learned adult-type volunteered response behavior, with the child verbalizing or signaling his responses by raising his hand, etc. Children 5 years of age and older are generally capable of responding to traditional adult audiometric test procedures.

While it is not in the purview of this chapter to detail normal development, clearly a suggestion from the developmental history that the child is delayed or retarded should cause an adjustment in test planning by the audiologist. Techniques and materials appropriate for a normal 4-year-old will not adequately test a retarded 4-year-old functioning at an 18-month level. Similarly, level three (above) test techniques should not be employed when testing a precocious 20-month-old whose functioning is at a 30-month level. Each level up yields increasingly definitive information, so it is desirable to test up to the child's level of functioning.

SOCIAL AND EDUCATIONAL HISTORY

Support programs (psychological, special educational, social/economic) may be needed. Their need can be determined and they can be arranged and coordinated most easily if the case history includes a careful social, behavioral and educational history.

Reports of poor adjustment to peers or teachers signal the need for attention and possibly intervention by qualified professionals. Counseling for parents and psychotherapy for the child may be indicated. Investigation of learning problems and special school placement or supportive tutorial programs may be warranted. The history should provide clues of any untoward behaviors the child demonstrates in his everyday life which may significantly impede his growth and adjustment. The principles of management by objective require that we first define the problems, and that task can be accomplished with the help of this social and educational information.

HEARING, SPEECH AND LANGUAGE

Of particular importance to the audiologist, both to enrich the diagnostic picture and to provide reliability checks for the formal testing, is the description of the child's hearing, language and speech. This description should include his developmental milestones of communication behavior, parental and any professional judgments of hearing and speech/language skills, and a record of any treatment or amplification use. It should include open-ended as well as specific questions so that parents' observations and impressions are elicited along with specific bits of information. Parents live 24 hours a day with their children; they know them best. We are often humbled by the astuteness of their observations, and we are well advised to listen carefully to what they have to say.

The case history may follow a format such as the one described below:

CASE HISTORY

Our evaluation of your child's difficulties will depend upon information about his past medical and developmental history. Please fill out this form as completely as possible and return it in the enclosed envelope.

NOTE: All information given is kept confidential.   Date_____

Person completing this form _____

Relationship to the child _____

I. IDENTIFICATION

Child's Name_____Birthdate_____Age_____

Address_____Phone_____

Mother's Name_____Mother's Age_____

Mother's Occupation_____

Father's Name _____Father's Age_____

Father's Occupation _____

Brothers and Sisters

	Name	Age	Sex	Grade in School	Speech, Hearing or Medical Problems
1.					
2.					
3.					
4.					
5.					

Referred by _____

Address _____

Name of child's doctor _____

Address _____

II. STATEMENT OF THE PROBLEM

A. Describe the problem _____

_____

_____

B. When was the problem first noticed? _____

By whom? _____

C. What do you think caused the problem? _____

_____

D. List people or clinics you have consulted about the problem.
   Date   Name and address   What you were told about the problem.

_____

_____

_____

_____

III. HISTORY

A. Family history
   1. List any relatives of child closer than second cousins who have or had a hearing loss. Indicate the cause, if it is known.

   Name _____Relationship_____Cause _____

   Name _____Relationship_____Cause _____

   Name _____Relationship_____Cause _____
   2. List any relatives of child closer than second cousins who have or had speech problems. Describe the problem briefly.
   Name _____Relationship_____Problem_____

   Name _____Relationship_____Problem_____

   Name _____Relationship_____Problem_____
   3. List any relatives of child closer than second cousins who have or had learning problems. Describe the problem briefly.
   Name _____Relationship_____Problem_____

Name _____Relationship_____Problem_____

Name _____Relationship_____Problem_____

B. Pregnancy and Birth History
   1. Did mother have any of the following? What month? Was hospitalization necessary?

Excessive vomiting?	Virus infection?
Bleeding?	German measles?
Swelling?	Diabetes?
High blood pressure?	Heart condition?
High fever?	Asthma?
Convulsions?	Thyroid condition?
Excessive weight gain or loss?	Kidney disease?
Toxemia?	X-rays?
Rh negative blood?	Accidents?
Medication (what)?	Surgery?

   2. Were mother's and father's blood types incompatible? _____
   3. What was the length of pregnancy? _____
   4. What was the length of hard labor? _____
   5. Type of delivery: (a) Vertex (head presentation) (b) cesarean (c) breech (d) dry (e) other
   6. Were there any unusual problems at birth? (If so, describe) _____
_____
   7. Were instruments used?_____ Bruises?_____
   8. Apgar score at 1 minute_____ At 5 minutes _____
   9. Were there any health problems during first 2 weeks of infant life?

Jaundiced?	Hemorrhage?
Blueness?	Infection?
Difficulty with breathing?	Feeding difficulty?
Convulsions?	Cry (strong, weak, high)?
Incubator or isolette?	Oxygen?
Transfusion?	Intravenous or intramuscular fluids?
Tube fed?	Medication?

  10. How long did child remain in the hospital nursery? _____

     Which hospital?_____
  11. Is there other information about the mother or baby which can help us evaluate your child?
_____
_____

C. Developmental History
Note the *ages* when the following occurred

1. Hold head erect?	Creep?
Follow objects with eyes?	Feed self with spoon?
Awareness of light?	Sit unsupported?
Roll over from back to stomach?	Stand alone?
Play with hands?	Walk alone?
Reach for objects?	Ride bike or tricycle?

. . . .

2. Dress self?	Tie shoes?
Button?	

   3. Toilet training completed?

	Bowel	Bladder
Day-time?	_____	_____
Night-time?	_____	_____

. . . .

4. Is he well coordinated or clumsy?
   Which hand does child prefer to use?
   Does child lose balance or fall easily?
   Has he had difficulty sucking_____chewing_____swallowing?_____
   Does he drool?

D. Medical History
   1. At what ages did any of the following illness or operations occur? Indicate severity and temperature.

	Age	Severity and Temperature		Age	Severity and Temperature
Whooping cough			Earaches		
Mumps			Running ears		
Scarlet fever			Chronic colds		
Measles			Head injuries		
Chicken pox			Asthma		
Pneumonia			Allergies		
Diphtheria			Epilepsy		
Croup			Encephalitis		
Influenza			Typhoid		
Headaches			Tonsillitis		
Sinus			Tonsillectomy		
Meningitis			Adenoidectomy		
Rickets			Mastoidectomy		
Rheumatic fever			Other		
Polio					

   2. Describe any operations your child has had_____
   _____
      Where was child hospitalized?_____When?_____
      Name and address of attending doctor _____
   3. Describe any serious illnesses child has had_____
   _____
   4. Has child had any convulsions?_____Under what circumstances did they occur?
      _____Was medication used?_____
      If so, which one? _____
   5. Describe any injuries_____
   _____
   6. Has the child's vision been examined?_____Date_____By Whom?_____
      Results_____
   7. Has the child's hearing been examined?_____Date_____By Whom?_____
      Results_____
   8. Is child presently taking any medication?_____For what reason? _____
      _____Name of medication_____

E. Social/Behavioral/Educational History
   1. Sleeping habits? _____
   2. Does child tend to play alone or with other children?_____Age of Play-
      mates?_____How does child get along with other children_____
      _____With adults?_____
   3. Is it difficult to discipline the child (Explain as fully as possible)_____
      _____
      _____
   4. Would you describe your child as happy or unhappy? _____
      Does your child have mood swings? _____

5. Is your child unusually quiet?_____Unusually active? _____
6. Does child have difficulty in concentrating? _____
7. What are child's favorite play activities? _____
_____
_____

8. Did child attend nursery school?_____Kindergarten? _____
   If so, where? _____
9. School attending_____Address_____
   Principal_____Grade_____Teacher_____
   What are child's average grades in the following subjects: Arithmetic _____
   Reading_____Spelling_____Grades failed_____Grades skipped_____
10. Is child frequently absent from school?_____Why?_____
11. How does child feel about school and about his teachers?_____
_____

F. Hearing, Speech and Language History
   1. At what age did child respond to his name?_____
   2. At what age could child identify objects by pointing?_____
   3. At what age could child identify pictures by pointing?_____
   4. At what age did child follow simple directions such as, "Give it to Mommy"?____
   5. At what age did infant babble and coo? _____
   6. When did child say his first word? _____
   7. When did child begin to use two word phrases?_____Sentences?_____
   8. Does child prefer to use speech or gestures? (Give examples if possible) _____
   _____
   9. Which does the child prefer to use: Complete sentences _____
      Phrases_____One or two words_____Sounds_____
   10. Do you question your child's ability to understand directions and conversation?_____
       Why? _____
   11. Do you question your child's ability to express himself?_____? Why?_____
   _____
   12. How well can child be understood: By parents_____By brothers and
       sisters_____By playmates_____By other adults _____
   13. Does child get stuck and/or repeat sounds or words?_____
   14. Do you think your child hears adequately?_____Do you think his hearing is constant
       or does it vary?_____
       What do you think may cause his hearing problem? _____
   15. Does your child wear a hearing aid(s)?_____Which ear?_____
       What kind?_____
       When did he begin to wear an aid(s)? _____
       Who recommended it?_____Does he like to wear the aid(s)?_____
       _____Does amplification help him? _____
   _____
   16. Has your child's voice seemed normal to you?_____
       If it is unusual, please describe_____
       What do you think causes it to be unusual? _____
   17. Has your child's speech and language ever been evaluated? _____
       By whom?_____When?_____What was reported to you
       about the evaluation?_____
   18. Has your child ever had speech, language or perceptual therapy? _____
       Where?_____When?_____

IV. ASSOCIATED SERVICES
    1. Intelligence testing_____Date_____Where_____
       Results_____
    2. Neurologic testing_____Date_____Where_____
       Results_____
    3. Physical therapy and/or evaluation_____Date_____By Whom _____
       _____Where? _____
    4. Occupational therapy and/or evaluation_____Date_____
       By Whom_____Where?_____

V. PLEASE ADD ANY INFORMATION OR COMMENTS YOU THINK MAY BE HELPFUL.
_____

REFERENCES

Ehrlich, C. H., Kimball, B. D., Shapiro, E., and Huttner, M., Communication skills in five-year-old children with high-risk neonatal histories. *J. Speech Hear. Res.*, 16, 1973.

Feinmesser, M., and Bauberger-Tell, L., Evaluation of Methods for Detecting Impairment in Infancy and Early Childhood. In *Proceedings of the Conference on Newborn Hearing Screening*, Public Health Service, 1971.

Fisch, R. O., Graven, H. J., and Engel, R. R., Neurological status of survivors of neonatal RDS. *J. Pediatr.*, 73, 395–403, 1968.

Hannah, J. E., and Sheeley, E. C., The audiologist's model for test selection. *ASHA*, 17, 83–89, 1975.

Johnson, J. D., Daely, W. J., Malachowski, R. G., and Sunshine, P., Personal communication, 1972.

Joint Committee, Policy statement circulated by the American Academy of Pediatrics, October 1973.

Katz, J., and Struckmann, S., A Case History for Children. In Katz, J. (Ed.), *Handbook of Clinical Audiology*. Baltimore: Williams & Wilkins, 1972.

Lubchenco, L. O., et al. Long term follow-up studies of prematurely born infants; 1. Relationship of handicaps to nursery routines. *J. Pediatr.*, 80, 501–508, 1972.

Lubchenco, L. O., Personal communication, 1973.

Northern, J. L., and Downs, M. P., *Hearing in Children*, p. 135. Baltimore: Williams & Wilkins, 1974.

Robertson, C., Neurological sequelae of RDS. *Am. J. Dis. Child.*, 117, 271–275, 1969.

Windle, W. F., Role of respiratory distress in asphyxial brain damage of the newborn. *Cerebral Palsy J.*, 27, 3–6, 1966.

chapter 33

TESTING INFANTS AND YOUNG CHILDREN

William R. Hodgson, Ph.D.

Considerable progress in testing the hearing of infants and children has been made in the past few years. At the same time, techniques for the management of young children with hearing loss have improved, making early detection doubly important. Both areas – detection and management – have far to go. It is the purpose of this chapter to discuss current clinical procedures for the measurement of hearing loss in infants and young children, and to review some of the experimental techniques which show promise. Three premises are developed underlying the testing of children:

1. *Simplicity*. The simplest method that will get the needed results is best.

2. *Flexibility*. Devotion to a particular test should not prevent use of another method more suitable for a given child. Flexibility should not be interpreted as anarchy; the examiner must retain control of the evaluation.

3. *Appropriateness*. Test procedures must be determined by the responses the child is capable of making.

Basic to all hearing testing is the acoustic signal used in the assessment. Common test stimuli are discussed in the following paragraphs.

THE TEST SIGNAL

Signals used to assess the hearing sensitivity of infants and children may be classified into two groups. One group consists of gross sounds which are either uncalibrated or for which only estimates of the frequency spectrum and intensity are known. Such sounds are generated by "noisemakers." Bells, whistles, drums and toy crickets have been popular. The other group consists of calibrated sound generators.

Gross Signals

Noisemakers, properly used, can be helpful in estimating hearing sensitivity. Objective estimates of their intensity and frequency should be made. To repeat the sound created by a noisemaker, care must be taken to activate it with the same force each time and to maintain the same distance between the noisemaker and the infant's ear. Even so, differences in intensity across presentations may result. It is difficult to compare results obtained by different examiners and standardization of tests with noisemakers is not possible.

The acoustic spectrum of the noisemaker may also be a problem, for most produce broad spectra. Bove and Flugrath (1973) analyzed 25 noisemakers and concluded that 20 had spectra too wide to be useful. The remaining 5 had the desirable features of concentrating energy primarily in the higher frequencies.

Despite the limitations of noisemakers, they are simple and inexpensive and can be used effectively by an experienced examiner. In difficult testing situations, a complicated test procedure sometimes breaks down under its own weight and obscures any minimal information available. Noisemakers are helpful in getting an initial quick estimate of hearing sensitivity, which is invaluable in determining the type of tests which should be used and the kind of response which can be expected. If the examiner knows the approximate level of response he is not entirely in the dark as he begins formal testing.

Practice in producing the sound with the noisemaker held a fixed distance from the microphone of a sound level meter may improve reliability. One may also monitor the signal during the actual evaluation. Even so, the examiner should realize that noisemakers are not as precise as properly controlled electronic signal generators.

Calibrated Signals

Electronically produced signals often used in auditory assessment of children are pure tones, warble tones and narrow bands of noise. These signals are easily controlled and give information about hearing sensitivity as a function of frequency. In addition, speech is often used for special purposes. Generally, the purposes and control problems using these signals are the same when testing children as adults, and the same calibration procedures should be followed.

"Abstract" signals such as pure tones have been criticized as not having meaning for children. Some have advocated the use of familiar sounds – barking dogs, train whistles or the cry of a baby. The rationale is that these sounds will have meaning for the child and he will respond to them. Actually, it is difficult to predict just what sounds will be meaningful to a given child. In addition, environmental sounds, necessarily recorded on tape or phonograph disc, are awkward to control. Therefore, for most children, it is probably better to "give meaning" to an abstract signal such as a pure tone, than it is to hope that an environmental sound will be interesting enough to elicit a stable response. Meaning can be given to a pure tone for most children by reinforcing the child's response.

NORMAL RESPONSE

Auditory evaluation of infants and children must be keyed to the responses that the child is capable of making. For this reason, a review of normal developmental responses appears below. These are only approximations since there is variability in the development of normal children, and various disorders may upset the developmental sequence.

The normal development of response to sound has been described by Ewing and Ewing (1944), Boone (1965), Kendall (1966) and Eisenberg (1970). Auditory responses which are useful in hearing evaluation are shown in Table 33.1 and will be discussed in the following section.

AUDITORY ASSESSMENT

The amount of information obtained from the auditory assessment of a given child will vary. Sometimes the clinician can produce an audiogram complete with air- and bone-conduction thresholds as well as speech test results. Unfortunately, the statements made about the auditory function of other children must be more limited.

Procedures used in the assessment of an

TABLE 33.1. *Developmental Response to Sound in Infants and Young Children*

Age		Response to Sound
years	*months*	
0	0	Reflexive responses—auropalpebral, startle. Generalized body movement; possibly cessation of movement
0	1	Reflexive responses may be inhibited
0	3	Localization efforts begin—eye or head movements toward source of sound
0	6	Localization response reasonably well developed
0	9	Sharp localization responses
1	0	Responds to simple speech (own name, "bye-bye," "no-no," "find mama")
1	6	Recognizes body parts or clothing when they are named (hair, mouth, nose, ears, hand, shoes)
1	9	Can select familiar objects when they are named (toy horse, dog, cow, airplane)
2	0	Points to familiar pictures when they are named. Conditioned play audiometry may be possible
3	0	Play audiometry should produce reliable thresholds

individual child are determined by the responses the patient is capable of making. The evaluation should be oriented toward obtaining the most pertinent information as quickly as possible, using the most sensitive test to which the child can respond. The sophistication of the child's response will depend on several factors:

1. His *mental age* — a determinant of his ability to learn new responses, as well as an indicator of the responses already present (for example, the language requisite for speech audiometry).

2. His *chronologic age* — relating primarily to adequate neuromuscular coordination plus limiting factors specific to disabilities which cause a difference between chronologic age and mental age.

3. His *neurologic status* — relating both to motor and perceptual ability to make the required response.

4. His *hearing level* — an important determinant of experience in auditory response and the ease with which the child learns to respond to new auditory signals.

5. His *willingness to perform*, influenced by the child's motivation, his fears, the rapport established by the clinician, and the skill with which the clinician operates.

6. The child's *prior experience* with auditory testing.

7. The *test environment* — the quality and flexibility of the equipment, the appearance of the room and the toys or other motivational devices that are available to interest the child.

It would appear that the clinician needs the skills of many professions — psychologist, neurologist and others — to assess these facets of the child. Fortunately, in some cases records of previous evaluations (auditory and others) will provide helpful information. These reports should describe the child's behavior, the test procedures and the responses he favored. Sometimes decisions about test procedure must be based solely on information obtained from the child's parents and the clinician's observations. In this case, start with the most sensitive test the child seems capable of performing, and as the evaluation progresses, revise the procedure upward if possible, or downward if necessary.

Because of the determinants mentioned above, there will be variations in which tests are appropriate, and the responses to be expected, from a child of a given age. With this qualification, procedures for auditory evaluation may be classified as follows according to the age of the child.

Age 0 to 6 Months

Auditory assessment, particularly during the early months of this age range, is primarily limited to the elicitation of reflexive responses to relatively intense auditory signals. The more useful responses are the auropalpebral reflex (APR), startle reflex and arousal (observable by generalized body movement). The APR represents contracture of the orbicularis palpebrae muscles, and is seen as a quick closing of the eyes (an eye blink), or a tightening of the lids if the eyes are already closed. Dennis (1934) described the Moro (startle) reflex: "In most cases the arms go apart, the fingers spread, the legs extend and the head is thrown backward." Less often than the classic Moro reflex, the startle response is seen as a small "jump" of the infant's body immediately following the stimulus. It is important that the infant be uncovered so that the entire body can be seen. Both the APR and the startle reflex tend to disappear quickly upon repeated presentations of the stimulus.

An infant lying quietly may be aroused to generalized movements by auditory signals. Unfortunately for our purposes, infants who are awake are seldom still and the examiner must be careful not to interpret random activity as responses. Some neonates, but more often infants later in the 0- to 6-month range, will halt motor activity on the presentation of an auditory signal. Bench (1970) emphasized the importance of considering the infant's prestimulus arousal state by discussing the "law of initial value": The lower the initial state, the greater the increase in level of activity on stimulation; the higher the initial state, the greater the decrease in level of activity.

The responses described above can also be elicited by visual and tactile stimuli, and the examiner must avoid such stimulation. Some problems may be avoided by testing the infant in a state of light sleep. This procedure reduces the probability of false positive responses. Of course, this conclusion joins the audiologist with parents in a primordial and vexing problem; trying to get the baby to sleep. When possible, it is helpful to observe the infant's responses both when sleeping and awake.

Thresholds for APR and the levels necessary for wakening were determined by Wedenberg (1963) using 20 normal infants age 1 to 10 days. The levels required to awaken the babies were 70 to 75 dB sound pressure level (SPL). APRs were elicited at 105 to 115 dB SPL for tones of 500, 1000, 1500, 2000 and 4000 Hz. In a follow-up study, Wedenberg (1972) concluded that an infant may have normal hearing if he responds with an APR to a tone of 105 to 115 dB SPL, or is awakened by a tone of 70 to 75 dB SPL, or less. A cochlear problem with recruitment may be suspected if the child gives an APR to 105 to 115 dB SPL, but requires greater than 75 dB SPL to be awakened. A conductive or retrococh-

lear disorder may be present if the child gives no APR to the 105 to 115 dB SPL sound, but is awakened by some signal greater than 70 to 75 dB SPL.

Assessment of hearing sensitivity during the first 6 months is generally qualitative not quantitative. An experienced observer should be able to identify normal infants who have normal hearing. Among unresponsive infants it is difficult to differentiate those who have hearing loss from those with other problems. However, there is a good possibility that those with profound hearing loss, characterized by consistent failure to respond to sound, can be correctly identified.

Identification Audiometry for Neonates

The desirability of early detection of hearing loss in infants has led to experimentation with mass auditory screening of neonates. Screening has been done in the hospital nursery, using trained volunteers as examiners, under the supervision of an audiologist. Portable sound generators are commercially available. Most of these deliver a high frequency (3000 Hz) warble tone or band of noise with available outputs of 70, 80, 90 and 100 dB SPL when the instrument is held at a standard distance from the infant's ear. Responses sought are the APR, other face or head movements, and the startle reflex, or other body movements. Infants who fail to respond receive audiologic follow-up.

Downs, at the University of Colorado Medical Center, has conducted an extensive experimental program in neonatal hearing screening. About 20,000 infants have been screened. The estimated false positive rate was 3%. That is, about 3% of the infants failed the screening but normal hearing was later verified. Three false negatives were found; three children who passed the screening were found to have hearing loss later, during the first year of life. Of course, the loss may have developed after the screening. Downs (1972) reports that, of the 20,000 screened, 12 deaf children were detected. These children would have been identifiable through use of a high risk register—a check list of familial, prenatal, and neonatal conditions known to be associated with deafness. For a thorough discussion of high risk registers and associated disorders, refer to Black et al. (1971) and Chapter 4 in Northern and Downs (1974).

Feinmesser and Bauberger-Tell (1972) reported on the screening of 17,708 neonates. Five deaf children were detected. By follow-up, 4 additional deaf infants were found, causing the authors to question the validity of the screening procedure. Eight of the 9 infants would have appeared on a high risk register.

Simmons and Russ (1974) and Simmons

(1976) described an automated procedure, the "crib-o-gram," for neonatal screening. A motion-sensitive transducer on the crib detects infant movements, which are recorded on a strip recorder. Twenty times in a 24-hour period, the recorder is activated for 16 sec. Halfway through each activation a signal is emitted from a test loud speaker. Auditory response is determined by comparison of movements recorded before and after the test signal. The authors reported that responses can be scored quickly, even by inexperienced readers. Of 7655 neonates screened, 777 failed. Of this group, 5 infants have documented hearing loss.

Altman, Shenhav and Schaudinischky (1976) also reported use of an automated screening device, the "accelerometer recording system." When 400 neonates were screened, all but 7 responded. Automated systems seem to have potential for use in routine neonatal screening. Efforts to improve their sensitivity and reduce false positive results should continue.

Concern about the efficiency of neonatal hearing screening programs led to the formation of a Joint Committee of the American Academy of Ophthalmology and Otolaryngology, the American Academy of Pediatrics, and the American Speech and Hearing Association. In 1970, this committee urged increased research efforts but did not recommend routine screening of neonates. In 1973, the committee issued a supplemental statement, recommending the use of a high risk register. The group suggested audiologic follow-up of infants with (a) familial history of hereditary childhood hearing loss; (b) history of prenatal maternal rubella or other viral infection; (c) defects of the ear, nose, throat, palate, or lip; (d) birthweight less than 1500 g; or (e) bilirubin level greater than 20 mg/100 ml serum. The committee recommended an in-depth audiologic evaluation during the first 2 months of life, and continued regular evaluations for those who passed, because of the possibility of hereditodegenerative disorders.

Recommendations resulting from a conference on early identification of hearing loss (Mencher, 1976) were that a high risk register be routinely utilized. Neonates at risk for deafness should receive professional evaluation. This group also recommended that a screening procedure may supplement the high risk register only if these high standards can be maintained: ambient noise levels during testing should be reported. Northern and Downs (1974) recommended that testing not be done in noise levels exceeding 60 dB SPL. Infants should be in a state of light sleep prior to the test. The stipulated test signal is to be predominately high frequency, with a sharp rise time. It should last 1/2 to 2 sec, with an interstimulus duration of at least 15 sec. The acceptable response is generalized body movement involving more than one limb, and accompanied by eye movement. Two or more responses out of eight signals constitute a passing score. A final recommendation of the conference was that "either the observer judge responses without knowing when signals are presented, or that a response be considered valid only when two observers independently agree on its presence."

Mencher (1974) obtained the greatest efficiency in detecting hearing loss in neonates through a combination of a simplified high risk register and use of narrow band noise to arouse the infant from light sleep. Follow-up evaluations of 80% of 10,000 infants originally observed found 9 to have hearing loss. Seven would have been identified by screening only, and 5 would have been detected by the high risk register. Two were not detected by either procedure. Efforts to improve the validity of neonatal screening should continue. In the meantime, careful attention should be given to neonates who, by their history, show a high risk for hearing loss.

Experimental Tests

The following paragraphs describe experiments investigating the auditory response of infants. By and large these techniques have not reached the stage of routine clinical use.

Classical and instrumental conditioning have been employed in hearing test procedures. Aldrich (1928) reported conditioning a 3-month-old baby by a pin scratch on the foot after the ringing of a bell. After 15 trials the baby raised the foot at the sound of the bell. Marquis (1931) attempted to condition 8 infants age 1 to 10 days by sounding a buzzer before the presentation of the infant's bottle. Eventually a sucking response was obtained from 7 of the 8 infants upon the sound of the buzzer. Butterfield and Hodgson (1969) found that, in normal neonates, when continuation of an auditory stimulus (music) was contingent on sucking, duration of sucks increased significantly over baseline sucking measures (without contingency). When maintenance of the signal was contingent on not sucking, the duration of sucks decreased compared to baseline activity.

Changes in rate of the heart beat following auditory stimulation have been investigated. Bartoshuk (1962) repeatedly elicited cardiac acceleration in response to intense auditory signals. Beadle and Crowell (1962) reported changes in pulse rate in one normal neonate following auditory stimulation, but with no consistent correlation of acceleration or deceleration with either frequency or intensity change. However, Bartoshuk (1964) obtained larger increases in heart rate for signals of successively greater intensity. Steinschneider, Lipton and Richmond (1966) reported increase of heart rate and decrease in latency of response with intensity increase. In general, these studies used relatively intense sounds and some used broad band noises.

Measurement of changes in respiration rate during tonal stimulation has been accomplished. Heron and Jacobs (1969) reported various changes in respiration of normal hearing infants following stimulation by frequency modulated tones. Bradford and Rousey (1972) summarized respiration audiometry procedures and studies. They concluded that it offers a useful diagnostic procedure.

Among others, Hardy and Bordley (1951) investigated galvanic skin response (GSR) audiometry with children. They reported problems conditioning uncooperative and neurologically impaired children. While some have had success testing children with GSR audiometry, it has not proved generally practical because of difficulty conditioning children who cannot be tested by other means. Unfortunately, these are the children for whom the procedure is needed.

The uses of electroencephalic response audiometry, electrocochleography, and impedance audiometry are discussed elsewhere in this book. Impedance audiometry, in particular, has made an enormous contribution. It affords previously unavailable information about middle ear status and sensory-neural function.

Age 6 Months to 2 Years

Some neonates show crude orientation responses to auditory stimuli (Wertheimer, 1961). There may be eye movement toward the sound source (cochleo-oculogyric reflex), and the head may turn also. However, localization responses can be expected to develop in normal infants only by 3 to 6 months of age. At first localization efforts are crude and limited by the infant's ability to control head movements. By 6 months the normal infant should make reasonably clear localization movements and these orientation responses are valuable in assessing auditory sensitivity of children generally between 6 months and 2 years of age (as well as older retarded children).

Suzuki and Ogiba (1961) utilized a "conditioned orientation reflex," and reported success in testing young children, as did Di Carlo and Bradley (1961). The usual arrangement for most localization audiometry is to place the child between two loudspeakers in a sound-treated room as shown in Figure 33.1. If the child responds by turning toward the loudspeaker when a signal is produced, an estimate of hearing sensitivity can be obtained by varying the intensity of the signal with subsequent presentations until the lowest level at which the child will respond is found. While various sounds have been used, perhaps warble tones or narrow bands of noise are best because they are easily controlled and provide information about sensitivity at different frequencies.

Because children tend to lose interest and stop responding to such sounds fairly quickly, reinforcement of localization responses is usually needed. One simple method is to mount animated mechanical toys near the loudspeakers. Inexpensive battery-powered toys can be rewired so that they may be operated from the examiner's control room. We have used at various times a dancing bear, a drummer boy and a bartender who mixed and consumed his own drink. After receiving a temperance lecture from the mother of one client, the audiologist put tape over the sign "bartender" painted on the toy and called him a "soda jerk." This change in procedure did not affect the quality of response noted in the children.

Each time the child responds to an auditory stimulus by looking toward the loudspeaker the toy is activated briefly to reinforce the response. With such reinforcement, most children will respond long enough for determination of hearing sensitivity at various frequencies. The noise made by the toys is of no consequence, since it is not activated until after the child has responded to the test signal.

Moore, Wilson and Thompson (1977) investigated the capacity of an animated toy animal to reinforce head turn responses in infants 4 months, 5 to 6 months, and 7 to 11 months of age. Compared to a control group, they found significantly increased responses only in the two older groups. This study supports the utility of localization audiometry in the age range being discussed.

If children have unilateral loss, it is usually assumed that they cannot localize sound well. However, Fisher and Freedman (1968) reported accurate sound localization among subjects with unilateral loss simulated by plugging one

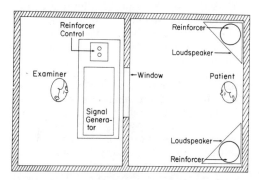

Fig. 33.1. Arrangement for localization audiometry.

ear. Gatehouse and Cox (1972) found that 8 subjects with severe to profound unilateral sensory-neural loss made horizontal localization of white noise bursts well above chance, but poorer than normal hearing subjects. In the usual test situation, with the child located between two loudspeakers, the localization task is simple. Even with unilateral loss, the child may be able to locate the sound source. Therefore, while some confusion in localization may suggest a unilateral loss, one can only be sure in most sound field audiometry that sensitivity of the better ear has been assessed. Interpretation of sound field testing should note this limitation.

A child who has a severe or profound hearing loss, even if it is bilaterally equal, will probably not have learned to localize, or perhaps even to respond consistently to sound. Therefore, in localization audiometry, as with most techniques, it is more difficult to assess the child with hearing loss than the child who has normal hearing. If confusion in localization is noted, it is best to use only one loudspeaker in testing. This way, the child learns that anytime he hears a sound it will come from a single source, and his task is made simpler. When using this technique, some provision should be made to distract the child's attention away from the loudspeaker between signals. Otherwise, he may look at the loudspeaker all the time. A distraction can be provided by mounting a third animated toy on the wall of the soundroom across from the child. Activating this toy distracts attention away from the loudspeaker between signals.

There are two reports of attempts to overcome the problem of testing the better ear only. Haug, Baccaro and Guilford (1967) described a procedure called the PIWI (puppet in the window illuminated) test. First, responses are obtained to localization audiometry in sound field, and each response is reinforced by the appearance of an interesting puppet behind a lighted window. Then earphones are placed on the child and the puppet is illuminated each time the child responds to a tone presentation by looking toward the window. They report success in establishing sensitivity levels on children under 3 years old.

Liden and Kankkunen (1969) reported a technique called visual reinforcement audiometry (VRA). Instead of limiting responses to orientation, they accept (1) reflexes, such as the APR, (2) investigatory responses, (3) orientation responses and (4) spontaneous responses, such as a smile or vocalization. Any response is reinforced by presentation of an interesting picture via a slide projector. Because small loudspeakers are placed close to the child's ear, a clear head-shadow effect is produced. In addition, a plug is placed in the ear canal of the nontest

ear and the ear is covered with a sound attenuating muff. These precautions permit monaural testing for children in whom the difference in sensitivity between ears is not as great as the attentuation provided by the head-shadow effect plus the plug and muff.

The question of whether to use one or two examiners when testing children will arise. For tests which can be conducted in one room, it is probably best to do so with only one examiner who has immediate contact with the child. However, tests in sound field generally require the use of separate examination and control rooms, and necessitate two examiners.

Age 2 Years to 6 Years

Play Audiometry

Localization audiometry, as described above, has some of the features of "play audiometry" (Barr, 1955). In common with play audiometry, localization testing makes provision to reinforce responses. The primary differences are that play audiometry requires a response other than looking and often uses procedures for stimulus presentation similar to those used with adults. By the age of 2 years, some children can be evaluated using play audiometry, and the probability of successful evaluation increases as the child approaches the age of 3 years.

An early example of play audiometry was reported by Dix and Hallpike (1947). In their "peep-show" technique, the child is taught to press a button upon the presentation of a simultaneous light and sound. An interesting picture is illuminated only if the button is pushed immediately after the stimulus presentation. When the child is responding well, the auditory signal is presented alone, and each appropriate response is reinforced until threshold is determined. Others have developed similar procedures: the "pediacoumeter" (Guilford and Haug, 1952), the "pup-show" (Green, 1958) and various mechanical toys suggested by Knox (1960).

The term play audiometry describes any test in which the child is taught a play response to the stimulus (for example, dropping a block into a box when the tone is heard). Regardless of the technique used, there are a number of principles which should be kept in mind. These are discussed below.

Frequently, the initial task of the examiner is to assess and attentuate the child's fear and to establish a good working relationship. O'Neill, Oyer and Hillis (1961) utilized a period of semistructured play prior to audiometric evaluation (1) to establish rapport with the child, (2) to observe reaction to gross sounds to get an idea of the level of response, (3) to establish the idea of responding to sound in a play audiometry setting and (4) to help the examiners select procedures and responses suited to the child's ability and interests. These four points are crucial to play audiometry and cannot be ignored. Of course, individual children will require varying amounts of attention to each of the points. The key to the procedure is astute observation of the child's behavior and appropriate reaction by the examiner. Skill and experience are required, as well as a thorough knowledge of the behavior of children and of the test equipment.

Once the child is in the test room and a test procedure decided upon, the next action which may cause an emotional crisis is placing the earphones on the child's head. Many children will not object, especially if the audiologist has done his preliminary work well, and the headset can be positioned without fuss. For children who are reluctant to accept the ear phones, the examiner can—to show the child what is expected of him—briefly wear the headset himself and illustrate the expected response. This action, valid as a training procedure, is usually not very successful as a motivation device. The child who is reluctant to accept the headset will usually be content to let the examiner wear it indefinitely. In some extreme situations it may help to let the problem child observe the testing of another cooperative child to convey the idea that there is nothing painful about the test and that it is fun. You might call this the Tom Sawyer approach to hearing evaluation. However, the most efficient approach to the child who will not accept earphones may be first to obtain responses in sound field. Thereby a general idea of hearing sensitivity will be obtained while the child is becoming more accustomed to, interested in and less fearful of the test. Usually it is not helpful to try to sneak the earphones onto the child's head, but rather to leave them in plain sight during the sound field conditioning and, eventually, without making a big thing of it, to place them on the child. Once the earphones are on, the child should be kept busy to reduce his tendency to remove them.

Because there is always the possibility that a young child will stop responding before the evaluation is completed, it is important to work quickly and to get the most important information first. The recommendation to work quickly must be interpreted with caution. While working too slowly may permit the child's attention to wander, proceeding too rapidly may confuse the child and encourage false responses. One is left with the lame recommendation to observe the rate at which a given child can work and proceed accordingly. For example, in play audiometry where the child is responding by dropping a block when he hears the signal, another block should be placed in his hand as soon as he has dropped the previous one. Keeping the child involved may prevent him from deciding just at that point that he is tired of playing and that the game is over.

The clinician must guard against accepting false responses. The criterion for the temporal relationship between signal and response must be observed rigidly and responses outside that relationship must be ignored. Only levels at which responses are repeatable should be accepted. Because threshold is usually defined as the level at which 50% response occurs, a further check may be made by presenting signals 5 dB above apparent threshold. At that level 100% response should occur.

Because the examiner must work quickly it is essential that he be completely familiar with the instruments used in testing. He must give only minimal attention to operation of the equipment and concentrate on the behavior of the child. Because the inexperienced clinician must devote most of his time to operation of the audiometer, his efforts at testing children may be quite unrewarding until manipulation of dials and switches becomes automatic.

Even if the clinician works quickly, some children will stop responding before the evaluation is completed. If this seems likely, it is desirable to get the most important information first. For example, it is better to obtain thresholds for those frequencies most important to the audibility and intelligibility of speech (500, 1000 and 2000 Hz) than to get a complete audiogram for one ear only. For some restless children, whose behavior indicates that they may cooperate for only a short time, it may be preferable first to obtain thresholds for speech. It is preferable to have speech thresholds for each ear than one or two pure tone thresholds for one ear. However, this philosophy should not be an excuse for obtaining less than complete results, and any report of a partial examination should be so labeled.

When the child gets restless and responses become unreliable, changing the method of response may introduce enough variety to renew his interest. That is, if the child has been dropping blocks in response to the signal, one might change to pegs in a pegboard or some other game. The game used for responding should not be too interesting in itself. For example, when attractive small animal toys were once supplied for the child to drop into a box, the toys were so interesting that most children wanted to examine each one before responding. The toys provided good material to interest the child, but were not appropriate for actual testing.

If the child is interested in some other activity, he may not respond to an audible sound. Therefore it is important to avoid distracting stimuli and have the child ready to respond when the auditory signal is presented. This set may be facilitated by the audiologist saying "Ready?" or "Listen" or by the audiologist's own attentive listening attitude.

The child with a marked hearing loss may have difficulty learning the expected response because he lacks experience responding to sound. Since he will have limited language or none at all, instructions must be by pantomime and demonstration. It is of course essential that he hear the signal during the conditioning process. In pure tone testing an intense 500 Hz is most likely to be audible. If difficulty in conditioning is encountered, two procedures have been suggested which may be helpful.

Lowell et al. (1956) suggested a technique for conditioning using sound generators which have a visual component. That is, they first condition the child to respond to a drum beat — to see and hear the production of the sound. Gradually the drum is moved out of the child's visual range. Hopefully he keeps responding to the sound alone. Once such conditioning is established, a pure tone is substituted for the drum beat. A potential problem with this method is the danger of overconditioning the child to respond to visual signals. The repeated presentation of the drum beat which the child can see may strongly condition the visual component, and he may never get the idea of responding to the sound.

Another helpful procedure was suggested by Thorne (1962). The vibrations of a 250 or 500 Hz signal sent through the bone oscillator can be easily felt when the audiometer is set to maximum output for bone conduction. For a child with profound hearing loss, this tactile stimulus may implement conditioning. Once the response is established, response to air-conducted tones can again be investigated. If the child responds readily to tactile signals at 250 and 500 Hz but responds to neither bone-conducted signals at 2000 or 4000 Hz nor to air-conducted tones, it is likely that he has no measurable hearing.

The generalization that play audiometry is appropriate for children 2 through 6 years of age will have many exceptions. For successful play audiometry with a 2-year-old, an exceptional child (and audiologist) is required. However, most children by 3 years should respond to this method. The fact that a 3-year-old cannot be tested with play audiometry by a skilled clinician may suggest some problem other than or in addition to hearing loss. Many children near the upper limits of this age range may not need (and may not prefer) to be tested with play audiometry, but prefer to respond by raising the hand or saying "yes." Remember that the test method is only a means to an end, and

the procedure which elicits the best responses is the method of choice.

Masking

When testing children, the use of masking to prevent the participation of the nontest ear is as necessary as it is in valid audiometry with adults. The same principles apply. In most cases, elaborate explanations to the child about the noise is unnecessary. If the child has sufficient language the examiner may explain that he is going to put a noise into one ear which the child should ignore, and that he should continue to respond to the test signal only. If, because of the age or language level of the child, such an explanation is not possible, the examiner should simply introduce the noise into the nontest ear. The onset of the noise will probably elicit a response. Leaving the noise on, the examiner by gestures indicates that the child should not respond to the noise. Then, presenting the test signal, the examiner should prompt the child to respond. This simple procedure may be sufficient to help the child differentiate between the masking noise and test signal. At any rate, more or less reconditioning may permit the test to continue. However, in some instances, when the examiner is just managing to maintain the test procedure (a situation not entirely foreign to audiologists), masking may not be possible. In such cases the examiner should report this fact so that the audiogram can be interpreted accordingly.

Speech Threshold Testing

Just as he would in good audiometry with adults, the audiologist will want to obtain speech thresholds to confirm pure tone results and give a direct measure of hearing for speech. Signals used for obtaining thresholds of intelligibility with children should meet the same criteria as those used with adults. That is, the words should be highly intelligible and of equal difficulty. Several investigators have suggested more or less formal techniques for obtaining speech thresholds with children (Keaster, 1947; Siegenthaler, Pearson and Lezak, 1954; Meyerson, 1956: Siegenthaler and Haspiel, 1966). In general, the test can be performed by selecting a few words within the child's vocabulary. If the child can repeat the words the test can proceed in approximately the same manner as adults. If not, pictures or objects must be found to represent the words. "Cowboy," "birthday (cake)" and "airplane" are good possibilities. The child points to the picture as he hears the word, and the intensity is varied until threshold is determined. Remember that if the test is limited to three or four words the child's task will be very easy and the resultant threshold may be closer to a threshold of detection than an ordinary speech reception threshold (SRT) would be. The test should be conducted under earphones so that each ear can be tested separately, but may be done in sound field if the child will not wear the headset.

Martin and Coombes (1976) described an attractive procedure for obtaining speech thresholds in young children. Test words are names of parts of a colorful clown, who awards the child with candy if the part named is pressed by the child. The investigators reported success in obtaining speech thresholds from children as young as 2½ years.

If the child does not know words which meet the criteria of intelligibility and equality usually required for threshold tests, other words within his vocabulary can be substituted ("Find mama," "Let's go bye-bye," "Where is your nose?"). In all of the procedures one must avoid giving visual clues which will help the child identify the words. Since this testing usually requires the flexibility afforded by live voice, a two-room test environment is necessary if the intensity of the signal is to be controlled carefully.

If language limitations prevent establishment of threshold of intelligibility (SRT), thresholds of detection for speech may be established with a procedure similar to that used in pure tone play audiometry. The child is conditioned to drop a block (or to make other appropriate response) when he hears the speech signal. It seems to have become conventional to use $[b_\wedge - b_\wedge - b_\wedge]$ as the speech signal. By varying the intensity, threshold is established. These speech awareness thresholds are as reliable as speech reception thresholds, and are reached at an intensity about 8 to 10 dB less than that required for SRT. If speech awareness thresholds are obtained, they should be labeled as such.

For some children, speech thresholds can be obtained when pure tone thresholds cannot. These results cannot be considered complete since they do not give information about hearing sensitivity as a function of frequency, but are sometimes the only information that can be obtained. For example, an older retarded child may have enough language to mediate speech thresholds although he cannot be conditioned easily to respond to play audiometry. Air-conduction speech thresholds give information about sensitivity, and bone-conduction speech thresholds give some diagnostic information about sensory-neural status. If the audiometer is not calibrated for bone-conduction speech signals, bone-conduction speech thresholds can be obtained by inserting the bone-conductor phone plug into one of the air-conduction earphone jacks. Recalibration of the system is then necessary by finding the point at which normal listeners can just repeat spondee words. If the speech audiometer is calibrated to 20 dB *re* 0.0002 dyne/cm², this point will be about 40 dB hearing threshold level (HTL), which then becomes 0 dB HTL for bone-conduction testing.

Word Discrimination Testing

While it is important to obtain SRTs for purposes of rehabilitation and comparison with pure tone findings, word discrimination scores provide a different type of measure which in many cases is more important than the SRT. A measure of word discrimination ability at a comfortably loud presentation level is used to determine the degree of clarity with which the child hears speech. Different criteria are used in the selection of materials for word discrimination than speech reception testing. Tests are usually lists of words whose phonetic composition covers the range of sounds in the language, with approximately the same frequency of occurrence as the sounds occur in the language. There are several auditory discrimination tests for children. The phonetically balanced (PB-K) list (K for "kindergarten") developed by Haskins (1949) is most like the PB word lists used with adults. These lists can be used with children who have enough language and intelligible speech to repeat the words of the test. Unfortunately, receptive language level affects discrimination scores. The role of word familiarity is discussed in Chapter 13, on word discrimination testing. Children with congenital hearing loss usually exhibit retarded language development which reduces discrimination scores. Results obtained under these circumstances must be interpreted with caution.

With very young or language-limited children, picture discrimination tests may be used. Such tests include those reported by Myatt and Landes (1963), Siegenthaler and Haspiel (1966), and the word intelligibility by picture identification (WIPI) test developed by Ross and Lerman (1970). In these closed set tests the child listens for the stimulus word while looking at a set of pictures, one of which represents the stimulus word. If he points to the proper picture, his response is scored correct.

Certain variables affect these scores. Lerman, Ross and McLauchlin (1965) reported considerable success in using the picture discrimination test of Myatt and Landes with hearing-impaired children, but noted that some pictures were not correctly identified as representing the stimulus word. Additionally, because the possible responses in picture tests are limited to a few words, the tests are easier than those which require the child to repeat the word he hears. Hodgson (1973) administered the WIPI to normal hearing children between 5 and 9 years of age. On one condition the WIPI was presented in the usual way as a picture discrimination test. In the other, WIPI words were presented as an open set test, without the picture, and the subjects repeated the words they heard. The mean score was better by 10% for the closed set test. Jones and Studebaker (1974) concluded that a closed set test may be more informative when used with older children with severe hearing loss. They presented closed and open set tests to 23 such children. They found the closed set test correlated better with tests of auditory sensitivity and teacher ratings.

Matkin (1977) recommends the PB-K lists for children with receptive language ages (RLA) between 6 and 12 years. He advocates the WIPI if RLA is from 4 to 6 years. Matkin describes an informal procedure to use if RLA is less than 4 years. Pictures or objects are used to represent words within the child's vocabulary to which pointing responses can be elicited. For completely nonverbal children, a discrimination test utilizing familiar environmental sounds has been developed (Hieber et al., 1975). To prevent misinterpretation of results, Matkin suggests that informal test scores be recorded as the ratio of correct responses out of number of trials, rather than in percent, as formal tests are reported.

An age effect has been reported in discrimination testing with young children. Siegenthaler and Haspiel (1966) found improvement in scores across an age range from 3 to 8 years. Smith and Hodgson (1970) presented PB-K lists to normal and to hearing-impaired children in three age ranges, 4-0 to 5-5, 5-6 to 7-0, and 7-1 to 8-5. For both normal and hearing-impaired children, scores improved with age.

Smith and Hodgson (1970) also reported consistent improvement in the discrimination scores of both normal and hearing-impaired children when correct responses were systematically reinforced using an operant conditioning approach. For example, in the group of hearing-impaired children mean scores improved with systematic reinforcement as follows: for the 4-0 to 5-5-year-old subgroup, from 39% to 65%; for the 5-6 to 7-0-year-old subgroup, from 66% to 82%, and for the 7-1 to 8-5-year-old subgroup, from 69% to 83%. A similar pattern of improvement appeared with reinforcement in the normal hearing children. These findings indicate that the unreinforced discrimination test may underestimate a child's potential for discriminating words in the PB-K lists. Reinforcement procedures in discrimination testing may be valuable in reducing variability caused by lack of motivation and attention.

Operant Audiometry

This term refers to the use of systematic tangible reinforcement in hearing evaluation. Operant procedures are discussed extensively by Fulton (1974). Bricker and Bricker (1969) presented a step-by-step program for operant audiometry. Operant procedures may be useful with difficult-to-test children of all ages. Fulton, Gorzycki and Hull (1975) reported moderate success obtaining pure tone thresholds on children between 9 and 25 months of age. Films illustrating this technique with severely retarded children and showing the procedures involved in operant audiometry have been produced at the Parsons, Kansas Research Center.*

It should be remembered that, as in any audiometric technique, operant audiometry is useful only when it obtains responses more quickly, precisely or inexpensively than other methods. Also, the procedure is only a technique for obtaining responses, and all of the precautions necessary for valid audiometry must be followed. Table 33.2 summarizes the test techniques most appropriate for various ages.

INTERPRETING TEST RESULTS

On the completion of the auditory assessment, test results must be interpreted and reported, and appropriate recommendations made. If medical problems, such as a conductive loss, are found, the child should be referred to a physician. The child's behavior during the evaluation may suggest the need for referral to speech, psychological, neurologic or educational specialists. The audiologist, in interpreting his test results, should describe the hearing impairment in terms of the handicap it causes, whether the loss is of sufficient magnitude to account for the deviation from normal behavior seen in the child, and make educational recommendations to minimize the effects of reduced hearing.

The effects of congenital loss are greater than those of a loss of the same magnitude acquired in an adult or older child. Those with congenital loss must learn language with an impaired auditory system, and even if the loss of hearing sensitivity is mitigated by hearing aid use, the dual distortion of the aid plus the impaired system makes learning doubly difficult. The child born with profound loss may not learn to respond to sound at all without training, and may not learn the meaningfulness and utility of sound.

For children with profound loss, particularly

---

* Available from the Audio-Visual Center, Film Rental Services, University of Kansas, 746 Massachusetts, Lawrence, Kansas 66044.

TABLE 33.2. *"Best Test" Techniques for Children*

Age	Test Procedure	Information Obtained
0–6 months	Impedance audiometry (useful for all ages)	Middle ear status and estimate of sensitivity
	Elicit reflexive responses with relatively intense signals. Perhaps elicit "listening" response with softer "meaningful" signals	Qualitative. Should differentiate between normal and profoundly hard of hearing
6 months–2 years	Sound field localization audiometry	Especially after 1 year of age, it is easy to identify normal hearing children with this method
		For those with hearing loss, a good approximation of the level of sensitivity in the better ear is possible
	Orientation response under earphones	For those children who will respond to this technique, good approximation of sensitivity in either ear can be obtained
	Response to speech	For children who have acquired language, good approximation of *overall* sensitivity is possible (for either ear if testing is done under earphones)
	Response to A/C and B/C speech	Estimate of cochlear response
2–6 years	Play audiometry. Pure tone A/C and B/C	Auditory thresholds
	TROCA	Thresholds for difficult-to-test children
	Speech awareness thresholds	Speech thresholds for children without language or loss too great to understand speech
	Speech reception thresholds	Speech thresholds for children with language
	Word discrimination score, PB-K	Measurement of discrimination ability for children with sufficient language and speech for formal testing
	Picture tests	Approximation of discrimination ability for children with language who have unintelligible speech

those with fragmented audiograms and audiometric response limited to the low frequencies, residual hearing—even with training—must remain a secondary channel supplementing visual clues. With such children hearing for speech cannot operate independently and the statement made years ago remains true: "There is no real evidence that profoundly deaf children were ever taught to discriminate speech sound" (Hudgins, 1954).

Downs (1974) maintains that some children have insufficient residual hearing to participate successfully in an auditory-oral training program. She has devised a "deafness management quotient" to help direct hearing-impaired children into appropriate educational settings. The quotient is derived from measures of residual hearing sensitivity, neurologic status, intelligence, support expected from the family, and socioeconomic situation. Children who rate high are recommended for an auditory-oral training program. Others are recommended for training in a setting where total communication is used.

Milder congenital losses have more subtle effects. Goetzinger (1962) reported that children with mild bilateral sensory-neural loss (approximately 30 to 45 dB re ANSI-1969 ISO norms for the speech frequencies in the better ear) were about 12 months retarded in speech and language acquisition at a chronologic age of 3 years. A study comparing school age children who had mild losses with a normal hearing control group showed the hearing-impaired to have reduced auditory discrimination ability, more articulation errors and, according to teachers' reports, poorer work habits and greater emotional variability (Goetzinger, Harrison and Barr, 1964).

Because certain disorders have symptoms in common with hearing loss, misdiagnosis of a hearing problem may result if auditory assessment is not a part of the diagnostic evaluation. Mental retardation, emotional disturbance, central dysacusis, auditory perceptual disability, as well as hearing loss, can cause language and speech retardation, reduced or inconsistent response to sound and inappropriate or hyperactive behavior. A review of the literature by Reichstein and Rosenstein (1964) shows the disagreement and confusion regarding differential diagnosis in these areas.

The danger of misdiagnosis of children with hearing loss has been emphasized by Merklein and Briskey (1962), Rosenberg (1966), Ross and Matkin (1967) and Hodgson (1969). Certain hearing losses cause behavior incongruent with the stereotype of the hearing-impaired child. On rare occasions, sudden bilateral hearing loss occurs in children without an obvious cause. In such instances the loss can be expected to cause catastrophic behavior, which may be interpreted as an emotional disorder unassociated with hearing loss if an auditory evaluation is not done. More commonly, confusion results with children who have enough hearing to respond to many sounds. These children may have a mild to moderate loss of hearing sensitivity, or they may have normal hearing for some frequencies and a loss for others (depressed sensitivity only for the low frequencies, or more often, a high frequency loss). They respond to sounds which are audible to them. Without knowledge of their hearing loss, their failure to respond to other sounds may suggest inappropriate and inconsistent behavior. The symptoms caused by the hearing loss may result in misdiagnosis of mental retardation, emotional disturbance or central language problems, without an adequate audiometric evaluation.

REFERENCES

Aldrich, C., A new test for hearing in the newborn; the conditioned reflex. Am. J. Dis. Child., 35, 36–37, 1928.

Altman, M., Shenhav, R., and Schaudinischky, L., Semi-Objective Method for Auditory Mass Screening of Neonates. In Mencher, G. (Ed.), Proceedings of the Nova Scotia Conference on Early Detection of Hearing Loss, pp. 181–189. Basel: S. Karger, 1976.

Barr, B., Pure tone audiometry for preschool children. Acta Otolaryngol. Suppl. 121, 1955.

Bartoshuk, A., Human neonatal cardiac acceleration to sound. Percept. Mot. Skills, 15, 15–27, 1962.

Bartoshuk, A., Human neonatal cardiac response to sound; a power function. Psychonomic Sci., 1, 151–152, 1964.

Beadle, K., and Crowell, D., Neonatal electrocardiographic responses to sound. J. Speech Hear. Res., 5, 112–123, 1962.

Bench, J., The law of initial value; a neglected source of variance in infant audiometry. Int. Audiol., 9, 314–322, 1970.

Black, F., Bergstrom, L., Downs, M., and Hemenway, W., Congenital Deafness: a New Approach to Early Detection of Deafness through a High Risk Register. Boulder, Colo.: Colorado Associated University Press, 1971.

Boone, D., Infant speech and language development. Volta Rev., 67, 414–419, 1965.

Bove, C., and Flugrath, J., Frequency components of noisemakers for use in pediatric audiological evaluations. Volta Rev., 75, 551–556, 1973.

Bradford, L., and Rousey, C., Respiration audiometry. Maico Audiol. Library Ser. 10, 22–24, 1972.

Bricker, D., and Bricker, W., A programmed approach to operant audiometry for low-functioning children. J. Speech Hear. Disord., 34, 312–320, 1969.

Butterfield, E., and Hodgson, W., Tools for the audiologic study of neonates. Scientific exhibit at the American Speech and Hearing Association Convention, 1969.

Dennis, W., A description and classification of the response of the newborn infant. Psychol. Bull., 31, 5–22, 1934.

Di Carlo, L., and Bradley, W., A simplified auditory test for infants and young children. Laryngoscope, 71, 628–646, 1961.

Dix, M., and Hallpike, C., The peep-show; a new technique for pure tone audiometry in young children. Br. Med. J., 2, 719–723, 1947.

Downs, M., Current Overview of Newborn Hearing Screening. In Public Health Service, Dept. HEW, Conference on Newborn Hearing Screening, pp. 112–118. Washington: A.G. Bell Association, 1972.

Downs, M., The deafness management quotient. Hear. Speech News 42, 8–28, 1974.

Eisenberg, R., The development of hearing in man; an assessment of current status. ASHA, 12, 119–123, 1970.

Ewing, I., and Ewing, A., The ascertainment of deafness in infancy and early childhood. J. Laryngol., 59, 309–333, 1944.

Feinmesser, M., and Bauberger-Tell, L., Evaluation of Methods for Detecting Hearing Impairment in Infancy and Early Childhood. In Public Health Service, Dept. HEW, Conference on Newborn Hearing Screening, pp. 119–125. Washington: A.G. Bell Association, 1972.

Fisher, H., and Freedman, S., Localization of sound during simulated unilateral conductive hearing loss. Acta Otolaryngol. 66, 213–220, 1968.

Fulton, R., Auditory Stimulus-Response Control, Baltimore: Park Press, 1974.

Fulton, R., Gorzycki, P., and Hull, W., Hearing assessment with young children. J. Speech Hear. Disord., 40, 397–404, 1975.

Gatehouse, R., and Cox, W., Localization of sound by completely monaural deaf subjects. J. Aud. Res., 12, 179–183, 1972.

Goetzinger, C., Effects of small perceptive losses on language and on speech discrimination. Volta Rev., 64, 408–414, 1962.

Goetzinger, C., Harrison, C., and Barr, C., Small perceptive hearing loss; its effect in school-age children. Volta Rev., 65, 124–131, 1964.

Green, D., The pup show; a simple, inexpensive modification of the peep-show. J. Speech Hear. Disord., 23, 118–120, 1958.

Guilford, F., and Haug, C., Diagnosis of deafness in the very young child. Arch. Otolaryngol., 55, 101–106, 1952.

Hardy, W., and Bordley, J., Special techniques in testing the hearing of children. J. Speech Hear. Disord., 16, 122–131, 1951.

Haskins, H., A phonetically balanced test of speech discrimination for children. Unpublished master's thesis, Northwestern University, 1949.

Haug, C., Baccaro, P., and Guilford, F., A pure-tone audiogram on the infant; the PIWI technique. *Arch. Otolaryngol.*, **86**, 101–106, 1967.

Heron, T., and Jacobs, R., Respiratory curve responses of the neonate to auditory stimulation. *Int. Audiol.*, **8**, 77–84, 1969.

Hieber, T., Matkin, N., Cherow-Skalka, E., and Rice, C., A preliminary investigation of a sound effects recognition test (SERT). Paper presented at the American Speech and Hearing Association Convention, 1975.

Hodgson, W., Misdiagnosis of children with hearing loss. *J. Sch. Health*, **39**, 571–575, 1969.

Hodgson, W., A comparison of WIPI and PB-K discrimination test scores. Paper presented at the meeting of the American Speech and Hearing Association, Detroit, October 1973.

Hudgins, C. Auditory training; its possibilities and limitations. *Volta Rev.*, **56**, 339–349, 1954.

Jones, K., and Studebaker, G., Performance of severely hearing-impaired children on a closed-response, auditory speech discrimination test. *J. Speech Hear. Res.*, **17**, 531–540, 1974.

Keaster, J., A quantitative method of testing the hearing of young children. *J. Speech Disord.*, **12**, 159–160, 1947.

Kendall, D., Pediatrics and disorders in communication; the audiological examination of young children. *Volta Rev.*, **66**, 734–740, 1966.

Knox, E., A method of obtaining pure-tone audiograms in young children. *J. Laryngol.*, **74**, 475–479, 1960.

Lerman, J., Ross, M., and McLauchlin, R., A picture-identification test for hearing-impaired children. *J. Aud. Res.*, **5**, 273–278, 1965.

Liden, G., and Kankkunen, A., Visual reinforcement audiometry. *Acta Otolaryngol.*, **67**, 281–292, 1969.

Lowell, E., Rushford, G., Hoversten, G., and Stoner, M., Evaluation of pure-tone audiometry with pre-school age children. *J. Speech Hear. Disord.*, **21**, 292–302, 1956.

Marquis, D., Can conditioned response be established in the newborn infant? *J. Genet. Psychol.*, **39**, 479–492, 1931.

Martin, F., and Coombs, S., A tangibly reinforced speech reception threshold procedure for use with small children. *J. Speech Hear. Disord.*, **41**, 333–338, 1976.

Matkin, N., Hearing Aids for Children. In Hodgson, W., and Skinner, P. (Eds.), *Hearing Aid Assessment and Use in Audiologic Habilitation*, Ch. 9, pp. 145–169. Baltimore: Williams & Wilkins, 1977.

Mencher, G., A program for neonatal hearing screening. *Audiology*, **13**, 495–500, 1974.

Mencher, G. (Ed.), *Proceedings of the Nova Scotia Conference on Early Detection of Hearing Loss*. Basel: S. Karger, 1976.

Merklein, R., and Briskey, T., Audiometric findings in children referred to a program for language disorders. *Volta Rev.*, **64**, 295–298, 1962.

Meyerson, L., Hearing for speech in children; A verbal audiometric test. *Acta Otolaryngol.*, Suppl. 128, 1956.

Moore, J., Wilson, W., and Thompson, G., Visual reinforcement of head-turn responses in infants under twelve months of age. *J. Speech Hear. Disord.* **42**, 328–334, 1977.

Myatt, B., and Landes, B., Assessing discrimination loss in children. *Arch. Otolaryngol.*, **77**, 359–362, 1963.

Northern, J., and Downs, M., *Hearing in Children*. Baltimore: Williams & Wilkins, 1974.

O'Neill, J., Oyer, H., and Hillis, J., Audiometric procedures used with children. *J. Speech Hear. Disord.*, **26**, 61–66, 1961.

Reichstein, J., and Rosenstein, J., Differential diagnosis of auditory deficits; a review of the literature. *Except. Child.*, **31**, 73–82, 1964.

Rosenberg, P., Misdiagnosis of children with auditory problems. *J. Speech Hear. Disord.*, **31**, 279–282, 1966.

Ross, M., and Lerman, J., A picture identification test for hearing-impaired children. *J. Speech Hear. Res.*, **13**, 44–53, 1970.

Ross, M., and Matkin, N., The rising audiometric configuration. *J. Speech Hear. Disord.*, **32**, 377–382, 1967.

Siegenthaler, B., and Haspiel, B., Development of two standardized measures of hearing for speech by children. Cooperative Research Program, Project No. 2372, United States Office of Education, 1966.

Siegenthaler, B., Pearson, J., and Lezak, R., A speech reception threshold test for children. *J. Speech Hear. Disord.*, **19**, 360–366, 1954.

Simmons, F., Automated Hearing Screening Test for Newborns. In Mencher, G. (Ed.), *Proceedings of the Nova Scotia Conference on Early Detection of Hearing Loss*, pp. 171–180. Basel: S. Karger, 1976.

Simmons, F., and Russ, F., Automated newborn hearing screening, the crib-o-gram. *Arch. Otolaryngol.*, **100**, 1–7, 1974.

Smith, K., and Hodgson, W., The effects of systematic reinforcement on the speech discrimination responses of normal and hearing-impaired children. *J. Audit. Res.*, **10**, 110–117, 1970.

Steinschneider, A., Lipton, E., and Richmond, J., Auditory sensitivity in the infant; effect of intensity on cardiac and motor responsivity. *Child Develop.*, **37**, 233–252, 1966.

Suzuki, T., and Ogiba, Y., Conditioned orientation reflex audiometry. *Arch Otolaryngol.*, **74**, 192–198, 1961.

Thorne, B., Conditioning children for pure-tone testing. *J. Speech Hear. Disord.*, **27**, 84–85, 1962.

Wedenberg, E., Objective audiometry tests on non-cooperative children. *Acta Otolaryngol.*, Suppl. 175, 1963.

Wedenberg, E., Auditory Tests on Newborn Infants. In Cunningham, G. (Ed.), *Conference on Newborn Hearing Screening*, pp. 126–131. Washington: A.G. Bell Association, 1972.

Wertheimer, M. Psychomotor coordination of auditory and visual space at birth. *Science*, **134**, 1692, 1961.

chapter 34

AUDITORY PERCEPTION IN CHILDREN WITH LEARNING DISABILITIES

Jack A. Willeford, Ph.D., and Joan M. Billger, M.A.

Traditional audiologic tests have been shown to be valid and reliable methods of evaluating the auditory system. Unfortunately, it is now recognized that the standard tests primarily evaluate the peripheral auditory mechanisms. The more subtle deficiencies of auditory functioning in many patients with brain lesions and learning disabilities (LD) may elude detection on standard hearing tests. The probable reason lies in the complexity of the auditory system and the highly transient nature of sound which, when combined, make audition difficult to study. Thus, although interest in central auditory behaviors has increased dramatically in recent years, our professional activity in this area is seriously lagging. Evidence may be found in the proceedings of a "state of the art" study conducted at the University of Arizona's Institute for Learning Disabilities Leadership Training (1972). Among the total of 846 pages in this two-volume report, there were numerous references on achievement, dyslexia, etc., but no full sections (or even pages) were devoted to auditory perception. A most revealing statistic is the fact that only 34 references on auditory perception were listed among the 1281 entries in the bibliography as compared to 482 references on visual problems, reading disorders, etc. In most LD literature, the discussion of visual-perceptual problems dominates the contents because relatively little is available on auditory deficits (Aten, 1972).

It became the purpose of this chapter to present a brief overview of the state-of-the-art in evaluation of auditory perceptual processes in children with LD. In so doing, it is the authors' intent to stimulate much wider interest in such evaluations among audiologists. Indeed, it is an unmet area of responsibility which demands our attention.

In view of the dichotomy of sophistication between peripheral and central auditory processes, it is useful to briefly review the anatomical and physiologic systems as they are presently understood.

ANATOMY AND PHYSIOLOGY OF THE CENTRAL AUDITORY PATHWAYS

The primary fibers of the auditory pathway arise in the spiral ganglion located in the modiolus at the foundation of the cochlea. Distal fibers of the spiral ganglion are stimulated by the organ of Corti and the proximal fibers extend to form the cochlear nerve. The fibers of the cochlear nerve bifurcate and then terminate at the dorsal and ventral tonotopically arranged cochlear nuclei after entering the brain stem at the junction of the medulla and pons (Everett, Sundsten and Lund, 1971; Matzke and Foltz, 1972; Whitfield, 1967; Butcher and Bueker, 1969; Carpenter, 1972). Messages have now been transferred to the ipsilateral cochlear nuclei for recoding of the neural signal (Carhart, 1969). The central auditory pathway begins at the synapse between the first- and second-order neurons of the afferent pathway in the cochlear nuclei (Jerger, 1973).

In nerve VIII and the lower brain stem region, the "bottleneck principle" is an important diagnostic concept to consider. This principle states that the transmission of complex stimuli such as speech comes across a labyrinth or "bottleneck" in nerve VIII and lower brain stem area. If a lesion occurs in this tract, marked reduction in the comprehension of speech messages will be observed (Jerger, 1960).

Researchers have reported test results for patients with brain stem lesions. However, the data are conflicting (Jerger, 1960, 1964; Eichel, Hedgecock and Williams, 1966; Parker, Decker and Richards, 1968; Miller and Daly, 1967; Shapiro, 1969). Jerger and Jerger (1975a), have recently reported that patients with carefully defined extra-axial lesions (outside of the brain stem) will usually exhibit decreased performance when administered the conventional differential diagnostic test battery. These patients demonstrated abnormal audiologic results for the ear ipsilateral to the confirmed extra-axial lesion. In contrast, lesions involving the intra-axial brain stem region (inside the brain stem) yielded fairly normal results. Decreased performance on a low redundancy speech test was evidenced for intra-axial lesions in the ear contralateral to the disorder. This finding would seem to explain the variation of results reported for lesions in the brain stem area. That is, those studies which report abnormal results on standard hearing tests may have included subjects with brain stem lesions that also involved nerve VIII. However, Katz (1976) and others have found patients with brain stem involvement, without nerve VIII lesions, to show sharply abnormal audiologic results on conventional differential tests. Thus, the controversy continues with seemingly reliable evidence to support each viewpoint.

From the cochlear nuclei, the complexity of

the central auditory system increases and the speech message can be transmitted to the auditory cortex by various routes. Because of these diverse paths and the redundant aspects of speech, lesions of the central auditory pathways tend not to manifest themselves on conventional audiometric tests. This has been referred to as the "subtlety principle" (Jerger, 1960). These factors are discussed in some detail by Bocca and Calearo (1963). They state that central auditory disorders are not evidenced on standard differential diagnostic tests of aural pathology. If there is a lesion in the central auditory system, the speech signal with its generic external redundant characteristics will be transmitted and interpreted in the auditory cortex. Therefore, a central auditory disorder can be best detected if the redundant factors of speech are minimized sufficiently to challenge the integrity of the higher auditory centers.

The majority of the fibers from the cochlear nuclei decussate and may terminate in the trapezoid body, the superior olivary complex, or the reticular formation (Carpenter, 1972). Because of the ipsilateral and contralateral routing of the fibers from the cochlear nuclei to the superior olivary complex and the trapezoid body, a binaural phenomenon is initiated at this level of the brain stem (Carhart, 1969). Localization ability is thought to occur at the superior olivary complex (Walsh, 1957; Galambos, Schwartzkopff and Rupert, 1959). However, Neff (1961) indicates that the temporal lobe is also an important contributor to localization ability.

At this stage in our discussion, a statement concerning the reticular formation is important in evaluating sensory integration and transmission. The reticular formation, also known as the reticular activating system (RAS), is a neural network in the central portion of the brain stem. The ascending RAS, which dispatches projections upward to the surface of the cerebral cortex, receives sensory input from every sensory modality and is influential in neural integration. French (1957) considers the reticular formation to be the principal control system in the central nervous system. This network has been described as a general alarm mechanism which, when activated by incoming sensory stimuli, arouses the cortex so that incoming information can be interpreted. Magoun (1963) refers to the RAS as discriminative, inferring that this system aids the cortex in selecting signals which are of focal importance while inhibiting others. Ayres (1972) has used this information to postulate that learning disabled children may have reticular systems which fail in the discrimination task and allow too many sensory signals to stimulate the child. This could preclude cognition of signals which carry pertinent information. We can hypothesize that a faulty RAS could also hinder the alerting process which is of paramount importance to the transmission of auditory information. An unalerted cortex is not prepared to perform efficiently. Perhaps it is the RAS itself which scrambles the impulses from any or all sensory systems. It is reasonable that inhibitory, facilitative and integrative functions may be disturbed in a variety of ways to account for the different types of behaviors observed in LD children. In some children their attention is continually interrupted as they are attracted to constantly changing signals in their environment. Other youngsters may suspend central nervous system (CNS) processing because of these changing stimuli. Such children seem to function efficiently only in the absence of competing sensory input. Moreover, sensory channels become "jammed" in unpredictable ways. In some cases competing sounds are the offenders, whereas, in others, visual stimuli seem to interfere with auditory processing more than ambient sounds. Goldstein (1967) has taken another position. He theorized that the reticular formation is not primarily a cortical alerting system. He believes the cerebral cortex is alerted via the "rapid transmission" lines of the central auditory system – the lateral lemnisci. When discriminatory action is necessary, efferent tracts from the cortex course through the RAS carrying auto-corrective and integrative messages.

From the trapezoid and superior olivary complex, the vast majority of ipsilateral and contralateral fibers extend to the appropriate lateral lemniscus, inferior colliculus, and medial geniculate body. At these levels, it is theorized that more recoding of binaural and monaural stimuli occurs (Carhart, 1969). Also, electrophysiologic studies disclose that the nucleus of the inferior colliculus might be an integration and reflex control center (Matzke and Foltz, 1972). In areas of the primary auditory projection pathway, tertiary fibers arise, such as in the superior olivary complex, decussations occur, and fibers terminate at various levels.

The medial geniculate body is the final subcortical level in the higher auditory system prior to fiber connections in the cortex. The synapse between the third- and fourth-order neurons in the medial geniculate bodies is considered the rostral termination of the brain stem (Carhart, 1969, and numerous classical sources).

A substantial body of evidence suggests that the human auditory system is finally represented by projections to both left and right temporal lobes from each ear (Sparks, Goodglass and Nickel, 1970; Kimura, 1961; Milner, Taylor and Sperry, 1968). It is also generally agreed that the crossed-pathways (contralateral) are the dominant pathways, and the same-side (ipsilateral) pathways serve a secondary role. Thus, each ear has a greater influence on its contralateral temporal lobe than it does on the direct ipsilateral temporal lobe. Basic to this discussion is the widely accepted fact that the left temporal lobe in most humans (consensus places the incidence at about 85%) is dominant for linguistic processes while the right temporal lobe is dominant for nonlinguistic functions. This characteristic is maintained even though there are important transverse connections between the two brain hemispheres via the corpus callosum. Thus, although both ears have representation in each hemisphere, the dominance characteristic significantly influences central auditory functions. These concepts are basic to understanding central auditory processes.

EVALUATION OF AUDITORY PERCEPTUAL PROCESSES

How many times have audiologists confidently told anxious parents, "I am pleased to tell you that our test results are absolutely normal. Any problem your youngster may have is not due to auditory factors." The basis for such statements is, of course, the finding that the child does have normal pure tone sensitivity and speech discrimination skills. These reassuring words are not warranted in many children with LD. Contemporary clinical audiology must go beyond the differential assessment of the peripheral auditory system if this population is to be adequately evaluated. One must include assessments of central auditory proficiency as well. To execute this task, a new set of clinical tools is required in order to identify the "hidden" dysfunctions of the central auditory nervous system (CANS). Unfortunately, we are still rather new at assessing the integrity of such anatomical mechanisms.

What sort of test constructions are necessary to tease out limited or disordered functions in the CANS? What is the influence, if any, on the child's behavior if test performance is depressed on a given site-of-lesion test? How do theoretical models and concepts compare with empirical clinical results and experimental data? What is the reliability of these measures of complex behavior? Is remediation possible? Feasible? Answers to these questions must await extensive research. For the present, however, considerable work has been done that can provide direction for future investigations. This work has been done, to a large extent, by our professional colleagues in other disciplines (speech pathology, psychology, and education). The work of audiologists constitutes an inordinately small part of these efforts, and should serve as a stimulus for concerted action by those of us whose major interest and expertise

is the science of hearing. The only audiologist (O'Neill, 1972) among 11 "specialists" at the Memphis State University First Annual Symposium on Auditory Processing and Learning Disabilities served simply as the program moderator for one session. O'Neill may have identified the reason why more audiologists have not contributed in the area of learning disabilities. He notes that some researchers (audiologists in our judgment) are concerned primarily with correlating central auditory deficits with the anatomical site-of-lesion in adults for diagnostic purposes. Others are interested in the relationships of central auditory function to academic and social behaviors. Both approaches contribute importantly, but a combination of the two is essential if we are to fully understand central auditory phenomena and to intelligently plan management strategies for the LD child. Thus, a plea is made for cooperative, interdisciplinary, research efforts.

EVALUATION OF CENTRAL AUDITORY FUNCTION

Numerous authors have identified what they feel to be the salient elements of audition, and have then devised a test or task which presumes to measure one or more of those elements. For example, Butler (1975) listed the following: (1) recognition of intonation pattern, (2) short and long term memory, (3) closure, (4) speech-sound discrimination, (5) auditory analysis, vigilance and synthesis and (6) association. She acknowledges that there are probably other characteristics, not yet thought of, which may be more important than those listed. Butler discussed the following sub-components of auditory perception:

1. Auditory vigilance
2. Figure-ground
3. Auditory analysis
4. Auditory discrimination
5. Auditory sequencing
6. Sequencing unrelated speech sounds
7. Intonation patterns
8. Auditory closure
9. Auditory synthesis
10. Auditory memory (for nonsense multisyllable words)
11. Auditory association.

These terms, and others used by Aten (1972), Witkin (1971), Wood (1972), Flowers, Costello and Small (1973), and Kirk, McCarthy and Kirk (1968) constitute a core of terms that attempt to define the complexities of audition. They stem largely from a variety of theoretical models and may, or may not, be important aspects of actual events occurring in human auditory perceptual experiences. More often than not, they are based on principles of language development and language use, and are difficult to isolate in clinical assessment. Witkin (1971) acknowledged that many of these concepts appear to overlap, or to occur in complicated simultaneous relationships, so that one does not know which concept is being evaluated. The APT (auditory perception training) training tapes* provide an excellent illustration of this problem. This series of tapes was created to train diverse aspects of audition, yet many involve tasks that are quite similar and overlap with requirements on other tapes that are supposed to train different auditory skills. Nonetheless, it is not uncommon for researchers to develop a single-feature test with little or no attempt to relate it to more global processes. It may also be that we simply do not know how to isolate or measure certain of these functions. At present, the degree to which any of these factors are important in themselves or in combination with other factors in some critical temporal or acoustical relationship is unknown. Despite the uncertainties, the literature provides stimulating reading for those interested in central auditory processes. Weener (1972) has recently presented an excellent review of theoretical models of auditory perception.

One of the most widely used tests for allegedly evaluating auditory perception is the Illinois Test of Psycholinguistic Abilities (ITPA). It contains a battery of five auditory subtests which were designed to measure reception, association, memory, closure, and sound blending (Kirk et al., 1968). It seems to be the "bible" for many speech clinicians in the sense that it is so widely used, either by itself or in conjunction with other tests — usually tests of speech discrimination (Wepman, 1958; Goldman, Fristoe and Woodcock, 1970; among others). Unfortunately, most tests of this type are administered by live voice and by different examiners in uncontrolled environments. Thus, we must question the reliability of these measures. Even when presented by tape, such as in the Goldman, Fristoe, Woodcock test (1970), the level, instrumentation, and environment are uncontrolled. The ITPA no doubt serves some useful functions, but we believe that its value in assessing auditory perception needs reevaluation. This view is also supported by Burns and Watson (1973) who, in a factor-analysis study of the ITPA, found little or no basis for the supposition that the Revised Edition of the ITPA measures the 10 distinct entities suggested by its 12 subtests. Rather, they suggest that no more than five abilities are measured

and that, if there are 10 distinct psycholinguistic abilities, the ITPA does not seem able to measure them separately and individually. One of the five factors which emerged from their analysis suggested a representation of general auditory language ability. This is an interesting finding in view of the fact that other recent data (Willeford, 1976a) have shown that many children with confirmed, auditory-based LD, score at normal or above age levels on the auditory subtests of the ITPA.

The Flowers-Costello tests of central auditory abilities (Flowers et al., 1973), the composite auditory perceptual test (CAPT) (Butler, Hedrick and Manning, 1973), the Goldman-Fristoe-Woodcock auditory skills test battery (GFWB) (Woodcock, 1976), are examples of recent tests that attempt to overcome some of the limitations of the earlier measures. At least stimulus generation can be held constant in these measures since all are recorded on magnetic tape. Other variables remain a problem, however. In the CAPT, for example, no mention is made of playback level or calibration of tape cassettes.

The GFWB manual has recommendations for use of their tapes which may be obtained in either reel-to-reel or cassette versions. The instructions with this battery merely state that the tapes should be played at "comfortably loud" levels. No calibration protocol is involved, and the examiner is advised to play the tapes on suitable equipment in environments which are quiet. Thus, again, a number of variables are subject to substantial changes in administering this battery. The CAPT and the GFWB were designed to test a series of theoretical auditory skills as shown in Table 34.1, which also includes the tests contained in the Flowers-Costello tapes.

It can be seen that the Flowers-Costello test is less comprehensive in the scope of functions it was designed to measure on the basis of the simple fact that it involves fewer tests than the other measures. However, its authors believe that their competing-message test evaluates an aspect of the CANS which other central auditory tests do not assess (Flowers et al., 1973). Moreover, they believe that this test alone could be utilized as a survey of overall development of auditory perceptual skills. On the basis of our experience, as shown in subsequent data, we feel that reliance on any single measure of central auditory function is ill-advised. However, the Flowers-Costello test can be recommended over the other tests, in our judgment, because of its superior design. Its creators stress the importance of controlling both the signal intensity and the test environment, an emphasis we strongly support. An electronic calibration system, and earphones set into protective earmuffs, may be obtained with, and

---

* Available from DLM (Developmental Learning Materials), 7440 Natchez Avenue, Niles, Illinois 60648.

TABLE 34.1. *Contents of the Flowers-Costello, Composite Auditory Perception Test (CAPT) and Goldman-Fristoe-Woodcock Battery (GFWB)*

Flowers-Costello	CAPT	GFWB
1. Low pass filtered speech (LPFS) 2. Competing messages (CM)	1. Selective listening 2. Figure-ground discrimination for dissimilar voices 3. Figure-ground discrimination for similar voices 4. Temporal sequencing 5. Speech sound analysis 6. Consonant discrimination 7. Vowel discrimination 8. Auditory closure 9. Auditory synthesis 10. Syllable recognition 11. Discrimination of linguistic forms 12. Discrimination of verb tense forms	1. Auditory selective attention against different noise backgrounds 2. Diagnostic auditory discrimination tests I, II, III 3. Auditory memory tests: Recognition memory Memory for content Memory for sequence 4. Sound-symbol tests: Mimicry Recognition Analysis Blending Speech symbol association Reading of symbols Spelling of sounds

are unique to, the Flowers-Costello tapes. Thus, much greater control of the test intensity level and the ambient noise level in the testroom (they still recommend that a quiet test room be used) can be exercised when the Flowers-Costello is administered by school clinicians. Clinic-based audiologists, of course, can play the tapes through calibrated playback units which are a part of sophisticated audiometers, and do so in sound-treated test rooms. This procedure would assure the highest degree of test standardization.

An interesting feature common to all three of the measures discussed above is the inclusion of a *competing-signal* task using various noises or speech as competition which is pitted against test items of speech signals. The test manuals present varying degrees of justification and rationale from research literature for including such a test in their respective batteries, ranging from none for the GFWB version to selected and limited references for the other two. One gets the impression in each case that such a procedure was chosen because it simulates a child's classroom and social experiences. The strongest case made for this point is found in the Flowers-Costello manual. The entire matter is treated very lightly in the other two test manuals. Witkin (1971) does discuss the work of Maccoby and Konrad (1966), and the classical experiments of Broadbent (1962) and Cherry (1953) which emphasize the marked differences between dichotic and diotic listening paradigms. However, after discussing those differences, the CAPT authors include only a diotic procedure without identifying which type it is, and offer no justification for its selection over a dichotic task. *Dichotic* tasks involve the simultaneous presentation of different signals to the two ears. *Diotic* tasks, on the other hand,

require the listener to decipher a signal which has been combined with a different signal in one or both ears.

The GFWB manual has some documentation as rationale for each of its tests *except* that of competing signals which the author (Woodcock, 1976) considers to be a test for "selective auditory attention." The point is of interest because of the wide attention given to dichotic listening tests in recent years (Berlin and McNeil, 1976; also see Chapters 22 and 23) as valid measures of cortical function and their well established relevance to the integrity of central auditory processes (Jerger and Jerger, 1975b; Lynn and Gilroy, 1975; and Katz, 1968). The Jergers have also shown that diotic tests, on the other hand, measure different central processes than do dichotic tests. This fact is not surprising since they are quite different tasks. Therefore, the exclusion of a dichotic test may be, in our judgment, a major omission from a central auditory test battery.

Some of the problems discussed above are illustrated in a study by Anderson and Novina (1973) who compared performances of 20 ethnic minority children on the ITPA auditory subtests (AST) and the Flowers-Costello test. For this population, a significant relationship was found between the competing message portion of the Flowers-Costello and three of the five ASTs of the ITPA (reception, association, and sound blending). There was no correspondence with the ASTs of memory and closure. The low-pass filtered speech (LPFS) portion of the Flowers-Costello, a presumed measure of closure, was not significantly related to the ITPAs closure subtest. Only "association" from the five ASTs of the ITPA was found to correlate significantly with the filtered subtest of the Flowers-Costello test. It appears that there are simply too many differences in the test construction, content, procedures and administration to draw meaningful comparisons between such diverse measures. However, the study did draw attention to the fact that there may be (and probably is) more than one type of closure process. One must also be wary of generalizing from a particular population. Moreover, we feel it is hazardous to rely on group data in drawing conclusions about the strengths or weaknesses of a given test in identifying a child with an auditory LD. Meaningful differences between LD children on single tests may range from very subtle to very dramatic, and reliance on group tendencies can often be misleading. Establishing a full range of performances on normal subjects seems to us to be the only feasible standard against which to judge whether an auditory processing problem exists in a given LD child.

Speech-in-Noise

One of the most common approaches to identifying the child with an auditory LD, according to limited literature and to audiologists of our acquaintance, is to measure the reception of speech in the presence of background noise or competing ambient speech. Some assess this very briefly by talking to a child in a soundfield while introducing white or complex noise as competition. This informal approach involves asking personal questions, presenting simple math problems, etc. A more formal approach which is used presents standard speech discrimination test lists in quiet and in the presence of fixed or varying levels of background noise. This may be done either in a soundfield or through earphones, but in the diotic mode. The presumption is that such an approach has been standardized on normal children.

A formal measure of speech-in-noise skill, which appears to be in fairly wide use by audiologists, speech pathologists, psychologists and otologists, is the taped Goldman-Fristoe-Woodcock (GFW) test of auditory discrimination (1970). Its stated purpose is for use as an index of a person's ability to discriminate speech under quiet and noisy conditions. This test is used by some clinicians as a screening measure for central auditory problems, but its lack of controls minimizes its value as a diagnostic clinical tool. This fact may be the reason why a variety of professionals have noted that some children score better on the noise subtest than they do on the quiet subtest.

Schubert, Meyer and Schmidt (1973) compared the noise-subtest (NS) of the GFW (NS-GFW) with Katz' staggered spondaic word (SSW) test on a group of normal young adults. The SSW has been found to reliably identify many patients with central auditory problems

(Katz, 1968), and its performance by normals has been well established (Brunt, 1972). Among the major findings by Schubert et al. were that subjects scoring in the normal range on the SSW (91 to 99%) ranged all the way from the first to the 99th percentile on the GFW (a range of 37 percentage points); little overlap was observed between the GFW test items found most difficult on the initial test versus a retest. They state that there is " . . . effectively zero correlation between test-retest on the NS-GFW. The NS-GFW cannot with our population be considered a reliable nor valid measure of central auditory function." In view of the different characteristics and natures of the two tests, one wonders whether meaningful comparison can be made between the SSW and the GFW. However, this study does raise some basic questions about the usefulness of the GFW.

Olsen, Noffsinger and Kurdziel (1975), Sinha (1959), Noffsinger et al. (1972), and Morales-Garcia and Poole (1972) have all suggested that speech discrimination deteriorates in the presence of white noise applied to the same ear in subjects with central auditory disorders. However, a major limitation of such tests would seem to be the wide range of scores observed among normal subjects and those with lesions at various anatomic sites. Morales-Garcia and Poole (1972) noted that bilaterally depressed scores were frequently found with subjects having brain stem lesions, but scores were always unilaterally diminished in temporal-lobe cases. However, they comment that since brain stem scores were *often* bilaterally depressed, any diagnostic significance attached to them depends on the clinician's ability to sort them out from normal behavior. Although the *majority* of their brain stem patients had much poorer scores than the *average* normal, a number of brain stem cases had comparable scores with those at the lower end of the normal discrimination range. Attention is directed to their use of the terms *majority* and *average*. We have already pointed out the limitations in using group data for clinical diagnosis.

Olsen et al. (1975) partially overcame this problem by attaching significance only to those scores which exceeded the normal "range of reduction" between the quiet and noise conditions. With a 0 dB signal-to-noise (S/N) ratio between Northwestern University Discrimination Test No. 6 and white noise the range was 56 to 94%. They ultimately considered differences greater than 40% as abnormal. On this basis, they found both normal and abnormal scores could be observed in noise trauma, Meniere's, eighth nerve tumor, temporal lobe, and multiple sclerosis populations, the latter two in spite of normal hearing sensitivity and excellent speech discrimination. Abnormal scores were observed in about 40% of their 24 subjects with temporal lobe lesions, and *always* in the ear contralateral to cortical insult. This laterality characteristic confirmed earlier observations by Sinha (1959) and Morales-Garcia and Poole (1972). Olsen et al. (1975) concluded that large differences in speech discrimination scores between quiet and noise conditions, especially when hearing sensitivity is normal or impaired only in the high frequencies probably reflect neural involvement of some portion of the auditory system. Therefore, they state that a speech-in-white noise test may have some value in identifying auditory dysfunction, but not in localizing the specific site of involvement.

Dayal, Tarantino and Swisher (1966) examined the discrimination-in-white-noise behavior of 14 patients with multiple sclerosis, and found 5 with reductions in discrimination which were out of proportion to their pure tone findings. They felt such scores could be attributed to CANS disturbance. It is difficult to draw comparisons between this study and others because they employed a S/N ratio of −10, and three different discrimination tests (CID W-22's, Rush Hughes—and there is a marked difference in the level of difficulty between these two tests, and two subjects were tested on a French test).

Heilman, Hammer, and Wilder (1973) evaluated a series of 18 subjects with temporal lobe dysfunction using W-22 word lists. However, they used *complex* noise at several S/N ratios as a competing signal. They also found that discrimination was reduced in noise in *both* ears of their subjects—but especially in the contralateral ear. They observed that subjects with temporal lobectomies had notably greater reduction with competing noise than did a group of subjects with temporal lobe seizures. This finding corresponds with that of Olsen et al. (1975) who compared temporal lobectomy patients with a group having suffered cerebrovascular accidents.

A major limitation of the speech-in-noise tests in each of these studies would seem to lie in the fact that only "portions" of each population studied had abnormal scores. Thus, it would appear that dependence solely on speech-in-noise tests represents a rather cavalier approach to the diagnostic process.

A final point of interest is found in the sharp contrast in results of the foregoing studies using white or complex noise competition, and findings of Jerger and Jerger (1975a) using competing speech. The latter produced a deficit in performance that was peculiar exclusively to *brain stem* dysfunction, particularly on the contralateral side. Stated differently, the Jer-

gers found normal performance bilaterally in their temporal lobe subjects, whereas the speech-in-noise studies found contralateral ear scores inordinately reduced in certain temporal lobe patients. Perhaps the difference is due to linguistic versus nonlinguistic competition. Heilman et al. (1973) did note that the discrimination defect caused by complex-noise competition did not appear to be related to language since there was no difference between patients with lesions in the dominant and nondominant hemispheres.

It seems evident that one should utilize speech-in-noise with appropriate caution, even as a screening device.

Other Procedures

Time-compressed speech has long been a phenomenon of interest to workers in speech science and perceptual processes. However, only in recent years has it been employed as a measure of documented central auditory processes (Bocca et al., 1954, 1955, and Bocca and Calearo, 1963; Calearo and Lazzaroni, 1957; Kurdzeil and Noffsinger, 1973) or linguistic behaviors (Orchik and Oeschlaeger, 1974; Ormson and Williams, 1975). One major thrust of recent studies has been to standardize accelerated-discrimination lists on children (Maki, Beasley and Orchik, 1974; Beasley, Schwimmer and Rintleman, 1972; Beasley, Forman and Rintleman, 1973; Sanderson and Rintleman, 1971). Another area of interest has been to compare the relationship of children with articulation disorders (Orchik and Oeschlager, 1974) and articulation disorders combined with reading deficiencies (Ormson and Williams, 1975) with speeded-speech performance. The evidence from these studies indicates the need for further investigation, but does suggest that time-compressed speech may be a useful method of looking at central auditory function.

One of the most effective and widely used approaches by audiologists is the staggered spondaic word (SSW) test mentioned earlier. This test, and its application to central auditory disorders—including those in children, has been thoroughly documented (Katz, 1968; Myrick, 1965; Lynn and Gilroy, 1975; Morrill, 1969; Brunt, 1972; Stubblefield and Young, 1975; Jerger and Jerger, 1975b). Recently, Schoenfeld (1975) has also used it successfully on a large population of children in the St. Louis Special School District.

Other approaches to the study and assessment of auditory perception in children with LD have been described in a variety of professional literature which has been reviewed in detail by Katz and Illmer (1972). Because of space limitations, no attempt will be made to rereview that information.

Northern and Downs (1974) have reviewed literature which focuses on the CANS mechanisms responsible for sound localization/lateralization. However, no standard clinical approach is yet available to measure these processes. The situation is similar for the "masking-level" differences phenomenon, although Noffsinger et al. (1972) have shown that the procedure has promise. Measurement of the acoustic reflex, especially since we now have ipsilateral measurement capabilities, also shows encouraging possibilities as a technique for identifying low brain stem pathology (Bosatra, Russolo and Poli, 1976; Jerger and Jerger, 1975a; Jerger and Jerger, 1975c). This approach is encouraging because of the appeal of objectivity, brevity and simplicity in reflex measurements, and because they can be administered to deaf and nonfluent subjects. It also has immediate utility for young children. Finally, a move toward the measurement of CANS integrity by electrophysiologic techniques such as brain-stem evoked response (BSER) is also gaining momentum. A review of this approach may be found in Mokotoff, Galambos, and Galambos, 1977.

AN EXPERIMENTAL BATTERY FOR LD CHILDREN

We have used a four-test battery of central auditory measures for the past 3 years with gratifying results. These tests, which have been described elsewhere (Willeford, 1976a, 1976b), involve procedures that challenge two aspects each of cortical and brain stem integrity as confirmed on adult patients with carefully defined lesions (Lynn and Gilroy, 1972, 1975; Lynn et al., 1972; Lynn, 1973, 1975). The battery involves tests of: (1) dichotically competing messages (sentences), (2) filtered consonant-nucleus-consonant (CNC) words, (3) a binaural-fusion technique involving the dichotic presentation of complementary portions of sharply filtered spondaic words and (4) an alternating speech task. Ivey (1969) recorded this version of the binaural fusion principle described earlier by Matzker (1959, 1962). Fortunately, these tests were designed so that the performances of "sick" patients and persons with limited literacy levels would not be penalized. The tests were subsequently found to be applicable to children down to the age of 5 years. Norms were established on youngsters who were judged to have adequate intelligence and health, and who were performing successfully in school.

Better than 90% of the children referred to us with suspected central auditory problems have failed one or more of the tests in our battery. The distribution and pattern of results on a population of 150 LD subjects are shown in Tables 34.2 and 34.3. Table 34.2 presents the number of children from that population who scored abnormally on each of the four tests, while Table 34.3 reveals the number of youngsters failing one or more of the tests as a function of inter-test combinations. For example Table 34.3 shows that 30 subjects failed the binaural fusion test alone, and that 23 subjects failed both the filtered-speech and binaural-fusion tests. This was the most frequently occurring combination followed by the competing sentence/filtered speech combination. At the other end of the scale, only one subject failed the alternating speech test by itself or in combination with either filtered speech or competing sentences. Table 34.2 indicates that binaural fusion is the task most often failed, and alternating speech is the task least often failed. Both tests, interestingly, are measures of auditory functions at the brain stem level. However, the data clearly suggest that these tests challenge different subcortical processes as demonstrated by Lynn (1975). Alternating speech always elicits the most dramatic subjective response of the four tests when played during demonstrations for parents, teachers, and others with normal central processing skills. However, the test presents a simple task for even normal five-year-olds. Binaural fusion, on the other hand, is a demanding task which requires ideal test conditions and great concentration in order for normals to perform adequately.

Table 34.4 presents data obtained on a series of 6-year-olds which illustrate the wide range of results that may be observed in children. Even the range of norms is wide and serves as testimony to the hazards of using means for clinical purposes. The binaural fusion test is arbitrarily labeled according to the ear receiving the low-band stimulus, whereas alternating speech is labeled according to the ear in which the stimulus sentence begins.

TABLE 34.2. *Distribution of Abnormal Results by Test (N = 150 Learning Disability (LD) Subjects)*

Competing Sentences	Filtered Speech	Binaural Fusion	Alternating Speech
73 (48%)	86 (57%)	96 (64%)	27 (18%)

TABLE 34.3. *Patterns of Abnormal Test Results on 150 Learning Disability (LD) Subjects*

	A	B	C	F	CF
–	1	30	7	19	20
A	–	9	1	1	3
B	–	–	13	23	14
AB	–	–	2	3	4

A, alternating speech; B, binaural fusion; C, competing sentences; F, filtered speech.

Tables 34.5 and 34.6 reflect similar trends in test performance with two older age groups.

We have recently added to our battery a test of compressed speech† and the synthetic-sentence-identification test with ipsilateral competing message (SSI-ICM) described by Jerger and Jerger (1975b). The latter test is discussed in detail in Chapter 22.

It is too soon for us to draw comparisons of the latter two measures with our current test battery, but their addition does provide us with three measures each of cortical and subcortical processes. Some interesting relationships are

† Supplied by Kerry Ormson, Amarillo Speech and Hearing Center, Texas.

evolving, but we are reserving judgments until we have accumulated more data.

IMPLICATIONS OF AN AUDITORY PROCESSING DISORDER

Over the years, parents, teachers and other school personnel have aided us in developing a behavioral profile of LD children with confirmed auditory processing problems. Educationally, these children are frequently non-achievers or "academic failures." This is often a perplexing problem for both teachers and parents because the child has been shown to have the native skills to achieve but has not performed up to his potential. As previously stated, a central auditory processing disorder

TABLE 34.4. *Data Illustrating Diversity of Results Observed in Younger Learning Disability (LD) Children*

Subject	Age	Competing Sentences L–R	Filtered Speech L–R	Binaural Fusion L–R	Alternating Speech L–R
AM	6.0	*20–30*	*0–0*	*10–30*	*60–50*
GT	6.0	90–100	*42–62*	*10–15*	100–100
TM	6.1	*10–80*	70–84	75–55	100–100
JS	6.2	*0–40*	52–52	*0–10*	*50–50*
HD	6.3	*70–40*	56–*36*	55–90	90–100
Range for normals age 6		0/100*	44/74†	40/95	90/100

* Developmental norms are discussed in detail in Chapter 22. Six-year-olds generally score 100% in one ear, but generally score very poorly in the other ear at this age.
† The range of performance is rather wide among normals at all age levels, but the two ears are generally within 10% of each other. Greater differences between ears are significant.
Abnormal scores, in percent, are shown in italics.

TABLE 34.5. *Data Illustrating Diversity of Results Observed in a Group of Intermediate-Age Learning Disability (LD) Children*

Subject	Age	Competing Sentences L–R	Filtered Speech L–R	Binaural Fusion L–R	Alternating Speech L–R
DL	9.0	90–90	*54–48*	*20–5*	100–100
JL	9.0	*0–30*	70–*54*	90–65	100–100
JA	9.2	100–100	76–72	*0–20*	*20–30*
RH	9.5	*20–10*	68–*48*	60–65	100–70
OW	9.11	*0–0*	*12–16*	80–80	*60–90*
Range for normals age 9		70/100	60/96*	40/90	90/100

* The two ears are generally within 10% of each other in this range, but both ears can be below the norm.
Abnormal scores, in percent, are shown in italics.

TABLE 34.6. *Data Illustrating Diversity of Results Observed in an Older Group of Learning Disability (LD) Subjects*

Subject	Age	Competing Sentences L–R	Filtered Speech L–R	Binaural Fusion L–R	Alternating Speech L–R
BH	13	90–100	94–88	*10–30*	100–100
DH	13	*40–90*	*34–36*	55–80	90–100
DSt	16	100–*50*	*18–2*	80–80	100–100
DSc	18	100–100	32–32	*50–35*	*80–80*
RP	20	100–*70*	*40–44*	*20–20*	100–100
Normals above age 10		90/100	70/100*	75/100	90/100

* The two ears are generally within 10% of each other in this range, but both ears can be below the norm.
Abnormal scores, in percent, are shown in italics.

hinders the reception and, therefore, the interpretation of auditory information, especially when presented in an environment which has auditory and visual distractions. Therefore, one can readily appreciate the frustration involved in trying to learn new concepts under such difficult conditions. One student recently reported to his teacher that his "brain was scrambling." Others, when in such an environment, would cover their ears with their hands or seek a quieter place in the classroom so they could attempt to complete their assignments. Observations have shown that the LD child seems to perform better in a traditional classroom than when placed in an open-type classroom with its multiple visual and auditory distractions.

Children with LD are commonly characterized as hyperactive. However, on the basis of our clinical observations, case histories, and discussions with parents and teachers, hyperactive children with auditory processing difficulties which result in LD simply represent one end of a pattern of kinetic activity. At the other end of the scale is the lethargic child who has trouble beginning academic assignments and seldom completes a given task. The latter child has poor motor skills, such as writing, and has a poor attitude toward motor tasks. Thus, children with auditory perception problems may be either hyperactive or hypoactive. The hyperactive child is also often termed a behavioral problem. This is the child that uses various antics to seek additional attention or relieve frustration in the classroom. He is the child who fails to comprehend instructions, and expresses his frustrations in physical ways. In contrast, the hypoactive child is passive, reserved, lethargic, and gradually struggles through school as a little noticed low achiever. He has been described as the child who "fades into the woodwork." These youngsters are typically fatigued, especially after school, according to parents. Such fatigue is the result of exhaustion in overcoming external distractions (Martin, 1976). He has to call upon a much greater supply of resources than other children in order to attend and to sort out the important auditory events in the classroom. In our judgment, the same may be true in daily living activities. However, the latter probably occurs to a lesser degree and with fewer adverse consequences.

Although these two groups are complete opposites with regard to activity levels, they have several attainment and conceptual attitudes in common. On a daily basis, teachers have noted that the youngster with reduced auditory perceptual skills often has difficulty following verbal instructions, completing class assignments and in attending to his classwork. An excuse is usually offered prior to even attempting a task,

such as "I can't do that." It appears that these children have experienced such frequent failure they are trapped in a failure cycle and commonly "give up" before trying to tackle assignments. If they do start an assignment, they may not understand it or else are easily distracted and usually do not complete the lesson. To illustrate this concept, a recent discussion with a teacher concerning a student with a confirmed central auditory processing problem disclosed that this first grader had never completed one assignment the entire year. He would usually "give up" and offer various excuses for the failure to complete his daily lessons. The parents of the child reported that he would come home from school extremely exhausted and would usually retire to his quiet room instead of going outside to play with the neighborhood children. We inferred that this behavior was a result of trying to isolate important auditory information amidst extraneous auditory and visual input, thus creating considerable fatigue and frustration. Already, at 6 years of age, this child was experiencing failure which was beginning to erode his self-concept.

We believe that children who perform poorly on tests of brain stem integrity may have their auditory attention diverted by visual distractions as well as by ambient auditory events. The basis for this assumption stems from classroom observations where movement or other visual stimuli appear to suspend or disrupt auditory processing. We believe this breakdown in the coordination of multisensory impulses may be due to dysfunctions in the reticular activating system, the thalamus, or other limbic system mechanisms (Schnitker, 1972; Ayres, 1972; Hernandez-Peon, 1961).

A discussion has been presented concerning the academic implications of a central auditory processing dysfunction; however, this section would not be complete without a statement regarding classroom acoustics. As gleaned from various studies (Sanders, 1965; Slater, 1968; Nober, 1973) the sound levels of unoccupied elementary classrooms far exceed the recommended sound level of 30 dBA. Nober (1973), for example, reported the average sound level in four elementary classrooms she analyzed to be about 65 dBA. Niemoeller (1968) indicates that sound levels of empty classrooms with normal surrounding activity should not exceed the NC-25 curve which is interpreted as a noise level not exceeding 30 dBA. Furthermore, Sanders (1965) reported that the S/N ratio found in classrooms ranging from elementary to high school levels was approximately +5 dB.

Mills (1975) has presented an interesting survey of research studies which relate the influence of noise on communication efficiency for both children and adults, and on language acquisition for children. Although he states that data concerning the effects of noise on a child's development of auditory perceptual skills are limited, Kryter (1970, p. 80) reported that sound levels of 60+ dBA interfered with auditory communication for normal hearing young adults when they were three feet from the speaker. Miller (1974) has reported similar values. In addition, Holm and Kunze (1969) indicate that periodic reduction in speech loudness levels can have a detrimental effect on the acquisition of speech and language in children. Mills (1975) also concludes that noise levels which do not interfere with the reception of speech by adults may do so significantly with the perception of speech by children. He states that these seemingly harmless noise levels may also interfere with their acquisition of speech, language, and language related skills.

The data from these noise surveys and subsequent adult performance demonstrate the need for reduced extraneous noise levels and acoustic treatment in our classrooms today. The additional distraction that ambient noise produces for the auditory LD child in the classroom can be dramatically illustrated by his unexplained sub-par performance in the educational setting. That is, they seem to have no problems other than auditory processing difficulties that could explain poor classroom achievement. However, when distractions are minimized or eliminated, these youngsters typically show marked improvement.

Psychological-Social Profile

Many of our referrals for central auditory testing have been initiated by psychologists in the surrounding area. With the majority of cases, parents have arranged for psychological consultation because their children have been failing academically without apparent cause, or have become behavior problems at home or at school. In some instances teachers recommend the psychological referral. Psychologists, in turn, request the central auditory processing evaluation if the youngster has shown inattentive behavior, decreased performance on verbal subtests in the psychological test battery, and decreased attainment on the Wide Range Achievement Test (WRAT) as compared to their intelligence quotients (Meyer, 1975). A common clue observed by parents and teachers is that the child simply does not seem to understand verbal instructions. Unlike some learning disabled children, they often do not have associated visual difficulties and their reading skills are acceptable. However, spelling and other memory tasks are frequently poor. These children range from 4 to 18 years of age, and the scale of their intellectual capacity spans dull normal to superior intellect.

The emotional and antisocial overlays associated with academic failure are oftentimes devastating for these children. Feelings of inadequacy, rejection, unacceptability, and depression saturate these children even as young as 9 years of age. At age 14, some of these individuals manifest intense emotional problems and resort to drugs, asocial acting out, destructive behavior, and fantasy suicides (Meyer, 1975). Perhaps the reason for these feelings and resultant behavior originated from perpetual failure associated with parental disappointment. The alarming factor when viewing the social-psychological implications of an auditory perception problem is that the failure cycle may commence during the first and second grade of school.

Interpersonal relationships are often difficult for these children. We find that such youngsters are often labeled "loners" by parents and teachers because of their inability to socialize adequately with other children their own age. This may be a product of shattered self-confidence, negative reinforcement and ridicule. These children often seek solace and companionship from older children, adults, or children younger than themselves. One such teenager occupied his time by developing explosives. His "hobby" was discovered when he destroyed a portion of the family residence.

Although some children may compensate for their difficulties and have normal interpersonal relationships and social development, others may have marked difficulties. In essence, a central auditory processing disorder might have negative effects on academic performance and social well being.

Medical Implications

There is a close correspondence between central auditory test results and confirmed CNS lesions in adults. However, most of the children with auditory LD problems appear neurologically normal or indicate only minimal dysfunction. Schoenfeld (1975) has found some of the same type of abnormal signs on the SSW test in children that are associated with CNS disturbances when found in adults. He has also shown a positive correlation between abnormal electroencephalographic (EEG) and SSW results for these children with auditory perceptual problems. The type of dysfunction one seeks to identify in some LD children may be subcortical or so subtle that it does not show up significantly on the EEG just as it may elude detection by the ITPA and the Wepman test. Early identification, extensive counseling and proper management are necessary for circumventing a detriment to the individual and his environment. However, if a child is experiencing headaches, black-outs, or sudden auditory-visual problems, an immediate referral for neurologic evaluation is indicated.

Remediation

Numerous pamphlets and books have been written on auditory perceptual training and remediation with the primary goal of improving the child's reading and language skills (Herr, 1968; Oakland and Williams, 1971; Barr, 1972; Eden, Green and Hansen, 1973; Reagan, 1973; Gillet, 1974; Heasley, 1974; Behrmann, undated). Therapy objectives such as environmental localization, sequencing, rhythm, awareness, discrimination (gross and fine) and memory tasks have been stressed in remediating auditory-based learning disabilities. Frankly, we have not found these techniques to dramatically improve the child's ability to consistently perceive and integrate auditory information. When considering remedial training it appears that we are focusing on two distinct categories of children: (1) language delay and (2) academic failure. If the child has a language delay, the therapy techniques are apparent. However, how does one remediate an "auditory perceptual disorder" without a concomitant language disorder? This child's problem has become obvious only after experiencing considerable academic difficulties or social acting-out which has led to psychological counseling. Therapy techniques such as loud-soft distinction, high-low pitch identification, noisemaker discrimination, rhythm drills (marching and clapping) do not seem appropriate for the youngster who has difficulty perceiving auditory information in a distracting environment. Can we actually remediate an organic-based problem affecting the brain stem or cortex regions so that a child can function normally in various acoustic environments? Again, we feel, the concept of language deficiency and a central auditory processing dysfunction must be isolated prior to implementing various therapeutic techniques.

It seems feasible that therapy techniques may one day be devised for helping the auditory-based LD child cope with his perceptual difficulties. Ayres (1972) indicates that the ultimate goal of a sensory therapeutic plan is for an individual to react and conduct himself meaningfully in response to the requirements of his environment. Once the child can cope with the various demands and succeed, he can then break the failure cycle. Undue structure, inappropriate developmental demands, and tasks that terminate in perpetual failure will not aid the child in coping with his problem, but will only add to his frustration. The child must learn to compensate for his disability, which may mean controlling himself so that various new experiences are not devastating.

Thus far, our discussion concerning remediation has presented therapy techniques which are not appropriate for the child experiencing academic difficulties at school and daily living conflicts at home. Fortunately, we have found an approach which can have a substantial effect on the child's ability to cope with various auditory environments in his daily life. This procedure involves counseling the child, family, and educational personnel concerning auditory perceptual problems and controls for coping with the auditory world.

We have developed some practical guidelines for teachers and parents based on our experience. These suggestions, summarized below, have resulted in optimistic reports, especially from parents. The suggestions are easier to implement at home than at school where teachers must be concerned with many other children. The guidelines are not equally applicable for each child. Therefore, flexibility and understanding are extremely important for success.

Suggestions for Teachers

1. Since children with central auditory processing deficiencies have difficulty listening, maintaining attention, or separating auditory figure-ground information, all extraneous noises and visual stimuli should be minimized especially when giving instructions or teaching new concepts. Teachers should always command the child's attention, if necessary, by either implementing verbal or physical cues such as calling his name prior to the instruction or lightly touching his shoulder.

2. Directions are best understood when presented in clear, well-articulated, and simply constructed sentences with an avoidance of complex or compound sentence structures. Also, new information should be separated into small, well-defined segments.

3. Periodic feedback should be required from the child to ensure that he is listening to the speech message. Such practice may also enhance his listening habits since he knows that he will be expected to recall the instructions or class material.

4. Instructions may need to be repeated following each class on an individual basis if the child has not been able to comprehend the material. The teacher is encouraged to have the child repeat what he thinks was said, rather than whether or not he understood the material. An assignment book may also be a helpful tool.

5. If the child also has visual-motor difficulties, reduce the amount of written responses you require of him. A tape recorder may be an ideal device in this teaching process in that you may record lessons or instructions on tape to be reviewed by the child at a later time. Also, the

child may use the tape recorder for verbal completion of assignments instead of traditional written exercises.

6. Move into new areas of academic instruction gradually, always reviewing past material so that the child can experience some degree of success.

7. Since memory is best for real-life events or occurrences, experiential approaches to learning would be beneficial. Parents can help supplement academic material in this manner if a coordinated liaison can be established between home and school.

8. New concepts and information can be complemented by providing reading material at his level.

9. Give the child praise and reinforcement for even minimal improvement. Encouragement and support are key factors in developing patterns of success.

10. Various seating arrangements in the classroom should be tried in order to locate an area of maximum auditory reception. This position has been found to vary according to a particular child's needs. For instance, front placement would seem to be a logical setting; however, some children perform best several rows from the front. It appears that certain youngsters can supplement their auditory deficiency with visual cues in monitoring both the teacher and their classmates. Seating away from frequent traffic areas, such as doorways and pencil sharpeners, is desirable. Finally, in those children showing asymmetry between ears on dichotic listening tests, seating with their strong ear toward the teacher (speaker) is helpful.

11. Sound-attenuating earmuffs and earplugs have been helpful in eliminating background noise when the child is working individually at his desk, or during any task where auditory competition is present. Ideally, several pairs of earmuffs should be available for students who wish to eliminate extraneous noise in order to concentrate on their assignments. If other children are free to use earmuffs the LD child will not be singled out. We have also observed that children who needed the muffs initially learned to compensate for the noisy conditions and therefore decreased the use of the device. School children have expressed a preference for American Optical's Model 1600 muffs over several types with which we experimented.

12. FM auditory training units have been used successfully with children who had central auditory deficiencies. These units provide favorable signal-to-noise ratios for enhanced reception of classroom instruction. Since these units are recommended only during select periods of instruction, their cost may discourage widespread use, but the Phonic Ear Model HC 421 has shown excellent results.

Many of the suggestions for teachers may also be implemented at home. For example, simply constructed sentences, minimal extraneous noise and reduced distractions are important in communicating effectively. Carrying on a conversation in the same room, eliminating various distractions such as TV, stereo, and obtaining the child's undivided attention will simplify the auditory demands placed on him. If the auditory environment cannot be controlled immediately, perhaps the conversation should be delayed until a better listening atmosphere can be maintained. This is particularly important when discussing specific duties or chores with the child. Care must be taken that disciplinary actions are not taken against a child when his misbehavior may have been due to auditory confusion. Specific recommendations for both teachers and parents may be found in Willeford (1976b).

In summary, these suggestions have been implemented by teachers, parents, and children with central auditory processing difficulties. Hopefully, in the future, therapy techniques and improved methods of modifying the child's auditory environment will be developed. In the meantime, most children with auditory-based LD can learn to compensate for their auditory deficiency.

We hope that this discussion will stimulate greater interest among audiologists in the area of central auditory processing disorders. A vast range of scientific and clinical inquiry should be launched to aid the LD child. We believe that audiologists in conjunction with other specialists have much to offer the LD child.

REFERENCES

Anderson, A., and Novina, J., A study of the relationship of the tests of central auditory abilities and the Illinois test of psycholinguistic abilities. *J. Learn. Disabil.*, 6, 167–169, 1973.

Aten, J., Auditory Memory and Auditory Sequencing. In *Proceedings of the First Annual Memphis State University Symposium on Auditory Processing and Learning Disabilities*, pp. 108–135, 1972.

Ayres, A., *Sensory Integration and Learning Disabilities*. Los Angeles, Calif.: Western Psychological Services, 1972.

Barr, D., *Auditory Perceptual Disorders*. Springfield, Ill.: Charles C Thomas, 1972.

Beasley, D., Schwimmer, S., and Rintleman, W., Intelligibility of time-compressed CNC monosyllables. *J. Speech Hear. Res.*, 15, 340–350, 1972.

Beasley, D., Forman, B., and Rintleman, W., Perception of time-compressed CNC monosyllables by normal listeners. *J. Aud. Res.*, 12, 71–75, 1973.

Behrmann, P., *Activities for Developing Auditory Perception*. San Rafael, Calif.: Academic Therapy Publications, undated.

Berlin, C., and McNeil, M., Dichotic Listening. In

Lass, N. (Ed.), *Contemporary Issues in Experimental Phonetics*, New York: Academic Press, 1976.

Bocca, E., Calearo, C., and Cassinari, V., A new method for testing hearing in temporal lobe tumors. *Acta Otolaryngol.*, **44**, 219–221, 1954.

Bocca, E., Calearo, C., Cassinari, V., and Migliavacca, F., Testing "cortical" hearing in temporal lobe tumors. *Acta Otolaryngol.*, **45**, 289–304, 1955.

Bocca, E., and Calearo, C., Central Hearing Processes. In Jerger, J., (Ed.), *Modern Developments in Audiology*, New York: Academic Press, 1963.

Bosatra, A., Russolo, M., and Poli, P., Oscilloscopic analysis of the stapedius muscle reflex in brain stem lesions. *Arch. Otolaryngol.*, **102**, 284–285, 1976.

Broadbent, D., Attention and the perception of speech. *Sci. Am.*, **206**, 143–151, 1962.

Brunt, M., The Staggered Spondaic Word Test. In Katz, J. (Ed.), *Handbook of Clinical Audiology*, Baltimore: Williams & Wilkins, 1972.

Burns, G., and Watson, B., Factor analysis of the revised ITPA with underachieving children. *J. Learn. Disabil.*, **6**, 371–376, 1973.

Butcher, E., and Bueker, E., *Concepts of Neuroanatomy*. New York: Hafner Publishing Co., 1969.

Butler, K., Hedrick, D., and Manning, C., In Witkin, R. (Ed.), *Composite Auditory Perceptual Test*. Hayward, Calif.: Alameda County School Department, 1973.

Butler, K., Short-course on auditory perception taught at the American Speech and Hearing Association convention, Washington, D.C., 1975.

Calearo, C., and Lazzaroni, A., Speech intelligibility in relation to the speed of the message. *Laryngoscope*, **67**, 410–419, 1957.

Carpenter, M., *Core Text of Neuroanatomy*. Baltimore: Williams & Wilkins, 1972.

Carhart, R., Special hearing tests for otoneurologic diagnosis. *Arch. Otolaryngol.*, **89**, 64–67, 1969.

Cherry, E., Some experiments on the recognition of speech with one and two ears. *J. Acoust. Soc. Am.*, **25**, 975–979, 1953.

Dayal, V., Tarantino, L., and Swisher, L., Neurootologic studies in multiple sclerosis. *Laryngoscope*, **76**, 1798–1809, 1966.

Eden, K., Green, J., and Hansen, J., *Auditory Training*. Iowa City, Iowa: University of Iowa Campus Stores, 1973.

Eichel, B., Hedgecock, L., and Williams, H., A review of the literature on the audiologic aspect of neuro-otologic diagnosis. *Laryngoscope*, **76**, 1–29, 1966.

Everett, N., Sundsten, J., and Lund, R., *Functional Neuroanatomy*, Ed. 6. Philadelphia: Lea & Febiger, 1971.

Flowers, A., Costello, M., and Small, V., *Flowers-Costello Tests of Central Auditory Abilities*. Dearborn, Mich.: Perceptual Learning Systems, 1973.

French, J., The reticular formation. *Sci. Am.*, **196**, 54–60, 1957.

Galambos, R., Schwartzkopff, J., and Rupert, A., Microelectrode study of superior olivary nuclei. *Am. J. Physiol.*, **197**, 527–536, 1959.

Gillet, P., *Auditory Processes*. San Rafael, Calif.: Academic Therapy Publications, 1974.

Goldman, R., Fristoe, M., and Woodcock, R., *Test of Auditory Discrimination*. Circle Pines, Minn.: American Guidance Service, 1970.

Goldstein, R., Paper presented at the University of Oklahoma Symposium entitled "Hearing Disorders in Children," January 1967.

Heasley, B., *Auditory Perceptual Disorders and Remediation*. Springfield, Ill.: Charles C Thomas, 1974. (Also see Book Review in *Asha*, **18**, 469, 1976.)

Heilman, K., Hammer, L., and Wilder, B., An audiometric defect in temporal lobe dysfunction. *Neurology*, **23**, 384–386, 1973.

Hernandez-Peon, R., Reticular Mechanisms of Sensory Control. In Rosenblith, W. (Ed.), *Sensory Communication*. Cambridge, Mass.: MIT Press, 1961.

Herr, S., *Teacher's Handbook of Perceptual Communication Skills*. Bountiful, Utah: Instructional Media, 1968.

Holm, V., and Kunze, L., Effect of chronic otitis media on language and speech development. *Pediatrics*, **43**, 833–839, 1969.

Ivey, R., Tests of CNS function. Master's thesis, Colorado State University, Fort Collins, Col., 1969.

Jerger, J., Audiological manifestations of lesions in the auditory nervous system. *Laryngoscope*, **70**, 417–425, 1960.

Jerger, J., Auditory Tests for Disorders of the Central Auditory Mechanism. In Fields, W., and Alford, B. (Eds.), *Neurological Aspects of Auditory and Vestibular Disorders*. Springfield, Ill.: Charles C Thomas, 1964.

Jerger, J., Diagnostic Audiometry. In Jerger, J. (Ed.), *Modern Developments in Audiology*, Ed. 2. New York: Academic Press, 1973.

Jerger, S., and Jerger, J., Extra- and intra-axial brainstem auditory disorders. *Audiology*, **14**, 92–117, 1975a.

Jerger, J., and Jerger, S., Clinical validity of central auditory tests. *Scand. Audiol.*, **4**, 147–163, 1975b.

Jerger, S., and Jerger, J., Recovery of crossed acoustic reflexes in brainstem auditory disorder. *Arch. Otolaryngol.*, **101**, 329–332, 1975c.

Katz, J., The SSW test—an interim report. *J. Speech Hear. Disord.*, **33**, 132–146, 1968.

Katz, J., and Illmer, R., Auditory Perception in Children with Learning Disabilities. In Katz, J. (Ed.), *Handbook of Clinical Audiology*, Ed. 1. Baltimore: Williams & Wilkins, 1972.

Katz, J., Personal communication, 1976.

Kimura, D., Cerebral dominance and the perception of verbal stimuli. *Can. J. Psychol.*, **15**, 166–171, 1961.

Kirk, S., McCarthy, J., and Kirk, W., *Illinois Test of Psycholinguistic Abilities*. Champaign, Ill.: University of Illinois Press, 1968.

Kryter, K., *The Effects of Noise on Man*. New York: Academic Press, 1970.

Kurdzeil, S., and Noffsinger, D., Performance of cortical lesion patients on 40% and 60% time-compressed speech materials. Paper presented at the American Speech and Hearing Association Convention, Detroit 1973.

Leadership Training Institute, Final Report, Department of Special Education, University of Arizona, Tuscon, 1972.

Lynn, G., Auditory correlates of neurological insult. Address delivered as part of "Guest Lectures in Science" series, Colorado State University, Fort Collins, Col., June 1973.

Lynn, G., Perception of rapidly alternating speech in patients with brainstem and cerebral hemisphere lesions. Paper presented at 9th Colorado Medical Audiology Workshop. Vail, Colo., March 1975.

Lynn, G., and Gilroy, J., Neuro-audiological abnormalities in patients with temporal lobe tumors. J. Neurol. Sci., 17, 167–184, 1972.

Lynn, G., and Gilroy, J., Effects of brain lesions on the perception of monotic and dichotic speech stimuli. Proceedings of a Symposium on Central Auditory Processing Disorders, University of Nebraska Medical Center, January 1975.

Lynn, G., Benitez, J., Eisenbrey, A., Gilroy, J., and Wilner, H., Neuroaudiological correlates in central hemisphere lesions; temporal and parietal lobe tumors. Audiology, 11, 115–134, 1972.

Maccoby, E., and Konrad, K., Age trends in selective listening. J. Exp. Psychol., 3, 113–122, 1966.

Magoun, H., The Waking Brain, 2nd Ed. Springfield, Ill.: Charles C Thomas, 1963.

Maki, J., Beasley, D., and Orchik, D., Children's perception of time-compressed speech using two measures of speech discrimination. Paper presented at the American Speech and Hearing Association convention, Las Vegas, 1974.

Martin, A., Personal communication, 1976.

Matzke, H., and Foltz, F., Synopsis of Neuroanatomy, Ed. 2. New York: Oxford University Press, 1972.

Matzker, J., Two new methods for the assessment of central auditory function in cases of brain disease. Ann. Otol. Rhinol. Laryngol., 68, 1185–1197, 1959.

Matzker, J., The binaural test. J. Int. Audiol., 1, 209–211, 1962.

Meyer, M., Paper presented at Symposium on Central Auditory Processing Disorders in Children with Learning Disabilities, Colorado State University, 1975.

Miller, J., Effects of noise on people. J. Acoust. Soc. Am., 56, 729–764, 1974.

Miller, M., and Daly, J., Cerebellar atrophy simulating acoustic neurinoma. Arch. Otolaryngol., 85, 383–386, 1967.

Mills, J., Noise and children; a review of literature. J. Acoust. Soc. Am., 58, 767–779, 1975.

Milner, B., Taylor, L., and Sperry, R., Lateralized suppression of dichotically presented digits after commissural section in man. Science, 161, 184–186, 1968.

Mokotoff, B., Schuman-Galambos, C., Galambos, R., Brainstem auditory evoked response in children. Arch. Otolaryngol., 103, 38–43, 1977.

Morales-Garcia, C., and Poole, J., Masked speech audiometry in central deafness. Acta Otolaryngol., 74, 307–316, 1972.

Morrill, J., A staggered spondaic word test as an indicator of minimal brain dysfunction in children. Master's thesis, Texas Technological College, 1969.

Myrick, D., A normative study to assess performance of a group of children ages seven through eleven on the staggered spondaic word test. Master's thesis, Tulane University, 1965.

Neff, W., Neural Mechanisms of Auditory Discrimination. In Rosenblith, W. (Ed.), Sensory Communication. Cambridge, Mass.: MIT Press, 1961.

Niemoeller, A., Acoustical design of classrooms for the deaf. Am. Ann. Deaf, 113, 1040–1045, 1968.

Nober, L., A study of classroom noise as a factor which affects the auditory discrimination performance of primary grade children. Doctoral thesis, University of Massachusetts, Amherst, Mass., 1973.

Noffsinger, D., Olsen, W., Carhart, R., Hart, C., and Sahgal, V., Auditory and vestibular aberrations in multiple sclerosis. Acta Otolaryngol., Suppl. 303, 1972.

Northern, J., and Downs, M., Hearing in Children. Baltimore: Williams & Wilkins, 1974.

Oakland, T., and Williams, F., Auditory Processing. Seattle, Wash.: Special Child Publications, Inc., 1971.

Olsen, W., Noffsinger, D., and Kurdziel, S., Speech discrimination in quiet and in white noise by patients with peripheral and central lesions. Acta Otolaryngol., 80, 375–382, 1975.

O'Neill, J., Perspectives in Auditory Processing: Questions to be Answered. In Proceedings of the First Annual Memphis State Symposium on Auditory Processing and Learning Disabilities, pp. 93–96, 1972.

Orchik, D., and Oeschlager, M., Time-compressed speech discrimination in children; its relationship to articulation ability. Paper presented at the American Speech and Hearing Association Convention, Las Vegas, 1974.

Ormson, K., and Williams, D., Central auditory function as assessed by time-compressed speech with elementary school age children having articulation and reading problems. Paper presented at the American Speech and Hearing Association Convention, Washington, D.C., 1975.

Parker, W., Decker, R., and Richards, N., Auditory function and lesions of the pons. Arch. Otolaryngol., 87, 228–240, 1968.

Reagan, C., Handbook of Auditory Perceptual Training. Springfield, Ill.: Charles C Thomas, 1973.

Sanders, D., Noise conditions in normal school classrooms. Except. Child., 31, 344–353, 1965.

Sanderson, M., and Rintleman, W., Performance of normal hearing children on three speech discrimination tests. Paper presented at the American Speech and Hearing Association Convention, Chicago, 1971.

Schnitker, M., The Teacher's Guide to the Brain and Learning. San Rafael, Calif.: Academic Therapy Publications, 1972.

Schoenfeld, S., The SSW test with children. Presented at Expanded SSW Workshop, Menorah Medical Center, Kansas City, Mo., July 1975.

Schubert, G., Meyer, R., and Schmidt, J., Evaluation of the noise subtest of the Goldman-Fristoe-Woodcock test of auditory discrimination. J. Aud. Res., 13, 42–44, 1973.

Shapiro, I., Progression of auditory signs in pontine glioma. *Laryngoscope, 79,* 201–212, 1969.

Sinha, S., The role of the temporal lobe in hearing. Master's thesis, McGill University, 1959.

Slater, B. Effects of noise on pupil performance. *J. Educ. Psychol., 59,* 239–243, 1968.

Sparks, R., Goodglass, H., and Nickel, B. Ipsilateral versus contralateral extinction in dichotic listening resulting from hemispheric lesions. *Cortex, 6,* 249–260, 1970.

Stubblefield, J., and Young, E., Central auditory dysfunction in learning disabled children. *J. Learn. Disabil., 8,* 89–94, 1975.

Walsh, E., An investigation of sound localization in patients with neurological abnormalities. *Brain, 80,* 222–250, 1957.

Weener, P., Toward a Developmental Model of Auditory Processes. In *Proceedings of the First Annual Memphis State Symposium on Auditory Processing and Learning Disabilities,* pp. 153–171, 1972.

Wepman, J., *Auditory Discrimination Test.* Chicago: Language Research Associates, 1958.

Willeford, J., Central auditory function in children with learning disabilities. *J. Audiol. Hear. Educ., 2,* 12–20, 1976a.

Willeford, J., Central Auditory Function. In Donnelly, K. (Ed.), *Communicative Disorders: Learning Disabilities.* Boston: Little, Brown & Co., 1976b.

Whitfield, I., *The Auditory Pathway.* Baltimore: Williams & Wilkins, 1967.

Witkin, R., Auditory Perception – Implications for Language Development. In *Language, Speech and Hearing Services in Schools, Monograph 4,* pp. 31–52. Washington, D.C.: American Speech and Hearing Association, circa 1971.

Wood, N., Auditory Closure and Auditory Discrimination in Young Children. In *Proceedings of the First Annual Memphis State Symposium on Auditory Processing and Learning Disabilities,* pp. 136–152, 1972.

Woodcock, R., *Goldman-Fristoe-Woodcock Auditory Skills Test Battery – Technical Manual.* Circle Pines, Minn.: American Guidance Service, 1976.

chapter 35

HEARING EVALUATION OF THE ELDERLY

Raymond H. Hull, Ph.D.

Many changes have taken place in this century, but scarcely any have been more significant than the achievement of a long life for most Americans. Factors contributing to greater longevity have been the discoveries of modern medicine which have reduced the death rate among the young and middle-aged and modern technology which has reduced the exhausting labor known by our grandparents. As a result, the population of individuals age 65 years and over has increased from 3.1 million in 1900 to 20 million in 1971 and, by the year 1980, it is estimated that they will number approximately 24 million (Department of Health, Education and Welfare, 1963).

The Metropolitan Life Insurance Company (1966) indicates that approximately 20% of that population is over age 65 years, accounting for 3 million hearing-impaired persons, or 150 persons out of every 1,000. These statistics, however, contradict more recent figures released by the National Center for Health Statistics (1975) which indicate that the incidence of hearing impairment among noninstitutionalized persons over age 65 years approximates a ratio of 72 out of every 1000. Other studies have shown that the incidence of hearing impairment among individuals age 65 years and older at all levels of severity greater than 26 dB (pure tone average in the better ear) may be as high as 32,269 in every 100,000 persons (Glorig and Roberts, 1965). The less conservative figures would appear to be in better agreement with those reported by currently practicing audiologists. Although a lack of similarity among incidence figures is evident, it is estimated that more than 15 to 20% of persons over age 65 are hearing impaired. Leutenegger and Stovall (1971) have indicated, that of the 20 million individuals over 65, 6% or 1.2 million, live in nursing/retirement homes. According to Chafee (1967), 90% of this confined population is hearing handicapped.

What does "old age" mean? Age 65 has been used for so long to denote retirement age that it is difficult to think of an individual over age 65 as anything but "aged." To a child of 6 years, a tall child of 13 years seems "old." To a teenager, a worker, age 30, is "old." To a "young adult," retirement seems to bring old age. Those in their 60s define "old age" as someone in the late 80s or 90s. To them old age implies being bedridden, dependent, and removed from an active, participating life (Shock, 1960). "Old age" then, is, indeed, arbitrarily defined. There are individuals who appear, at age 50 years, to be "old" in regard to their activity, vitality, and their state of health. On the other hand, there are individuals at age 70 years who appear to be young in terms of their health, social activity, and general vitality. Because health statistics on hearing and aging use 65 years as a reference point for aging, information in this chapter will also use that age. However, this reference point will be for convenience sake since we know that the beginnings of aging in relation to the auditory mechanism start much before age 65. It is interesting to consider that although people are living longer, this does not necessarily mean that the aging process has been reversed or slowed appreciably. Rather, better and/or more frequent medical attention has averted more of the situations which would have been fatal in the past.

The multitude of problems associated with the elderly individual's ability to function auditorily are encompassed in the term "presbycusis." Presbycusis includes (a) the pathology of the aging ear, (b) the related auditory discrimination difficulties, and (c) the many other associated social-psychological problems encountered by the individual.

Schuknecht (1974) views aging as a "complex integration of inherited defects, injury, environmental exposure, accumulation of DNA errors (causing a decline in capability of mitosis for repair), genetic makeup, accumulation of pigment, and chemical changes in the cells." Presbycusis is presented as an accumulation of degenerative changes in the auditory system determined by aging but depending upon heredity, diet, environment, and use. He feels it is difficult to distinguish between heredity factors in aging as it relates to hearing impairment and presbycusis.

To look at the possible locus for the structural degenerative changes in regard to the aging auditory mechanism, the following areas will be discussed individually and then as a whole: (a) the outer ear, (b) the middle ear, (c) the cochlea, and (d) the eighth nerve and central auditory system.

THE OUTER EAR

A typical characteristic of the pinna of the elderly individual is an increase in size and a decrease in elasticity. The rough appearance, scaliness, dryness, and inelasticity, with loss of rebound in the epithelium are the result of degenerative processes (Johnson and Hadley,

1964). Loose, unpadded skin covering falls at the mercy of gravity. Greater growth of hair within the folds of the auricle is often seen among elderly individuals, especially among men.

No matter to what extent the aging process affects the outer ear relative to structure and appearance, those changes, in all probability, do not reflect themselves auditorily. However, the flaccid pinna can cause a false conductive hearing loss if the ear phones are not placed properly. The pressure on the soft tissue of the pinna can force it to occlude the orifice of the external auditory meatus.

THE MIDDLE EAR

Structural changes of the middle ear appear to be more specific and in all probability may be related to auditory difficulties experienced by some aged individuals. Among the changes that appear to occur with aging are those described by Rosenwasser (1964) including ossicular atrophy predominant in the joint of the stapes and caudal joint of the malleus. There may be atrophy of the tensor tympani muscle, along with a thinning of the tympanic membrane. Rosenwasser indicates that since many conditions of aging depress general body functions, this could explain the high incidence of infection and hearing difficulties in the elderly. Leake (1963) reports that auditory impairment seen in presbycusis may include middle ear muscle dysfunction. Acoustic signals were delivered to the ears of cats in whom electrodes were implanted within the reflex loop of the middle ear muscles. Leake found that since these muscles may contribute significantly to auditory signal analysis and attentiveness, the reduction of hearing in aging may not be so much a disturbance in the sensory-neural mechanism itself, but a gradual reduction of muscle function in the middle ear.

Glorig and Davis (1961) investigated the involvement of the conductive mechanism in presbycusis using 164 businessmen and residents of a home for old soldiers. The subjects did not have a prior history of excessive noise exposure. They ranged from 25 to 80 years of age. Air- and bone-conduction threshold measurements were conducted at frequencies of 500, 1k, 2k, and 4k Hz. The older subjects had a noticeable air-bone gap at 4k Hz along with a general absence of loudness recruitment. The authors attributed this phenomenon to loss of function of the conductive mechanism and referred to it as "conductive presbycusis."

In view of conflicting reports regarding the existence of conductive presbycusis, Satoloff, Vassalo and Menduke (1965) tested men and women between 62 and 82 years of age. They found little, or no, discrepancy between air conduction and bone conduction, thus failing to support the conductive element noted by Glorig and Davis. Satoloff's findings support the majority of research which shows that presbycusis is primarily a sensory-neural phenomenon.

Goodhill (1969) provides information about an elderly patient which might support the possibility of a conductive element in presbycusis. A 71-year-old male patient, who was generally in good health, had complained of a 30-year progressive bilateral mixed hearing loss. There were no indications of childhood ear infections and no family history of deafness. In 1958, the patient had a right stapes operation which resulted in no improvement and the progressive loss continued. In 1962, an aid was fitted unsuccessfully. In 1967, he was diagnosed as having a primary malleal fixation with no otosclerosis. The audiogram, however, was that of cochlear presbycusis, demonstrating probable cochlear pathology but with some conductive element. Following surgery, the audiometric picture was reversed. His loss was then found to be primarily conductive with only a slight sensory-neural involvement, the conclusion being that there appeared to be a real relationship between the mass and stiffness of a fixed malleus and depression of bone conduction acuity. The author concluded that presbycusis may be not only sensory-neural but also conductive due to senescent ossicular chain atrophy.

THE COCHLEA

Research into the anatomic locus of presbycusis has generally supported the area of the cochlea as a primary site of the degenerative processes involved. Conditions of the outer and middle ear are usually minimized, if mentioned at all. Most of the literature on presbycusis deals with the hearing test results for elderly patients and the histologic changes of their cochleas found at autopsy. Despite extensive studies of the cochlea, spiral ganglion, midbrain, and cortex, there is no universal agreement as to the correlation between decreased hearing sensitivity, the loss of auditory discrimination ability, and the site of lesion for patients diagnosed as having presbycusis.

There are approximately 35,000 nerve fibers in the cochlea which send coded information into the auditory cortex. These cells are fixed in number and cannot regenerate or reproduce themselves. A study by Schuknecht and Woellner (1955), found that up to 75% of the spiral ganglion cells in cats must be damaged before threshold elevations occur, so a gradual diminution in these cells, especially over an extended period of time, would probably not be perceptible to the person until considerable pathology was present.

Clinically, presbycusic changes in the cochlea probably start at birth. As Schuknecht (1974) has stated, "This is deafness of aging, not of the aged."

After detailed studies of human temporal bones, Schuknecht (1964) noted four distinct types of presbycusis. They are as follows:

1. *Sensory presbycusis* – caused by atrophy of the organ of Corti and degeneration of hair cells, beginning at the basal end of the cochlea and moving toward the apex. Hearing test results in these cases show an abrupt hearing loss at 8000 Hz and above. This is the least common of the four types.

2. *Neural presbycusis* – results from the loss of neurons in the auditory pathways and cochlea. This usually becomes noticeable when 30 to 40% of the neurons are lost or damaged. There is a relatively more severe speech discrimination problem than with the first type. Although 90% of the cochlear nerves can be destroyed without affecting pure tone thresholds, speech discrimination is affected much more quickly. Amplification frequently does not benefit these persons.

3. *Stria vascularis atrophy or metabolic presbycusis* – is often seen where there is a family history of hearing loss and an insidious onset in the third or fourth decade of life. Degeneration takes place in the apical area of the cochlea and causes a flat pure tone hearing loss to about 50 dB, at which point speech discrimination is affected. Schuknecht feels this is probably a genetically determined condition. Amplification is often found to benefit these persons.

4. *Inner ear conductive-type presbycusis* (somewhat theoretical) – although there are no evident histologic changes, Schuknecht feels an increase in the stiffness in the supporting structures of the cochlear duct may cause a mechanical-type "conductive" loss. The greatest impairment is produced at the basal end of the basilar membrane where it is the thickest, while the fewest changes occur near the apical end where it is thinnest. Although in his 1964 account Schuknecht was somewhat vague and uncertain when describing this type, during his 1974 presentation he spoke with more confidence regarding the existence of this conductive phenomenon. He indicated that, when each of these four types occur alone, they can be specifically identified.

Proctor (1961) compiled information on findings related to the cochlear pathology involved in the aging ear. He stated that in the case of presbycusis, the "etiologic mechanism is assumed to be an atrophy of the basal coil of the cochlea." Arteriosclerosis and high blood cholesterol might be predisposing factors. It was surmised that progressive deafness due to aging might be caused by atrophy of nerve fibers. Degeneration of the specific elements in the labyrinth (spiral ganglion) would be regarded as a secondary factor. He felt that contributory factors involved in the causation of presbycusis could be "the processes of the middle ear, arteriosclerosis, toxic influences, avitaminosis, and hormonal deficiencies." Senile hyperostosis of the cranial bones is to be considered as the primary cause of pure idiopathic presbycusis.

Kirikae, Sato and Shitara (1964) describe presbycusis as resulting from epithelial and neural atrophy. They define the causes of presbycusis as lesions of the inner ear, especially the organ of Corti and the spiral ganglion cells. They list two types of degenerative changes: (1) atrophy of the spiral ganglion (neural atrophy), and (2) angiosclerotic degeneration of the inner ear (epithelial atrophy).

Jorgensen (1961), while conducting histologic studies of 25 temporal bones from patients ranging in age from 2 months to 80 years of age, discovered a loss of ganglion cells in the basal portion of the cochlea among older patients along with thickening of the capillary walls in the stria vascularis. The pathology involving the stria vascularis was thought to be related to arteriosclerosis. Jorgensen felt that the thickening could affect not only the oxygen levels of the cochlear duct, but correspondingly, the electrical potentials. Miller and Ort (1965) contend that clinical studies do not yet confirm the effect of arteriosclerosis on the cochlea.

Researchers of the pathology of presbycusis are becoming increasingly aware that it is difficult, if not impossible, to separate the effects of noise and the use of drugs for medication from the normal process of aging when attempting to discover the locus of presbycusis (Johnson and Hawkins, 1972). They discovered hair cell degeneration in infants and newborns a few hours old. Thus, "in some instances, the hair cell degeneration must have begun in the uterus." There was clear evidence of nerve degeneration secondary to hair cell degeneration by the early teens in the extreme basal turn of the cochlea. This degeneration progressed steadily with advancing years.

Hawkins (1973) feels that the effects of ototoxicity on the ear and the degenerative changes leading to presbycusis are so similar that it is difficult to differentiate between them. Since noise exposure and/or ototoxic injury are such common occurrences during one's lifetime, he postulates that purely metabolic presbycusis must be a rare occurrence. Hawkins, then refers to presbycusis as the cumulative effects of noise, drugs, as well as time.

Even though one of the primary sites of lesion for the degenerative process observed in presbycusis appears to be the cochlea, special emphasis in research regarding the phenomenon of the devastating discrimination problems encountered by the older individual has been focused on the eighth nerve and central auditory mechanism.

EIGHTH NERVE, BRAIN STEM, AND AUDITORY CORTEX

Simple atrophy of the eighth nerve has been observed by Rosenwasser (1964), Schuknecht and Woellner (1955), Schuknecht (1964), Harbert, Young and Menduke (1966), Matzker and Springhorn (1958), Rosen et al. (1964), and others. In an investigation conducted by Taniewaki (1963), the concept of nerve deterioration was further substantiated. He found that defective hearing in senile patients depends either on the changes in the sensory epithelium of the cochlea or changes in the eighth nerve. Taniewaki concluded that it is difficult to determine how much the loss of hearing of the aged depends on the extensive use of tissue and how much is the expression of a true pathological process.

Research involving the central auditory pathways has provided information in understanding the auditory difficulties of the aged. Kirikae et al. (1964) conducted histopathologic studies of nuclei of the auditory pathways, i.e., the superior olive, inferior colliculus, and the medial geniculate nuclei at autopsy. For all older subjects, premortal speech discrimination was impaired as compared with younger subjects when subjected to frequency distortion of speech (low pass filter) and interrupted speech. Elevation of auditory threshold, especially the high frequencies, was also revealed. There appeared to be no question that presbycusis is caused in part by degeneration of tissues within the inner ear, however, senile changes of nerve cells of the central auditory pathway was also considered important. They concluded that the auditory characteristics seen in presbycusis are probably the result of degeneration of the central auditory mechanism compounded by the results of pathology within the cochlea.

An investigation conducted by Hansen and Reske-Nielsen (1965) demonstrated results similar to the study above. Ten subjects aged 80 years and older were evaluated. Two other subjects were age 60 and 69 years. All were affected by symmetrical hearing loss for the high frequencies. For 10 of the subjects, histologic examinations showed alterations in the basal cochlear pathways which could explain hearing loss for the high frequencies. Hearing loss for the low frequencies was assumed to be exclusively centrally located. One subject with a normal cochlea showed deterioration in the cochlear branch of the eighth nerve as well as in the central auditory pathways. In another, a hearing loss on the right side was thought to be caused by peripheral as well as central pathological alterations. The causes of the degenerative alterations were found to be partially due to arteriosclerosis and partially senile atrophy.

Hinchcliffe (1962), in an exhaustive investigation regarding the anatomical location of presbycusis, has found that even though degenerative changes are seen throughout the auditory system and apparently all contribute to the phenomenon of presbycusis, "it seems more likely that changes in the brain are primarily responsible for the overall audiologic picture of presbycusis." Jerger (1973) further investigated the concept of phonemic regression by comparing the responses of young normally hearing individuals, young subjects with sensoryneural hearing loss, and elderly individuals with equal hearing loss to various auditory tasks. The tests utilized included auditory discrimination tasks in quiet, at a 5-dB sensation level, in a competing message condition, and with 50% signal compression. Jerger concluded that when comparing the results of young and elderly individuals with essentially equal pure tone thresholds, "we must look beyond the cochlea to explain the loss in speech discrimination unique to the elderly." Jerger concurs with Hinchcliffe (1962) that central auditory system dysfunction is the primary locus of presbycusis.

RESPONSE TO STANDARD AUDITORY MEASURES BY THE ELDERLY CLIENT

There are certain characteristic auditory responses observed by the audiologist when assessing the aged client. A compilation of typical audiometric results seen among the elderly are presented here.

Pure Tone Audiometric Configurations

As stated by Jerger (1973), "The aging process produces systematic changes in each of the two critical dimensions of hearing impairment—loss in threshold sensitivity and loss in the ability to understand suprathreshold speech."

A principal auditory symptom of the phenomenon described as "presbycusis" is seen as an inability of the elderly individual to understand the speech of others when auditory sensitivity appears adequate for communication purposes. A typical statement by the elderly often noted by the audiologist is, "I can hear you, but I cannot understand what you are saying." The elderly client is probably relating a very accurate description of the situation. The sensory mechanism may be impaired but not so much that a younger individual would not be able to function with it adequately. The central auditory mechanism may not allow the elderly person to utilize well what he/she receives auditorily. It is up to the audiologist to interpret the audiometric results, differentiating between the effects of the peripheral sensory-neural element and the effects of the central involvement that hinder efficient auditory perception and, thereby, communication.

The pure tone test results generally reveal a bilateral sensory-neural hearing loss sloping downward through the frequencies above 2k Hz. Miller and Ort (1965) found this slope in 88% of a group of individuals over age 65. Average hearing loss ranged from 16 to 60 dB bilaterally. Generally, the loss is greater for men in frequencies above 4k Hz, whereas women show a greater loss toward the lower frequencies (Department of Health, Education and Welfare, 1975). Miller and Ort attribute the difference in the high frequencies to greater noise exposure in men than in women. Hinchcliffe (1962) reaffirms the location of a more marked impairment in the higher frequencies. The characteristic high frequency hearing loss in the elderly was also reported by early investigators such as Bunch (1931) and Beasley (1938).

Glorig et al. (1957) reported average pure tone thresholds of individuals ranging from 10 to 79 years of age. These composite thresholds are shown in Figure 35.1. The greatest impairment is in the higher frequencies, beginning with a slight degree at ages 10 to 19 years. At ages 60 to 69, some decrease in auditory sensitivity begins to appear in the lower frequencies.

Hinchcliffe (1959) plotted median pure tone thresholds as a function of age in Figure 35.2. Thresholds for a wider range of frequencies show the dramatic impact of aging on high frequency hearing.

Traynor and Hull (1974) obtained mean pure tone thresholds for 120 confined elderly individuals between the ages of 65 and 90. Their findings were compared with those of Miller and Ort (1965) who investigated hearing function in a similar population. The results of both studies are presented in Figure 35.3. The averaged thresholds of the two studies show good agreement. The audiometric configuration is relatively flat but slopes gradually toward the high frequencies above 2k Hz. The impact of presbycusis cannot be appreciated, however, without considering speech reception and discrimination capabilities.

Speech Perception

It is difficult to imagine that the high frequency sensory-neural hearing loss noted in presbycusis is the sole cause of the auditory discrimination disabilities noted in the elderly. Jerger (1973) concluded that the locus of "phonemic regression" (Gaeth, 1948) or the loss of ability to understand speech in light of relatively good peripheral hearing appears to be a

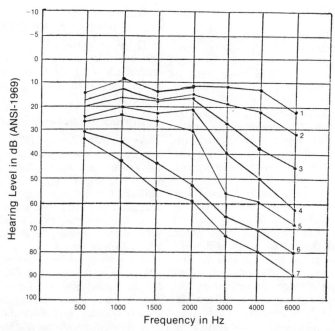

Fig. 35.1. Median hearing losses for males ages 10 to 79 (*1*, 10–19; *2*, 20–29; *3*, 30–39; *4*, 40–49; *5*, 50–59; *6*, 60–69; *7*, 70–79). Data are converted to the ANSI-1969 reference. (Adapted from Glorig et al. (1957).)

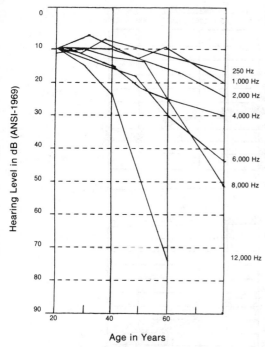

Fig. 35.2. Threshold sensitivity for hearing as a function of age. Median hearing losses in decibels *re* median threshold at 21.5 years of age. Threshold levels have been converted to ANSI-1969. (Adapted from Hinchcliffe (1959) as cited in Hinchcliffe (1962).)

central rather than a peripheral phenomenon. Whether the locus of phonemic regression is peripheral or central, the phenomenon is present in many elderly individuals and constitutes one of their greatest handicaps.

To the lay person, the confusions of auditory messages seen among the elderly may become synonymous with the term "senility." The confusion may be amusing to some as in the case of "Old Uncle Joe" who confuses "Sue is buying a new gown" with "We're all going to town." To Uncle Joe, however, the confusion is embarrassing and can result in withdrawal from other possible communication situations. He may be a bright, alert elderly person but with a devastating auditory discrimination problem. Willeford (1971) cites an interesting doctoral dissertation (Gaeth, 1948). Gaeth approached this investigation with "the observation . . . that certain patients show much greater difficulty in discriminating the phonemic elements of speech than would be expected on the basis of their pure-tone scores" (Willeford, 1971). He describes the characteristics of phonemic regression as follows:

1. Audiologically there is a mild or moderate sensory-neural loss.

2. The decrease in the speech average for pure tones is consistent with the threshold drop in responding to connected speech.

3. There is more difficulty in speech discrimination tests than expected from the pure tone loss.

4. Phonemic perception difficulty does not parallel a general decay in mental capacities.

5. The patient tends to blame his deficiency in auditory sensitivity for his trouble.

6. Phonemic regression appears more frequently in individuals over 50 years of age, but a substantial number of older individuals with hearing losses do not display the difficulty. Therefore, age alone cannot be considered the sole cause.

Jerger (1973) investigated the ability of the elderly to discriminate auditorily by studying the performance-intensity function for phonetically balanced monosyllabic words. He was thus able to determine a maximum phonetically balanced (PB) score (PB max) for each ear of each subject. His investigation was based on 4095 ears of 2162 patients ranging in age from 6 to 89 years. The number of ears in each decade ranged from a maximum of 740 in the 60- to 69-year range, to 109 in the decade from 80 to 89. All PB test materials were National Defense Research Council (NDRC) lists one through six recorded on magnetic tape. Average PB max as a function of age and hearing level can be seen in Figure 35.4. There is a dramatic drop in auditory discrimination scores with both advancing age and decreased averages.

When the data are averaged across hearing levels for each age group, the change in auditory discrimination for PB words is dramatic as can be seen in Figure 35.5. The effect is somewhat exaggerated because the older subjects had poorer hearing.

RESPONSES BY THE ELDERLY TO SPECIAL AUDITORY ASSESSMENT TECHNIQUES

Tests for Recruitment

The presence of recruitment in a patient with sensory-neural impairment is indicative of cochlear pathology and lack of it is a sign of pathology along the neural pathways. Investigators have studied recruitment in presbycusis. Studies by Jerger (1960) indicated that recruitment is not necessarily present in presbycusis despite sensory-neural hearing loss.

Pestalozza and Shore (1955) studied loudness recruitment in presbycusics with a monaural loudness balance procedure. Twenty-four elderly individuals were tested. Twenty percent of the subjects demonstrated complete recruitment, 30% showed partial recruitment, and

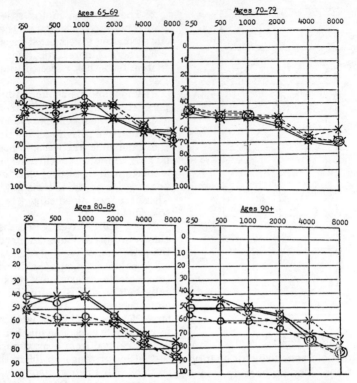

Fig. 35.3. Comparative mean pure tone thresholds for confined elderly persons. All thresholds have been converted where necessary to ANSI-1969. -----, Miller and Ort; ——, Traynor and Hull; O, right ear; ×, left ear. (Adapted from Traynor and Hull (1974) and Miller and Ort (1965).)

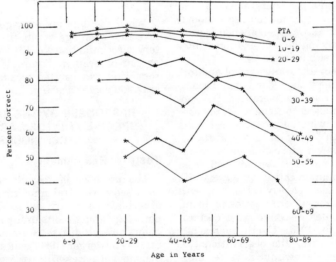

Fig. 35.4. Average phonetically balanced (PB) max as a function of age with pure tone average (PTA) held constant. Note systematic decline in PB max with advancing age (2162 patients, 4095 ears). (Adapted from Jerger (1973).)

50% showed none. Since the phenomenon of loudness recruitment is found to be characteristic of cochlear pathology, these results support the view that in many cases, presbycusis is due to pathology of higher auditory centers. Hinchcliffe (1962) concludes that the absence of recruitment indicates that degenerative changes in the cochlea are not wholly responsible for

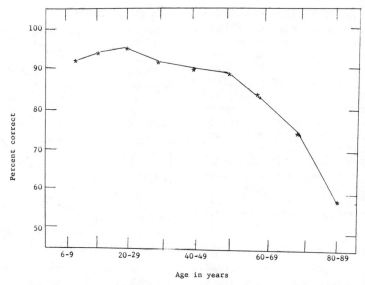

Fig. 35.5. Average PB max as a function of age (2162 patients, 4095 ears; pure tone average (PTA) ; 0 to 69 dB. (Adapted from Jerger (1973).)

threshold shifts in presbycusis. Goetzinger et al. (1961), however, found only 15% of the male patients to have a lack of recruitment.

More recent investigations of loudness recruitment have utilized acoustic reflex measurements. Alberti and Kristensen (1970) report that loudness recruitment as measured by the loudness balance technique correlates well with the middle ear reflex procedure. The clinical value of acoustic reflex measurement has been demonstrated. There are, however, no studies which present normative data relative to the strength of the acoustic reflex among aged clients. It would seem logical that if recruitment is not observed in large numbers of elderly clients, then the same would hold true with regard to the acoustic reflex. Traynor (1975), in an unpublished doctoral dissertation, studied the reliability of the use of impedance audiometry for assessment of elderly individuals in the health care facility environment compared to standard air- and bone-conduction evaluation techniques. The subjects ranged in age from 78 to 92 years, and all were confined elderly persons. During that investigation, acoustic reflexes were elicited in individuals with moderate sensory-neural hearing losses. Twenty percent of the subjects demonstrated such rapid fatigue that acoustic reflex measurements could not be made, while another 20% revealed absent reflexes in at least one ear. Sixty percent of the subjects did not show acoustic reflexes that would be indicative of recruitment, while 40% did demonstrate reflexes at normal or near normal intensity levels. If acoustic reflex measures do, indeed, indicate loudness recruitment when there is a

sensory-neural hearing loss, then the majority of these subjects could not be considered as having primarily sensory disorders. It must be noted, however, that subjects in this investigation were quite elderly.

Some authors have indicated auditory discrimination scores may indicate the presence of recruitment. Hirsh, Palva, and Goodman (1954) found that a reliable relationship can exist between low discrimination scores and recruitment if the hearing loss is greater than 20 dB. Pestalozza and Shore (1955), however, report this not to be true of older individuals and suggest that phonemic regression may be present in the absence of cochlear damage. They indicated that the absence of recruitment might indicate lesions in the spiral ganglion cells or nerve fibers which are most commonly responsible for presbycusis. These authors also suggest that since discrimination scores in presbycusis are generally poor, tests for recruitment should be used as the deciding factor in diagnosis.

Jerger (1973) conducted an interesting investigation concerning the effect of loudness recruitment on auditory discrimination capabilities among the elderly. Acoustic reflex measurements were utilized to determine the presence of recruitment as opposed to traditional loudness balance procedures. Discrimination scores were compared for two groups of 12 elderly individuals, each with presbycusis; one group demonstrating recruitment and one without. A third group of subjects, as controls, consisted of 12 young persons with recruitment. Three measures were compared between groups: (1) the pure tone audiogram, (2) the

PB max score and (3) the sensation level of the acoustic reflex. Presence or absence of recruitment was defined by the sensation level at which the acoustic reflex was elicited for frequencies of 500, 1k, 2k, and 4k Hz. Acoustic reflex levels and air-conduction thresholds for the three groups were not substantially different. Jerger concluded that "the disproportionate loss in speech understanding in aging patients is apparently not strongly related to the loudness recruitment phenomenon."

In summary, despite the pure tone configuration which would suggest cochlear involvement, in many elderly patients there is an absence of loudness recruitment indicating the likelihood of complicating involvement beyond the cochlea.

Tests for Tone Decay

Goetzinger et al. (1961), in an extensive investigation of auditory response in presbycusis, found virtually no correlation between the existence of presbycusis and tone decay. Decay varied from 0 to 5 dB for frequencies of 500 through 2k Hz for individuals with normal functioning cochlea or mild sensory-neural hearing loss. Hinchcliffe (1962) states that in reviewing data regarding decreased hearing and tone decay, nerve VIII and cochlear degeneration are not the dominant factors in developing presbycusis.

Jerger (1960) used Bekesy audiometry (see Chapter 18) with patients having various types of hearing impairment. There were 44 elderly persons labeled as presbycusics. The presbycusic subjects had more Type I than Type II tracings with two subjects demonstrating Type IVs. Three subjects gave responses that did not fit any of the four patterns. Since Type I tracings generally indicate a normal auditory mechanism or conductive impairment, Type II patterns a cochlear problem and Type IV tracings a retrocochlear disorder, presbycusis does not appear to fall into a definite category. It appears that significant tone decay is not a predominant factor in presbycusis.

The SISI Test

Site of lesion testing through the use of the short increment sensitivity index (SISI) was conducted as part of a classic investigation by Jerger, Shedd and Harford (1959). As in the case of other special tests, the performance of the elderly on the SISI test is quite unpredictable. Presbycusic subjects do not fit into any definite category.

Although studies of the central auditory mechanism (the brain stem pathways and auditory cortex) are scarce, nevertheless they provide important information about presbycusis.

Degraded Speech

Jerger (1973) studied the response of 18 elderly subjects to a variety of suprathreshold tasks involving speech understanding in difficult listening conditions. Five younger subjects demonstrating sensory-neural hearing loss were assessed under the same conditions as controls. All hearing impaired subjects revealed the same degree and configuration of sensory-neural hearing loss. Five normally hearing subjects were also exposed to all experimental conditions. Suprathreshold tasks included: (1) PB max, (2) PB score at 5 dB sensation level (SL), (3) sentences in competition (see Chapter 22) and (4) time-compressed sentences. Average scores for all three groups are shown in Figure 35.6. Jerger presents his conclusions as follows:

We see that, for the relatively easy task of repeating back PB words at a level well above threshold (PB max), there is little difference among the three groups. When the task is made somewhat more difficult, however, by simply presenting the words at a very faint level (5 dB SL), the presbycusic group has more difficulty than either the normal or the control groups. Sentence identification in the presence of ipsilateral competing message (SSI-ICM) shows an even more pronounced effect. Con-

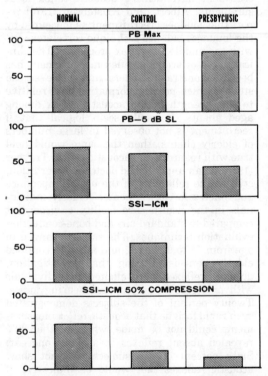

Fig. 35.6. Average scores on four speech understanding tasks for three patient groups. (Adapted from Jerger (1973).)

trols break down relative to normals, but presbycusics show an even greater loss.

Finally, subjecting the SSI sentences to time compression accentuates the effect even more. Both the control and presbycusic groups show a severe breakdown in comparison with the normal group. . . . Presbycusics show a slightly greater effect than the younger controls (pp. 121–122).

Jerger concludes that among the elderly there is a disproportionate breakdown in understanding speech when compared to their pure tone threshold.

In summarizing the literature, the following is revealed:

1. Typically there is a bilateral hearing loss by air and bone conduction. The general configuration is sensory-neural in appearance, sloping gently into the high frequencies.

2. The effects of noise and ototoxic drugs cannot be separated well from true presbycusis.

3. Speech understanding is generally worse than one would expect from observing the pure tone audiogram.

4. Site of lesion tests are inconsistent from person to person; however, recruitment is seldom seen in presbycusis whether measured by traditional means or by acoustic reflex measurements.

5. Tests of higher auditory function show noticeable differences when the presbycusic client is compared with a younger individual with equal sensory-neural hearing loss.

6. Since elderly patients have considerably more difficulty in understanding verbal messages than would be suggested by their pure tone thresholds or performance on other site of lesion tests, then one must conclude that the problem involves primarily the higher auditory centers.

DISCUSSION

Presbycusis appears to be a disorder of central processing that is compounded by peripheral sensory-neural hearing loss. The amount of hearing loss noted in the elderly would not present itself as an overwhelming disorder to a younger person, but the elderly person has a great auditory disability. For example, a decrease in the speed of processing auditory/linguistic symbols at higher auditory centers would compound the peripheral auditory difficulties of the elderly client. Problems in sorting auditory information, i.e., separating a structured set of phonemic symbols from background noise would also prove difficult.

The devastation encountered by the elderly client who can hear what people are saying but cannot make any sense of it must be overwhelming. For individuals who once were able to hear at church, able to communicate around a large dinner table, talk to their grandchildren, go to a movie, watch television, listen to the radio, go to social gatherings, or understand the words to music, the effect is dehumanizing. The individual is no longer able to participate in social activities and gradually eases himself out, or is eased out, of meaningful contact with the world around him. Self-isolation, depression, and withdrawal from family and society are the common consequences of severe auditory dysfunction in the elderly.

ROLE OF THE AUDIOLOGIST IN DEALING WITH THE ELDERLY

Although elderly clients make up a great percentage of the audiologist's case load, the complexity of their auditory difficulties has caused many audiologists to avoid the challenge. Busse (1960) has stated that audiologists have realized that phonemic regression and related disorders in the elderly present a formidable problem in diagnosing and treating, not to mention the interference and frustration felt by the elderly person. Aging clients do not understand why they cannot make sense out of what they hear, nor do they understand why someone cannot provide them with the tools to make use out of what they receive auditorily. According to Rossenwasser (1964), the adult over age 65 faces a greater handicap with equal hearing impairment because of the complex psychological problems common to the aged and the adjustments he must make to his environment. In order to avoid the difficulties of working with the elderly client, it is easy for the audiologist to dismiss his responsibility with, "Your ears have grown older," or "Your ears are old, and there is nothing medically that can be done for you." This eliminates the possibility that the individual will receive rehabilitative services which could benefit him.

The audiologist is the proper professional for the elderly to discuss the impact of their hearing impairment as it affects them communicatively, socially, and occupationally. It is easy for the alert elderly person to realize his severe limitations when the auditory confusions cause him to miss parts of messages, and therefore respond inappropriately. When this occurs frequently enough; it not only alarms him but concerns his family and other associates as well. These are unfortunate experiences for the elderly person who is feeling less than useful anyway, and who is not as active as he feels capable of being. They will, in most instances, cause embarrassment and anger. If these situations occur frequently enough, the elderly person may retire into self-exile to maintain his pride and avoid further embarrassment.

Audiologists have a responsibility to help the presbycusic patient as they would any other patient who is in need of their help. This might be in the form of diagnosis, counseling or rehabilitation. The elderly individual generally comes to the audiologist out of desperation. Of any other handicapping condition related to aging, the inability to communicate with family and friends must be the most devastating. If the elderly individual is confronted by an audiologist who turns him away because "there is nothing that can be done," then that audiologist may have pushed him sharply in the direction of isolation. We are finding that many of the elderly with presbycusis who were thought to be beyond rehabilitation can be helped to communicate more efficiently (Hull and Traynor, 1975). Many can learn to communicate at least to the point of being able to relate more efficiently with their family. The skilled diagnostic evaluation is the first step toward successful rehabilitation of the elderly client. Together with skilled diagnosis, an understanding of the devastating effects of presbycusis on the aging individual is necessary. Without that understanding, a complete diagnosis will not be made. An audiologist who does not understand or who does not have a real desire to deal with the elderly person will be doing a disservice to those clients by going through the motions of evaluation only to dismiss his rehabilitative responsibility.

AUDIOLOGIC ASSESSMENT OF THE ELDERLY

The successful audiologic evaluation is the first step toward successful rehabilitation of the elderly. When evaluating the hearing of the aged person, the audiologist is dealing with someone who probably heard and understood well at one time. For reasons unknown to him, his hearing gradually decreased until he was concerned enough to seek the aid of an audiologist who might help him or at least give him counsel.

According to Alpiner (1965), the elderly person might complain that he cannot "understand" people as well as he used to. Or, he might state that he feels that his family and friends are mumbling lately, but that he is afraid that it might be because he is not hearing as well as he should. He might say that he feels that he is able to hear all right, but that he has difficulty "making out" what people say. One frequent comment is that he can hear well when he is talking to one or two persons, but as soon as he must communicate with a group of people he has difficulty understanding what is being said to him. Because he does have difficulty understanding what people say, he will often confuse the content of messages. If he also has typical high frequency hearing loss, the difficulty in understanding speech is compounded. He may hear messages incorrectly and, thus, answer inappropriately. Some family members, friends, and especially those unfamiliar to the individual, may then diagnose senility in the geriatric. This diagnosis may be inaccurate since senility has been confused with inability to understand auditory messages. The case history may reveal nothing except the fact that the person being evaluated has grown older.

The tests utilized during the audiologic evaluation and the manner in which they are administered are dependent upon the particular client being evaluated and his/her individual temperament. Such factors as fatigue, frustration tolerance, along with the motivation of the individual are necessarily taken into consideration when assessment techniques are chosen. Alpiner (1965) suggests that it is oftentimes best if the testing period can be extended to two separate sessions on different days. Because of the transportation difficulties for many elderly individuals, however, as much information should be derived during the first assessment period as possible. It may not be possible to do the complete hearing aid evaluation during the first visit.

Depending upon the physical capabilities of the elderly client, the following tests should be considered in whatever modified form the audiologist deems necessary for the purpose of acquiring needed information for either medical referral or rehabilitative efforts:

1. Pure tone air-conduction thresholds.
2. Pure tone bone-conduction thresholds.
3. Speech reception thresholds under phones with and without visual clues.
4. Auditory discrimination under phones with and without visual clues for:
   a. Phonetically balanced monosyllabic words; and
   b. Sentences (C.I.D. Everyday Speech).
5. Impedance audiometry including acoustic reflex measurements for determining the presence of recruitment.

THE CASE HISTORY

Prior to the audiometric evaluation, case history information should be taken. Since, in most cases, such items as those referring to childhood illness are not pertinent to the elderly individual, modifications may be desirable. Information regarding the handicap they experience in various communication situations is important, as is the approximate time of onset of the hearing loss itself and the onset of its handicapping effects. A sample of an extension of the traditional case history form utilized at the University of Northern Colorado Audiology Clinic specifically for elderly patients is seen in Figure 35.7.

UNIVERSITY OF NORTHERN COLORADO

AURAL REHABILITATION EVALUATION FORM

Date_____

Name_____ Age_____ Sex_____

Present occupation_____ Previous occupation_____

Reason for seeking audiometric assessment_____

_____

Does the utilization of visual clues help you understand what people are saying?

_____

Do you think learning to use visual clues will help you?_____

In what way/ways?_____

How do you compensate in difficult conversation situations?_____

_____

Please indicate the situations in which you communicate best and those which

give you the most difficulty:

	No Problem	Problem
Socially.	_____	_____
Dinner Table.	_____	_____
Telephone	_____	_____
In the Home	_____	_____
With Males.	_____	_____
With Females.	_____	_____
With Children	_____	_____
Groups.	_____	_____
Individuals	_____	_____
At Work	_____	_____
Other (Please Indicate)	_____	_____

Fig. 35.7. Extension of standard case history form adapted for the elderly client and utilized in the Audiology Clinic, University of Northern Colorado.

Skillful interviewing techniques are necessary when dealing with many elderly clients. The question, "When did you first begin to notice that your hearing was not as good as it should be?" can bring about a lengthy discussion on the part of the elderly individual beginning with information regarding childhood experiences or an oration on the topic of the lack of clarity of speaking habits by young people today. The skillful clinician will be able to guide the elderly client into specific topics related to not only the onset of hearing loss but specific difficulties experienced in various communication situations. The audiologist must take the time necessary to listen to the elderly client. In many instances, the information being given by the client has been told to no one else; for example, the client's concerns in making sense out of conversations or understanding what his grandchildren are saying. The resolution "not to be a bother by asking their friends or relatives to repeat what they said so Grandma can be a part of the conversa-

tion" was undoubtedly a traumatic one and needs airing. Tears will often be shed by the elderly client during the case history interview. The audiologist should listen well but also guide the conversation toward pertinent topics. Most importantly, however, the audiologist must listen and learn about that client, not only about the auditory impairment and the resulting handicap, but also his/her desire for work toward rehabilitation.

PURE TONE EVALUATION

After the case history interview is completed, the audiologic evaluation is initiated to determine the type and extent of the auditory impairment. Instructions for all auditory tests must be explicit. On occasion, directions must necessarily be given several different ways until the individual understands them. Patience on the part of the audiologist is the key here. The concept of responding by raising one's hand or pushing a button whenever a barely audible signal is heard is a difficult concept for many elderly persons. They will often wait until the pure tone signal is comfortably loud and then nod their head to acknowledge its presence and also raise their hand or sometimes not raise their hand. When the audiologist asks the client if the tone was heard, he/she will state confidently that it was. Careful instructions regarding correct response along with the purpose of the test are then given once more. If a manual response is requested by the audiologist, the reaction time by the elderly must be kept in mind. The elderly person will often respond more slowly than the younger individual simply because age has slowed voluntary motor response. On occasion, manual response (raising the hand or pushing a response button) will come several seconds after the pure tone signal is presented. The audiologist must wait for such a delayed response before presenting the next signal at a higher intensity or what seems to be a response to the more intense signal may actually be a delayed response to the previous one, thus not only confusing the client but also resulting in false information regarding that person's sensitivity for puretones.

A verbal response is utilized through the Community-wide Program in Geriatric Aural Rehabilitation (Hull and Traynor, 1975, and Traynor, 1972). Verbal response by the elderly client has been found to be an effective technique for those clients who either have difficulties grasping the concept of a manual response to a barely audible pure tone signal or have very delayed responses. The elderly person will often converse regarding the intensity of the signal during the evaluation period. The verbal response procedure capitalizes on the client's natural inclination to speak to the audiologist. The signal is presented, for example, at 60 dB. If the client does not respond, the intensity is increased by 10 dB and the client is asked once again if the signal was heard. If at that point the response is positive, the intensity is decreased by 5 dB. As the audiologist nears the client's threshold, the usual response is a verbal one, that the signal is "very faint," or "very weak," or is "very far away." Thresholds for frequencies of 250, 500, 1k, 2k, 4k and 8k Hz are thus established utilizing that procedure. This usually results in more reliable responses, less confusion for the client and less frustration for the audiologist. Much positive reinforcement is used throughout the evaluation.

EVALUATION OF SPEECH RECEPTION

Procedures for speech audiometry are generally less confusing for the elderly client. For speech audiometry as in pure tone audiometry, the audiologist must learn patience if it does not come as an innate quality. During assessment of the speech reception threshold, the audiologist must give explicit instructions such as, "You will hear some words such as baseball, hotdog, and airplane. I would like for you to repeat them after me. Some may be very soft but try to tell me what they are the best you can." On occasion, the elderly client will describe the relative intensity of the word rather than repeat it. Such responses may be, "That was very soft," or "Turn it down, it is too loud," or "Yes, I can hear you." This may be a carryover from the verbal response utilized for pure tone audiometry. If this does occur, clients should be asked if they can hear your voice; if they say, "Yes," then ask, "Can you understand me?" If the response is, "Yes, I can," then repeat the instructions and allow the client to practice on several of the words before continuing the test.

A point should be stressed here. When instructions for all test procedures are given, remove the client's head phones and face him. Ask the client if he can hear and understand you and then proceed with the instructions. The audiologist, then, avoids the confusions that can arise from auditory discrimination difficulties when visual clues cannot be utilized by the client.

After speech reception thresholds are obtained, the test is repeated with the client able to see the audiologist's face. This procedure is utilized to determine how the client is able to utilize visual clues.

EVALUATION FOR SPEECH DISCRIMINATION

Assessment for auditory discrimination may be conducted utilizing lists of both monosyllabic phonetically balanced words and sentences (C.I.D. Everyday Speech) with and without visual clues. For either type of assessment, the audiologist is warned against placing the client in an inevitable situation of failure. If, for example, the client is obviously unable to receive and respond to any stimulus item, the client's frustration can spell disaster for future rehabilitative efforts or other professional contacts if the audiologist continues on through the lists of words or sentences blindly ignoring that frustration. If the client appears unable to respond to any test item and is quickly arriving at the point of extreme frustration, the audiologist may ask the client to face him to test the client's ability to utilize visual clues for the same monosyllabic words or sentences. If the client is more successful with this mode of presentation, then frustration is lowered and some very valuable information can be obtained for future rehabilitative efforts.

IMPEDANCE AUDIOMETRY

Impedance audiometry appears to be an efficient tool for assessment of peripheral auditory function to rule out the existence of conductive impairment when air-conduction thresholds indicate hearing loss. Traynor (1975) studied the efficiency of impedance audiometry in assessing the nonambulatory elderly person when compared with traditional air- and bone-conduction tests, conducted both in a sound-treated environment and in the non-sound-treated health care facility. Results of that investigation indicated the following:

1. There is a significant difference in thresholds when pure tone air and bone conduction are assessed in a non-sound-treated environment as compared to the evaluations in a sound-treated environment. However, bone conduction is affected more than air conduction. These data suggest that air conduction could be evaluated outside of a sound-treated room with reasonable accuracy.

2. Prediction of the type and extent of hearing loss was better using pure tone air-conduction audiometry and acoustic impedance measurements than by traditional air- and bone-conduction audiometry conducted in a sound-treated environment.

3. The average amount of time required to administer air- and bone-conduction tests versus air conduction and impedance measurements was essentially the same.

From these results, several conclusions seem reasonable:

1. Air-conduction evaluations can be conducted outside of a sound-treated environment with reasonable accuracy in the elderly population.

2. Bone-conduction evaluations should not be conducted outside of a sound-treated environment.

3. A skilled clinician can obtain accurate conclusions from pure tone air-conduction and electro-acoustic impedance testing in a non-sound-treated environment. This includes whether there is a hearing loss, the degree of loss, and the type even in a nonambulatory geriatric population.

CONCLUSIONS

Beyond the Audiogram

Accurate evaluation of auditory function of the elderly client requires a skilled and adaptable audiologist, who has considerable patience. The rapport established with the older individual plays a large part in the success of the entire diagnostic and rehabilitative effort. If the elderly client views a younger audiologist as "flippant," or "arrogant," or "intolerant" of his elders, then it is very difficult to salvage any type of professional relationship. On occasion, those feelings by the client can arise simply by the general appearance of the audiologist or a side comment that was not understood by the elderly person. All comments and all communication about the elderly client should be made directly to the client and not privately to a family member. The suspicious nature oftentimes seen in the hearing-impaired elderly person may be simply a defense mechanism to help him cope in an uncertain environment. To avoid complications of this nature, the client must be involved in all verbalization regarding the results of the evaluation and should be made to feel free to ask questions. The environment should be a good one for open communication between the audiologist and the client; relaxed, but professional in climate. The audiologist must develop a feeling of trust between himself and the client. Without it the diagnostic evaluation and aural rehabilitation program may be doomed.

The audiologist must be able to look beyond the audiogram and the anatomic pathology of presbycusis when dealing with the elderly person. The audiologist should have a clear understanding of the handicapping effects of presbycusis on communicative function in the "real world" outside of the audiology clinic. The audiologist should try to understand the desperation of the elderly individual and what it must mean to see one's communicative skills dwindle in the face of mandatory retirement, low income and decreasing physical capabilities. Gradually the one avenue of contact with his world (hearing/communication) is degenerating. In conducting the audiometric evaluation, the hearing aid evaluation, and in initiating and maintaining that individual's aural rehabilitation program, the audiologist must look to the handicapping effects of presbycusis on the elderly person and the individual's concerns and goals. The goal of the audiologist should be to guide the elderly to develop a better understanding of their auditory impairment and to use this knowledge in establishing the most communication possible.

For information regarding the specific aural rehabilitation processes for the elderly including the hearing aid evaluation, counseling techniques, and utilization of speechreading auditory training techniques, see Chapter 49 of this text.

REFERENCES

Alberti, P., and Kristensen, R., The clinical application of impedance audiometry. *Laryngoscope,* 80, 735–746, 1970.

Alpiner, J., Diagnostic and rehabilitative aspects of geriatric audiology. *ASHA*, 7, 455–459, 1965.

Beasley, W., Generalized Age and Sex Trends in Hearing Loss. In *National Health Survey, Hearing Study Bulletin No. 7*, Washington, D.C.: Public Health Service, 1938.

Bunch, C., Further observations on age variations in auditory acuity. *Arch. Otolaryngol.*, 13, 170–180, 1931.

Busse, E., Aging and Personal Relations. In Shock, N. W. (Ed.), *Aging: Some Social and Biological Aspects*. Washington, D.C.: American Association for the Advancement of Science, 1960.

Chafee, C., Rehabilitation needs of nursing home patients—a report of a survey. *Rehabil. Lit.*, 18, 377–389, 1967.

Department of Health, Education and Welfare, Health Resources Administration. *Health Resources*, 2, 9, 1975.

Department of Health, Education and Welfare, Vocational Rehabilitation Administration. *Information Service Series No. 63–11*, Washington, D.C., 1963.

Gaeth, J., A study of phonemic regression associated with hearing loss. Dissertation, Northwestern University, Chicago, 1948. (Cited by Willeford, 1971.)

Glorig, A., and Davis, H., Age, noise and hearing loss. *Ann. Otol. Rhinol. Laryngol.*, 70, 556–571, 1961.

Glorig, A., and Roberts, J., Hearing Levels of Adults by Age and Sex: United States 1960–1962. *Public Health Service Publication No. 1000*, Series 11, No. 11, Washington, D. C., 1965.

Glorig, A., Wheeler, D., Quiggle, R., Grings, W., and Summerfield, A., 1954 Wisconsin state fair hearing survey. *Am. Acad. Ophthalmol. Otolaryngol. Monograph*, 1957.

Goetzinger, C., Proud, G., Dirks, D., and Embrey, J., A study of hearing in advanced age. *Arch. Otolaryngol.*, 73, 662–674, 1961.

Goodhill, V., Bilateral malleal fixation and conductive presbycusis. *Arch. Otolaryngol.*, 90, 6, 759–764, 1969.

Hansen, C., and Reske-Nielsen, E., Pathological studies in presbycusis. *Arch. Otolaryngol.*, 82, 115–132, 1965.

Harbert, F., Young, I., and Menduke, H., Audiologic findings in presbycusis. *J. Aud. Res.*, 6, 297–312, 1966.

Hawkins, J., Comparative otopathology; aging, noise, and ototoxic drugs. *Adv. Otorhinolaryngol.*, 20, 125–141, 1973.

Hinchcliffe, R., The threshold of hearing as a function of age. *Acoustica*, 9, 303–308, 1959.

Hinchcliffe, R., The anatomical locus of presbycusis. *J. Speech Hear. Disord.*, 27, 301–310, 1962.

Hirsch, I., Palva, T., and Goodman, A., Difference limen and recruitement. *Arch. Otolaryngol.*, 60, 525–540, 1954.

Hull, R., and Traynor, R., A community-wide program in geriatric aural rehabilitation. *ASHA*, 14, 33–34, 47–48, 1975.

Jerger, J., Bekesy audiometry in analysis of auditory disorders. *J. Speech Hear. Res.*, 3, 275–287, 1960.

Jerger, J., Audiological findings in aging. *Adv. Otorhinolaryngol.*, 20, 115–124, 1973.

Jerger, J., Shedd, J., and Harford, E., On the detection of extremely small changes of sound intensity. *Arch. Otolaryngol.*, 69, 200–211, 1959.

Johnson, L. G., and Hawkins, J., Sensory and neural degeneration with aging, as seen in microdissections of the human inner ear. *Ann. Otol. Rhinol. Laryngol.*, 81, 179–193, 1972.

Johnson, J., and Hadley, R., The Aging Face. In Converse, J. (Ed.), *Reconstructive Plastic Surgery*, pp. 1306–1342. Philadelphia: W. B. Saunders, 1964.

Jorgensen, M., Changes of aging in the inner ear. *Arch. Otolaryngol.*, 74, 161–170, 1961.

Kirikae, I., Sato, T., and Shitara, T., Study of hearing in advanced age. *Laryngscope*, 74, 205–221, 1964.

Leake, C., Study of the components of deafness. *Geriatrics*, 18, 506, 1963.

Leutenegger, R., and Stovall, J., A pilot graduate seminar concerning speech and hearing problems of the chronically ill and aged. *ASHA*, 13, 61–66, 1971.

Matzker, J., and Springhorn, E., Richtungshoren and lebensalzer. *Z. Laryngol. Rhinol. Otol.*, 37, 739–745, 1958.

Metropolitan Life Insurance Company, Hearing impairment in the United States. *Statist. Bull.*, 47, 3, 1966.

Miller, M., and Ort, R., Hearing problems in a home for the aged. *Acta Otolaryngol.*, 59, 33–44, 1965.

National Advisory Council for Neurological Diseases and Stroke, Report of the Subcommittee on Human Communication and Its Disorders, National Institutes of Health Report, D.H.E.W., 1969.

National Center for Health Statistics, Prevalence of Selected Impairments, 1971. Vital Health Statistics, Rockville, Md., Health Resources Administration, D.H.E.W., 1975.

Pestalozza, G., and Shore, I., Clinical evaluation of presbycusis on the basis of different tests of auditory functions. *Laryngoscope*, 65, 1136–1163, 1955.

Proctor, B., Chronic progressive deafness. *Arch. Otolaryngol.*, 73, 444–499, 565–615, 1961.

Rosen, S., Plester, D., El-Mofty, A., and Rosen, H., High frequency audiometry in presbycusis; a comparative study of the Mabaan tribe of the Sudan with urban populations. *Arch. Otolaryngol.*, 79, 18–32, 1964.

Rosenwasser, H., Otitic problems in the aged. *Geriatrics*, 19, 11–17, 1964.

Sataloff, J., Vassalo, L., and Menduke, H., Presbycusis; air and bone conduction thresholds. *Laryngoscope*, 75, 889–901, 1965.

Shock, N., Aging; some social and biological aspects. American Association for the Advancement of Science, Washington, D. C., 1960.

Schuknecht, H., Further observations on the pathology of presbycusis. *Arch. Otolaryngol.*, 80, 369–382, 1964.

Schuknecht, H., The pathology of presbycusis. Unpublished presentation at a Workshop on Geriatric Aural Rehabilitation, Denver, Colo., 1974.

Schuknecht, H., and Woellner, R., An experimental and clinical study of deafness from lesions of the cochlear nerve. *J. Laryngol. Otol.*, **69**, 75–97, 1955.

Taniewaki, J., Hearing in senility. *Wiad. Lek.*, **16**, 337–339, 1963.

Traynor, R., The aural rehabilitation of geriatric patients. Unpublished honors project, University of Northern Colorado, Greeley, Col., 1972.

Traynor, R., A method of audiological assessment for the non-ambulatory geriatric patient. Unpublished dissertation, University of Northern Colorado, Greeley, Col., 1975.

Traynor, R., and Hull, R., Pure-tone thresholds among a confined elderly population. Unpublished research, University of Northern Colorado, Greeley, Col., 1974.

Willeford, J., The Geriatric Patient. In Rose, D. (Ed.), *Audiological Assessment.* Englewood Cliffs, N. J.: Prentice-Hall, 1971.

Introduction to the Management of the Hearing Impaired

chapter 36

INTRODUCTION TO AURAL REHABILITATION

J. Curtis Tannahill, Ph.D., and Walter J. Smoski, M.S.

Audiologic habilitation (ASHA, 1974), rehabilitative audiology (Oyer and Frankmann 1975), and aural rehabilitation (Sanders, 1971; Ross, 1972; O'Neill and Oyer, 1973) are current terms which refer to those evaluation and therapy procedures designed to bring about maximum communication skills among the hearing impaired. A survey of modern textbooks dealing with the management of hearing related communication handicaps shows a prevalence of the use of the term "aural rehabilitation." Therefore, we have chosen to use this more traditional term.

Aural rehabilitation is initiated following thorough audiologic evaluation and completion of medical care. There is a well established relationship between hearing, language acquisition and speech development. Clinicians engaged in aural rehabilitation must clearly understand the deleterious impact hearing impairment has on these behaviors. Specific management is dependent on the individual needs of each client and may include hearing aid evaluation/selection and follow-up care, speechreading training, auditory training, and speech therapy. In addition, there are tangential aspects to aural rehabilitation such as associated language problems, educational needs, and psychosocial considerations which the clinician must integrate into the total rehabilitating scheme (Mindel and Vernon, 1971; Myklebust, 1964.) Although aural rehabilitation may be carried out by a number of different professionals, the clinical audiologist is often considered the major provider of such services.

The importance of aural rehabilitation to the hearing impaired cannot be overemphasized. Although handicapping hearing impairment may be accompanied by many problems, the most outstanding is the breakdown in communication. Helping the hearing impaired individual overcome this problem is the task of aural rehabilitation clinicians. As Ross (1972, p. 3) has pointed out, "Our immediate therapy goal is the improvement of communicative abilities; our eventual goal is a well-adjusted and productive individual." Early identification, thorough measurement, and good medical care are essential to remediation of hearing impairment. However, if verbal communication, either expressive or receptive, remains inadequate, aural rehabilitation is necessary.

Practically all children with handicapping hearing losses require aural rehabilitation. Two major factors determine specific type of treatment. First is the degree of loss which differentiates deaf children from hard of hearing children. The second is age of onset of the hearing loss. From an aural rehabilitative point of view, it is common to establish onset as *pre-* or *postlingual* rather than congenital or adventitious. Prelingual means "prior to language acquisition". Postlingual implies that basic language skills have been developed.

The primary effect of severe, prelingual deafness is the handicap of retarded language development and, therefore, communication skills (Levine, 1960). Although these children must rely heavily on vision for learning, the value of even limited residual hearing must not be overlooked. For these children all aspects of aural rehabilitation are essential. Children with lesser degrees of hearing impairment experience less language deficit and aural rehabilitation is focused on developing and maintaining hearing as the major avenue for communication. Almost all hearing-impaired children display some degree of difficulty in speech development and production. Therefore, considerable effort is directed at improving these skills.

For the most part, adults who are seen for aural rehabilitation have acquired hearing loss some time during adulthood as a result of disease, noise exposure, and/or aging. Most are beyond the age of 50. Many are retired and experience a more limited life style. Often plagued by reduced mobility and limited financial resources, these adults come to the audiologist in need of improved receptive communication skills. Unlike congenitally hearing-impaired adults, the adventitiously hearing-impaired adult usually does not have a speech and/or language problem. For the most part, their expressive skills are well developed and intact. Their primary handicap is broadly related to the auditory reception. Specifically, they want to hear and understand speech.

HEARING AIDS

If permanent hearing impairment exists following medical care, the first and most logical step in the aural rehabilitative process is a hearing aid evaluation. For some individuals, successful use of amplification resolves the communication handicap; however, for many others the acquisition of a hearing aid is the first in a long line of aural rehabilitation procedures.

Successful hearing aid use is dependent on competent hearing aid evaluation, selection of an appropriate aid, and supervision of the adjustment period. Audiologists have the primary role in this aspect of aural rehabilitation but may work closely with a hearing aid dealer regarding delivery of the aid to the client.

Based on the hearing aid evaluation, the audiologist will determine potential benefit to be derived from amplification and often which aid is most appropriate. An examination of current literature indicates no clear consensus among professionals in the field as to the specific procedures which should be used in the hearing aid evaluation. There is diverse opinion not only concerning the specific tests, but also how many aids should be evaluated (Millin, 1975).

Some audiologists feel that their responsibility is only to determine hearing aid candidacy. Selection of the specific aid is left up to the hearing aid dealer. When this approach is taken, the audiologist usually reserves the right to make the final decision as to appropriateness of the aid and manages the post-fitting period. Other audiologists assume responsibility for both hearing aid evaluation and selection of a specific aid. Since several aids are usually evaluated, this procedure requires the maintenance of a large stock of hearing aids. Even though actual hearing aid evaluation

procedures vary among audiologists, the common goal is to provide each individual with the hearing aid that will maximize his reception and discrimination of speech.

The combined efforts of audiology and the hearing aid industry have promoted rapid changes in hearing aid technology. Clinicians in the field must constantly keep abreast of new developments. Recent trends favor fitting children with aids at earlier ages. Advancements in hearing aid design and earmold acoustics make it possible to fit individuals with unusual losses previously considered unaidable. Finally, the dispensing of hearing aids by clinical audiologists appears to be well on its way to becoming a permanent aspect of aural rehabilitation (ASHA, 1976).

COMMUNICATION TRAINING

When the hearing-impaired person has been properly fitted with a hearing aid or hearing aid use has been ruled out, therapeutic management of the remaining communication handicap is initiated. Such management may include speechreading, auditory training, and speech therapy.

Speechreading

A common approach to speechreading training is based on the premise that "practice makes perfect." This approach is founded on the notion that speechreading is a behavior which can be taught (O'Neill and Oyer, 1961). Therapy often entails repetitious drills which require the client to identify a visual signal produced by the clinician. Clinicians favoring a synthetic approach will use materials presented in differing linguistic contexts. A progression from isolated words to phrases, and then to conversational speech, is often used. Clinicians favoring an analytic approach will initiate drill activities using isolated sounds and nonsense syllables, therefore eliminating semantic requirements. Practice begins by identifying highly visible sounds such as /p/, /θ/, /ʃ/, etc., and works toward identification of low visibility sounds such as /k/, /g/, and /h/. The eclectic approach to speechreading training involves the clinician choosing aspects from both the synthetic and analytic approach. Here, the client may be drilled on sounds in isolation and also words in context.

A second approach to speechreading training is based on the premise that speechreading is a complex behavior which is difficult to modify by direct practice. This approach stresses the need for informational and tutorial counseling. That is, the clinician teaches the client "about" speechreading rather than having the client practice speechreading. Counseling may include information about sounds that look alike on the lips (homophenous sounds), the need to pay visual attention, the importance of relying on situational and contextual clues, and the value of proper lighting, distance and angle of vision. A certain amount of drillwork may be included in order to illustrate and support each area of counseling.

Speechreading training for the very young hearing-impaired child is designed to teach the child that lip movement and other visual signals associated with communication have meaning. Their speechreading skills are acquired simultaneously with language skills. Speechreading for the older hearing-impaired child is often accomplished by applying the drill methods previously described.

For adults, speechreading skills are often improved by drill work and/or the informational and tutorial counseling method. Use of the latter method is more common among adults than children.

Auditory Training

Auditory training is essential even for those individuals with profound hearing loss. Such training is designed to maximize the use of residual hearing regardless of the degree of hearing loss.

Auditory training methods for children start with developing an awareness of and sensitivity to meaningful acoustic signals and increase to encompass discrimination and perception of speech. This training is almost always carried out with the use of amplification. An overall plan of auditory training for children was described by Carhart (1960). He suggested beginning by teaching the child to identify the presence or absence of sound. The plan called for progression through the identification and discrimination of environmental sounds and concluded by switching to speech sounds in isolation and eventually to words and phrases.

Auditory training for older hearing-impaired children focuses on the "problem" sounds of each child; that is, those sounds the child mishears or confuses with other sounds. Drill work techniques are used to increase the child's skill in discriminating particular sounds in isolation and in context.

Auditory training for adults tends to focus on two areas: discrimination of speech and increasing tolerance for loud speech and environmental sounds. The latter is almost exclusively associated with new hearing aid users who initially cannot tolerate amplified sound (Tannahill, 1973). Speech discrimination training relies heavily on drill work and often includes listening in the presence of background noise. Consideration of the fact that most hearing impaired listeners, even when using a hearing aid, receive a less than desirable auditory signal, has led to the inclusion of training

in auditory closure. Clients are encouraged to use their knowledge of linguistic constraints to "guess" what was said based on partial information.

Combined Methods

Many professionals feel that speechreading training and auditory training administered separately are not as productive nor as realistic as the bisensory approach. The bisensory approach includes procedures similar to those previously mentioned; however, the client is provided both the visual and auditory information simultaneously. Sanders (1971) has dealt effectively with the philosophy supporting bisensory stimulation. He states (p. 6): "We must, however, constantly bear in mind that maximum communication for the hard-of-hearing individual occurs when the auditory and visual pathways act in an integrative manner."

Speech Therapy

Speech therapy for hearing-impaired children employs similar techniques applied to normal hearing children with speech problems. That is, the clinician provides the model which the client is required to imitate. Unfortunately, hearing impairment tends to distort the clarity and perception of the model. Therefore, speech therapy for the hearing-impaired child stresses the development of motor and tactile feedback as well as auditory feedback (Carhart, 1970).

Since most hearing impaired adults have developed normal speech prior to the onset of their hearing loss, the resulting speech problems tend to be minor. They often omit sibilant sounds in the final position of words and show some tendency to run words together. Where hearing loss is more severe, there may be an associated problem of speaking too loudly (Ewing and Ewing, 1938). Management of these minor speech problems is appropriately labeled "speech conservation." In many cases, simply making the client aware of the problem will eliminate it. Where a problem still exists, limited speech therapy will enable the hearing impaired adult to maintain socially acceptable speech patterns.

Whether communication training is directed at children or adults, and regardless of the techniques used, the goal is to facilitate maximum expressive and receptive communication skills. There seems to be no best strategy and the clinician must co-mingle his bias and skills with the individual requirements of each client.

TOTAL MANAGEMENT

The hearing-impaired individual may be introduced into the aural rehabilitative process by a number of different professionals. Because measurement of the loss and need for amplification are recognized as fundamental to aural rehabilitation, the audiologist becomes involved early in the process. Depending on the involvement of other professionals, the audiologist must be prepared to develop and coordinate ongoing management. It is important to be sensitive to the fact that no single professional can provide the total rehabilitation needs of hearing impaired individuals. Thus, the clinician must be acquainted with the services in many professional areas. A total rehabilitation program could involve one or all of the following services:

Medical referral
Audiologic evaluation
Hearing aid evaluation, selection, and procurement
Communication training
Family counseling
Educational, psychosocial, and vocational counseling and planning
Financial planning and assistance.

Children

Total management for infants must necessarily begin with identification and measurement of the hearing loss. Following medical care, hearing aid evaluation and selection are initiated for those infants with medically irreversible losses. Concurrently, regular parent counseling is provided along with appropriate referral to supportive agencies and other professionals, particularly the parent-infant educator. The parent-home educator, often a teacher of the hearing impaired, specializes in teaching parents how to manage hearing related problems of their child with a special emphasis on development of communicative skills. This training usually takes place in the child's home or a model home set up to simulate the child's home environment. (See: *A guide to early education of the hearing impaired, Wisconsin Department of Public Instruction Bulletin, 1971* and Connor, 1967.)

For the preschool age hearing-impaired child, total management includes introduction into a formal educational setting. Special attention is given to the development of specific communication skills. This is supported by regular staffings. These staffings are essential in order to develop long range programs which fit the needs of each individual child.

Children with mild losses or those with greater losses who have been "mainstreamed" into regular classrooms require less comprehensive management. However, communication training is essential and is usually provided by the speech pathologist or audiologist in the regular school setting.

Adults

Total management for adults is facilitated by grouping clients based on the amount of hearing loss and the resulting communication handicap.

Minimal Loss/Minimal Handicap. Many hearing-impaired adults fall into this group. These are people who have slight hearing losses; just enough to be aggravating in difficult listening situations. Usually they are seeking confirmation that they do not need a hearing aid. Informational counseling following a hearing evaluation is often sufficient. A clear explanation of the loss, confirmation that they indeed would receive little if any benefit from amplification, and guidance related to improving communication in difficult listening situations provide the confidence needed to deal with their hearing loss.

Potential Hearing Aid Users. This group includes those adults with enough hearing loss to warrant hearing aid use. Many do not readily accept the recommendation that they need a hearing aid. Therefore, a simple hearing aid evaluation and acquisition of a hearing aid may result in limited and unsuccessful use of the aid. Careful follow-up management is often essential. It should include a supervised trial period with counseling for the hearing aid user as well as his family. For this group, successful hearing aid use will eliminate much of the hearing handicap.

Poor Hearing Aid Users. A large number of hearing-impaired adults find that, although a hearing aid is beneficial, their aided communication skills are not adequate for social and vocational needs. Among the more common facets of their loss are poor word discrimination and/or tolerance problems. When this is the case, the clinician must provide additional aural rehabilitation focusing on speechreading and aided auditory training. The likelihood of completely eliminating the communication problem is tenuous. Therefore, it is important that the clinician focus on maximum communication rather than perfect communication.

Non-Hearing Aid Users. A few hearing-impaired adults simply cannot benefit from hearing aid use even though they have a handicapping hearing loss. This group, perhaps more than any other, requires patience and skill from the clinician. Often, auditory training yields limited improvement due to very poor auditory discrimination. Therapy efforts are then concentrated on speechreading and use of non-speech cues. An appropriate objective may be to achieve acceptable performance for essential communication such as purchasing daily needs, understanding directions and instructions.

Profound Congenitally Deaf Adult. It is highly unusual for this population of hearing impaired adults to seek aural rehabilitation services. It seems that when they finish formal education they adjust to a communication process which serves their needs. Occasionally assistance is sought when a replacement hearing aid is needed or when hearing evaluation is required for employment purposes. Beyond this, formal aural rehabilitative services are rarely requested.

Summary

The audiologist must keep in mind that total management involves more than the hearing and hearing aid evaluation. Regardless of the age of the hearing-impaired person or the degree of loss, each individual must be considered in light of his background, current needs and life style, and anticipated demands on his communication skills.

SYNOPSIS OF FOLLOWING CHAPTERS

The remaining chapters in this book provide a broad spectrum of information related to the various aspects of aural rehabilitation. Practicing clinicians and graduate students will find these chapters to be both theoretical and practical.

Chapter 37, "The Psychology of Hearing Impairment," provides information related to the impact hearing loss has on the intellectual, educational, and psychosocial development and function of the hearing impaired. Such information is vital to counseling and careful therapeutic planning.

Chapter 38, "Classroom Acoustics and Speech Intelligibility", contains rather specialized information pertaining to the environment in which hearing-impaired children must learn. Such information may be difficult to obtain and is often overlooked until the special building is finished or the classroom remodeling is completed. This chapter should provide the impetus to ensure adequate sound treatment for classrooms used by the hearing impaired.

Since the hearing aid plays a very important role in aural rehabilitation, it is appropriate that several chapters be devoted to this topic. Chapters 39, 40, and 41 deal with a review of historical and technical hearing aid information and with philosophies about specific types of aids and their use. Chapter 42 presents both theoretical and practical information concerning earmolds. This chapter includes a discussion concerning modification of earmolds which alters the acoustic output of the aid to the best advantage of the user. Hearing aid evaluation methods and consultation procedures are the general topics of Chapters 43 and 44.

The detail necessary for planning and initiating comprehensive training for the hearing impaired is dealt with in Chapters 45 to 49. These chapters encompass general background information as well as specific therapeutic strategies for children and adults. Recent work in educational and geriatric audiology are presented in the last two chapters.

Finally, each chapter is supported by an extensive bibliography. These references will be useful to clinicians, teachers, and researchers.

REFERENCES

American Speech and Hearing Association, The Audiologist: Responsibilities in the Habilitation of the Auditorily Handicapped. *ASHA*, 16, 68–70, 1974.

American Speech and Hearing Association, Ethical Practice Board Interpretations of Principles Governing the Dispensing of Products to Persons with Communicative Disorders. *ASHA*, 18, 237–240, 1976

Carhart, R., Auditory training. In Davis, H., and Silverman, S. R. (Eds.), *Hearing and Deafness*, Ed. 2. New York: Holt, Rinehart & Winston, 1960.

Carhart, R., Development and Conservation of Speech. In Davis, H., and Silverman, S. R., (Eds.), *Hearing and Deafness*, Ed. 3. New York: Holt, Rinehart & Winston, 1970.

Connor, L. Recent trends in education of the deaf. *In* McConnell F., and Ward, P. H. (Eds.), *Deafness in Childhood*. Nashville, Tenn.: Vanderbilt University Press, 1967.

Ewing, I. R., and Ewing, A. W., *The Handicap of Deafness*. London: Longmans, Green & Co., 1938.

Levine, E. S., *The Psychology of Deafness*. New York: Columbia University Press, 1960.

Millin, J. P., Practical and Philosophical Considerations. In Pollack, M. C. (Ed.), *Amplification for the Hearing Impaired*. New York: Grune & Stratton, 1975.

Mindel, E. D., and Vernon, M., *They Grow in Silence*. Maryland: National Association of the Deaf, 1971.

Myklebust, H. R., *The Psychology of Deafness*, Ed. 2. New York: Grune & Stratton, 1964.

O'Neill, J. J., and Oyer, H. J., *Visual Communication for the Hard of Hearing*. Englewood Cliffs, N. J.: Prentice-Hall, 1961.

O'Neill, J. J., and Oyer, H. J. Aural Rehabilitation. In Jerger, J. (Ed.), *Modern Developments in Audiology*, Ed. 2. New York: Academic Press, 1973.

Oyer, H. J., and Frankmann, J. P., *The Aural Rehabilitative Process*, Ch. 1. New York: Holt, Rinehart & Winston, 1975.

Ross, M., *Principles of Aural Rehabilitation*. Indianapolis: Bobbs-Merrill Co., 1972.

Sanders, D. A., *Aural Rehabilitation*. Englewood Cliffs, N. J.: Prentice-Hall, 1971.

Tannahill, J. C., Hearing aids: trial and adjustment by new users. *Audecibel*, 22, 90–97, Spring 1973.

chapter 37

THE PSYCHOLOGY OF HEARING IMPAIRMENT

Cornelius P. Goetzinger, Ph.D.

BACKGROUND OF THE PROBLEM

Interest concerning the impact of hearing impairment upon the psychological development of children arose in the United States in the latter part of the 19th century. Greenberger in 1889 proposed the use of picture books and a number test for the elimination of feebleminded deaf children from schools for the deaf. He also advocated block building and the perception of form and color as a test of a child's ability.

Around the turn of the century several studies were conducted comparing deaf and hearing children on a number of abilities and skills such as free association spelling (Taylor, 1897), bodily strength and agility, manual dexterity, memory and observation (Mott, 1899, 1900) and immediate and delayed recall (Smith, 1903).

However, the first study of the deaf employing standardized psychological tests was that of MacMillan and Bruner (1906). These investigators administered mental and physical tests to 184 hearing-impaired children attending the public schools of Chicago. The mental tests included the cancellation of As test, perception of size and weight differences, and visual memory span for numbers. There was also a tapping test to measure motor ability. The deaf subjects were found to be inferior to the hearing on all of the tests with the exception of the perception of weight differences.

After the Goddard revision of the Binet-Simon intelligence test in the United States, Kilpatrick (1912, 1914) suggested that either the test or a modification be used to evaluate the mental ability of the deaf. Furthermore, he proposed that a commission be appointed to study the problem.

Pintner and Paterson (1915) investigated the use of the Goddard revision of the Binet-Simon IQ scale with deaf children. They concluded that the test was not suitable for use with the deaf. This finding gave rise to a series of studies in schools for the deaf by Pintner and his associates. In addition, they developed a performance scale of intelligence (Pintner and Paterson, 1923), a group non-language mental test (Pintner, 1929) and an educational achievement test. These tests were used in investigations of the deaf (Pintner, Eisenson and Stanton, 1946).

During the past 50 years there has been a substantial amount of research devoted to the effects of hearing impairment upon psychological development. However, there are still incredible gaps in our knowledge. Therefore, the purpose of this chapter is to present the psychological implications of hearing impairment as revealed by research and clinical experience, to foster a better understanding of the impact of deafness upon behavior, and to suggest avenues for future study.

PREVALENCE OF HEARING IMPAIRMENT

Schein and Delk (1974) recently released the results of a census concerning the prevalence of hearing impairment in the United States. The data indicate that there are 13.6 million people with hearing impairment. This number includes 410,522 individuals who cannot hear and understand speech, and who became deaf before 19 years of age. However, when age of onset is disregarded, the number increases to 1.7 million deaf persons. In addition, the prevalence of deafness is higher in urban than in rural areas, and in the North Central region as compared to the Northeast, South and West. Furthermore, there are as many deaf people in the birth to 17-year age range as in the 17- to 44-year age range.

With respect to children enrolled in schools and classes for the deaf in the United States, a total of 53,009 (28,472 males and 24,537 females) is reported as of October, 1974 (American Annals of the Deaf, 1975).

FACTORS ASSOCIATED WITH AUDITORY IMPAIRMENT

Degree of Hearing Loss

Degree of hearing loss is related to hearing handicap. Hearing loss refers to the increase in the intensity of sound above the normal level which is required to reach threshold. Table 37.1 presents the classification of hearing levels according to Eagles, Hardy and Catlin (1968) after conversion to ANSI-1969 thresholds. Also included in the table are the relationships of hearing level to understanding of speech, psychological impact, need for a hearing aid, and the percent of children within each classification from the Pittsburgh study (Eagles et al., 1968).

Age at Onset of Hearing Impairment

The age at which hearing impairment occurs is important to subsequent language development. Children who suffer hearing loss after

TABLE 37.1. Classification of Hearing Handicap for the Better Ear Relative to the Speech Frequencies (500 to 2000 Hz)

ANSI	Handicap	Speech Discrimination[1]	Psychological Implications	Hearing Aid Need[2]	Pittsburgh Study, 4064 Subjects, 5–10 Years of Age
dB					
0	None	Excellent	None	None (the CROS with unilateral cases at times)	Number in class was 3996 (98.3% of total)
25	Mild (slight)[4]	Difficulty with faint speech	Children may show a slight verbal deficit	Occasional use	Number in class was 36 (0.9%)
40	Moderate (mild)	Trouble frequently with normal speech at one meter (SPL of 65–70 dB)	Psychological problems are measurable in children. The beginning of social inadequacy in adults	Hearing aids are needed frequently	Number in class was 19 (21)[3] (0.5%)
55	Moderately severe (marked)	Frequent difficulty with loud speech	In general, children are retarded educationally if they do not receive special help. Emotional and social problems are frequent. Psychological problems are measurable in adults	Generally the area of greatest satisfaction from an aid	Number in class was 9 (0.2%)
70	Severe	Might understand shouted or amplified speech, but this will depend upon other factors as type of impairment etc.	Congenitally and pre-lingually deaf children usually show marked educational retardation. Emotional and social problems may obtain in children and adults	Generally, good results, but benefits depend on auditory discrimination, etc.	Number given as 2 (0.05%). It includes the profound class
90	Profound (extreme)	Generally, no understanding of speech, even amplified	Congenitally and prelingually deaf may show severe educational retardation and emotional underdevelopment. Deafened adults may have personal and social problems	Help from aid depends on objectives. Lipreading, voice quality are often helped	

[1] Modified from Davis and Silverman (1970); Eagles et al. (1968) and Goodman (1965).
[2] Modified from the lectures of Dr. Raymond Carhart. The Pittsburgh study provides an estimate of the percentages of children in the public schools who fall within the various hearing impairment classifications.
[3] The original table was in error. Should be 21 instead of 19.
[4] In parenthesis, Davis and Silverman's terminology.

the acquisition of spoken language have a definite educational advantage over those with congenital deafness. Early research (Pintner and Paterson, 1917; Reamer, 1921; Day, Fusfeld and Pintner, 1928) showed that children who were either congenitally deaf or acquired severe hearing loss prior to the age range 4 to 6 years were retarded in language and eventual educational achievement compared to children who lost their hearing at later ages. Thus, adventitiously deaf children benefited by virtue of their earlier hearing.

Now, 3 years of age is considered the critical time at which a child acquires a hearing loss. This is primarily because of the beneficial effects which may be ascribed to early diagnosis, parent and infant programs and preschools for the deaf. Of interest in this connection is the research in linguistics which indicates that the elements of one's native language are mastered by ages 3 to 4½ years (McNeill, 1965). Northern and Downs (1974) discuss critical periods for hearing and language learning. Clearly, the age of onset of deafness has important educational and psychological implications.

The deleterious effects of hearing impairment vary depending on the locus of the lesion. The ability to discriminate speech clearly is usually normal in conductive hearing loss of the external and middle ear. Conversely, speech may be severely distorted in hearing impairment of cochlear or eighth nerve etiology. Generally, speech distortion is related to degree of hearing loss, but is less pronounced in patients with cochlear as compared to eighth nerve lesions. Cochlear or eighth nerve deafness may be extreme or total while the maximum conductive hearing loss does not exceed 60 to 70 dB (ANSI-1969).

As shown in Table 37.1 the majority of children with hearing impairment in the Pittsburgh study had thresholds in the better ear within the 25-to 70-dB range. The primary avenue for the acquisition of language and education for these children is through the auditory channel with or without a hearing aid. Thus they are likely to develop functional hearing. Conversely, when hearing loss in the better ear exceeds the 70-dB hearing level, vision is likely to develop as the primary channel for the acquisition of language and education, particularly, as in the case of congenital deafness. Children with hearing losses of 70 dB and greater in the better ear are usually classified as educationally deaf.

PSYCHOLOGICAL AND EDUCATIONAL FACTORS RELATED TO HEARING IMPAIRMENT IN CHILDREN

The early psychological investigators concentrated on intelligence and educational achievement in their comparisons of children with normal and impaired hearing. By selecting children in schools for the deaf they were able to study the effects of profound hearing impairment which could be determined reasonably well with the crude hearing tests of that day. As a consequence, psychological studies of hard of hearing children with hearing losses within the 40-to 70-dB range were not seriously pursued until the development of the first commercial audiometers and the recorded numbers tests in the 1920s (Bunch, 1943).

Intelligence

Hard of Hearing Children. An early study by Waldman, Wade and Aretz (1930) comparing the intelligence of normal and hard of hearing children found the latter to be retarded slightly as measured by a group verbal intelligence test. About the same time Madden (1931), administering mental and hearing tests, also reported some retardation for hard of hearing as compared to normal hearing children.

In a comprehensive study Pintner and Lev (1939) compared more than 1100 normal and hard of hearing children in grades five through eight on the Pintner IQ test (a group verbal test). The subjects with hearing levels within the 10- to 40-dB range by today's ANSI standards were found to be retarded by 5 IQ points. Pintner and Lev divided their subjects into two groups, one with 10 to 25 dB and the other with 25- to 40-dB thresholds. The former were not significantly different in IQ from normal hearing subjects. The latter, however, were retarded by 8 IQ points. Hence, hearing losses between 25 and 40 dB induced a retardation in verbal skills which was reflected in the verbal IQ test. Pintner and Lev concluded that the difference, though significant, was not large, and indicated that their hard of hearing subjects were within the normal range of intelligence. When a smaller sample of the same two groups was tested with the Pintner Non-Language Mental Test, a significant difference was not found. They recommended the use of nonlanguage tests for assessing the mental ability of hearing impaired children.

Within the last 25 years there have been no published reports of large studies of the intelligence of hard of hearing children. Deficits for hard of hearing children in verbal, as compared to non-verbal intelligence, are likely to be a function of degree, type and age of onset of hearing loss rather than mental retardation. Thus, the reduced verbal scores will reflect the hearing problem rather than the lack of innate ability.

Deaf Children. Pintner and Paterson (1915) demonstrated conclusively that verbal tests of intelligence were not suitable for measuring the mental ability of deaf children. Pintner and Paterson (1923) developed an individual performance scale of intelligence and a group non-verbal mental test (Pintner, 1929). These tests were not dependent upon language, and could be used with the deaf. Research with the Pintner Non-Language Mental Test, as well as with the Digit-Symbol and Symbol-Digit Tests found deaf children to be 2 to 3 years retarded in intelligence (Pintner, 1915; Pintner and Paterson, 1916, 1918; Reamer, 1921; Day et al. 1928). Only the study by Newlee (1919) reported deaf children to be normal in intelligence. She administered the Digit-Symbol and Symbol-Digit tests to 85 deaf children in the Chicago School System and found them to be equal to the norms for hearing children. Her results were criticized on the basis of selectivity of sample and the small number of cases.

In 1928, Drever and Collins (1936) in England using their own individual performance scale of intelligence found the deaf to be equal to or better than their normal hearing subjects. As the results were in conflict with those of Pintner and his associates using the non-verbal tests, a number of studies were conducted subsequently comparing the two types of mental tests.

During the next 25 years several investigations were conducted utilizing a number of non-verbal and performance tests of intelligence. In general, the deaf were found to be retarded in intelligence on some non-verbal group tests, (Lyon et al., 1933; MacKane, 1933; Zeckel and Van der Kolk, 1939; Oleron, 1950; Levine and Iscoe, 1955; Goetzinger, Wills and Dekker, 1967). However, the deaf were not found to be subnormal in intelligence when the Chicago Non-Verbal Test was used (Streng and Kirk, 1938; Goetzinger, 1946; Johnson, 1947, 1948; Myklebust, 1960; Goetzinger et al., 1967).

Deaf children have invariably tested within normal limits on performance scales of intelligence (Lyon, et al., 1933; MacKane, 1933; Schick, 1934; Petersen, 1936; Streng and Kirk, 1938; Burchard and Myklebust, 1942a; MacPherson and Lane, 1948; Kirk and Perry, 1948; Goetzinger, 1950; Birch and Birch, 1951; Goetzinger and Rousey, 1957).

In view of the discrepancy in the performance of deaf children on many group non-verbal intelligence tests as compared to individual performance scales it appeared that the former were more abstract and that the retarded language development of deaf children contributed to their inferiority on such tasks (Oleron, 1950).

Furth (1964) began a series of studies about 1958 which ultimately demonstrated that the inferiority of deaf children on many non-verbal cognitive tasks was not observed in deaf adults.

He attributed the inferiority in children to experiential deficit rather than to retardation per se, as the latter should have persisted into adulthood if the condition had been permanent. He also concluded that the retarded language development of deaf children did not deleteriously affect their performances. His conclusions agreed with the later position of Oleron as reported by Levine (1963) that language is less significant in problem solving and relational learning than formerly entertained.

In 1960, Goetzinger and his associates (1967) began a series of studies using the 1938 Raven's Standard Progressive Matrices. Research with this test by Oleron (1950) and Levine and Iscoe (1955) found deaf children to be retarded by about 2 years. Goetzinger and his associates confirmed the expected 2-year retardation for deaf children whose average age was 13½ years. However, the deficit was no longer observable in older children whose average age was 18½ years. The findings were identical for the Terman Non-Language Multi-Mental Test.

Goetzinger et al. (1967) also studied the relationship between the mental tests and vocabulary and paragraph meaning of the Stanford Achievement Test. The latter tests measure indirectly the language ability of deaf children. Correlations between the IQ and achievement tests were significant but low. In addition, the older when compared to the younger children were less than 6 months superior on the achievement tests even though they had been in school for 5 more years. Hence, there was only a weak relationship between language, as measured here, and the non-verbal mental tests. The retardation of the younger children on the IQ tests was interpreted as being the result of experiential deficit. The results supported Furth's (1966) conclusions.

During the last two to three decades much research has centered on the perceptual and conceptual abilities of deaf children. The results from studies on visual perception have been controversial. Myklebust and Brutten (1953) reported deaf children to be inferior to hearing children in visual foreground-background differentiation. A number of subsequent studies have not confirmed this finding (Embrey, 1955; Hayes, 1955; Larr, 1956).

The research pertaining to the verbal conceptualization of deaf children has found them to be inferior to hearing children. Templin (1950) showed that deaf children's explanations of physical phenomena were characteristic of hearing children at a much younger age. Other researchers have reported on different aspects of verbal conceptualization with essentially the same results (Heider and Heider, 1940, 1941; Larr, 1956; Myklebust, 1960; Kates, Kates and Michael, 1962; Rosenstein, 1960, 1964).

Conversely, on non-verbal tests of conceptualization the deaf perform as well as the hearing. Differences which may occur are related to lack of experience.

One could expect the deaf to show a deficit in abstract concepts particularly if exposure to the concept is contingent upon language. Blake, Ainsworth and Williams (1967) compared deaf and hearing subjects on concept attainment when the concepts were presented through verbal material by the methods of induction-discovery, induction-demonstration and deduction. The hearing were superior to the deaf in the recognition and use of concepts. However, the groups did not differ in their responses to the methods of concept attainment. Deduction was more effective than induction for both groups, and there were no differences in effectiveness of the two inductive methods between groups. The investigators maintained that their results were consistent with past research, and attributed the differences in concept attainment which were demonstrated between the groups to the deaf subjects' less adequate language facility.

Although language is not regarded as being as important as once maintained in non-verbal cognitive reasoning and conceptualization of the deaf, nevertheless, the acquisition and extension of knowledge, and the higher levels of conceptualization are severely circumscribed unless a verbal language is developed. This follows because without a verbal language, a rich and extensive written language is not likely to evolve. Without a written language for the storage and retrieval of information it is questionable that higher levels of conceptualization would be possible. One of the most important characteristics of advanced cultures is a written language. Hence, the congenital or prelingual deaf cannot realize their full potential for mental growth until they have developed sufficiently a basic verbal language which is a prerequisite for access to the stored knowledge of the culture through the written language.

The impact of severe congenital or prelingual deafness upon language acquisition is usually not well understood except by individuals associated with the education of the deaf. The young hearing child develops the basic language and speech of his culture essentially by the time he is 4 to 4½ years of age. He is constantly exposed to a barrage of verbal language from those around him, in addition to the informal teaching efforts of the parents. The important point is that the child acquires language through the ear essentially from countless incidental exposures, and not from direct teaching.

Conversely, the deaf child's incidental contacts with the language are minimal and largely meaningless. This is because his defective auditory system is incapable of processing even amplified speech signals sufficiently for the development of language. Unfortunately, the visual system, which is the primary channel in the acquisition of language for the deaf, provides little opportunity for incidental learning. Furthermore, the imprecision of lipreading as a method of communication, not to mention its inadequacies as the primary vehicle in the acquisition of language, clearly delineates the language difficulties either of the congenital or the prelingual deaf.

Therefore, there is need to develop a visual method for language development in deaf children which is superior to speechreading, and/or speechreading plus amplified speech by means of a hearing aid. Cornett's (1967) cued speech in conjunction with speechreading and amplification could conceivably serve this purpose. More will be addressed to this point under the section on learning.

In summary, deaf children manifest normal intelligence on most non-verbal cognitive tests. When retardation occurs it is related to a lack of experience and underdevelopment, and as such it is amenable to better educational procedures.

Educational Achievement

Hard of Hearing Children. A child's success or failure in school is obviously of importance to the psychologist as well as to the educator. Hence, there have been a number of studies comparing normal and hard of hearing children on such educational indicators as grade repetition (Caplin, 1937) and scores from standardized educational achievement tests (Pintner et al., 1946). Many of the large investigations were conducted before 1941. Generally, it was found that the hard of hearing repeated more grades and were likely to be retarded in educational achievement.

Later, Henry (1947) studied the impact of low, middle and high frequency hearing loss upon educational achievement. Significant differences in threshold between the best and poorest readers were found for those subjects with middle and high frequency losses. Low tone loss was not related to proficiency in reading.

Fisher (1966) in England studied vocabulary and basic school subjects in 83 hard of hearing children in the public schools. They had a mean hearing level of 38 dB with a range of 20 to 64 dB (British Standard which is in close agreement with ANSI-1969). Their mean chronologic age was 10.1 years. Although these children were normal in intelligence as measured with the Raven's Progressive Matrices, nevertheless, they were substantially retarded in vocabulary and in basic school subjects.

In another study Young and McConnell (1957) compared normal and hard of hearing children, equated for age, sex, grade and socioeconomic status, in intelligence using the standard 1938 Raven's Progressive Matrices, a nonverbal test, and in vocabulary with the Ammon's Full-Range Picture Vocabulary Test. The hard of hearing subjects had a mean hearing loss of 61 dB (ANSI-1969) in the better ear. The results indicated that the groups were equal in non-verbal intelligence, but significantly different in vocabulary, with the normal subjects evincing a distinct superiority.

The effects of slight to mild hearing loss, usually congenital, upon language development in children has received but little attention by researchers. Goetzinger (1962) after longitudinal observation of children with sensory-neural hearing losses of 30 to 45 dB (ANSI-1969) in the better ear tentatively concluded that such losses induce a language lag of 12 to 18 months at age 3 years when intelligence is normal. Hearing losses of this degree do not preclude the development of language, but frequently cause a speech defect. Children between 2 and 4 years of age with small sensory-neural hearing losses are often misdiagnosed as being emotionally disturbed, aphasic, retarded, or as having learning disabilities when there is an absence of hearing test information.

Deaf Children. Approximately 50 years ago Pintner and Paterson (1917, 1918), Reamer (1921), Day et al. (1928) found deaf children to be retarded in educational achievement by about 4 to 6 years. Later, Pugh (1946), Goetzinger (1950), Miller (1958), Goetzinger and Rousey (1959) and Boatner (1965) reported educational retardation of deaf children which was not markedly different from the Pintner era.

Myklebust (1960) found progressive retardation with age for deaf children using the Columbia Vocabulary Test. At age 16 years the deaf were more than 6 years below the level of hearing children.

The limited educational success of the deaf has recently been emphasized by the Babbidge (1965) report. Furthermore, the Gentile and Di Francesca study (1969) of educational achievement in hearing-impaired children provided the most recent evidence of their retardation. The implication of the foregoing is that we have not as yet developed methods to alleviate appreciably the deleterious effects of profound congenital and prelingual deafness upon language development.

Personality and Emotional Adjustment

Hard of Hearing Children. There have been a number of studies comparing normal and

hard of hearing children in emotional adjustment. Habbe (1936) administered a battery of behavior rating and adjustment scales to normal and hard of hearing adolescent boys equated for chronologic age, school, grade, nationality, intelligence and socioeconomic level. His hard of hearing subjects had mean hearing losses (ANSI-1969) of 39 and 37 dB, respectively, in the left and right ears. Although the subjects with normal hearing obtained better ratings on five of the six scales, none of the differences was significant. However, the hard of hearing tended to be more introvertive and submissive than those with normal hearing.

In an important study Pintner (1942) compared normal and hard of hearing children in several areas of adjustment. Although the two groups did not differ in ascendant-submissive behavior, there was a tendency for aggression to appear in subjects with hearing losses of greater than 40 dB (ANSI-1969). The groups did not differ statistically in introversion-extroversion, yet, there was a trend to better adjustment in the normal subjects. Children with greater hearing loss appeared to be less emotionally stable. As a result of his investigations Pintner concluded that hard of hearing children were not as well adjusted as normal hearing children, and were inclined to be introverted.

During the past 20 years there have been a number of small studies of normal and hard of hearing children concerned with such factors as personal and social adjustment (Reynolds, 1955; Goetzinger, Harrison and Baer, 1964; Fisher, 1966), ability to handle frustration, (Kahn, 1957), and their acceptance and rejection by classmates (Elser, 1959). Suffice to say that differences in personal and social adjustment favoring the normals were observed when hearing losses were about 40 dB (ANSI-1969) (Goetzinger et al., 1964; Fisher, 1966) but not at lesser levels (Reynolds, 1955). Although hard of hearing children were not accepted as well by their classmates (Elser, 1959), there was a great deal of overlap. Finally, Kahn's study suggested that his hard of hearing subjects handled their frustration more constructively than his normal hearing controls.

Deaf Children. Early studies into the personality and adjustment of deaf children were conducted by Brunschwig (1936), Bradway (1937), Springer (1938), Kirk (1938), Heider and Heider (1940, 1941), Burchard and Myklebust (1942b). More recently Avery (1948), McAndrew (1948), Levine (1956), Bindon (1957), Myklebust (1960), Goetzinger et al. (1966) and Vegely and Elliott (1968) have investigated the effects of deafness upon emotional and personality development. These studies have utilized personality tests of the paper and pencil variety, projective techniques such as the Rorschach and MAPS (Make A Picture Story), inventories and drawings.

In general, the majority of the research has indicated that deaf children are not as well adjusted as their hearing peers. In addition, there is a higher incidence of immaturity among the deaf, and they tend to be more egocentric, rigid and neurotic. Yet, much that is negative in the behavior of deaf children may be improved through educational and character-forming procedures. Behavior modification is being increasingly used with deaf children and is effective.

Rehabilitation

Auditorily Impaired Children – Unimodal Versus Bimodal Approaches. Gaeth (1967) during the last decade conducted a number of significant studies with reference to learning in hearing-impaired children. Using a paired associates paradigm, he compared unimodal and bimodal methods of presenting materials to be learned. The three methods were the visual, the auditory and the auditory-visual combined.

Gaeth's normal hearing children did not show any significant differences with the three methods of learning. His hard of hearing subjects with average hearing losses in the better ear from 26 to 70 dB (ANSI-1969) did not differ significantly on the visual and audiovisual methods. However, both the visual and audiovisual methods were superior to the purely auditory approach. Gaeth felt the results suggested the need for changes in the educational management of hearing-impaired children. When the three methods were compared with children within the 71- to 85-dB (ANSI-1969) hearing range, the visual method was superior to the audiovisual and the auditory methods.

Gaeth rechecked his results by the repetition of experiments and by the use of new materials, hypothesizing that the bimodal presentation is critical when either normal or hearing-impaired children are learning new words and concepts. In the new experiments he used nonverbal and non-meaningful symbols, nonsense syllables, simple meaningful words and non-meaningful sounds. He concluded as a result of a variety of experiments that the child learns originally either through one or the other channel (visual or auditory) but not through both simultaneously. Furthermore, the child selects the channel with the more meaningful material. With reference to the deaf child Gaeth wrote:

"Interestingly the same conglomeration of experiments presented to deaf children suggest that the preceding statement must be reinterpreted, since with them the predominance of performance in the visual modality is so strong it tends to override the more usual definition of meaningfulness. Finally, our current inference is that when individuals do show benefit from a bimodal presentation, such as in the apparent combination of lipreading and hearing through a hearing aid, it is being done, not from the integration of simultaneous bimodal presentation, but the integration of rapidly alternating unimodal stimulation. It would appear that these data have implications for the educational management of the hard of hearing and deaf child." (Gaeth, 1967, p. 292)

Gaeth's reference to bimodal improvement for lipreading and hearing through a hearing aid is amply supported by the research findings of Heider (1943), Numbers and Hudgins (1948), Hudgins (1951), Prall (1957), Purcell and Costello (1970) and Sanders (1971). These investigators have demonstrated that a bimodal presentation as discussed is significantly superior to unimodal visual presentation for hearing-impaired children.

The apparent conflict between Gaeth's results (that is, the finding of a nonsignificant difference between the visual and the combined auditory-visual or bimodal method) and the studies of Hudgins, Prall, Purcell and Costello, and Sanders showing superiority of the bimodal over the visual method is simply related to the stimulus which was used in the visual modality.

Gaeth employed either words, nonsense symbols or nonsense syllables, all of which were in printed form, in contrast to the other investigators whose stimuli were lip or speech movements. The former (printed forms) are precise and reliable methods for conveying messages to be understood via the visual channel. The latter (lip or speech movements) are comparatively imprecise and unreliable because of ambiguity of homophenous words and sounds (which look alike on the lips as man-pan or du-tu) and variations in the formation of words and sounds from speaker to speaker. Hence, on the one hand Gaeth's subjects concentrated on the relatively precise and stable visual stimuli (the printed form) to the exclusion of the distorted auditory stimuli. On the other hand the subjects of the other investigators were exposed to lip movements (lipreading) as the visual stimuli which are often as distorted, imprecise and variable as the auditory stimuli, particularly in the case of educationally deaf children. However, in the bimodal approach, when lip movements (lipreading) are the visual stimuli, additional cues to understand are available, as the visual and auditory stimuli are received simultaneously. Hence, the bimodal representation, as described, is usually superior either to the visual (lip movements, namely, lipreading) or the auditory reception alone.

The extent of superiority is dependent upon a number of variables, two of which relate to the subject's lipreading and auditory discrimination abilities. For example, it is not unusual in the clinic to observe improvement in communication for patients under a bimodal approach who have poor auditory discrimination and are poor lipreaders. Scores of say, 20% each for lipreading and auditory discrimination, frequently increase to 60 to 70% when the two are combined. As a matter of fact, it has been standard practice in our clinic (Kansas University Medical Center Audiology-Electronystagmography Clinic) during the past 20 years to evaluate the auditory and visual modalities separately, and also, in combination (Goetzinger, 1963) in the assessment of hearing aid performance.

However, the point at which a difference in scores between modalities (visual and auditory) results in an absence of improvement when there is bimodal reception has not been determined conclusively, although O'Neill (1954) has reported data in this regard. It will be recalled that in Gaeth's experiments there was some evidence that the bimodal was poorer than the unimodal visual approach when printed words and syllables were the visual stimuli. Recently research was conducted at the National Technical Institute for the Deaf (NTID) dealing with the relative efficacy of lipreading, sign language and printed material as media in conveying information to deaf students (Gates, 1970 as reported by Stuckless, 1971). Gates selected 140 subjects in the beginning class at NTID and randomly assigned them to 7 groups of 20 each. Criteria for selection were the absence of any serious visual defects, and at least an eighth grade reading ability. Each group was presented with the same 2000-word test passage under 7 different presentation conditions utilizing a video tape, split screen technique. All presentations were at a rate of 125 words per min. A 39-item multiple choice test was devised to test their comprehension. The 7 presentations were: (1) spoken without sound (i.e., lipreading); (2) manual communication only; (3) the printed form of the lecture; (4) a combination of the spoken and signed lectures; (5) a combination of the spoken and printed lectures; (6) a combination of the signed and printed lecture; and (7) a combination of the spoken, signed and printed lecture. The results were as follows:

	Mean	S.D.
1. Spoken (lipreading, L.R.) only	13.50	3.73
2. Manual (seemingly) only	15.05	3.87
3. Printed symbol (graphic or reading) only	26.05	7.70
4. Spoken (L.R.) and signs combined	13.70	2.43
5. Spoken (L.R.) and graphic (reading) combined	25.65	7.36
6. Sign and graphic (reading) combined	23.95	6.87
7. Spoken (L.R.), signed and graphic (reading) combined	25.65	10.05

Several of the findings are of more than passing interest in the context of this discussion. First, the spoken message (#1, lipreading) and the sign language (#2) resulted in low scores. Both are imprecise methods of communication. Combining the two (#4) did not increase intelligibility. Simultaneous reception through the visual channel of two dissimilar signals does not improve understanding as is the case when a distorted visual and distorted auditory are receptively processed. However, there is a significant increase in the mean score when the printed symbol (#3) is used. The addition of sign language (#6) or lipreading (#5) to the printed symbol does not improve performance. Furthermore, combining the three modes of transmission (#7) does not improve reception over the printed symbol (#3) alone. These findings indicate that neither sign language, lipreading nor a combination of the two are as effective as the printed word for conveying information. In addition, combining sign language, lipreading and the printed word does not improve reception over the printed word alone. Apparently, the organism can attend only to one visual presentation mode. That mode is used which provides the maximum information. Reading, in this case being the superior one, is utilized.

With reference to the hearing impaired in the 71- to 85-dB range as well as the profoundly deaf, Gaeth (1967) demonstrated the superiority of the visual over the combined auditory-visual mode when the former (visual) was the printed word. In short, adding severely distorted auditory signals to clear visual signals reduced information. However, when the visual mode is lipreading, the combined auditory-visual approach is superior (Numbers and Hudgins, 1948; Hudgins, 1951; Prall, 1957; Purcell and Costello, 1970; Sanders, 1971). Regardless of the superiority of bimodal over the unimodal presentation when lipreading is the visual mode, it is unlikely that the bimodal as described would be superior to the unimodal when the latter is the printed symbol. This brings up the question utilizing an aid to lipreading such as cued speech (Cornett, 1967) in conjunction with auditory amplification to improve reception during communication. There is need for research in this area. However, the use of total communication (i.e., using either the sign language, the manual alphabet or both in conjunction with lipreading and auditory amplification) is not likely to be any more effective than the bimodal visual-auditory consisting of lipreading and hearing through amplification.

A recent study by Carson (1974) lends credence to this statement. She investigated the learning of nonsense syllables in deaf children whose age range was 8 to 10 years. The experimental conditions were as follows: lipreading alone, auditory alone, signs alone, lipreading and auditory, lipreading and signs, signs and auditory, and lipreading, auditory and signs. There was no significant difference between the lipreading-auditory condition and the lipreading-auditory-signs condition (essentially, total communication) relative to mean number of correct responses. The lipreading-auditory condition was superior to the signs alone, the auditory alone and the auditory-signs conditions at the 0.01 level of confidence. The lipreading-auditory-signs condition was superior to the auditory alone, and the auditory-signs conditions, but at the 0.05 level. Lipreading alone did not differ significantly from signs alone. Furthermore, lipreading-signs did not differ either from lipreading or signs alone.

In short, the organism cannot process two visual signals simultaneously (signs and/or finger spelling plus lipreading). One or the other would become essentially noise and, hence, would either be suppressed or ignored. There is also the possibility of one or the other constituting a distraction, which could actually lower the information received. The aforementioned possibilities are not likely to occur when Cornett's cueing gestures are used in conjunction with lipreading and auditory stimulation. The reason for this postulation is that the "cues" are just that and nothing more. In addition, they are executed essentially at the lips and, as a consequence, are incorporated into the ongoing lip motion to assist in the comprehension of obscure movements.

Although the sign language was not anymore effective than lipreading for the transmission of information as shown previously, nevertheless the former appears to be a more basic method of communication than speech and its visual correlative, lipreading. For example, it has been customary for years among educators of the deaf to refer their oral-aural failures to state schools for the deaf where the sign language and finger spelling are usually the principal methods of communication. The recent scientific experiments associated with teaching apes to communicate by means of the sign language (Gardner and Gardner, 1969) appear to point up the basic nature of signs for communication. It will be recalled that the earlier experiments at the Yerkes laboratories concerned with teaching apes to communicate through vocalizations resulted in failure (Yerkes and Learned, 1925). Conversely, the studies employing sign language appear to be bearing a modicum of success not hitherto realized.

Auditorily Impaired Children – Language. In the Pittsburgh study (Eagles et al., 1968) more than one-half of the children with hearing problems in the age range 5 to 10 years had hearing levels of 25 to 40 dB (ANSI-1969) in the better ear. This amount of loss would be classified by Davis and Silverman (1970) as slight, or by Goodman (1965) as mild. As pointed out earlier Pintner and Lev (1939) found an 8-point deficit in verbal intelligence for such children.

It has been the practice in the past to recommend hearing aids only sparingly for individuals with mild (Goodman's classification) hearing loss in the better ear. The recommendations for children usually consisted of lipreading and placement in the front row of the classroom when the deficit in the better ear was 25 to 30 dB. It is likely with the advances which are being made in ear-level instruments and open earmolds that more frequent use of amplification will be encouraged for these children. Patterns of hearing loss vary in this classification and must be taken into consideration in the rehabilitative process. Of greater importance is that teachers and parents understand the nature of the child's problem. Children with mild to moderate hearing losses frequently give the impression of inattention and stubborness in the classroom thus triggering reprimand with the subsequent development of psychological problems.

Sensory-neural hearing loss of about 40 dB induces a language lag of 1 to 1½-years at age 3 years when intelligence is normal (Goetzinger, 1962) and greater emotional problems (Pintner, 1942; Goetzinger et al., 1964; Fisher, 1966). The Pittsburgh study showed that almost a third of the total number of cases with hearing loss had hearing levels of 40 to 55 dB and can be considered to have moderate hearing losses. Generally speaking, these children require hearing aids as soon after diagnosis as possible. It is not unusual for a diagnosis of hearing loss in the mild and moderate classifications to be confirmed during the first year of life. Thus, remedial procedures may be initiated to overcome the language retardation. This statement does not imply the use of highly formalized procedures with very young children. A natural approach which emphasizes the usual "mother to child talk" is effective.

As the child reaches age 3 the parents should make copious use of story telling with appropriate picture books. Correction of speech production and auditory discrimination errors are better taken care of incidentally as children at this age level have limited attention span.

After the child enters preschool more formal work in lipreading and auditory training is usually necessary. The objective is to reduce the language lag as effectively as possible before the child enters the regular school. In the past children with moderate hearing losses have too frequently been left to struggle for themselves. With just a minimum of effort these children should be able to get along in the regular school. They will require special placement in the classroom, a teacher who understands their problems, special efforts by teachers to educate classmates about the implications of hearing loss, and individualized help with classwork. There is no reason why children with hearing losses of 40 to 55 dB should not succeed in the regular classroom, providing intelligence and adjustment are normal and there is no learning problem.

Table 37.1 shows that 2 out of 1000 children had hearing levels of 55 to 70 dB in the better ear. There is no question about the need for amplification in these cases. Research indicates that children with such losses are often found to be retarded in educational achievement (Young and McConnell, 1957). In addition, social and emotional problems are more frequent. These children almost always require additional help in the classroom and at home. The hearing conservationist or speech correctionist/hearing specialist in the schools should have an understanding of the deleterious effects of marked hearing loss on education and behavior. Children with moderately severe hearing levels require the services of a trained teacher of the hard of hearing. In many instances they will require special classrooms for the hard of hearing. Children with moderately severe losses should have emphasis on a unimodal visual approach utilizing the printed symbol, if Gaeth's findings are to be utilized. This statement does not imply that the visual (lipreading)-auditory modality should be neglected, but merely recognizes the inherent superiority of the printed symbol in educating children with this degree of handicap.

In the Pittsburgh study only 2 of 4064 children had hearing losses in the better ear of 70 dB or greater—hence less than 1 in 1000 children in the public schools are classified as educationally deaf. However, there are 53,009 children in schools and classes for the deaf in the United States (*American Annals of the Deaf*, 1975). For the majority of these children, the visual channel is the primary avenue through which they will acquire language. The child who is either born deaf or who suffers deafness before the acquisition of language is cut off from the spoken word through which language is learned. Since hearing is omnidirectional, and a sense for perceiving at distances, the child with normal hearing is continuously saturated with incidental language from everyone in the vicinity and, in addition, may be exposed to an incidental teaching situation with the mother even though she is not in the same room. Unfortunately, the deaf child does not have such exposure to incidental learning. His language experiences which are mainly through the visual channel are comparatively meager, and his incidental contacts are almost nil, unless the speaker is in his direct line of vision. Therefore, the need is great to expose the child to language continuously during the formative years (birth to 5 or 6 years) and to provide him with the best possible medium for acquiring facility in language.

As suggested previously, Cornett's Cued Speech in conjunction with speechreading and auditory amplification may provide a very effective system. The cues consist of 12 hand positions centered around the face which give additional information in the auditory-visual modality. It does not constitute the addition of a second visual method, such as for example, the sign language (or a combination of signs and finger spelling) used in conjunction with speechreading and auditory amplification. Such combination would not be expected to facilitate comprehension or the acquisition of language for the reasons which were previously presented. To the contrary the addition of a few visual cues, such as those of Cornett, should enhance rather than deter understanding and language development because of their location and moderate use.

It was noted previously that the language of signs plus finger spelling has been utilized in this country for deaf children who have not experienced success with an oral-aural approach and that sign language is being used with apes with a modicum of success. Therefore, the sign language cannot be discounted as a method for the development of basic language in prelingually deaf children. However, the sign language as traditionally used by the deaf in the United States is not based on English. As a result it contributes minimally to language growth. In England, Gorman and Paget (1969) began to develop a systematic sign language a number of years ago which had been originated by Sir Richard Paget in the early 1930s. Sir Richard Paget died in 1955, but had published several papers describing his "New Sign Language." By 1969 Dr. Gorman and Lady Paget had developed the system to a point where it included 2000 signs. It is unlikely that they will develop more than 3000 signs. Therefore, signs do not constitute a rich medium for the conveyance of thought.

Recently a number of manual systems have been devised which relate well to English syntax. Cokely and Gawlik (1973) have presented a critical review of three manual English systems and their relationship to signs. The three systems are: Seeing Essential English (S.E.E. I), Anthony (undated); Signing Exact English (S.E.E. II), Gustason, Pfetzing, and Zawolkow (1972); Linguistics of Visual English (L.O.V.E.), Wampler (undated).

Obviously, the language of signs is circumscribed. It is not well suited either for abstract thought or for expressing shades of meaning. Yet it appears to be endowed sufficiently for the development of a basic language to serve eventually as a foundation for language growth through the printed word for the prelingually deaf.

It follows then that there is need of a technique to present systematically either vocalized speech plus the cues of Cornett (cued speech plus auditory amplification) or a grammatically correct sign language to deaf children between birth and 5 to 6 years of age which will compensate somewhat for the loss of incidental learning contingent upon the defective auditory system. Systematization either of the former or the latter is possible through modification of a technique currently used by Winitz (1973) to expedite the learning of German by college students. Essentially, his method consists of the development of an understanding of spoken German to the exclusion of any mastery of expression, i.e., speaking the language. His rationale is that facility in speaking the language will be expedited if one develops a high level of comprehension of the spoken language. In fact, Winitz does not formally teach his students to speak German, but permits speaking ability to develop as a corollary of comprehension. Therefore, he systematically develops auditory comprehension of spoken German through multiple choice picture exercises to build vocabulary, language principles, phrases, sentences and topic work. For example in teaching vocabulary a four-picture display (presented in quadrant format) appears on the video screen in conjunction with the spoken word for one of the pictures. The student marks one of four squares or quadrants on a response sheet which he considers to be correct. If his choice is correct the square turns a specific color. Succeeding displays are designed to teach the correct response and also to provide sufficient repetitions to assure learning. With ap-

propriate modifications of this simple technique, language principles such as plurals, prepositions, verb tense and so forth, as well as phrases, idioms, sentences and situational language could be taught to children with severe hearing impairment.

Obviously, the approach must be informal for children under 3 years of age. The vocabulary, phrases and short sentences which normal hearing children of this age range learn to understand are available in the literature (Lillywhite, Young and Olmstead, 1970; Perkins, 1971) and should provide the foundation for language development in children with hearing impairment. Teachers of the deaf have stressed for many years that the hearing-impaired child should be "bombarded" with language. However, the concept here is that there should be "controlled bombardment" to develop receptive language. By "controlled bombardment" is meant the provision of sufficient contacts with words and phrases to assure that learning takes place. Obviously, the child must also acquire expressive language, but the implication is that expressive language will be expedited if the child first of all has some understanding of language or a framework of comprehension. In the child with normal hearing expressive language appears to emerge concomitantly with receptive language. However, the hearing child's receptive language and inner speech are likely to precede expressive language (Myklebust, 1960).

Although a number of training programs are available in the country today for parents of children who are under 3 years of age (see each January issue of the *American Annals of the Deaf*), it does not seem amiss to suggest the need for a commission to review the studies of early language development in children in order to devise controlled language procedures which could be used by parents. In fact, one might go a step further and recommend the use of video tape recordings involving the parents and other members of the family—in short, using video tape as a supplement in presenting controlled language to the child. For example, depending upon one's methodologic persuasion, action verbs such as "run," "jump," short sentences as "Open the door," appropriate nouns, language principles as "under," "over" and so forth could be systematically presented to the child in gamelike fashion to assure adequate learning experience for receptive language development. Furthermore, the child could be video taped in the role of teacher to develop his expressive skills.

After the child reaches the age of 3 years a more formal approach to the development of receptive language should begin. This could consist of working with children in groups of 4 or 5, and progressing to objects and pictures as representations. For example, utilizing a modification of the technique of Winitz, the children would be provided with response sheets which were divided into four quadrants or boxes, each of which contained a different picture. The children would be required to identify the correct stimulus as initiated by the teacher or parent. Again, video tape presentations would be an excellent adjunct at this level for developing receptive as well as expressive language. It should be recalled that teachers of young deaf children have used similar approaches for many years. However, not infrequently, the systematic presentation of language principles and vocabulary to develop comprehension becomes of secondary consideration in relation to expression.

After the child reaches a mental age of about 6 years, introduction to the printed word should begin in earnest. The same technique as previously described may now be employed to attach either vocalized speech, signs, finger spelling or a combination of them to corresponding printed symbols, If a basic language comprehension has been established previously, the transfer to the printed symbol and, consequently, reading should be somewhat analogous to that of the child with normal hearing. Since it is only through reading that the congenitally deaf may hope to reach eventually that level of cognitive development and verbal abstract functioning of which they are inherently capable, it is imperative that research be directed toward language development during the first 5 or 6 years.

Obviously, the foregoing recommendation is not a new idea. At the present time, there is a concerted effort to foster the use of "total communication" with the deaf. The method advocates the use of the full spectrum of language modes such as speech reading, auditory stimulation, sign language, manual alphabet, and reading in teaching the deaf (Kent, 1971). Essentially, total communication means the simultaneous uses of auditory amplification of speech, lipreading and a combination of signs plus manual alphabet in teaching the deaf and in communication.

Teaching the deaf child to communicate utilizing a number of modalities is laudable. However, even though the organism can process simultaneously visual and auditory stimuli in vocalized speech, nevertheless, it cannot handle concurrently two visual inputs. As a consequence, when multiple modes of communication are used simultaneously by a sender, the receiver will select the modality to which he has been accustomed or else from which he obtains maximum comprehension. In total communication, where there is simultaneous presentation (Katz, Mathis and Merrill, 1974) of vocalized speech and a sign-manual alphabet combination, the receiver is likely to attend either to the former or the latter but not to all signals simultaneously. Although one may attend to the auditory input in conjunction with sign-fingerspelling, nevertheless, synchronization is likely to be poor as compared to an auditory-visual input of vocalized speech.

The Gardners had apparent success in using sign language with the chimpanzee, Washoe. Fouts (1972) has contributed additionally to their findings. Equally exciting is the work of Premack (1970, 1971); Premack and Premack (1972), and more recently, of Rumbaugh, Gill and von Glassersfeld (1973). Premack used plastic, geometric shapes of different color, and Rumbaugh et al. used a special typewriter of 50 keys with a geometric design on each one in their experimental programs with chimpanzees. The fact that both the sign language and the sequencing of geometric shapes have proven fruitful with apes suggests their appropriateness for use with children with special language problems such as the congenitally deaf.

During the past 10 to 15 years there have been a number of studies which purport to show that deaf children reared in a manual communication environment are more advanced educationally than those from an oral background. For example, Stuckless and Birch (1966), Meadow (1968) and Vernon and Koh (1970) compared deaf children of deaf parents with deaf children of hearing parents and reported superiority of the former over the latter in a number of educational areas. However, such studies, although of great importance, are not infrequently open to criticism by virtue of the number of confounding variables inherently present in descriptive research. Actually, experimental studies are rare in the field of auditory impairment.

Auditorily Impaired Children—Adjustment. As noted earlier, emotional and adjustment problems become evident when hearing loss in the better ear reaches a level of about 40 dB. In many instances, audiologic habilitation which includes the use of hearing aids, lessons in lipreading, placement in the front of the classroom, and the education of the parents, teachers and the children's classmates is effective in alleviating problems and in bringing about better adjustment. When psychotherapy is indicated the conventional techniques, involving environmental manipulation, insight, emotional release from tension, supportive relationship and socialization, may be employed (Hadley, 1958).

More recently, behavior modification techniques have been used with hearing impaired children. With regard to the deaf, many residential schools now include counselors and psychologists on their staffs. At the Kansas School for the Deaf, psychiatric, psychological and counseling services are provided for the children. Psychiatric therapy as well as behavior modification are utilized in working with the students. In addition, the psychiatrist periodically presents a series of lectures on therapeutic techniques to the house parents and supervisors. Furthermore, the majority of the teaching staff have taken courses in counseling and guidance as well as in behavior modification, as the latter is extensively used.

The number of tests which are available for use with hearing impaired individuals varies somewhat as a function of age, age at onset, degree and type of deafness. On the one hand there are the tests of the paper and pencil variety, inventories and behavior rating scales. On the other hand there are the projective tests such as the Rorschach, Thematic Apperception Test (TAT), sentence completion tests, Make A Picture Story Test (MAPS), human figure drawings, Bender Gestalt test and projective play.

The Rorschach, TAT and MAPS have been useful with the adolescent and the adult deaf. However, for young deaf children, because of the language problem, there is virtually a void with the exception of projective play. While at times exceedingly pertinent information can be obtained from the human figure drawings and the Bender Gestalt tests, yet the paucity of the young child's language poses severe problems of interpretation. A number of such tests and the age levels at which they are useful appear in the Appendix.

Auditorily Impaired Children – Motor and Locomotor Ability. Motor ability and locomotor coordination are usually regarded as primary aspects of maturation and development. The latter as noted by the age at which a child begins to walk, is taken often as supportive confirmation in the diagnosis of mental retardation. That there is not a clear-cut relationship between motor and mental abilities even at early ages, but instead, much overlapping of functions has been emphasized by Bayley (1935) and Gesell and Amatruda (1948). However, Myklebust (1946, 1949, 1954), has pointed out the importance of a motor evaluation in contributing to the differential diagnosis of aphasia, deafness, autism and mental retardation in children.

Motor tests for clinical use were developed by Bayley (1935), Oseretsky (Doll, 1946) and Heath (1942, 1943, 1944). Heath devised a rail-walking test to measure gross locomotor ability and published norms for children and adults. Goetzinger et al. (1961) reevaluated the Heath

test for male and female children, 8 to 16 years of age, and obtained excellent agreement with Heath's data.

In discussing equilibrium as associated with the rail-walking test Heath (1944) stressed that both sensory and motor pathways are involved. The sensory pathways indicate to the subject that he is off balance; the motor enable him to regain balance. Poor performance is often difficult to attribute either to motor or sensory deficit, or to central coordinating mechanisms such as the cerebellum. In conjunction with the vestibular apparatus consisting of the semicircular canals, the utricle and the saccule, vision and the kinesthetic senses also contribute to equilibrium. Myklebust (1946), and Scanlon and Goetzinger (1969) have supplied evidence pertaining to the inferior ability of deaf children on the Heath Rail Walking Test. Scanlon and Goetzinger (1969) also reported poorer performance for the deaf on the Fukuda Vestibular Tests. However, both studies reported great variability among subjects which would have been anticipated because of differences in etiology and degree of the hearing loss. For example, subjects who suffer deafness as a result of meningitis would have more disturbance in locomotor ability than those with Scheibe's deafness. It is well known that the vestibular and cochlear divisions of the eighth nerve as well as the utricle and saccule are often destroyed in meningitis, whereas in Scheibe's deafness, the semicircular canals and utricle are normal (Lindsay, 1967; Omerod, 1960; Schuknecht, 1967; Whetnall and Fry, 1964). Furthermore, Sandberg and Terkildsen (1965) studied subjects in a school for the deaf and reported a higher incidence of abnormal calorics for those with greater than 90 dB loss through the speech range (500 to 2000 Hz) as compared to those with less than 90 dB loss. It is clear therefore, that tests of locomotion and balance have a place in the diagnosis, treatment and education of hearing-impaired children.

A recently reported instrument which is particularly appropriate for screening is the Floor Ataxia Test Battery by Cunningham and Goetzinger (1972). Essentially these investigators developed normative data for male and female children, ages 8 through 18 years, on four of the most discriminative subtests of the Graybiel and Fregly (1956) Ataxia Test Battery for adults. The subtests are conducted with eyes closed and are as follows: (1) the sharpened Romberg, (2) standing on the right leg, (3) standing on the left leg and (4) walking toe to heel. The test is easy to administer and requires only about 6 min. The only equipment essential for administration is a stopwatch or a watch with a second hand.

The Multiply Handicapped. Within the last 10 to 15 years there has been increasing concern over the multiply handicapped child. Hardy (1969) has pointed out the magnitude of the problem as related to rubella. In the 6-month period after September 1964, thousands of "rubella babies" were born in the United States as a result of a German measles epidemic the previous year. This one epidemic left 20,000 to 30,000 children with various handicapping conditions. The triad of congenital heart disease, cataracts and deafness has long been associated with rubella.

Vernon (1967a) reported on the psychological, educational and physical characteristics of 129 applicants for admission to the California School for the Deaf at Riverside from 1954 to 1964. He found 53% of them to be multiply handicapped. Furthermore, their educational achievement was below other groups of deaf children even when IQ level was considered. Their poor educational achievement was due partly to the high prevalence of aphasia (22%) in rubella children. Vernon postulated that central nervous system lesions were at the basis of their aphasia and other disabilities (87% were mentally retarded—below 70 IQ). There was also a high prevalence of severe emotional disturbances in the group. As compared to children with hereditary Rh factor, premature birth and meningitis etiologies, the post-rubella cases had the highest incidence of psychological maladjustment.

Vernon (1967b) also studied 114 post-meningitic deaf children. Their mean IQ was about 96. Thirty-eight percent of them had multiple handicaps. In addition, 24% were emotionally disturbed. Educationally, these children achieved at $2/3$ the rate of deaf children of deaf parents.

In the same sample of children Vernon (1967c) isolated 46 cases of definitely established Rh factor deafness. Of this number about 71% were multiply handicapped. The mean IQ of the group was 94. Educationally the Rh deaf achieved at about $1/2$ the rate of normal children and about $5/7$ the rate of the hereditary deaf. However, the figures are biased and do not reflect the fact, as explained by Vernon, that 14% of the Rh children who had applied for admission to the school were rejected because of inadequate potential—the highest rejection rate of the handicapped who were studied. This group also showed the highest degree of neurologic impairment. In addition, 12% were diagnosed as being severely disturbed.

Vernon (1967d) investigated the premature deaf for whom there was no other cause of deafness. The mean IQ for this group was 89 with 16% being mentally retarded (IQs below 70). These children progressed academically at $1/2$ the rate of normal children and about $2/3$ the rate of the hereditarily deaf. With reference to adjustment, 34 of 117 had been diagnosed as having severe problems.

Thus the hereditarily deaf were significantly superior to the rubella, meningitic, Rh factor and premature deaf groups educationally, intellectually, emotionally and in a lower incidence of secondary handicaps.

Recently, Jensema (1974) reported a study involving 43,946 students enrolled in special educational programs for the auditorily impaired during the 1972–1973 school year. A total of 7,739 subjects suffered hearing loss as a result of rubella. Jensema noted that children for whom the etiology was reported to be maternal rubella had a more severe hearing impairment than children with other causal factors. They also had a higher incidence of visual, behavioral and heart related disorders. A higher proportion of these children were enrolled in full-time special education programs. This was felt to be a result of the more severe hearing losses and the additional handicaps.

Hereditary Deafness. There are numerous causes of hereditary deafness in man. Konigsmark (1969) has written a comprehensive review of the subject. However, psychological studies of the various etiologic categories are sparse. Owsley (1962) surveyed intelligence and educational achievement of children in schools for the deaf who showed symptoms of Waardenburg's syndrome. This is a hereditary disease characterized by unilateral or bilateral congenital deafness, a white forelock, lateral displacement of the inner canthi of the eyes and of the inferior lacrimal puntae producing a broad, nasal root, by heterochromia of the iris, and by confluence of the eyebrows with hypertrichosis of the medial ends. Owsley's findings indicated that his subjects had normal intelligence, and educational achievement in accordance with other studies of the deaf.

THE PSYCHOLOGY OF HARD OF HEARING AND DEAF ADULTS

Hard of Hearing and Deaf Adults

Numerous articles have appeared concerning the psychological adjustment of hard of hearing and deaf adults (Barker et al., 1953). These views have diverged widely, ranging from those who regard the hearing impaired as markedly different in personality to those who consider them as indistinguishable from the normally hearing. Some of the personality characteristics attributed to the hard of hearing and deaf include: introversion, despondency, hopelessness, sense of inferiority, fear, supersensitivity, bitterness, brooding, persecution complex, suspicion, apathy and listlessness.

Cruelty, egocentrism, selfishness, and lack of sympathy are also used generously in descriptions of the hard of hearing and deaf. Factors said to contribute to adjustment problems of the hearing impaired include the extra effort which must be exerted to meet the demands of the environment, head noises, the absence of sound itself, the threat of limited employment opportunities and second class citizenship.

Three of the early studies of the hard of hearing used the Bernreuter Personality Inventory (Welles, 1932; Pintner, 1933; Pintner, Fusfeld and Brunschwig, 1937) which measures self-sufficiency, neurotic tendency, introversion and dominance. However, according to Barker et al. (1953) some of the items of the inventory tend to put the hearing impaired in a poor light. The hard of hearing were found to be slightly more neurotic, introverted and submissive than the hearing. However, the large overlap between groups was more significant than the differences.

Ingalls (1946) using psychiatric interviews studied hearing impaired patients at Borden General Hospital during World War II. He reported that 27% were diagnosed as psychoneurotic and less than 5% as psychotic. The latter were mostly of the anxiety type. Ingalls classified his patients on the basis of chronic and acute hearing losses. The former referred to deafness which had obtained from birth; the latter, to hearing impairment which had been acquired recently. Cases with chronic hearing loss were said to feel injured, defective, isolated, hostile and depressed. Audiologic habilitation which included hearing aids, auditory training and lipreading, was reported to be helpful for them, but it was no substitute for psychotherapy. Conversely, the patients with acute hearing loss responded well to audiologic therapy, which was effective in relieving depressed feelings.

Knapp (1960) conducted psychiatric studies on patients admitted to Deshon Hospital during World War II. Some patients with the more severe hearing impairments reacted neurotically to the constricting effects of the deafness by overcompensating in outgoing activities, by denial of impairment, by withdrawal from society or by exploitation of the deficit. Knapp noted that adjustment was poorer when impairment obtained from childhood. However, he concluded that the study showed "no one psychology of deafness."

An intensive investigation pertaining to the psychology of the hard of hearing and the deaf was conducted by Myklebust (1960). The subjects were asked also to write an autobiographical account on the topic "What my hearing loss means to me." The hard of hearing emphasized the increased stress of everyday life, the patience required of the family in handling their (hard of hearing) telephone messages, the problems in obtaining employment, maintaining friends, social isolation, despondency and the need to identify with other hard of hearing individuals.

Myklebust also administered the Minnesota Multiphasic Personality Inventory (MMPI) both to his hard of hearing and deaf subjects. The hard of hearing males were found to have more emotional maladjustment than normal hearing males. They also manifested poorer emotional adjustment than their female counterparts. However, the use of a hearing aid was conducive to better adjustment both for the deaf as well as the hard of hearing. Neither the hard of hearing nor the deaf showed a high incidence of schizophrenia on the scale.

Myklebust administered the MMPI to 194 deaf students at Gallaudet College as well as to 94 hard of hearing subjects. He made numerous comparisons such as between the deaf and hard of hearing, the meningitic and non-meningitic deaf and the sexes. He found a correlation between sensory deprivation (deafness) and emotional adjustment which was related to degree of deafness, age at onset of deafness and sex. The profoundly deaf showed the largest emotional deviations. Males, irrespective of degree of loss and age at onset, manifested more personality disorders than females. Also the deaf appeared unaware of their handicap. They lacked insight into the significance of hearing loss. The hard of hearing estimated hearing loss to be a greater handicap and manifested more depression because of the disability. However, the deaf's naivete with regard to their handicap could not be regarded as an index of better adjustment. To the contrary those deaf who maintained that their deafness was no handicap were found to be the most disturbed emotionally. Myklebust stated "the primary conclusion to be drawn from this study, therefore, is that deafness, particularly when profound and from early life, imposes a characteristic restriction on personality but does not cause mental illness" (Myklebust, 1960, p. 158).

It is clear from the literature that many of the negative characteristics associated with deafness are the result of environment and training. Levine (1956) in her study of adolescent girls in a residential school for the deaf found immature and atypical responses in comparison to the normal, nevertheless, she interpreted her results as representative of adequate adjustment in the context of the particular environmental setting.

Fusfeld (1955) had over 100 deaf adults of both sexes list the disadvantages and advantages of being deaf. Disadvantages included the inability to hear warning sounds, absence of ordinary social minglings, limitations of educational opportunities outside the school, slowness in learning problems related to employment, feelings of inadequacy and frustration, inability to enjoy music and recreation dependent upon hearing. The advantages stressed were freedom from discord thus contributing to mental rest and repose, the development of enduring friendships, inner poise and contentment, numerous social and recreational activities, aesthetic values from sensitivity to vibrations and "the harmony of rhythm in the phenomena of action in the life around them."

Despite the fact that the disadvantages outweighed the advantages Fusfeld notes that the deaf on the whole present a satisfactory social picture, establish homes of satisfying standards, hold a successful place in the occupational world when given the opportunity, have a strong group consciousness, manifest a zest for life in recreation and travel, maintain religious affiliation, achieve well in art and make good citizens.

The most comprehensive psychiatric study of the deaf in this country was conducted in New York (Rainer, 1963). Altshuler (1962a) reporting the New York group's observations on about 500 persons with varying degrees and kinds of disorders has listed certain personality characteristics common to the deaf. The findings from these psychiatric observations are remarkably in agreement with projective and psychometric investigations.

With reference to mental illness in the hospitalized deaf, Altshuler (1962b) reported that schizophrenia is the most common form of psychosis. It accounts for slightly more than 50% of the cases which is similar to the hearing population statistics. The disease is no more severe in the deaf than in the hearing, but is characterized by aggressive, impulsive acts which might be associated with the deaf's orientation toward action. The most common reasons for referral to the outpatient clinic were poor work adjustment, acute psychiatric illness, social conflicts, homosexuality and family disturbances in connection with the handicap.

Myklebust (1960) noted that hard of hearing adults have particular anxiety regarding employment. The second class citizenship of the deaf adult (Vernon, 1969) may be inferred from the comparison of their job status with that of the general population. Fifty percent of the deaf are employed in manual labor as compared to 28% of the total population.

In summary, deaf and hard of hearing adults manifest deviations from the normally hearing in some areas of personality and adjustment which are related primarily to their difficulty in communication. Many of their tendencies are amenable to improvement through a realistic approach to their problems. This includes education, mental health programs for acceptance of their plight, the education and sensitization of the public concerning the nature of the handicap as well as the potential and capabilities of the hearing impaired.

SUMMARY

1. Research tends to indicate that children with hearing levels within the 0- to 25-dB range (ANSI-1969) do not manifest any measureable psychological deficiencies either in verbal intelligence or adjustment.

2. Children with hearing loss within the 25- to 40-dB range in the better ear may show significant retardation on group verbal tests of intelligence but will still fall within the limits of normalcy. Their reduction in IQ reflects the language lag due to the hearing loss.

3. Children approximating a 40-dB hearing loss in the better ear, particularly if it obtains from birth and is of sensory-neural origin, may be significantly retarded in educational achievement in comparison to normal hearing children, and may give evidence of emotional and social maladjustment. Such children will require help in compensating for their problems.

4. Children with congenital or prelingual sensory-neural hearing loss approximating 40 dB in the better ear for the speech frequencies appear to be retarded in language development by about 12 to 18 months at 3 years of age. They are often diagnosed as aphasic, brain injured or as having learning disabilities.

5. Educational guidelines are discussed with reference to degree of hearing loss.

6. There is unequivocal evidence that children who are born deaf or who suffer profound deafness before the acquisition of language are severely retarded in educational achievement. Their intelligence is normal as measured by performance scales. On some non-verbal group tests of intelligence about a 2-year retardation in mental ability has been observed in young deaf children. However, the deficit disappears with age which indicates that it is attributable to an earlier underdevelopment and an experiential deficit rather than to mental retardation per se.

7. Deaf children compare favorably with their normal hearing peers on abstract verbal reasoning tasks when the language is within their understanding and facility. Inferiority of the deaf on verbal tasks is related to lack of facility and breadth of language rather than to any mental deficit contingent upon deafness.

8. When the cause of deafness is associated

with rubella, meningitis, the Rh factor and prematurity, the prevalence of other handicaps is reported to be increased.

9. The combined auditory-visual modality is superior to either one alone when the visual stimuli are lip movements or lipreading. However, when the visual modality is the printed word it is equal or superior to either the auditory or the combined auditory-visual modality.

10. Methods for reducing the language retardation of deaf children which consist of controlled experiences are outlined.

11. A number of tests which are appropriate for use in the diagnosis and treatment of emotional problems in hearing-impaired persons are listed.

12. The Cunningham-Goetzinger test of locomotor ability and equilibrium is discussed. It is easily administered and norms are provided for ages 8 to 18 years.

13. Psychological problems associated with hearing impairment in adults are presented. Basically, these problems are the same as those encountered in normal hearing individuals.

APPENDIX

A. Psychological Tests Appropriate for Use with the Hearing Impaired (Children and Adults)

Tests	Standardization Years
Individual Performance Scales:	
Leiter International Scale (Original)[1]	2 through adult
Leiter International Scale (Grace Arthur Restandardization)[1]	3 to 8
Merrill-Palmer Pre-School Performance Tests (19 subtests of non-verbal abilities)[1]	Preschool through primary grades
WPPSI (Wechsler Pre-School and Primary Scale of Intelligence)[2]	4 to 6½
WISC (Wechsler Intelligence Scale for Children)[2]	5 through 15
WISC-R (revised)[2]	5 through 15
WAIS (Wechsler Adult Intelligence Scale)[2]	16 to 75+
Wechsler-Bellevue Intelligence Scale (Form II is the retest for WAIS)[2]	10 through 59
Arthur Point Scale of Performance (Revised Form II)[2]	5 to 15
Arthur Point Scale of Performance (Form I)[3]	5 through 15
Hiskey-Nebraska Test of Learning Aptitude[4]	3 to 16
Group Non-Verbal Tests of Intelligence:	
Revised Army Beta Test[2]	16 to 59
Raven Progressive Matrices (Colored-1947)[1,2]	5 through 11
Raven Progressive Matrices (Standard-1938)[1,2]	8 through 65
Raven Progressive Matrices (1947 and 1962)[1,2]	For above average adolescents and adults
Chicago Non-Verbal Examination[2]	8 to adult
Science Research Associates, Inc. (SRA Non-Verbal Form)[5]	Adult

B. Personality and Emotional Adjustment Tests (Must Be Used With Caution with the Deaf)

Adjustment Tests:	
Make A Picture Story (MAPS Test)[2]	Projective. Children and adults
Thematic Apperception Test (TAT)[2]	Projective. Adolescents and adults
Rorschach Technique Tests[2]	Projective. Adolescents and adults
Psychological Evaluation of Children's Human Figure Drawings (Elizabeth Koppitz) (Also Developmental Norms)[6]	5 to 12
California Personality Tests[7]	Kindergarten through adult
The Hand Test (E.E. Wagner) (Used experimentally by C.P.G.)[1]	Projective. Adolescents and adults
Buttons: A Projective Test for Pre-Adolescents and Adolescents (Esther Rothman and Pearl Berkowitz) (Used experimentally by C.P.G.)[1]	(See Title)
Group Personality Projective Test (GPPT) (R.N. Cassell and T.C. Kahn) (Used experimentally by C.P.G.)[8]	Projective. Adolescents and adults
Other Tests:	
Benton Revised Visual Retention Test (A. Benton) (Visual Memory Test)[2]	8 through adults
Bender Gestalt (Elizabeth Koppitz) (Organicity, Development, Adjustment)[6]	5 to 12

[1] Western Psychological Services, 12031 Wilshire Blvd., Los Angeles, California 90025.

[2] The Psychological Corporation, 304 East 45th St., New York, New York 10017.

[3] C. H. Stoelting Co., 424 North Homan Ave., Chicago, Illinois 60624.

[4] Union College Press, Lincoln, Nebraska 65806.

[5] Science Research Associates (SRA) Inc., 259 East Erie St., Chicago, Illinois 60611.

[6] Grune & Stratton Inc., 381 Park Ave. South, New York, New York 10016.

[7] California Test Bureau, 5916 Hollywood Blvd., Los Angeles, California 90028.

[8] Psychological Test Specialists, Box 1441 Missoula, Montana 59801.

REFERENCES

Altshuler, K. A., Psychiatric considerations in the school age deaf. *Am. Ann. Deaf,* 107, 553–559, 1962a.

Altshuler, K. A., Psychiatric considerations in the adult deaf. *Am. Ann. Deaf,* 107, 560–561, 1962b.

American Annals of the Deaf, 120, 175, 1975.

Anthony, D. A., *Seeing Essential English.* Center for the Hearing Impaired, Community College of Denver, 1001 62nd Ave., Denver, Colorado, 80216.

Avery, C., Social competence of pre-school acoustically handicapped children. *J. Except. Child.,* 15, 71–73, 1948.

Babbidge, H., Education of the deaf. A report to the Secretary of Health, Education and Welfare by his advisory committee on the education of the deaf. Washington, D.C.: U.S. Dept. of Health, Education and Welfare, 1965.

Barker, R. G., Wright, B. A., Meyerson, L., and Gonick, M., Adjustment to physical handicap and illness; a survey of the social psychology of physique and disability. Bulletin 55, New York: Social Science Research Council, 1953.

Bayley, N., The development of motor abilities during the first three years. Washington, D.C.: Society for Research in Child Development, National Research Council, 1, 1935.

Bindon, M., Make-A-Picture-Story Test findings for rubella deaf children. *J. Abnorm. Soc. Psychol.*, 55, 38–42, 1957.

Birch, J. R., and Birch, J. W., The Leiter International Performance Scale as an aid in the psychological study of deaf children. *Am. Ann. Deaf*, 96, 502–511, 1951.

Blake, K. A., Ainsworth, S. H., and Williams, Charlotte, L., Effects of induction and deduction on deaf and hearing individuals' attainment of first-order concepts. *Am. Ann. Deaf*, 112, 606–613, 1967.

Boatner, E. B., The need for new vocational-technical programs for the deaf. In *Report of the Proceedings of the 42nd Meeting of the Convention of American Instructors of the Deaf*, No. 71, pp. 201–206. Washington, D.C.: U.S. Government Printing Office, 1965.

Bradway, K. P., The social competence of deaf children. *Am. Ann. Deaf*, 82, 122–140, 1937.

Brunschwig, L., A study of some personality aspects of deaf children. New York: Columbia University, Teachers College Contributions to Education, No. 687, 1936.

Bunch, C. C., *Clinical Audiometry*. St. Louis, C.V. Mosby Co., 1943.

Burchard, E. M., and Myklebust, H. R., A comparison of congenital and adventitious deafness with respect to its effect on intelligence, personality and social maturity (Part I). *Am. Ann. Deaf*, 87, 140–152, 1942a.

Burchard, E. M., and Myklebust, H. R., A comparison of congenital and adventitious deafness with respect to its effect on intelligence, personality and social maturity (Part II: Social Maturity). *Am. Ann. Deaf*, 87, 241–251, 1942b.

Caplin, D., A special report of retardation of children with impaired hearing in New York City schools. *Am. Ann. Deaf*, 82, 234–243, 1937.

Carson, P. A., A comparison of learning by deaf children through seven conditions of communication. Unpublished master's thesis, University of Kansas, 1974.

Cokely, D. R., and Gawlik, R., Options; a position paper on the relationship between manual English and sign. Washington, D.C.: Kendall Demonstration Elementary School for the Deaf, 1973.

Cornett, R. O., Cued speech. *Am. Ann. Deaf*, 112, 3–14, 1967.

Cunningham, D. R., and Goetzinger, C. P., Floor ataxia test battery. *Arch. Otolaryngol.*, 96, 559–564, 1972.

Davis, H., and Silverman, S. R., *Hearing and Deaf-ness*. New York: Holt, Rinehart & Winston, 1970.

Day, H. E., Fusfeld, I. S., and Pintner, R., A survey of American schools for the deaf. Washington, D.C.: The National Research Council, 1928.

Doll, E. A., *The Oseretsky Test of Motor Proficiency*. Minneapolis, Minn.: Educational Test Bureau, 1946.

Drever, J., and Collins, M., *Performance Test of Intelligence*. London: Oliver & Boyd, 1936.

Eagles, E. L., Hardy, W. G., and Catlin, F. I., NINDB Monograph No. 7. Human Communication: The Public Health Aspects of Hearing, Language and Speech Disorders. Washington, D.C.: Public Health Service Publication No.1745, U.S. Government Printing Office, 1968.

Elser, R. P., The social position of hearing handicapped children in the regular grades. *Except. Child.*, 25, 305–309, 1959.

Embrey, R., A study of visual perceptual responses of congenitally deaf children. Unpublished master's thesis, University of Kansas, 1955.

Fisher, B., The social and emotional adjustment of children with impaired hearing attending ordinary classes. *Br. J. Educ. Psychol.*, 36, 319–321, 1966.

Fouts, R. S., Use of guidance in teaching sign language to a chimpanzee. *J. Comp. Physiol. Psychol.*, 80, 515–522, 1972.

Furth, H. G., Language and the development of thinking. In: *Report of the Proceedings of the International Congress on Education of the Deaf and of the 41st Meeting of the Convention of American Instructors of the Deaf*. (Held at Gallaudet College, Wash., D.C. in 1963.) No. 106, pp. 475–483, Washington, D.C.: U.S. Government Printing Office, 1964.

Furth, H. G., *Thinking Without Language*. New York: The Free Press, 1966.

Fusfeld, I. S., Counseling the Deafened. In Frampton, M. E., and Gall, E. D. (Eds.), *Special Education for the Exceptional; Vol. II. The Physically Handicapped and Special Health Problems*, pp. 209–218. Boston: Porter Sargent, 1955.

Gaeth, J. H., Learning with Visual and Audiovisual Presentations. In McConnell, F., and Ward, P. H. (Eds.), *Deafness in Childhood,* pp. 279–303. Nashville: Vanderbilt University Press, 1967.

Gardner, R. A., and Gardner, B. T., Teaching sign language to a chimpanzee. *Science*, 165, 664–672, 1969.

Gates, R. R., The differential effectiveness of various modes of presenting verbal information to deaf students through modified television formats. Unpublished doctoral dissertation, University of Pittsburgh, 1970.

Gentile, A., and Di Francesca, S., Academic achievement test performance of hearing impaired students. Washington, D.C.: U.S. Office of Demographic Studies, Gallaudet College, 1969.

Gesell, A. L., and Amatruda, C.S., *Developmental Diagnosis*. New York: Paul B. Hoeber Inc., 1948.

Goetzinger, C. P., A study of intermediate department deaf children with the Chicago Non-Verbal Test (unpublished), 1946.

Goetzinger, C. P., Relationship between school achievement and intelligence test data for deaf adolescents. Unpublished master's thesis, University of California, Berkeley, 1950.

Goetzinger, C. P., Effects of small perceptive losses on language and on speech discrimination. *Volta Rev., 64*, 408–414, 1962.

Goetzinger, C. P., Management of hearing problems in persons of advanced age. *Eye Ear Nose Throat Mon., 42*, 38–41, 1963.

Goetzinger, C. P., and Rousey, C. L., A study of the Wechsler Performance Scale (form 2) and the Knox Cube Test with deaf adolescents. *Am. Ann. Deaf, 102*, 388–398, 1957.

Goetzinger, C. P., and Rousey, C. L., Educational achievement of deaf children. *Am. Ann. Deaf, 104*, 221–231, 1959.

Goetzinger, C. P., Ortiz, J. D., Rousey, C.L., and Dirks, D. D., A re-evaluation of the Heath Railwalking Test. *J. Educ. Res., 54*, 187–191, 1961.

Goetzinger, C. P., Harrison, C., and Baer, C. J., Small perceptive hearing loss; its effects in school-age children. *Volta Rev., 66*, 124–131, 1964.

Goetzinger, C. P., Ortiz, J. D., Bellerose, B., and Buchan, L. G., A study of the S. O. Rorschach with deaf and hearing adolescents. *Am. Ann. Deaf, 111*, 510–522, 1966.

Goetzinger, C. P., Wills, R. C., and Dekker, L. C., Non-language I.Q. tests used with deaf pupils. *Volta Rev., 69*, 500–506, 1967.

Gorman, P., and Paget, G., A systematic sign language. Originated by Sir Richard Paget, London, England, 1969. (An unpublished handout obtained from Dr. Kevin Murphy of the Royal Berkshire Hospital in Reading.)

Goodman, A., Reference zero levels for pure tone audiometer. *Asha, 7*, 262–263, 1965.

Graybiel, A., and Fregly, A. R., A new quantitative ataxia test battery. NSAM-919, NASA R-93, Pensacola, Fla.: Naval School of Aviation Medicine, 1956.

Greenberger, D., Doubtful cases. *Am. Ann. Deaf, 34*, 93–99, 1889.

Gustason, G., Pfetzing, D., and Zawolkow, E., *Signing Exact English: Seeing Instead of Hearing*. Rossmoor, Calif.: Modern Signs Press, 1972.

Habbe, S., Personality adjustment of adolescent boys with impaired hearing. New York: Columbia University, Teachers College Contributions to Education, No. 697, 1936.

Hadley, J. M., *Clinical and Counseling Psychology*. New York: Alfred A. Knopf, 1958.

Hardy, J., Rubella and its aftermath. *Children, U.S. Department of Health, Education and Welfare, 16*, 91–93, 1969.

Hayes, G. M., A study of the visual perception of orally educated deaf children. Unpublished master's thesis, University of Massachusetts, 1955.

Heath, S. R., Clinical significance of motor defects with military implications. *Am. J. Psychol., 57*, 482–499, 1944.

Heath, S. R., Railwalking performance as related to mental age and etiological type among the mentally retarded. *Am. J. Psychol., 55*, 240–247, 1942.

Heath, S. R., The military use of the railwalking test as an index of locomotor coordination. *Psychol. Bull., 40*, 282–284, 1943.

Heider, F., Acoustic training helps deaf children. *Volta Rev., 45*, 135, 1943.

Heider, F., and Heider, G. M., A comparison of sentence structure of deaf and hearing children. *Psychol. Monogr., 52*, 42–103, 1940.

Heider, F., and Heider, G. M., Studies in the psychology of the deaf. *Psychol. Monogr., 53*, 1–158, 1941.

Henry, S., Children's audiograms in relation to reading attainments; III. Discussion, summary and conclusions. *J. Genet. Psychol., 76*, 49–63, 1947.

Hudgins, C. V., Problems of speech comprehension in deaf children. *Nerv. Child., 9*, 57–63, 1951.

Ingalls, G. S., Some psychiatric observations on patients with hearing defects. *Occup. Ther. Rehabil., 25*, 62–66, 1946.

Jensema, C., Post-rubella children in special education programs for the hearing impaired. *Volta Rev., 76*, 466–473, 1974.

Johnson, E. H., The effect of academic level on scores from the Chicago Non-Verbal Examination for primary pupils. *Am. Ann. Deaf, 92*, 227–233, 1947.

Johnson, E. H., The ability of pupils in a school for the deaf to understand various methods of communication. *Am. Ann. Deaf, 93*, 258–314, 1948.

Kahn, H., Responses of hard of hearing and normal hearing children to frustration. *Except. Child., 24*, 155–159, 1957.

Kates, S., Kates, W., and Michael, J., Cognitive processes in deaf and hearing adolescents and adults. *Psychol. Monogr., 76*, 1962.

Katz, L., Mathis, S. L., and Merrill, E. C., *The Deaf Child in the Public Schools: A Handbook for Parents of Deaf Children*. Danville, Ill.: The Interstate Printers & Publishers, 1974.

Kent, S., Total communication at Maryland School for the Deaf. *Maryland Bull., 91*, 69–86, 1971.

Kilpatrick, W. M., Comparative tests. *Am. Ann. Deaf, 57*, 427–428, 1912.

Kilpatrick, W. M., The Binet-Simon tests and the establishment of age and class year norms. *Am. Ann. Deaf, 59*, 394–398, 1914.

Kirk, S. A., Behavior problem tendencies in deaf and hard of hearing children. *Am. Ann. Deaf, 83*, 131–137, 1938.

Kirk, S. A., and Perry, J., A comparative study of the Ontario and Nebraska tests for the deaf. *Am. Ann. Deaf, 93*, 315–323, 1948.

Knapp, P. H., Emotional aspects of hearing loss. In Barbara, D. A. (Ed.), *Psychological and Psychiatric Aspects of Speech and Hearing*, pp. 396–439. Springfield, Ill.: Charles C Thomas, 1960.

Konigsmark, B. W., Hereditary deafness in man. *N. Engl. J. Med., 281*, 713–720, 774–778, 827–832, 1969.

Larr, A. L., Perceptual and conceptual abilities of residential school deaf children. *J. Int. Council Except. Child., 23*, 63–66, 1956.

Lennan, R.K., Use of programmed instructions with emotionally disturbed deaf boys. *Am. Ann. Deaf, 114*, 906–911, 1969.

Levine, E. S., *Youth in a Soundless World*. New York: New York University Press, 1956.

Levine, E. S., Studies in psychological evaluation of the deaf. *Volta Rev.*, 65, 496–512, 1963.

Levine, B., and Iscoe, I., The Progressive Matrices (1938), the Chicago Non-Verbal and the Wechsler-Bellevue on an adolescent deaf population. *J. Clin. Psychol.*, 11, 307–308, 1955.

Lillywhite, H. S., Young N. B., and Olmsted, R. W., *Pediatrician's Handbook of Communication Disorders*. Philadelphia: Lea & Febiger, 1970.

Lindsay, J. R., Congenital Deafness of Inflammatory Origin. In McConnell, F., and Ward, P. H. (Eds.), *Deafness in Childhood*. Nashville, Tenn.: Vanderbilt University Press, 1967.

Lyon, V. W., Stein, S., Levin, A., Johnson, E., Fogwell, D., and Brown, A. W., Report of the 1931 survey of the Illinois School for the Deaf. *Am. Ann. Deaf*, 78, 157–175, 1933.

MacKane, K., A comparison of the intelligence of deaf and hearing children. New York: Columbia University, Teachers College Contributions to Education, No. 585, 1933.

MacMillan, D. P., and Bruner, F. G., Experimental studies of deaf children. Special Report of the Department of Child Study and Pedagogical Investigation. Chicago: Chicago Public Schools, 1906.

MacPherson, J. G., and Lane, H. S., A comparison of deaf and hearing on the Hiskey Test and on performance scales. *Am. Ann. Deaf*, 93, 178–184, 1948.

Madden, R., The school status of hard of hearing children. New York: Columbia University, Teachers College Contributions to Education, No. 499, 1931.

McAndrew, H., Rigidity and isolation; a study of the deaf and blind. *J. Abnorm. Soc. Psychol.*, 43, 476–494, 1948.

McNeill, D., The capacity for language acquisition. In: *Research on Behavioral Aspects of Deafness. Proceedings of a National Research Conference on Behavioral Aspects of Deafness. U.S. Department of Health, Education and Welfare*, pp. 11–28. Washington, D.C.: Vocational Rehabilitation Administration, 1965.

Meadow, K., Early manual communication in relation to the deaf child's intellectual, social and communicative functioning. *Am. Ann. Deaf*, 113, 29–41, 1968.

Miller, J. B., Educational achievement. *Volta Rev.*, 60, 302–304, 1958.

Mott, A. J., A comparison of deaf and hearing children in their ninth year. *Am. Ann. Deaf*, 44, 401–412, 1899; also, 45, 33–39, 1900.

Myklebust, H. R., Significance of etiology in motor performances of deaf children with special reference to meningitis. *Am. J. Psychol.*, 59, 249–258, 1946.

Myklebust, H. R., The relationship between clinical psychology and audiology. *J. Speech Hear. Disord.*, 14, 98–103, 1949.

Myklebust, H. R., *Auditory Disorders in Children*. New York: Grune & Stratton, 1954.

Myklebust, H. R., *The Psychology of Deafness: Sensory Deprivation, Learning and Adjustment*. New York: Grune & Stratton, 1960.

Myklebust, H. R., and Brutten, M., A study of the visual perception of deaf children. *Acta Otolaryngol. Suppl.* 105, 1–126, 1953.

Newlee, C. E., A report of learning tests with deaf children. *Volta Rev.*, 21, 216–223, 1919.

Northern, J., and Downs, M., *Hearing in Children*, pp. 71–74. Baltimore: Williams & Wilkins, 1974.

Numbers, M. E., and Hudgins, C. V., Speech perception in present day education of deaf children. *Volta Rev.*, 50, 449–456, 1948.

Oleron, P., A study of the intelligence of the deaf. *Am. Ann. Deaf*, 95, 179–195, 1950.

Omerod, F. C., Pathology of congenital deafness. *J. Laryngol. Otol.*, 74, 919–950, 1960.

O'Neill, J., Contributions of the visual components of oral symbols to speech comprehension. *J. Speech Hear. Disord.*, 19, 429–439, 1954.

Owsley, P. J., A study of intelligence and achievement among children exhibiting symptoms of the Waardenburg syndrome. *Volta Rev.*, 64, 429–431, 1962.

Perkins, W. H., *Speech Pathology: An Applied Behavioral Science*. St. Louis: C.V. Mosby, 1971.

Petersen, E. G., Testing children with the Kohs Block Design. *Am. Ann. Deaf*, 81, 242–254, 1936.

Pintner, R., A class study with deaf children. *J. Educ. Psychol.*, 6, 591–600, 1915.

Pintner, R., *The Pintner Non-Language Mental Test*. New York: Columbia University, Bureau of Publications, 1929.

Pintner, R., Emotional stability of the hard of hearing. *J. Genet. Psychol.*, 43, 293–311, 1933.

Pintner, R., Some personality traits of hard of hearing children. *J. Genet. Psychol.*, 60, 143–151, 1942.

Pintner, R., and Lev, J., The intelligence of the hard of hearing school child. *J. Genet. Psychol.*, 55, 31–48, 1939.

Pintner, R., and Paterson, D. G., The Binet Scale and the deaf child. *Am. Ann. Deaf*, 60, 301–311, 1915.

Pintner, R., and Paterson, D. G., Learning tests with deaf children. *Psychol. Monogr.* 20, No. 88, 1916.

Pintner, R., and Paterson, D. G., A measure of the language ability of deaf children. *Am. Ann. Deaf*, 62, 211–239, 1917.

Pintner, R., and Paterson, D. G., Some conclusions from psychological tests of the deaf. *Volta Rev.*, 20, 10–14, 1918.

Pintner, R., and Paterson, D. G., A Scale of Performance Tests. New York: Appleton-Century-Crofts, 1923.

Pintner, R., Fusfeld, I. S., and Brunschwig, L.: Personality tests of deaf adults. *J. Genet. Psychol.*, 51, 305–327, 1937.

Pintner, R., Eisenson, J., and Stanton, M.: *The Psychology of the Physically Handicapped*. New York: F. S. Crofts, 1946.

Prall, J., Lipreading and hearing aids combine for better comprehension. *Volta Rev.*, 59, 64–65, 1957.

Premack, D., A functional analysis of language. *J. Exp. Anal. Behav.*, 14, 107–125, 1970.

Premack, D., Language in chimpanzee? *Science*, 172, 808–822, 1971.

Premack, A. J., and Premack, D., Teaching language to an ape. *Sci. Am.*, 227, 92–99, 1972.

Pugh, G. S., Summaries from "Appraisal of silent reading abilities of acoustically handicapped children." *Am. Ann. Deaf,* **91**, 331–349, 1946.

Purcell, G., and Costello, M. R., Multisensory stimulation and verbal learning. *Bull. Am. Org. Educ. Hear. Impaired,* **1**, 66–68, 1970.

Rainer, J. D., *Family and Mental Health Problems of a Deaf Population.* New York: New York Psychiatric Institute, 1963.

Raven's Standard Progressive Matrices of 1938. (See Appendix.)

Reamer, J. C., Mental and psychological measurements of the deaf. *Psychol. Monogr.* No. 132, 1921.

Reynolds, L. B., The school adjustment of children with minimal hearing loss. *J. Speech Hear. Disord.,* **20**, 380–384, 1955.

Rosenstein, J., Cognitive abilities of deaf children. *J. Speech Hear. Res.,* **3**, 108–119, 1960.

Rosenstein, J., Concept Formation Problems. In: *Report of the Proceedings of the International Congress on Education of the Deaf and of the 41st Meeting of the Convention of American Instructors of the Deaf.* (Gallaudet College, 1963). No. 106, pp. 518–523. Washington, D.C.: U.S. Government Printing Office, 1964.

Rumbaugh, D. M., Gill, T. V., and von Glassersfeld, E. C., Reading and sentence completion by a chimpanzee. *Science,* **182**, 731–733, 1973.

Sandberg, L. E., and Terkildsen, K., Caloric tests in deaf children. *Arch. Otolaryngol.,* **81**, 350–354, 1965.

Sanders, D. A., *Aural Rehabilitation.* Englewood Cliffs, N.J.: Prentice-Hall, 1971.

Scanlon, S. L., and Goetzinger, C. P., The Heath Rails and Fukuda Vestibular Tests with deaf and hearing subjects. *Eye Ear Nose Throat Mon.,* **48**, 29–39, 1969.

Schein, J. D., and Delk, M. T., The Deaf Population of the United States. National Association of the Deaf, 814 Thayer Ave., Silver Spring, Maryland, 1974.

Schick, H. F., A performance test for deaf children of school age. *Volta Rev.,* **36**, 657–658, 1934.

Schuknecht, H. F., Pathology of sensorineural deafness of genetic origin. In: McConnell, F., and Ward, P. H. (Eds.), *Deafness in Childhood,* pp. 69–91. Nashville, Tenn.: Vanderbilt University Press, 1967.

Smith, J. L., Mental characteristics of pupils. *Am. Ann. Deaf,* **48**, 248–268, 1903.

Springer, N., A comparative study of the behavior traits of deaf and hearing children of New York City. *Am. Ann. Deaf,* **83**, 255–273, 1938.

Streng, A., and Kirk, S. A., The social competence of deaf and hard of hearing children in a public day-school. *Am. Ann. Deaf,* **83**, 244–254, 1938.

Stuckless, E. R., Assessing and supporting linguistic development in deaf adolescents. Hearing and Speech Conference at Kansas University Medical Center, February, 1971. Kansas University Medical Center Postgraduate Medical Study Handout, pp. 7–13, 1971.

Stuckless, E. R., and Birch, J. W., The influence of early manual communication on the linguistic development of deaf children. *Am. Ann. Deaf,* **111**, (part I) 452–460, (part II) 499–504, 1966.

Taylor, H., A spelling test. *Am. Ann. Deaf,* **42**, 364–369, 1897.

Templin, M., *The Development of Reasoning in Children with Normal and Defective Hearing.* Minneapolis: The University of Minnesota Press, 1950.

Vegely, A. B., and Elliott, L. L., Applicability of a standardized personality test to a hearing-impaired population. *Am. Ann. Deaf,* **113**, 858–868, 1968.

Vernon, M., Characteristics associated with post-rubella deaf children; psychological, educational, and physical. *Volta Rev.,* **69**, 176–185, 1967a.

Vernon, M., Meningitis and deafness; the problem, its physical, audiological, psychological, and educational manifestations in deaf children. *Laryngoscope,* **77**, 1856–1874, 1967b.

Vernon, M., Rh factor and deafness; the problem, its psychological, physical, and educational manifestations. *Except. Child.,* **33**, 5–12, 1967c.

Vernon, M., Prematurity and deafness; the magnitude and nature of the problem among deaf children. *Except. Child.,* **34**, 289–298, 1967d.

Vernon, M., Social and psychological factors associated with hearing loss. *J. Speech Hear. Res.,* **12**, 541–563, 1969.

Vernon, M., and Koh, S. D., Early manual communication and deaf children's achievement. *Am. Ann. Deaf,* **115**, 527–536, 1970.

Waldman, J. L., Wade, F. A., and Aretz, C. W., *Hearing and the School Child.* Philadelphia: Volta Bureau, 1930.

Wampler, D., Linguistics of Visual English, 2322 Maher Drive, #35, Santa Rosa, Calif., 95405.

Welles, H. H., The measurement of certain aspects of personality among hard of hearing adults. New York: Columbia University, Teachers College Contributions to Education, No. 545, 1932.

Whetnall, E., and Fry, D. B., *The Deaf Child.* London: William Heinemann Medical Books Limited, 1964.

Winitz, H., Problem solving and the delaying of speech as strategies in the teaching of language, *Asha,* **15**, 583–586, 1973.

Yerkes, R. M., and Learned, B. W., *Chimpanzee Intelligence and its Vocal Expression,* p. 53. Baltimore: Williams & Wilkins, Co., 1925.

Young, C., and McConnell, F., Retardation of vocabulary development in hard of hearing children. *Except. Child.,* **23**, 368–370, 1957.

Zeckel, A., and Van der Kolk, J. J., A comparative intelligence test of groups of children born deaf and of good hearing by means of the Porteus Maze Test. *Am. Ann. Deaf,* **84**, 114–123, 1939.

chapter 38

CLASSROOM ACOUSTICS AND SPEECH INTELLIGIBILITY

Mark Ross, Ph.D.

The average classroom is a noisy place where 30 or more children shuffle their feet, scrape their chairs and tables on hard floors, crumple paper, drop books and scratch on their desks with pens and pencils. The footsteps, conversational babble and horseplay of exuberant youngsters echo through the corridors and into the classrooms. On the street outside the school, vehicular traffic rumbles incessantly, while noisy jets streak overhead. Into this environment we place approximately 300,000 hard of hearing children, and we expect them to hear, understand and learn. Studies concerned with the academic performance of these youngsters show that we have not succeeded. The acoustical environment in which these children are being educated may be one of the major factors responsible for their poor performance.

The acoustics of the average classroom permit normal hearing children to receive and understand the teacher's speech. Any gross interference with speech intelligibility for these children should be apparent to the teacher, who could then make every effort to rectify or adjust the situation. The negative effects of classroom acoustics for the hearing-impaired child, however, are not usually apparent to a normal hearing teacher. Under the same conditions of noise, reverberation or distortion, the relative effects upon speech intelligibility are much greater for the hearing-impaired individual than for the normal hearing person (Tillman, Carhart and Olsen, 1970). Thus, a teacher may assume that because the acoustics are adequate for the normal hearing children, they are also adequate for the hearing-impaired children in the same classroom. When it is obvious that a hearing-impaired child cannot understand the oral material presented in a classroom, his inability is either considered to be a direct consequence of the hearing loss or it is dismissed as inattentiveness. By definition, a congenital sensory-neural hearing loss precludes normal auditory functioning. For hearing-impaired children, however, their "normal" limitations in understanding speech are compounded by the poor speech signal they receive and by the erroneous expectations of

their teachers. In view of these additional factors, it is hardly surprising that they demonstrate academic and behavioral problems. Indeed, it would be remarkable if they did not.

NOISE

Noise Levels in Classrooms

A classroom should be sufficiently quiet to permit a teacher's voice to be heard with little difficulty. The goal is to achieve sound levels of 30 to 35 dB on the A scale of a sound level meter in an empty classroom which has normal activity in adjacent areas (Niemoeller, 1968). In a recent study (McCroskey and Devens, 1974), it was found that the sound levels of only 1 of the 9 elementary schools evaluated were within 5 to 10 dB of the recommended limits, with the older schools being the greatest offenders in this respect.

Other studies which have measured the noise levels in classrooms have used either the B or C scales of a sound level meter, and thus precise comparisons with the recommended minimum A scale figures are not possible. Sanders (1965) found that the average sound level ranged from 55 dB on the B scale to 58 dB-B in a number of empty classrooms which had normal activity in surrounding areas. With the children at their desks, but with the teacher silent, sound level readings of 69 dB-B in kindergarten, 59 dB-B in elementary and 62 dB-B in high school were obtained. In a similar study (Paul, 1967), an average sound level of 63 dB-C was measured in a number of elementary school classes. These findings indicate that the ambient noise in classrooms is greater than the desirable level.

Speech-to-Noise Ratios

The most important consideration for speech intelligibility is not the absolute noise level existing in classrooms, but rather the intensity ratio at the child's ear (or hearing aid microphone) between the teacher's voice and the ambient noise. When this signal-to-noise ratio is highly favorable, the child will perceive the teacher's voice as clearly as his auditory system permits. The studies which investigated signal-to-noise ratios in schools found consistently unfavorable results. Sanders (1965) found ratios that ranged from +1 dB in kindergarten classrooms to +5 dB in elementary and high school classrooms. Paul (1967) found an average signal-to-noise ratio of +3 dB in the classrooms and instructional settings he examined. Contrary to expectations, he found a poorer signal-to-noise ratio at a 4-foot instructional setting than at an 8-foot setting; this was attributed to the reduction in the intensity of the teacher's voice when she was engaged in small group instruction at the 4-foot distance as opposed to large group instruction at the 8-foot distance. These findings appear to be valid estimates of the speech-to-noise ratios in the classroom, and they reveal listening conditions particularly difficult for hearing-impaired youngsters.

Noise Reduction

The time to begin reducing noise in a classroom is when a new school is in the planning stages. Choice of a proper site, away from heavy road, rail or air traffic; control of vibrations and impact noise by the use of discontinuous constructions; selection and installation of the proper type of ventilation and heating systems; placement of the classrooms away from noise-producing activities within the school; use of compound walls, double windows, and well fitting, heavy and rigid doors; these and other considerations must be weighed by the architect whose responsibility it is to meet the noise level requirements necessary in an educational setting (Knudsen and Harris, 1950; Niemoeller, 1968; John and Thomas, 1957; Davis, 1965).

However, it is rare that one has the opportunity to consult with the architect in the planning stages of a new school. Most often, teachers and therapists are confronted with existing classrooms (with "built-in" acoustical problems) in which they have to teach. Fortunately, there are a number of simple steps which can be taken to reduce the trasmission of noise into, and the generation of noise within, a classroom. A significant amount of noise reduction can be accomplished by lining door frames with rubber or felt to ensure a tight seal in the frame. The corridors outside a classroom can be carpeted and treated with acoustical tile to reduce the noise level generated right outside the classroom. The classrooms themselves can be treated with acoustical tiles, and drapes hung on the windows. If it is not possible to carpet the floors, felt or rubber stoppers can be used to cover the legs of the movable tables and chairs. In the classrooms for the younger children in particular, the wood top desks and tables can be covered with such resilient material as hard rubber. In classrooms with noisy fans, air conditioners or open windows, it is desirable to seat the hearing-impaired child as far from the noise source as possible, with the teacher making every effort to present her oral material from the child's side of the room.

REVERBERATION
Sound Reflections in a Room

In an open field or an anechoic chamber, sound waves follow the inverse square law, decreasing 6 dB in sound pressure level (SPL) with every doubling of distance. Thus a sound which is 80 dB SPL 1 foot from a speaker's lips would be reduced to 74 dB 2 feet away and 68 dB 4 feet away. In a room, the boundaries confine the sound energy and do not permit it to escape. Therefore, the noise level in a room can be much greater than it would be in an open field. The sound waves travel spherically from the source at approximately 1100 feet per sec. As they strike a surface they are reflected back into the room, in the opposite direction but at the same angle at which they struck the surface. They then travel at the same speed until another surface is encountered which produces another reflection into the room. The original spherical wave is quickly broken up into many segments traveling in all different directions. Depending upon the dimensions and types of surfaces in a room, several hundred such reflections may occur before the sound is rendered inaudible. This prolongation of sound in a room after the source has ceased vibrating is the definition of reverberation. At any given instance in time, the sound pressure at a listener's ears is a combination of the sound issuing directly from the speaker's lips and that due to the repeated reflections of the original sound wave (plus, of course, ambient noise from sources other than the speaker).

The amount of reverberation depends upon the type of surface the sound waves strike. Perfectly rigid and smooth surfaces reflect most of the incident sound waves (the sound waves which strike the surface), thus increasing the degree of reverberation. Interior finish material such as concrete, hard plaster, glass and wood are examples of nearly perfect sound reflectors. They absorb little of the incident sound energy. On the other hand, acoustical tile, carpets, drapes, overstuffed furniture and a large number of occupants in a room considerably reduce sound reflections by absorbing much of the incident sound energy.

Sound Absorptions in a Room

Reflection and absorption of incident sound waves are reciprocally related to one another. Sound energy which is not reflected back is absorbed by the surfaces, furnishings or occupants of the room. Absorption occurs when the incident sound energy is converted into heat by vibrations and friction in the minute interspaces of the surface. The more porous the material, the more absorption which occurs.

The absorption and reflection of incident sound energy are frequency dependent; that is, different types of materials tend to absorb differing degrees of energy at various frequencies. With most carpets, for example, absorption is usually greatest at the higher frequencies. The height, weight and type of backing of a particular carpet are variables which will affect the specific absorption curve obtained. Drapes are also useful absorbers of sound energy. The absorption depends upon their extent, weight and amount of gather; it can be increased at the low frequencies by extending the distance at which the drapes are hung from the walls. This may be useful, since it is usually more difficult to arrange adequate low frequency absorption than middle and higher frequency absorption. Most acoustical tiles, for example, are not very efficient absorbers of low frequencies. Tables are available which rate the absorption characteristics of different types of acoustical materials (Knudsen and Harris, 1950; Sabine, 1957). This information can assist the clinician in approaching the goal of a relatively balanced absorption curve across frequency.

Ratings of Absorption Characteristics

The fraction of sound energy that is absorbed when a sound wave encounters a surface is called the sound absorption coefficient. If a sound surface absorbs only 5% of the incident sound wave, as would be the case with a plaster wall, the sound absorption coefficient is 0.05. If the surface is composed of acoustical tile, 60 or 70% of the incident sound waves may be absorbed, producing a sound absorption coefficient of 0.60 or 0.70. The sound absorption coefficient depends not only on the nature of the material, but also upon the frequency and angle of the incident sound wave. Usually, the coefficient is an average of all angles of incidence, and it is termed the random incidence coefficient as distinguished from the normal incidence coefficient. For convenience, random incidence coefficients are frequency averaged at 250, 500, 1000 and 2000 Hz and this average is called the noise reduction coefficient (NRC) (Sabine, 1957).

The amount of absorption necessary to produce desirable acoustic qualities in a room has been worked out in nomogram form by Knudsen and Harris (1950, pp. 162 and 163). It depends upon the size of the room and the reduction in reverberation required; the less the reverberation desired, the more acoustical treatment necessary. In the average classroom, it is not necessary or desirable to completely cover all room surfaces with acoustical material.

Distribution of Sound in a Room

Reflections due to a continuing sound source, such as speech, will spread rapidly throughout a room and, except in the immediate vicinity of the speaker, will result in an approximately equal distribution of energy in the room. The intensity level of this sound energy is a function of the amount of absorption. The more the absorption in a room, the less the sound pressure level of the uniform sound field. An example of this relationship is given in Figure 38.1. Rooms A, B and C represent three rooms that differ only in the degree of sound treatment. There is little treatment in room A, more in room B and still more in room C. The distance versus intensity relationship of the direct sound path has been included for comparison to demonstrate what the relationship would have been had the inverse square law been applicable. Note that, at 1 foot from the speaker's lips, the direct sound predominates in all three rooms. In room A, however, the reverberant sound already exceeds the direct sound at the 2-foot distance, with a stabilization of the sound energy becoming apparent at the 4-foot distance. In room B, the reverberant sound does not predominate until the 4-foot distance, with the stabilization of sound level occurring at the 8-foot distance. In room C, the reverberant sound does not exceed the direct energy until the 8-foot distance, with the stabilization occurring at about 16 feet. In all three curves, the difference between them and the direct sound path is an indication of the increase in sound pressure due to the reflection characteristics in the rooms.

The uniform distribution of sound energy in rooms with different absorption characteristics is based upon the assumption of a diffuse sound field. In a perfectly diffuse field, the sound pressure would be equal everywhere in the room, with an equal probability at any point in the room that the sound waves are traveling in every direction. This condition does not completely hold in the average classroom, nor would we want it to. In a classroom, the intensity of the direct sound is greater in the vicinity of the speaker than the intensity of the diffuse

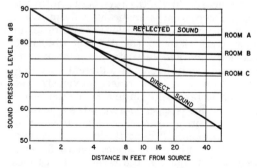

Fig. 38.1. The relationship between differing amounts of sound absorption in three otherwise similar rooms and the sound pressure level (SPL) of the same sound source as a function of distance.

field. In addition, the wave fronts of the direct sound travel in a predictably spherical fashion; they do not become randomly distributed until after a large number of reflections have taken place. Indeed, to anticipate a later discussion, it is these two factors, the intensity of the direct versus the reflected sounds and their relative times of arrival, which are the most important determiners of speech intelligibility in a room. A certain amount of diffusion in a room is very desirable, however. Otherwise, the sound energy would be concentrated in one area or surface of a room with much less energy at other locations in the room.

Examples of the kinds of rooms which do not have relatively diffuse sound fields are those with one dimension very different from the other (such as a long, narrow room), those which have domed ceilings or concave or convex surfaces, those which are odd shaped (elliptical, circular or "L" shaped), and those which have all the absorptive treatment concentrated on one surface. A classroom 25 feet wide by 30 feet long and 12 feet high, increases the likelihood of a diffuse field in the room. The same proportions would apply to smaller or larger rooms (Knudsen and Harris, 1950). It is possible to increase the diffusion of a room by such devices as scattering the sound treatment around the room, by increasing the amount of absorption and by overcoming large irregularities in the room shape by the use of false walls and dropped ceilings (with the advice of an architectual acoustician).

Reverberation Time

Reverberation time is considered to be the single most important factor determining the acoustical qualities of a room (Lochner and Burger, 1964). It is defined as the time required for a specified sound to decrease 60 dB in SPL after the source has been stopped. Thus, if it takes 1 sec for a 100 dB noise burst in a room to decrease to 40 dB, the reverberation time is 1 sec. The concept is applicable only in rooms in which the sound distribution is diffuse. In other types of rooms the decay of the sound may show marked fluctuation in intensity and rate and be different at different locations within the room. As noted previously, the amount of reverberation and hence the reverberation time is dependent upon the amount of absorption in a room. Generally, the higher the absorption coefficient, the less the reverberation time. Since the absorption coefficients vary with frequency, the reverberation times are also frequency dependent. It is necessary, therefore, to know the applicable frequency or range of frequencies when reverberation time is considered. Citing reverberation time at a single frequency to describe the reverberation

qualities of a room can be deceptive. It is possible to have a desirable reverberation time at 2000 Hz, for example, and an extremely lengthy and undesirable reverberation time at other frequencies.

The optimum reverberation time for any room is that time which results in the highest speech intelligibility scores. Smaller rooms, require shorter reverberation time to maintain equal intelligibility. This is understandable since in a small room there will be many more reflections of any given sound wave, and thus an increased masking effect, than in a larger room with the same reverberation time. For normal hearing listeners the optimum time in a classroom 32 feet long by 27 feet wide by 12 feet high is approximately 0.75 sec at 500 Hz and higher frequencies, and slightly longer at lower frequencies (Knudsen and Harris, 1950, pp. 194 and 195). We shall see that this "optimum" reverberation time for normal hearing individuals is too large for the hearing-impaired and may actually be too large for even the person with normal hearing (Moul, 1974).

Localization, Integration and Masking in Reverberant Rooms

In an ordinary classroom, the sound waves which reach a listener's ears are reflected from the different surfaces of the room and from many directions. Yet the normal hearing person is able to correctly pinpoint the source. To him it seems as if all the sounds were emanating directly from the speaker. The perceived sound source is fixed by the time and intensity differences at the listener's two ears of the first direct pulses of the speech sounds before reflection takes place. This is known as the Haas or Precedence Effect (Gardner, 1968).

The reflections of a specific direct sound which arrive at the ears of a listener within about 50 msec are masked by the direct sound. Although a listener may not be aware of these reflections, their energy is integrated with the direct sound to increase the loudness and the intelligibility of speech (Lochner and Burger, 1964). However, in the average size classroom with a reverberation time of about a second, there will be relatively few such reflections which arrive at the listener's ears within the 50-msec period compared to the number of reflections which arrive after this period.

The reflections which arrive after the integration period are responsible for most of the difficulty in understanding speech in a reverberant situation. The persistence of energy from previously uttered sounds overlaps and masks speech sounds. In a two- or three-syllable word, the last syllable may be perceived simultaneously with strong reflections from the first and second syllable of the same word.

This overlapping will affect consonants and their transitions more than vowels for two reasons. First, the consonants are generally weaker and shorter than vowels, and thus more susceptible to strong reflections; and second, they are usually of higher frequency, and thus more easily absorbed by the average room surface. Tests of the intelligibility of speech in reverberant conditions have shown that listeners do indeed make many more errors on consonant than vowel discriminations (John, 1957). The place features of consonants, which depend greatly upon high frequency cues for correct perception, are more adversely affected than either the manner or voicing features of consonants, (Nabelek and Pickett, 1974a, 1974b).

The point of view has been expressed that it is the amplitude and time of arrival of these reflected sound patterns rather than reverberation time per se which determine intelligibility under reverberant conditions (Lochner and Burger, 1964). The reverberation time and room volume "set the stage" while the sound reflections do the acting. These reflections of an ongoing speech signal are a particularly deceptive masking source. They are timelocked in an overlapping manner to the speech and they occur only when speech is being emitted. A room may appear to have good acoustic qualities because of a low ambient noise level, but this factor cannot predict the masking effect of reflected speech sounds.

EFFECTS UPON INTELLIGIBILITY

Normal Versus Hearing-impaired Listeners

The acoustical acceptability of a classroom is evaluated in terms of the normal hearing pupils in it, and not in reference to the hearing-impaired children in the same classroom. A classroom with an ambient noise level of 60 dB SPL, with an average reverberation time of 0.9 sec, and with the students seated approximately 8 feet from the teacher, will permit normal hearing children to receive an acceptable (although not optimal) speech signal. These same conditions will produce an unacceptable signal for the hearing-impaired children in the same classroom.

The normal hearing listener has two good ears, one of which is always favorably oriented toward a sound source (the monaural direct condition). The precedence effect permits him to focus on the direct sound and suppress the reverberant sound, with binaural hearing per se adding auditory information not supplied even in the best monaural listening condition (Olsen and Carhart, 1967; Moncur and Dirks, 1967). The hearing-impaired individual, on the other hand, usually has a basic speech intelligibility problem to which is added the distor-

tions produced by the average hearing aid. If this person wears a monaural hearing aid (or if he has a unilateral hearing loss and does not wear a hearing aid), he is deprived of the substantial advantages of binaural hearing. His situation should be improved if he wears a binaural hearing aid, although he is still faced with the communication problems inherent in a pathological auditory system and the negative effects of an imperfect amplifying system.

The point that must be emphasized again is that the same acoustical environment will have different effects upon speech intelligibility for normal and for hearing-impaired children. What is an acceptable situation for one group will not necessarily be acceptable for the other group.

Reverberation Time and Intelligibility

Using normal hearing subjects, Moncur and Dirks (1967) compared intelligibility scores obtained monaurally and binaurally in four different reverberation times, with and without a simultaneous competing signal. The competing signal consisted of newspaper articles read by a male and female speaker. The phonetically balanced (PB) words and competing message (at a 0 signal-to-noise ratio) were delivered to microphones mounted on the ears of a dummy head from loudspeakers placed 6 feet from the center of the head. The competing message speaker was located at a 0° azimuth, while the primary speaker was located at a 45° angle from the midline of the dummy head. Half the recordings were made with the primary speaker to the right of the midline and half to the left of the midline. Their results indicated considerable decrements in intelligibility scores as the reverberation time was increased from 0.0 to 0.9 to 1.6 to 2.3 sec, with greater decrements in the monaural than in the binaural condition. The drop in intelligibility scores was much greater in the monaural condition when the speech emanated from the far side of the head, and even more so in the presence of competing signals. The authors selected the 0.9-sec reverberation time as representing for normal hearing listeners "a time typical of optimal liveness for speech." It is instructive to see what intelligibility effects were produced for normal hearing listeners with this "optimal" reverberation time. Under quiet conditions, the average binaural score was 79.7%, the average monaural near ear score was 72.6%, and the average monaural far ear score was 54.9%. Under competing message conditions, these same scores were, respectively, 41.2, 28.7 and 3.8 %.

The binaural scores, with and without competing noise, are an indication of the intelligibility scores which would result for normal hearing pupils in a classroom with an "optimal" reverberation time. They are approximately 20% poorer than the scores which would be obtained with no reverberation present. The monaural near and far ear scores suggest the kind of results which would occur with a unilateral hearing loss pupil not using a hearing aid. Under the best condition in quiet, such a pupil would obtain a 72.6% score; under the poorest condition in noise, he would receive a 3.8% score. The scores would be even poorer for the hearing-impaired pupil listening to the speech signal as it is processed through a monaural hearing aid. These results imply that a smaller reverberation time than 0.9 sec is necessary for hearing-impaired students.

John (1960) suggests that reverberation times for classrooms in which hearing-impaired pupils are placed should not exceed 0.5 sec. He recorded speech at reverberation times of 0.3, 0.5 and 0.7 sec, and obtained subjective preferences and objective word discrimination scores from a group of hearing-impaired adults. They overwhelmingly preferred the 0.5- to the 0.7-sec time, and expressed little preference between the 0.3- and 0.5-sec conditions. In a discrimination test, their scores fell from 70% at the 0.5-sec time to 52% at the 0.7-sec condition.

Moul's (1974) results with 12 normal hearing children supported the work of John (1960). The children whom Moul tested had superior intelligibility scores in the room with 0.35-sec reverberation time but considerably poorer results at 0.80 sec. Niemoeller's (1968) suggestions for a 0.4-sec reverberation time for small classrooms and a 0.6-sec time for larger classrooms are in accord with these experimental results.

In two companion studies, Nabelek and Pickett (1974a, 1974b) evaluated the effects of reverberation and noise on monaural and binaural intelligibility for both normal hearing and hearing-impaired listeners. Using the relatively short reverberation times of 0.3 and 0.6 sec, they found (a) decreased intelligibility scores with increased reverberation time, (b) sensory-neural hearing-impaired listeners were more sensitive to the effects of increased reverberation than normal hearing subjects, (c) hearing-impaired listeners are also more sensitive than normal hearing subjects to noise effects in reverberant rooms, with a signal-to-noise ratio of +10 dB as the lowest which permits hearing-impaired listeners to function auditorily under such conditions, and (d) binaural intelligibility scores were higher than monaural scores under all conditions for both the normal hearing and the hearing-impaired listeners.

Crum and Tillman (1973) investigated the effects on the intelligibility scores of 12 normal hearing subjects of different reverberation times (0, 0.4, 0.8 and 1.2 sec), signal-to-noise ratios (+6 and 0 dB), and distances (6, 12 and 24 feet). Under quiet conditions, they found that a significant reduction in intelligibility scores occurred only at the longest reverberation time and the greatest distances. In contrast, they found that the introduction of noise in a reverberant situation drastically decreased the intelligibility scores, with significant reductions occurring as a function of both distance and reverberation time. Except for the anechoic condition, their subjects achieved their highest intelligibility scores with a reverberation time of 0.4 sec at the 6-foot distance.

Using the same basic design, Finitzo-Hieber (1975) extended the above study to include 12 hearing-impaired children. She found poorer performance by the hearing-impaired group under every condition of noise and reverberation, with their scores dropping even further as the speech signal was processed through a hearing aid rather than high fidelity speakers. The combined effects of noise and reverberation produced larger decrements in performance than either factor did singly. As would be expected, the highest speech intelligibility scores were obtained under quiet conditions with no reverberation. The scores decreased both as a function of decreasing signal-to-noise ratio and increasing reverberation time, relatively more so for the hearing-impaired than the normal hearing group.

The actual reverberation times in classrooms do not conform to levels which would provide for the best intelligibility based on the experimental results reviewed above. As measured in a number of classrooms, the reverberation time in one study averaged 1.2 sec (Tolk, 1961), and in another study, it ranged from 1.3 to 3.4 sec (Thomas, 1960). Considering the effects that even smaller reverberation times have upon the intelligibility of speech, we can safely assume even greater decrements at these larger times. The situation does seem to be improving, however. McCroskey and Devens (1974) found that the reverberation times in classrooms of school buildings constructed 40 or more years ago usually exceeded 1.0 sec, while those constructed more recently demonstrated average reverberation times of about 0.65 sec.

Microphone-Ear Distance and Intelligibility

Perhaps the best technique for improving the hearing-impaired student's intelligibility score is to reduce the distance between the speaker and the listener (or between the speaker and the microphone of a hearing aid or auditory trainer). The closer the listener is to the speaker, the more favorable the relationship between the direct and the reverberant sounds. Conversely, the further the distance, the poorer the signal-to-noise ratio. The most important determiner of speech intelligibility in classrooms is just this intensity relationship between the teacher's speech and the noise (which is a combination of both the time-muddled reverberant sounds and the ambient noise). The distance in which the direct sounds retain a favorable relationship to the reflected and ambient sounds is greater in rooms with shorter reverberation times; the poorer the room, the closer the listener has to be to the speaker in order to achieve a favorable relationship (see Fig. 38.1).

Table 38.1 summarizes the research on the effects upon speech intelligibility of increased distance between the speaker and the listener. One observation is quite clear despite the use of different types of subjects, intelligibility tests and rooms of different dimensions and reverberation characteristics: the greater the distance, the poorer the intelligibility. The relative drop in intelligibility was much greater for hearing-impaired subjects than for normal hearing subjects, when both groups were tested under the same conditions (Watson, 1964). When a group of hearing-impaired children were tested at different distances in sound-treated and untreated rooms, the children achieved lower intelligibility scores in the untreated rooms (Dale, 1968; Fisher, 1964). When the intelligibility scores of the same group of children were compared monaurally and binaurally (two body worn aids side by side on the chest), the scores were superior in the binaural condition (Fisher, 1964). It is interesting to note that the binaural advantage at the maximum distance (15 feet) is present only in the sound-treated and not in the untreated room.

CLINICAL IMPLICATIONS

Clinical services currently stressed for hearing-impaired children include speech and language therapy, speech reading, auditory training and academic tutoring. Without minimizing the need for any of these services, the first objective should be to ensure a favorable signal-to-noise ratio at the children's ears. This will permit them to function auditorily up to the limits imposed by their impaired auditory systems. Once this is accomplished, our therapies can then be aimed at the children's real deficiencies and not just those which reflect intelligibility problems secondary to poor classroom acoustics.

There are a number of ways to improve the signal-to-noise relationship, and thus speech intelligibility, in a classroom. The application of a minimum amount of sound treatment can shorten the reverberation time of a room and lower its ambient noise level. If this is not possible because of penurious or ignorant school officials, then the signal-to-noise ratio can be improved by reducing the distance between the teacher and the child (or microphone). It will be recalled from Figure 38.1 that the closer one is to a sound source, the more the intensity of the direct sound predominates over the reverberant sound. The better the sound treatment, the further one can be from the source and still obtain a favorable signal-to-noise relationship. No matter what the sound treatment is, there should always be some point at which the intensity of the direct sound predominates over the indirect sound. In many classrooms, it is pedagogically possible for a teacher to place herself 3 to 6 feet from a hearing-impaired child while giving instruction to the entire class. This should help to some degree, and any help for these children cannot be minimized.

The best possible signal-to-noise ratio can be obtained with the teacher's lips within 6 to 8 inches of a child's ear or hearing aid. In essence, this is what occurs when a wireless FM microphone-transmitter with its associated receiver unit is used. The teacher wears the microphone-transmitter around her neck, and the child wears the FM receiver around his neck. The reduced microphone-teacher distance results in a favorable signal-to-noise ratio for the hearing-impaired child, while permitting the usual instruction for the normal hearing children in the same classroom. An environmental microphone on the receiver unit enables the child to monitor his own voice and to receive direct communication from the other children. In a recent study (Ross, Giolas and Carver, 1973), intelligibility scores were 36% higher with the wireless microphone over the standard method. This improvement was noted for most hearing-impaired children whether or not they normally used hearing aids.

Speech intelligibility in a classroom can be improved with the use of a binaural as opposed to a monaural hearing aid (assuming the child is a binaural hearing aid candidate). The article by Fisher (1964) is the only one which has directly tested this statement in a classroom environment, but there is a developing accumulation of literature which supports binaural versus monaural amplification for both children and adults (see Nabelek and Pickett, 1974a, 1974b, for an extensive list of references regarding adults; and Ross et al., 1974, for references pertaining to children).

Finally, our focus on audition should not blind us to the contribution that vision makes when combined with audition. Bisensory intelligibility scores are typically better than single modality scores (Sanders, 1970). In Fisher's (1964) study, for example, the binaural intelligibility scores of his subjects at the 9-foot dis-

TABLE 38.1. *Relationship between Speech Intelligibility and Distance from Speech Source*
Shilling entries indicate that testing was accomplished under two conditions, with the scores for the poor condition(s) on the left and those for the good condition(s) on the right.

Investigator	Distance from Source									Subjects
	3 inches	6 inches	12 inches	18 inches	3 to 4 feet	5 feet	9 to 12 feet	14 to 15 feet	22 feet	
John and Thomas (1957)	96	94		77	70		65		39.2/64	Normal hearing university students
Dale (1968)			/84		54.4/70.8			44.8/		12 partially deaf children
Watson (1964)					84.8		35.2			19 partially hearing children
Watson (1964)					98.6		53.3			Normal hearing adults
Watson (1964)					91.8		28.3			Partially hearing adults
Fisher (1964)		/87.3			/68		54.7/57.3	42.7/50.7		9 partially hearing children (monaural)
Fisher (1964)		/98			/82		64.6/80.7	44/58.7		9 partially hearing children (binaural)
Miller and Niemoeller (1967)		25/34				4/20				One elderly Ménière's patient
Ross and Giolas (1971)		59					32			13 hard of hearing children
Ross, Giolas and Carver (1973)		58					22			11 hard of hearing children

tance improved from 64% to 93% when students were permitted to both see and hear the speaker. It should be recalled that maximum communication efficiency is attained when vision is utilized as a supplemental channel, to add information not available under optimal auditory conditions, and not as a substitute channel, because negative classroom acoustics prevent the maximum utilization of auditory cues.

DISCUSSION

Clinical audiologists have been accused of being overly enthusiastic about the benefits of amplification with hearing-impaired children. It is suggested that we view hearing aids and auditory trainers as a panacea with little attention paid to the developmental and educational problems these children present. The poor results attained after more than 20 years of widespread use of amplification certainly lend credence to this accusation. The average hearing-impaired child is still sorely deficient in his speech, language and educational achievements. The responsibility for much of the failure is not inherent in the concept of amplification. Rather, it is a consequence of the unskilled application of the concept. We do not know how far we can go with the use of amplified sound because, generally speaking, we have not used it appropriately. Optimum training and use of residual hearing require the best possible signal consistent with the hearing loss. The evidence clearly indicates that this is a rare rather than a frequent occurrence. When systematic checks of hearing aids are made (Gaeth and Lounsbury, 1966; Zink, 1972; Northern et al., 1972; Porter, 1973), it is the exception rather than the rule to find a child's hearing aid working properly. Similar findings are obtained when classroom auditory trainers are examined (Matkin and Olsen, 1970a, 1970b, 1973). Finally, even if we assume that the amplifying systems are working properly, the acoustical environment in a classroom often precludes the best possible auditory signal. Unless we ensure that hearing-impaired children receive an excellent signal, the advantages of amplification will tend to be more of theoretical than practical significance.

One not unusual example of the practical misuse of amplification was a preschool program located in a basement with plaster walls, ceiling and floor. About 20 hearing-impaired children, most of whom wore hearing aids, were noisily and happily engaged in free play. The teacher was only a few feet away from me and I could not understand a word she was saying through my own hearing aid. The children were taken into a separate room for individual tutoring. Each child's hearing aid was removed and he was fitted with the receiver unit of an FM loop system. During the entire tutoring period for each of the children, the teacher did not use her microphone. In addition, when the child's receiver unit was checked, it was found that its microphone was inoperable.

Similar observations were made on other occasions in other programs. Rooms were poorly sound-treated; teachers often adjusted the preamplifier of the auditory training system too high or too low; there would be several open microphones scattered throughout a room hooked to the single loop system; or a single centrally placed microphone was placed too far from everybody for anybody to hear clearly. In one program, the supervisor noted that it was against the policy of the school for the children to hear themselves, that it would just "confuse" them. These observations are not new or original with me (Hirsh, 1968; Ling, 1966; Ross, 1969; Calvert, Reddell, Donaldson and Pew, 1965). What is disturbing is the snail's pace at which these problems are being recognized and rectified. Whole generations of children are being maleducated while presently available information slowly filters down to the classroom. The recognition and correction of the negative effects of classroom acoustics is an example of one such area.

REFERENCES

Calvert, D. R., Reddell, R. C., Donaldson, R. J. and Pew, L. G., A comparison of auditory amplifiers for the deaf. *Except. Child.*, 31, 247–253, 1965.

Crum, M. A., and Tillman, T. W., Effects of speaker-to-listener distance upon speech intelligibility in reverberation and noise. Paper presented at ASHA Convention, Detroit, 1973.

Dale, D. M. C., *Applied Audiology for Children*, Ed. 2. Springfield, Ill.: Charles C Thomas, 1968.

Davis, D., *Acoustical Tests and Measurements*. New York: Bobbs-Merrill Co., 1965.

Finitzo-Hieber, T., The influence of reverberation and noise on the speech intelligibility of normal and hard of hearing children in classroom size listening environments. Dissertation, Northwestern University, Evanston, Ill., 1975.

Fisher, B., An investigation of binaural hearing aids. *J. Laryngol.*, 78, 658–668, 1964.

Gaeth, J. H., and Lounsbury, E., Hearing aids and children in elementary schools. *J. Speech Hear. Disord.*, 31, 283–289, 1966.

Gardner, M. B., Historical background of the Haas and/or precedence effect. *J. Acoust. Soc. Am.*, 43, 1243–1248, 1968.

Hirsh, I. J., Use of amplification in educating deaf children. *Am. Ann. Deaf*, 113, 1046–1055, 1968.

John, J. E. J., Acoustics and efficiency in the use of hearing aids. In Ewing, A. W. G. (Ed.), *Educational Guidance and the Deaf Child*. Manchester: Manchester University Press, 1957.

John, J. E. J., The efficiency of hearing aids as a function of architectural acoustics. In Ewing, A. W. G. (Ed.), *The Modern Educational Treatment of Deafness*. Manchester: Manchester University Press, 1960.

John, J. E. J., and Thomas, H., Design and construction of schools for the deaf. In Ewing, A. W. G. (Ed.), *Educational Guidance and the Deaf Child*. Manchester: Manchester University Press, 1957.

Knudsen, V. C., and Harris, C. M., *Acoustical Designing of Architecture*. New York: John Wiley & Sons, 1950.

Ling, D., Loop induction for auditory training of deaf children. *Maico Audiol. Library Ser.*, 5, Report 2, 1966.

Lochner, J. P. A., and Burger, J. F., The influence of reflections on auditorium acoustics. *J. Sound Vib.*, 1, 426–454, 1964.

Matkin, N. D., and Olsen, W. O., Response of hearing aids with induction loop amplification systems. *Am. Ann. Deaf*, 115, 73–78, 1970a.

Matkin, N. D., and Olsen, W. O., Induction loop amplification systems; classroom performance. *Asha*, 12, 239–244, 1970b.

Matkin, N. D., and Olsen, W. O., An investigation of radio frequency auditory training units. *Am. Ann. Deaf*, 118, 25–30, 1973.

McCroskey, R. L., and Devens, J. S., Acoustic characteristics of public school classrooms constructed between 1890 and 1960. Paper presented at ASHA Convention, Las Vegas, 1974.

Miller, J. D., and Niemoeller, A. F., Hearing aid design and evaluation for a patient with a severe discrimination loss for speech. *J. Speech Hear. Res.*, 10, 367–372, 1967.

Moncur, J. P., and Dirks, D., Binaural and monaural speech intelligibility in reverberation. *J. Speech Hear. Res.*, 10, 186–195, 1967.

Moul, M. J., Effects of classroom reverberation levels on hearing-aid transduced speech. Paper presented at ASHA Convention, Las Vegas, 1974.

Nabelek, A. K., and Pickett, J. M., Reception of consonants in a classroom as affected by monaural and binaural listening, noise reverberation and hearing aids. *J. Acoust. Soc. Am.*, 56, 628–639, 1974a.

Nabelek, A. K., and Pickett, J. M., Monaural and binaural speech perception through hearing aids under noise and reverberation with normal and hearing-impaired listeners. *J. Speech Hear. Res.*, 17, 724–739, 1974b.

Niemoeller, A. F., Acoustical design of classrooms for the deaf. *Am. Ann. Deaf*, 113, 1040–1045, 1968.

Northern, J. L., McChord, W., Fischer, E., and Evans, P., Hearing services in residential schools for the deaf. *Maico Aud. Library Ser.*, 11, Report 4, 1972.

Olsen, W. O., and Carhart, R., Development of test procedures for evaluation of binaural hearing aids. *Bull. Proc. Res.*, 10, 22–49, 1967.

Paul, R. L., An investigation of the effectiveness of hearing aid amplification in regular and special classrooms under instructional conditions. Unpublished doctoral dissertation, Wayne State University, 1967.

Porter, T. A., Hearing aids in a residential school.

Am. Ann. Deaf, 118, 31–33, 1973.

Ross, M., Loop auditory training systems for preschool hearing-impaired children. *Volta Rev.,* 71, 289–295, 1969.

Ross, M., and Giolas, T. G., The effect of three classroom listening conditions on speech intelligibility. *Am. Ann. Deaf,* 116, 580–584, 1971.

Ross, M., Giolas, T. G., and Carver, P. W., Effect of classroom listening conditions on speech intelligibility. *Lang. Speech Hear. Serv. Schools,* 4, 72–76, 1973.

Ross, M., Hunt, M. F., Kessler, M., and Heniges, M., The use of a rating scale to compare binaural and monaural amplification with hearing impaired children. *Volta Rev.,* 76, 93–99, 1974.

Sabine, H. J., Acoustical materials. In Harris, C. M. (Ed.), *Handbook of Noise Control.* New York: McGraw-Hill Book Co., 1957.

Sanders, D., Noise conditions in normal school classrooms. *Except. Child.,* 31, 344–353, 1965.

Sanders, D., *Aural Rehabilitation: Within a Communication Framework.* Englewood Cliffs: Prentice-Hall, Inc., 1970.

Thomas, H., Architectual acoustics as a fundamental factor in the design of schools for the deaf. In Ewing, A. W. G. (Ed.), *The Modern Educational Treatment of Deafness.* Manchester: Manchester University Press, 1960.

Tillman, T. W., Carhart, R., and Olsen, W. O., Hearing aid efficiency in a competing speech situation. *J. Speech Hear. Res.,* 13, 789–811, 1970.

Tolk, J., Acoustics, intelligibility of speech and electro-acoustic systems in classrooms. In *Proceedings of the 2nd International Course in Paedo-Audiology,* pp. 103–109. The Netherlands: Groningen University, 1961.

Watson, T. J., The use of hearing aids by hearing-impaired children in ordinary schools. *Volta Rev.,* 66, 741–744, 787, 1964.

Zink, G. D., Hearing aids children wear; a longitudinal study of performance. *Volta Rev.,* 74, 41–51, 1972.

Hearing Aids

chapter 39

A HISTORICAL AND TECHNICAL REVIEW

William F. Carver, Ph.D.

One could say (and it has been said) that the first hearing aid was used when man cupped his hand behind his ear to enhance the sound gathering function of his auricle. Throughout history* a variety of devices have been used to make sounds louder, most taking the form of the well known ear trumpet. Ear trumpets took the general form of a tapered horn, a large opening at one end and a small one at the other, effectively concentrating the energy at the large end into a smaller area. Additional increases in energy were obtained through resonance in a part of the frequency range. However, since there was no power supply, resonance was achieved at the expense of a reduction in energy at some other part of the frequency spectrum. Some of the unusual shapes of ear trumpets were a hearing vase, one which was built into a hat and one in a cane. Another model had a long (about 4 feet) flexible tube which enabled one-to-one conversation at a comfortable distance. There were also acoustic fans which were held in the teeth for bone conduction. The large variety of shapes, many designed to hide the trumpet, show that, even before electronic hearing aids, the hard of hearing attempted to conceal their handicap.

The development of the electrical hearing aid probably began with Alexander Graham Bell's attempt which, as everybody knows, resulted in the telephone. Early electrical hearing aids were cumbersome boxes which were hardly portable. Instead, they were placed in the most advantageous place and left there.

Then in the early 1930s the first wearable electronic hearing aids were introduced. These early hearing aids did not require a separate

---

* For a more complete early history, the reader is referred to Berger (1970), Davis (1947) and Watson and Tolan (1949).

battery pack and thus were the "first" one piece body worn electrical hearing aids. These aids used a carbon granule "transmitter." Small granules of carbon have the property of changing resistance to current flow in proportion to the pressure exerted on them. This is the principle which was utilized in the first wearable hearing aid. Figure 39.1 is a diagram of a microphone using this principle. A diaphragm, responding to the alternating pressures of sound waves, exerted corresponding pressure on the small balls of carbon. An electrical current from a battery was connected to the diaphragm and the base of the microphone. The current traveled through the carbon in varying amounts relative to the sounds at the diaphragm. These changing currents were fed to a magnetic receiver (earphone) where the electrical signal was transduced into sound waves.

With one microphone, very little amplification was obtained. However, additional amplification could be obtained by the use of two microphones. With two, approximately 20 dB gain was obtained. Then carbon amplification was added. In a sense, carbon amplification was accomplished through a receiver-microphone combination (Fig. 39.2). The addition of carbon amplification required a separate pack to hold the carbon amplifier and batteries, but as much as 30 to 35 dB peak gain was realized.

Carbon aids were, however, extremely noisy with very sharp resonant peaks and antiresonant valleys and they had the annoying property of "going off the air" when the user bent over or, when worn in one's pants pocket, sat down, separating the carbon granules from contact with the diaphragm. These aids were notoriously poor, having a great amount of distortion, but nevertheless many people with conductive losses wore them successfully.

The first wearable vacuum tube aids, introduced in the mid 1930s, were made possible when radio tube manufacturers were able to reduce the size of the tubes significantly, making it possible to build an amplifier into a comparatively small package. However, the size of the power supply had to be increased because two batteries had to be used. An "A"

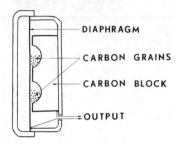

Fig. 39.1. Diagram of a carbon microphone.

battery with low voltage and high amperage was needed to heat the filaments of the tubes and a "B" battery with high voltage and low amperage to drive the plate of the tube for amplification. The power supply had to be placed in a separate package, usually worn by men in their hip pockets or on their torso and by women, strapped to their leg or torso. These hearing aid wearers were literally wired for sound! Nevertheless most hearing aid users were willing to go to vacuum tube amplification, since the aids were much less noisy, had a better frequency response and less distortion.

The next major improvement in wearable hearing aids was the introduction of the piezoelectric microphone using a rochelle salt crystal. These microphones had a flat frequency response from an extremely low frequency to a resonant peak somewhere in the higher frequencies. To avoid amplifying the resonant peak of the microphone, hearing aid manufacturers chose receivers whose sensitivity dropped out at a frequency below the high frequency peak of the microphone.

Another breakthrough in hearing aid manufacturing came with the introduction of the mercury battery in the early 1940s. These were comparatively small but long lasting. Because the manufacturers were still confined to tubes (which had been further reduced in size), they still needed a "B" battery.

The reduction of battery size allowed manufacturers to return to one piece hearing aids. The hearing aids of the 1940s were quite good. They had wide, essentially flat frequency responses with comparatively little distortion, but they were still being worn on the body.

In one attempt to make hearing aids less conspicuous, ear molds were made with long polyethylene tubes allowing the receivers to be hidden in a woman's hair or under the wearer's shirt. The long tube had the effect of reducing the gain considerably, especially in the higher frequencies.

While transistors had been in use for some time, it was not until 1952 that they were marketed in hearing aids. The early transistors were of the point contact type and were not too

suitable for hearing aids partly because they were fragile. Thus, manufacturers had to wait for the introduction of the junction transistor before it was possible to further reduce the size of hearing aids. These transistors were considerably smaller than radio tubes (which were then quite small; smaller than the little finger). But most important, it was no longer necessary to have a battery to heat a filament. Also, transistors do not need the comparatively high voltage of the "B" battery but will amplify with the 1.35 volts produced by the mercury batteries.

While rochelle salt microphones were excellent in terms of frequency response, they also had problems. In excessive heat or humidity, or in a climate that was too dry, they would not function. The introduction of the very small but efficient balanced armature magnetic microphone solved this problem, however, bandwidth was reduced.

All of these innovations made it possible to design a hearing aid which would fit into the temple frame of an eyeglass. The first eyeglass aid had the microphone on one side of the head and the amplifier and receiver on the other side. Soon thereafter, however, a hearing aid was produced which had the entire aid on one side. Compared to today's head worn hearing aid, it was bulky, but it worked and it made possible true, on the head, binaural aids.

The trend since introduction of the eyeglass aid, and shortly thereafter, behind the ear aids, has been toward miniaturization. Transistors have been reduced considerably in size. This plus other innovations such as the hybrid amplifier, the integrated circuit, smaller and smaller batteries, volume controls, transducers and very small tantalum capacitors has resulted in hearing aids which are small enough to fit in the concha and entrance of the ear canal.

Recently, significant advances in microphone design have improved performance markedly. First, the ceramic microphone was introduced, again employing the piezoelectric effect as did the rochelle salt crystal microphone. The improvements were extended band width (compared with the magnetic microphone) while eliminating the problem with moisture. Ce-

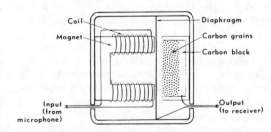

Fig. 39.2. Diagram of a carbon amplifier.

ramic microphones, however, were sensitive to shock. Soon the electret microphone (a type of condenser microphone with a permanent charge on the plates) entered the market. This microphone has the advantages of a broad flat frequency response, good shock resistance and excellent resistance to humidity.

It is difficult to predict the future for hearing aids. At the present state of the art, miniaturization has about reached its ultimate. One hearing aid manufacturer mentioned that when designing a hearing aid they plan for the two transducers (microphone and receiver), the volume control and the battery compartment. Then, because the amplifier is so small, they merely look for any small leftover space in which they can insert it.

TECHNICAL NOTES

The configurations of hearing aids have taken many shapes, but all electronic aids are basically the same. Hearing aids are simple amplifiers, a sort of "private" public address system. Each hearing aid has a microphone (transducer), an amplifier, a battery to drive the amplifier, usually a volume or gain control (variable resistor) to adjust the level of amplification and another transducer which is called a receiver.

Presently there are two general classes of hearing aids which are commercially available. One is worn on the body, usually on the chest, with an external receiver. The other is worn on the head with an internal (in the case) receiver. The head worn hearing aids are either in the temple and/or paddle of eyeglass frames, or hang behind the ear or fit in the ear canal and concha of the pinna.

Electronics

At the present time microphones are magnetic or electret. In the magnetic microphone an armature moves in a magnetic field which develops or induces a small electrical current. To varying degrees this current matches electrically the acoustic properties of the sound impinging on the diaphragm of the microphone.

The electret microphone is a miniature condenser type microphone. In condenser microphones, there are two plates separated by a dielectric (air in condenser microphones, clay in electrets). These plates have opposite electrical charges on them, and as the distance between the plates varies when sound impinges on the top plate, the flow of current varies. The minute changes in current flow are then amplified by the amplifier. With most condenser microphones, the charge on the plates must be applied continuously from an outside source. The electret, however, has a permanent charge which is applied when it is manufactured. The amplifier, using power from the battery, builds up or increases the electrical signal produced by the microphone. The process goes through several stages of amplification and, in general, the more stages of amplification, the more intense the electrical signal reaching the receiver. The receiver transduces or changes the electrical signal into sound waves by varying the current of a coil in a magnetic field which alternately pulls a diaphragm in and lets it go out in close approximation to the alternating strength of the electrical signal.

Hearing aids are commonly described in terms of gain, frequency response, bandwidth, and maximum output in addition to various kinds of distortion.

Gain

The gain of any amplifying system is simply the difference in dB between the input and output of the system. Thus, if an input of 60 dB is at the microphone and 100 dB is measured at the output, the gain is 40 dB. However, hearing aids do not provide the same gain throughout the entire frequency range. The Hearing Aid Industry Conference has established that the gain of the hearing aid will be expressed as average gain; this is the average gain at the three frequencies of 500, 1000 and 2000 Hz. These measurements are made with the volume control full-on. For additional information on standards and other procedures, see Chapter 40.

Frequency Response

Since gain is not uniform throughout the frequency range, a chart is made of the aid's response or gain for all frequencies where it does amplify. The resulting curve represents the particular aid's gain per frequency or frequency response. Figure 39.3 is an example of a frequency response. Note that below 100 Hz there is no appreciable amplification. Then as the input increases in frequency the aid begins to progressively amplify the signal. After about 3600 Hz amplification progressively decreases. The average gain (Hearing Aid Industry Conference, HAIC) of this aid would be about 40 dB or the mean of the gains at 500 (33 dB), 1000 (48 dB) and 2000 Hz (39 dB).

Bandwidth

In an attempt to provide, in numbers, the frequencies in which the aid effectively amplifies, HAIC has provided a bandwidth calculation procedure. Simply, a line is drawn across the graph 15 dB below the average gain of the aid. The frequencies where the line intersects the frequency response are the lower and upper

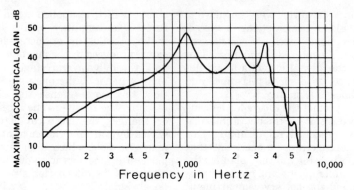

Fig. 39.3. Representative frequency response of a modern head worn hearing aid.

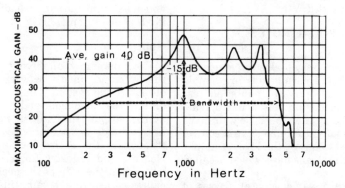

Fig. 39.4. A frequency response illustrating the method for the derivation of bandwidth according to HAIC (Hearing Aid Industry Conference).

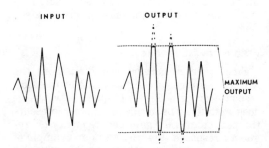

Fig. 39.5. An illustration of peak clipping.

limits of the bandwidth. In Figure 39.4, which is the same hearing aid as in Figure 39.3, the frequency response is again depicted. Recall that this particular aid's average gain was about 40 dB. A line has been drawn 15 dB below 40 dB which is 25 dB. Note that this line intersects the frequency response at 230 Hz at the low end and 4800 Hz at the high end. Therefore, this hearing aid's bandwidth is 230 to 4800 Hz.

Maximum Output

No hearing aid or amplifying system will continue to amplify more and more intense inputs. Somewhere along the line, the output will become nonlinear with respect to the input. That is, after some point, no additional output will be obtained no matter what the input. All amplifying systems have a maximum output beyond which they will not amplify. Thus if a signal of 60 dB is the input, with 40 dB gain the output would be 100 dB. If the input is increased to 100 dB, 140 dB would be expected at the output with 40 dB gain. Usually this much output is not desirable, therefore the system will limit the output somewhere below 140 dB. Most often limiting is achieved by peak clipping. That is, the amplitude of the amplified signals are flattened at their peaks. Figure 39.5 demonstrates peak clipping. Note that the output is distorted by this method of limiting.

Hearing aid manufacturers often provide curves of their hearing aids' maximum outputs. They are obtained by setting the volume control full-on, raising the input until no further amplification is noted and reading the output in dB *re* 0.0002 microbar. The HAIC average maximum output is again the average of 500, 1000 and 2000 Hz. Maximum output is constant. That is, reducing the volume control will not reduce the maximum output.

Automatic Gain Control

While most hearing aids' maximum output is accomplished by peak clipping, some hearing aids have another system which is called automatic gain control (AGC) or compression amplification. In essense, the device limits amplification by reducing the gain as input overshoots a specified level. That is, the gain of the instrument is automatically reduced when the input to the aid goes beyond some predetermined or preset level. One characteristic of AGC is that there is a short time lag between the overshoot of the input and resultant reduction in amplification or gain, and there is also a lag when the input drops below the preset compression level. These lags are called the attack and release times, respectively, and are usually quite short. Figure 39.6 shows an example of this type of limiting. Note that after the input reaches a high level, the gain is reduced after a short lag. The effect, when listening, is quite unusual and when the time constants are comparatively slow the effect becomes quite noticeable.

The advantage of AGC is that low inputs can be given comparatively high amplification, while very loud sounds are not given as much amplification. This affords some protection to a person with a severe tolerance problem without the distortion inherent in peak clipping.

Manufacturer's Published Data

The performance characteristics of specific model hearing aids which are published by most hearing aid companies represent an average of many aids and not a single aid. Therefore, as in any averaging process, individual characteristics are averaged out. Each aid differs from the next aid of the same model. The degree of deviation depends on the quality control exerted by the particular manufacturer.

Other Methods of Measurements

There are other methods of measurement of hearing aid performance which can be used. The Veterans Administration, in conjunction with their hearing aid program, has the National Bureau of Standards (NBS) measure hearing aid performance. Presently the NBS obtains a frequency response in the manner previously described. To obtain a single measure of gain, however, they use a broad band noise of specified characteristics as the input. The difference between output and input is specified as gain. They also use the same noise to specify maximum output, noting the sound pressure level (SPL) at which no further increase is obtained as the noise level is increased. They also measure distortion.

Distortion

Neither the microphone nor the receiver are capable of producing an exact copy of the signal (acoustic or electrical) which impinges upon them. No amplifying system reproduces perfectly. Distortion is caused by the transducers and the amplifier. The results are decreased bandwidth, resonant peaks and antiresonant valleys, all of which are types of distortion. That is, if the acoustic properties of the input are not reproduced exactly, the output is distorted when compared to the input. Two types of distortion are amplitude distortion and frequency distortion. Amplitude distortion occurs when the response is nonlinear as a function of amplitude. That is, the output in terms of amplitude is not a faithful reproduction of the amplitude of the input. This can occur at any or all frequencies. Frequency distortion occurs when the response is nonlinear as a function of frequency; that is, when the system performs better at some frequencies than others. How distortion affects intelligibility of speech is very important.

Harmonic Distortion. Harmonic distortion occurs when signals other than the input are produced. For example, if a 500-Hz (the fundamental or first harmonic) tone is presented to the microphone, ideally only 500 Hz should be at the output. However, other products will often be found which are integral multiples of the fundamental. Therefore, in addition to 500 Hz, the frequencies 1000, 1500, 2000, 2500, 3000 and 3500 may also be at the output in varying degrees. Harmonic distortion is usually expressed in percentage of distortion and is derived through the use of the formula:

$$\% \text{ distortion} = \frac{\sqrt{f_2^2 + f_3^2 + f_4^2 \cdots f_n^2}}{f_1} \times 100$$

INPUT

OUTPUT

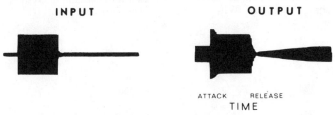

ATTACK   RELEASE
TIME

Fig. 39.6. Illustration of automatic gain control (AGC).

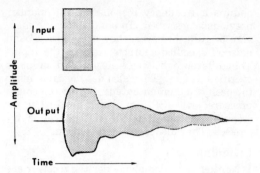

Fig. 39.7. Illustration of transient distortion and "ringing."

where f_1 is the fundamental and f_2, f_3, f_4 and f_n are the second, third, fourth and nth harmonics. Obviously a large amount of harmonic distortion will change the output signals in relation to the input in a harmful manner, that is, speech (or other inputs) will be distorted and speech intelligibility will be progressively poorer.

Transient Distortion. A second type of distortion is called transient distortion. Here the output "rings" as transient signals are presented to the system. If we present a square wave (a click, for instance) to the hearing aid, it would produce at the output a longer pulse than was at the input. Figure 39.7 illustrates transient distortion. Note that the input has a very sharp or quick rise time, remains on for a short period and then decays with equal rapidity, while the *output* does not reproduce the sharp rise time and further, does not decay for an appreciable time after the input has stopped. The latter part of the output is called "ringing." Ringing or transient distortion varies with the system and often appears to be directly related to the presence of sharp resonant peaks in the frequency response. Even the best loudspeaker systems will have a small amount of ringing. Since much of speech is highly transient in nature, ringing can and will distort speech and reduce intelligibility.

Intermodulation Distortion. Transient and harmonic distortion are easily seen, described and quantified; a third type of distortion, intermodulation distortion is more difficult to describe and measure. Again, the output contains more components that the input. When the output contains frequencies which are arithmetical additions or subtractions of two or more frequencies, the product is called intermodulation distortion. For instance, if the inputs were 500 and 800 Hz (f_1 and f_2, respectively), intermodulation distortion might create an output of 1300 Hz ($f_1 + f_2$) and/or 300 Hz ($f_2 - f_1$) in addition to 500 and 800 Hz.

Batteries

Another important part of a hearing aid, not directly related to its acoustic performance, is the power supply. The batteries used in hearing aids vary greatly in size which governs to a great degree the length of usable service a battery will provide, current drain being held constant. Batteries are specified in terms of nominal voltage and life, the latter in terms of milliampere hours at a specified current drain.

Hearing aids are usually designed for a specific voltage. The comparatively new silver oxide batteries have an average open circuit voltage of about 1.6 volts while the old carbon zinc batteries have 1.5 volts. Mercury batteries, on the other hand, have a voltage of 1.35. Important to the hearing aid user, however, is how long the battery will maintain the required voltage. Each of the two batteries (mercury and silver oxide) which are used in today's hearing aids have comparatively good characteristics over most of their life span. Under load conditions they will maintain approximately the same voltage until exhausted, when the voltage drops rapidly. In this respect, of the two batteries, the silver oxide has the best performance. Fresh full voltage batteries are important to the proper function and performance of a hearing aid. When voltage drops, not only does the gain decrease, but worse, distortion often increases.

REFERENCES

Berger, K. W., *The Hearing Aid: Its Operation and Development.* Detroit: National Hearing Aid Society, 1970.

Davis, H. (Ed.), *Hearing and Deafness,* Ch. 7. New York: Rinehart, 1947.

Watson, L. A., and Tolan, T., *Hearing Tests and Hearing Instruments,* Ch. 13. Baltimore: Williams & Wilkins Co., 1949. (Out of Print). Reprint Facsimilie, Hafner Publishing Co., New York, 1967.

chapter 40

STANDARDS AND STANDARD HEARING AIDS

Roger N. Kasten, Ph.D.

Any discussion of ear level and body type hearing aids must take into consideration the measurement of the electroacoustic characteristics of the aids. Without a detailed description of the performance characteristics, the aids cannot be compared with the reported curves or the literature in the manufacturers' specifications. The technical discussion in this chapter will be from an audiologist's rather than an engineer's point of view. For special techniques and problems of hearing aid measurement, many very competent engineers are available within the hearing aid industry from whom assistance should be sought.

This chapter will discuss the two major types of hearing aids, body worn instruments which historically preceded the other instruments, and the ear level aids which are the most popular form of amplification at the present time. The ear level instruments include those worn behind the ear, in the eyeglasses and those worn in the ear. This chapter will exclude a consideration of binaural and cross amplification which will be covered in another chapter.

ELECTROACOUSTIC REQUIREMENTS

The International Electrotechnical Commission (IEC-1959) and the American National Standards Institute (ANSI-1960; R-1971) have specified detailed procedures for the measure of physical performance of hearing aids. In addition, the American National Standards Institute (ANSI-1967; R-1971) and the Hearing Aid Industry Conference (HAIC-1961 and HAIC-1975) specify standardized procedures for the graphic display and expression of these data. More recently, the American National Standards Institute and the Acoustical Society of America have approved a new and much improved specification of hearing aid characteristics, ASA STD7-1976 (ANSI S3.22-1976). This new document deals in detail with both the specification and tolerances of hearing aid performance characteristics. Prior to measurements of any of these characteristics, individuals should thoroughly familiarize themselves with the contents of each referenced specification. A rather detailed accounting of the recommendations included in the earlier documents has been presented elsewhere (Kasten,

1968, 1972; Pollack, 1975). Individuals without an extensive academic or experiential background in the measurement of the electroacoustic characteristics of hearing aids are strongly encouraged to investigate these narrative descriptions before they attempt to tackle the standards or specifications themselves. In addition to the above mentioned references, it would be helpful for the beginner in measurement procedures to carefully examine additional existing literature such as: Lybarger (1961, 1965), Briskey, Greenbaum, and Sinclair (1966), Holden (1975) or Heide (1977). Often the audiologist, the hearing aid dispenser or the student who is beginning the measurement of electroacoustic characteristics commits a number of unthinkable mistakes during the first period of measurement. Much of the frustration and the grief brought about during this initial time could be alleviated by familiarity with appropriate methods and techniques and with a knowledge of the problems most commonly encountered by others.

As stated earlier, good reviews of the original standards and specifications can be obtained from the existing literature. This chapter will review the standard that has been developed during the past few years. It has been developed primarily by the American National Standards Institute Working Group (S-3-48) for Hearing Aids in cooperation with audiologists, hearing aid industry members, component part manufacturers and government representatives to achieve a comprehensive, workable and meaningful set of recommendations.

The test requirement described in the new standard is similar to that originally specified in ANSI S3.3-1960 (R-1971). One particular change that should be noted is that input sound pressure level is specified at the microphone opening of the hearing aid rather than at some control point in the sound field. This change can be accomplished within the test space by placing the control microphone leading to the microphone amplifier approximately 1/8 to 1/4 of an inch away from the microphone opening of the hearing aid to be measured. This calls for a sizable departure in the procedure from the earlier measurement technique, and will be appropriate for all types of amplification systems other than those with directional microphones. Measurement of systems with directional microphones will still require free field techniques in an anechoic chamber.

Fig. 40.1 provides the basic components necessary for a measurement scheme. The space marked "Anechoic Chamber" may be a true anechoic chamber, or a pressure type test space available with some of the more portable commercial type hearing aid test units. Regardless of the system, an oscillator will provide a pure tone signal to a loudspeaker within the test space. The sound intensity in the test space will be picked up by a monitor microphone, carried through a form of microphone amplifier, and fed back to a compressor unit within the oscillator circuitry. This feed back loop will have the task of controlling the intensity of the input sound pressure level into the test space.

The hearing aid under test will be located at a predetermined test point immediately adjacent to the control microphone. The hearing aid will be coupled directly to a hard walled steel coupler of the type specified in the American National Standard S3.7-1973, Method for Coupler Calibration of Ear Phones. These are the same coupler systems that have been in conventional use for several years. The receiver portion of the body type hearing aid will snap directly onto the surface of the type HA-2 coupler. Behind the ear and eyeglass hearing

aids will also utilize the type HA-2 coupler but will be attached to it by means of a rigid metal tube. In the ear hearing aids will be measured using the type HA-1 coupler. These three coupler arrangements are shown in Figure 40.2.

The output of the hearing aid coupler leads directly to an audio frequency spectrometer or some other visual readout instrument. This will provide the individual making the measurements with an instantaneous display of the hearing aid output. The output of the visual measurement display instrument is then fed to some type of graphic level recorder to obtain a permanent record of the characteristics in question. A frequency counter may be located between the final two components in order to ensure accurate agreement between the sound source and the print-out mechanism.

The test space, where the hearing aid is located during measurement, should be an enclosure with high sound absorption. It should be constructed in such a way that ambient

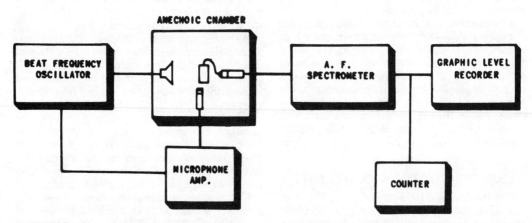

Fig. 40.1. Simplified block diagram of a basic hearing aid measurement system. (From R. N. Kasten, S. H. Lotterman and E. D. Burnett, Paper presented before convention of the American Speech and Hearing Association, 1967.)

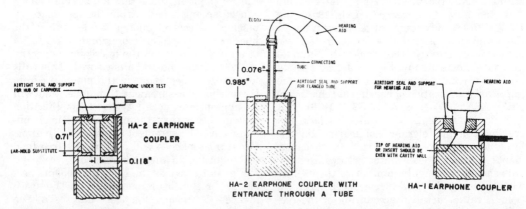

Fig. 40.2. Three coupler arrangements. (Reprinted by permission from S. F. Lybarger, *Hearing Instruments,* February 1977, © 1977 Harcourt, Brace Jovanovich.)

noise or stray electrical or magnetic field shall be sufficiently weak that their effect on the test result is no greater than 0.5 dB.

As described earlier, the sound source consists of an oscillator, loudspeaker, control microphone, amplifier and generally a compressor circuitry to compensate for imperfections within the system. This complete sound source should be capable of maintaining a constant sound pressure level at the hearing aid microphone opening within ± 1.5 dB in the range from 200 to 2000 Hz and within ± 2.5 dB in the range from 2000 to 5000 Hz. This sound source should also have the capability to deliver to the hearing aid microphone sound pressure levels from 50 to 90 dB. The total harmonic distortion of the sound source shall not exceed 2% when the system is being used for general hearing aid response measurements, and shall not exceed 0.5% when the system is being used for the measurement of harmonic distortion. Since the control microphone has the task of monitoring the sound pressure level at the hearing aid microphone, the frequency response of this portion of the sound source system shall be flat within ± 1 dB in the range between 200 and 5000 Hz.

Since the sound source will be delivered pure tones, and the output of the hearing aid will be specified according to these pure tones, the indicated frequency from the sound source shall be accurate within ± 2%. This means that the actual frequency output of the sound source shall be within 2% of the dial or face reading of the sound source at all times. Furthermore, the indicated frequencies on the printout device should be within ± 5% of the indicated frequency of the pure tone source. When a level recorder is used as the printout device, there is considerable difference of opinion regarding the paper and pen speeds needed for the most accurate output measurements. For example, a very rapid paper speed with a very slow pen speed can provide an extremely broad and flat frequency response that would give an erroneous representation of the hearing aid output. The available equipment provides different paper and pen speeds and thus, an absolute numerical designation did not seem appropriate. As a result, the standard recommends that the paper and pen speeds be such that their output indications do not differ by more than 1 dB from those of steady state measurements over the entire frequency range.

Finally, the frequency response of the pressure microphone used within the measurement coupler, along with its associated measurement system, should be uniform within ± 1 dB over the frequency range from 200 to 5000 Hz. In addition, the calibration of this output system should be accurate at any frequency between 200 to 1000 Hz to within ± 1 dB.

In an attempt to obtain uniformity across the great variety of geographical and atmospheric conditions, the standard also stipulates the acceptable atmospheric conditions at a test site. Measurements are to be conducted at temperatures between 64 to 82° Fahrenheit; relative humidity should be between 0 and 80%; and, atmospheric pressure should fall between 725 and 910 mm of mercury. The actual conditions at the time measurements are made should be recorded for validation of the test conditions.

The specific settings on the hearing aid itself at the time of measurement will, of course, be determined by the individual making the measurement. For the purposes of hearing aid specification sheet, however, the hearing aid should be set to give the widest possible frequency response. Other available control settings should then be selected to provide the highest output and the greatest amplification that the instrument is capable of delivering. If these particular settings are not compatible, then the hearing aid should be set to provide the highest possible output. If an aid has varying degrees of automatic gain control (AGC), the measurements should be made with the greatest amount of AGC, even if that particular setting results in a reduced output for the instrument.

Once again it should be noted that the comments in this text are a summary of the recommendations from the standard. An individual desiring to begin electroacoustic measurements of hearing aids is urged to obtain a copy of the standard in its entirety and study it carefully prior to the initiation of measurements.

ELECTROACOUSTIC MEASUREMENTS

Several changes in electroacoustic measurement technique and specification have been made in the new standard. A summary of these specifications is presented in Table 40.1. It is particularly important to note that the new standard, for the first time, not only specifies the method by which measurements are to be made, but also stipulates the tolerances that specific characteristics may have in their deviation from the information given on the manufacturer's specification sheet. Inasmuch as instruments may technically be rejected if they exceed these tolerances, great care must be taken to ensure that each individual's separate measurements are made exactly in accordance with the recommendations of the standard. More than one response curve will need to be plotted. Therefore, it is recommended that all output versus frequency curves be plotted on a grid having a linear decibel ordinate scale and a logarithmic frequency abcissa scale with the length of one decade equal to the length of 50

TABLE 40.1

SUMMARY OF SPECIFICATIONS AND TOLERANCES
ASA STD 7-1976
(ANSI S3.22-1976)

SPECIFICATIONS	TOLERANCE
1. SSPL 90 Curve	Maximum value of SSPL90 shall not exceed specified value.
2. HF-Av. SSPL 90	Must be with ± 4dB of specified value.
3. Full-On Gain Curve	No tolerances.
4. HF-Av. Full-On Gain	Must be within ± 5dB of specified value.
5. Frequency Response Curve (See Note A)	See Note B below.
6. Harmonic Distortion (See Note A)	Must not exceed specified values at 500, 800 and 1600Hz.
7. Equivalent Input Noise Level (See Note A)	Must not exceed specified maximum value.
8. Battery Current (See Note A)	Must not exceed specified maximum value.
9. Induction Coil 1000Hz Sensitivity	Must be within ± 6dB of specified value.
10. AGC Input-Output Characteristic	Match measured and specified curves at 70dB input. Measured values @ 50 and 90dB must be with ± 4dB of specified values.
11. AGC Attack and Release Times	Must be within ± 5 Ms. or ± 50% (whichever is larger) of specified values.

NOTE A

Reference test gain control position is used in items 5, 6, 7 and 8. Gain control must be set 17dB (± 1dB) below HF-average SSPL90 for each individual instrument.

NOTE B

FREQUENCY RESPONSE CURVE

    a. From the manufacturer's specified frequency response curve, determine the average of the 1000, 1600 and 2500Hz response levels.
    b. Subtract 20dB.
    c. Draw a line parallel to the abcissa at the reduced level.
    d. Note the lowest frequency, f_1, at which the response curve intersects the straight line.
    e. Note the highest frequency, f_2, at which the frequency response curve intersects the straight line.

Frequency range. For information purposes, but not for tolerance purposes, the frequency range of the hearing aid shall be considered as being between f_1 and f_2.

Frequency response tolerance. The tolerances in two bands shall be as follows:

	Frequency Limits	Tolerance
Low Band	$1.25f_1$ to 2000Hz	± 4dB
High Band	2000 to 4000Hz or $0.8f_2$ whichever is lower.	± 6db

(Reprinted courtesy of Zenith Hearing Instrument Corp.)

± 2 dB on the ordinate. By plotting all characteristics on the same grid, an easier and more accurate comparison of results may be accomplished. An example of the same response curve plotted on two different scales is given in Figure 40.3. The untrained viewer might easily assume that these were two totally different hearing aids.

SSPL 90

The characteristic that had been previously called saturation sound pressure level is now given the term saturation sound pressure level 90 (SSPL 90) and is pictured in Figure 40.4. This particular characteristic is to be measured with the gain control of the hearing aid turned to full-on and with an input to the hearing aid microphone of 90 dB SPL. With these settings, a saturation curve of coupler output will be measured through the range from 200 to 5000 Hz. A single numeric value for saturation can then be computed by determining the average of saturation values at 1000, 1600 and 2500 Hz. This single numeric value will be referred to as "HF-average SSPL 90." This HF-average SSPL 90 for any given instrument shall fall within ± 4 dB of the manufacturer's specified value for that model and the maximum value of the SSPL 90 curve shall not exceed that specified by the manufacturer.

It should be noted that there will no longer be any necessity for individual point by point measurements of saturation as was the case with the old standard. Occasionally, the constant 90 dB SPL signal may not drive a hearing aid to saturation, or may drive the hearing aid beyond saturation. Nevertheless, the rapid determination of a saturation curve and an average value could be more accurate than the more tedious measurements. The reader should also note the change in frequencies for the computation of an average saturation value. The three frequencies recommended in the new standard are significantly higher than the fre-

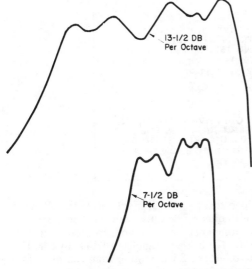

Fig. 40.3. Frequency response curves of the same hearing aid traced on two different standard recording devices. (The 13-¹/₂ dB per octave scale approximates that recommended by S3.22-1976.) (Reprinted by permission from R. J. Briskey, W. H. Greenbaum and J. C. Sinclair, Pitfalls in hearing aid response curves. *Journal of the Audio Engineering Society,* **14,** 4, October 1976.)

quencies previously used. These frequencies more accurately represent the most important operating conditions of the hearing aid. In an attempt to eliminate confusion, the prefix "HF" has been added to the designation so that the reader will have no difficulty in determining the specified method.

Gain

The hearing aid will be measured with the gain control maintained at the full-on setting. The input to the hearing aid microphone should be 60 dB SPL, or 50 dB SPL if a lower input is needed to obtain linear input-output conditions. Regardless of which setting is used, the specific input level should be recorded. In addition, when measurements are made with instruments having automatic gain control, the input sound pressure level should always be held at 50 dB.

A single numeric value can be obtained by averaging the gain values at 1000, 1600 and 2500 Hz. This value will be referred to as "HF-average full-on gain." The HF-average full-on gain for a particular hearing aid should be within ±5 dB of the manufacturer's specification. Individuals are cautioned that rigid adherence to the standard was maintained before making comparative statements.

Reference Test Gain

The concept of a reference test gain is totally new in this standard and is summarized in Table 40.2. The reference test gain setting is achieved using an input SPL of 60 dB and adjusting the gain control of the hearing aid so that the average of the 1000, 1600 and 2500 Hz

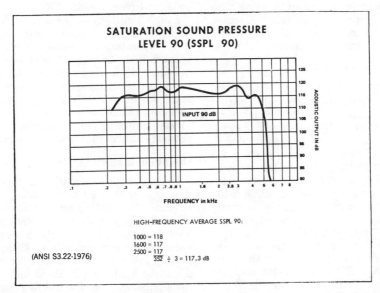

Fig. 40.4. (Reprinted Courtesy of Zenith Hearing Instruments Corporation.)

TABLE 40.2

```
REFERENCE TEST GAIN
CONTROL POSITION


INPUT : 60dB


        VOLUME
        CONTROL: ADJUST
                SO THAT EARPHONE
                SPL AVERAGE AT 1000,
                1600 AND 2500 IS
                17dB LESS THAN THE
                HF-AVERAGE SSPL 90.


                        IF GAIN AVAILABLE WILL NOT
                        PERMIT THIS , AND FOR AGC
                        AIDS, USE THE FULL-ON GAIN
(ANSI S3.22-1976)       CONTROL POSITION OF AID.
```

values of coupler output are 17 ± 1 dB less than the HF-average SSPL 90 value. If a hearing aid does not have enough gain to permit this particular adjustment, then the gain control should be set to full-on. Instruments with automatic gain control should also be set to full-on.

The rationale for the reference test gain setting is that the long term average SPL for speech at a distance of 1 meter is approximately 65 dB with speech peaks typically occurring 12 dB above this average level. When a hearing aid gain control is adjusted to give an output SPL 12 dB below saturation with a 65-dB input level, it is assumed that the speech peaks typically will not exceed the SSPL of the aid. This situation can be duplicated by using a 60-dB input SPL with a 17-dB gain reduction. These latter settings will be easier to achieve with most of the current equipment.

Frequency Response Curve

The new standard calls for the measurement of a single frequency response curve rather than the cumbersome family of frequency response curves previously measured. The frequency response curve shall be measured with an input SPL of 60 dB and the hearing aid gain control set to the reference test position as shown in Figure 40.5. Instruments with automatic gain control will be measured using an input SPL of 50 dB. Frequency response will typically be traced and plotted through the range from 200 to 5000 Hz.

The tolerance for frequency response is to be computed by subtracting 20 dB from the average of the 1000-, 1600-and 2500-Hz response levels. From this 20-dB down point, a line is drawn parallel to the abcissa and the point at which this parallel line intersects the skirts of the frequency response will be considered the low frequency limit (f_1) and the high frequency limit (f_2). In the range from $1.25\, f_1$ to 2000 Hz, the tolerance for deviation from the manufacturer's recommended response curve will be ± 4 dB. In the range from 2000 to 4000 Hz, or $0.8\, f_2$, whichever is lower, the tolerance from the manufacturer's specified curve will be ± 6 dB.

Using the above scheme, a hearing aid with a low frequency limit of 200 Hz and a high frequency limit of 5000 Hz would have to satisfy tolerance limits only in the region from 250 to 4000 Hz. It is particularly important to realize that the tolerance in the high frequency region does not extend beyond 4000 Hz, regardless of the high frequency response of the hearing aid. This decision was made in order not to penalize those manufacturers who attempt to build greater high frequency emphasis into their hearing aids. Realizing that the high frequency region of the response curve is the most difficult region to accurately control, it was felt that every effort should be made at this time to allow manufacturers the freedom to construct new extended high frequency instruments.

Harmonic Distortion

Harmonic distortion will be measured with the gain control of the hearing aid in the reference test setting and an input SPL of 70 dB at the frequencies of 500, 800 and 1600 Hz. Measurement will be made in terms of total harmonic distortion which can be accomplished rapidly and efficiently with most commercial distortion analyzers. In those instances where the frequency response curve rises 12 dB or more between any of the distortion test frequencies and their second harmonic, the distortion test at that frequency may be omitted in order not to contaminate the measurement with artifact caused solely by the shape of the frequency response curve. Total harmonic distortion for any given hearing aid shall be the same or less than that specified by the manufacturer for that model. Distortion products should never exceed those specified by the manufacturer.

Automatic Gain Control

The input-output characteristics of AGC hearing aids are measured at the frequency of 2000 Hz with input SPL in 10-dB steps from 50 to 90 dB. Coupler output from the hearing aid is then plotted against the input SPL on a grid having equal linear decibel scales on both the ordinate and the abcissa. When the measured and the manufacturer's specified curves are equated at the 70 dB input sound pressure level point, the measured curve at the two input extremes should not differ from the manufacturer's specified curves by more than ± 4 dB.

The dynamic AGC characteristics are to be measured at the frequency of 2000 Hz with the hearing aid gain control set full-on and a square wave modulated pure tone used as the input signal. This input signal is alternated abruptly between the sound pressure level of 55 and 80 dB. Attack time is defined as the time between the onset of the abrupt increase and the point where the level has stabilized to within 2 dB of the steady state value for the 80-dB input. Release time carries the same definition except measurement is made as the

signal strength is decreased from 80 to 55 dB. The tolerance allowed on attack and release time is ± 5 msec or ± 50%, whichever is greater.

The above characteristics are those most commonly associated with hearing aid performance. A great many other characteristics are also available for measurement, some of which are mentioned in the new standard. These characteristics, while seemingly very important to hearing aid performance, typically have not been measured in the field and have remained primarily within the realm of the hearing aid engineer or a few dedicated audiologic researchers. These would include such items as the characteristic of the gain control, the effect of gain control positions on frequency response, the effect on acoustic gain of variations of battery or supply voltage, the effect on acoustic gain by variation of internal resistance of the battery or supply, the frequency response and electrical impedance of the earphone, the effect on harmonic distortion of variation of battery or supply voltage, the random noise from the hearing aid and battery current. It should again be apparent that individuals desiring to undertake hearing aid measurements must be conversant with all aspects of the existing standards in order to properly evaluate the accuracy of their measurements.

Two additional characteristics not specifically covered in the standards have received attention in the recent literature. These are transient distortion and intermodulation distortion. The measurement of transient distortion involves the analysis of the response of the hearing aid to a square wave or click of acoustic energy. Olsen and Wilber (1967), have

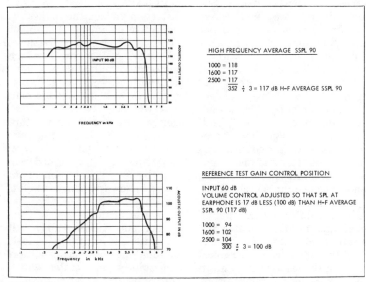

Fig. 40.5. (Reprinted Courtesy of Zenith Hearing Instruments Corporation.)

pointed out the difficulty in interpreting the results of these measurements. Intermodulation distortion has been examined using a variety of techniques. The International Telephonic Consultative Committee (1937) procedure appears to be most appropriate for use with hearing aids, however, it is somewhat cumbersome and time consuming, and the choice of input signals has not been standardized. Both Burnett (1967) and Bang (1962) have proposed methods which utilize a notched white noise as an input signal. These methods appear to have promise as measurement techniques, but little published research is presently available regarding the appropriateness of these measurements.

We should be aware that the above listing of measurement procedures is not exhaustive. No researcher has yet identified that elusive characteristic that is primarily responsible for most successful hearing aid performance with the hearing-impaired individual. Indeed, characteristics not yet fully recognized may be found to be of great importance.

INFLUENCE OF ELECTROACOUSTIC CHARACTERISTICS

A major investigation, conducted by Harris et al. (1961), involved comprehensive measurements of physical performance. They utilized several aids, several talkers and several listening conditions. Harmonic distortion appeared to be the major contributor to the degradation of speech intelligibility. Intermodulation distortion was also important, but to a lesser degree than harmonic distortion.

At approximately the same time, Jeffers (1960) reported on the relation between quality judgments and acoustic characteristics. She stated that when aids are rated in terms of ". . . the relative linearity of the frequency response with respect to gain," the judgments of conductively impaired individuals will reflect differences in physical performance. It should be noted that she did not examine either of the distortions discussed by Harris et al.

Jerger, Speaks and Malmquist (1966) examined the word discrimination scores of both normal hearing persons and subjects with sensory-neural hearing loss with harmonic distortion being the prime characteristic measured. Subjects listened to tape recordings of PAL-8 lists in the presence of competing speech. These materials were processed through three hearing aid systems which differed according to frequency response and harmonic distortion. They state, "Analysis of individual performance data showed that most listeners ranked the three conditions in the same order (i.e., in inverse proportion to per cent harmonic distortion)." Jerger (1967) also examined the influ-

ence of intermodulation distortion in a "nonspeech" procedure. He suggested that such a type of evaluation might be beneficial in detecting differences between aids with widely differing characteristics. Jerger and Thelin (1968) suggested that the influence of these distortions is not as great as was previously reported. They also pointed out that the latency of the subject's response to synthetic sentence speech materials was essentially as accurate in rank ordering the performance of aids with different characteristics as were the actual responses to the speech materials.

In 1967, Olsen and Wilber reported the results of an extensive investigation of the influence of various electroacoustic characteristics. They concluded that the effective bandwidth of the instrument was the only measured characteristic which ranked the aids in the same order as did speech intelligibility performance. Olsen and Wilber (1968) also studied the specific influences of bandwidth, harmonic distortion and intermodulation distortion on hearing aid processed monosyllables in the presence of competing speech. They again concluded that bandwidth was more important to intelligibility than either of the distortions.

The influence of total nonlinear distortion upon intelligibility, when hearing aid bandwidth is held constant, was examined by Kasten, Lotterman and Burnett (1967). Distortion was measured using a notched noise method (Burnett, 1967) and one body type aid was driven to four different levels to create distortion differences. They reported a systematic and significant deterioration of intelligibility as distortion levels increased.

Witter (1971) examined subjective quality judgments of normal listeners for hearing aid processed speech and reported that transient distortion yielded the highest correlation with subjective judgments. On the other hand, Del Polito (1967) reported that low frequency cutoff of the response correlated most highly with subjective intelligibility judgments from subjects with sensory-neural losses. Interestingly, of the six aids used in his paired comparison task, the three body aids were preferred significantly more often than the three ear-level instruments. It appears that this preference reflects the fact that the body aids were more capable of providing a broad frequency response with better amplification of the low frequencies. The low frequency cut-off of the body aids tended to be 100 Hz or more lower than that of the ear level aids.

Bode and Kasten (1971), utilizing a closed set consonant identification task, reported that intelligibility of hearing aid processed speech consistently deteriorated with systematic increases in harmonic distortion. They also reported that hearing aid bandwidth may be a contributing factor in the control of intelligibility. Smaldino (1975a, 1975b) utilized 7 different speech discrimination materials and related them to 42 different hearing aid performance measurements. Although he presents intriguing results in the sizeable investigation, he was hesitant to identify dominant characteristics and rather referred strongly to the influence of interactions among various characteristics.

Miller and Niemoeller (1967) reported a reduction in intelligibility as the hearing aid microphone was moved away from the talker when testing in the presence of noise. They relate this to distortion caused by reflective waves and recommended the detachable microphones that can be held close to the talker's lips in order to improve speech-to-noise ratios.

The exact influences of the various electroacoustic characteristics are still far from understood. Some of the more definitive findings appear to be in direct contradiction to other equally definitive findings. It appears likely that future research dealing with the intelligibility of hearing aid processed speech will need to involve some intricate manipulations of varieties of characteristics rather than concentrate on the influence of a single characteristic. Also, as most researchers have demonstrated, it is essential to conduct the speech intelligibility investigations, regardless of the stimulus material, in the presence of some type of competing message. Conventional intelligibility testing in quiet is notoriously unsuccessful in demonstrating differences between or among aids with differing characteristics.

BODY VERSUS EAR-LEVEL AIDS

The single most obvious difference that typically differentiated body and ear-level instruments was the amount of power that the aids were capable of delivering. Traditionally, body type aids were capable of providing significantly greater gain and saturation sound pressure level than the ear-level instruments. In the past 5 years there has been a major change in hearing aid technology and hearing aid performance. Indeed, many ear-level hearing aids are presently available that are capable of delivering the same levels of acoustic gain and acoustic output as body type instruments. This would particularly hold true with ear level instruments of the behind-the-ear and eyeglass type. Although some hearing aid advertising and hearing aid literature report excellent results fitting severely hearing impaired individuals with in-the-ear hearing aids, the success rate with this type of instrument is still questionable. Indeed, this writer has never been able to find a severely hearing-impaired individual who could be considered a successful user of in-the-ear hearing aids.

Physical structure appears to be the major determinant of the power delivering capacity of the ear level hearing aids. The body aid has the microphone and the receiver as two physically separated components. In actual use, these components are often as much as 8 to 15 inches from each other. This physical separation does much to reduce the probability of acoustic feedback. With the ear-level instruments, both the microphone and the receiver are built into the same small unit. This means that the two components are physically less than 1 inch apart. Also, the microphone is frequently much less than 1 inch away from the user's earmold. With many in-the-ear aids, the microphone is actually located inside the user's earmold. Thus, not only is there an increased chance for acoustic feedback, but because the components are in the same case, there is also the possibility of generating mechanical feedback.

The above comments are not made to discourage the use of ear-level aids with those individuals who have severe to profound hearing losses. Rather, they point up the critical nature of the earmold as an actual component of the hearing aid. No attempt will be made at this time to discuss earmolds in detail since that discussion is covered in another chapter. It should be kept in mind, however, that the high gain and high powered ear-level hearing aid can be as useful as the fit of the earmold will allow it to be.

The versatility and usability of ear-level hearing aids are reflected by the fact that many clinical programs have eliminated the use of body type aids except with real problem cases. This writer does not foresee a future in which body aids will be totally eliminated since they serve a real need in special cases, but it is likely that their use will be even more restricted in the future.

Other purely physical features often dictate the type of instrument that must be used with a given individual. Body aids, even with their bulk, unsightly cord connecting amplifier and receiver, and button type receiver, are frequently preferable for young children. These aids can be firmly anchored to the body by means of a cloth carrier, and are less likely to be seriously damaged or lost. Ear-level aids are much less conspicuous and therefore do not call as much attention to the hearing loss. For some people this is the most important factor in hearing aid selection. Body aids are particularly susceptible to noises generated by clothing rubbing against them. This clothing noise can be partly relieved by using a cloth carrier that fits fairly tightly around the aid and does not slide back and forth over the surface of the aid. Also, many body aids are constructed with the microphone on the top surface of the instrument so that clothing cannot rub against the microphone grill.

Eyeglass type aids also present special problems. Since the aid is built into the temple of the glasses, the aid will be taken off every time the glasses are taken off. The eyeglass hearing aid user must be prepared to use his glasses whenever he uses his aid, and he obviously must use only one pair of glasses. If reading glasses or sunglasses are also used, the aid will be necessarily disconnected while they are in use. On the other hand, there is generally no problem in wearing standard eyeglasses and a behind-the-ear aid. These two devices do not interfere with each other and they can be used independently as the needs of the individual demand. The power handling capabilities of eyeglass aids and behind-the-ear aids are essentially the same and the selection of which type of instrument to use can be made on the basis of individual preference.

Many ear-level aids are now constructed with forward facing microphones. This particular microphone orientation is often preferred in that it tends to partially eliminate the unwanted sound generated behind the head. The clear reception of this unwanted sound was a frequent complaint from the users of aids with back facing microphones. Finally, body type aids are often mandatory for those individuals who are physically unable to manipulate the small controls of ear-level instruments. Even when only mild powered amplification is required, it is often necessary to modify body aids to the required needs so that the user is capable of controlling his amplification system. This must be kept in mind, particularly when working with the physically handicapped or the geriatric population.

With the decrease in usage of body type hearing aids, a significant increase in usage has been noted for behind-the-ear aids with directional microphones and in-the-ear aids. The directional hearing aid provides the user with a focused acoustic pick-up that allows the user to literally point the hearing aid microphone to the area of interest. Not only does this permit him to concentrate on the signal of interest, but also the directional microphone greatly reduces the amount of noise generated from other areas in the environment. An example of a typical directional characteristic is shown in Figure 40.6 (from manufacturers specifications for Danavox Model 735 DV). The manufacturer provides the single ear directional characteristics taken from Fletcher's work along with the measured directional characteristics of their hearing aids.

It should be noted that, with the directional hearing aid on the right ear, the field of maximum sound reception is in the 0 to 90° azimuth range. In most listening situations the hearing aid user will be primarily interested in the acoustic events occurring within that azimuth range. At the same time, as pictured in Figure 40.6, the area of maximum signal attenuation occurs between 180 and 270° of azimuth. Stated more simply, the signals emanating from the rear of the head are attenuated significantly in relation to those signals emanating from the front of the head.

When one closely examines the two directional plottings in Figure 40.6, it becomes apparent that the directional hearing aid actually accomplishes two effects simultaneously. To begin with, it provides reasonably uniform amplification throughout the complete semicircle to the front of the head. A somewhat greater sound pickup is seen in the anterior quadrant ipsilateral to the hearing aid, but a more uniform total anterior pickup can be seen with the hearing aid in place than with the human ear unaided. At the same time, greater degree of sound attenuation is noted through the posterior semicircle with the directional hearing aid than with the unaided ear. This is particularly true through the posterior quadrant contralateral to the directional aid.

Clearly, this type of response characteristic would appear to be extremely beneficial to the hearing aid user who finds it necessary to attend to only one incoming signal at a time. This method of amplification would also appear to be highly beneficial to the hearing aid user who is annoyed, bothered or distracted by a variety of incoming environmental sounds emanating from diverse areas in the environment. The hearing aid user utilizing a directional instrument for the first time frequently comments that it is refreshing to be able to carry on a conversation with individuals in front of them without having to also listen in to conversations going on behind them. Particular care should be taken however, since some potential directional hearing aid users will rather vigorously complain that the directional aid cuts off a complete dimension of sound and tends to make their environment a great deal more one dimensional.

A great deal of additional research is needed in order to better identify those individuals who might be good candidates for directional amplification, and those circumstances in which directional amplification might prove more beneficial. While substantial research regarding the efficiency of directional microphones has been sparse, user reactions and fitter reports have been highly enthusiastic regarding this type of instrument. The directional hearing aid appears to be particularly useful for individuals who must frequently communicate in either noisy or chaotic environments.

At the same time, the hearing aid industry

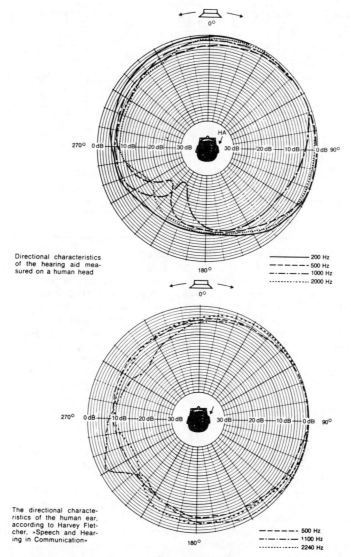

Fig. 40.6. Directional characteristics for the Danavox Model 735 DV, taken from manufacturer's specifications. (Reprinted by courtesy of Danavox, Inc., Minneapolis, Minnesota.)

has made outstanding developments with in-the-ear hearing aid technology. A truly exceptional series of reports by Griffing and Preves (1976a, 1976b) and Preves and Griffing (1976a, 1976b) has detailed the versatility and usability of this type of instrument. Their reports have provided a great deal of comprehensive technical information regarding the operation and utilization of in-the-ear aids, and they have demonstrated, perhaps for the first time, the real utility of this type of instrument. There is little doubt that the in-the-ear aid will continue to occupy an ever increasing share of the hearing aid sales market. Many individuals, including this writer, have tended to function as "doubting Thomases" regarding the usability

of in-the-ear aids. The type of information provided by Preves and Griffing can do much to advance the cause for utilization of in-the-ear aids. One should look at the results of probe tube microphone measurements made at the microphone inlet of a typical behind-the-ear aid and an in-the-ear aid as shown in Figure 40.7. It is readily apparent that the in-the-ear hearing aid user can experience a real sound enhancement in the total range from 200 through 5000 Hz. Throughout this complete frequency range the sound pressure levels measured at the microphone inlet of the in-the-ear aid are uniformly greater than those measured at the microphone inlet of the behind-the-ear aid.

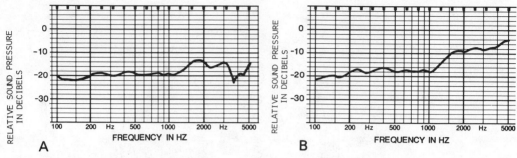

Fig. 40.7. (A) Probe MIC measurement on real ear at frontal MIC inlet of BTE aid—0° incidence. (B) Probe MIC measurement at ITE MIC inlet on another real ear—0° incidence. (Reprinted with permission from T. S. Griffing and D. A. Preves, *Hearing Instruments, 27*, 22–24, 1976a.)

Perhaps a more realistic method of picturing this phenomenon would be that displayed in Figure 40.8. Here we have a more common type of response chart comparing the SPL at the microphone inlets of both an in-the-ear and behind-the-ear instrument. This particular set of measurements clearly demonstrates the superior high frequency response that can be obtained simply through advantageous positioning of the microphone inlet. Preves and Griffing thoroughly discuss the many modifications that can be made on in-the-ear aids to further alter the frequency characteristics.

An example of versatility that can be achieved is given in Figure 40.9. Here we have a frequency response and a saturation curve from an in-the-ear instrument with a medium diameter vent, a relative short canal portion and a wide range receiver. Although this set of measurements was made using a Zwislocki coupler and a Knowles Electronic Mannequin for Acoustic Research, the instrument involved has a significant high frequency emphasis with an extended high frequency-range. Virtually no amplification exists below 1000 Hz, and the instrument exhibits a primary peak at approximately 2000 Hz with a secondary peak at approximately 6000 Hz. The saturation curve also exhibits the same two peaks, and it also has only limited output in the low frequency region. In an era when those individuals engaged in hearing aid fitting are trying valiantly to achieve true high frequency emphasis, it would appear that these authors have clearly pointed out a meaningful method of accomplishing this goal.

Once again, it behooves all individuals involved in the fitting of in-the-ear instruments to be aware of the technical information regarding the use of these complex amplification systems. The development of the in-the-ear aids once again points up the fact that the hearing aid fitter needs to be much more than an instrument manipulator. It is becoming increasingly apparent that the successful fitting of the many different combinations of ear level amplification systems can come only through detailed knowledge of parameter manipulations that are available through these various combinations.

One final word of caution appears appropriate regarding in-the-ear aids. It has become fashionable in recent years for manufacturers of ear-level aids to construct custom units for each individual user. The hearing aid fitter is encouraged to make a lengthy series of pure tone, speech and impedance measurements and forward this information to the manufacturer. From these data, the manufacturer then constructs a custom instrument according to some "company secret." The finished product is then returned to the fitter for final evaluation or delivery to the user. Each manufacturer tends to keep their construction methods as privileged information, and recent attempts to obtain either the method or the rationale for the methods have been fruitless. To this writer, this appears to be a most unfortunate state of affairs. At a time when technologic advances in the state of the art have been great, the withholding or masking of psychoacoustic advances seems perplexing. It would appear that increased cooperation, joint research and combined information sharing among the many members of the hearing aid fitting team could not help but result in marked improvements for the hearing aid user. It is hoped that this type of information sharing may be developed in the near future to the benefit of all members of the fitting team, but particularly to the benefit of the hearing aid user.

DISCUSSION

It should be clear that any individual desiring to measure or interpret the measurements of hearing aid characteristics must be thoroughly familiar with the existing documents specifying measurement procedures. This does not mean that the tester must restrict himself to existing procedures. Indeed, there is a good rationale for conducting measurements at settings other than those specified in the regulating documents. Measurements carried out at the input and gain settings normally encountered by a specific user will be much more valuable in describing the performance of an aid than those conducted according to standard methods. This philosophy does not invalidate the standard methods, it simply points out the necessity for additional measurements. For an individual who must function in a relatively noisy environment, it would seem more appropriate to measure hearing aid performance with a relatively high input level. This may very well result in frequency response, gain and distortion values that are different from those obtained using the settings specified in the standards. Another method of user oriented measurement would involve specifying performance as a function of volume control seting rather than precise gain settings. It has been reported (Kasten and Lotterman, 1969) that some aids will demonstrate a much greater change in gain during rotation of the first half of the control than during rotation of the second half as shown in Figure 40.10. Thus, an instrument with 60 dB gain might deliver 45 to 50 dB with the gain control set at half on. It also has been reported (Lotterman and Kasten, 1967) that some instruments will produce relatively high levels of distortion when the gain control is advanced beyond the one-half to three-quarters positions as pictured in Figure 40.11. With this in mind, it would be particularly meaningful if performance characteristics could be specified at various known positions of the volume control. These types of user oriented measurements could then provide valuable information

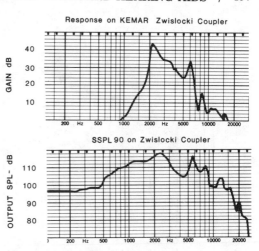

Fig. 40.9. High frequency emphasis ITE aid with medium vent, short canal, wide range receiver and low frequencies filtered out electronically. (Reprinted by permission from D. A. Preves and T. S. Griffing, In-the-ear aids, Part IV, *Hearing Instruments*, September 1976, © Harcourt Brace Jovanovich, Inc.)

which would serve to supplement or augment the data collected via standard measurement procedures.

Even with an excellent knowledge of the electroacoustic performance of aids the actual selection of the type of aid for a given individual must be based upon a variety of factors. While it might be desirable for every hearing-impaired individual to use an ear level instrument, this is frequently not possible. The specific selection of body or ear level type aids must consider power requirements, vanity, age, physical dexterity and the psychological state of the hearing aid user.

One final item deserves mention at this time. The Food and Drug Administration (1977) has recently published rules and regulations that govern hearing aid devices. This is the first major step on the part of a federal governmental agency to dictate conditions surrounding hearing aid fitting, sales and usage. Other governmental agencies are considering the publication of additional regulations that will further regulate and restrict the conditions surrounding the fitting and sales of hearing aids. As with most regulations, portions appear to be extremely beneficial to the hearing aid user while other portions are very questionable. Obviously, the true value of these regulations will be revealed only after a period of enforcement.

Effective August 1977, a hearing aid purchaser will need to be seen by a licensed physician (preferably an ear specialist) before a hearing aid dealer may consummate the sale

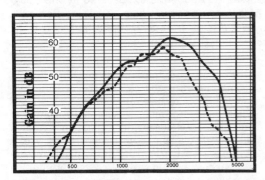

Fig. 40.8. Response of ITE (———) vs. BTE (---) microphone inlets using same amplifier and receiver on KEMAR. (Reprinted by permission from D. A. Preves and T. S. Griffing, In-the-ear aids, Part III, *Hearing Instruments*, July 1976, © Harcourt Brace Jovanovich, Inc.)

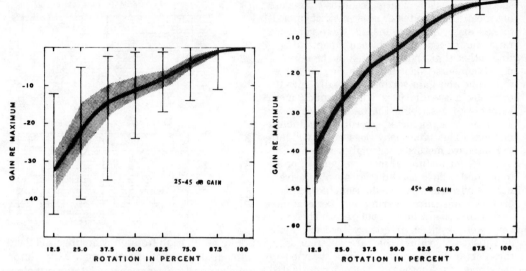

Fig. 40.10. (*A, left*) Median taper characteristics for aids with 25 to 45 dB gain. Interquartile range shown by shaded area, full range depicted by vertical bars. (*B, right*) Median taper characteristics for aids with 45 + dB gain. Interquartile range shown by shaded area, full range depicted by vertical bars. (Reprinted by permission from R. N. Kasten and S. H. Lotterman, *The Journal of Auditory Research*, **9**, 35–39, 1969.)

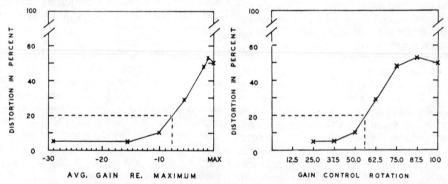

Fig. 40.11. Nonlinear distortion at 500 Hz, plotted in two manners, observed in one body-type instrument. (*A*) Distortion as a function of average acoustic gain. (*B*) Distortion as a function of gain control position. (Reprinted by permission from S. H. Lotterman and R. N. Kasten, *Journal of Speech and Hearing Research*, **10**, 3, September 1967.)

of a hearing aid. The user may sign a waiver to keep from seeing a physician, but the wording of the waiver makes it clear that the medical evaluation is definitely in the best interest of the hearing aid user. Following clearance from the physician, the user should be referred to either an audiologist or a hearing aid dealer. In the case of children, the regulation makes it clear that the hearing aid evaluation should be conducted by an audiologist. The regulation further stipulates very clear and concise information regarding the hearing aid that must be provided to the user at the

time of purchase. Information must be provided on maintenance and care of the hearing aid, replacing or recharging batteries, how and where to obtain repair service, a description of undesirable conditions, identification of known side effects associated with hearing aid use, a statement that a hearing aid will not restore normal hearing and will not prevent or improve an organic hearing impairment, a statement that infrequent hearing aid use in most cases does not allow attainment of full benefit from the aid and a statement that hearing aid use is only part of hearing habilitation. Hearing aid users are also advised to seek prompt medical attention if they have any of the following conditions:

1. Visible congenital or traumatic deformity of the ear.
2. History of active drainage from the ear within the previous 90 days.
3. History of sudden or rapidly progressive hearing loss within the previous 90 days.
4. Acute or chronic dizziness.
5. Unilateral hearing loss of sudden or recent onset within the previous 90 days.
6. Audiometric air-bone gap equal to or greater than 15 dB at 500, 1000 and 2000 Hz.
7. Visible evidence of significant cerumen accumulation or a foreign body in the ear canal.

The FDA regulation warns:

Special care should be exercised in selecting and fitting a hearing aid whose maximum sound pressure level exceeds 132 dB because there may be risk of impairing the remaining hearing of the hearing aid user.

This type of warning is long over due, particularly with regard to young hearing-impaired children. This warning will not eliminate the manufacture or sale of high powered hearing aids, but it will make it clear to the purchaser that greater than ordinary care must be taken for the protection of the hearing aid user.

With the advent of federal regulations, it becomes necessary for all individuals associated with hearing aid evaluation, fitting and sales to also become fully conversant with the regulations and their implications. Hopefully, a highly informed and highly motivated hearing health team will be able to provide even more efficient amplification for the hearing impaired public.

REFERENCES

American standard methods for measurement of electroacoustic characteristics of hearing aids, S3.3-1960 (R-1971). New York: American National Standards Institute, 1960.

American standard methods of expressing hearing aid performance, S3.8-1967 (R-1971). New York: American National Standards Institute, 1967.

American standard method for coupler calibration of earphones, S3.7-1973. New York: American National Standards Institute, 1973.

American national standard for specification of hearing aid characteristics, ASA STD7-1976 (ANSI S3.22-1976). New York: American National Standards Institute, 1976.

Bang, B. E., Nonlinear distortion measurement by wide band noise. Paper presented before Fourth International Congress on Acoustics, 1962.

Bode, D. L., and Kasten, R. N., Hearing aid distor-

tion and consonant identification. *J. Speech Hear. Res.*, 14, 323–331, 1971.

Briskey, R. J., Greenbaum, W. H., and Sinclair, J. C., Pitfalls in hearing aid response curves. Paper presented before the 13th Annual Spring Convention of Audio Engineering Society, 1966.

Burnett, E. D., A new method for the measurement of nonlinear distortion using a random noise test signal. *Bull. Prosthetics Res.* (BPR 10-7), 79-92, 1967.

Del Polito, G. A., A new method of subjective and objective intelligibility performance with hearing aid processed speech. Unpublished master's thesis, Purdue University, 1967.

Food and Drug Administration Rules and Regulations Regarding Hearing Aid Devices: Professional and Patient Labeling and Conditions for Sale, Part IV, Federal Register, 9286-9296, February 15, 1977.

Griffing, T. S., and Preves, D. A., In-the-ear aids, Part I. *Hearing Instruments*, 27, 22–24, 1976a.

Griffing, T. S., and Preves, D. A., In-the-ear aids, Part II. *Hearing Instruments*, 27, 12–14 and 56, 1976b.

H.A.I.C. standard method of expressing hearing-aid performance. New York: Hearing Aid Industry Conference, 1961.

H.A.I.C. standards for hearing aids. New York: Hearing Aid Industry Conference, 1975.

Harris, J., Haines, H., Kelsey, R., and Clack, T., The relation between speech intelligibility and the electroacoustic characteristics of low fidelity circuitry. *J. Aud. Res.*, 1, 357–381, 1961.

Heide, J., Hearing aid testing: an analysis of the new specifications of hearing aid characteristics. *Hearing Instruments*, 28, 12–13 and 36, 1977.

Holden, S. D., The hearing aid: an engineer's perspective. Excerpts from *Acoustics for Amplification*, pp. 1–17, 1975.

IEC Recommended methods for measurement of the electro-acoustical characteristics of hearing aids, Publication 118. Geneva: International Electrotechnical Commission, 1959.

International Telephonic Consultative Committee, Document No. 11 of the meeting of the "Commission Mixte" CCIF/UIR, 1937.

Jeffers, J., Quality judgment in hearing aid selection. *J. Speech Hear. Disord.*, 25, 259–266, 1960.

Jerger, J., Behavioral correlates of hearing-aid performance. *Bull. Prosthet. Res.*, 10, 62–75, 1967.

Jerger, J., Speaks, C., and Malmquist, C., Hearing-aid performance and hearing-aid selection. *J. Speech Hear. Res.*, 9, 136–149, 1966.

Jerger, J., and Thelin, J., Effects of electroacoustic characteristics of hearing aids on speech understanding. *Bull. Prosthet. Res.*, 11, 159–197, 1968.

Kasten, R. N., Electroacoustic measurement of hearing aids. Paper presented at the American Speech and Hearing Association Convention, 1968.

Kasten, R. N., and Lotterman, S. H., The influence of hearing aid gain control rotation on acoustic gain. *J. Aud. Res.*, 9, 35–39, 1969.

Kasten, R. N., Lotterman, S. H., and Burnett, E. D., The influence of nonlinear distortion on hearing aid processed speech. Paper presented at the American Speech and Hearing Association Convention,1967.

Kasten, R. N., Body and over the ear hearing aids. In J. Katz (Ed.) *Handbook of Clinical Audiology*. Baltimore: Williams & Wilkins Co., 1972.

Lotterman, S. H., and Kasten, R. N., The influence of gain control rotation on nonlinear distortion in hearing aids. *J. Speech Hear. Res. ,* 10, 593–599, 1967.

Lybarger, S. F., Standardized hearing aid measurements. *Audecibel,* 10, 8–10 and 24–25, 1961.

Lybarger, S. F., Performance measurements on ear-level hearing aids. Paper presented at the 17th Annual Fall Convention of Audio Engineering Society, 1965.

Lybarger, S. F., A profile of ASA STD7-1976. *Hearing Instruments,* 28, 10–11 and 36, 1977.

Miller, J., and Niemoeller, A., Hearing aid design and evaluation for a patient with a severe discrimination loss for speech. *J. Speech Hear. Res.,* 10, 367–372, 1967.

Olsen, W., and Wilber, S., Physical performance characteristics of different hearing aids and speech discrimination scores achieved with them by hearing impaired persons. Paper pre-sented at American Speech and Hearing Association Convention, 1967.

Olsen, W., and Wilber, S., Hearing aid distortion and speech intelligibility. Paper presented at American Speech and Hearing Association Convention, 1968.

Pollack, M. C., Electroacoustic Characteristics. In M. Pollack (Ed.) *Amplification for the Hearing Impaired*. New York: Grune & Stratton, 1975.

Preves, D. A., and Griffing, T. S., In-the-ear aids, Part III. *Hearing Instruments,* 27, 16–17, 1976a.

Preves, D. A., and Griffing, T. S., In-the-ear aids, Part IV. *Hearing Instruments,* 27, 16–17 and 32, 1976b.

Smaldino, J., Prediction of speech understanding through hearing aids. Paper presented at the American Speech and Hearing Association Convention, Washington, D.C., 1975a.

Smaldino, J., Estimation of speech intelligibility from electroacoustic characteristics of hearing aids. Paper presented at the American Speech and Hearing Association Convention, Washington, D. C., 1975b.

Witter, H. L., Quality judgments of hearing aid transduced speech. *J. Speech Hear. Res.,* 14, 312–322, 1971.

chapter **41**

BINAURAL HEARING AIDS AND NEW INNOVATIONS

Robert J. Briskey, M.A.

BINAURAL HEARING

Binaural hearing is the ability of a person to receive a signal through both ears. It has been the subject of experimentation for over a century. The type of signal, defined by the acoustic properties of frequency, intensity, time, phase or other measurements, may not be as critical as the fact that some part of the acoustic characteristics must be sensed through each ear. The ability of a person to use binaural hearing effectively in an acoustic environment appears to be a subjective and psychological experience supported by objective test data.

Studies in binaural hearing have concentrated on the advantages of two ears which produce measurable differences. By measurable difference we mean improvement observed when two ears are compared to the results obtained using only one ear or monaural stimulation.

If we consider threshold audiometry as a basic test and the results fundamental to the understanding of the performance of each ear as a separate sense organ, we might look at the results for the two ears at pure tone threshold levels. At threshold using pure tones there is a difference in hearing which has an advantage of approximately 3 dB of sensitivity when comparing binaural to monaural listening (Keys, 1947; Shaw, Newman and Hirsh, 1947). This advantage has been observed when the two ears are identical. If one ear is better than the other by any noticeable degree then this improvement is insignificant as the two ears perform in a manner similar to the better one alone. A similar threshold advantage has been reported for speech as well (DiCarlo and Brown, 1960). Although a binaural threshold difference is important it is not as meaningful as the increased binaural dB advantage observed at higher levels of loudness. Others have reported a binaural summation which results in a loudness difference of 10 to 12 dB as the signal is increased to suprathreshold levels (Fletcher and Munson, 1933). Levels of sound pressure up to 90 dB appear to enhance the binaural advantage of loudness over monaural.

Binaural listening provides a greater sensitivity to difference limens (DL) for frequency and intensity (Licklider, 1951; Shower and Biddulph, 1931; Stevens and Davis, 1938). The DLs are smaller for each, however, they are dependent on frequency and intensity. The smallest DLs appear with the higher frequencies and, as noted earlier, at higher intensities. At this early point in our discussion of binaural hearing we can observe that this summation effect results in the processing of different information by the two ears. The differences become the first noticeable point to remember when considering binaural hearing, as they combine into an advantage of two ears over one. In considering the binaural advantage we may also consider earedness, in which one ear is superior to the other in processing certain forms of acoustic information (Liberman et al., 1967). This advantage can be measured by using various dichotic presentation procedures (Berlin et al., 1973; Studdert-Kennedy and Shankweiler, 1970; Beiter and Sharf, 1976; and Danaher and Pickett, 1975). Each ear, through a greater capacity to react to one acoustic cue or several, would then be able to provide a combined difference resulting in enhanced binaural information. Two ears and their combining characteristic produce differences which are of a greater magnitude than the one acoustic dimension measured monaurally.

Without binaural hearing, complete localization of all sound sources would not be possible. This is a basic function of our two ears. The ability to localize will vary depending on the signal, its duration and of course its intensity (Searle et al., 1975; Butler, 1970; Bosatra and Russolo, 1976).

We already know that binaural hearing has provided some advantages for intensity. Binaural hearing also provides difference information in duration or time. An acoustic signal will be received by one ear earlier than the other. The arrival of a signal at one ear will tend to lead the individual in the direction of that sound.

This directional ability is further influenced by the nature of the signal. If the signal is of long duration it takes a longer time to localize the sound and it requires a head movement to optimize the head shadow effect. This does not appear to be true in sounds of short duration. The short signal provides clues that result in a perception of localization based on the combination of different auditory information, mediated in the brain (Matykeo, 1959). While intensity may be one of the primary characteristics for localizing on a continuous sound, time and phase differences appear to provide the basic information with signals of short duration (Thompson, 1877; Licklider, 1948; Hirsh, 1948;

Guttman, 1962; David, Guttman and Van Bergerijk, 1958; Perrott and Nelson, 1969; Deatherage and Evans, 1969).

Localization on a sound source has been used as a technique in audiometry (Jerger et al., 1969). In using directional audiometry it is noted that individuals with sensory-neural impairments have very little difficulty in localizing on the correct angle or direction of a signal. Persons with retrocochlear lesions reportedly have greater difficulty (Nordlund, 1964). This form of audiometry would appear to provide additional diagnostic information.

Localization testing using both horizontal and vertical sound sources has indicated some directional patterning with the hearing impaired. With the subjects investigated a confusion was created when the two directions of horizontal and vertical sources were combined. This acoustic environment was created by mounting 24 speakers in a large cage called the LTA (localization testing apparatus). The positioning of the speakers and the programming of the stimulus allowed for angular directional changes combining both horizontal and vertical sound sources. When the short duration signal was presented at a sufficiently high level to offset the hearing level of the individual and then compared with the score when using binaural hearing aids at a reduced signal level, the pattern of the localgram was similar (Briskey and Sundquist, 1966).

Localization is based on the detection of interaural time differences. The interaural time differences sensed by the two ears will vary depending on the acoustic characteristics of the signal (Perrott and Nelson, 1969; Perrott, 1974). Time differences of as little as 0.5 msec will provide an improvement in the word discrimination score (Schubert and Schultz, 1962). This improvement increases as the time difference is increased. The interaural time advantage is further enhanced by frequency selection. The higher the frequency the greater the information provided by the interaural difference (Hirsh, 1950).

The auditory system is designed to favor binaural over monaural hearing. This is vividly illustrated when we note the use of intensity and time difference information in the processing of the complex acoustic signals of speech.

The unique acoustic signature of individual speech sounds is as complex in its elements as each of the separate measurements made in binaural hearing studies. The complex signal is significantly different as it arrives at the two ears. The frequency characteristics of an artificial head in an azimuth study show the influence of the angle of incidence (Nordlund and Fritzell, 1963). The greatest influence is on frequencies above 1 to 1.5 kHz. Sonograms of speech recorded in this study at various angles clearly demonstrated the influence of the head on higher frequencies. Frequencies from 2 kHz and up showed the greatest difference. The sentence material selected included several voiceless fricatives. The sonograms demonstrated the influence of the head on high frequencies represented in the fricative consonant phonetic elements. The vowels were influenced very little. The signal occurred within an azimuth change of as little as 30°.

Word discrimination scores with masking present were obtained monaurally for the ear near the sound source and the far ear. These scores obtained under headphones were higher for the near ear than for the far ear. In the presence of a masking signal the information contributed by the far ear was very little. Nevertheless, there was a significant improvement in intelligibility when both ears were used than when either of the ears was tested alone. Individuals with unilateral hearing losses demonstrate considerably reduced word discrimination scores when tested in a noisy environment (Nordlund and Fritzell, 1963).

The summation of binaural information was demonstrated by Bocca (1955). Monaural discrimination in one ear was reduced by the acoustic filtering while the other ear showed a poor word discrimination score (WDS) due to a faint level of presentation. When these separate signals were presented binaurally the discrimination score was nearly perfect. The two partial and dissimilar signals are mediated at higher levels than the sense organ resulting in a perception of the whole. The amount of acoustic information necessary to be added by a second ear appears to be infinitely small to achieve good intelligibility of speech (Huizing and Taselaar, 1961).

An example of this small difference producing a meaningful cueing may be found in the careful study of the interaural phase difference performance of the two ears. In studies performed using speech and noise in phase and out of phase, intelligibility was superior when the antiphasic signals were presented under earphones (Schubert, 1956). If we consider the reverberation in a typical real life acoustic environment, we can add the factor of interaural phase difference as another infinitely small bit of information supplementing the binaural combination of differences. Masking is also affected by the phase relationship binaurally (Wightman, 1969). A practical observation of this difference apparently providing the hearing impaired more information is noted by merely supplying a person with binaural hearing aids that are 180° out of phase with each other. Individuals experience a greater capacity for processing the binaural information in this antiphasic condition and accept the use of amplification more readily (Briskey, 1975).

The complex physical differences in the signals arriving at the two ears are compared. When this difference is mediated at higher levels of the auditory system, the person will have a better spatial separation resulting in a greater ease in attending to the preferred acoustic signal. The differences resulting from the combination of two-ear-hearing produce the cueing and clueing necessary to select out of a multiple acoustic array the one signal to which we wish to attend. Once we have been able to select the signal the higher brain centers continue to selectively process that part of the signal and we are able to listen more effectively to the wanted or primary signal with binaural hearing (Spieth and Webster, 1955; McSayers and Cherry, 1957; Perrott, Briggs and Perrott, 1970; Findlay and Schuchman, 1976).

The literature further describes a neurophysiologic action of suppression which adds to the total difference between ears (Klinke, Boerger and Gruber, 1969; Koenig, 1950). This suppression tends to reduce the sensitivity of one ear. This reduction of the background noise in the ear that is not attending to a primary signal will provide an enhancement of discrimination or localization on the part of an individual in conversation. What this suggests is that one ear is capable of ignoring or suppressing signals that are unwanted. This squelch may also result in an improvement in intelligibility in a reverberant environment binaurally when compared to monaural listening (Gelfand and Hochberg, 1976). The system is capable of taking a multiple input and ferreting out, as a result of a storing and sorting, the identifying characteristics in certain environments which the individual wishes to follow. Angle of incidence or free head movement further enhance this situation with head shadow.

The reduction of the intensity on the far ear assists in the spatial separation. This spatial separation of complex auditory signal in an environment might very well be compared to the interaural phase or intensity differences observed when in an experimental condition. When we listen to two individuals speaking, it is easier for us to shift our attention from one voice to the other and distinguish them as the two voices are separated in space. In this spatial separation of binaural hearing it should be noted that the individual must shift his attention from one source to another. Although the two ears may function independently it is necessary for the individual to select, on the basis of some quality of difference, the signal that he wishes to monitor. Although each ear functions as an independent sense organ and can be measured as an independent unit it is not

possible for an individual to separately listen to two independent signals as a result of the summation of the binaural act (Cherry and Taylor, 1954; Bilsen, 1976).

Included in these factors of differences is the discussion of an ear dominance. Although each sense organ is capable of receiving all auditory information, there is evidence that one ear may process certain of the small dimensional characteristics of the signal differently than the other. Through the combination of the differences we are able to use auditory clues in a meaningful way (McFadden and Pasanen, 1976).

BINAURAL AMPLIFICATION FOR THE HEARING IMPAIRED

Binaural hearing aids make it possible for an individual to be able to listen to someone on either side without having the head shadow effect interfere with hearing the information. This becomes particularly important in conferences and meetings where the one eared listener is at an extreme disadvantage.

When we discuss a wearable binaural hearing aid we mean two complete hearing aids or one for each ear. The sound patterns striking the microphones of the two hearing aids are not identical in time, phase or intensity, therefore the sequence of excitatory events reaching one ear is not only independent of, but also different from the sequence reaching the other ear. It is this fact that gives the binaural system its potential for sharp superiority over either a monaural system or an arrangement where one amplifier supplies stimuli to both ears.

The conventional Y cord should not be considered as binaural hearing as it uses only a single amplifier divided to two earphones. The Y cord provides bilateral stimulation but not binaural.

The utilization of CROS (contralateral routing of signals) amplification provides still a different form of directional aid to the user (Harford and Dodds, 1966; Rintelman, Harford and Burchfield, 1970). The application of the CROS on the unilateral loss does give the person an awareness of the sound source on the otherwise impaired side by the presence of the microphone on that side. However, the signal is amplified and presented to the normal or near normal ear providing a monaural fitting with a cueing resulting in a directional ability not normally experienced by the person with a unilateral loss. These people will report an ability to know the signal is coming from the side where the microphone is located by an awareness of a different sound quality amplified by the aid. This appears to provide binaural hearing, but instead it is giving directional assistance to the person.

CROS amplification has made a significant contribution to the hearing impaired not only providing hearing to the classical unilateral loss but providing assistance to many other types of losses. The most important aspect of the fitting is the use of the open ear mold. The CROS provides information for many types of sloping losses with feedback being reduced as a result of the placement of the microphone on the side of the head opposite the receiver and open mold.

This same type of assistance can be achieved with binaural instruments using open molds. The determinant is the amount of gain necessary to provide the person with the high frequency clueing supplied by the aid. If the gain need is great, a monaural CROS fitting may be necessary. If, on the other hand, the gain requirements are not too great, a binaural fitting using open molds will result in a satisfactory fitting.

BICROS (bilateral CROS) amplification utilizing two microphones, one amplifier and presenting the signal to only one ear is another form of the same amplification. Some BICROS users will experience difficulty in the use of the amplifying system. This appears to occur as a result of the slight differences created by the two microphones in the various dimensions of sound being amplified to only one ear.

These variations of bilateral stimulation and monaural stimulation through a variety of placements of the microphone should not be considered binaural amplification. In some instances of CROS/BICROS fitting the person may have an ability to localize a sound source with greater ability enhancing their directional hearing, but the hearing aid systems do not provide a true binaural stimulation.

The binaural system utilizing two aids generally requires less gain and less power output than one instrument alone. The additional sensitivity is noted with the use of a second ear which produces a summing effect resulting in the need for less stimulation. This suggests that binaural instruments with less gain may be used beneficially and generally result in a more normal rehabilitation of an individual.

The primary purpose of rehabilitation is to give the hard of hearing person a greater understanding of speech. Binaural hearing has been found to be superior to monaural hearing in noisy environments (Belzile and Markle, 1959). When speech was delivered at a level higher than the ambient noise there appeared to be no significant advantage to binaural hearing. However, when speech was lowered to a level approximating the sound pressure level of the noise binaural hearing did, in fact, provide cues resulting in improved discrimination scores. This position has been supported by other individuals indicating that binaural hearing does provide the ability to separate out one signal as a result of the multiple cues from acoustic inputs received by the two ears (Koenig, 1950; Harris, 1965; Gelfand and Hochberg, 1976; Carhart, 1958). The binaural user can localize and attend to the particular signal more easily and, therefore, improve his proficiency in understanding what is being said.

In the fitting of hearing aids for children, audiologists have revised their thinking and many now recommend a hearing aid for each ear. In a survey of clinical audiologists 44% indicated that binaural hearing aid fittings were always beneficial with children and an additional 39% supported binaural fittings under selected conditions (Zenith, 1971). Although two body type instruments may not provide accurate localization or directionality because of their proximity on the body, they are recommended because with binaural stimulation the child is receiving additional information of sufficient magnitude to warrant their use. In order to enhance directional training, instruments have been placed on the front and the back of the child.

Several studies have attempted to evaluate the reports of subjects using binaural hearing aids. The users tend to report such things as speech being subjectively more clear or easier to understand or greater fidelity or greater ease or less effort to listen. The reports are all subjective inasmuch as it has been difficult to actually measure these reported improvements. Possibly directional audiometry may assist in differentiating significant discrimination scores using binaural hearing or some form of localization testing can measure a more practical application of the two aids.

Binaural hearing may be demonstrated best by using two hearing aids with somewhat different acoustic characteristics. The variation between the two aids will enable the individual to summate the two signals and thereby produce a noticeable enhancement (Danaher and Pickett, 1975).

The benefits of binaural hearing may be demonstrated more easily with a different approach to the testing procedure. The testing should come closer to simulating that which is experienced in real life. The value of binaural hearing can be noted with the placement of one hearing aid on an individual and testing in the presence of a variety of different ambient noise situations and then adding the second aid. This testing procedure provides the person with the opportunity of experiencing the value of the aided auditory information in a more life-like situation.

During the testing the person should be allowed free head movement. The movement of the head will provide the natural adjustment of the angle of incidence of the selected sound enhancing the binaural condition. Utilizing a multidirectional source of competing inputs and adding the free movement of the head will evaluate a binaural hearing aid as binaural hearing is utilized by normal hearing individuals. It is difficult to evolve a test measurement that will clearly indicate the advantage of two hearing aids.

Binaural hearing is the optimal method of rehabilitating hearing-impaired individuals. Binaural, therefore, becomes the basic premise upon which future hearing amplification should be based. There are many auditory events which are processed binaurally that are interrelated and produce the difference of the combination. Binaural hearing aids should be analyzed and designed with the difference of either ears or instruments as the basic consideration. As indicated earlier, phase difference used in binaural amplification through hearing aids appears to be subjectively different to the individual. This phase difference may be slight when we consider the complexity of the speech signal. However, to the individual it becomes a different signal and the brain is capable of processing the differences apparently resulting in a greater ease in attending. This is one way to change the characteristics of the acoustic signal of an aid leaving the frequency response, gain and power output unchanged on instruments.

Binaural hearing combines two acoustic signals. This combination is then analyzed for differences. These differences provide the person with bits of information that add to the basic acoustic signal the dimensions of localization, foreground, background, separation and other subjective reactions to binaural hearing. The person with a bilaterally symmetrical hearing loss may benefit, therefore, if the differences of the acoustic signal are made larger at the time they are presented binaurally. Providing the person with two signals different in gain, power output, frequency response or any other characteristic of the hearing aids would stimulate the auditory mechanism to react in a more normal way and process the difference information. This would provide a more complementary acoustic signal making it different at the ears. To attempt to select amplification to "replace" that which is impaired in shape and gain is virtually impossible and may also be the least desirable way of serving the total auditory mechanism. This is a different approach in the assessment of binaural function with amplification.

Even with standard test procedures a review of the results will give a general profile of the individual who can benefit from binaural hearing aids. Satisfaction will be predicated on the

selection of hearing aids with the correct saturation sound pressure level (SSPL) to prevent acoustic insult. Standard clinical procedure will provide several general areas which will assist in making the initial decision regarding binaural hearing aid selection.

1. The average of 500, 1000 and 2000 Hz should be 15 dB or less between ears.
2. Two of the three frequencies—500, 1000 or 2000 Hz—must be 15 dB or less between ears.
3. The discrimination scores should be within 8% of each other.
4. The dB value of the uncomfortable listening (UCL) on the two ears should be within 6 dB of each other.
5. The dB value of the most comfortable listening (MCL) on the two ears should be within 6 dB of each other.
6. There should be a high activity index.

It is not necessary to obtain agreement in all 6 of these areas. Experience indicates that a successful binaural fitting can be achieved by considering either 1 or 2; any two of 3, 4 and 5; and always have 6. There are exceptions to this recommendation but they are generally extreme cases. These recommendations are designed to provide a practical and workable guide which are applicable in a majority of the situations.

After the initial selection it is important to fit the appropriate combination of slopes. Generally the ear advantage is optimized with a higher frequency emphasis slope to the right ear and with a less high, or medium slope to the left ear. These variations may be achieved either through the alteration of the tone positions on the aid, or through acoustic modification of the earmold. The acoustic modifications dictating an "open mold" or "tube" fitting on the right ear and a small parallel vent on the left achieves maximum user satisfaction when listening in noise or a highly reverberant environment.

The discussion in this chapter does not permit a full expansion of a specific activity index. The concept is easily understood if the dispenser considers an active, dynamic, mobile, hearing-impaired person as having a high index as opposed to an isolated recluse type. The basic idea is to include an assessment of the individual's life style. This observation is generally made when taking a complete case history. Successful binaural users are people who are able to maintain an active and productive life with the hearing aids.

New concepts in hearing aids require new approaches in their assessment. The change in the designs of aids must be evaluated as suprathreshold signals as they are received at the ear in a more natural setting. In the typical audiologic assessment variations of time, phase and intensity normally found in life situations plus multiple signals received by the normal hearing binaural system are generally not simulated. The individual may use one set of difference information in one listening situation while a different set of difference information is important in another situation. If we consider these differences as the contributory factors to good localization and the ability to discriminate in the presence of noise then the hearing aids should be designed to compensate with a dissidence in one or several of the dimensions sensitive to the binaural system.

HEARING AIDS OF THE FUTURE

In the design of future hearing aids some new thinking may be necessary. The amount of gain that is necessary for a hard of hearing individual may become a relatively constant figure. The amount of improvement that can be achieved through this gain can be a function of frequency response and have a certain physiologic limitation.

Power output and peak clipping become a very important part of the processing of information. Evidence has been generated in the past years to suggest that peak clipping actually enhances intelligibility in some cases. The traditional thinking of hearing aid amplification has indicated that peak clipping should be considered as undesirable. Forms of peak clipping in communication systems do enhance discrimination in the presence of noise. Peak clipping, therefore, is a method whereby we may improve the intelligibility of the signal to an ear by eliminating unwanted and unneeded acoustic information.

Studies have indicated that information in low frequencies is meaningful to individuals in providing the necessary tonal quality for voice reproduction (Briskey and Sinclair, 1966; Briskey et al., 1967). Frequencies from 100 Hz to approximately 500 Hz appear to influence the development of more normal voice quality in profoundly deaf individuals. In individuals with mild to moderate losses the frequencies from 500 to 700 Hz appear to provide a subjective quality of smoothness. In the development of the instrument, therefore, some consideration should be made in terms of the relative value of the energies between 500 to 700 Hz and 2000 Hz for mild to moderate losses. If we consider that 70% of the intelligibility of speech is in the information provided in the second formant of the speech signal from approximately 700 to 3000 Hz, it might be possible to supplement this acoustic information in one ear with some dissimilar cueing system in the other. This analysis of the differences between the ears may aid the individual's ability to use

binaural hearing (Franklin, 1975). This would also aid us in knowing how to use monaural hearing more effectively if we understood the function of one ear in relationship to the other in some dimension other than sensitivity.

REFERENCES

Beiter, R. C., and Sharf, D. J., Influence of encoding and acoustic similarity on the ear advantage and lag effect in dichotic listening. *J. Speech Hear. Res.*, 19, 78–92, 1976.

Belzile, M., and Markle, D. M., A clinical comparison of monaural and binaural hearing aids worn by patients with conductive or perceptive deafness. *Laryngoscope*, 69, 1317–1323, 1959.

Berlin, C., Lowe-Bell, S., Cullen, J., Thompson, C., and Hughes, L., Dichotic signs of right ear advantage and temporal offset effects. *J. Acoust. Soc. Am.*, 53, 699–709, 1973.

Bilsen, F. A., Pronounced binaural pitch phenomenon. *J. Acoust. Soc. Am.*, 59, 467–468, 1976.

Bocca, E., Binaural hearing; another approach. *Laryngoscope*, 65, 1164–1171, 1955.

Bosatra, A., and Russolo, M., Directional hearing, temporal order and auditory pattern in peripheral and brain stem lesions. *Audiology*, 15, 141–151, 1976.

Briskey, R. J., U. S. Patent 3,894,196, 1975.

Briskey, R. J., and Sinclair, J., The importance of low frequency amplification in deaf children. *Audecibel*, Winter, 7–20, 1966.

Briskey, R. J., and Sundquist, J. H., Procedures and experimental application of localization tests. *Proceedings of the Symposium on Biomedical Engineering*, Vol. I. Milwaukee: Marquette University, 1966.

Briskey, R. J., Garrison, M. J., Owsley, P., and Sinclair, J., Effects of hearing aids on deaf speech. *Audecibel*, Fall, 173–188, 1967.

Butler, R. A., The effect of hearing impairment on locating sound in the vertical plane. *Int. Audiol.*, 9, 117–126, 1970.

Carhart, R., The usefulness of the binaural hearing aid. *J. Speech Hear. Disord.*, 23, 41–51, 1958.

Cherry, E. C., and Taylor, W. K., Some further experiments upon the recognition of speech with one and with two ears. *J. Acoust. Soc. Am.*, 26, 554–559, 1954.

Danaher, E. M., and Pickett, J. M., Some masking effects produced by low-frequency vowel formants in persons with sensorineural hearing loss. *J. Speech Hear. Res.*, 18, 261–271, 1975.

David, E. E., Jr., Guttman, N., and Van Bergerijk, W. A., On the mechanism of binaural fusion. *J. Acoust. Soc. Am.*, 30, 801–802, 1958.

Deatherage, B., and Evans, T., Binaural masking; backward, forward and simultaneous effects. *J. Acoust. Soc. Am.*, 46, 362–371, 1969.

DiCarlo, L. M., and Brown, W. J., The effectiveness of binaural hearing for adults with hearing impairments. *J. Aud. Res.*, 1, 35–76, 1960.

Findlay, R. C., and Schuchman, G. I., Masking level difference for speech; effects of ear dominance and age. *Audiology*, 15, 232–241, 1976.

Fletcher, H., and Munson, W. A., Loudness-Its definition, measurement and calculations. *J. Acoust. Soc. Am.*, 5, 82–106, 1933.

Franklin, B., The effect of combining low- and high-frequency passbands on consonant recognition in the hearing impaired. *J. Speech Hear. Res.,* 18, 719–727, 1975.

Gelfand, S. A., and Hochberg, I., Binaural and monaural speech discrimination under reverberation. *Audiology,* 15, 72–84, 1976.

Guttman, N., A mapping of binaural click lateralizations. *J. Acoust. Soc. Am.,* 34, 87–92, 1962.

Harford, E., and Dodds, E., The clinical application of CROS. *Arch. Otolaryngol.,* 83, 455–464, 1966.

Harris, J. D., Monaural and binaural speech intelligibility and the stereophonic effect based on temporal cues. *Laryngoscope,* 75, 428–446, 1965.

Hirsh, I. J., The influence of interaural phase on interaural summation and inhibiton. *J. Acoust. Soc. Am.,* 20, 536–544, 1948.

Hirsh, I. J., The relation between localization and intelligibility. *J. Acoust. Soc. Am.,* 22, 196–200, 1950.

Huizing, H. C., and Taselaar, M., Experiments on binaural hearing. *Acta Otolaryngol.,* 53, 151–154, 1961.

Jerger, J., Weikers, N., Sharbrough, F., III, and Jerger, S., Bilateral lesions of the temporal lobe. *Acta Otolaryngol.* Suppl. 258, 1–51, 1969.

Keys, J. W., Binaural versus monaural hearing. *J. Acoust. Soc. Am.,* 19, 629–631, 1947.

Klinke, R., Boerger, G., and Gruber, J., Alteration of afferent, tone-evoked activity and neurons of the cochlear nucleus following acoustic stimulation of the contralateral ear. *J. Acoust. Soc. Am.,* 45, 788–789, 1969.

Koenig, W., Subjective effects in binaural hearing. *J. Acoust. Soc. Am.,* 22, 61–62, 1950.

Liberman, A. M., Cooper, F. S., Shankweiler, D. P., and Studdert-Kennedy, M., Perception of the speech code. *Psychol. Rev.,* 74, 431–461, 1967.

Licklider, J. C. R., The influence of interaural phase relations upon the masking of speech by white noise. *J. Acoust. Soc. Am.,* 20, 150–159, 1948.

Licklider, J. C. R., Correlates of auditory stimulus. In Stevens, S. S. (Ed.), *Handbook of Experimental Psychology,* p. 1031. New York: John Wiley & Sons, 1951.

Matykeo, J., Attempts at explanation of directional hearing on the basis of very fine time differences registration. *Translation Beltone Inst. Hear. Res.,* 12, 4–5, 1959.

McFadden, D., and Pasanen, E. G., Lateralization at high frequencies based on interaural time differences. *J. Acoust. Soc. Am.,* 59, 634–639, 1976.

McSayers, B. A., and Cherry, E. C., Mechanism of binaural fusion in the hearing of speech. *J. Acoust. Soc. Am.,* 29, 973–987, 1957.

Nordlund, B., Directional audiometry. *Acta Otolaryngol.,* 57, 1–18, 1964.

Nordlund, B., and Fritzell, B., The influence of azimuth on speech signals. *Acta Otolaryngol.,* 56, 632–642, 1963.

Perrott, D. R., Auditory apparent motion. *J. Aud. Res.,* 14, 163–169, 1974.

Perrott, D., Briggs, R. and Perrott, S., Binaural fusion, its limits as defined by signal duration and signal onset. *J. Acoust. Soc. Am.,* 47, 565–568, 1970.

Perrott, D., and Nelson, M., Limits of the detection of binaural beats. *J. Acoust. Soc. Am.* 46, 1477–1481, 1969.

Rintelman, W., Harford, E., and Burchfield, S., A special case of auditory localization. *Arch. Otolaryngol.,* 91, 284–288, 1970.

Schubert, E. D., Some preliminary experiments on binaural time delay and intelligibility. *J. Acoust. Soc. Am.,* 28, 895–901, 1956.

Schubert, E. D., and Schultz, M. C., Some aspects of binaural signal detection. *J. Acoust. Soc. Am.,* 34, 844–849, 1962.

Searle, C. L., Braida, L. D., Cuddy, D. R., and Davis, M. F., Binaural pinna disparity; another auditory localization cue. *J. Acoust. Soc. Am.,* 57, 448–455, 1975.

Shaw, W. A., Newman, E. B., and Hirsh, I. J., The difference between monaural and binaural threshold. *J. Exp. Psychol.,* 37, 229–242, 1947.

Shower, E. G., and Biddulph, R., Differential pitch sensitivity of the ear. *J. Acoust. Soc. Am.,* 3, 275–287, 1931.

Spieth, W., and Webster, J. C., Listening to differentially filtered competing voice messages. *J. Acoust. Soc. Am.,* 27, 866–871, 1955.

Stevens, S. S., and Davis, H., *Hearing, Its Psychology and Physiology.* New York: John Wiley & Sons, 1938.

Studdert-Kennedy, M., and Shankweiler, D., Hemispheric specialization for speech perception. *J. Acoust. Soc. Am.,* 48, 579–594, 1970.

Thompson, S. P., The phenomena of binaural audition. I. *Philosophy Magazine,* 4, 274–276, 1877.

Wightman, F., Binaural masking with sine-wave maskers. *J. Acoust. Soc. Am.,* 45, 72–78, 1969.

Zenith, *Collection of Shared Letters,* Vol. II, Number 2, 1971.

chapter 42

EARMOLDS

Samuel F. Lybarger, B.S.

The total performance of a hearing aid is determined by the interaction of the microphone, amplifier and the earphone-earmold characteristics modified by the acoustical properties of the body, head and ear canal.

By earmold is meant not only the plastic plug made to fit a particular ear, but also its drilling, venting, damping and any associated sound conducting tubes which carry sound from the exit nub of the hearing aid or hearing aid earphone (receiver) to the ear canal.

EARMOLD MATERIAL

The principal earmold materials (Caine, 1974) and some of their major characteristics are as follows.

Hard Acrylic. This is by far the most used material. The usual form is crystal clear, which is very good cosmetically. Acrylic accepts a high polish and is comfortable to wear if correctly made. Tubing can be easily and firmly cemented. It is largely free from allergic affects.

Flexible Acrylic. This is used where a softer material is needed for comfort, safety and/or a better seal. It is very useful for small children's earmolds. The durability of this type of material is less than for hard material.

Combination hard acrylic outer portion with flexible acrylic tip. This combination gives the good cosmetic and mechanical properties of hard acrylic outside and provides a flexible tip which may give greater comfort when a tight seal is required in the canal.

Silicone. A flexible material that is quite inert and that is used primarily where a very tight seal is required for high gain aids. It also is very useful for infant's and children's earmolds where softness is important. Silicone is the most frequently used material for "make-it-yourself" earmolds. Tubing attachment and replacement are not as easy as on acrylic earmolds.

Polyethylene. Rarely used except where a user has an allergy problem with other materials. It is difficult to polish to a smooth finish.

Because all earmold material, in comparison with air, is relatively heavy and nonyielding, sound transmission through the earmold hole is not significantly affected by the choice of material (Lybarger, 1958). The wall thickness of the plastic tubing on earmolds can affect transmission slightly and sound radiation moderately if too thin.

EARMOLD TUBING

Earmold tubing is almost universally made from special formulations of polyvinyl chloride compounded to give the needed flexibility and color and to reduce the leaching out of plasticizers by perspiration as much as possible. Eventually, perspiration causes tubing to stiffen and discolor.

The National Association of Earmold Laboratories (Radcliffe, 1974) standardized a series of earmold tubing diameters to reduce the wide assortment of sizes. Table 42.1 lists the NAEL sizes. Earmolds can be specified with any of the NAEL sizes of tubing from most earmold laboratories.

For convenience, sizes are given in both inches and millimeters. European practice appears to be to use the same tubing numbers as in the United States, but to round off the inside diameter to tenths of millimeters (e.g., #13 = 1.9 mm, #16 = 1.4 mm).

EARMOLD CONFIGURATIONS

While various proprietary names are in use to identify earmold types, most earmolds can be classified by the terminology proposed by the NAEL (Coogle, 1970). The terms skeleton, ³/₄ skeleton, semiskeleton, canal, canal-lock, shell and half-shell applicable to tubing type molds refer primarily to the cosmetic and comfort aspects of the earmold design rather than to the acoustic properties. NAEL uses the term high frequency mold, for one having a short tip to allow a maximum of air volume between the mold and the eardrum, and the term nonoccluding mold for one which holds the tubing in or at the ear canal but leaves the ear canal open. These types have significantly different acoustic effects than the types first mentioned. The receiver type mold is generally a solid type mold provided with a snap ring to accept the nub of the receiver of a body-type hearing aid. All of these various NAEL earmold configurations are illustrated and described in detail by Delk (1975).

From an acoustical standpoint, the important features of an earmold are its tip length, the length(s) and diameter(s) of the hole(s) and/or tubing leading back to the earphone. With regard to vented mold, importance is attached to the distance from the tip back to the exit surface of a vent (for parallel vents), the size of the vent channel and the application, if any, of various adjustable or variable vents.

For acoustical classification purposes, the

simplified earmold types shown in Figure 42.1, *A* and *B*, are suggested. The dimensions given are such that the medium length tip matches the length of the coupler extension canal in the KEMAR manikin (Burkhard and Sachs, 1975). The short and long length tips are typical of actual earmolds. The distances from the tip to the outer faces of the molds were determined from the examination of typical molds. The short-hollowed configuration is usually used in "high frequency" molds, which typically have rather short, large diameter vents. The configuration in Figure 42.1*B* simulating a receiver mold with a medium tip length has the same hole length as the standard HA-2 coupler. The nonoccluding mold is not shown, but will be discussed later under venting.

TABLE 42.1 *Earmold Tubing Sizes*

NAEL Standard Size	Nominal Inside Diameter		Nominal Outside Diameter	
	inches	*mm*	*inches*	*mm*
No. 12 Standard	.085	2.16	.125	3.18
No. 13 Standard	.076	1.93	.116	2.95
No. 13 Medium	.076	1.93	.122	3.10
No. 13 Thick	.076	1.93	.130	3.30
No. 14 Standard	.066	1.68	.116	2.95
No. 15 Standard	.059	1.50	.116	2.95
No. 16 Standard	.053	1.35	.116	2.95
No. 16 Thin	.053	1.35	.085	2.16

COMPARISON OF EARPHONE AND EARMOLD RESPONSE ON 2-cc COUPLER ZWISLOCKI COUPLER AND ON REAL EARS

Sachs and Burkhard (1972a), have shown that, for closed earmold systems, the response measured on a Zwislocki coupler (e.g., as used in the KEMAR manikin) is extremely close to that measured on real ears and that it bears a rather constant relationship to the response on a 2-cc coupler for earphones typically used in hearing aids. For a given receiver and closed earmold with a constant electrical input, the sound pressure level (SPL) developed in a Zwislocki coupler is about 4 dB higher than in a 2-cc coupler for frequencies up to 800 Hz. Above this the SPL in the Zwislocki coupler rises with frequency in relation to that in the 2-cc coupler and is about 17 dB higher at 8 kHz, as shown in Figure 42.2. Thus, the performance on a Zwislocki coupler can be reasonably well predicted from the 2-cc response for a typical closed earmold situation. Lybarger (1975a) has shown that this constant relationship no longer is applicable when vents of substantial openings are used. When using venting, the Zwislocki coupler gives results that are very similar to the results of subjective or real ear measurements.

Generally, we are concerned in this chapter with the effects of changes in performance

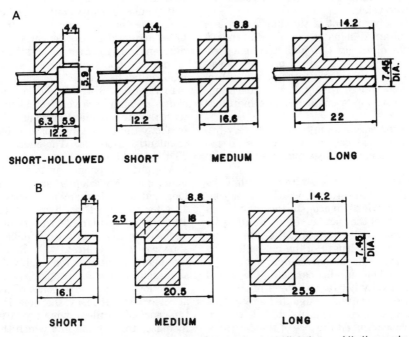

Fig. 42.1. (*A*) Suggested tubing-type earmold length classifications. All dimensions are in millimeters. (*B*) Suggested receiver-type earmold length classifications. All dimensions are in millimeters.

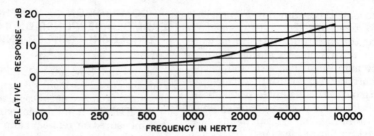

Fig. 42.2. Curve showing amount by which the response in a Zwislocki coupler exceeds that in a 2-cc coupler for a typical earphone and closed earmold situation. Data from Sachs and Burkhard (1972a).

when earmold changes are made. For closed mold conditions, the difference in results would be the same for either coupler. For vented conditions, data in this chapter are all based on Zwislocki coupler measurements.

CONVENTIONAL EARPHONE (RECEIVER) SYSTEM

Figure 42.3 shows a sectional view of the earphone-earmold-ear system when a "button" or "conventional" earphone is used. The transduction mechanism of the earphone (usually of the magnetic type) produces a vibratory force on the diaphragm, which can be most simply represented as having an effective area (S), a vibratory mass (M_D), a mechanical compliance (C_D) and some amount of mechanical resistance (R_D), all of which affect the response characteristics of the system.

Immediately in front of the diaphragm is a volume of air designated as V_1 that has a substantial effect on the high frequency response of the earphone. Sound pressure developed in cavity V_1 travels through the nub of the earphone, the relatively narrow hole diameter which acts as a small acoustic inertance (M_1).

Beyond the earphone nub, there is very frequently a second cavity (V_2), which, if too large, can adversely affect high frequency response.

The sound is then transmitted through the drilled hole in the earmold, which can be considered primarily as an acoustic inertance. This hole, because of the friction of the vibrating air with its walls, also has acoustic resistance. The diameter and length of the hole affect the response of the system materially.

From the hole in the earmold, the sound enters the cavity between the end of the earmold and the eardrum, designated as V_3. This cavity ranges from about 0.4 to 1.0 cm³ in volume, depending on the size of the ear canal and the length of the earmold tip. A value of 0.6 cm³ is probably typical for the standard type of earmold.

One wall of cavity V_3 is formed by the ear-

drum, whose effect is large in the total acoustic system under consideration. A compliant membrane such as the eardrum is the acoustic equivalent of a volume of air. For many years, the sum of V_3 and the equivalent volume of the eardrum compliance was considered to average about 2 cm³. The eardrum also includes a substantial amount of acoustical resistance.

In recent years, the acoustical impedance of the eardrum has been more accurately defined. Zwislocki (1971) designed a coupler which is comprised of acoustic networks that simulate both the compliance and resistance of the eardrum and ear canal for the frequency range of interest in hearing aids. This coupler has been further refined by Sachs and Burkhard (1972b) and is currently the subject of national and international standardization.

It should be pointed out that when a hearing aid is used on a pathologic ear, the impedance presented by the eardrum can be substantially different from the average and the performance of the earphone-earmold-ear system may be materially affected.

In Figure 42.3, the hole designated as $M_3 R_3$ shows a small-bore vent connecting cavity V_3 with the air outside. Earmolds seldom have a perfectly tight fit to the ear so a "built-in" vent frequently exists also. The effects of vents will be discussed later in this chapter.

A typical earphone-earmold response curve made on a 2-cc coupler using a hole 18 mm long and 3 mm in diameter is shown in Figure 42.4, for an "insert" or "button" type earphone. There is a considerable variety of insert earphone response curves available. The one shown is fairly typical, with the design objective being to obtain a reasonably flat response· as measured on a 2-cc coupler.

The low frequency response of the system is affected very little by the hole in a receiver type earmold, unless it is very large and thus increases the volume into which the earphone works.

The volume of air beyond the tip of the earmold (cavity V_3 in Fig. 42.3) and the impedance of the eardrum influence the low frequency response level. The greater the effective air volume is, the lower the level. If one increases V_3 by shortening the earmold tip to nearly nothing, the low frequency response might be expected to drop about 2 dB, other factors remaining constant. If one decreases V_3 by increasing the earmold length to its practical maximum, the low frequency response might be expected to increase about 2 dB. Obviously, the ear canal diameter can affect the size of cavity V_3.

The comments above concerning the effect of V_3 on the low frequency response also apply to the response at higher frequencies. Increasing V_3 will lower the whole response curve and decreasing it will raise the whole response curve, other conditions remaining the same.

In the mid-frequency range from about 800 to 2000 Hz, the earmold hole diameter and length, as well as acoustic damping inserts, affect the response. The effect of reduced hole diameter (relative to 3 mm) is indicated in Figure 42.4 by the *dashed line* curve.

When an insert earphone already has a substantial peak in the mid-range, as is often employed to obtain very high output (accompanied by a reduced high frequency cutoff), a smaller diameter hole in the earmold will lower the frequency of the peak; a larger earmold hole diameter will raise it. Similarly, a longer hole length will reduce the frequency of the peak and a shorter hole will increase it.

The earmold hole size has a considerable influence on the system response in the high frequency region near the cutoff frequency of the earphone, as can be seen in Figure 42.4. A hole smaller than the design size of 3 mm will usually reduce the cutoff frequency of the earphone. A hole larger than this will extend the range, but will usually cause a drop in output level at the high frequency end of the earphone's pass band.

The "real-world" earmold very frequently differs from the "ideal" of the 3-mm diameter by 18-mm long earmold hole and the very small cavity in front of the earphone nub (V_2), in

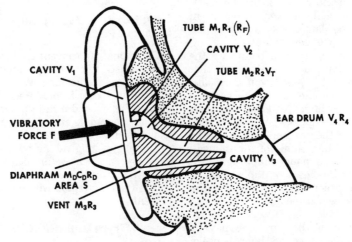

Fig. 42.3. Sectional view of conventional earphone system.

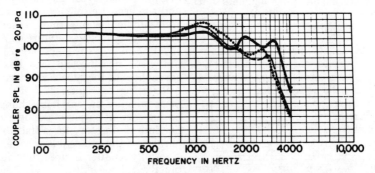

Fig. 42.4. Response curves of conventional earphone on 2-cc coupler with closed earmold condition. *Solid curve*, standard HA-2 hole 3-mm diameter by 18 mm long. *Dashed curve*, hole 1.5 mm diameter by 18 mm long. *Dotted curve*, hole 2.44 mm diameter by 23.4 mm long plus enlarged cavity in front of nub of 0.057 cm³ (0.250-inch diameter by 0.071 inch long).

that the hole often has to be smaller to avoid weakening the earmold tip and also a very substantial volume of air is left beyond the earphone nub in order to permit the sharply angled drilling from the outer face of the earmold usually needed. The dotted line of Figure 42.4 shows the effects observed on a typical earphone for these two departures from the "ideal" conditions. Receiver type earmolds would have significantly better high frequency response if the cavity V_2 in front of the nub were reduced to virtually no cavity at all.

When extreme increases are made in cavity V_2, both the low frequency and high frequency response can drop markedly (Lybarger, 1958). Figure 42.5 shows what happened when the entire interior of an earmold was hollowed out, practically eliminating the drilled hole in the ear mold. The high frequency peak disappeared, along with much of the output above 2000 Hz. Low frequency response also suffered because of the greatly increased air volume into which the earphone was operating. The mid-frequency peak increased markedly in frequency because of the reduction in the inertance of the earmold hole, and increased in height because the damping provided by the earmold hole was no longer present.

The example of Figure 42.5 points up the fallacy of certain types of generalizations that have been made in the past about earmolds, such as the one that the larger the earmold hole, the better the high frequency response. Actually, the high frequency response is usually dependent on the resonant action of the earmold hole and the volume of air immediately in front of the earphone diaphragm (V_1) and the hole should be of suitable size, as anticipated by the earphone designer, if the best results are to be obtained.

Acoustic damping devices, "filters" or "discs" placed in the nub of the earphone have a substantial smoothing effect on the response of a peaked earphone. Currently, however, earphones contain internal damping elements that give nearly flat responses over the earphone's passband. The selection of a suitable earphone

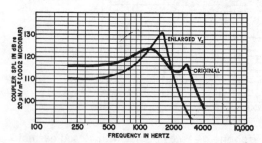

Fig. 42.5. Effect of extreme enlargement of cavity V_2 (conventional earphone).

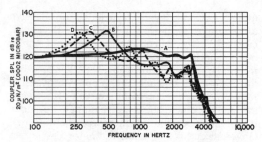

Fig. 42.6. Effects of long lengths of tubing (conventional earphone). *Curve A,* ear phone response on 2-cc coupler, 3-mm diameter by 18-mm long tube; *Curve B,* 3-inch length of tubing with inner diameter of 0.077 inch added to *Curve A* system; *Curve C,* 6-inch length of tubing with inner diameter of 0.077 inch added to *Curve A* system; *Curve D,* 9-inch length of tubing with inner diameter of 0.077 inch added to *Curve A* system.

is generally preferable to the use of damping devices in conventional type earphones.

Long Length of Tubing with Conventional Earphone

Occasionally a conventional earphone is coupled acoustically to the earmold via a plastic tube several inches long. When this is done, a substantial peak is produced in the low frequency region and a multiplicity of peaks appear in the middle and high frequency regions, as is shown in Figure 42.6.

The use of long tubing with a conventional earphone can be a useful means of maximizing performance in the low frequency region when this is the only region where usable hearing is present.

INTERNAL EARPHONE SYSTEM

When the hearing aid is of the eyeglass or behind-the-ear type, the earphone is internal and the acoustic connection is through a substantially longer tube than is used than for the conventional receiver. Figure 42.7 is a diagram of a typical acoustical system of this sort. The in-the-ear hearing aid also has an internal earphone, but the tube is shorter.

Referring to Figure 42.7, the transduction mechanism of the earphone changes the alternating current output of the hearing aid amplifier into a vibratory force that drives the diaphragm of the internal earphone, usually substantially smaller in area than in the conventional earphone.

Sound is generated in cavity V_1 adjacent to the diaphragm. The size of this cavity is important in determining the high frequency response of the system. From cavity V_1, the sound is transmitted through an exit tube leading from the earphone to the external nub of the hearing aid, the point at which the tubing or the elbow and tubing to the earmold is attached.

Between the exit tube and the hearing aid nub are a number of acoustic elements. There is always a length of very flexible tubing to isolate the earphone vibrationally from the hearing aid housing to prevent feedback to the microphone. There can be a substantial length of tubing between the earphone and the external nub if the earphone is located a distance from the nub. The external nub itself is a short length of small tubing. There may be an acoustic resistance permanently placed in the nub or in the connection between the earphone and the nub to give a desired response characteristic. Since most of these elements between the earphone and the nub are relatively short, small diameter tubes, their effects may be approximated by lumping them into an acoustic inertance (M_1) and an acoustic resistance (R_1) (Fig. 42.7).

It should be pointed out that all of the acoustic elements from the earphone to the external nub of the hearing aid are inaccessible except to the hearing aid manufacturer and cannot be used in the field as control elements. The fact that different earphones and different acoustic conditions exist inside different hearing aids also means that changes in earmold tubing size and the addition of external filters do not have identical effects on different hearing aids.

From the nub of the hearing aid, sound is transmitted through a plastic tube, often on the order of 2-mm diameter and 60 mm long. This tube is an acoustical transmission line, but can be represented acoustically by a few low pass filter "T" sections (Bauer, 1965). It

may be approximated at low and medium frequencies by an inertance and acoustical resistance in series (M_2R_2 in Fig. 42.7). At middle and high frequencies, this tube produces a series of response peaks (Carlson, 1974).

Acoustic "filters" or "chokes" may be placed just outside the nub of the hearing aid for the purpose of smoothing earphone response peaks and coincidentally for reducing the saturation output of the hearing aid. Such filters are primarily acoustic resistances, although most also have a small or moderate amount of acoustic inertance. In Figure 42.7, a filter is shown just outside the hearing aid nub and designated as R_F.

The sound passing through the tubing enters cavity V_3 between the earmold tip and the eardrum. Typically, this cavity has a volume of about 0.6 cm³. The eardrum, closing one end of V_3, is very roughly equivalent to a volume of 0.8 cm³ in series with an acoustic resistance of about 350 ohms, although it is better represented by a more complex acoustic network (Zwislocki, 1971).

Finally, in this system there can be a leak or vent from cavity V_3 to the outside. Since this vent is relatively short, it acts acoustically like an inertance (M_3) in series with an acoustic resistance (R_3). At its maximum opening, such as is used in CROS (sound picked up on one side of head, delivered to open ear canal on opposite side) and IROS (sound picked up on one side of head, delivered to open ear canal on same side) applications, the vent may be regarded as almost as large in cross section as the ear canal and equal in length to the depth of insertion of the tubing into the ear canal.

As in the case of the conventional earphone, the elements that have the greatest effect on low frequency response are the effective size of the cavity V_3 and the venting. The larger the

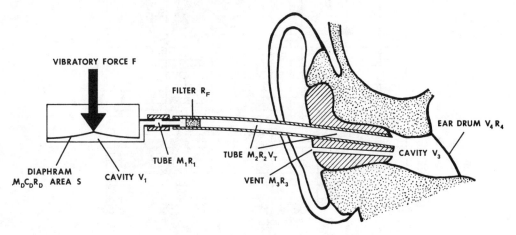

Fig. 42.7. Sectional view of internal earphone system.

cavity V_3, the lower will be the general level of response and vice-versa.

The element offering the greatest possibility of control of response (other than venting) is the diameter of the tubing employed. In Table 42.1, inside tubing diameters from 1.35 mm (0.053 inch, #16) to 2.16 mm (0.085 inch, #12) are listed as NAEL standard sizes. To obtain the response planned by the designer of the hearing aid, the specified tubing size should be employed. To change the response, other sizes may be used.

The effects of changing tubing diameter are indicated in Figures 42.8 and 42.9. The curves shown are constant available power response curves for two typically used earphones mounted in behind-the-ear hearing aid cases for two sizes of tubing. An earhook was used that had a length of 23 mm along its axis and an average inside diameter of 1.8 mm. The net

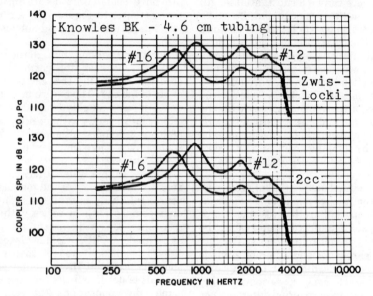

Fig. 42.8. Effect of tubing diameter on internal earphone response. Knowles BK receiver in hearing aid case plus earhook plus 4.6 cm of tubing.

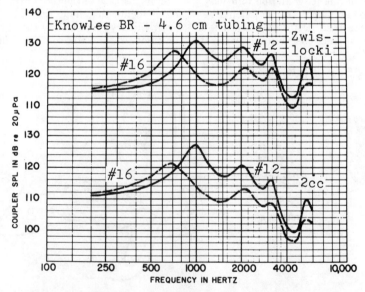

Fig. 42.9. Effect of tubing diameter on internal earphone response. Knowles BR receiver in hearing aid case plus earhook plus 4.6 cm of tubing.

tubing length was 4.6 cm. Figure 42.8 is for an earphone of usual bandwidth (Knowles BK); Figure 42.9 is for a wide range earphone (Knowles BR).

The effects of tubing diameter are similar for the two earphone types on both the 2-cc and the Zwislocki couplers. As the tubing decreases in diameter, the first response peak moves downward in frequency with an accompanying reduction in middle and high frequency response. Thus the tubing diameter can be used as a means of shifting emphasis from higher to lower frequencies or vice-versa. The use of smaller tubing can also be employed as a means of reducing average saturation output and gain.

The option of changing tubing length is generally not available, since a certain length of tubing is required to reach from the hearing aid to the earmold tip. However, the effects of such length changes are indicated in Figure 42.10. Starke (1971) points out the downward shift in the frequency of the first resonant peak and the addition of resonance peaks at higher frequencies as the tubing length is increased.

Acoustic Damping

Acoustic damping added to the transmission system has the effect of smoothing and lowering the response peaks that are generated in the earphone-earmold system. Acoustic damping in the tubing will not affect the sharpness of peaks that occur in the microphone response, however. Figure 42.11 shows the smoothing of response relative to the original response of an earphone (*Curve A*) when an acoustic resistance is placed at the sound exit nub of the hearing aid case (*Curve B*). When the acoustic resistance is placed at the earmold end of the tubing, a much stronger smoothing effect occurs, as shown by *Curve C*. Acoustic filters are often sintered stainless steel or plugs with small holes in them. If these are placed at the earmold end of the tubing, they have a tendency to become clogged in a few weeks.

Correct use of damping elements in a hearing aid with an internal earphone is very important, because it provides a means of controlling

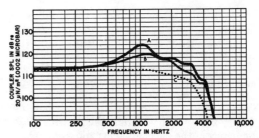

Fig. 42.11. Effect of filter placement. *Curve A*, original earphone response; *Curve B*, filter placed at nub of hearing aid; *Curve C*, filter placed at coupler end of tubing.

smoothness of response, gain and particularly of saturation output of an aid. It should not be assumed that a particular filter will give the same results on different types of hearing aids; generally this will not be true. The manufacturer's response curves should be consulted to determine the effects of various recommended filters.

Acoustic damping elements employed successfully are discs with a small hole or holes, fine screens and porous sintered stainless steel plugs.

Special Tubing Systems

Knowles (1970) has pointed out the improvement in high frequency response obtained by the use of dual bore tubing. A small diameter tubing, for example 0.062 inch, is connected from the hearing aid toward the earmold. About an inch or slightly less from the earmold tip, the bore is increased abruptly to 0.094 or 0.125 inch and kept at the larger diameter to the tip of the mold. The result of the discontinuity in the tube diameter and the action of the larger bore section opening into the ear cavity as a quarter wave resonator will produce a response several dB higher in the frequency region above 2000 Hz.

This dual bore effect is present in the coupler first adopted by International Electrotechnical Commission (IEC) as Amendment 1 to the IEC 118 hearing aid standard. This coupler was later specified in Section 4.5.2.3 of American National Standard S3.7-1973, method for coupler calibration of earphones, and is also employed in the recent American National Standard S3.22-1976 (ASA Std. 7-1976), method of specifying hearing aid performance. Such an arrangement is convenient, because it merely requires the addition of tubing to the 2-cc coupler used for measuring conventional earphones, but is should be borne in mind that some enhancement of the high frequencies, compared to the response with a single tubing diameter, occurs on the coupler but may not be present in the practical hearing aid.

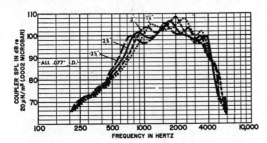

Fig. 42.10. Effect of tubing length on response with diameter constant.

Killion (1976) has extended the dual bore idea to a multiple bore concept that makes the tubing connection from the hearing aid to the earmold almost like a small horn. He describes two earmold designs that make possible extended high frequency performance of hearing aids using wide band earphones (such as Knowles BP). The first design is labeled the "6R10" because it extends the upper cutoff frequency of the earphone-earmold system to 6 kHz and enhances the response in the 2.5- to 6-kHz region by 10 to 15 dB. This earmold has three tubing diameters: 1.9 mm for 22 mm of length, 2.8 mm for 8 mm, and 3.8 mm for 10 mm at the tip end of the mold. The two latter sections are produced by appropriate drilling of the earmold; the first section is flexible plastic tubing. Two 560-ohm acoustic damping resistances are employed, one at the nub end of the 1.9-mm section and the other at its opposite end.

Carrying this same idea further, Killion also describes a "9 kHz" earmold, that provides good response to 8.5 or 9 kHz. This design employs four enlargements of the tubing diameter from the hearing aid earhook to the tip of the earmold. The dimensions of the sections are: 1.9 mm for 27 mm of length, 2.8 mm for 6 mm, 3.8 mm for 4 mm and 5.3 mm for 3 mm, the latter three presumably being achieved by appropriate drilling of the earmold. In this design, a 560- and a 1200-ohm acoustical resistance are placed at appropriate locations in the 1.9-mm section of tubing. Killion's results were determined using a Zwislocki type coupler.

Another very innovative type of earmold tubing arrangement, having the property of giving a response free from the usual tubing resonances, was developed by Carlson (1974). In Carlson's arrangement, a closed tubing stub is added to the system. Also two acoustic resistances equal to the characteristic impedance of the tubing transmission line are employed. This concept is borrowed from well known electrical transmission line theory. The action is to "cancel out" the tubing effects and to obtain the same freedom from resonance in the tubing that would occur if the earphone were connected directly to the ear canal cavity. The effect works for any length tubing. There is a tradeoff between average output level and smoothness of response in Carlson's system; some output level will be sacrificed. The extra closed end tubing stub can be concealed in several fairly simple ways.

RECEIVER-EARMOLD SYSTEM — IN-THE-EAR HEARING AIDS

In currently popular in-the-ear aids, the entire device is constructed in an earmold shell and the acoustic connections from the earphone to the earmold tip are internal. The tube from the earphone to the earmold tip (corresponding to $M_2R_2V_T$ in Fig. 42.7) is usually much shorter than in eyeglass or behind-the-ear aids. A length of 1 cm is typical. As a result, the primary resonant peak may be in the area of 1500 to 2000 Hz. Some control of the primary response peak is obtainable at the time of manufacture by choice of the earmold tip length or by the addition of extra tubing length within the housing.

Venting is used extensively in in-the-ear aids to reduce low frequency response, or, in some cases, to increase low frequency response near 500 Hz. The true increase in low frequency response (if any) will be much less than indicated by a 2-cc coupler measurement.

To obtain significant reduction in low frequency response, a short, large diameter (3 to 4 mm) vent is desirable. To obtain this, the tip length of the hearing aid must be quite short if the vent channel traverses the tip. By making the vent extremely large in diameter, approaching the size of the ear canal, a condition approaching the IROS arrangement can be obtained.

Small "select-a-vent" plugs are available for use with in-the-ear aids.

Basic venting principles are the same for in-the-ear aids as for behind-the-ear or eyeglass aids.

EARMOLD VENTING

An earmold vent is an opening between the cavity adjacent the eardrum (V_3, Fig. 42.7) and the outside air. For many years, vents have been employed in an effort to make hearing aids more acceptable to the wearer who objected to a closed mold. With the trend in recent years for most hearing aids to be used with persons who have sensory-neural hearing loss that often increases rapidly with frequency, correct venting of earmolds has become a very important fitting tool. It is not always possible to establish clearly what venting accomplishes for a hearing aid user who reports better results with a vent, but there appear to be three major effects.

1. Any size vent provides equalization of atmospheric pressure to the cavity V_3 between the earmold tip and the eardrum and can sometimes relieve a "feeling of pressure." Only a very small hole is needed for pressure equalization; often there is enough leakage around the earmold tip to accomplish this. Very constricted leaks or vents will cause a roll-off of extremely low frequency response, but will not usually cause any noticeable effect on the performance of a hearing aid. For very high gain aids, even small vents can cause acoustic feedback.

2. Moderate size vent holes are often used with the idea that they cut low frequencies.

They do cut very low frequencies, but they may not cut the middle lows where the reduction is desired. Even a slight increase in low frequency response can occur. This is because the inertance of the vent resonates with the acoustic capacitance of the ear canal cavity to produce a low frequency peak. Such peaks are usually damped by the acoustical resistance of the ear (Studebaker and Zachman, 1970). Medium size vents can present a serious feedback problem on other than a low or moderate gain hearing aid.

3. For really significant reduction in low frequency response, a wide, short vent is needed. Tabular information later in the chapter will indicate the effects of various lengths and diameters of vents as measured on a Zwislocki coupler. The use of large vents definitely limits the usable gain of a hearing aid if acoustic feedback is to be avoided. A large vent permits the direct entrance into the ear canal of low frequency sound, useful when the hearing loss is small in the low frequencies.

Measurement of Venting Effects

It has been recognized for some years that the 2-cc coupler did not accurately show how a vent affected response in real ears. The lack of damping in the 2-cc coupler gives rise to a large resonant peak due to venting that is not observed in real ears. More recent work (Lybarger, 1975a; Studebaker, Cox and Wark, 1976; Cox and Wark, 1976; Preves, 1977) compares the results of venting in the 2-cc coupler, the Zwislocki coupler and real ears. The 2-cc coupler was found unsatisfactory for venting measurements. The Zwislocki coupler appears to give results reasonably close to those reported for real ears, although any resonant peak due to venting may be slightly more emphasized than it is in real ears.

Measurements have been made by the author on several earmold configurations using different diameters and lengths of parallel and diagonal vents. A typical internal earphone (Knowles BK) was employed, mounted in a behind-the-ear hearing aid case with typical internal "plumbing." An earhook 23 mm long with an average diameter of 1.8 mm was used. The tubing was #13 (1.93 mm, 0.076 inch) 4.6 cm long, as measured to the tip of the "medium" earmold configuration (see Fig. 42.1A). The simulated earmold was inserted into a Zwislocki type coupler (DB-100) manufactured by Industrial Research Products, Inc., to which had been added an 8.8 mm (0.346 inch) extension of the canal portion. This makes the canal length the same as used in the KEMAR manikin. However, the manikin portion was not present.

TABLE 42.2. *Vented Minus Unvented Response in Decibels for Simulated Earmold on DB100 Coupler* Tubing type earmold, short-hollowed tip, parallel vent.

Vent Diameter (mm)	Frequency (Hz)									
	200	250	315	400	500	630	800	1000	1250	1600
1.0	−8	−3	4	8	6	3	1	1	1	0
2.0	−22	−18	−13	−9	−2	6	5	4	3	2
3.0	−29	−24	−20	−16	−11	−5	1	1	4	3

TABLE 42.3. *Vented Minus Unvented Response in Decibels for Simulated Earmold on DB100 Coupler* Tubing type earmold, short tip, parallel vent.

Vent Diameter (mm)	Frequency (Hz)									
	200	250	315	400	500	630	800	1000	1250	1600
1.0	−2	4	7	5	3	2	−1	1	0	0
2.0	−17	−13	−8	−2	6	9	3	3	2	1
3.0	−25	−20	−16	−12	−6	1	4	3	4	3

TABLE 42.4 *Vented Minus Unvented Response in Decibels for Simulated Earmold on DB100 Coupler* Tubing type earmold, medium tip, parallel vent.

Vent Diameter (mm)	Frequency (Hz)									
	200	250	315	400	500	630	800	1000	1250	1600
1.0	0	6	6	4	2	1	1	1	0	0
2.0	−15	−11	−6	0	9	5	2	3	2	1
3.0	−23	−19	−14	−10	−4	4	3	3	4	2

TABLE 42.5. *Vented Minus Unvented Response in Decibels for Simulated Earmold on DB100 Coupler* Tubing type earmold, long tip, parallel vent.

Vent Diameter (mm)	Frequency (Hz)									
	200	250	315	400	500	630	800	1000	1250	1600
1.0	2	6	5	3	2	1	0	0	0	0
2.0	−14	−10	−4	3	9	5	1	2	1	1
3.0	−22	−18	−13	−8	−2	6	1	2	3	2

TABLE 42.6. *Vented Minus Unvented Response in Decibels for Simulated Earmold on DB100 Coupler* Tubing type earmold, medium tip, diagonal vent.

Vent Diameter (mm)	Frequency (Hz)									
	200	250	315	400	500	630	800	1000	1250	1600
1.0	−6	0	6	6	3	1	0	−1	−1	−1
1.5	−15	−11	−4	3	6	2	0	−1	−2	−2
2.0	−21	−17	−11	−5	2	3	−1	−2	−4	−5

TABLE 42.7. *Vented Minus Unvented Response in Decibels for Simulated Earmold on DB100 Coupler* Tubing type earmold, long tip, diagonal vent.

Vent Diameter (mm)	Frequency (Hz)									
	200	250	315	400	500	630	800	1000	1250	1600
1.0	−8	−2	4	5	2	0	−1	−1	−2	−3
1.5	−17	−13	−6	1	4	0	−2	0	−4	−5
2.0	−23	−20	−13	−7	2	−1	−3	−4	−6	−8

TABLE 42.8a. *Vented Minus Unvented Response in Decibels for Simulated Earmold on DB100 Coupler* "Positive venting valve" earmold, short-hollowed tip, 1.5 mm diameter parallel vent channel.

Vent No. and Hole	Frequency (Hz)									
	200	250	315	400	500	630	800	1000	1250	1600
1 (.125″)	−18	−15	−9	−4	4	9	5	3	2	1
2 (.094″)	−18	−14	−9	−3	4	9	4	3	2	1
3 (.062″)	−18	−13	−8	−3	5	8	4	3	2	1
4 (.031″)	−15	−11	−5	1	8	6	3	2	1	1
5 (.020″)	−9	−5	0	4	5	3	1	1	1	1

Tables 42.2 to 42.11 show the simulated earmold configuration at the left. The numbers in the body of the table are the *changes* in response with the vent open compared to the sealed condition (vent hole completely filled for Tables 42.2 to 42.7). A negative number means that the venting decreased the level measured by the Zwislocki coupler; a positive number means that the venting increased the level. Frequencies used in the tables are preferred one-third octave values from 200 to 1600 Hz. All dimensions shown in the table diagrams are in millimeters. Note that in Tables 42.6 and 42.7 both low and high frequencies are reduced by diagonal vents (the lows much more, of course), whereas parallel vents (see Tables 42.2 to 42.5) do not appear to reduce high frequency response.

Adjustable and Variable Venting

One of the most convenient ways to control venting for a given situation is to make an earmold with a vent channel leading to a socket on the face of the earmold into which can be pressed vent inserts having holes of different diameters. At least two types of inserts are in widespread use, the "positive venting valve" (Blue, 1972; Briskey and Wruk, 1974) and the "select-a-vent." The former is a cup-shaped insert made from polyethylene plastic with its thin bottom wall pierced with holes of various diameters. The length of the holes is negligible. The "select-a-vent" is made of soft plastic in the form of a plug about 4.3 mm (0.170 inch) long with the vent hole running through the full length. The venting actions will be somewhat different for the same diameter of vent hole because of the difference in hole lengths.

The venting action of these inserts is a function of the vent channel leading through the earmold to the socket where the vent inserts are placed. If the channel is relatively long or rather small in diameter, it will have the controlling effect on the venting and only the

TABLE 42.8b. *Vented Minus Unvented Response in Decibels for Simulated Earmold on DB100 Coupler* "Positive venting valve" earmold, short-hollowed tip, 3.0 mm diameter parallel vent channel.

	Vent No.	Frequency (Hz)									
		200	250	315	400	500	630	800	1000	1250	1600
(Refer to Table 42.8a for diagram)	1	−28	−24	−19	−15	−4	2	1	4	3	2
	2	−27	−23	−19	−14	−3	3	2	4	3	2
	3	−25	−21	−16	−12	0	4	3	4	3	2
	4	−20	−16	−11	−6	6	4	3	2	2	1
	5	−11	−8	−3	1	3	2	1	1	1	0

TABLE 42.9a. *Vented Minus Unvented Response in Decibels for Simulated Earmold on DB100 Coupler* "Positive venting valve" earmold, long tip, 1.5 mm diameter parallel vent channel.

Vent No.	Frequency (Hz)									
	200	250	315	400	500	630	800	1000	1250	1600
1	−9	−3	4	9	6	3	1	1	1	1
2	−9	−3	4	9	6	3	1	1	1	1
3	−9	−3	4	9	6	3	1	1	1	1
4	−8	−2	5	9	5	3	1	1	1	1
5	−5	0	5	6	4	2	0	1	1	1

TABLE 42.9b. *Vented Minus Unvented Response in Decibels for Simulated Earmold on DB100 Coupler* "Positive venting valve" earmold, long tip, 3.0 mm diameter parallel vent channel.

	Vent. No.	Frequency (Hz)									
		200	250	315	400	500	630	800	1000	1250	1600
(Refer to Table 42.9a for diagram)	1	−21	−17	−12	−6	−1	7	1	3	4	3
	2	−21	−16	−12	−6	0	7	1	3	4	3
	3	−20	−15	−11	−5	1	8	1	3	3	2
	4	−17	−14	−8	−1	5	7	1	3	3	2
	5	−12	−8	−3	3	4	3	0	2	2	1

TABLE 42.10a. *Vented Minus Unvented Response in Decibels for Simulated Earmold on DB100 Coupler* "Select-a-vent" earmold, short-hollowed tip, 1.5 mm diameter parallel vent channel.

	Vent No. and Hole	Frequency (Hz)									
		200	250	315	400	500	630	800	1000	1250	1600
	1 (.156″)	−19	−15	−10	−5	2	8	4	3	2	1
	2 (.125″)	−19	−14	−10	−4	3	9	4	3	2	1
	3 (.100″)	−18	−14	−9	−3	4	9	4	3	2	1
	4 (.054″)	−12	−8	−2	6	9	5	2	2	1	1
	5 (.031″)	1	3	3	3	2	1	0	0	0	0

TABLE 42.10b. *Vented Minus Unvented Response in Decibels for Simulated Earmold on DB100 Coupler* "Select-a-vent" earmold, short-hollowed tip, 3.0 mm diameter parallel vent channel.

	Vent No.	Frequency (Hz)									
		200	250	315	400	500	630	800	1000	1250	1600
(Refer to Table 42.10a for diagram)	1	−28	−24	−20	−15	−11	−5	1	1	4	3
	2	−26	−22	−18	−13	−8	−2	4	2	4	3
	3	−25	−20	−16	−12	−6	0	5	3	4	3
	4	−15	−11	−5	1	8	7	3	2	2	1
	5	0	3	3	3	2	1	1	0	0	0

TABLE 42.11a. *Vented Minus Unvented Response in Decibels for Simulated Earmold on DB100 Coupler* "Select-a-vent" earmold, long tip, 1.5 mm diameter parallel vent channel.

	Vent No.	Frequency (Hz)									
		200	250	315	400	500	630	800	1000	1250	1600
	1	−9	−4	3	9	7	3	1	2	1	1
	2	−9	−4	3	9	7	3	1	2	1	1
	3	−9	−4	4	9	6	3	1	2	1	1
	4	−6	−1	7	8	5	2	1	1	1	1
	5	1	4	4	3	2	1	0	1	1	0

TABLE 42.11b. *Vented Minus Unvented Response in Decibels for Simulated Earmold on DB100 Coupler* "Select-a-vent" earmold, long tip, 3.0 mm diameter parallel vent channel.

	Vent No.	Frequency (Hz)									
		200	250	315	400	500	630	800	1000	1250	1600
(Refer to Table 42.11a for diagram)	1	−21	−17	−12	−7	−1	6	1	3	4	3
	2	−20	−16	−11	−6	0	7	2	3	4	3
	3	−20	−15	−11	−6	1	8	2	3	3	3
	4	−14	−9	−4	3	9	5	1	2	2	2
	5	−1	2	4	3	2	1	0	1	1	0

smaller diameter inserts will make a noticeable difference. In fact, the larger diameter vent inserts could well be eliminated in favor of a better selection of those with smaller diameters. For example, in Table 42.8a, the first three diameters of vent inserts listed give the same results as if no insert were present. The 0.031-inch diameter vent hole starts to make a difference.

Tables 42.8 to 42.11 were made using the short-hollowed tip and the long tip earmold configurations. In Tables 42.8 to 42.11, "unvented" means that the vent insert had no hole and closed the channel.

Also available are variable vents (Griffing (1972) "variable venting valve"; Feingold (1972) "variable vent"). These have knobs that allow the user to adjust the amount of venting he requires for various situations. In one type, the amount of venting is set by the dispenser by means of a screw adjustment rather than having the user change it. The range of venting action is similar to that for the vent inserts.

NONOCCLUDING EARMOLDS

The nonoccluding or open canal earmold system was used originally with CROS hearing aids. The head separation provided by having the microphone on one side and the earphone on the other allowed more gain to be used. However, the use of nonoccluding earmolds on IROS (same side) hearing aids has become widespread and successful where only low gains are required.

A number of studies have demonstrated improved speech intelligibility using an open or partially open earmold for high frequency losses. Dodds and Harford (1968, 1970) report on the clinical results and later generally favorable reaction to open earmolds. Jetty and Rintelmann (1970) report substantially better discrimination scores for open and partially open earmolds for subjects with sensory-neural hearing losses with precipitous or gradual slopes. Hodgson and Murdock (1970) found improved speech discrimination for subjects with high frequency sensory-neural loss when vented and open molds were compared with standard molds.

The nonoccluding mold may consist simply of a piece of tubing projecting into the ear canal, or a skeleton earmold designed to hold the tubing in place without blocking the ear canal appreciably. The importance of not reducing the canal size with this type of mold is pointed out by Hewitt (1977). If no mold is employed, a heavy wall tubing is ordinarily used to give the necessary mechanical strength. Delk (1975) shows various nonoccluding earmold arrangements.

The nonoccluding earmold may be considered as working into cavity V_3 of size similar to the one in a closed mold, but with a huge vent present. The large vent acts almost like a short circuit at low frequencies and little sound pressure is developed below 500 Hz. As the frequency increases, the acoustic reactance of the vent rises and the sound pressure at the eardrum gradually increases. Berland (1975) has investigated the effects of nonoccluding earmolds on real ears and found that the diameter of the tubing from the earphone has a strong effect on the frequency at which the response rises. With #13 tubing the response starts to rise at about 1000 Hz; by using #16 or #18

tubing, the rise did not start until about 2000 Hz. With the latter, persons who have nearly normal hearing to 1500 or 2000 Hz can be assisted without excess gain in the transition frequency range.

Figure 42.12 (Lybarger, 1974) shows the effect of tubing diameter on the response of a CROS aid with the tubing projecting into the simulated ear canal of a Zwislocki coupler. Figure 42.13 (Knowles and Burkhard, 1975) shows responses of a CROS hearing aid with nonoccluding earmolds as measured on a KEMAR manikin.

EARMOLD LEAKAGE

Even with a perfect seal, sound is radiated from an earmold because the whole mold is vibrated by the sound pressure acting on it from the inside. However, most earmolds leak sound around the periphery because they do

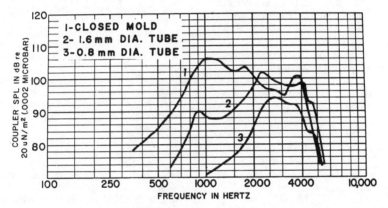

Fig. 42.12. CROS hearing aid response measured on Zwislocki coupler. *Curve 1,* closed earmold condition; *Curve 2,* 1.6-mm diameter tube from hearing aid; *Curve 3,* 0.8-mm diameter tube from hearing aid. Tube inserted 13 mm into simulated ear canal of coupler.

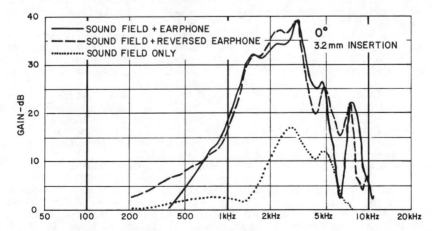

Fig. 42.13. Response of a laboratory CROS hearing aid measured on a KEMAR manikin. Predicted functional gain is the difference between the upper curves and the sound field only curve. (From H. S. Knowles and M. D. Burkhard: *Hearing Instruments,* **26,** 19–41, 1975.)

not fit perfectly. Johansen (1975) has calculated that the leakage around a typical earmold is equivalent to that through a hole roughly 1.4 mm (0.055 inch) in diameter by 22 mm (0.866 inch) long. Using this value, he both calculated and measured the SPL at a point 3 cm distant from the outer face of the earmold, which simulates a typical behind-the-ear hearing aid microphone location. The results were in good agreement and the levels were found to be about 58 to 66 dB lower than the SPLs at the earmold tip. This would represent the maximum allowable gain in the range from about 2000 to 4000 Hz.

When the leakage hole was replaced with a vent 3 mm in diameter by 22 mm long, the level difference dropped to about 53 dB in the 2000- to 4000-Hz range. This imposes a definite limit on usable gain when venting is used.

Grover and Martin (1974) have experimented on the practical gain limit for behind-the-ear hearing aids using silicone rubber earmolds on real ears. They found that the earmold attenuation averaged 66.5 dB at 500 Hz and fell gradually to 57 dB at 3 kHz.

Experiments reported by Lybarger (1975b) indicate a difference, compared to a closed mold condition, of about 14 dB for a #4 PVV vent insert (0.031 inch) and 18 dB for a #1 PVV vent insert (0.125 inch). Curves of leakage sound pressure level vs. frequency indicated that the most critical range for feedback was from 1500 to 3000 Hz. That is, the gain for the vented condition in the "feedback range" would have to be reduced by these amounts compared to the closed mold condition.

REFERENCES

Bauer, B. B., Equivalent circuit of a tube or spring. J. Acoust. Soc. Am., 38, 882, 1965.

Berland, O., No-mold fitting of hearing aids; earmoulds and associated problems. Scand. Audiol., Supp. 5, 173–193, 1975.

Blue, J. V., Positive venting valve concept. Hear. Dealer, 23 (No. 10), 23, 1972.

Briskey, R., and Wruk, K., Acoustic influence of insert vents. Hear. Instruments, 25 (No. 10), 12–14, 1974.

Burkhard, M. D., and Sachs, R. M., Anthropometric manikin for acoustic research. J. Acoust. Soc. Am., 58, 214–222, 1975.

Caine, M., Plastics and materials utilized in earmolds. Hear. Instruments, 25 (No. 12), 17, 1974.

Carlson, E. V., Smoothing the hearing aid frequency response. J. Audio Eng. Soc., 22, 426–429, 1974.

Coogle, K. L., NAEL standard terms for earmolds. Hear. Dealer, 21 (No. 12), 13, 1970.

Cox, R. M., and Wark, D., Effects of earmold modifications on auditory thresholds and on earcanal and coupler spectrum levels. Paper presented at annual meeting of American Speech and Hearing Association, November 20, 1976.

Delk, J. H., Comprehensive dictionary of audiology. Hearing Aid Journal, Sioux City, Iowa, third printing, 1975.

Dodds, E., and Harford, E., Modified earpieces and CROS for high frequency hearing losses. J. Speech Hear. Res., 11, 204–218, 1968.

Dodds, E., and Harford, E., Follow-up report on modified earpieces and CROS for high frequency hearing losses. J. Speech Hear. Res., 13, 41–43, 1970.

Feingold, A., Variable vent earmolds. Nat. Hear. Aid J., 25 (No. 6), 33, 1972.

Griffing, T. S., Variable venting valve technique for custom earmolds. Nat. Hear. Aid J., 25 (No. 4), 11, 1972.

Grover, B. C., and Martin, M. C., On the practical gain limit for post-aural hearing aids. Br. J. Audiol., 8, 121–124, 1974.

Hewitt, C., New "free-field" earmold. Hear. Aid J., 30 (No. 5), 10–32, 1977.

Hodgson, W. R., and Murdock, C., Jr., Effect of the ear mold on speech intelligibility in hearing aid use. J. Speech Hear. Res., 13, 101–114, 1970.

Jetty, A. J., and Rintelmann, W. F., Acoustic coupler effects on speech audiometric scores using a CROS hearing aid. J. Speech Hear. Res., 13, 290–297, 1970.

Johansen, P. A., An evaluation of the acoustic feedback damping for behind the ear hearing aids. Report, Research Laboratory for Technical Audiology, State Hearing Centres, Odense, Denmark, 1975.

Killion, M. C., Earmold plumbing for wide-band hearing aids. J. Acoust. Soc. Am., 59, Supp. 1, S62 (A), 1976.

Knowles, H. S., Private communication, 1970.

Knowles, H. S., and Burkhard, M. D., Hearing aids on KEMAR. Hear. Instruments, 26 (No. 3), 19–41, 1975.

Lybarger, S. F., The earmold as a part of the receiver acoustic system. Pamphlet, Radioear Corporation, McMurray, Pa., 1958.

Lybarger, S. F., The acoustical engineer's viewpoint of hearing aid design. Bull. N.Y. Acad. Med., 50, 917–930, 1974.

Lybarger, S. F., Comparison of earmold characteristics measured on the 2-cc coupler, the Zwislocki coupler and real ears; earmoulds and associated problems. Scand. Audiol., Supp. 5, 65–85, 1975a.

Lybarger, S. F., Sound leakage from vented earmolds; earmoulds and associated problems. Scand. Audiol., Supp. 5, 260–270, 1975b.

Preves, D. A., Effects of earmold venting on coupler, manikin and real ears. Hear. Aid J., 30 (No. 5), 9–47, 1977.

Radcliffe, D., NAEL helps to "mold" the future. Hear. Aid J., 27 (No. 5), 9–32, 1974.

Sachs, R. M., and Burkhard, M. D., Insert earphone pressure response in real ears and couplers. J. Acoust. Soc. Am., 52, 183(A), 1972a.

Sachs, R. M., and Burkhard, M. D., Zwislocki coupler evaluation with insert earphones.

Knowles Electronics, Inc., Report 20022-1, 1972b.

Starke, C., About acoustic measurements on earmolds. *J. Audiol. Tech.*, 10, 142–158, 1971.

Studebaker, G. A., and Zachman, T. A., Investigation of the acoustics of ear mold vents. *J. Acoust. Soc. Am.*, 47, 1107–1115, 1970.

Studebaker, G. A., Cox, R. M., and Wark, D. J., Effect of earmold modifications measured by coupler, threshold and probe techniques. *J. Acoust. Soc. Am.*, 60, Suppl. No. 1, S105 (A), 1976.

Zwislocki, J. J., An earlike coupler for earphone calibration. Report LSC-S-9, Laboratory Sensory Communication, Syracuse University, 1971.

chapter 43

HEARING AID EVALUATION

Mark Ross, Ph.D.

Over twenty-five years ago, Carhart (1950) began an article regarding hearing aid selection by saying that, "The problem of hearing aid selection is currently the most controversial aspect of clinical audiology." In spite of (and sometimes because of) the large body of literature which has since accumulated, this statement is probably as appropriate now as it was then. Audiologists disagree on the methods to be used in a hearing aid evaluation, on the type and reliability of the signals to be employed, on the electroacoustic characteristics suitable for different hearing-impaired populations, and on whether the dividends in present day selection procedures justify the clinical efforts. Some areas of disagreement perhaps can be resolved, or at least clearly defined, with a close examination and discussion of the relevant literature. Other areas of disagreement cannot be resolved even by the most careful and extensive review of the literature, since they are rooted in differing conceptions of the audiologist's role regarding hearing aid recommendations. Much of the information in this chapter will reflect my conception of the audiologist's responsibilities in adult hearing aid evaluations; that of selecting and making a specific hearing aid recommendation. Where the experimental literature is scanty, I have abstracted from my and other clinician's practices to make the indicated suggestions. For the important counseling and adjustment factors which must be considered whenever a hearing aid is recommended see Chapter 44.

PRESELECTION PROCEDURES

Hearing Aid Candidacy

The first decision to be made is whether or not the client is a candidate for a hearing aid. The most frequently quoted audiometric criterion in the older literature was 30 dB (ASA-1951) or more hearing threshold level (HTL) in the better ear. Individuals with sensory-neural, minimal, high frequency or unilateral hearing losses were not considered hearing aid candidates (Ross, 1969). The development of ear level and CROS hearing aids (see Chapter 41), the utilization of earmold characteristics for "selective amplification" (see Chapter 42) and the acceptance of a supervised trial hearing

aid period for questionable cases (Ross, Barrett and Trier, 1966; Rassi and Harford, 1968) have rendered obsolete the old audiometric criterion for hearing aid candidacy. Provided the client reports significant communicative difficulty, and provided further that he is motivated to objectively evaluate the effects of amplification in personally significant communicative situations, then very few hearing-impaired individuals are not prospective hearing aid candidates. This should not be construed to mean that all these people can successfully adjust to or benefit from amplification. The question which must be answered is whether the client is able to communicate more effectively with than without the hearing aid. Perhaps an improvement is noted in only one or two situations, but, if these are crucial to the client, then a hearing aid trial is warranted. Much of this decision must be based on the subjective impressions of clients as they experience amplified sound in everyday circumstances. The clinician's decision becomes less tentative the more severe a client's hearing loss; in these instances, we can often predict sufficient communicative difficulty to warrant a hearing aid recommendation. The less severe a client's hearing loss, the more we must attend to the particular situations in which he has communicative difficulty. In all cases, recommendations regarding a hearing aid have to consider the client's motivation as well as audiometric suitability and communicative needs. A poorly motivated, institutionalized geriatric client is, for example, a poor candidate for amplification no matter what degree of loss he manifests (Alpiner, 1967).

Otologic Examination

Once it has been determined that a client is a prospective hearing aid candidate, then it is important to ensure that he has received an otologic examination no more than a few months prior to the hearing aid selection. This is required for a number of reasons. The first is the possibility that the client has a medical condition which requires treatment, either for health reasons or for the possible alleviation of the hearing loss. The recommendation of a hearing aid for such a client, without informing him of the possible alternatives, is neither ethically defensible nor in the client's best interests. Sometimes a medically reversible condition can coexist with a medically irreversible condition; the amplification needs of a client may be different depending upon whether treatment is or is not instituted. The most prosaic reason for requiring a prior otologic examination is the necessity to remove cerumen before taking an ear impression. The soft ear impression material will either flow around the cerumen or push it further back into the ear canal. In either case, the result is likely to be an ill-fitting earmold and acoustic feedback. Clinically, it is the consequences of just this type of apparently mundane and pica-yune event which often preclude the most effective use of amplification by our hearing-impaired clients.

Earmolds

Earmolds are an integral part of the electroacoustic chain that begins at the hearing aid microphone and ends in the client's ear canal. When the physical dimensions of the mold are modified, the acoustic signal which a client receives is changed. When the molds do not fit well, an acoustic squeal occurs at lower gain levels than would otherwise occur. In view of the undoubted importance of the earmold, it is advisable to fabricate one for every client undergoing a hearing aid evaluation. This can be accomplished by scheduling hearing aid evaluations in two stages; one for the audiologic evaluation and the taking of an ear impression, and the other, a week or so later, for the hearing aid evaluation itself. The widespread use of ear-level hearing aids makes it possible for the audiologist to fabricate the entire earmold ("instamold"). This sharply reduces any need for use of stock earmolds. Stock molds should be used only when no other alternative is possible (Konkle and Bess, 1974), as with body aids.

Ear Selection

The use of a binaural hearing aid is strongly recommended whenever possible (see Chapter 41). For audiologic and personal reasons, however, some clients may not be candidates for binaural amplification, and for them it is necessary to select the one ear which can benefit most from amplification.

Generally speaking, the ear chosen is the one with the best speech discrimination function and the widest dynamic range (the difference between the speech reception threshold [SRT] and the threshold of discomfort [TD]. The tests used to evaluate the speech discrimination function must be sufficiently sensitive to reflect differences in intelligibility between the two ears. For example, about 60% of the individuals administered the CID W-22 test in quiet score above 90% (Carhart, 1965); meaningful differences between the ears cannot be assessed when the scores in both ears are close to the upper limit (ceiling effect). The utilization of a competing noise signal can often

separate the discrimination functions of two ears not differentiated under quiet conditions (Ross et al., 1963). The same objective can be achieved by administering the tests at a number of sensation levels.

When not contraindicated by a narrow dynamic range or poor speech discrimination, it is advisable to fit the poorer ear in instances when the HTL in the better ear is not greater than 30 or 40 dB (ANSI-1969). This will permit the unaided better ear to contribute to the total auditory signal received by a client. An example of this would be a client with a 60-dB HTL in his poorer ear, with a TD in excess of 100 dB, and word discrimination score (WDS) of 90%, while the better ear displays an HTL of 30 dB, a TD of 90 dB, and a WDS of 90%. By aiding the poorer ear in this case, both ears are now able to make an auditory contribution. The better ear should be utilized when the poorer ear is not a good candidate for amplification because of the severity of the loss, the poor discrimination function or a narrow dynamic range. (The possibility of a CROS or BICROS fitting for such a client is discussed in Chapter 41.)

When both ears are similar in terms of degree of loss, dynamic range and speech discrimination scores, then a comparison of the pure tone threshold configurations of the two ears can assist in determining which one is the most suitable for amplification. The ear with the flattest configuration is ordinarily selected (Miller, 1967). This ear is chosen on the possibility that the overall discrimination function is superior, although the scores under phones may have been similar for the two ears. In cases of rising threshold configurations, the ear with the flattest configuration is selected because of the possible contribution to intelligibility the higher frequencies can make in the unaided ear.

There are a number of instances when it is not possible to choose between the ears because of similarities in all the measured auditory dimensions. In these cases, it is advisable to make an earmold for each ear and suggest that the client rotate use of the aid between the two ears. After such a trial, the client will frequently express a preference for one ear. The nonpreferred ear should still be used on occasion in the event of a temporary incapacity in the preferred ear, such as an ear infection or abrasions due to an ill-fitting earmold, and in preparation for possible binaural amplification in the future. Also, while it has never been conclusively demonstrated that a nonused ear will become "rusty," we have seen a sufficient number of instances wherein word discrimination in two otherwise similar ears is poorer in the nonused ear to justify explicit directions regarding rotating hearing aid usage from ear to ear.

It is sometimes advisable to make an earmold for each ear, although the hearing levels in the two ears differ considerably, when the conditions under which a client uses a hearing aid may dictate the use of one ear in one type of situation and the other ear in another type of situation. An example of this would be the client with a 60-dB HTL in the poorer ear and a 30-dB HTL in the better ear, with both ears manifesting adequate discrimination and dynamic ranges. In noisy situations this client may find it advisable to aid the poorer ear, thus achieving a certain degree of binaural functioning. The increased speech signal occurring in noisy situations (the Lombard effect) will help him overcome the residual bilateral loss. In quiet situations he may find it helpful to aid the better ear, thus achieving a lower overall aided threshold level.

Body-Worn Versus Ear-Level

Approximately 90% of the hearing aids sold today are ear-level instruments; the majority of these are postauricular aids. Although their initial acceptance may have been produced by their cosmetic appeal, their continued popularity is probably also due to certain favorable acoustic effects relative to body-worn hearing aids. However, not all clients are candidates for ear-level hearing aids. Prior to selecting the specific aids to be tested during a hearing aid evaluation, it is necessary to determine which type of hearing aid is to be evaluated. This choice is made on the basis of the audiologic results and the relative advantages and disadvantages of each type of hearing aid for any given client.

Audiologic Considerations. The rough audiometric guideline (degree of hearing loss) used in the past no longer seems appropriate in deciding whether or not an individual is a candidate for an ear-level aid. From an electroacoustic point of view, some of the current models of ear-level instruments are quite comparable to body-worn aids. If one is aware of the pattern of amplification desired, then it is quite possible to select an ear-level aid which can provide the proper signal. For some clients, whose tympanic membranes reflect an abnormally large amount of energy back into the external auditory meatus, it may be necessary to select a body aid so that the distance between the microphone and the receiver can be increased and thus reduce the possibility of acoustic feedback. Feedback can also be reduced with ear-level aids through a power-CROS arrangement, in which the microphone on one side feeds the receiver on the contralateral side, and for binaural cases a CRIS-CROS arrangement (though the presumed reduction of feedback has never been investigated directly).

Relative Advantages and Disadvantages. The placement of the hearing aid at the ear rather than on the body provides most of the advantages accruing to ear-level hearing aids. When worn on the body, the body-baffle effect tends to increase the response of the aid at the lower frequencies and decrease it at the higher frequencies (Byrne, 1972). The high frequency response is depressed further when the aid is covered by a shirt or jacket. Baffle effects also occur with ear-level hearing aids, but they are of a lesser magnitude (Kasten, Lotterman and Hinchman, 1967/1968). Head shadow effects, however, may in the most unfavorable azimuth positions decrease the high frequency response by as much as 14.5 dB between 3000 and 4000 Hz. The hearing-impaired person can reduce head shadow effects in ear-level aids by moving his head slightly, but he cannot eliminate the baffle effect of a body-worn aid, nor easily dispense with the clothing covering the microphone.

Another major advantage of ear-level rather than body placement of a hearing aid is the elimination of "clothing noise," the noise produced when the body aid rubs against the clothing. This can be quite disturbing and may interfere with speech intelligibility. One of the most frequent comments made by the client who changes from a body to an ear-level aid concerns the elimination of clothing noise. Modern body aids are designed to minimize this noise by mounting the microphone on top, by isolating the microphones with nonvibratory material and by utilizing different case materials, but the problem has not been eliminated. The absence of clothing noise in the use of ear-level hearing aids must be balanced by the presence of "wind noise." This refers to air turbulence generated around the margins of the aid when it is worn outdoors on a windy day. This noise is detected by the microphone and amplified as any other sound.

The recent development of directional microphones incorporated in ear-level aids provides another possible advantage for them as compared to body-worn instruments. Although the research reports are somewhat mixed, there seems to be good evidence that at least some hearing-impaired adults can improve their communication ability in noise with the use of this type of hearing aid (Lentz, 1972; Sung, Sung and Angelelli, 1974).

Some geriatric clients, although audiometrically suitable for ear-level amplification, may be more appropriately fitted with a body-worn instrument. If they have poor motor control of their hands, they will find it more difficult to seat the ear-mold, to change the batteries and to manipulate the gain control of an ear-level aid than they would with a body-worn aid. If they are not particularly mobile, then the clothing noise factor should not be too disturbing.

Gain and Output Requirements

Up to this point, the clinician has had to select the appropriate ear and general type of hearing aid for the client. From his supply of hearing aids, he now has to select a number of aids which meet the client's needs in terms of gain and output. See Chapter 39 for the electroacoustic description of these factors.

Output. A client whose hearing aid delivers sound in excess of his TD is not apt to be a happy or successful user. For this reason, the output of the aid must be less than the client's TD. On the surface this appears to be a straightforward proposition; there are, however, a number of complications which must be considered.

Usually TD measures are made under phones using speech as the stimulus, with the zero reference level set at 20 dB sound pressure level (SPL). A TD of 90 dB under phones would thus be equivalent to 110 dB SPL. The definition of the maximum power output of a hearing aid, on the other hand, is defined in terms of the SPL of pure tones. In order to keep the output of a hearing aid within the limits imposed by a client's TD, it is necessary to reconcile both the different reference levels and the different signals.

Some authors suggest accomplishing this by measuring a client's TD across frequency, using either pure tones or narrow band noises calibrated to the same reference level which defines the output of the hearing aid (Victoreen, 1960; Wallenfels, 1967; Zink and Alpiner, 1968; Ross, 1975). This is an instructive technique for measuring individual variations in TD across frequency. It is still necessary to compare the complex speech signals to which a client listens with the pure tones or narrow band noises used to measure his TD. A TD of 120 dB across frequency as measured by pure tones does not signify that the client can tolerate a 120 dB speech signal; the peak pressures of a speech signal which averages 120 dB may be far in excess of his tolerance level. Whether the output of a hearing aid is indeed less than the TD for speech is checked during the hearing aid evaluation by measuring aided TD levels for speech with the different hearing aids.

McCandless (1973) has suggested using the stapedial reflex threshold as an objective assessment of the TD. He reports a close correlation between the TD and the stapedial reflex threshold and states that we have typically been guilty of overamplifying clients. Based on the results of his study, he suggests that mild losses require maximum power output limits of about 100 dB SPL, to about 120 dB SPL for the more severe losses. He cautions that the instructions given a client during the measurement of the TD are crucial, and suggests that we evaluate the point of beginning discomfort rather than a definite discomfort level.

There is no general agreement on the best method for limiting the output of a hearing aid. Peak clipping acts instantaneously to limit the output, but harmonic distortions are thereby produced. A compression system retains the identify of the signal once the threshold of compression has been reached (Davis and Silverman, 1960), but the most effective time constants for speech intelligibility are still questionable (Kretsinger and Young, 1960; Lynn and Carhart, 1963; Caraway and Carhart, 1967). Some compression systems act almost instantaneously over the entire operating range of the instrument (linear and curvilinear compressors) to modify the gain of various input levels to reach a predetermined output level. The problem with these systems is that the hearing aid does not differentiate between noise and speech; during pauses in the conversation, the ambient noise is amplified to reach the predetermined output. The time constants are so fast that they can operate within phonemes. If the intensity of a fricative is less than the ambient noise, it will be the noise which is processed by the hearing aid, while the situation is immediately reversed for a more intense subsequent vowel. Under quiet conditions, linear or curvilinear compressions appear to have a great deal of merit; under noisy conditions, however, the complex intensity variations in time of the noise and the speech present problems which have not been fully evaluated.

Gain. In selecting hearing aids with reference to gain, a common clinical procedure is to compensate for the hearing loss with an aid whose gain approximates the unaided sound field SRT. The aid producing the aided SRT closest to 0 dB is considered the most desirable. Unfortunately, the problem is not so simple. The gain of a hearing aid operates on the auditory signal and not the auditory threshold (Markle and Zaner, 1966). For the average hearing-impaired person, it is more important that the gain provide maximal understanding of average intensity speech than a lower aided SRT. Sometimes these goals are mutually exclusive.

Markle and Zaner (1966) compared intelligibility scores at three different HTLs of speech input (35, 50 and 65 dB) when the gain of the aid was set to be equivalent to the unaided SRT and when it was set 50 dB below the unaided most comfortable listening (MCL) level (gain = unaided MCL − 50 dB). This gain setting was chosen so as to deliver an average speech input (50 dB HTL) to the MCL of a client. At the average (50 dB) and loud (65 dB) speech inputs, WDSs were superior when the gain was set in reference to the unaided MCL level. At the low (35 dB) speech input, WDSs were superior when the gain was set to be equivalent to the unaided SRT.

Yantis, Millin and Shapiro (1966) kept the input constant (60 dB SPL) and varied the gain setting of the hearing aid around the "preferred" gain setting of their subjects (in essence, the MCL level). They found higher WDSs at the preferred gain settings, with generally lower scores at higher and lower gain settings, in other words settings which would result in lower and higher aided SRTs. The "preferred" gain setting usually exceeded by no more than 10 dB the point where aural harmonics were produced in the ear. The lower WDSs resulting from the higher gain settings were attributed mainly to the distortion products of aural overload, although the effect of amplitude distortion in the hearing aid at high gain levels was also considered a contributing factor.

These studies suggest that the aids selected for a hearing aid evaluation should provide sufficient gain to enable a client to reach a "preferred gain" or MCL level, rather than being set to be equivalent to the client's unaided SRT. If it is necessary to rotate the gain control close to its maximum in order to reach this point, the large increase in distortion which occurs near the maximum gain setting of aids (see Chapter 40) will make the particular aid unsuitable. Conversely, an aid can be considered unsuitable if its lowest gain setting delivers an average input above the client's MCL level. The optimal setting, that which permits an average input to reach a client's MCL or "PB Max" (frequently, but not necessarily the same), appears to be about midway between the lowest and highest possible gain settings. Some recently accumulated evidence suggests that the "preferred" or "use" gain setting is adjusted by patients to deliver a gain which represents approximately half their measured hearing loss. Thus patients with HTLs of 60 dB set the gain at 30 dB while those with 90 dB HTLs set their gain at 45 dB (Brooks, 1973; Martin, 1973; McCandless, 1975; Byrne and Tonisson, 1976; Morris, 1977).

Selective Amplification

Background. Another consideration for the clinician is the frequency response of the aids to be tested. If the audiologist selects a number of hearing aids with widely divergent responses, then the results of the evaluation may reflect either these or other electroacoustic differences between the aids. Much of the hearing aid evaluation controversy has occurred because the goal has been defined in terms of hearing aids rather than in terms of electroacoustic systems. The analysis of this point will be deferred until the discussion. For the present, we will be concerned only with the clinical practice of changing the frequency response characteristics of aids to conform to the presumed needs of the client.

The concept of "selective amplification," that is, tailoring the frequency response curve of a hearing aid in conformance with the client's audiogram, has been with us since the early days of vacuum tube hearing aids (Watson and Tolan, 1949). Taken to its extreme, selective amplification led to the concept of "mirror imaging," in which the precise degree of loss a client displayed at different frequencies was built into the response curve of the hearing aid. The theoretical result of such a practice is presumed to be normal aided pure tone thresholds. In the classic "Harvard report" (Davis et al., 1946), some of the problems inherent in the concept of selective amplification were noted. The concept deals with thresholds, while listening is a suprathreshold phenomenon. At suprathreshold levels, the equal loudness contours tend to normalize and a relatively low sensation level may result in a fairly high loudness level. Another problem pointed out in the report was the technical difficulty in designing a hearing aid which would precisely reflect the hearing loss across all the frequencies, and which would not be unduly altered by gain, baffle and ear mold characteristics. Watson and Tolan (1949) provide an extensive review of the relevant literature in the years preceding 1949. They generally agree with the conclusions of the Harvard report, namely that either a flat or a high pass 6-dB per octave response is most appropriate for most subjects, but they cite a number of individual exceptions wherein the response of the aid had to be tailored more selectively for the best results.

Recent Research. Considering the significance of the question, it is somewhat surprising that few studies in recent years have directly evaluated the effects of frequency response on discrimination scores. In the Reddell and Calvert (1966) study, WDSs in quiet and noise were compared for two aids selected by the experimenters, with one "custom adjusted" in slope of amplification curve by the manufacturer to roughly conform to each subject's threshold configuration. Scores with the custom-adjusted aid were statistically superior to those obtained with the standard clinic aids. The objective scores were supported by the subjective preferences of most of the subjects for the experimental aid. The authors do point out, however, that while they selected frequency response as the basic difference between the experimental and the control aids, differences in other electroacoustic dimensions may also have been present. Their findings, therefore, do not necessarily reflect only the variable under investigation.

Thompson and Lassman (1969) selected 30 subjects with similar high frequency sensory-neural hearing losses and administered several discrimination tests with earphones under conditions of flat and selective amplification. The response curve of the playback system in the selective (filtered) condition approximately "fit" the average hearing loss configuration of the subjects. The group as a whole showed no difference in discrimination scores between the flat and filtered conditions when the W-22s were administered in quiet. Differences in favor of the filtered condition did emerge when the W-22s were administered in noise and when a nonsense syllable discrimination test was used. The subjects were further divided into high, middle and low distortion groups on the basis of their performance on three different types of Bekesy tests, a short increment sensitivity index (SISI) test and a tone decay test. For the low distortion group in particular, the selective amplification condition resulted in higher scores with the W-22s in noise and with the nonsense syllable discrimination test. They point out that the feasibility of selective amplification may depend upon the degree of endogenous distortions in the auditory system and that it will be reflected only under certain conditions of testing.

Thomas and Sparks (1971) presented 17 hearing-impaired listeners with both processed speech signals, in which high-pass filtering (cutoff of 1100 Hz) with a slope of 12 dB per octave was combined with infinite amplitude clipping, and an unmodified version of the same signal at sensation levels (SL) of 20, 30 and 40 dB. They found that 13 of the 17 subjects achieved significantly higher discrimination scores at the 20 and 30 dB SLs, with little difference at the 40 dB SL. They attribute the improvement to a possible reduction in the masking effects of high intensity low frequency sounds, a psychoacoustic phenomenon explored in detail by Danaher, Osberger and Pickett (1973) and further verified by Sung, Sung, and Angelelli (1971) in speech discrimination testing with hearing-impaired listeners.

Perhaps the most complete, and convincing, demonstration of "selective" amplification was achieved by Pascoe (1975). He compared word intelligibility scores with five different frequency responses, two defined in a coupler

(uniform coupler gain, and a 6-dB per octave rise), two defined behaviorally, as the difference between the aided and unaided narrow-band sound-field thresholds (uniform functional gain and uniform hearing level) and one simulated commercial aid. The one response with which the eight sensory-neural hearing-impaired subjects obtained the highest WDS was with the one which provided sufficient amplification at all frequencies to produce an aided narrow-band threshold curve paralleling the normal audibility curve (the uniform hearing level condition). Since the unaided threshold configuration of these subjects was moderately sloping, it follows that the aided response provided more amplification in the high frequencies than the lows. Moreover, since the frequency response was defined in terms of each individual wearing the aid (the difference between the aided and the unaided sound-field thresholds), we have in this study the elimination of a major variable which has confounded much of the previous research, that is, defining the response as that measured in a coupler rather than that occurring in a particular ear.

A special application of selective amplification is the utilization of earmold acoustics to alter the frequency response of the signal reaching the client's ear. These alterations are made by producing vents of differing diameters in the earmold, by changing the length and diameter of the bore and by using an open or nonoccluding type earmold (see Chapter 42). A very dramatic attenuation of the frequencies below 1000 Hz occurs, for example, when an open earmold is used. A number of studies have demonstrated improvements in word discrimination resulting from these variations in earmold acoustics.

McClellan (1967) compared scores in quiet and noise with vented and unvented earmold for five subjects with precipitous high frequency hearing losses. Under the same signal-to-noise conditions, he found higher WDSs with the vented than with the unvented mold. Jetty and Rintelmann (1970) measured speech discrimination in quiet for three groups of hearing-impaired subjects: a group of 10 with conductive losses, a group of 10 with precipitous sensory-neural hearing losses and 10 with gradual slope sensory-neural hearing losses. The vented mold did not improve the WDSs of the conductive group, but did result in an approximately 10% improvement for both groups of sensory-neural subjects. On the other hand, Hodgson and Murdock (1970), Revoile (1968), Dodds and Harford (1968a) and Northern and Hattler (1970) could find no consistent differences in WDSs for any group of subjects under any conditions when they compared earmolds with different size vents and bores to a standard earmold. All four of these studies, however, point out that their subjects often expressed a subjective preference for the vented over the standard mold.

The results are less equivocal when discrimination scores obtained with open or nonoccluding molds are compared to those obtained with standard or vented molds. It will be recalled that the acoustical effect of an open mold is to sharply attenuate frequencies below 1000 Hz. Thus this type of earmold provides a form of selective amplification, particularly appropriate for subjects with precipitous high frequency hearing losses. Hodgson and Murdock (1970), Dodds and Harford (1968a), Jetty and Rintelmann (1970) and Frank and Karlovich (1973) all found that their subjects achieved higher WDSs with the use of the open earmold than with standard molds. In two of these studies (Hodgson and Murdock, 1970; Dodds and Harford, 1968a), the scores obtained with the open molds were also significantly higher than those obtained with the vented molds.

These findings imply that the clinician must consider earmold variations as an integral part of his preselection procedures. If a modified earmold is clearly indicated for a particular client, then all the aids should be evaluated with the modified earmold. If there is a question whether a modified earmold is indicated, then one or more aids can be evaluated with and without the modified earmold.

Specifying Frequency Response. A number of hearing aid companies provide fitting manuals which purport to relate specific adjustments on their aids to the amplification requirements of a particular client. Other companies will build or alter circuits to fit as nearly as acoustically possible the client's hearing loss configuration. In essence, these are a priori judgments, since experimental verification of the effects of these adjustments on word discrimination has not been forthcoming. For most hearing-impaired clients, one can demonstrate some improvement in speech discrimination with almost any standard frequency response simply as a function of gain; the ultimate criterion, which is not yet with us, is to demonstrate that a particular formula for specifying frequency response produces the most possible improvement in discrimination. This is not to say that these formulas are erroneous or valueless; only that they have not been rigorously investigated. Two published examples of such formulas will be briefly reviewed.

Both methods (Victoreen, 1960; Wallenfels, 1967) plot hearing loss on an SPL scale rather than an audiogram. On this scale, the normal threshold appears on the bottom and is plotted in terms of the SPL necessary to reach the "normal" threshold at the different frequencies. An abnormal threshold is displaced upward by an amount equivalent to the degree of hearing loss (exactly the same downward displacement which would appear on an audiogram). The plot of the abnormal threshold is considered to be the lower limits of the scale when determining the required frequency response. In one method (Victoreen, 1960), the upper limit is considered to be 130 dB SPL unless specifically measured otherwise. In the other method (Wallenfels, 1967), the upper limit is the measured TD across frequency. The use of this scale permits a direct comparison of the abnormal threshold configuration and the response of the hearing aid, since they are now both plotted with the same reference level. Essentially, both methods bisect the upper and lower limits in order to specify the frequency response characteristics of the "prescribed" hearing aid. The necessary gain is considered to be the difference between a 65-dB SPL input at 1000 Hz and the SPL of the bisection point at the same frequency. Neither method (nor any other) incorporates the alterations in the frequency response produced by variations in ear canals, earmolds, baffle effects, microphone placement and tubing size and diameter.

The recommendation of specific frequency responses for certain classes of clients is also widely practiced by professional audiologists. Generally, these recommendations are rather broad, i.e., extreme high tone emphasis for a client with a sharply sloping loss or a moderate high tone emphasis for a gradually sloping loss. There are numerous clinical reports which suggest that these broad changes in frequency response do result in superior discrimination over that obtained with either flat response hearing aids or flat response earphones (Menzel, 1964; Miller, 1967; Dodds and Harford, 1968a). Until demonstrated otherwise, there appears to be merit in continuing the practice of tailoring the response curve to roughly conform to the audiometric configuration. However, it would be wise for the clinician to keep his options open by arranging for comparative testing, trial periods, and, in particularly difficult cases, such further audiometric measures as the assessment of the suprathreshold loudness function.

A system of modifying amplification characteristics which appears to have a great deal of merit is that suggested by Villchur (1973). In his procedure, two separate bands of a speech signal (an upper and lower with overlap in the middle) are compressed and then filtered to conform to either a measured or computed equal-loudness contour. The ratio and threshold of compression in the two bands can be independently adjusted as can the contour of the compressed speech. Villchur reports significant increases in intelligibility with this method as compared to a conventional signal processing system. His results have been corroborated and extended by Yanick (1976) who used a similar multiband compression and equalization procedure.

Preliminary Evaluation

There are numerous clients for whom a definite recommendation regarding a hearing aid cannot be made, and for whom a trial period cannot be arranged. Clients in this category are usually elderly people or individuals with precipitous threshold configurations. The problem in getting geriatric clients to accept and utilize amplification has been recognized for some time (Alpiner, 1967). An audiometric demonstration of improved communicative efficiency wrought by amplification can assist both these categories of clients to accept a hearing aid, as well as giving the clinician some objective evidence that a hearing aid is indeed indicated.

A common clinical method of achieving this result is by administering discrimination tests in the sound field at a constant HTL, usually 40-to 50-dB, under both aided and unaided conditions. The difference in discrimination scores for the two conditions reflects the contribution made by hearing aid amplification. For a more exacting comparison, the tests can be administered with and without a competing signal. Consider a typical example of an adult with a bilateral high frequency hearing loss, with an unaided sound field SRT of 20-dB, and with an unaided WDS of 56% obtained with a 40-dB HTL signal. With an ear-level hearing aid adjusted to moderate high tone emphasis, his aided WDS with the same 40-dB HTL signal improved to 82%. The objective improvement is apparent. This objective improvement was subjectively confirmed by the client when he was permitted to listen to the constant signal with and without the hearing aid.

Dodds and Harford (1968b) describe a bisensory approach to determine whether clients with low discrimination scores, mild losses or poor motivation can benefit from amplification. Both forms of the Utley lipreading test are administered face-to-face, with and without the hearing aid. For some clients with poor or borderline auditory capability, the tests can demonstrate the auditory contribution in a bisensory presentation mode. In one example, the subject achieved an aided sound field WDS of 20%, thus suggesting a poor prognosis for successful hearing aid usage. Without the hearing aid, his lipreading score was a poor 23%. With the hearing aid, however, his lipreading score increased to 78%, indicating the addi-

tional communicative ability due to amplification. In another example, they describe using the technique to motivate hearing aid usage for an elderly lady who insisted that she could hear as well without the aid as with it. Her lipreading score without amplification was 32%, but with amplification it was 100%. This was sufficient to demonstrate to her the benefits of a hearing aid. In addition to the contribution this simple technique can make in a preliminary evaluation, its application can serve to remind us that communication efficiency for the hearing impaired depends not only on audition, but also upon the interacting contribution of visual clues.

SELECTION PROCEDURES

Introduction

The clinician is now almost ready to select the aids with which the client is to be tested. He has determined that the client is a hearing aid candidate, verified a prior otologic examination, made arrangements to secure the proper earmold(s), chosen the ear and type of hearing aid, and considered what general electroacoustic characteristics are required. He has, however, several other decisions to make before he can select the aids to be evaluated.

If the client is a candidate for an ear-level aid, then the question arises whether an eyeglass aid or a behind-the-ear aid is more suitable. A hearing aid built into an eyeglass frame ties together vision and hearing; if the client has several sets of glasses, or uses glasses only occasionally, then a behind-the-ear aid is more suitable. For some clients, telephone usage is an important factor in their lives; for them a telephone attachment on the hearing aid is indispensable. The physical dimensions of postauricular aids are an important consideration for the client whose pinna is smaller or lies flat against the mastoid process. The ease in rotating the gain control and the accessibility of the battery compartment may support the use of certain aids for elderly or physically handicapped clients. Frequently, financial and maintenance considerations obviate the inclusion of certain aids. All of these factors must be weighed by the clinician in determining which aids are to be included.

The usual practice is to evaluate from three to six hearing aids. The clinician must be thoroughly familiar with the published characteristics of each; some clinics are able to supplement and confirm the manufacturer's specifications with their own instrumentation. Each aid has to be checked to ensure that it is working properly. The required electroacoustic adjustments must be made, e.g., high tone emphasis and output limits set. Fresh batteries must be available because reductions in gain and output will occur and distortions increase as the battery voltage drops (Lotterman, Kasten and Majerus, 1967). By making these determinations and preparations in advance, the clinician can concentrate his attention on the client.

Carhart Method

Thirty years ago, Carhart (1946a) described the procedures used to evaluate hearing aids at the Deshon General Hospital. With some variations and refinements, these procedures are still widely practiced (ASHA, 1967; Burney, 1972). Four dimensions of hearing aid performance were explored: effective gain, tolerance limit, efficiency in noise and word discrimination.

In step one, the subject's unaided sound-field SRT, tolerance limit and discrimination score (PB-50s at 25 dB SL) were measured. These scores served as the reference for comparison with aided performance.

In step two, the gain control of the first instrument was adjusted until the subject reported that a 40-dB HTL speech signal was at the MCL level. An aided SRT and TD were then measured.

In step three, the aid was set on maximum gain and the aided SRT and TD were again measured.

In step four, the gain control was adjusted to permit the subject to reach an MCL level with a 50-dB HTL input speech signal. Two signal-to-noise ratios were obtained, one with white noise and the other with sawtooth noise. The intensity of the noise was alternately increased and decreased until a point was reached where the subject could barely repeat several test words. The difference between the speech and the noise levels at this point defined the signal-to-noise ratios.

In step five, the aid was again adjusted to permit the subject to reach an MCL level, this time with a 40-dB HTL input speech signal. The aided SRT was again measured for a reliability check against step two. A 50-word intelligibility test was administered at a 25-dB SL.

Steps two through five were repeated for each of the preselected hearing aids. These tests permitted the aids to be compared in terms of effective gain (the lowest SRTs), widest dynamic range (the difference between the aided SRTs and the aided TDs), signal-to-noise ratios (tolerating higher levels of noise before discrimination was disrupted) and the relative word discrimination scores. The selection of a specific aid was made on the basis of the composite results. Many subjects performed equally well with several of the aids on one or more of the dimensions, but their performance could be differentiated on the basis of other dimensions. When several of the best performing aids gave similar results on several dimensions, the selection was made on the basis of size, weight and esthetic preferences. In a different setting, other factors such as cost, warranty, repair availability would have been considered.

Modifications of the Carhart Method

Individual clinics and clinicians have modified the procedures described by Carhart, but, in tribute to his original insights, essentially the same four dimensions of hearing aid performance are still being investigated. In the following paragraphs, some of the more common modifications of the basic Carhart method will be discussed.

The effective gain of an aid is still assessed by comparing the client's unaided and aided SRTs, with the client adjusting the gain to reach his MCL level. It has been shown that subjects can replicate this same gain setting upon retest (Carhart, 1946b; Walden and Kasten, 1969; Kopra and Blosser, 1968).

It is no longer common to measure SRT and TD with the aid set at maximum gain. First, these measures provide little practical information regarding a client's use of the aid; second, if a client did have to utilize the maximum gain setting of an aid fairly often, he undoubtedly would require a more powerful aid; and third, except for some body aids, most of which are probably placed on a baffle board some distance from the client, the occurrence of acoustic squeal at high gain levels will prevent this setting with the average aid.

The most extensive modifications relate to the measurement of discrimination under noise conditions. In the original method, the noise level was varied until a point was reached where the constant speech signal was barely intelligible. Currently, this test is accomplished by measuring discrimination against a competing signal, which may be either noise or speech. The signal-to-noise ratio is predetermined, usually at a level which depresses discrimination scores for normal listeners below their maximum performance. The competing signal and the speech emanate from two physically separated loud speakers. Open ended monosyllabic word lists still appear to be the most common stimuli for aided discrimination testing. Some investigators have noted the increased information and sensitivity which can be derived from other types of speech signals, such as a rhyme type test (Bode and Kasten, 1971) and a synthetic sentence test (Jerger and Thelin, 1968). This aspect will be more fully discussed in a later section.

The level at which intelligibility tests are

administered has also undergone revision. In the original method, the tests were administered at a 25-dB SL. While some clinicians still administer discrimination lists at a fixed SL (e.g., 25 to 40 dB), other clinicians prefer to present the lists at a fixed HTL (approximately 40 to 50 dB). The relative performance of hearing aids can be compared at any level. The rationale for a fixed HTL input is that the most pertinent input to assess the relative performance of various aids is the level equivalent to average conversational speech.

Hood (1970) has taken this reasoning one step further. He administers discrmination tests, in quiet and noise, at two or three HTLs (varying somewhat from client to client) roughly representing soft, average and loud conversational speech. He reports a number of instances in which the performance of different aids could not be differentiated at one input level, but could be differentiated at other input levels. Since this method is rather time-consuming, only a limited amount of aids can be evaluated. He points out, however, that he would rather evaluate fewer aids thoroughly, than more aids less thoroughly.

The most recent modification of the original Carhart procedure was described by Jerger and Hayes (1976), and it is a welcome new addition to the literature. The authors' procedures preclude a number of the problems which will be discussed later. They use recorded versions of the synthetic sentence identification (SSI) test, objective scoring procedures on the closed response task (1 out of 10 possible sentences are identified), and administer the lists ordinarily from a frontally placed speaker at a 60-dB SPL level, while another loudspeaker in the rear presents the competing stimuli at different intensity levels. A number of message competition ratios (MCRs) are generated, ranging from very easy (plus 20 dB, to very difficult, minus 20 dB), and the subject's scores across all aids and/or combinations can be compared at the different MCRs. Thus differences in performance are teased out which may not be apparent at one MCR. The subject's scores can be viewed in terms of the aided improvement wrought by a particular aid or fitting, and in terms of the residual deficit, by comparing the scores to the function obtained by normal listeners.

This procedure has a number of appealing points, and a few potential pitfalls. The location of the primary speaker directly in front of the listener and the secondary speaker directly in back presents the speech and the competing signal in phase at the two ears. This orientation does not seem suitable for comparing binaural versus monaural hearing aids; the in-phase location of the speech and the competition minimizes the capacity of the binaural system to act upon and differentiate the signal from the noise. The other possible pitfall deals with using a closed response synthetic sentence as the stimulus, which, while permitting the relative comparison of aids and/or fittings, provides an overoptimistic view of the individual's performance with an aid (100% score on the SSIs says little about how a person will really function in a communicative situation in his real life environment). The same procedure, utilizing the SPIN test (see below) would appear to preclude this difficulty, while the addition of another speaker (or cassettes presenting predetermined levels of noise) would obviate the first pitfall.

Other Methods

Zerlin (1962) used a paired comparison method to evaluate differences among six hearing aids. He taped 30-sec passages of conversational speech in the presence of recorded cafeteria noise, using a 65-dB SPL input for the speech and a 60-dB input for the noise. The 21 sensory-neural hearing loss subjects listened to the recordings through an earphone, and, by manipulating a two-position selector switch, they could listen alternately to either one of a pair of aids. Each of the six aids was paired during the recordings with every other aid, resulting in 15 recorded pairs. The subjects were asked to rate which aid appeared to make the speech most intelligible. In the event of a tie, they expressed their preferences in terms of the relative comfort of the auditory experience. Following the paired comparison test, the subjects were administered a 25-word monosyllabic test list in quiet which had been recorded through the aids in the same manner as the conversational speech. His results indicated that the paired comparison preference method produced definite discriminations among five of the six aids, while the aids could not be differentiated with the WDS results. Furthermore, upon retest, the paired comparison preferences were fairly reliable.

Many clinicians commonly ask their clients to express relative preferences among aids. The advantage of the Zerlin method is that it permits rapid comparisons, thus minimizing memory and adaption factors. A major problem in a clinical setting is that the method requires the recorded pairing of each aid with every other aid. Even if only the aids in the same general category were paired with one another, the problems of recording, storage, rapid retrieval and playback would still have to be surmounted. The fact that clear-cut and reliable distinctions among hearing aids could be made with a paired comparison preference method, but not with the WDSs is, nevertheless, a noteworthy result. One wonders if speech discrimination distinctions among the aids would not have also been apparent had a 50-word test list been used and administered under the same noise conditions existing in the paired comparison method (Carhart, 1965).

Jeffers (1960) also used a quality judgment paired comparison method to assess differences among hearing aids. She selected five aids, encompassing a range of good, fair and poor acoustic characteristics and arranged them in four pairs. The 34 conductive hearing loss subjects listened to a 1-min recording of cold running speech reproduced through a sound-field speaker, first while wearing one aid of a pair and then while wearing the other. The subjects were asked to comment on their preferences and describe any apparent differences in the aids. The results indicated that the subjects definitely and unambiguously preferred the aids with the more desirable acoustic characteristics. All the subjects considered the 1-min listening time adequate. No problems were experienced in retaining the auditory impressions of the first aid for comparison to the second aid, although there was an unspecified interval between their listening trials.

In Jeffers' (1960) study, only two aids with contrasting acoustic characteristics were directly compared subjectively. The experimental instrumentation did not permit rapid listening comparison between the aids, as did the Zerlin (1962) study, and whether the same clear-cut distinctions would have been made if three or more aids had been subjectively compared is not known. Jeffers' report that subjective hearing aid preferences were related to the "desirability" of the electroacoustic system was confirmed by Witter and Goldstein (1971), who found that better transient responses, extension of the upper frequency range, and less harmonic distortion were both preferred subjectively and generally resulted in higher intelligibility scores. Hendry and Rupp (1973) found similar results in that subject-selected frequency responses coincided with subjective preferences and superior intelligibility scores.

Jerger (1967) describes an intermodulation distortion test (IDT) for differentiating among hearing aids. He recorded two pure tones, one at 1000 Hz and the other at 1600 Hz, on each channel of a two-channel tape recorder. On one of the channels, the two frequency signal was "clean"; on the other channel, it was recorded after being processed through a hearing aid. The subjects listened alternately to the signal pairs under four signal-to-noise conditions. Their task was to determine whether they heard the clean signal or the hearing aid processed signal first. Three hearing aids were used: aid "A" characterized by a flat response and minimal harmonic distortion, aid "B" by a peaked frequency response and moderate distortion, and aid "C" by considerable harmonic distortion. Performance with these three aids had previously been differentiated with the same subjects using a sentence intelligibility test (PAL-8) in a −6-dB signal-to-competing speech ratio (speech 6 dB weaker than noise). The results indicated that the IDT procedure and the sentence intelligibility tests produced the same rankings among the aids. The signals processed through aid "A" could be differentiated from the clean signal only in the most favorable signal-to-noise conditions; for aid "B," the differentiation clearly occurred at all signal-to-noise ratios, although less so under higher levels of noise; aid "C," on the other hand, could be clearly differentiated from the clean signal at all signal-to-noise ratios. Two advantages are ascribed to the IDT procedure over speech materials. First, for any given aid, the performances of the different subjects are more alike, i.e., the standard deviations were smaller; and second, the stimuli, being pure tones, are precisely specifiable.

Zink (1969), Zink and Alpiner (1968) and Ross (1975) suggest that an electroacoustic hearing aid evaluation supplement, and sometimes substitute for, conventional hearing aid evaluations. Each new aid is assessed electroacoustically to determine if the instrument meets basic standards in respect to gain, gain control linearity, frequency response, frequency range, distortion and output. Only those aids which meet the electroacoustic standards (not explicitly specified) are included in the conventional hearing aid evaluation. For children whose language inabilities make conventional procedures impossible, the electroacoustic hearing aid evaluation is used to directly select the aids which conform to their presumed needs. Considering the paucity of electroacoustic information supplied in many hearing aid specifications, the variability of electroacoustic characteristics among aids of the same make and model, and the necessity to check aids over time, the routine use of electroacoustic instrumentation can give the clinician a firmer foundation on which to base and modify his clinical judgments.

Selection of Speech Stimuli

Although a number of methods for selecting among hearing aids have been suggested, the primary criterion is still the relative scores obtained on word discrimination tests. Thus the effectiveness of any such method depends upon the type of speech signal and the condition under which it is utilized. The material must be sufficiently sensitive to reflect electroacoustic differences among hearing aids, and sufficiently reliable so that the error of measurement is less than intelligibility score variations produced by the electroacoustic differences.

Sensitivity. There is growing agreement among audiologists that the open ended monosyllabic word test in quiet conditions is not sufficiently sensitive. That is, real differences among subjects and hearing aids may be obscured since the tests and test conditions lack resolving power (Carhart, 1965; Jerger, Malmquist and Speaks, 1966a; Thompson and Lassman, 1969; Cooper and Cutts, 1971). This was confirmed in four different studies (Jirsa and Hodgson, 1970; Orchik and Oyer, 1972; Dodds and Bode, 1972; Foust and Gengel, 1973). Each of the studies noted that, while small differences could be found when testing under quiet conditions, the tests employing noise interference were able to differentiate the aids much more clearly.

The most common procedure entails delivering a competing signal (either noise, voice babble or other discrimination material) from a secondary speaker placed at a 45° angle to one side of the client, while the primary speaker is placed at a 45° angle at the other side of the client. This physical arrangement of the loud speakers necessitates awareness of the varying effects the head shadow can have upon the perceived signal-to-noise relationship and thus upon the resulting discrimination score (Olsen and Carhart, 1967). In a monaural ear level hearing aid evaluation, the effect can be eliminated by seating the client sideways, so that the sound field from both speakers has equal access to the hearing aid. The most common speech material utilized with this arrangement still appears to be one of a number of open ended monosyllabic word lists (see Chapter 13). The face validity of this procedure can be increased by locating the loudspeaker from which the primary signal is delivered directly in front of the client, with the competing signals being delivered from speakers located on one or both sides of the client, or from a ceiling speaker with the client located directly under the cone of sound. Hearing-impaired individuals almost invariably try to face the source of a desired signal, and so they should, and the practice of locating the desired source at a 45° angle in hearing aid evaluations does not appear to be very realistic.

The next most common speech discrimination material utilized in hearing aid research appears to be sentences. The basic rationale for their use lies in the similarity of the test to conditions facing the hearing aid user in everyday life (Harris et al., 1961). Furthermore, sentence tests can be distorted in ways which have less relevance for monosyllabic words, e.g., reverberation, filtering and time compression and expansion. Their sensitivity

has been further increased through the multiple use of these distortions (Harris, 1960) and through the use of competing speech signals (Jerger et al., 1966a). Speaks and Jerger (1965) used an SSI test for hearing aid research. Jerger and Thelin (1968) used the SSI test in research relating electroacoustic characteristics of hearing aids to speech discrimination. They concluded that "the basic technique of sentence identification coupled with the competing message concept can well be recommended as a point of departure for the design of new approaches to hearing aid evaluation in the clinical context." These investigators also found that response latency was strongly related to the subject's SSI score, the poorer the score the longer the latency. This finding corroborates a long held clinical impression; namely, that the length of time it takes a client to respond is an important indicator of his skill. It is possible that the sensitivity of all discrimination tests can be increased by incorporating response latency measures in hearing aid evaluations (Hecker, Stevens and Williams, 1966).

To the author's knowledge, the most complete, and rationalized, sentence test ever developed was just recently published (Kalikow, Stevens and Elliot, 1977). It is called the SPIN test (Speech Intelligibility in Noise), and it tests a listener's ability to utilize both the linguistic situational information contained in sentences with the acoustic-phonetic discriminations which must be made to identify low probability words embedded in sentences. This test deserves to (and no doubt soon will) gain widespread acceptance.

For a more analytical assessment of the effects of hearing aid characteristics upon a speech signal, a monosyllabic word rhyme discrimination test can be used. A number of these have been developed (House et al., 1965; Kreul et al., 1968; Schultz and Schubert, 1969) since the original test was developed by Fairbanks (1958). The test permits evaluation of phonemic errors because of the rhyming closed set response format. Bode and Kasten (1971) used a modified rhyme test to evaluate the effects of hearing aid distortion on consonant discrimination. Their results indicated that the test accurately differentiated among relatively minor increases in distortion. For this reason, and because of the "closed set response format with increased reliability of responses and emphasis on consonantal discrimination," they suggest that the test would be desirable to use in hearing aid evaluations.

Reliability. One major criticism of conventional hearing aid evaluations concerns the lack of resolving power of discrimination tests. As we have seen, however, the evidence suggests that it is possible to differentiate the performance of hearing aids, given appropriate test material and test conditions. A related criticism of conventional hearing aid evaluations deals with the apparent lack of test reliability, i.e., variations in retest scores which can change the rank ordering of a number of aids.

The study by Shore, Bilger and Hirsh (1960) was the first which seriously questioned the reliability of repeated hearing aid measurements. Fifteen hearing-impaired subjects, five in each of three diagnostic categories, were tested with four different hearing aids on four occasions comparing aided SRTs and aided discrimination scores in quiet and noise. Half-lists of the Rush-Hughes recording of the PB-50 test were administered at a 40-dB SL. Under the noise conditions, the speech and the noise emanated from the same loudspeaker at a 0 signal-to-noise ratio. The large variations in test-retest scores that they found for different aids, settings and days led them to conclude "that the reliability of these measures is not good enough to warrant the investment of a large amount of clinical time with them in selecting hearing aids."

Shortly after the above study was published, McConnell, Silber and McDonald (1960) reported high correlations when they compared the aided WDS obtained in quiet conditions by one clinician to that obtained by another clinician with the same aid on the same day. They also found a high correlation when the time span between the test and the retest sessions was delayed for two or more weeks. While the results of this study showed excellent reliability, it should be noted that only the discrimination results for the selected aid were compared. The study was not designed to evaluate whether the rank ordering of the aids would have changed if all the aids initially tested were all retested. But this is the crucial question upon which rests much of the rationale of current hearing aid evaluation procedures.

Although not designed for this purpose, the study by Olsen and Carhart (1967) includes some information relevant to this point. As part of a larger investigation, each of their three groups of subjects participated in two identical test sessions. Thus the aided test-retest monosyllabic word reliability could be computed for the three modes of testing (monaural direct, monaural indirect and binaural), the two types of competitive signals (sentences and noise), the four primary-to-secondary ratio levels (+6 dB, +12 dB, +18 dB and in quiet), and the three hearing aids incorporating known electroacoustic differences. Their results indicated high test-retest reliability, i.e., the scores achieved in the test session were closely repeated during the retest session for all three hearing aids. The same rank ordering among the aids found in the first session also occurred in the retest session. The only exception to this finding concerned the reliability coefficients for the conductive hearing loss group; for this group, significant coefficients were found only in the more difficult listening conditions. Olsen and Carhart point out that "it was only when the task was sufficiently taxing to produce an appreciable spread in the scores obtained by these subjects that systematic individual differences in scores were distinctive enough to manifest themselves through a high coefficient of correlation." To demonstrate reliability, then, it is necessary to ensure a sufficient range of scores.

Indirect evidence regarding the reliability of aided discrimination scores can be adduced from the hearing aid research in which the scores rank themselves in accordance with the variable being investigated. When, for example, discrimination scores are inversely related to progressive increases in distortion (Bode and Kasten, 1971; Kasten, Lotterman and Burnett, 1967) or increasing irregularities in the response curve (Jerger and Thelin, 1968), then it follows that the inherent variability of the discrimination tests are less than the variability produced by the electroacoustic modification. We can, in other words, assume sufficient sensitivity and reliability in these test instruments and test conditions to reflect at least the range of electroacoustic variations under investigation.

The evidence supporting reliability of aided intelligibility measures is based on research studies in which experimenters carefully controlled signal presentation and test conditions. Thus, the closer the clinician can approximate this kind of control, the more assurance he will have of the reliability of his discrimination measures. Live voice testing, without specified conditions of competing signal, and with variations in number of test words, introduces variables hardly conducive to reliable test measures. It is not a question of whether it is possible to achieve reliable and sensitive measures, but rather whether the clinician is willing to avail himself of the prerequisite conditions.

A learning or practice effect may occur to complicate a reliable hearing aid evaluation. Using the PAL-8 sentences, Jerger, Speaks and Malmquist (1966b) found that their subjects' performance improved with each trial. Performance evaluated on a six trial average ranked the aids differently than that obtained on only a single trial. If this type of an effect occurs in a clinical hearing aid evaluation, then the last aid evaluated may show higher intelligibility scores just on this basis. Since it is not known what the magnitude of this effect is with different types of test material and different conditions of testing, clinicians must individually assess this factor when performing hearing aid evaluations. An occasional retest of the first aid evaluated would seem to have merit.

FOLLOW-UP PROCEDURES

Hearing Aid Orientation and Counseling

Orientation and counseling usually begin at the conclusion of the hearing aid evaluation. Too often, this is the extent of these services which are offered, or accepted, by the client. Rassi and Harford (1968) noted that 38% of the hearing aid users they queried experienced problems adjusting to their new aids. Although three-fourths of these clients were interested in a short orientation and counseling course, the difficulties in scheduling and the dwindling attendance led them to view its utility with "more than a small amount of skepticism." The value of the service is not questioned by them or by others (ASHA, 1967), simply our success in convincing our clients of its utility.

Finally, it should be recalled that as clinicians our responsibilities encompass more than the selection of a particular aid. The client's need for aural rehabilitative and vocational rehabilitative services of all kinds must be assessed and made available, whether or not the audiology center can provide all of them (ASHA, 1967). The audiologist is uniquely equipped to understand the communication problems wrought by a hearing loss, with all of its ramifications, and his contribution to the rehabilitation of the hearing-impaired client can be borne by no one else.

Hearing Aid Rechecks

Most clinics conduct hearing aid evaluations using instruments consigned by hearing aid dealers or companies for this purpose. Until recently it was rare that a client purchased the exact instrument with which he was evaluated and on which he attained superior performance. The Veterans Administration audiology clinics have been a major exception and more recently some audiologists have begun to evaluate and dispense the same hearing aid. The assumption is made that the electroacoustic characteristics of the purchased instrument will closely conform to the characteristics of another instrument of the same make and model (see Chapter 40), and that any variations which do occur are not sufficient to negatively affect the aid's speech processing capability. It is further assumed that the audiologist's recommendations regarding specific type and adjustments of the aid and earmold were honored by the dealer and followed by the client. To test these assumptions, clients are frequently asked to return to the clinic for a hearing aid recheck. The recheck can be routinely scheduled some weeks after the delivery of the aid or requested by the client after he has overcome the initial adjustment problems.

The audiometric aspects of the recheck ordinarily consist of the same performance tasks used in the initial evaluation. The results obtained with the client's new aid are compared to the results obtained with the clinic consigned aid at the time of the hearing aid evaluation. Since only the one aid is tested, the recheck session can be relatively brief. If performance with the new aid is measurably inferior to the performance with the clinic aid, then the clinician must investigate and attempt to resolve the discrepancy. The problem may be simply an erroneous adjustment or a clogged earmold. In some cases, it may be necessary to retest the client with the clinic aid in order to obtain a direct performance comparison. In the event the new aid is definitely inferior to the clinic aid, the dealer is contacted and steps taken to either repair the new aid or exchange it for another one.

Several studies have investigated this aspect of clinic hearing aid evaluations. In a study reviewed earlier, McConnell et al. (1960) compared the aided SRTs and intelligibility scores at the time of the initial evaluation to these same measures obtained some time later with a new aid of the same make and model. They found an extremely high correlation in discrimination measures and a moderate correlation in aided SRTs. Haug et al. (1963) reported similar findings. For the 20 subjects they examined, the aided SRTs between the two aids agreed within 5 dB in all instances, while WDSs varied more than 4% in only one instance.

These findings notwithstanding, a number of clinicians have a contrary impression regarding the performance similarities between the clinic and the purchased aid. Many audiologists, and I am one, can cite a number of examples where the performance of the purchased aid proved to be markedly inferior to that of the clinic aid. Part of the value of the hearing aid recheck lies in just such instances. For example, in the one case cited by Haug et al. (1963) where the subject's score with the new aid was much poorer than that obtained with the clinic aid, the instrument was replaced and a later test demonstrated the resulting improvement. The assumption behind this comparison is that the measures used to evaluate the hearing aid are adequately reliable; without this assurance, the audiometric aspects of the hearing aid rechecks would be of questionable value.

The recheck appointment has several nonaudiometric purposes. At this time, the client has been wearing his hearing aid for at least several weeks. If he is wearing his first aid, he should have already experienced some of the more common problems associated with hearing aid usage. Perhaps he is having difficulty understanding in noisy situations, or is unable to utilize the telephone attachment, or cannot insert the earmold by himself, or is bothered by clothing or wind noise, or is using a stock or improperly fitted earmold, or does not know that hearing aids cannot function without batteries (this has actually occurred!), or any one of a number of other related problems. The clinician now has the opportunity to instruct and counsel the client on problems which directly relate to his own experiences. He is focusing the discussion on that which most interests the client: his own unique problems. This aspect of the hearing aid recheck can make a significant contribution to a client's adjustment to his aid.

Unfortunately, of the clients queried by Rassi and Harford (1968) only 25% returned for a recheck; similar experiences are reported by Shore and Kramer (1963) in their follow-up questionnaire study. The results of both these studies point out the need to emphasize and re-emphasize to the client the necessity for keeping the recheck appointment. That it is possible to attain almost 100% attendance at a recheck appointment was pointed out to me by Green (1970). The client is scheduled for the recheck at the time of hearing aid evaluation; the fee he pays includes this service. The recheck is considered a "doctor's appointment" and the patient is instructed to return for it, with no alternate option "if everything is going all right." The recent trend toward hearing aid dispensing by audiologists may improve the follow-up situation (Cutler, 1975).

ORGANIZATION AND ADMINISTRATION OF HEARING AID SELECTION PROGRAM

The most complete description of the organization and administration of a clinical hearing aid selection program was given by Harford and Musket (1964). Additional information appeared in the publication of the Conference on Hearing Aid Evaluation Procedures (ASHA, 1967, Chapter 3). The following discussion is essentially a brief summary of these two sources.

Hearing Aid Inventory

A hearing aid inventory must contain a representative selection of the different types of hearing aids, including those with special features such as low frequency emphasis and automatic volume control (AVC). The make, model and serial number of each aid placed in the clinic is entered on an invoice. It is sometimes convenient to abbreviate the manufac-

turer's specifications on a separate index card for each reference. To ensure maximum utilization of the information supplied by the manufacturer, however, it may be desirable to refer directly to the printed specifications rather than an abbreviation. Each new aid is submitted initially for a trial period; the length of time will vary somewhat, being less in clinics which perform few hearing aid evaluations and more in active clinics.

During the trial period, the number of times each aid is evaluated and recommended is tabulated. At the conclusion of the trial period, those aids which demonstrate relatively low recommendation-trial ratios are assessed for possible replacement. Some aids with special features may be kept in an inventory in spite of a low ratio. The tabulation helps to minimize biases toward and against certain aids, since a visible record is kept of the trials and recommendations of each aid. It also provides assurance to the dealer that their aids are being given a fair shake. Dealers are encouraged to periodically place new models in the clinic, thus assuring an up-to-date representation of the current market. The number of aids in an inventory varies from clinic to clinic, depending upon their philosophy, activity and function; the modal value appears to be between 10 and 20.

Industry Cooperation

It should be remembered that clinic aids represent a substantial financial investment on the part of the hearing aid industry and individual dealers. It behooves audiologists to treat this investment with respect and to try to foster close working relationships with dealers who supply clinic aids. They should be encouraged to make periodic visits to the clinic to check on the performance of their aids, to consult with the clinicians regarding any problems and to discuss the placement of new aids. In some clinics, when a specific aid is recommended, the client is given a card to present to the hearing aid dealer. This card summarizes the audiometric results, and specifies the aid and adjustments recommended. Dealers are encouraged to call the clinic if they have any questions or if they think that some modification of the recommendation will improve the client's performance. The clinician's major responsibility is to his client; if by cooperating with the dealers we can better meet this responsibility, then it is incumbent upon us to do so. Cooperation is a two-way street, however; dealers who are found to indulge in shady or unethical practices should not be permitted to consign their aids in clinics.

Since a growing number of audiologists are now dispensing hearing aids they have more direct communication with the hearing aid industry. This should eliminate some of the problems noted in the past and will provide a greater input from audiologists to the industry.

DISCUSSION AND CONCLUSIONS

Resnick and Becker (1963) described an approach to hearing aid evaluations which they felt to be more defensible than conventional selection procedures. They thereby initiated a public controversy (healthy, in my opinion) which still seems to be unresolved (Millin, 1963; Jeffers and Smith, 1964; Resnick and Becker, 1965; Jerger et al., 1966b). They gave the three assumptions of conventional procedures as (1) "that there are significant differences among hearing aids in terms of how they enable the user to understand everyday speech," (2) "that these differences change from one user to the next, that is, that there is an interaction between people and hearing aids" and (3) "that these differences can be demonstrated reliably by monosyllabic word (PB-50) intelligibility scores." In their estimation, the second and third assumptions were not then being met, thus weakening the underlying rationale for comparative hearing aid evaluations. The third assumption has already been discussed in an earlier section.

There do not appear to be any serious differences of opinion regarding the first assumption. There are indeed differences among hearing aids which do enable hearing aid users to differentially understand speech signals. A number of studies have shown a negative relationship between various indices of distortion and speech intelligibility (Bode and Kasten, 1971; Harris et al., 1961; Jerger and Thelin, 1968; Kasten et al., 1967; Olsen and Carhart, 1967); the point is that, while there were differences among these studies in terms of the relative significance of specific distortions, in all of them the "best" and the "worst" aids were usually ranked similarly for all classes of populations. Or, as one study concluded, "that whatever factors operated to produce performance differences among aids in subjects with hearing loss operated to at least the same extent in the normal listeners" (Jerger et al., 1966b). These findings apparently contradict the second assumption of conventional hearing aid selection procedures, i.e., no interaction could be demonstrated between people and aids.

If we turn, however, to another body of evidence we find that interactions have been demonstrated between people and hearing aid characteristics. In the studies reviewed earlier under "selective amplification," we find that, by tailoring the frequency response, either electroacoustically or through earmold modifica-

tions, we can increase WDSs; and furthermore, that this result seems to be dependent upon the type and slope of the loss, and the degree of other endogenous distortions. These studies have clearly demonstrated that certain acoustic characteristics are more desirable than other characteristics for some categories of the hearing impaired. We also have some evidence that other physical performance indices of hearing aids (response irregularity, bandwidth and harmonic distortion) have less consequence for speech discrimination the steeper the slope of the audiometric contour (Jerger and Thelin, 1968).

How do we resolve these apparently contradictory bodies of evidence that, on the one hand, there is no interaction between aids and people, and, on the other hand, that there is such an interaction? It should be recalled that the studies which demonstrate similar rankings from the "best" to "worst" aid for all groups do so by characterizing "best" and "worst" in terms of such electroacoustic features as harmonic distortion, intermodulation distortion and bandwidth (Harris et al., 1961; Kasten et al., 1967; Jerger et al., 1966b; Olsen and Carhart, 1967). When one deviates from the "ideal" amplifier in these dimensions, the consequences do appear to be progressively negative for all population groups. That is, with some contradictory evidence regarding the significance of the audiometric slope (Jerger and Thelin, 1968), a poor amplifying system is poor no matter who uses it. Deliberate variations in the response curve, although strictly speaking also a distortion since the output is nonlinear with regard to input, are different because of the possible favorable interaction between the slope of the loss and slope of the amplification curve. Thus, rather than available information being degraded, as in harmonic distortion, more information is made accessible to the client.

In my opinion, this controversy may be resolved if it is made clear whether one is talking about hearing aids or electroacoustic systems. It is not reasonable to assume that one electroacoustic system will provide maximum speech intelligibility for all hearing-impaired clients; clearly, changes have to be made depending upon individual differences with regard to degree of loss, slope, tolerance, discrimination function and so on. Clearly, too, we are far from certain what specific electroacoustic modifications would be the most applicable for the large variety of hearing problems we see in our clinics. In addition, we are handicapped in not knowing what discrimination function can best predict an individual's performance in everyday life. When we have adequately resolved these questions, and further, when we can describe the electroacoustic performance of aids in terms of real ears rather than 2-cc couplers, audiologists will have reached the millennium of the "prescribed" hearing aid-electroacoustic system. Hearing aid evaluations as we now know them will become unnecessary, for we will know exactly what is necessary for whom.

Until then, we are confronted in our clinics with a bewildering variety of individual hearing aids, representing a continuum of physical performance on a number of dimensions. Typically, the manufacturer's specifications do not provide sufficient electroacoustic information, and what is included does not always conform to reality because of insufficiently rigorous quality control procedures. Furthermore, while we recognize the desirability of minimizing some distortions, others may exist whose presence and effect are as yet unknown. For example, how do aids differ in following a rapid frequency shift over time, such as during a formant transition? In these and other uncertainties lies much of the rationale for conventional hearing aid evaluations. It seems that we can best detect these differences among hearing aids with a comparative aided evaluation. By virtue of training and experience, granting the wide overlap between competent dealers and incompetent audiologists, the audiologist is the most qualified to perform this service. Resnick and Becker (1963) pointed out that there are problems in their approach, but on balance it seems the most effective method of continuing and enhancing the audiologist's responsibilities to his clients. Probably the theoretically "best" aid rarely if ever gets recommended; this result awaits the electroacoustic millennium, but until then the hearing aid evaluation seems to offer the best hope of approaching this goal.

REFERENCES

Alpiner, J. G., Aural rehabilitation and the aged client. *Maico Audiol. Library Ser.* 4, 9–12, 1967.

American Speech and Hearing Association. A Conference on Hearing Aid Evaluation Procedures. ASHA Reports No. 2, 1967.

Bode, D. L., and Kasten, R. N., Hearing aid distortion and consonant identification. *J. Speech Hear. Res.*, 14, 323–331, 1971.

Brooks, D., Gain requirements of hearing aid users. *Scand. Audiol.*, 2, 199–204, 1973.

Burney, P. A., A survey of hearing aid evaluation procedures. *ASHA*, 14, 439–444, 1972.

Byrne, D. J., Some implications of body baffle for hearing aid selection. *Sound*, 6, 86–91, 1972.

Byrne, D., and Tonisson, S., Selecting the gain of hearing aids for persons with sensorineural hearing impairments. *Scand. Audiol.*, 5, 51–62, 1976.

Caraway, B., and Carhart, R., Influence of compressor action on speech intelligibility. *J. Acoust. Soc. Am.*, 41, 1424–1434, 1967.

Carhart, R., Tests for selection of hearing aids. *Laryngoscope*, 56, 780–794, 1946a.

Carhart, R., Volume control adjustment in hearing aid selection. *Laryngoscope*, 56, 510–526, 1946b.

Carhart, R., Hearing aid selection by university clinics. *J. Speech Hear. Disord.*, 15, 105–113, 1950.

Carhart, R., Problems in the measurement of speech discrimination. *Arch. Otolaryngol.*, 82, 253–260, 1965.

Cooper, J. C., and Cutts, B. P., Speech discrimination in noise. *J. Speech Hear. Res.*, 14, 332–337, 1971.

Cutler, W. D., Dispensing Systems. In Pollack, M. (Ed.), *Amplification for the Hearing-Impaired*. New York: Grune & Stratton, 1975.

Danaher, E. M., Osberger, M. J., and Pickett, J. M., Discrimination of formant frequency transitions in synthetic vowels. *J. Speech Hear. Res.*, 16, 439–451, 1973.

Davis, H., and Silverman, S. R., *Hearing and Deafness*, Rev. Ed., pp. 317–320. New York: Holt, Rinehart & Winston, Inc., 1960.

Davis, H., Hudgins, C. V., Marquis, R. J., Nichols, R. H., Jr., Peterson, G. E., Ross, D. A., and Stevens, S. S., The selection of hearing aids. *Laryngoscope*, 56, 85–115, 135–163, 1946.

Dodds, E., and Bode, D. L., An evaluation of clinical hearing aid selection procedures. Paper presented at the American Speech and Hearing Convention, 1972.

Dodds, E., and Harford, E., Modified earpieces and CROS for high frequency hearing losses. *J. Speech Hear. Res.*, 11, 204–218, 1968a.

Dodds, E., and Harford, E., Application of a lipreading test in a hearing aid evaluation. *J. Speech Hear. Disord.*, 33, 167–173, 1968b.

Fairbanks, G., Test of phonemic differentiation; the rhyme test. *J. Acoust. Soc. Am.*, 30, 596–600, 1958.

Foust, K. O., and Gengel, R. W., A comparison of aided speech discrimination using four different hearing aids in conditions of quiet and noise. Paper presented at the American Speech and Hearing Association Convention, 1973.

Frank, T., and Karlovich, R. S., Ear-canal frequency response and speech discrimination performance as a function of hearing-aid mold type. *J. Aud. Res.*, 13, 124–129, 1973.

Green, D. Personal communication, 1970.

Harford, E., and Musket, C. H., Some considerations in the organization and administration of a clinical hearing aid selection program, *ASHA*, 6, 35–40, 1964.

Harris, J. D., Combinations of distortions in speech. *Arch. Otolaryngol.*, 72, 227–232, 1960.

Harris, J. D., Haines, H. L., Kelsey, P. A., and Clack, T. D., The relation between speech intelligibility and the electroacoustic characteristics of low fidelity circuitry. *J. Aud. Res.*, 5, 357–381, 1961.

Haug, C., Guilford, F. R., Battin, R. R., and Baccaro, P., A comparison of hearing aid evaluation test instruments and aids purchased from dealers. *Volta Rev.*, 65, 26–29, 1963.

Hecker, M. H. L., Stevens, K. N., and Williams, C. E., Measurements of reaction time in intelligibility tests. *J. Acoust. Soc. Am.*, 39, 1188–1189, 1966.

Hendry, C. J., and Rupp, R., Subject-adjusted frequency response settings; a new concept in hearing aid evaluations. *Mich. State Speech Hear. Assoc. J.*, **9**, 44-52, 1973.

Hodgson, W. R., and Murdock, C., Jr., Effect of the earmold on speech intelligibility in hearing aid use. *J. Speech Hear. Res.*, **13**, 290-297, 1970.

Hood, R. B., Modifications in hearing aid selection procedures. *Acad. Rehabil. Audiol. Newsletter*, **3**, 7-10, 1970.

House, A. S., Williams, C. E., Hecker, M. H. L., and Kryter, K. D., Articulation testing methods; consonantal differentiation with a closed response set. *J. Acoust. Soc. Am.*, **37**, 158-166, 1965.

Jeffers, J., Quality judgement in hearing aid selection. *J. Speech Hear. Disord.*, **25**, 259-266, 1960.

Jeffers, J., and Smith, C. R., On hearing aid selection—in part a reply to Resnick and Becker. *ASHA*, **6**, 504-506, 1964.

Jerger, J., Behavioral correlates of hearing-aid performance. *Bull. Prosthet. Res.*, **10**, 62-75, 1967.

Jerger, J., and Hayes, D., Hearing aid evaluation. *Arch. Otolaryngol.*, **102**, 214-225, 1976.

Jerger, J., and Thelin, J., Effects of electroacoustic characteristics of hearing aids on speech understanding. *Bull. Prosthet. Res.*, **10**, 159-197, 1968.

Jerger, J., Malmquist, C., and Speaks, C., Comparison of some speech intelligibility tests in the evaluation of hearing aid performance. *J. Speech Hear. Res.*, **9**, 253-258, 1966a.

Jerger, J., Speaks, C., and Malmquist, C., Hearing-aid performance and hearing-aid selection. *J. Speech Hear. Res.*, **9**, 136-149, 1966b.

Jetty, A. J., and Rintelmann, W. F., Acoustic coupler effects on speech audiometric scores using a cross hearing aid. *J. Speech Hear. Res.*, **13**, 101-114, 1970.

Jirsa, R. E., and Hodgson, W. R., Effect of harmonic distortion in hearing aids on speech intelligibility for normal and hypacusics. *J. Aud. Res.*, **10**, 213-217, 1970.

Kalikow, D. N., Stevens, K. N., and Elliot, L. L., Development of a test of speech intelligibility in noise using sentence materials with controlled word predictability. *J. Acoust. Soc. Am.*, **61**, 1337-1351, 1977.

Kasten, R. N., Lotterman, S. H., and Burnett, E. D., The influence of non-linear distortion on hearing aid processed signals. Paper presented at the American Speech and Hearing Association Convention, 1967.

Kasten, R. N., Lotterman, S. H., and Hinchman, S. J., Head shadow and head baffle effects in ear level hearing aids. *Acoustica*, **19**, 154-160, 1967/1968.

Konkle, D. F., and Bess, F. H., Custom-made vs. stock earmolds in hearing aid evaluations. *Arch. Otolaryngol.*, **99**, 140-144, 1974.

Kopra, L. L., and Blosser, D., Effects of method of measurement on most comfortable loudness level for speech. *J. Speech Hear. Res.*, **11**, 497-508, 1968.

Kretsinger, E. A., and Young, N. B., The use of fast limiting to improve the intelligibility of speech in noise. *Speech Monogr.*, **27**, 63-69, 1960.

Kreul, E. J., Nixon, J. C., Kryter, K. D., Bell, D. W., Lang, J. S., and Schubert, E. D., A proposed clinical test of speech discrimination. *J.*

Speech Hear. Res., **11**, 536-552, 1968.

Lentz, W. E., Speech discrimination in the presence of background noise using a hearing aid with a directionally-sensitive microphone. *Maico Audiol. Library Ser.*, **10**, Report 9, 1972.

Lotterman, H. S., Kasten, R. N., and Majerus, D. M., Battery life and non-linear distortion in hearing aids. *J. Speech Hear. Disord.*, **32**, 274-278, 1967.

Lynn, G., and Carhart, R., Influence of attack and release in compression amplification on understanding of speech by hypoacusics. *J. Speech Hear. Disord.*, **28**, 124-140, 1963.

Markle, D. M. and Zaner, A., The determination of "gain requirements" of hearing aids; a new method. *J. Aud. Res.*, **6**, 371-378, 1966.

Martin, M. C., Hearing aid gain requirements in sensorineural hearing loss. *Br. J. Audiol.*, **7**, 21-24, 1973.

McCandless, G., Loudness discomfort and hearing aids. In *Proceedings of the 3rd Oticongress*, pp. 39-44, Copenhagen, 1973.

McCandless, G. A., Lexington Hearing Aid Conference, Lexington School for the Deaf, New York, N. Y., 1975.

McClellan, M. E., Aided speech discrimination in noise with vented and unvented earmolds. *J. Aud. Res.*, **7**, 93-100, 1967.

McConnell, F., Silber, E. F., and McDonald, D., Test-retest consistency of clinical hearing aid tests. *J. Speech Hear. Disord.*, **25**, 273-280, 1960.

Menzel, O. J., Hearing aids for "problem" cases. *Audecibel*, **13**, 150-164, 1964.

Miller, M. H., Clinical hearing aid evaluation. *Maico Audiol. Library Ser.*, **3**, 24-33, 1967.

Millin, J. P., "Conventional" hearing aid selection. *ASHA*, **5**, 880-881, 1963.

Morris, T., An approach to calculating gain requirements for severely deaf children as a function of hearing loss which is independent of frequency response. *Scand. Audiol.*, **6**, 21-26, 1977.

Northern, J. L., and Hattler, K. W., Earmold influence on aided speech identification tasks. *J. Speech Hear. Res.*, **13**, 162-172, 1970.

Olsen, W. O., and Carhart, R., Development of test procedures for evaluation of binaural hearing aids. *Bull. Prosthet. Res.*, **10**, 22-49, 1967.

Orchik, D. L., and Oyer, H. J., A modified traditional hearing aid evaluation procedure. *J. Aud. Res.*, **12**, 8-13, 1972.

Pascoe, D. P., Frequency responses of hearing aids and their effects on the speech perception of hearing-impaired subjects. *Ann. Otol. Rhinol. Laryngol.*, **84**, Suppl. 23, 5-40, 1975.

Rassi, J. and Harford, E., An analysis of patient attitudes and reactions to a clinical hearing aid selection program. *ASHA*, **10**, 283-290, 1968.

Reddell, R. C., and Calvert, D. R., Selecting a hearing aid by interpreting audiologic data. *J. Aud. Res.*, **6**, 445-452, 1966.

Resnick, D. M., and Becker, M., Hearing aid evaluation—a new approach. *ASHA*, **5**, 695-699, 1963.

Resnick, D., and Becker, M., A brief reply to '. . . in part a reply . . .' *ASHA*, **7**, 31, 1965.

Revoile, S. G., Speech discrimination ability with ear inserts. *Bull. Prosthet. Res.*, **10**, 198-205, 1968.

Ross, M., Changing concepts in hearing aid candidacy. *Eye Ear Nose Throat Mon.*, **48**, 27–34, 1969.

Ross, M., Hearing Aid Selection for the Preverbal Hearing-Impaired Child. In Pollack, M. (Ed.), *Amplification for the Hearing-Impaired.* Grune & Stratton: New York, 1975.

Ross, M., Huntington, D. A., Newby, H. A., and Dixon, R. F., Speech discrimination of hearing-impaired individuals in noise; its relationship to other audiometric parameters. *U.S. Air Force Sch. Aerospace Med.,* Technical Document Report No. 62-130, 1963.

Ross, M., Barrett, L. S., and Trier, T. R., Ear-level hearing aids for motivated patients with minimal hearing losses. *Laryngoscope,* **76**, 1555–1561, 1966.

Schultz, M. C., and Schubert, E. D., A multiple choice discrimination test (MCDT). *Laryngoscope,* **79**, 382–399, 1969.

Shore, I., and Kramer, J., A comparison of two procedures for hearing aid evaluation. *ASHA,* **28**, 159–170, 1963.

Shore, I., Bilger, R. C., and Hirsh, I., Hearing aid evaluation; reliability of repeated measurements. *J. Speech Hear. Disord.,* **25**, 152–170, 1960.

Speaks, C., and Jerger, J., Method for measurement of speech identification. *J. Speech Hear. Res.,* **8**, 194–195, 1965.

Sung, G. S., Sung, R. J., and Angelelli, R. M., Effect of frequency-response characteristics of hearing aids on speech intelligibility in noise. *J. Aud. Res.,* **11**, 318–321, 1971.

Sung, G. S., Sung, R. J., and Angelelli, R. M., Effect of directional microphones in hearing aids on speech discrimination in noise. Paper presented at the American Speech and Hearing Association Convention, 1974.

Thomas, I. A., and Sparks, D. W., Discrimination of filtered/clipped speech by hearing-impaired subjects. *J. Acoust. Soc. Am.,* **49**, 1881–1887, 1971.

Thompson, G., and Lassman, F., Relationship of auditory distortion test results to speech discrimination through flat versus selective amplifying systems. *J. Speech Hear. Res.,* **12**, 594–606, 1969.

Victoreen, J. A., *Hearing Enhancement.* Springfield, Ill.: Charles C Thomas, 1960.

Villchur, E., Signal processing to improve speech intelligibility in perceptive deafness. *J. Acoust. Soc. Am.,* **53**, 1646–1657, 1973.

Walden, B. E., and Kasten, R. N., Test-retest reliability and inter-aid consistency of two methods of setting hearing aid gain control. Paper presented at the American Speech and Hearing Association Convention, 1969.

Wallenfels, H. G., *Hearing Aids on Prescription.* Springfield, Ill.: Charles C Thomas, 1967.

Watson, L., and Tolan, T., *Hearing Tests and Hearing Instruments.* Baltimore: Williams & Wilkins Co., 1949.

Witter, H. L., and Goldstein, D. P., Quality judgements of hearing aid transduced speech. *J. Speech Hear. Res.,* **14**, 312–322, 1971.

Yanick, P., Effects of signal processing on the intelligibility of speech in noise for persons with sensorineural hearing loss. *J. Am. Audiol. Soc.,* **1**, 229–238, 1976.

Yantis, P. A., Millin, J. P., and Shapiro, I., Speech discrimination in sensory-neural hearing loss; two experiments on the role of intensity. *J. Speech Hear. Res.,* **9**, 178–193, 1966.

Zerlin, S., A new approach to hearing-aid selection. *J. Speech Hear. Res.,* **5**, 370–376, 1962.

Zink, G. D., Hearing aids: an incidence study of faulty functioning. Paper presented at the American Speech and Hearing convention, 1969.

Zink, G. D., and Alpiner, J. G., Hearing aids; one aspect of a state public school hearing conservation program. *J. Speech Hear. Disord.,* **33**, 329–344, 1968.

chapter 44

HEARING AID COUNSELING AND ORIENTATION

William R. Hodgson, Ph.D.

Prospective purchasers of hearing aids may approach their initial amplification experiences showing astounding naivete regarding hearing, hearing loss and hearing aid use. Adults with acquired loss or parents of hearing-impaired children may know little about the advantages and limitations of amplification. They may not understand the principles of effective hearing aid use. Examples are numerous. Recently, one lady was convinced that her hearing aid battery was powered by solar energy and, that in Arizona's sunny climate, it would never need replacing. Parents of a child with a newly discovered loss were eager to procure aids immediately to implement regenerative exercises for the auditory nerve. An elderly patient was unaware that the binaural aids in her eyeglasses consisted of two separately adjustable units.

The successful hearing aid user must understand what his aid is for and how to use it. Without advice, the new hearing aid owner is likely to first try it out in places where he has the most difficulty, not the least. He may want to learn how much he benefits in noisy and difficult circumstances where he really needs help. He may be horrified by the amplified noise and resultant poor function.

The adult with hearing loss must learn why he can hear sounds but does not always understand. It may in fact be necessary to convince him of the very presence and organic nature of his disorder if he has been overreacting and blaming his problems on mental incapacity. On the other hand, he may have attributed his difficulty in understanding to the mumbling speech of others.

The implications underlying these problems are obvious. It is not sufficient that the audiologist only recommend appropriate amplification. In addition he must explain to his patients the nature, advantages, and limitations of hearing aids. He must also orient his patients to effective hearing aid use.

UNDERSTANDING HEARING LOSS

Parents must accept and learn to deal effectively with their child's hearing loss. During the process, they may experience a sequence of emotional reactions. Disbelief may be their understandable first reaction when told their young child is hearing impaired. If so, the parents must be convinced. An independent second opinion may be helpful in verifying the loss and convincing the parents. In the initial counseling session, little more than communicating the fact of the loss may be possible. Even if the parents have strongly suspected a loss previously, they are now being asked to accept and acknowledge it as certain. The emotional impact of this information may preclude absorbing any additional information.

A similar situation may occur during the initial counseling of adults with an acquired hearing loss. The adult seeking help may deny or minimize his hearing problem when the audiologist verifies it. In these cases the loss must be explained and its effects demonstrated.

The audiologist must clarify for the patient, or the parents of the hearing-impaired child, the nature and extent of the hearing loss. The explanation must be undertaken using terms familiar to the patient. He must not be overwhelmed with technical jargon. To the patient, Hertz is a commercial firm whose name is apparently being mispronounced. The audiologist should speak simply, use redundancy, get feedback. However, he should not talk down to the patient. Because the patient is uninformed about hearing does not mean he cannot learn.

Acceptance of the presence of the hearing loss is often followed by a natural desire to treat and correct the disorder. Competent medical examination and explanation of the disorder should be obtained. A second opinion should be encouraged if necessary. It is essential that the irreversibility of the sensory-neural loss be accepted. If not, time which might be important for rehabilitation will be lost, as a cure is continuously sought. Unscrupulous practitioners may victimize the patient with ineffective treatment.

Other avenues of treatment must be clarified. This consideration is particularly pertinent to the parents of the child with newly discovered hearing loss. They will probably know nothing of the effect of congenital hearing loss on language and speech development, or the educational implications of deafness. They must be helped to understand and accept these implications. If the loss is severe, they may need to make a decision, eventually, about the language system the child will use. They deserve to learn the available facts, not propaganda, on which to base their decision.

All of these things are prerequisite to counseling about the nature and use of hearing aids.

UNDERSTANDING NATURE, ADVANTAGES, AND LIMITATIONS OF HEARING AIDS

Realistic expectations are crucial to successful hearing aid use. It should be understood, before hearing aid use is undertaken, that a hearing aid is similar to a miniature public address system. That is, it functions to make sounds louder, not clearer except for the improved intelligibility associated with the increased loudness. It must be understood that hearing aids do not correct all the problems associated with hearing loss. The prospective user must understand that a properly fitted hearing aid will make soft sounds comfortably loud and that no sounds will exceed tolerable loudness. Further, that maximum amplification will be delivered for those frequencies where hearing loss is greatest. Beyond that, the benefits from the aid will be a function of how well the patient's ear can differentiate, or learn to differentiate, sound. The success of this latter function depends on the patient and his ear, and not on the properly functioning hearing aid.

It must be realized that hearing aids function poorest in situations where the majority of hearing-impaired individuals need them most. Persons with sensory-neural hearing loss suffer a disproportionate drop of discrimination ability in noise, relative to normal hearing individuals (Watson, 1964; Olsen and Tillman, 1968; Ross and Giolas, 1971).

The prospective hearing aid candidate should know whether he ought to wear the aid full time or part time. The answer to this question will be determined by the magnitude of loss, the demands on the patient's hearing, and the acoustic circumstances under which he listens. Generally people with slight or mild hearing losses benefit from part-time use, and wear their aid in quiet surroundings where people talk softly. Those with moderate loss are likely to wear the aid most of the time, but may remove it in "cocktail party" listening situations. There, the combined babble of many voices overwhelms their discrimination ability and amplification may contribute only irritation. Listeners with severe loss and those with profound loss who use amplification are likely to be full-time wearers of hearing aids. In those difficult listening circumstances when their reduced discrimination does not permit understanding of speech, their aid at least keeps them in contact with the environment. Appropriate counseling in this area should prevent problems such as those of the steelworker with noise-induced loss who once came to the clinic seeking help adjusting to his powerful body-worn hearing aid. He explained, "Doc, I'm determined to get my money's worth from this thing, so I turn her up full, but when those rivet guns get started, I have a helluva time keeping her on."

Misconceptions must be removed. Considering hearing aid use, some think the aid may improve or decrease hearing sensitivity. They should be informed that, while auditory attentiveness and functional ability should certainly increase with hearing aid use, exercising the ear via amplification will not improve sensitivity. Conversely, there are sporadic reports of threshold shift associated with amplification (Harford and Markle, 1955; Kasten and Braunlin, 1970; Jerger and Lewis, 1975; Darbyshire, 1976). While these reports are not common, they justify instructing the new hearing aid user to be alert for apparent change in hearing, and to obtain regular audiologic evaluations. Routine testing should probably be done yearly for adults and semi-annually for children who wear hearing aids. In short, there is no rationale for rushing into, or avoiding, initiation of amplification because of concern over change in sensitivity in either direction.

Many adult hypacusics express the concern that the use of a hearing aid will make the wearer dependent on amplification to the extent that unaided hearing will subsequently not be useful. They should be assured that such is not the case. Further, it should be explained that if amplification does in fact prove useful enough for the wearer to become dependent on his hearing aid, there is certainly no good reason why he should deprive himself of the benefit.

Other prospective hearing aid users may have been misinformed that the nerve in their ear is dead or damaged and a hearing aid will not be helpful. They should be told that, while the aid will not restore the damaged sensory mechanism, the great majority of people who wear and benefit from hearing aids have sensory-neural loss. A similar situation may exist for those with unilateral disorder, precipitous high frequency loss, or others not historically considered good hearing aid candidates. They may have been told they cannot benefit from hearing aid use. Innovations described elsewhere in this book may offer successful hearing aid use, and at least a trial should be considered. In summary, the audiologist should listen to the patient's misconceptions, answer his questions, explain and reassure. Literature that will help parents understand hearing aids includes that written by Dodds and Harford (1970) and Israel (1975).

LEARNING TO USE A HEARING AID

The patient should understand that he must learn to use the hearing aid properly for greatest benefit. There are several facets to learning efficient hearing aid use. These include such physical aspects as learning to insert and remove the aid, manipulating the controls, putting in and removing the battery. Care and maintenance of the aid are involved. Most importantly, learning to accept the aid and listen through it are features in hearing aid orientation.

Physical Aspects of Hearing Aid Use

The beginning hearing aid user will have trouble putting his hearing aid on. He should be assured that, with practice, this act will become effortless and automatic. He should be shown how to hold the hearing aid, how to insert the earmold into the canal, and how to place the aid over the ear. He should practice before a mirror. Stress should be placed on the importance of seating the earmold correctly and completely. The patient should be reminded to turn the aid off before removing it, to avoid feedback. He should be told to remove the aid by grasping the earmold, not the aid itself, or the tubing.

He must know the type of battery the aid requires and how to insert the battery properly. He should be reminded that the aid will not function if the battery is inserted backward. He must learn how to remove the earmold from the aid, and how to wash the earmold in warm soapy water. It is important to remove accumulated wax. The mold must be dried carefully after washing to prevent water in the canal from blocking sound.

The audiologist should explain the various controls that the patient must learn to use, and how they operate. He should be told where the controls should be set. It is essential that the patient learn to manipulate the gain control quickly and accurately while wearing the aid, so he can adjust it in different acoustic environments for optimum amplification. Lack of physical dexterity, such as that caused by arthritis, may prevent the patient from making these adjustments. It may be necessary to recommend an easier to manipulate body type aid.

Some or all of the following controls are found on hearing aids, and the patient should be taught their purpose and operation:

1. The off-on switch is variously located. It may be incorporated in the gain control. On some aids, it is associated with the telephone switch. Most commonly, behind-the-ear aids are turned off by partly opening the battery compartment.
2. An input selector is present on some aids. Usual settings are telecoil, microphone, and—sometimes—combined telecoil and microphone inputs. The patient must understand the purpose of these settings and their efficient use.
3. When the hearing aid is on the ear the gain control wheel of some aids must be rotated upward to increase amplification. On other aids, the control is rotated downward to increase gain. Controls on still other aids are horizontal when the aid is in its use position. The patient must be taught the particular details of his own aid.
4. There may be a tone control which effects some change in frequency response. The preferred setting, or the acoustic circumstances in which the setting should be changed, should be taught to the patient.
5. Some hearing aids have preset controls which should not be manipulated by the patient. Instruction about these controls should be duly given.

Care and Maintenance

Causes of feedback should be explained to the patient. The audiologist should mention the effects of poorly fitting earmolds, occluded sound channels, and loose tubing. He should indicate that feedback will result from too much gain or from the presence of sound reflecting surfaces close to the aid.

The patient should be instructed to buy a voltage tester and shown how to use it to check his batteries. He should check the battery daily at the end of the day and discard it if it falls below its specified voltage. A new battery should be tried if speech sounds faint or unclear, or if it is necessary to rotate the gain control more than usual for adequate loudness. He should not expect to use the battery until it is absolutely dead, since harmonic distortion tends to increase toward the end of battery life (Lotterman, Kasten, and Majerus, 1967). Perhaps the new hearing aid user should record for a time the hours of use obtained from each battery after daily use of the aid has stabilized. The resultant average can serve to alert him to replacement time. Gaeth and Lounsbury (1966) demonstrated that parents are not always aware of this need. In a questionnaire asking how long children's batteries lasted, 9% of the parents indicated that the batteries lasted 12 months or more. Another 14% were apparently more honest and admitted that they had no idea.

Elements of hearing aid care should be considered. The patient should be told not to subject the aid to excessive heat (radiators or sunlight) or humidity (hair spray or vaporizers). He should be alerted to kinked (occluded) tubing and broken cords on body aids, which cause intermittent function.

Parents of hearing-impaired youngsters should listen to the child's aid daily. To do this, they will need an individual earmold or a hearing aid stethoscope. Either can be obtained from hearing aid dispensers, or the latter can be ordered from the Hal-Hen Company, 3614 11th Street, Long Island City, New York 11106. Parents should be sure that speech through the aid has its usual loudness and clarity, that the aid is not generating extraneous noises, and that it is not intermittent in operation. Regular audiologic evaluations, including assessment of hearing aid function, are an important part of the program.

Learning to Use a Hearing Aid

The patient must first learn how to set the gain control for best listening. This setting should be made by ear, not by eye. The criterion should be comfortable loudness for existing acoustic conditions. No single gain setting can provide adequate and comfortable amplification for all daily listening conditions. The patient should learn to turn the gain up when it is quiet and down when it is noisy. He should not continuously fiddle with the gain control in an attempt to equalize loudness of each incoming signal. Rather, as he moves from one general acoustic condition to another, he should adjust the gain to compensate for the overall change. The audiologist should determine a gain setting for optimum listening in quiet. He should assist the patient in learning to make intelligent adjustments from that setting as listening conditions change. He should not put a mark on the gain control to indicate a setting which the patient will never vary.

Children who wear aids should learn, as soon as possible, to adjust the gain control for themselves. Until then, someone has to do it for them. For most people, a gain setting that gives an aided speech reception threshold (SRT) of 25 to 30 dB (or an aided speech awareness threshold of 15 to 20 dB) will provide comfortable and effective listening for conversational level speech. The audiologist should determine the gain control setting needed for that aided level. Parents should learn to reduce gain in noise and increase it in the presence of low level speech in quiet, and teach the child to make his own adjustment as soon as possible.

Hearing aid users must acclimate themselves to the unaccustomed loudness and quality of aided listening. During their first amplification experience, patients usually comment about the audibility of forgotten background noises and the loudness and peculiar quality of their own voice. To implement the adjustment, the patient should begin practice hearing aid use in a quiet place, listening to simple signals. The listening situation should be structured and controlled. He should progress gradually to listening in noisy places to complex signals.

That is, his goal is performance in non-structured, uncontrolled situations. A possible hierarchy of listening experiences is suggested below:

1. A good beginning place might be a quiet home living room. One person should talk about familiar, everyday things. For a child, a toy might be used which makes a sound accompanied by a visible movement. Practice listening with the sound source in different positions and at varying distances.
2. Next, the listener might move to the kitchen, where the acoustics are not quite as good. Listen to one person talking, or to water running at different levels, but not too loud. With children, stress the visual-auditory association.
3. Next the patient might try listening to television in a quiet room. He should begin with easier situations; the news, programs of familiar music.
4. The aid should be worn next at a quiet dinner table.
5. Engage in conversation in a quiet room with two, then three or four other people.
6. The aid should be worn outside in a quiet place, perhaps the back yard. The goal is to acclimate to wind noise.
7. The aid may be used at church, a lecture, or at a play. The patient should get as close to the speakers as possible, the first time. Next time, he may try listening at a little greater distance.
8. The wearer should take a quiet drive in the country, with the windows up.
9. The patient should walk along the street in a quiet neighborhood.
10. The patient should take a drive with the car windows open.
11. A shopping trip should be arranged.
12. The patient should try wearing the aid at a party or in a room where a number of people are talking.

At some point along this route, the patient may discover he gets along as well or better without the aid. This discovery does not mean he cannot benefit from an aid, but that he may choose not to wear it under certain conditions. A careful program of experimentation will not only orient the individual to wearing a hearing aid, but will help him become an efficient and intelligent hearing aid user.

While the above program of experiences is being carried out, the patient should also practice listening to and identifying sounds. There are many sounds he will not have been hearing at all before using the aid. He should relearn to identify these soft sounds, or, in the case of a child with congenital loss, strive to learn them for the first time. There may be other sounds that could be heard without the aid. Now they will be louder and have a different quality, and the patient should practice listening to them also. At the same time, he should get reacquainted with the sound of his voice. He should strive to reestablish correct loudness control. Someone should listen to him as he practices. He should also practice adjusting the gain control quickly, unobtrusively, and accurately for comfortable loudness under different listening conditions.

Concurrently, the patient should consider other avenues of rehabilitation. For children, there are multiple concerns; language, speech and educational considerations. Adults should consider lipreading instruction. In some cases, concern for the conservation of speech is warranted. Penn (1955) reported voice and articulation deviations developing in association with acquired hearing loss.

Additional steps in learning to use an aid are necessary for young children, especially those with severe or profound congenital loss. The much more extensive problems of training necessary for listening, language or speech development are not considered here except as they are interrelated with learning to use a hearing aid.

The first problem may be keeping the aid on the child. If the child has a lot of residual hearing, the meaningfulness and utility of sound may already be obvious to him. Otherwise, the benefits of a hearing aid will not be immediately noticeable and the child may object to the foreign, noisy device.

Parents themselves must be convinced and committed. Sometimes parents make only a half-hearted attempt to get the child to wear the aid. The aid is a constant reminder of the defect. Some parents are not ready to tolerate this advertisement to themselves and others of the existence of the problem. Additionally, a good habilitation program is a lot of work, and some parents may not be capable of the effort. Failure of the child to adapt to the aid may constitute a concrete point at which the burden of responsibility and effort can be unloaded. To prevent these problems the audiologist must effectively explain the loss and the need for the aid. He must answer the parents' questions and support their involvement in the habilitation program. He must help them see the long term implications of a training program, or the lack of it.

Downs (1967) recommended a step-by-step procedure for helping a child learn to accept and use an aid. With adjustments in particular cases for age, magnitude of loss, and other individual problems, it should be very useful. The essence of the program is presented below.

The instructions are addressed to the parents of the hearing impaired child.

During the first week, indicate to your child that you plan for him to wear the aid for four 5-min periods each day. Then do it; be in charge of the situation. Put in the earmold without turning the aid on. If he does not object, play quietly for 5 min and remove the aid. If he resists, gently immobilize him, recruiting whatever help you need. Proceed as before. As soon as the child tolerates the aid, turn it up to a low gain setting, talk quietly, play with his favorite toy for the 5-min period.

For the second week, extend each period to 15 min. Set the volume control a little higher. Play quietly for 5 min then take your child exploring around the house. Point out sounds. Make it clear you hear them.

During the third week, extend the periods to 30 min each. Turn the volume control up a little more. Place the child near you and call his attention to sounds that occur.

In the fourth week, extend the listening periods to 45 min. Turn the gain control almost to the level recommended by the audiologist for listening in quiet.

For the fifth week, utilize four 1-hour periods of hearing aid use. Use the gain control recommended by the audiologist.

Thereafter, increase hearing aid use until, by the end of the second month, he is wearing the aid during all waking hours, unless part time use has been specified by the audiologist. Exceptions might be three 10-min rest periods per day and during rough play outdoors. In addition to the suggestions of Downs above, other recommendations for orienting children to hearing aid use may be found in Seligman (1962), Pollack and Downs (1964), Ross and Lerman (1966), Pollack (1970), Northern and Downs (1974), Kasten and Warren (1977), and Oyer and Hodgson (1977).

With the onset of adolescence, a long-time hearing aid wearer may reject the aid, becoming more aware of appearance and concerned about being different. In such instances, the following suggestions may help. The importance of the problem to the child should not be belittled. An atmosphere of understanding and concern is important. Prevention, of course, is better than cure. A good training program and a history of successful hearing aid use may reduce the tendency to reject the aid. Efforts should be made to help the child see that he is less different with the aid than without it. Cosmetic appearance should be improved when possible. A mother recently brought her crew-cut-topped son to the clinic because he would not wear his behind-the-ear aid. Hair length was the crucial issue. It took a lot of talking to convice her it was better to have a long haired hippie in the family temporarily than a straight but stupid permanent dependent. Parental attitudes and parent-child relationships are important. Adolescents (and other people) need a lot of support.

As implied in the preceding program, young children with severe and profound loss may not respond consistently to sounds they hear. They must be taught the meaning and utility of sound. They must learn (1) the relationship between environmental happenings (movement) and sound, (2) how they can get information via sound and (3) how they can control their environment with sound. These stages must be completed before the child is a hearing aid user. The hearing aid may be used for amplification during training. If the training is not accomplished, the child may become a hearing aid wearer rather than a hearing aid user.

CONCLUSION

Different individuals approach hearing aid use with different levels and sources of motivation. The motivation of children to wear hearing aids must initially be supplied by parents. Some adults are actively interested in improving their hearing and approach hearing aid use positively. Others have a real aversion stemming from cosmetic concern or admission of the handicap associated with hearing aid use. Still others are pushed to trial hearing aid use more by the urging of relatives than by their own concern. For all these individuals, effective counseling and orientation are needed. Otherwise initial unsatisfactory experiences with amplification may prevent successful hearing aid use.

Perhaps it makes sense to divide potential hearing aid users into three groups. There are children born with hearing loss who face the prospect of learning language and speech with defective hearing. There are elderly people who, because of hearing loss, suffer social isolation in addition to the other problems of aging. There is another group, in between, who may be faced with the threat of failing to get an education, losing a job, or changing a life style, because of developing hearing loss. Amplification has potential for assisting each group with its particular problem. The audiologist has a role in helping each group realize this potential.

REFERENCES

Darbyshire, J., A study of the use of high power hearing aids by children with marked degrees of deafness and the possibility of deteriorations in auditory acuity. *Br. J. Audiol.*, 10, 74–82, 1976.

Dodds, E., and Harford, E., *Helpful Hearing Aid Hints,* Washington, D.C.: A. G. Bell Association for the Deaf, Inc., 1970.

Downs, M., The establishment of hearing aid use; a program for parents. *Maico Audiol. Library Series 4,* Report 5, 1967.

Gaeth, J., and Lounsbury, E., Hearing aids and children in elementary schools. *J. Speech Hear. Disord.*, 31, 283–289, 1966.

Harford, E., and Markle, D., The atypical effect of a hearing aid on one patient with congenital deafness. *Laryngoscope,* 65, 970–972, 1955.

Israel, R., The hearing aid. *Volta Rev.*, 77, 21–26, 1975.

Jerger, J., and Lewis, N., Binaural hearing aids; are they dangerous for children? *Arch. Otolaryngol.*, 10, 480–483, 1975.

Kasten, R., and Braunlin, R., Traumatic hearing aid usage; a case study. Paper presented at the American Speech and Hearing Association Meeting, New York, 1970.

Kasten, R., and Warren, M., Learning to Use the Hearing Aid. In Hodgson, W., and Skinner, P. (Eds.), Ch. 11, *Hearing Aid Assessment and Use in Audiologic Habilitation,* Ch. 11, pp. 188–205. Baltimore: Williams & Wilkins Co., 1977.

Lotterman, S., Kasten, R., and Majerus, D., Battery life and nonlinear distortion in hearing aids. *J. Speech Hear. Disord.*, 32, 274–278, 1967.

Northern, J., and Downs, M., *Hearing in Children,* Baltimore: Williams & Wilkins Co., 1974.

Olsen, W., and Tillman, T., Hearing aids and sensorineural loss. *Ann. Otol. Rhinol. Laryngol.*, 77, 717–727, 1968.

Oyer, H., and Hodgson, W., Aural Rehabilitation through Amplification. In Hodgson, W., and Skinner, P. (Eds.), *Hearing Aid Assessment and Use in Audiologic Habilitation,* pp. 206–220. Baltimore: Williams & Wilkins Co., 1977.

Penn, J., Voice and speech patterns with the hard-of-hearing. *Acta Otolaryngol.*, Suppl. 124, 1955.

Pollack, D., *Educational Audiology for the Limited Hearing Infant.* Springfield, Ill.: Charles C Thomas, 1970.

Pollack, D., and Downs, M., A parent's guide to hearing aids for young children. *Volta Rev.*, 66, 745–749, 1964.

Ross, M., and Giolas, T., Effect of three classroom listening conditions on speech intelligibility. *Am. Ann. Deaf,* 116, 580–584, 1971.

Ross, M., and Lerman, J., Hearing aid selection and usage in young children. *Conn. Med.*, 30, 793–795, 1966.

Seligman, D., Hearing aid orientation for young hard of hearing children. *Except. Child.*, 29, 268–270, 1962.

Watson, T., The use of hearing aids by hearing impaired children in ordinary schools. *Volta Rev.*, 66, 741–744, 787, 1964.

Communication Training

chapter **45**

LANGUAGE AND SPEECH TRAINING

Vincent H. Knauf, Ph.D.

Adequate hearing is essential for normal language and speech development. So interrelated are these processes that Fletcher (1953) states, "we speak with our ears." While talking, hearing serves as a monitor for our speech sounds, loudness, pitch, quality, inflection, rhythm, and stress patterns. In addition, hearing systems monitor our pronunciation and grammar. Other sensory systems do supply some feedback information while we talk, but the auditory sense is dominant for most of us. We do play our speaking instrument by ear.

These functions of the auditory monitoring process assume the person already has acquired the speech sounds of the language, the vocabulary, the rules of grammar and skills involved in listening and talking. Most importantly in relation to the discussion in this chapter, *hearing serves as the basic sensory channel for the learning of language and speech skills. The speech models must be heard consistently and clearly and the speech patterns must be heard completely for the normal receptive and expressive language processes to develop*. The understanding of speech (listening skills) develops before talking (speaking skills). Receptive skills precede and exceed in quantity and complexity expressive skills. The language to be spoken must be understood.

It follows, then, that a general relationship exists between hearing sensitivity and the normal spontaneous development of language in a child; between hearing sensitivity and the individual's speech quality. These general relationships help determine the emphasis in various educational programs and the appropriate placement of the hearing impaired person within these programs.

HEARING IMPAIRED: CLASSIFICATION

Audiologists and teachers of the deaf categorize the hearing impaired by the extent of hearing loss with consideration for the time of onset and the functional use of the residual hearing, particularly as it affects language and speech. Although hearing impairments have never been defined to the satisfaction of all authorities, the White House Conference on Child Health and Protection as early as 1931 emphasized speech and language development relative to the hearing impairment.

The most widely known and generally accepted definitions for the hearing impaired were developed in 1937 by the Committee on Nomenclature of the Conference of Executives of American Schools for the Deaf. It serves as a broad frame of reference and emphasizes functional hearing and time of onset:

The *deaf*: those in whom the sense of hearing is nonfunctional for ordinary purposes of life. This general group is made up of two distinct classes based entirely on the time of the loss of hearing:

(a) The *congenitally deaf*—those who are born deaf;

(b) The *adventitiously deaf*—those who are born with normal hearing but in whom the sense of hearing became nonfunctional later through illness or accident.

The *hard of hearing*: those in whom the sense of hearing although defective is functional with or without a hearing aid (Conference of Executives, 1938).

Since the values of faint, average and loud speech are approximately 55, 65 and 75 dB sound pressure level (SPL), respectively, the impact of different hearing impairments on speech and language behavior can be grossly described. Hearing-impaired children may be conveniently divided into six groups for describing the impact of their hearing loss and their special needs. The decibel values relate to speech reception threshold levels or the average hearing threshold level in the better ear for 500, 1000 and 2000 Hz (ANSI-1969).

Group 1: 25 dB or Better—No Significant Hearing Involvement. Hearing for speech will be adequate except in some special listening situations. There will be no significant delay in speech. Children with very slight hearing losses should be identified and their progress in language related skills monitored. These slight hearing losses are frequently conductive and variable but may adversely affect auditory perceptual abilities (Katz and Illmer, 1972; Lewis, 1976).

Group 2: 26 to 40 dB – Mild Hearing Loss. Children with hearing losses in this range have difficulty hearing faint speech, speech at a distance as in a classroom or speech in background noise. Their language and speech developments are within normal limits.

Children with these mild losses benefit from special seating in the classroom. Hearing aids should be considered in each case. Parents and teachers need to be alerted to the hearing loss and its effects so that they can react appropriately when the child has difficulty understanding. Some educational retardation is likely.

Group 3: 41 to 55 dB – Moderate Hearing Loss. Without amplification these children have frequent difficulty understanding and the talker must be either nearer or speak louder to be understood. Language skills are mildly affected. They have difficulty with infrequently used words, subtleties of meaning and idioms. Articulation is usually defective but speech is intelligible. Voice quality and inflection are normal. Reading and writing skills are delayed.

These children respond well to amplification. Early language and speech instruction as well as parent counseling are indicated. Their speech and language development requires monitoring by the speech and hearing therapist. These children can attend regular classes and frequently do well so long as they have preferential seating and an understanding teacher who appreciates the effect of a hearing loss. Special attention with reading and writing skills and deliberate vocabulary development are indicated.

Group 4: 56 to 70 dB – Moderately Severe Hearing Loss. For children in this group the talker must be nearby and speak loudly. They are frequently confused by language. Their grammar, vocabulary, articulation and voice are usually defective. Their speech and language development is definitely delayed and early speech is unintelligible.

Even with hearing aids these children will have difficulty understanding in many school situations. Some will benefit from the regular class placement along with special assistance. Many require speech and language training during their preschool years and special classes, particularly in the early grades, to develop their basic language skills and to learn to read and write. Later they will need tutorial assistance in academic subjects.

Group 5: 71 to 90 dB – Severe Hearing Loss. These children are aware of loud voices and moderate sounds at 1 foot from the ear. They do not develop language and speech spontaneously. Their voices and articulation will be defective.

Initially these children should be considered educationally deaf. Hearing aids, auditory training, language development, speechreading, speech therapy and special classrooms for the hearing impaired are indicated for this group. Enrollment in preschool programs is essential for language development. Some may enter regular classes later and, hopefully, more will matriculate in the regular high schools.

Group 6: 91 dB and Greater – Profound Hearing Loss. These children may respond to some loud sounds but generally they do not rely on hearing as their primary channel for communication.

These children do benefit from hearing aids through which they are able to monitor their own voices as well as discriminate the loudness, inflection and rhythm patterns of other talkers. Hearing aids tie these children to the world of speech and sounds.

These children are "educationally deaf." Their language and speech are developed through consistent and prolonged training. Special classes or schools are necessary for their elementary education and a select few may attend regular high school classes. Others will participate in high schools for the deaf or vocationally oriented programs.

The hearing threshold level is perhaps the primary variable for estimating the impact of a child's hearing impairment and it frequently is the first measurement available. It is not surprising then that judgments and classifications of the hearing impaired are sometimes based only on this criterion. While classifications based on hearing level are valuable in estimating the impact of a certain hearing level on an average child and in the early counseling of parents, there are many exceptions. Some unusual children with profound losses of 90 dB perform better in language and academic skills compared to other children with average intelligence and moderately severe to severe losses of 70 dB. Similar individual variations will be found along the entire continuum of hearing levels.

Other factors, in addition to hearing level are significantly related to this individual variation. Without undue elaboration some of these factors will be mentioned. The hearing level and communication system of the parents are important. Children of deaf parents usually are well adjusted and come to school at 5 or 6 years of age with an established language of signs. They learn the oral and written communication and academic skills as well as or better than a matched group of children with hearing parents (Stevenson, 1964; Meadow, 1968). The attitude of the parents toward the child and the hearing impairment is critical. It will largely determine the child's outlook toward himself, his impairment, hearing aid, special needs and problems. The parents also control his early developmental environment and, to some extent, his educational setting. The intelligence and personality of the child are obviously related to his success. Differing etiologies have differing organic residua accounting for both psychotic and lesser mental disorders (Vernon, 1961, 1967a–d, 1968). Time of onset of hearing loss particularly in relation to language development is critical. The greater the child's competency in language skills before the onset of the loss, the greater advantage he has. The age at which amplification was first used, its quality and the consistency of its use are important. When training was begun is similarly significant. Then there are the many variables related to peripheral and central hearing which influence the functioning level of the child. A conductive hearing loss, for instance, related to bilateral, congenital atresia generally responds well to amplification by bone conduction and these children learn language and speech quite normally. On the other hand some sensory-neural losses do not respond well to amplification. The difference could be due to cochlear distortions and limited tolerance for high intensities or central auditory deficits with difficulty processing auditory information. These variables, operating singly or in combination can affect the progress of speech and language development and significantly influence the impact of the hearing impairment.

Because progress is dependent on many variables and is highly individualistic, evaluation of the hearing impaired should be an ongoing process and should reflect the changes in the child. More complete and reliable evaluations can be made as the child matures and has had a relatively prolonged exposure to concept development, language and speech training.

PRINCIPLES FROM NORMAL LANGUAGE AND SPEECH DEVELOPMENT

The normal language and speech acquisition process serves as the model for all teaching techniques designed to improve the oral communication skills for the preschool hearing impaired. It may serve as the referent for evaluating the special remedial techniques. Rather than describe the normal process here, the reader is referred to several of the many excellent references (McCarthy, 1954; Saporta, 1961; Smith and Miller, 1967; Carroll, 1964; Mussen, 1963; Brown, 1973). However, some pertinent principles from the normal acquisition literature will be developed briefly.

General Developmental Sequence

Speech and language emerge in relation to many other developments. These include neurophysiologic, motor, psychologic, intellectual and social developments. There is a species-determined regularity in the development of children, and language and speech are a part of this total behavior matrix.

It is not because all parents suddenly begin teaching speech when children are 12 to 15 months old that first words emerge. Rather the fact that speech development follows a lawful time pattern, almost regardless of environmental differences and in many cases in spite of the parents, strongly suggests a dependency on the development of the nervous system (Lenneberg, 1967). The gross developmental schedule for language and speech is: single words are used between ages 1 and 2 years, phrases and sentences between 2 and 3 years, with occasional grammatical errors between 3 and 4 years, and basic language skill established between 4 and 5 years.

The critical period for language acquisition is between 1 and 5 years with diminishing potential until adolescence. The beginning is limited by lack of maturation and the end seems to be related to a loss of adaptability and inability for reorganization in the brain (Lenneberg, 1967). Environmental factors play an important role in language acquisition.

The speech and language process is also dependent upon the child's reaching levels of self-realization, interest in his environment and the development of interpersonal relationships. All aspects of development progress simultaneously at different rates and are interrelated.

Acquisition of Language Rules

Language acquisition can be regarded as a process in which the child abstracts a finite number of rules from the language he hears. With these rules he can generate an infinite number of utterances (Berko, 1958; McNeill, 1966; Menyuk, 1969). Although the child cannot verbalize these rules, he can apply them in his language and speech.

Child Language Is Not Miniature Adult Language

Child language at different stages of development may be regarded as internally consistent language and speech systems rather than defective or inadequate adult language. He structures sentences that conform to the rules which he has abstracted (Brown and Fraser,

1963; Ervin, 1964; McNeill, 1966; Menyuk, 1969). The system is an idiolect which is related to a child's experiences and adequate for his needs. In child-adult communication the adult-listener rather than the child-talker makes the accommodation and the adult participates in the child's world. Child language also serves different functions as apparent in Piaget's ego-centric speech or in the naming and questioning stages. Children's experiences are less universal or standardized and their meanings of words and sentences will reflect these differences. Different language rules apply to progressive stages in language development and adult language always influences the direction of change.

Discrimination and Comprehension

The auditory system in a neonate is functioning and infants can make fine discriminations among speech sounds as early as one month (Eisenberg, 1969; Menyuk, 1972; Trehub and Rabinovitch 1972; Morse, 1972). Before infants are 6 months, they obviously discriminate speech forms. They respond discriminatingly to intonation and stress patterns that communicate the feelings and desires of adults. By the age of 1 year, most infants respond to expressions like "No, no!" or "Give me that!" Northern and Downs (1974) present a complete review of auditory development. At all stages of language development, discrimination and comprehension precede talking, receptive skills develop before expressive skills. Apparently language competency is developed through listening rather than talking.

Language, a Creative Process

Use of language is a creative rather than an imitative process. A child does not memorize all possible word combinations but rather as he talks he invents or generates unique utterances that conform to his rules. This inventive aspect of language enables a child to string words together in new patterns. It accounts for expressions such as, "The flower has sharp whiskers," when he touches the rose stem, or "The paint has cry drops," when he sees a thickly painted surface for the first time. These child utterances are evidence that he uses language to express concepts in an original way.

Phonologic Development

A child learns the speech sounds of the language over an extended period of time and a pattern of development is noted (Templin, 1957). Adult articulation skill is acquired by most children by the age of 8 years. In the early years, diphthongs, vowels, consonant elements, double consonant blends and triple consonant blends are learned in that order. Among consonants the order from most to least accurate progresses from nasals through plosives, fricatives and combinations to semivowels. Consonants in the initial position in words are more accurately produced than those in the medial and final positions. The final consonants are last to be acquired. Omitted sounds tend to be followed by substituted sounds. In the later stages of articulation development only distortions of speech sounds will usually be found.

According to one theory (Jakobson and Halle, 1961), the gradual evolution of a child's phonologic system is correlated with the development of auditory discrimination of the various distinctive features among as well as within classes of speech sounds.

Another possible explanation is that children begin to identify and discriminate only the most prominent auditory features of the word. This might explain why vowels are mastered first followed by initial consonants. Medial and final consonants tend to be unstressed and learned later. Redundancy might also be a factor in this phonologic acquisition process. Initially, the child tends to discriminate those speech sounds which are most significant for identifying the message. Similarly, in speaking, he produces not all of the speech sounds in words, but rather, only those which were auditorily significant for him. These significant sounds which the child uses in his receptive and expressive language are usually adequate so long as the messages are simple, the possible messages are limited and contextual clues are present.

Vocabulary

Frequently a 12-month-old child uses a nucleus of several words and it may be several months before many new words are added. Then the child learns that everything has a name and he says, "Horse, daddy?" or "Book, mommy?" as if checking to see whether the parents also call it that. At this stage the child is concerned about labels and asks questions like "What's that?" "What's that called?" and "What does that mean?" In these early stages his vocabulary is related to his needs, his activities and his environment. Later, words take on additional denotations and connotations through usage. He always understands more words than he uses.

Grammar and Syntax

The manner in which a child acquires his skill in grammar and syntax is at this time partially understood. A fairly high level of proficiency in application of grammar rules has been demonstrated among children as young as 4 years of age (Berko, 1961). An inductive process for applying rules by analogy to word classes takes place (Ervin, 1964). For past tenses he generalizes from "have" to haved," from "do" to "dood" while contractions might generalize from "am not" to "amn't" although he never has heard these modifications. He classifies words and applies the rules.

Syntax usually develops through stages from the one word naming stage at about age 12 months through the several word phrase stage at age 18 months, to simple sentence stage with as many as 10 words at age 36 months. His early two- and three-word strings usually consist of nouns and verbs or nouns with adjectives (McNeill, 1966, Menyuk, 1969). These word combinations preserve the word order of the model he hears and are classified as "content" words. Also noteworthy is the observation that these words are stressed in the adult model utterances (Brown and Bellugi, 1964). The unstressed words which show grammatical relationship and are sometimes called "functors" are added later. This latter group includes auxiliary verbs, articles, prepositions and conjunctions. Children learn syntax, partly by analogy of word classes and rules. This process undergoes gradual change under the influence of the adult model. Expansion of utterances seems to be related to and follows growing comprehension and ability to plan the structure.

The Speech Model

Mothers in talking to their young children use a simple repetitive and idealized dialect (Brown and Bellugi, 1964). Sentences are short and perfectly grammatical. Generally the conversation is very much "here and now." There is no speech about other times and other places. It concerns the ongoing activities and objects within the view or grasp of the child.

The mother tends to repeat with expansions or corrections the child's phrases. For example, "Milk, mommy?" might be expanded to "Does Jimmy want milk?" or "Home now, mommy?" to "Yes, we're going home now." The model includes the kinds of sentences the child will produce as much as a year later. The mother corrects, repeats and expands the syntactic structures the child uses as they verbalize ongoing experiences.

Interpersonal Relationships

According to the "autism" theory, in the initial stages of speech development, children reproduce and perfect human speech, not because of its objective utility but rather because of the subjective comfort and satisfaction the sounds provide (Mowrer, 1952). The sounds themselves have acquired secondary reinforcing properties since they are associated with pleasant and satisfying contacts with the adult, usually the mother. Initially the use of the sounds by the child provides comfort, security and satisfaction; later they are used functionally in communication.

This notion suggests the importance of a warm, friendly, positive relationship between the child and the mother or mother substitute. This person supplies the motivation and reinforcement for talking by being a responsive listener for any attempted message. Speech is a social phenomenon and experiencing good interpersonal relationships is an important part of learning to talk.

PRESCHOOL PROGRAMS

Child psychologists and psycholinguists regard the first 5 years as the most critical for development of language, perception and cognition. Programs for the parents of hearing-impaired babies and toddlers have been established (Miller, 1965; Simmons, 1966; Luterman, 1967; Ling, 1968; Horton, 1968). The focus of these programs is on the adjustment of the parents to the handicapped child and information relative to language development. In the classes for parents basic information about hearing, causes of hearing losses, the use of hearing aids and some aspects of child development are taught. Also, techniques for developing lipreading and listening skills are described and demonstrated in simulated homes so that language and speech stimulation can take place early in the natural and meaningful home setting with the parents as teachers. The topics are developed as the parents need and want the information. The parents bring assigned observations of their children to class. They receive encouragement from each other and learn that their child's problems are not unique. If training is to begin early, the home is the appropriate setting and many parents are excellent teachers.

In some programs parents receive training in the use of signs as part of the "total communication" approach, which will be discussed later. It should be emphasized here that the simultaneous use of signs and speech is a difficult task but if early language development and communication are the goals the parent will have to assume some role as model and communicator. Without parent participation the child might establish a language in a nursery program but have little opportunity to use it meaningfully at home. The psychological space between a deaf child and his parents will be bridged when they can communicate with each other.

For the parents of very young deaf children, the correspondence course of the John Tracy Clinic (807 W. Adams Blvd., Los Angeles, California 90007) has been available since the 1940s. It has enjoyed very wide use by parents from countries around the world. It is particularly appropriate for parents who cannot receive counseling directly from audiologists or at schools for the deaf. Like all correspondence courses, it requires feedback by the parents before additional lessons are sent. Cooperation and persistence are necessary to carry out the step by step procedures. These include matching colors and pictures, imitating body movements as well as language readiness tasks that a deaf child can perform. The approach is psychologically sound and it helps establish a cooperative and understanding relationship between the child and his parents.

Nursery school programs for hearing-impaired children as young as 2½ or 3 years are generally available. In these programs the child receives language stimulation and readiness activities which the parents observe. In this way the mother sees that her child is like the other children and she is encouraged to apply, supplement and expand the school learning experience in the home.

A philosophy emphasizing socialization in the management of preschool hearing impaired comes from England (Whetnall and Fry, 1964) where these children are encouraged to attend regular nursery programs in which a special teacher trained in oral methods is on the staff. The hearing impaired are exposed to normal children's loud and simple speech uttered at the level of the child's ear. All play together and the child learns to socialize and acquire language in a natural setting.

Another more recent philosophy affecting the nursery school programs comes from experiences of the Head Start programs for the disadvantaged children in the United States. The traditionally socially oriented programs were found to be less effective than those which emphasized academic approaches to cognitive learning in meeting the needs of the disadvantaged (Di Lorenzo, 1969). Specific skills involved in language readiness, reading readiness and number concepts are stressed.

In all preschool programs the focus should be on the parent as well as the child. The parent needs orientation and guidance so that he can adjust to his unusual and unexpected role and make intelligent decisions concerning the child's immediate and long-term needs.

In addition to the training goals just alluded to, the preschool programs include "diagnostic training" or "diagnostic teaching." Although the study of every child in the program continues, some will be singled out for more careful scrutiny because their behavior or progress cannot be accounted for by the hearing loss alone. The same agents or conditions precipitating the sensory-neural hearing loss could affect different levels of the nervous system. Maternal rubella and encephalitis, for example, sometimes affect other systems in addition to the cochlea.

Brain damage with specific learning problems, mental retardation and emotional disturbance are not uncommon among the hearing impaired. Diagnostic teaching for these special children calls for varying teaching techniques and making specific and detailed behavioral observations. It may also call for a more elaborate case history and special psychological, audiologic or medical evaluations to aid in understanding the lack of progress.

When the child is ready to leave the oral preschool program, recommendations for immediate educational placement are made consistent with his language achievement, social development, academic readiness and hearing. Communities vary widely in the available programs for hearing impaired. Attitudes of parents, school administrators and teachers also influence the placement selection process. No simple criteria will cover all of the possibilities. Placements out of the preschool programs range from the regular classrooms, programs for the hard of hearing, day classes, day schools for the deaf to residential schools and other special education programs.

RECEPTIVE COMMUNICATION

The normal child learns language through hearing and comprehending the speech of others. In order to exploit the hearing-impaired child's potential to receive spoken language, the use of amplification is an important consideration along with auditory training and speechreading.

Hearing Aids

The use of amplification should be considered for each hearing-impaired child as soon as the hearing loss is identified and assessed as completely as possible. Selecting the personal hearing aid should be done as soon as practicable (see Chapter 43). The hearing aid is the single development that makes the biggest improvement in the lives of the hearing impaired. This does not imply that all will benefit equally from a hearing aid. But the earlier and the more speech and language that can be gotten through the auditory channel the better will be the child's potential for oral communication.

The proper functioning of each child's hearing aid should be checked at least daily. Malfunctioning hearing aids are very common

(Gaeth and Lounsbury, 1966; Zink, 1972). Not only should the hearing aids be checked subjectively daily to see that they are operating, but a regular electroacoustic evaluation of their function ensures optimum performance.

Auditory Training

Some children readily adjust to a hearing aid. They accept it, tolerate the sound and easily learn to use the auditory information. On the other hand, for some children a tolerance for a hearing aid will have to be developed more gradually beginning with ideal and controlled conditions for short periods of time (see Chapter 44). As soon as practical, however, a child should be wearing his personal, optimally functioning hearing aid during his waking hours. Only with the consistent availability of the best amplified sound for the child will he have the opportunity to learn to discriminate speech and language cues. The people in the child's environment also learn to adjust to his auditory participation and they develop consistent levels of expectancy for performance when they speak to the child.

Audition can serve different functions in varying degrees. These include the psychological coupling of the person to his environment, receiving signal and warning cues, enjoying music, monitoring one's own voice and articulation, learning speech and language and finally speech perception. The person's residual hearing, intelligence, personality, hearing aid, and environment will partly determine to what extent he will be able to use his hearing. Auditory training includes the techniques for developing the greatest participation of the auditory sensory channel in these processes, particularly in the understanding of speech.

Speechreading

For some children the auditory code for speech reception is incomplete. Some may be able to discriminate loudness, pitch and stress patterns of voices and some vowels. Others may be able to identify most of the speech sounds in stressed syllables under ideal listening conditions. To help compensate for the inadequacies of audition, the hearing impaired learn to use visible speech cues as well as the contextual and situational cues. This is speechreading (see Chapters 46 and 47).

For the normal hearing person the visual cues are generally redundant and are used only to confirm the auditory message. For the hearing impaired, however, these visual cues provide essential information and complement the residual hearing. The phonologic systems of languages depend upon auditory contrasts rather than distinctive visual features. The visual code may be regarded only as a fairly consistent accompaniment to the basic auditory pattern. Visual characteristics do not provide voice-voiceless contrasts nor reliable differences for many speech sounds at the same point of articulation and some have no visible features. The visible features of speech sounds are also masked in some contexts and a wide range of variation of visible cues exists among different talkers. Some talkers have minimal movement of their jaws and lips. These kinds of limitations have broadened the scope of "lipreading" to include cues from facial expressions and gestures as well as the language and situational contexts and is now called "speechreading."

Various speechreading methods were developed with adults before the use of hearing aids. For many people speechreading offsets the effect of the hearing losses which occurred after the language and social skills were developed. These skills enabled the adults to anticipate conversational topics and language structures. During this period visual discrimination of speech sounds was universally taught and different methods evolved around various techniques. The Nitchie method emphasized the positive attitude of the speechreader and the training of the mind in intuition, synthesis, quickness, alertness and concentration. The Jena method stressed the rhythmic and kinesthetic aspects of talking and applied them to listening. The Mueller-Walle method emphasized rapid and rhythmic syllable drills. Generally in teaching speechreading to adults and those who already have language, there are advantages to unisensory approach, that is, allowing the person only to see but not to hear the speaker. The person then is forced to observe, discriminate and interpret the visible cues. Without the unisensory stimulation, the adult tends to persevere in his usual listening habits.

But these methods which have been used successfully with adults are not readily transferred to teaching children who have no language or speech. These children need all available auditory and visual information as they acquire language. Speechreading complements audition and is not usually isolated as a separate skill to be taught. Rather it is an integral part of the total receptive process involved in language learning. The young child is encouraged early to watch the talker's face so that he sees and hears speech simultaneously. In this way, although the separate sense modalities receive incomplete cues, together they may supply enough consistent information to enable the child to organize and interpret the speech and language cues.

EXPRESSIVE COMMUNICATION

Speech and language differences frequently are the only observable behavior characteristics of the severely hearing impaired. Their speech is characterized by a high pitched monotone which is frequently too loud and has a breathy and nasal quality. Stress, rhythm and intonation patterns are wanting and generally their voices lack emotional color and variety. Misarticulation tendencies are also present. Vowels are often prolonged and distorted but still recognizable. Sometimes syllables are added. Consonant differences cover a wide range but omissions of final consonants and slower articulation development are common. All standard methods for improving voice and articulation skills are pertinent with the hearing impaired.

Most importantly the teacher needs a thorough understanding of the speech mechanism and the functions of the larynx, resonators and articulators in producing voice and speech sounds. With this information, she knows which cues are significant and available to the different senses. In teaching speech all available sensory cues are used to help the child learn to produce adequate voice and speech sounds. These involve the auditory, visual, tactile and kinesthetic senses.

The best amplification available should be used to augment hearing in trying to improve a child's speech. Most children will be able to hear and recognize the rhythm pattern of sentences, perhaps the pitch inflection patterns and the voice-voiceless contrasts in consonants. If they can recognize these patterns in the auditory model, they attempt imitation which is also amplified.

The visual sense should receive undistorted information through speechreading but in later attempts at improving the speech, the movements are exaggerated by the teacher making the focal articulation points as visible as possible. Again the child attempts imitation and his own performance might be visually monitored in a mirror. Some clinicians find the visual feedback from electroacoustic filters attached to different colored lights helpful in aiding children to discriminate and produce the correct sound by matching the light pattern of the model.

The tactile sense is used by placing the child's hand on the teacher's face while she produces a speech sound. Contact of the fingers at the larynx picks up the voice-voiceless contrast, at the nose the nasal resonance contrast, along the mandible picks up that movement while the part of the hand in front of the mouth picks up the distinctive extraoral pressure pattern of the escaping air stream.

The kinesthetic sense is involved grossly through rhythmic movements of hands, for example, accompanying talking. In this way an awareness of rate and rhythm of a sentence might be created. Also, the teacher might manipulate the child's jaw and place the tongue in the position for a particular sound with a tongue depressor assuming the child is getting kinesthetic cues and will be able ultimately to repeat the movement without the manipulation.

In all speech improvement it is helpful to establish a baseline of speech behavior through testing. Through an analysis of the speech, it is possible to establish a priority of needs for change so that significant progress is made early. Also through the evaluation, the skills which the child can readily learn early, skills that are at his threshold of learning are determined. The minimal goal for the hearing impaired should be intelligible speech with as much progress toward normal speech as possible.

ORTHOGRAPHY AND SPEECH

In an ideal orthographic system there is a one to one correspondence between the written letters or symbols and the speech sounds they represent. Since there are approximately 43 speech sounds in the English language and 26 letters in the alphabet, the lack of correspondence is apparent. It should be noted that the letters c, q and x duplicate the function of other letters, that digraphs are common, that the same letters represent different speech sounds, that the same sounds have different spellings and finally, that the vowel sounds have more variations in spellings than the consonants. The problems of using the English written code as an aid in speech development and pronunciation become apparent. The situation has challenged the ingenuity of teachers to devise more adequate orthographic systems.

In an article published as early as 1872, Alexander Graham Bell pointed up the advantage of "visible speech" as a means of communicating articulation information to the deaf. This visible speech consists of a "minute analysis of speech sounds, complete for all languages and phonetic effects, and coupled with a scheme of symbols expressive to the eye, of the organic formation of the sounds they represent" (Bell, 1916). His vowel symbols show the voicing, the relative height of the tongue, whether it is a front, mixed or back vowel, the opening between the teeth and the rounding of the lips. His consonant symbols have markers for place and manner of articulation as well as voicing. Included in this schema are supplementary symbols for stress on a syllable or emphasis on a word. Pitch inflection markers are available to show level tone, simple rise or fall, compound rise or fall, pitch height relative to the preceding syllable and others. The visible speech of the Bell family is ideal so far as available information is concerned but far too complex and detailed for practical use by the child. The use of visible speech was abandoned and teachers of the deaf began modifying the alphabet to serve the pupil's needs.

The Northampton speech sound charts evolved out of the practical experiences of many teachers at the Clarke School for the Deaf. The basic organization of the charts dates back to 1885 when Alice Worcester, a special teacher of speech at that school, stated her objections to the use of visible speech and diacritical markings and first described her methods (Yale, 1946). Later Caroline Yale, for many years principal at Clarke School, improved this original system.

The Northampton speech sound charts (Fig. 45.1, *A* and *B*) contain the most common spellings for speech sounds found among frequently occurring words in a child's vocabulary. Primary or most common spellings are in bold print with secondary spellings appearing in small print below. If the same letter represents more than one sound the number above the letter designates the intended sound. For example, $\overset{2}{s}$ represents the sound in *sun*, $\overset{}{s}$ the sound in *is* and $\overset{3}{s}$ the sound in *measure*. Also, it should be noted that in the vowel group, the final *e* marker which affects the value of the preceding vowel is shown by *a-e* as in *pane* in contrast to -*a*- as *pan* or -*a sofa*.

The chart is used in the early stages of language and speech development to enable the child, after he is familiar with the sound value of the spellings, to pronounce the words he sees in print. It is a tool to teach the

A. CONSONANT SOUNDS

h—

wh   w—

p   b   m

t   d   n   l   r—

k $\overset{2}{g}$ ng
c   n(k)
ck

f   v
ph

$\overset{1}{th}$ $\overset{2}{th}$

$\overset{1}{s}$ z
c(e) $\overset{2}{s}$
c(i)
c(y)   y—

sh   zh
      $\overset{3}{s}$
      $\overset{2}{z}$ x=ks

ch   j
tch $\overset{2}{g}$—
     —ge   qu=kwh
     dge

B. VOWEL SOUNDS

$\overset{\cdot}{oo}$ $\overset{2}{oo}$ o–e   aw   –o–
(r)u–e   oa   au
(r)ew   —o   o(r)
          $\overset{2}{}$
          ow

ee   –i–   a–e   –e–   –a–
—e   —y   ai $\overset{2}{}$
$\overset{2}{}$ ay   ea
ea
e–e

      a(r)   –u–   ur
           —a   er
               ir

a–e   i–e   o–e   ou   oi   u–e
ai   igh   oa $\overset{2}{ow}$ oy   ew
ay   —y   —o
          $\overset{2}{}$
          ow

Fig. 45.1. (*A*) The Northampton Consonant Chart categorizes the voiceless speech sounds in the 1st column; the voiced cognates are in the 2nd column; and the three nasals are listed in the 3rd column. The *horizontal lines* generally classify the consonants according to place of articulation. A *dash following a letter* indicates that the sound is initial in a word or syllable.

(*B*) The Northampton Vowel Chart categorizes the back vowels in the 1st horizontal line; the front vowels in the 2nd line and the remaining vowels in the 3rd line. The diphthongs appear in the 4th line. The /e/ and /o/ speech sounds occur with both the pure vowels and the diphthongs. The *dash* indicates consonants relative to the vowel in the syllable or word. (From C. A. Yale, *Formation and Development of Elementary English Sounds.* Northampton, Mass.: The Clarke School for the Deaf, 1946.)

pronunciation of the child's basic vocabulary. Later the diacritical markings are taught in relation to dictionary use.

Some years ago Sir James Pitman devised the Initial Teaching Alphabet (ita) which was intended to teach the phonic approach to reading (Pitman and St. John, 1969; O'Halloran, 1973). The ita consists of a modified alphabet which has a discrete symbol for each speech sound. As many letters from the alphabet as possible were assigned their usual sound value. For the rest of the sounds he ingeniously devised variations of fairly standard symbols and digraphs so that they have a visual similarity to common spellings. In learning to read the child is taught to associate the sounds with the symbols and shortly he can phonically produce any word written in ita system. According to some reports, the normal hearing child readily makes the transition from the ita to conventional spellings. Since beginning reading materials are commercially available and the system has discrete symbol-sound relationships, it satisfies some of the needs of an ideal orthographic system for teaching speech to the hearing impaired.

Teachers of the hearing impaired have devised many other systems the most common of which is color coding the letters to indicate some feature of articulation or production. Red usually represents the sonants and blue the surds. To this some add particular colors to indicate nasals, plosives, fricatives, vowels and diphthongs. This code gives additional articulation cues which aid the speech performance.

SPECIAL METHODS FOR TEACHING GRAMMAR AND SYNTAX

Many hearing impaired, even with the use of amplification and speechreading, do not discriminate language patterns adequately enough for them to formulate their rules of grammar and syntax through use alone. They benefit from a system which categorizes their vocabulary items as they are acquired and, later, the ordering of these words into sentences through the use of a visible, structured outline. This programmed system of teaching language is sometimes called the grammatical or analytical method.

A number of language teaching systems have been used with the deaf but only one method is adopted for one particular program so that there is continuity and consistency in the language training as the child progresses through the program. An early and simple method which demonstrates the grammar and syntax principles of all systems is known as the "Five Slate System" described by Barry (1899). The analysis of sentences is done with five large wall slates or blackboards divided by lines into five columns. These slates are numbered consecutively. The children also have their individual slates ruled into five columns. The first slate or column is reserved for the subject of the sentence, the second for the verb and its complement, the third for the object of the verb, the fourth for the preposition and the fifth for the object of the preposition. Later a sixth column is added to the slate to accommodate the adverbial time concept "when." Initially the children analyze every written sentence by acting it out and putting the person or objects in front of the appropriate wall slates. For example, the action of the sentence, "Mary threw the ball into the basket," is first demonstrated. Then Mary stands before slate 1, "threw" is written on slate 2, the ball is put before slate 3, "into" is written on slate 4 and the basket is put before slate 5. The class visualizes the sentence and each child writes it on his slate by substituting the words for the person and objects. This is a typical sample of the early visualization stage of language learning with this method.

The system most widely used to teach grammar and syntax to the deaf today is the Fitzgerald Key (Fitzgerald, 1949). Edith Fitzgerald, the author of the Key, was a congenitally deaf teacher who believed that language could not be acquired by memorizing correct sentences. She also observed that early language progress did not continue in higher grades. The deaf needed a sense of grammar which the normal child acquires through hearing sentences spoken. The Key provides a visible sentence pattern so that the child can generate his own acceptable sentences and recognize and correct his own mistakes.

The Fitzgerald Key consists of a series of interrogative pronouns and adverbs which along with six symbols form the headings under which the sentences are cast. Symbols are used because no appropriate question can be framed to elicit the verb or to clarify the grammatical functions of some words. Hence the verb, adjective, connective words, infinitives, present participle and predicate noun have symbols.

The Key must be seen as a part of the Fitzgerald system of teaching language. It begins by having the children classify people and things under "who" or "what." The concepts of animate and inanimate and human and nonhuman are acquired this way. Both words as well as pictures of people, animals and objects are placed under the appropriate headings, "How many?" "What color?" and "What?" Later some verbs are added and sentences are formed. The Key is expanded with the language development of the child and accommodates indirect and direct objects, adverbial phrases, as well as compound and complex sentences.

Like all teaching systems the success of the method depends on the skill of the teacher. The method can become a mechanical frame for limited stereotyped sentences. Or it can be a reference for natural and creative language as advocated by Mildred Groht (1958). She recommends that language principles should be introduced through usage in speech and writing as is the case in normal children so the principle has functional and practical value rather than only academic interest. After the principle is used and understood it is drilled in many meaningful childlike situations. In this way the language skills acquired in the classroom have a direct applicability to their daily communication needs.

The Fitzgerald Method and Key for teaching straight language are practical and complete. The Key will be found on the blackboards of schools and in the language workbooks of the deaf across the country. Teachers continue to expand and refine its use (Buell, 1952; Pugh, 1955). Teaching language to the deaf need not be a choice between the grammatical and natural language approaches. Many hearing impaired need both methods and the ingenious and knowledgeable teacher ties language in the classroom with the lives of the students through such activities and topics as the family and home, daily activities, the calendar, weather, vacations, field trips, experience charts, news events, conversations and planned activities. The teacher's confidence in the deaf child's ability and her enthusiasm for teaching add a natural atmosphere and motivation to the use of language.

MANUAL COMMUNICATION

The manual method of communication, which is widely used in many public residential schools for the deaf, is the preferred medium among the adult deaf and is now used in some television newscasts. Many deaf teenagers and adults prefer manual communication in spite of having been exposed to excellent speech training in school. They claim it is their natural language since it involves their vision and motor dexterity which are usually intact. They also point out that facility in speaking and speechreading skills varies widely in any group of deaf and for the most proficient, speechreading has inherent ambiguities. Because sign language is so generally used among the deaf and because of the several contrived language systems which have been based on a combination of the American Sign Language for the Deaf and the English language, some familiarity with sign language is desirable.

The American Sign Language for the deaf (ASL) is based on natural gestures and pantomime with many obvious relationships between sign and meaning. It is a less arbitrary system than spoken languages and is entirely independent of and different from English. The gestures are made with the hands and arms with time and space as basic parameters. Facial expression, vigor of movement and body position are important. For example, a pleasant expression on the face combined with the sign for "pleasure" indicates one is enjoying something. However, a frown or shaking of the head negatively while making the same sign shows that one has no pleasure or does not like something. The sign for "request" is identical with the sign for "demand" with the difference indicated by vigor of movement (Riekehof, 1963). It is a language in its own right with its own morphology, syntax and semantics (Stokoe, 1970). Plurals, tenses and word endings are not indicated except through context or by adding the sign for "finish" to indicate past tense.

The gross syntax of sign language in conversation might be described as consisting of four steps: (1) a gesture, touch or tap of the foot on the floor to get the visual attention of the group, (2) a sign indicating the topic, (3) the message and (4) a closure consisting of an evaluative gesture expressing the signer's reaction like, "Funny, isn't it?" or "Sad, isn't it?" (Tervoort, 1961).

In the above description ASL was referred to as if it were a single, homogeneous language. This is not the case. ASL has many dialects showing varying degrees of influence by the English language. Pidgin Sign English is the name for the many distinct dialects with varying combinations of ASL and English language syntax and morphology. If ASL would be at one end of the continuum and Sign English at the other, many dialect forms of Pidgin Sign English would fall between (Bornstein, in press). A schematic of this continuum is presented in Figure 45.2.

Sign English at the opposite pole from ASL is English rendered visible with signs. It is a contrived language used in teaching deaf children the English language through signs. Signs from ASL are employed in English syntax and the signs represent words or parts of words, morphemes. Past tense markers and plurals are shown. This system would not be attractive to the native user of ASL because of the redundancies from English (Bornstein, in press).

Exactly where on a Pidgin Sign English continuum a person can and does perform depends on a variety of circumstances. Skill in the use of ASL is rare among the hearing people. Conversely a large proportion of deaf

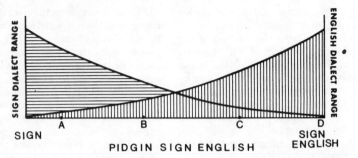

Fig. 45.2. A schematic with the various dialects of American Sign Language at the "Sign" pole and the various contrived language learning systems at the "Sign English" pole and the varieties of "Pidgin Sign English" falling on a continuum between the poles. The relative influence of American Sign Language and the English Language in each variety of Pidgin Sign English on the continuum is shown. (With permission from H. Bornstein, in I. M. Schlesinger and L. Namir (Eds.), *Current Trends in the Study of Sign Language of the Deaf,* in press.)

have difficulty with English structures and vocabulary (Bornstein, in press). Some people, therefore, will be able to send and receive at all points, *A, B, C, D,* along the continuum in Figure 45.2. Others will have their communication limited from point *B* to the "Sign" end of the continuum or from *C* to the "Sign English" end, for example.

In educational settings in which hearing people prevail and which emphasize participation in the "hearing" world and reading and writing skills, the Pidgin English variety is usually much closer to Sign English than ASL (Bornstein, in press).

Fingerspelling is another system of signs which employs the manual alphabet. Finger and hand configurations and movements represent the 26 letters of the alphabet. In application the sequences of letters spelling words are presented by serial positions and movements with one hand with slight pauses in movements separating the words. It is frequently used in sign English for proper names and specific words.

The combined use of fingerspelling every word as it is spoken is known as the "Rochester method." Zenas F. Westervelt, a former superintendent of the Rochester School for the Deaf in New York, advocated that fingerspelling be used consistently in the classrooms to supplement lipreading as early as 1878 (McClure, 1967).

The "simultaneous method" is another communicative mode in which the speaker-signer simultaneously encodes the message in speech and a variant of Sign English. The sender either speaks or only mouths the words (no voice) but rhythm and rate differ from normal speech in this method. This method is widely used in the upper grades of schools for the deaf as well as at Gallaudet College for the deaf.

TOTAL COMMUNICATION

In the mid-1960's several publications focused attention on the failure of the oral deaf programs in the United States that had continued in the philosophy espoused by the International Congress of Teachers of the Deaf in Milan in 1880. At that Congress a resolution was passed declaring "that the oral methods ought to be preferred to that of signs for the education and instruction of the deaf and dumb" (for the complete resolution see Bender (1970)). Generally these articles and reports (Babbidge, 1965; Boatner, 1965; McClure, 1968; Wrightstone, Aronow and Muskowitz, 1962) show that the average reading ability of deaf students, aged 16 years or older, was at a grade level of 5.3 or below. The average gain in reading from age 10 to age 16 was 8 months. Finally the median score on the Stanford Achievement Test of all deaf students as they left school was at the 5.9-grade level. These results were based on large samples of deaf students including over half of the total enrollment in this country. This relatively low academic achievement is especially remarkable in view of the normal intelligence found in the deaf population.

The positive effect of early exposure to manual-visual language has also received emphasis. Perhaps the Russian experimentation with "neo-oralism" prepared the way. The Russians, dissatisfied with the results of the traditional oral methods, initiated programs similar to the Rochester method in the United States in which fingerspelling accompanied speech in the home and nursery schools beginning when the child was 2 years old. Children from these programs were reported to have vocabularies of several thousand words by 6 years of age (Morkovin, 1960). The Russians reported the unexpected observation that the combined use of fingerspelling with speech enhanced speech and speechreading skills (Moores, 1972).

A number of studies show the modest academic superiority of deaf children with deaf parents who were exposed to manual communication from infancy. Stevenson (1964), Stuckless and Birch (1966), Meadow (1968), Quigley and Frisina (1961), and Vernon and Koh (1970) showed between 1- and 2-year superiority specifically in arithmetic, reading, written language, fingerspelling and vocabulary. There were no significant differences in speech and speechreading skills in these comparisons of deaf children from deaf parents with deaf children from hearing parents. From these studies one can generalize at least to the extent that organized manual communication at this time is the method of choice for deaf children with deaf parents. Quigley's research (1969) compared 16 orally educated preschool deaf children with 16 children trained with the Rochester method—fingerspelling simultaneously presented with speech. The Rochester method students were superior in fingerspelling, speechreading, 5 of 7 measures of reading and 3 of 5 measures of written language. The oral only students were superior in 1 of 5 measures of written language. For a more complete coverage of research on manual communication, see Moores (1971).

This, briefly, is the background for the introduction of the manual methods into the education of the deaf during the 1960s to the present time. The emphasis of the movement was to teach language by making available all forms including signs, fingerspelling, auditory information, speechreading and reading. It combines the oral, manual and auditory methods. The use of amplification and speech is to be encouraged as is the use of manual communication. The model is always to be simultaneously and completely spoken and signed. This simultaneous, multisensory and dual language presentation is to provide an unambiguous language (the manual) with which the child would learn to associate oral English. Language is learned and the child ultimately selects his optimum mode of communication with some proficiency in both oral and manual communication.

The "total communication" approach as it is frequently referred to has two purposes: (1) to teach language to the child and (2) to provide a communication system so that he can communicate with his parents, teachers and classmates. Total communication is consistent with the concept that language cannot be taught directly through drills with sounds of the language, vocabulary lists and memorizing the rules of grammar. Rather it emphasizes that children learn language through experience and contact with it, by the free interchange with others in meaningful contexts so that the child is able to extrapolate his own language rules from these exposures.

In addition to the simultaneous fingerspelling and talking (the Rochester method) four other systems of manual presentation have developed: "Signed English" (Bornstein, 1974), "seeing essential English" (Anthony, 1971), "linguistics of visual English" (Wampler, 1972), and "signing exact English" (Gustason, Pfetzing and Zawolkow, 1972). None of these are languages and the names of these systems are most descriptive. They are substitutes for neither the ASL nor English. Rather all are similar contrived systems. They are combinations of ASL and the English language in which both languages lose their identity. The signs taken from ASL become semantic equivalents for words. A particular system may have particular signs for more or fewer bound morphemes. All have invented signs for plurals, possessives, tense, participle, the adverbial and adjectivial markers and comparative and superlative forms. The signs a child sees are the parallel of the English spoken by the model. The Sign English and spoken English will be very similar at the semantic and syntactical levels. All are attempts to make English morphemes and syntax visible.

Total communication has enjoyed wide acceptance since its recent introduction. When ideally used it can be regarded as the best oral-aural program implemented by Sign English.

Some comments might help put the movement in perspective. Considerable practice and high level of skill are required for parents and teachers to become proficient in the complete, simultaneous and consistent presentation of language in the two modalities, oral English and Sign English. Further, teachers of the deaf will need all of the previously prescribed competency related to speech and hearing in addition to the complete fluency in Sign English and some expertise in ASL. Also, they will need the ability to teach Sign English and perhaps ASL to parents and the hearing public generally. The parents should be encouraged in every way to learn Sign English so that the child-parent relationship can be established through communication without the usual frustrations related to limited "home gestures."

The initial purpose of Sign English is to make available a consistent visible language from which the deaf child can learn his English morphology and syntax in normal communication settings for children. Hopefully, the child will develop his speech, speechreading and auditory skills at the same time. The experience with Sign English also facilitates all communication processes including reading and writing. But Sign English hypothetically has different utility for different children. For example, the child who learns to understand speech readily and to talk clearly would have no further use for Sign English and would matriculate in school with hearing children. For those deaf children with hearing parents who have varying levels of proficiency in speech, utility for Sign English would be high during the language acquisition and early elementary school periods as shown in Figure 45.3 (Bornstein, in press). On the other hand, ASL would be the first language for the child with deaf parents. Sign English has high utility during the period when the child acquires the English language as a second language. After he acquires some proficiency in English, he also uses Pidgin Sign English as shown in Figure 45.4 (Bornstein, in press).

Sign English is another resource, which, along with nursery programs for the hearing impaired, amplification, and speechreading, is now available to close the gap between potential and performance for the deaf. While the "perfect" solution to the communication problem of the deaf still eludes us, Sign English certainly is appropriate for many. But the introduction of signs alone will improve neither a poor teacher nor a poor program.

Kent (1973) reflects the judgment of many when she states:

Signs are the easiest means of getting the very young congenitally deaf child to communicate in the true sense of the word, that is, expressing his own ideas. When this happens we see positive changes in behavior and in interpersonal relationships. The deaf child joins the family at home and at school.

CONCLUSION

Teaching speech and language to the hearing impaired is still an art and the results as seen in the performance of many hard-of-hearing and deaf leave much to be desired. The outlook is brighter today, perhaps, because of the advent of total communication and the focus of

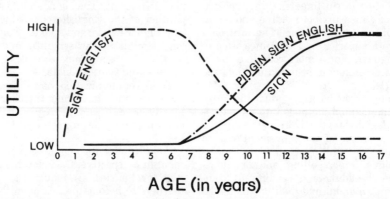

AGE (in years)

Fig. 45.3. Hypothetical curves showing utility for Sign, Sign English and Pidgin Sign English in general communication and in education for deaf children born of hearing parents. (With permission from H. Bornstein, in I. M. Schlesinger and L. Namir (Eds.), *Current Trends in the Study of Sign Language of the Deaf,* in press.)

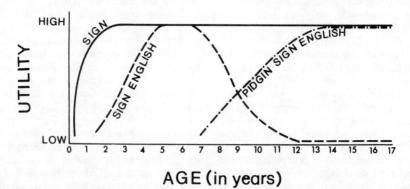

AGE (in years)

Fig. 45.4. Hypothetical curves showing utility for Sign, Sign English and Pidgin Sign English in general communication and education for deaf children born of deaf parents. (With permission from H. Bornstein, in I. M. Schlesinger and L. Namir (Eds.), *Current Trends in the Study of Sign Language of the Deaf,* in press.)

attention on the language learning problems by psychologists, psycholinguists, teachers of the deaf, speech pathologists and audiologists. But total communication is not a panacea. It is a contrived language of signs designed to implement and facilitate the development of language and speech as well as to make early communication possible. Although still unproven, it is one more available language approach for the deaf.

REFERENCES

Anthony, D. A., and Associates, Seeing Essential English. 1-2. P.O. Box 3520, Anaheim, Calif.: Education Services Division, Anaheim Union High School District, 1971.

Babbidge, H. D., Education of the Deaf: A Report to the Secretary of Health, Education and Welfare by His Advisory Committee on the Education of the Deaf. Washington, D.C.: U. S. Department of Health, Education and Welfare, 1965.

Barry, K. E., The Five Slate System: A System of Objective Language Teaching. Philadelphia: Sherman & Co., 1899.

Bell, A. G., Visible speech as a means of communicating articulation to deaf mutes. Am. Ann. Deaf, 17, 1-21, 1872.

Bell, A. M., Principles of Speech and Dictionary of Sounds. Washington, D. C.: Volta Bureau, 1916.

Bender, R. E., The Conquest of Deafness. Cleveland, Ohio: The Press of Case Western Reserve University, 1970.

Berko, J., The child's learning of English morphology. Word, 14, 150-177, 1958.

Berko, J., The Child's Learning of English Morphology. In Saporta, S. (Ed.), Psycholinguistics: A Book of Readings. New York: Holt, Rinehart & Winston, 1961.

Boatner, E. B., The need for a realistic approach to the education of the deaf. A paper presented to a joint convention of Parents of Deaf and Hard-of-Hearing Children, California Association of Teachers of the Deaf and Hard-of-Hearing, and California Association of the Deaf, November 6, 1965.

Bornstein, H., Signed English; a manual approach to English language development. J. Speech Hear. Disord., 39, 330-343, 1974.

Bornstein, H., Sign Language in the Education of the Deaf. In Schlesinger, I. M., and Namir, L. (Eds.), Current Trends in the Study of Sign Language of the Deaf, in press.

Brown, R., A First Language—The Early Stages. Cambridge, Mass.: Harvard University Press, 1973.

Brown, R., and Bellugi, U., Three Processes in the Child's Acquisition of Syntax. In Lenneberg, E. H. (Ed.), New Directions in the Study of Language. Cambridge, Mass.: M.I.T. Press, 1964.

Brown, R., and Fraser, C., The Acquisition of Syntax. In Cofer, C. N., and Musgrave, B. (Eds.), Verbal Behavior and Learning. New York: McGraw-Hill, 1963.

Buell, E. M., Outline of Language for Deaf Children. Books I and II. Washington, D. C.: Volta Bureau, 1952.

Carroll, J. B., Language and Thought. Englewood Cliffs, N.J.: Prentice-Hall, 1964.

Conference of Executives of American Schools for the Deaf. Report of the Committee on Nomenclature. Am. Ann. Deaf, 83, 1-3, 1938.

Di Lorenzo, L., Prekindergarten Programs for the Disadvantaged. Albany, N. Y.: New York State Office of Research and Evaluation, 1969.

Eagles, E., The Survey, Proceedings of the Conference on the Collection of Statistics of Severe Hearing Impairments and Deafness in the United States. Public Health Service Publication 1227, 1964.

Eisenberg, R., Auditory behavior in the human neonate; functional properties of sound and their ontogenetic implications. Int. Audiol., 8, 34-45, 1969.

Ervin, S. M., Imitation and Structural Change in Children's Language. In Lenneberg, E. H. (Ed.), New Directions in the Study of Language. Cambridge, Mass.: M.I.T. Press, 1964.

Fitzgerald, E., Straight Language for the Deaf. Washington, D. C.: Volta Bureau, 1949.

Fletcher, H., Speech and Hearing in Communication. New York: D. Van Nostrand Co., 1953.

Gaeth, J. H., and Lounsbury, E., Hearing aids and children in elementary school. J. Speech Hear. Disord., 31, 551-562, 1966.

Groht, M. A., Natural Language for Deaf Children. Washington, D. C.: The Volta Bureau, 1958.

Gustason, G., Pfetzing, D., and Zawolkow, E., Signing Exact English. Rossmore, Calif.: Modern Signs Press, 1972.

Horton, K. B., Home Demonstration Teaching for Parents of Very Young Deaf Children, Reprint 903. Washington, D. C.: A. G. Bell Association for the Deaf, Inc., 1968.

Jakobson, R., and Halle, M., Phonemic Patterning. In Saporta, S. (Ed.), Psycholinguistics: A Book of Readings. New York: Holt, Rinehart & Winston, 1961.

Katz, J., and Illmer, R., Auditory Perception in Children with Learning Disabilities. In Katz, J. (Ed.), Handbook of Clinical Audiology. Baltimore: Williams & Wilkins Co., 1972.

Kent, M. S., Total Communication at the Maryland School for the Deaf. In Watson, S. (Ed.), Readings on Deafness. New York: Deafness Research and Training Center, New York University School of Education, 1973.

Lenneberg, E. H., Biological Foundations of Language. New York: John Wiley & Sons, 1967.

Lewis, N., Otitis media and linguistic incompetence. Arch. Otolaryngol., 102, 387-390, 1976.

Ling, A. H., Advice for Parents of Young Deaf Children: How to Begin, Reprint 912. Washington, D. C.: A. G. Bell Association for the Deaf, Inc., 1968.

Luterman, D. M., A Parent-Oriented Nursery Program for Preschool Deaf Children, Reprint 890. Washington, D. C.: A. G. Bell Association for the Deaf, Inc., 1967.

McCarthy, D., Language Development in Children. In Carmichael, L. (Ed.), Manual of Child Psychology. New York: John Wiley & Sons, 1954.

McClure, W. J., The Revival of the Rochester Method. In Fusfeld, I. S. (Ed.), A Handbook of Readings in Education of the Deaf and Postschool Implications. Springfield, Ill.: Charles C

Thomas, 1967.

McClure, W. J., Current problems and trends in the education of the deaf. *Deaf American*, 18, 8–14, 1968.

McNeill, D., Developmental Psycholinguistics. In Smith, F., and Miller, G. (Eds.), *The Genesis of Language: A Psycholinguistic Approach*, pp. 15–48. Cambridge, Mass.: M.I.T. Press, 1966.

Meadow, K., Early communication in relation to the deaf child's intellectual, social, and communicative functioning. *Am. Ann. Deaf*, 113, 29–41, 1968.

Menyuk, P., Sentences Children Use. In *Research Monograph 52*. Cambridge, Mass.: M.I.T. Press, 1969.

Menyuk, P., *The Development of Speech*, pp. 11–13. Indianapolis, Ind.: Bobbs-Merrill Co., 1972.

Miller, J., Speech and the Preschool Child, Reprint 747. Washington, D. C.: A. G. Bell Association for the Deaf, Inc., 1965.

Moores, D., Recent Research on Manual Communication. Occasional Paper No. 7, Project No. 332189, Department of Health, Education and Welfare, U. S. Office of Education, 1971.

Moores, D., Language Disabilities of Hearing-Impaired Children. In Irwin, J. V., and Marge, M. (Eds.), *Principles of Childhood Language Disabilities*. Englewood Cliffs, N. J.: Prentice-Hall, 1972.

Morkovin, B., Experiment in teaching deaf preschool children in the Soviet Union. *Volta Rev.*, 62, 260–268, 1960.

Morse, P. A., The discrimination of speech and non-speech stimuli in early infancy. *J. Exp. Child Psychol.*, 14, 477–492, 1972.

Mowrer, O. H., Speech development in the young child; 1. The autism theory of speech development and some clinical implications. *J. Speech Hear. Disord.*, 17, 263–268, 1952.

Mussen, P. H., *The Psychological Development of the Child*. Englewood Cliffs, N. J.: Prentice-Hall, 1963.

Northern, J. L., and Downs, M. P., *Hearing in Children*. Baltimore: Williams & Wilkins, Co., 1974.

O'Halloran, G., *Teach Yourself ita, Initial Teaching Alphabet*. Belmont, Calif.: Lear Siegler, Inc./ Fearon Publishers, 1973.

Pitman, J., and St. John, J., *Alphabets and Reading: The Initial Teaching Alphabet*. New York: Pitman Publishing Corp., 1969.

Pugh, B., *Steps in Language Development for the Deaf, Illustrated in Fitzgerald Key*. Washington, D. C.: Volta Bureau, 1955.

Quigley, S., *The Influence of Fingerspelling on the Development of Language, Communication and Educational Development in Deaf Children*. Urbana, Ill.: University of Illinois Press, 1969.

Quigley, S., and Frisina, R. D., Institutionalization and Psycho-Educational Development in Deaf Children. Council for Exceptional Children Monograph No. 3, 1961.

Riekehof, L. L., *Talk to the Deaf*. Springfield, Mo.: Gospel Publishing House, 1963.

Saporta, S. (Ed.), *Psycholinguistics, A Book of Readings*. New York: Holt, Rinehart & Winston, 1961.

Simmons, A. A., Language Growth for the Pre-Nursery Deaf Child, Reprint No. 853. Washington, D. C.: A. G. Bell Association for the Deaf, Inc., 1966.

Smith, F., and Miller, G. A. (Eds.), *The Genesis of Language: A Psycholinguistic Approach*. Cambridge, Mass.: M.I.T. Press, 1967.

Stevenson, E., A study of educational achievement of deaf children of deaf parents. *California News*, 80, 142, 1964.

Stokoe, W. C., Jr., Center for applied linguistics conference on sign language. *Linguistic Reporter*, 12, 5–8, 1970.

Stuckless, E. R., and Birch, G. W., The influence of early manual communication on the linguistic development of children. *Am. Ann. Deaf*, 111, 452–462, 1966.

Templin, M. C., *Certain Language Skills in Children*. Minneapolis, Minn.: University of Minnesota Press, 1957.

Tervoort, B., Lecture at Indiana University, 1961.

Trehub, S. E., and Rabinovitch, M. S., Auditory-linguistic sensitivity in early infancy. *Dev. Psychol.*, 6, 74–77, 1972.

Vernon, M., The brain injured child; a discussion of the significance of the problem, its symptoms, and causes in deaf children. *Am. Ann. Deaf*, 106, 239–250, 1961.

Vernon, M., Tuberculosis meningitis and deafness. *J. Speech Hear. Disord.*, 32, 177–181, 1967a.

Vernon, M., Characteristics associated with post-rubella deaf children; psychological, educational, and physical. *Volta Rev.*, 69, 176–185, 1967b.

Vernon, M., Prematurity and deafness; the magnitude and nature of the problem among deaf children. *Except. Child.*, 34, 289–298, 1967c.

Vernon, M., Meningitis and deafness. *Laryngoscope*, 77, 1856–1874, 1967d.

Vernon, M., Current etiological factors in deafness. *Am. Ann. Deaf*, 115, 106–115, 1968.

Vernon, M., and Koh, S., Early communication and deaf children's achievement. *Am. Ann. Deaf*, 116, 527–536, 1970.

Wampler, D. W., Linguistics of Visual English. Booklets: Morpheme List One, An Introduction to the Spatial Symbol System, Questions and Answers. Santa Rosa, Calif., 1972.

Whetnall, E., and Fry, D. B., *The Deaf Child*. New York: William Heinemann Medical Books Limited, 1964.

White House Conference on Child Health and Protection. Special Education: The Handicapped and the Gifted, Report of the Committee on Special Classes, Section III, Education and Training, Vol. III F. New York: Appleton-Century-Crofts, 1931.

Wrightstone, J. W., Aronow, M. S., and Muskowitz, S., *Developing Reading Test Norms for Deaf Children*. Test Service Bulletin, No. 98. New York: Harcourt, Brace & World, 1962.

Yale, C. A., *Formation and Development of Elementary English Sounds*. Northampton, Mass.: The Clarke School for the Deaf, 1946.

Zink, G. D., Hearing aids children wear; a longitudinal study of performance. *Volta Rev.*, 74, 41–51, 1972.

chapter 46

VISUAL AND AUDITORY TRAINING FOR ADULTS

Donald G. Sims, Ph.D.

Audiologists might ask, "Does aural rehabilitation exist?" They could question its existence because the preponderance of audiologic effort is medically oriented and is associated with the literature which is dominated by diagnostic research. Aural rehabilitation does exist. In fact, it is alive and well in private practices, in leagues or societies for the hard of hearing, in Chicago, New York, and other cities. It fares nicely within the Veterans Administration and Army audiology services (Northern et al., 1969). It is also flourishing within many schools for the deaf and/or hard of hearing (Fellendorf, 1973).

The purpose of this chapter is to describe an aural rehabilitation program as it exists at an institution for educationally deaf young adults. It is hoped that this description will be of benefit in three ways: (1) as encouragement for audiologists to enter the area of aural rehabilitation (AR) for the deaf as the deaf can achieve great improvement in their communication skills; (2) to describe some specific procedures in an AR program and (3) to demonstrate how an AR program can be accountable in demonstrating its effectiveness. The reader should not be "turned off" by the word *deaf* as he will recognize that any and all of this material is easily adaptable to the hard of hearing adult.

Sanders (1971) and O'Neill and Oyer (1973) have reviewed the state of the art in AR. They were not able to find much evidence of the success or failure of AR procedures. This chapter will focus on the pretraining baseline evaluation, therapy techniques and applied research as well as the results of auditory and visual training with hearing-impaired adults.

EVALUATION AND REHABILITATION

After the audiologist completes a routine audiometric assessment (including aided speech audiometry) other information should be obtained to guide the therapy process. The client's speechreading abilities with and without sound should be evaluated, as well as his speech intelligibility and articulation errors (particularly with more severe hearing losses). His language skills should be evaluated in terms of reading comprehension, writing skills, and vocabulary level, when the hearing loss developed during the language developmental years.

If the person's schooling was in a deaf education environment, his expressive and receptive skills in sign language should be tested. At the National Technical Institute for the Deaf (NTID) a small percentage of entering students appear unable to benefit from either aural-oral (sound and speechreading) or sign language. Up to 10% of the students have had scores of 10% or less when they were given the CID Everyday Sentence Test (Davis and Silverman, 1970) via the simultaneous method. Obviously, they represent students with very limited abilities to receive information in the classroom. The rehabilitation of a client should take into account the effects that the hearing loss has had on the individual's social and emotional relationships at home and at work (High, Fairbanks and Glorig, 1964). After the wide range of test scores and other information are obtained, they can be so voluminous that the therapist cannot routinely use the information. Various types of profile systems which summarize the client's communication skills have been used to overcome this problem (Johnson, 1976b; Alpiner, 1975; Gochnour, 1973). Figure 46.1 shows a sample of the NTID profile summary sheet.

A profile system provides a summarized reference of the communication skills of the client upon entry, and therefore one can easily pinpoint the areas of rehabilitative need. Once a significant number of clients have received training, the interrelationships among the entering profile levels can be summarized and studied to determine whether they have any value for establishing the prognosis for therapy. For example, one might study whether clients with poor language profiles and speech intelligibility are less likely to benefit from speechreading training. This is indeed the case. Subtelny (1975) found that low profile scores in language and speech intelligibility predict poor speechreading profiles. This type of study allows the clinician to predict which clients are likely to make significant gains in communication skills and which methods would be most appropriate to obtain at least a minimum level of competence. Thus, the profile system can lead to a systematic means of referring clients into a complex therapeutic process on the basis of need and expectation for success.

The NTID Communication Profile is made up of 10 areas of receptive and expressive skills (Fig. 46.1). Receptive skills include (1) hearing discrimination (speech-sound discrimination), (2) speechreading without sound, (3) speechreading with sound, (4) manual reception (sign language), (5) simultaneous reception (speechreading with sound and sign language), (6)

Division of Communication Programs

Name

Student #

Date of Birth

Date of Entry

Projected Termination

Major Program

Comm. Advisor

PHOTO

Hearing Aid Information

Own Hearing Aid: ___ Yes ___ No
Uses Hearing Aid: ___ All the Time
___ Most Times
___ Seldom
___ Never

Uses Telephone: ___ Yes ___ No
___ All People ___ Most People
___ Some People ___ Relatives and Friends

Check List

___ Parental Info Form
___ Personal References
___ Entering Audio Rec
___ Discrim Response Sheet
___ NTID Audiogram
___ HA Info Sheet
___ ENT Evaluation
___ Visual Evaluation
___ Comm Aids Survey
___ Speech Survey
___ Speech Diagnostic
___ Fisher-Logeman Test
___ Drama Interest Sur

NTID Communication Performance Profile

RECEPTIVE

Hearing Discrimination — Date / Ear (HA) / HA file / % Correct / Pro-file / Test/List

Speechreading w/o Sound — Date / Pro-file / % Correct / Test/List

Speechreading w/Sound — Date / HA (HA) / Pro-file / % Correct / Test/List

Manual Reception — Date / Pro-file / % Correct / Test/List

Simultaneous Reception — Date / HA (HA) / Pro-file / % Correct / Test/List

Vocabulary — Date / Pro-file / Score / Test Form

Reading Comp. — Date / Pro-file / Score / Test Form

EXPRESSIVE

Speech — Date / HA (HA) / Mean Rating / Pro-file / Test

Writing — Test Date / Pro-file / Score / Test Form

Non-Verbal Kinetic — Date / HA / Aver. Profile (✓) / Test

PHYSICAL EXAMS

Otological — ___ Yes ___ No
Anomalies ___ Yes ___ No
Treatment Needed ___ Yes ___ No
Medical Approval For HA Fitting ___ Yes ___ No
Comments:

Laryngeal — ___ Yes ___ No
Medical Contraindications For Therapy ___ Yes ___ No
Follow Up Comments:

Visual Screening
Vis. Screen: ___ Pass ___ Fail
Date:
SHS Referral: ___ Yes ___ No
Date SHS:
SHS Rx: ___ Yes ___ No
Date SHS Rx Completed:
Off-Campus Med: ___ Yes ___ No
Date Med:
Off-Campus Rx:
Off-Campus Rx Completed ___ Yes ___ No
Comments

Fig. 46.1. Summary profile face sheet for individual student folders at the National Technical Institute for the Deaf.

vocabulary and (7) reading comprehension. The expressive profiles consist of (1) speech intelligibility, (2) writing and (3) nonverbal kinetic ability (the use of body language and natural gesture without sign language).

Clients are rated on a 5-point scale with 5 representing no difficulty and 1 representing poor ability in the specific skill. Ratings are derived from raw scores, percentage scores, or averages of the most common subjective readings by a number of trained judges depending on the parameter in question (Johnson, 1976b).

Two of the profile parameters will be described to demonstrate the methods used to establish them and show their value. The speechreading profile without sound is obtained by administering an NTID produced color film version of the CID Everyday Sentence Test

TABLE 46.1. *Profile Ratings, Percentage Ranges, and Functional Descriptors For Assessment of Speechreading Ability of NTID Students*

Profile Rating	Range	Functional Descriptor
	%	
5	70–100	Client understands the complete message.
4	52–69	Client understands most of the content of the message.
3	28–51	Client understands with difficulty about one-half of the message (follows the gist of the conversation).
2	16–27	Client understands little of the content of the message, but does understand a few words or phrases.
1	0–15	Client does not understand the message.

(Davis and Silverman, 1970; Jeffers and Barley, 1971). Each list of 10 sentences contains 50 key words. The client writes word-for-word what he is able to understand and the scoring is based on the percentage of key words which are correctly identified. Table 46.1 presents the conversion of raw score, percent correct into the 1 to 5 ratings of general speechreading skill.

Sims (1976) in some ongoing research has noted that the subjective ratings of speechreading (without sound) by five judges using the functional descriptors were significantly correlated ($r = 0.77$) with the scores obtained on the CID Everyday Sentence Test.

The Hearing Discrimination Profile is based on results obtained from the CID Everyday Sentence Test and selected spondee words from the CID W-1 test. The test materials are presented at the most comfortable listening level. Figure 46.2 shows the sequence of tests and the resulting profiles. Progressively easier tests are needed when evaluating the severely hearing impaired. Fully 75% of the students cannot respond to the CID W-22 PB Test. The Spondee Discrimination Test is given first. One of 10 selected spondiac words is presented randomly via audio cassette. The student then selects his answer on a 10-choice response box (Johnson and Yust, 1976). If the student is not able to correctly identify 50% of the 20 test words, he is given the Same-Difference task. This test uses the same selected spondiac words but they are now paired; for example, "baseball-cowboy" or "rainbow-rainbow." The student decides whether the words paired were the same two words or two different words and indicates his decision on the response box (Fig. 46.3) by pushing a button marked "same" or "different."

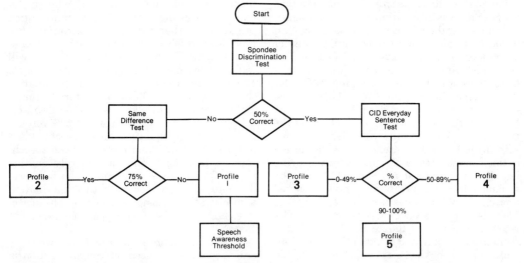

Fig. 46.2. Flow chart of the auditory speech sound discrimination profile testing system.

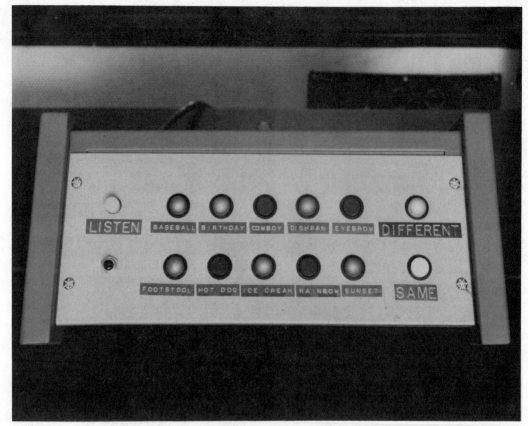

Fig. 46.3. Student response station for auditory speech sound discrimination testing.

Seventy-five percent correct identification on this task is equivalent to a student profile of 2 for that ear. If the student scored less than 75% correct, he would be assigned a profile of 1.

For a student who scores 50% or better on the Spondee Discrimination Test, the flowchart indicates that the CID Everyday Sentence Test would be given in order to determine whether the student should receive a 3, 4 or 5 profile. The CID Everyday Sentence Test is administered at most comfortable listening (MCL) for sentence-length material via audio tape cassette. The student writes down the sentence he heard and the test is scored on the basis of the percent of 50 key words correctly identified within the list of 10 sentences. The validation of this sentence test with the severely hearing impaired is discussed by Sims (1975). If the student scores 0 to 49% correct, he is assigned a profile 3, 50 to 89% is a profile 4, and 90 to 100% is a profile 5. The research at NTID which is geared to validate the Hearing Discrimination Profile and the descriptors of communication behavior may be of considerable value. If these tests which are used in profiling

are sensitive enough to detect changes in communication behavior it will help the audiologist to know when his therapy program has been successful. At long last, one will be able to quantitatively describe the change in communication behavior due to training, when a student improves his profile. The communication program will then have a valid accountability procedure which is based on whether a meaningful change in behavior occurred. This will tell us much more than simply stating that a student improved his speech discrimination score, for example, 10% after auditory training.

Summary statistics for the profiles are interesting to study. Approximately 50% of the NTID student population have speechreading profiles of 1, 2 or 3 and therefore need speechreading training if they are to rely on this ability for successful communication in everyday situations. Armed with this information administrative decisions regarding the objectives and level of staff effort can be made more easily.

A summary of profile information across several modalities of receptive communication is also interesting to study. In Figure 46.4, speechreading *with* sound and speechreading *without* sound are compared. The addition of sound to the speechreading of the CID Everyday Sentences enabled most students to substantially improve their scores in spite of the fact that the average hearing loss for this group was 94 dB. Consideration must also be given to individual needs in setting up a therapeutic plan. Approximately 9% of the 254 students tested achieved poorer scores in the speechreading *with* sound condition, 35% remained unchanged and 56% improved (Smith, 1975).

After 3 years of utilization of these profiles, a flowchart system of referral was established at NTID for placing clients into rehabilitation curricula. Figure 46.5 presents the basic flowcharting system of symbols and an example of one of the charts which enables the therapist to conclude whether a client could benefit from speechreading instruction. In this example, a clinician is asked to decide, first, whether the instructor or advisor's recommendations (Rx) for speechreading have been completed, then whether he has a score of 53% or more in speechreading and his priority for speech therapy *before* considering whether the client should concentrate his effort on an intensive series of speechreading lessons. The flowchart system at first glance appears to be complex, but once the "squares, arrows and diamonds" are explained, these charts simplify and clarify the sequence of events that should take place without having to refer to long written explanations. Note also, that flowcharts can include *objective* criteria on which an action should be taken. For example, a student must have less than 53% correct on a pretest in order to benefit from a *basic* speechreading curriculum. We have also used flowcharts for stating referral and follow-up procedures for ear, nose and throat examination. The use of an organized

system such as this allows for stability within a program sequence to establish a sense of direction for the clinicians and eventually to provide an easy mechanism for change in the therapy program when it is needed. If the decision "diamonds" of the flowchart is proved to be valid, the profile and flowchart systems can be combined to allow a nonprofessional person (or computer) to select clients who qualify for the various training courses.

Once a client has been selected for a therapeutic sequence, it is important to obtain more detailed, analytic information regarding auditory and visual phoneme perception capabilities. Hutton (1960), Walden, Prosek and Worthington (1974), Binnie (1976), Binnie, Montgomery and Jackson (1974), and Erber (1972) have suggested and utilized this approach successfully to pinpoint specific analytical training requirements of their clients' perception of acoustics and/or visual distinctive features. Erber (1972) found that, for instance, normal and profoundly deaf children categorize consonants *visually* by place of articulation (bilabial, alveolar and velar). Most of their visual recognition errors occur within each place category. *Auditorily* severely hearing-impaired children were able to categorize the eight consonants tested according to voicing and nasality classes. Danhauer and Singh (1975b) found voicing, sibilancy, nasality and stop/continuant as "distinctive features" for both the hard of hearing and deaf subjects. However, when the severely hearing-impaired group in Erber's 1972 study were ". . . permitted to look *and* listen simultaneously, auditory (mainly *voicing/nasality*) and visual (mainly place) cues complement one another and nearly perfect recognition . . . [was] the result . . . " (p. 419). The *profoundly* impaired subjects, however, did not improve their performance as much when the auditory

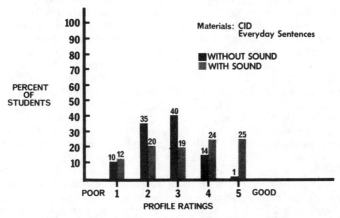

Fig. 46.4. Summary of results of tests of speechreading ability (administered with and without sound) for NTID students entering summer, 1974 (*N*=254).

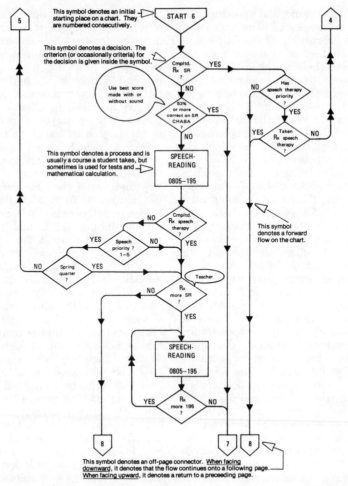

Fig. 46.5. Flow chart for planning speechreading training as a course within a total therapy program.

and visual modes were combined. Thus, perceptual distinctive features are subject to variation among subjects who are hearing impaired depending on the amount of hearing loss, the configuration of the loss, the amount of noise present, and the ability of the subject to use a feature perception process rather than a simple peripheral analysis of the acoustic-phonetic event. Some of Danhauer and Singh's (1975a) subjects "track the feature of sibilancy when their pure tone audiograms indicated a severe lack of sensitivity for the high frequencies." They explained that the subjects' ability to do this might be based on the knowledge of their language and phonemes. It is possible that high frequency, sibilant sounds are perceived as a void. Temporal processing provides the necessary closure to determine the correct word based on the silent interval. Thus the audiologist should measure the distinctive feature detection capabilities of each of his clients in

order to establish a therapeutic regimen rather than estimate the needs of the client based on the audiometric contour. Note that we have disregarded the concept of simply recording the percentage of words correctly identified. We are now concerned with distinctive feature identification of the articulatory and acoustic factors in the phoneme analysis (Miller and Nicely, 1955). This system provides meaningful data for individuals with severe discrimination problems. Following therapy the improvement in feature detection can be documented. Jones and Whitehead (1975) have shown that although the percent scores on auditory-visual phoneme perception tasks do not change a great deal after therapy, the percentage of responses of the subjects within a distinctive feature class improves substantially. Similar results with a visual phoneme perception task have been reported by Sims (1976), Montgomery (1976), and Binnie (1974).

HEARING AID EVALUATION

The follow-up is a critical part of the hearing aid evaluation. One method of accomplishing this type of ongoing evaluation procedure is by the use of loaner hearing aid fittings. The client should be allowed to use an aid for a short period of time and report his impressions. This is particularly useful when dealing with clients having severe to profound hearing impairments and when absolute thresholds and uncomfortable loudness levels are only 5 to 10 dB apart. The client can use a rating scale during the week of hearing aid use in different acoustic environments. Galloway (1975) designed a complete rating and hearing aid information booklet which has been useful for documenting a client's responses to each aid in his own environment. Noble and Atherly (1970) and Alpiner (1975) have also described hearing environment questionnaires for the hearing impaired.

Forty-five to 50% of the school age population with severe to profound hearing impairments do not use hearing aids consistently (Gaeth and Lounsbury, 1966; Zink, 1972; Porter, 1973). At NTID, 43% of the entering class of students (average age 19 years) do not use hearing aids at least 5 hours or more per day (Johnson, 1976b). This may be due in part to excessive gain in many hearing aid fittings. The most frequent complaint of students is that their hearing aids are uncomfortable and cause headaches, dizziness or pain. The Tullio effect has often been observed. That is, the low frequency sound pressure levels (SPLs) generated by the hearing aid result in tinnitus or mild vertigo (Tullio, 1929; Dohlman and Monay, 1963). McCandless (1976) and Millin (1971) indicate that the majority of hearing aid users adjust the gain of their aids so that the aid amplifies a 60-dB input by about one-half of the obtained speech reception threshold (SRT). For example, if a listener had an SRT of 50 dB, he would probably set his aid to give 85 dB average output for the frequency range of 500 to 2000 Hz (i.e., 60 dB SPL input + 25 dB = 85 dB SPL). If no SRT can be obtained due to the severity of the hearing impairment, usually MCL for speech is only 10 dB SL *re* the Speech Detection Threshold for severe to profound hearing loss (Rubin and Ventry, 1975). Loftiss and O'Neill (1964) demonstrated that a MCL level for the hearing aid fitting also results in best speech discrimination scores.

Obviously, when fitting with amplification according to the client's preferred loudness, the need for high gain amplification is relatively rare (at NTID only 5% of the recommendations for deaf students are for body aids).

Typically, our young deaf adults who do not own hearing aids or are not using aids most of the time are encouraged to try amplification during the course of an adjustment and/or hearing aid evaluation process which occurs within a 10-week academic quarter and includes 10 hours of individual work with an audiologist, 6 to 8 hours of programmed self-instruction, and 2 hours of group evaluation. During the 10 hours of individual work, 3 hearing aids are selected, adjusted and fit via sound-field, hearing aid evaluation techniques. These techniques have as their basis the establishment of a fitting which (over the broadest frequency spectrum) provides greatest gain without eliciting uncomfortable listening levels (Ross, 1975, Erber, 1973, Gengel, Pascoe and Shore, 1971). The hearing aid recommendation is made by considering which aid provides (a) the greatest range between threshold, MCL and uncomfortable listening (UCL) through the speech frequencies; (b) the best speech discrimination score (if measurable) and; (c) the client's preferences after a 1-week trial period with each. The 6 to 8 hours of programmed, self-instruction is concurrent with the individual hearing aid evaluation and is directed toward improvement of the client's understanding of the hearing aid selection process, tone and volume control adjustments, care, repair, warranties, and the purchase of an aid. Any questions that arise from the self-instruction readings are handled by the audiologist during the individual sessions of the evaluation process. The final 2 hours of this program are taken up with assessment of speechreading with sound skills and an attitudinal survey regarding amplification. The success of this program has been outstanding in that 85 to 100% (depending upon the quarter studied) of the NTID students enrolled have elected to use a hearing aid on a regular basis in spite of severe or even profound hearing losses.

One case study is especially illustrative of the success of this type of approach: In 1970, Alex was 20 years old and was one of the 10% of our population who had *no measurable hearing via air or bone conduction*. He had used a hearing aid in high school intermittently. The audiologist who first saw him on intake indicated that due to the severity of his hearing loss he would be unable to benefit from the use of a hearing aid. In addition, his speechreading and speech were poor. After completing the 20-hour program called Orientation to Hearing Aids, another audiologist reported that Alex was able to localize sounds using binaural aids. He was also aware of his own voice and other voices at average conversational levels and could make some discriminations among vowel sounds. His aided sound-field thresholds were 50 dB at 0.5 and 1 kHz and 45 dB at 2 kHz. By

1973 he had improved 20% on the Utley speech-reading test (live voice) for a final score of 66% correct. Alex was able to understand the gist of a familiar message with repeated exposures in a one-to-one speech situation. Without the advantages of long-term trial fittings, it is doubtful that Alex would have been fitted with an aid.

AUDITORY TRAINING

Houchins (1974) and Binnie (1976) reviewed traditional and new approaches to auditory and visual training. The following is a description of the philosophy and approach to auditory training at NTID. Auditory training, speechreading, and speech therapy are provided via separate curricula, each designed to cover 20 hours of therapy (2 hours per week for 10 weeks). It was set up this way to enable the speech pathologists to concentrate on speech production skills and the audiologists to concentrate on receptive skills. This approach enforces concentrated effort within one modality of expression or reception. While one seldom communicates via a single modality in real life, systematic evaluation and training of the individual elements of oral-aural communication allow for a prescriptive and individualized approach to AR.

At NTID, individualization of AR is considered an absolute necessity because of the range of speech sound discrimination ability exhibited by our students (Fig. 46.6). It is not practical to provide individual therapy for the 750 students at NTID. Consequently, our first attempt at auditory training was in groups of 6 or 8 students who were at the profile 2 level. That is, those students who scored 0% on the CID Everyday Sentence Test (sound only condition), but who could reliably identify whether a series of paired spondaic words were the

same or different. This grouping of students proved to be much too gross. When training drills, designed to improve suprasegmental feature detection such as juncture, stress, and pitch were attempted, we had difficulty because of the differing amount of practice needed by students to achieve the requisite skill levels (Lehiste, 1970).

Programmed self-instruction was then used in auditory training so that each student could obtain the amount of drill and practice required to learn the materials at his own pace. Also, our experiences with the suprasegmental training materials suggested that the students did not see the value of the drills no matter how many linguistic demonstrations we used to explain how suprasegmental features can change meaning. Consequently motivation lagged.

Materials

A self-instruction auditory training program was assembled by Aiello and Moore (Moore, 1975). Job-related, short sentence length materials were recorded on an audio-flash card reader. Recently, Erber (1976) described a program of auditory training using this type of approach. The materials were obtained from the technical fields offered at NTID. In some cases, on-site recordings were made of conversations between employees within a technical field. Other technical materials were gathered from the NTID instructors in these areas. The materials used had the constraint of being of a short sentence length and actual "on-the-job" communication. For example, among the materials developed for data processing, one of the sentences is, "The CPU is down today." (The CPU is the Central Processing Unit, or brain of a computer.)

Sentences were also developed in three non-

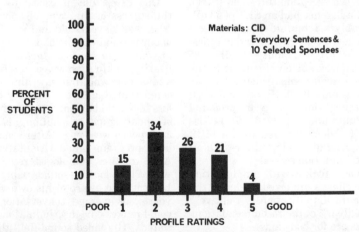

Fig. 46.6. Summary of results on test of hearing discrimination for NTID students entering summer, 1974 (N=248).

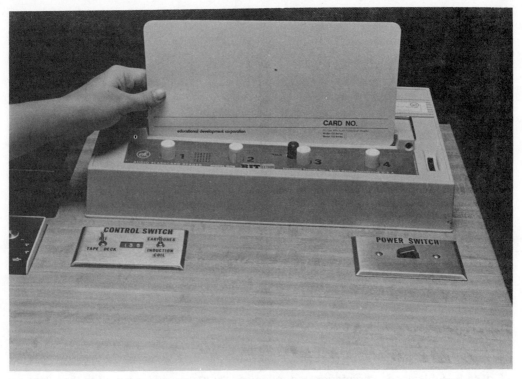

Fig. 46.7. An audio-tape card-reader.

technical areas: (a) On-the-Job Social (e.g., "Let's go on coffee break"); (b) Campus Social (e.g., "Do you have a date tonight?"); and (c) Survival Communication (e.g., "Let me see your driver's license."). These materials appear very useful to the students who as a result are well motivated to learn them.

For each of 20 technical areas, 10 units containing 10 sentences each were developed. Definitions were provided for all of the key-technical words by the instructors to ensure that students understood the materials. When students are able to reach an 80% criterion for matching key words to their definitions they can undertake the auditory training on these materials.

Equipment

The heart of this self-instruction program is the audio tape flash-card reader. The particular one which is used plays back a recording of four separate messages (tracks 1, 2, 3 and 4) from the strip of magnetic tape across the back of the flash card (Fig. 46.7). A Siemens "Phonoduct" induction coil is mounted on an inexpensive earphone headband (Fig. 46.8) or taped onto a strip of Velcro to make a headband so that the students with a telecoil on their hearing aids can practice with their own amplification without disturbing others in the classroom. On the audio flash-cards one technical/vocational sentence is recorded on track 1. The key word (the most important or technical word in the sentence) is recorded on track 2. On track 3, the student can record his or her own voice, listen to it and compare it with the model on track 1 and/or track 2. On track 4, the same sentence is recorded in a background noise which is related to that particular job environment. For example, in data processing, a keypunch machine noise is recorded at +4 dB signal-to-noise ratio.

Procedures

A programmed, self-instructional procedure was developed which tells the student, step-by-step, how to manipulate the training materials and equipment (Snell and Managan, 1976). The first step is to determine the student's pretraining level of discrimination for the particular sentences in the training unit. To accomplish this, the student shuffles the 10 cards in a unit, listens to track 1, and writes down what he hears for each card. After this pretest, the student begins training by listening to the key words on track 2. When he can understand the words, he tests himself on them by shuffling the 10 cards again, listening to track 2, and writing the word he thinks he hears for each card. If the student obtains a score of 80% or better, he may proceed. Otherwise, he must repeat the key word practice and testing until

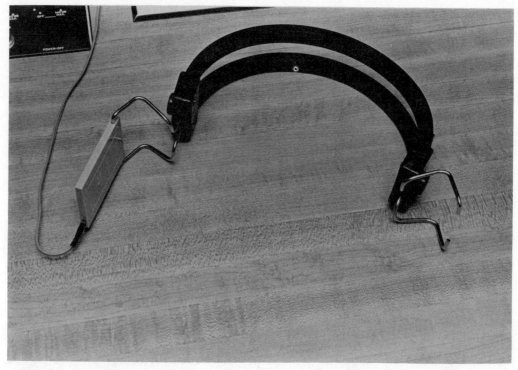

Fig. 46.8. A Siemens "Phonoduct" induction coil for linking audio output to the telephone coil input of a hearing aid.

an 80% score is achieved. The student then proceeds to practice and test on the sentences in quiet (track 1). After achieving 80% mastery on these items, the student practices and tests on the sentences in noise (track 4). The cards are numbered on the back so that for each test in the training unit, the student can shuffle the cards and listen to them in a new random order.

Scoring

For each test within the training unit, the students score themselves by checking their transcription of the audio sentences or key words with the unit list of 10 sentences or key words. Sentences are scored correct or incorrect based on the "general meaning" (whether the student understood the meaning of the sentence, even if he did not get every word exactly correct). Later, the students' tests are rescored by the instructor for "general meaning" (to check the accuracy of the student's scoring), for the number of key words correct in the sentence, and the total number of correct words in the sentence. Each of these scoring procedures was shown to be highly correlated; therefore, the student scoring for general meaning was adapted for grading purposes because of its efficiency. When the student completes a

test in the training unit, he determines whether to repeat the practice or go on.

Results of Training

Figure 46.9 shows the results of this training with 55 students in terms of improvement exhibited on the pre- versus post-test for each of the students' 100 technical sentence materials. After 20 hours of training, 1 hour twice a week for 10 weeks, the mean improvement on these materials was 30%, ranging from −13% to +83%. One student with no measurable hearing beyond 750 Hz with 0% correct on the CID Everyday Sentence Test obtained a pretest score of 0% correct on the training materials and a post-test score of 78% correct. Recall that these are highly technical sentences with regard to vocabulary. It is probable that the student was making maximum use of the suprasegmental features of the acoustic speech "envelope" such as pauses and intensity versus time patterns to be able to identify the sentences.

Preliminary analysis of the performance of students with "intermediate" hearing abilities (30 to 60% CID Sentence Test scores) suggests that this type of auditory training drill is most often successful for students who have used their hearing aids at least 15 years, wear it all the time, have hearing thresholds through 2,000 Hz and who have hearing better than 95 dB (Snell and Managan, 1976). The prognosis is substantially improved as the speech discrimination scores on the CID Sentence Test exceed 30%. These CID sentences yield a score approximately 30% better than the usual PB word list scores (Sims, 1975).

Further analysis of the data relevant to long-term retention of the sentence length training material was completed by Snell and Managan (1976). They found: (1) pretest scores were significantly worse than all other scores, (2) test scores obtained immediately after practice were significantly better than all other scores, but (3) 5-, 10-, 15- and 20-week post-test scores were not significantly different from one an-

other. Also, no differences were found between the rates at which technical versus social-type sentences were forgotten. Figure 46.10 shows the number of sentences retained over a time period 15 weeks after training was completed. Approximately 16 hours of self-instruction were needed to achieve these results.

This concept of auditory training can be applied to any adult or child therapy situation by selecting the subject matter to be recorded on the basis of the interest and needs of the client. If the client is having difficulty, limit the number of choices in the response set until he begins to respond. Limitation of the response set can take the form of restricting the language to survival type materials such as "the bank teller" or by restricting the number of

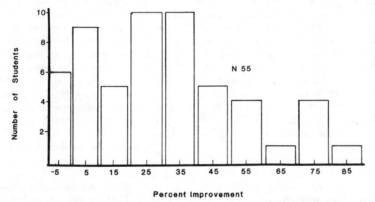

Fig. 46.9. Results of training as measured by pre- to post-test percent improvement in identification of 100 technical-vocational sentences after approximately 20 hours of auditory training.

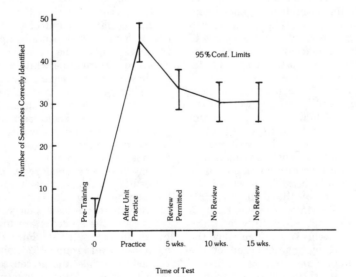

Fig. 46.10. Sentence retention for students before and periodically after completion of auditory training.

alternative answers the client has to choose from. The difficulty of this task can also be regulated by the rate of speaking, the length of the sentences, male versus female voice, and the amount of background noise. The possibilities for manipulation of the materials to an appropriate level of difficulty (about 80% correct responses) are endless, and the beauty of the audio flashcard reader format is that recording the cards for the exercises is a very simple and quick task.

SPEECHREADING

Monographs and books which review the research relevant to speechreading are numerous (Jeffers and Barley, 1971; O'Neill and Oyer, 1961, 1973; Berger, 1972). Although speechreading is not a substitute for hearing in that 60% of what is said is obscure or invisible (Jeffers and Barley, 1971), there are many totally deaf individuals who are able to function within the hearing world because of their speechreading skills. In fact, one's speechreading skills do not need to be great in order to aid in understanding a conversation. Preliminary results of an NTID study (Sims, 1976) indicate that among the deaf students a speechreading score of approximately 28 to 51% on the CID Everyday Sentence Test (no sound) is sufficient to follow the gist of a message.

The present speechreading program at NTID has a three-phased approach as designed by Jacobs (1975). First, association training is given in which the student predicts the speaker's following sentences on the basis of environmental cues. For example, the student might be presented with a common situation in Rochester: "You slip and fall on some ice and you report to the hospital emergency room. What are the nurse and doctor going to ask you?" A small group (6) of the students will then work with the teacher to construct the appropriate language and practice speechreading the teacher and each other.

The second phase of the program is more analytic in nature and consists of work in the recognition of individual vowels and consonants. Students with very little speech often lack knowledge of the basic lip positions for production of speech sounds. Consequently, these students require an introduction to these movements. As soon as possible, however, the instructor will structure the drill materials into word length elements. The emphasis is also on creating the ability to rapidly recognize the elements of speech. The difficulty of the drill can be varied by manipulation of the number of alternative answers, e.g., a list of 20 sentences from which to choose a response, or a list of 4 words, or the speaker can become a variable by having the students themselves

give the drill material to the other students in the class. The drill can be intensified by requiring multiple or chained responses, e.g., the student must speechread and repeat words with contrasting initial phonetic elements like, "dish, wish, fish, wish, fish." This exercise may also help build visual memory which is probably helpful in the central processing of the message. Finally, during any and all exercises the student is encouraged to follow the speakers' articulatory movements with his own speech mechanism in order to have the advantage of his motor-kinesthetic memory in the recognition of the message.

The third phase of training is accomplished with videotaped materials for self-instruction. These materials were needed because the poorer speechreaders with low motivation do not experience enough success in the group situation to build confidence in their ability. Some of the poorer speechreaders need instruction in an anxiety-reducing situation free from pressure before they can handle this in class. Thus each student can have the advantage of getting the amount and kind of practice that he needs at the pace which is most comfortable. Everyday sentences and survival communication materials are introduced to this type of client.

The materials developed for self-instruction on videotape with students in advanced lipreading (scores better than 50% on CID Everyday Sentence Test) are similar to those in auditory training. That is, they are technical, job related sentences. The videotapes were recorded on 20-min cassettes for ease of student use. There are 25 expressions on each tape. Different tapes have different speakers. The speaker says the sentence twice and then the student is given an appropriate amount of time to respond in one of four ways depending upon his speechreading ability. The speaker then says the sentence a third time while a written caption is shown on the screen for the student to immediately correct his response. Students may use one of four worksheets with the videotapes: (1) multiple choice response, (2) completion of sentence, (3) key words to give associational cues and (4) write the complete sentence (Jacobs, 1975). Approximately 175 videotape lessons have been developed to date.

Results of this approach to training have been encouraging. There has been substantial improvement on tests before and after the course and the students are highly motivated by job-related materials. For example, with an advanced level group of 52 students using job-related materials, the precourse scores were 0 to 50% correct. After completing 20 hours of self-instruction, the post-test scores ranged from 58% to 100% correct. A complete description of the results of each of the training phases is provided by Sims and Jacobs (1976).

TELECOMMUNICATION TRAINING

The importance of the telephone can be illustrated by trying to think of a white collar manager who does not use the telephone during a business day. The use of the telephone is an upward mobility factor for the already underemployed hearing-impaired community (Adler, 1970). Johnson and Rubenstein (1972) surveyed 130 hearing-impaired students. Forty-seven percent of the students who did not use the telephone wanted to learn how to use it. Also, more significantly, of those students who do now use the telephone occasionally, 48% stated they would like to learn how to use it better. For example, many of the students did not know the meaning of some of the telephone signals such as the busy signal or the misdial (cry baby) tone. They were also unsure about the accessories available such as the hard-of-hearing telephone amplifier. Fully 25% of NTID students had 50% or greater speech

sound discrimination scores on the CID Everyday Sentence Tests, had hearing through 3000 Hz, and had intelligible speech. Since 300 to 3300 Hz is the bandwidth of most telephone systems, these students had potentially sufficient oral-aural communication skills to be able to use the telephone for two-way conversation. Consequently a teletraining program has been developed within a specially designed laboratory (Johnson, 1976a) for learning about and practice using telephones. Castle (1976) described the procedures used with this group as not being auditory training on the telephone but of strategy training to improve the student's ability to get accurate information over the phone. For example, after students have learned basic telephone equipment and dialing procedures, they practiced a strategy of instructing the long distance directory assistance operator to repeat the telephone number slowly digit by digit, and then confirmed the information by repeating the number back to the operator. Preliminary results with this approach indicate that although the deaf person takes

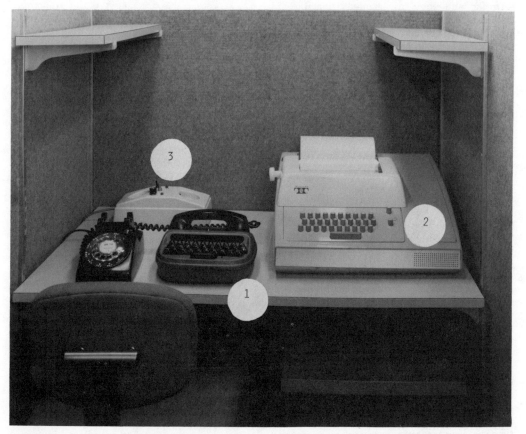

Fig. 46.11. Representative teletypewriter equipment for the deaf. (1) Fully electronic MCM unit with a "Times Square" type of read out. (2) Teledyne electromechanical hard copy type printout. (3) The acoustic coupler for the type 2 unit.

longer to get the message, his accuracy is greatly improved.

Among the NTID students who have no speech discrimination or speech production skills, there was still a desire to know more about the inexpensive teletypewriter networks for the deaf. The teletypewriter (Fig. 46.11) used is acoustically coupled to normal telephone equipment (Dicker, 1974; Jamison and Crandall, 1974; Rupp, 1974; Santos, 1975). Therefore, a second program is under development which will inform and instruct those students with no speech and hearing capabilities in the use of the teletypewriter and other non-voice telephone compatible communication equipment such as the Vistaphone (television telephone) and the "Electrowriter" which produces a facsimile of handwritten messages.

THE GERIATRIC PATIENT

At the beginning of this chapter, the author noted that AR for adults was alive and well in guilds and leagues for the hard of hearing. The bulk of this adult population being served is made up of the geriatric patient who is being seen for audiologic assessment, hearing aid evaluations, and speechreading lessons. Harless and Rupp (1972), Alpiner (1965), and Willeford (1971) have described their activities with this important clientele. As audiologists begin to dispense hearing aids they will assuredly find that the vast majority of hearing aids will be sold to senior citizens. Thus, the ultimate accountability for the involvement of audiologists in dispensing of hearing aids may very well rest on whether the older hearing impaired person experiences successful audiologic rehabilitation.

SUMMARY

This chapter has presented current rationales, practices and results associated with an adult rehabilitation program for the deaf. A major point of emphasis was the establishment of a methodology for describing the client population in a functional manner with a profile system. This enables the clinic to plan individual approaches to therapy and to obtain information needed for clinical accountability and management in a form that is not overly technical. Our approaches to speechreading, auditory training and the hearing aid evaluation were described and estimates of their success tabulated. It is hoped that the audiologist can use these descriptions to get started in aural and visual rehabilitation with the adult, keeping in mind that a combination of analytical type training for improvement in phoneme distinctive feature recognition is important but that it is also important to synthesize this skill

into vocationally and socially related sentence length recognition tasks for the hearing impaired listener in order to maintain motivation and improve the face validity of the drill materials.

REFERENCES

Adler, E. P. (Ed.), *Research Trends in Deafness: State of the Art*. Washington, D. C.: Department of Health, Education and Welfare, Social and Rehabilitation Service, Office of Research Demonstrations, 1970.

Alpiner, J. G., Diagnostic and rehabilitative aspects of geriatric audiology. *ASHA*, 7, 455–459, 1965.

Alpiner, J. G., Hearing Aid Selection for Adults. In Pollack, M. C. (Ed.), *Amplification for the Hearing Impaired*. (Appendix A The Denver Scale of Communication Function.) New York: Grune & Stratton, 1975.

Berger, K. W., *Speechreading*. Baltimore: National Educational Press, 1972.

Binnie, C. A., Relevant Aural Rehabilitation. In Northern, J. L. (Ed.), *Hearing Disorders*. Boston: Little, Brown & Co., 1976.

Binnie, C. A., Montgomery, A. A., and Jackson, P. L., Auditory and visual contributions to the perception of consonants. *J. Speech Hear. Res.*, 17, 619–630, 1974.

Castle, D., A telecommunications training course for the deaf adult. Paper presented at the A. G. Bell Convention, Boston, 1976.

Danhauer, J. L., and Singh, S., A multidimensional scaling analysis of phonemic responses from hard of hearing and deaf subjects of three languages. *Lang. Speech*, 18, 42–64, 1975a.

Danhauer, J. L., and Singh, S., *Multidimensional Speech Perception by the Hearing Impaired: A Treatise on Distinctive Features*. Baltimore: University Park Press. 1975b.

Davis, H., and Silverman, R., *Hearing and Deafness*, Ed. 3, pp. 492–495, Appendix 10, Everyday Sentences. New York: Holt, Rinehart & Winston, 1970.

Dicker, L., Suggested procedures for using telecommunications devices. *Deaf American*, 27, 9, 1974.

Dohlman, G. F., and Monay, K., Experiments on the Tullio vestibular fistula reaction. *Acta Otolaryngol.*, Suppl. 183, 34–35, 1963.

Erber, N. P., Auditory, visual and auditory-visual recognition of consonants by children with normal and impaired hearing. *J. Speech Hear. Res.*, 15, 413–422, 1972.

Erber, N. P., Body-baffle and real-ear effects in the selection of hearing aids for deaf children. *J. Speech Hear. Disord.*, 38, 224–231, 1973.

Erber, N. P., The use of audio tape cards in auditory training. *Volta Rev.*, 78, 209–218, 1976.

Fellendorf, G., Regional conference on the auditory approach; summary of proceedings and interviews with conference participants. *Volta Rev.*, 75, 344–358, 1973.

Gaeth, J., and Lounsbury, E., Hearing aids and children in elementary schools. *J. Speech Hear. Disord.*, 31, 283–289, 1966.

Galloway, A. L., A review of hearing aid fittings on young adults with severe to profound hearing impairment. *J. Acad. Rehabil. Audiol.*, **8**, 95-100, 1975.

Gengel, R. W., Pascoe, D., and Shore, I., A frequency-response procedure for evaluating and selecting hearing aids for severely hearing-impaired children. *J. Speech Hear. Disord.*, **36**, 341-353, 1971.

Gochnour, E. A., Evaluating the communication skills of the adult deaf. *ASHA*, **15**, 687-691, 1973.

Harless, E. L., and Rupp, R. R., Aural rehabilitation of the elderly. *J. Speech Hear. Disord.*, **37**, 267-273, 1972.

High, W., Fairbanks, G., and Glorig, A., Scale for self-assessment of hearing handicap. *J. Speech Hear. Disord.*, **29**, 215-230, 1964.

Houchins, R. R., Auditory Training and Speechreading; Suggestions for the Clinician. In Cozad, L. (Ed.), *The Speech Clinician and the Hearing Impaired*. Springfield, Ill.: Charles C Thomas, 1974.

Hutton, C., A diagnostic approach to combined techniques in aural rehabilitation. *J. Speech Hear. Disord.*, **25**, 267-272, 1960.

Jacobs, M., Programmed self instruction in speechreading. *J. Acad. Rehabil. Audiol.*, **8**, 106-109, 1975.

Jamison, S., and Crandall, J., Telephone communication assistance devices for deaf people. *PRWAD Annual: Deafness*, 1974.

Jeffers, J., and Barley, M., *Speechreading*. Springfield, Ill.: Charles C Thomas, 1971.

Johnson, D. D., Communication characteristics of NTID students. *J. Acad. Rehabil. Audiol.*, **8**, 17-32, 1975.

Johnson, D. D., Laboratory design for instruction in Telecommunication for the deaf. *Info Series 2* NTID—Rochester Institute of Technology, Rochester, N. Y., 1976a.

Johnson, D. D., Communication characteristics of a young deaf adult population: techniques for evaluating their communication skills. *Am. Ann. Deaf*, **121**, 409-424, 1976b.

Johnson, D. D., and Rubenstein, C., Communication aids course; rationales, problem statements, and objectives. Unpublished report, NTID Communication Center, December 1972.

Johnson, D. D., and Yust, V., Rationale and design for a student response system. *Info Series 2*, NTID—Rochester Institute of Technology, Rochester, N. Y., 1976.

Jones, K. O., and Whitehead, R., A multidimensional test of auditory perception used for student placement into communication center courses at the National Technical and Hearing Association, Washington, D. C., November 1975.

Lehiste, I. *Suprasegmentals*. Cambridge, Mass.: M.I.T. Press, 1970.

Loftiss, E., and O'Neill, J. J., Estimation of acoustic gain in fitting of hearing aids. Summary Report, NIH Grant NB 04307-01. University of Illinois, Urbana, Ill., 1964.

McCandless, G., Special Considerations in Evaluating Children and the Aging for Hearing Aids.

In Rubin, M. (Ed.), *Hearing Aids Current Developments and Concepts*. Baltimore: University Park Press, 1976.

Miller, G., and Nicely, P. E., An analysis of perceptual confusions among some English consonants. *J. Acoust. Soc. Am.*, **27**, 338-352, 1955.

Millin, J. P., Speech discrimination as a function of hearing aid gain; implications in hearing aid evaluation. Masters thesis, Cleveland Ohio, Western Reserve University, as cited in Berger, K., and Millin, J. P., Hearing Aids. In Rose, D. (Ed.), *Audiological Assessment*. Englewood Cliffs, N. J.: Prentice-Hall, 1971.

Moore, E., Programmed self-instruction in auditory training. *J. Acad. Rehabil. Audiol.*, **8**, 90-94, 1975.

Neely, K. K., Effect of visual factors on the intelligibility of speech. *J. Acoust. Soc. Am.*, **28**, 1275-1277, 1956.

Noble, W. G., and Atherly, G. R. C., The hearing measurement scale; a questionnaire for the assessment of auditory disability. *J. Aud. Res.*, **10**, 229-249, 1970.

Northern, J. L., Ciliax, D. R., Roth, D. E., and Johnson, R. J., Military patient attitudes toward aural rehabilitation. *ASHA*, **11**, 391-395, 1969.

O'Neill, J. J., and Oyer, H., *Visual Communication for the Hard of Hearing*. Englewoods Cliffs, N. J.: Prentice-Hall, 1961.

O'Neill, J. J., and Oyer, H., Aural Rehabilitation. In Jerger, J. (Ed.), *Modern Developments in Audiology*, Ed. 2. New York: Academic Press, 1973.

Porter, T. A., Hearing aids in a residential school. *Am. Ann. Deaf*, **118**, 31-33, 1973.

Ross, M., Hearing Aid Selection for Children. In Pollack, M. C. (Ed.), *Amplification for the Hearing Impaired*. New York: Grune & Stratton, 1975.

Rubin, M., and Ventry, I., Speech detection thresholds and comfortable loudness levels for speech in children with limited hearing. *Am. Ann. Deaf*, **120**, 564-567, 1975.

Rupp, R., Commercially available products to assist the hearing impaired individual. *Mich. State Speech Hear. Assoc. J.*, **10**, 81-90, 1974.

Sanders, D. A., *Aural Rehabilitation*. Englewood Cliffs, N. J.: Prentice-Hall, 1971.

Santos, K. D., Telephone-teletype communication for the deaf; an exploratory study of purpose and means. Unpublished masters thesis, San Diego State University, 1975.

Sims, D. G., The relationship of the CID everyday sentences test to functional descriptions of receptive speechreading ability with a deaf population. Unpublished research, in progress, 1976.

Sims, D. G., The validation of the CID everyday sentences test for use with the severely hearing impaired. *J. Acad. Rehabil. Audiol.*, **8**, 1975.

Sims, D. G., and Jacobs, M., Speechreading evaluation at the National Technical Institute for the Deaf. Paper presented at the Annual Convention, A. G. Bell Association for the Deaf, Boston, 1976.

Sims, D., Whitehead, R., Bancroft, J., and Jones, K. O., The performance of students at the

National Technical Institute for the Deaf on an auditory perception test. Paper presented at the American Speech and Hearing Association Annual Convention, Houston, November 1976.

Smith, J. (Ed.), What are the characteristics of entering students? *NTID Focus*. NTID — Rochester Institute of Technology, Rochester, N. Y., April–May 1975.

Snell, K., and Managan, F., The effectiveness of auditory training at the National Technical Institute for the Deaf. Paper presented to the Annual convention of the American Speech and Hearing Association, Houston, 1976.

Subtelny, J., An overview of the communication skills of NTID students with implications for planning of rehabilitation. *J. Acad. Rehabil. Audiol.*, 8, 33–50, 1975.

Tullio, D., Das ohr und die entstehung der sprache und schrift. *Urban und Schwartzenberg*, Wein, 1929.

Walden, B. E., Prosek, R. A., and Worthington, D. W., Predicting audiovisual consonant recognition performance of hearing impaired adults. *J. Speech Hear. Res.*, 17, 270–278, 1974.

Willeford, J. A., The Geriatric Patient. In Rose, D. (Ed.) *Audiological Assessment*. Englewood Cliffs, N. J.: Prentice-Hall, 1971.

Zink, G. C., Hearing aids children wear; a longitudinal study of performance. *Volta Rev.*, 74, 41–51, 1972.

chapter 47

VISUAL AND AUDITORY TRAINING FOR CHILDREN

Michael Rodel, M.A.T.

The habilitative needs of children with hearing impairments present a formidable challenge to the audiologist. Although our concern focuses primarily on the impact which an auditory deficit imposes upon a child's speech and language skills, one cannot ignore numerous research studies which have investigated the effects that this communication handicap also has on a child's social, emotional, educational and vocational development (see Chapter 37). Our task in structuring an aural habilitation program for a young hearing-impaired child is to develop and employ techniques for auditory and visual training that will facilitate the acquisition and growth of oral communication skills and thereby minimize the influence which the sensory deficit has on his overall development.

In order to establish an appropriate auditory and visual training program, it is necessary to understand the function which these two senses serve for the normal hearing individual. Hearing and vision serve as the primary sensory modalities through which we maintain an awareness of our surroundings. Furthermore, they are the avenues through which we acquire and refine our communication skills. Because the majority of our communication competence rests in our ability to comprehend and use verbal language, audition is considered to be the primary channel for language learning. The presence of a significant auditory impairment alters the functions of these two sensory modalities and limits the amount of information which can be gained through oral communication.

To offset the disabling effects of a hearing loss, visual and auditory training programs for young children must be designed to serve two purposes. First, these programs must train the child to perceive a wide variety of environmental sounds which will allow him to alert to unexpected changes in his environment and thus ensure his safety and well being. Secondly, these programs must train the child to perceive verbal signals, to acquire the linguistic rules of his language and to develop his speech skills so that he will ultimately be able to exchange thoughts and ideas with others using oral communication.

SHORT-RANGE OBJECTIVES

The dual goals of environmental sound recognition and verbal language learing can be achieved only if several short-range objectives are met. As soon as the initial diagnosis of hearing loss has been confirmed, the young hearing-impaired child should be provided with appropriate amplification. It may be necessary to try different hearing aids over an extended series of sessions during which time the audiologist and parents carefully observe and record the child's response to sound. Attention must be given to selecting amplification which has the most favorable frequency response for the child based upon the residual hearing he exhibits at the various frequencies.

A comprehensive guidance program must be provided to the parents of the hearing-impaired child. The importance of this aspect of the auditory and visual habilitation program cannot be overemphasized since parents constitute the primary influence on the child during his formative years and will, in large measure, determine the attitudes that he will develop toward his hearing handicap. One should not assume that a single explanation of the child's hearing loss following the initial evaluation is sufficient to properly orient the parents to their child's communication handicap. Follow-up visits with the audiologist are necessary to explain the nature of the hearing loss and the effects which it will have on the child's communication skills, as well as his daily living experiences. Recorded materials, such as *Getting Through** and *How They Hear,*† are useful adjuncts for demonstrating the effect which the hearing loss has on the intensity and clarity of speech. Since, as discussed later, parents assume a major role in auditory and visual training, it is imperative that they have a clear understanding of their child's auditory deficit. A counseling procedure which has met with a favorable response from parents of the hearing-impaired infant is one that provides an opportunity for them to talk with the parents of older hearing-impaired children. Through this contact, parents receive the emotional support they urgently need during the initial months after their child has been diagnosed as having a hearing loss. Parent meetings also allow the participants the opportunity to share experiences and exchange ideas concerning discipline

---

* Edited by Aram Glorig, M.D., and produced by Zenith Radio Corp., Chicago, Illinois.

† By Earl Harford, Ph.D., and produced by Gordon N. Stowe and Associates, Northbrook, Illinois.

and toilet training, as well as eating and sleeping habits.

If the young hearing-impaired child is to accept amplification and obtain maximum benefit from its use, a thorough hearing aid orientation program must be implemented. Care should be taken to explain to the parents how the hearing aid operates, how to check the aid when it is malfunctioning, and how to clean and insert the earmold properly. Providing them with written tips for troubleshooting a hearing aid, such as the booklet *Caring for a Child's Hearing Aid,*‡ is also useful. It is essential for parents to understand that a hearing aid will make sounds louder for their child, but that it cannot correct the problem he will have in perceiving speech intelligibly. This point often needs to be reiterated to parents, especially as their child grows older and he continues to experience difficulty understanding speech.

The establishment of a training program for the hearing-impaired child at a young age is another short-range objective which must be met if we are to achieve success in helping the child develop adequate communication skills. The importance of early intervention during the critical period of time when the child is biologically programmed for learning language is well recognized by researchers (Tervoort, 1964; Lenneberg, 1967a, 1967b; Bronfenbrenner, 1975). If we hope to minimize the negative effect which a hearing loss imposes on a child's communication capabilities, then the auditory and visual training program must be initiated as soon after the hearing loss has been identified as possible.

Early intervention programs which stress the active involvement of the parents in the auditory and visual training procedures have been gaining popularity in recent years (McConnell, 1968). Centers around the country have established nursery programs for hearing-impaired infants which train parents, under the close supervision of audiologists and deaf educators, to utilize everyday work and play activities in the home as a means of developing rudimentary speech and language skills. Parents are encouraged to constantly draw their child's attention to sounds heard in the home environment (i.e., telephone, kitchen appliances, doorbell, piano, etc.) as a means of teaching him to alert to sound and to attach meaning to what he hears. These and other types of home management programs have been developed on the premise that "the center of learning for every young child is in the home and that the parents are his natural, informal teachers" (Northcott, 1972, p. iv).

‡ By Charlotte Dempsey, Zenith Hearing Aid Sales Corp., Chicago, Illinois.

Therapy programs which take place in the home rather than at a speech and hearing center constitute another vehicle for early intervention (Northcott, 1972; Rollins, 1972). Here the audiologist or educator of the deaf may schedule regular visits to the home to demonstrate therapy techniques, answer questions and review the reports which the parents make on their child's progress.

The John Tracy Clinic Correspondence Course (1968) is yet another program which can be employed to assist parents in structuring language learning experiences in the home. Although this program is designed primarily for parents who reside in areas where professional help is not readily available, these lessons can be used by teachers and parents to supplement activities carried out in the above mentioned programs.

Having met these aforementioned short-range objectives, it is then appropriate to focus our attention on the auditory and visual training programs themselves. For ease of discussion, these two components of a comprehensive aural habilitation program are dealt with individually. Despite this artificial separation, it should be recognized that our objective in working with hearing-impaired children is to design therapy procedures which will allow these two sensory modalities to complement one another. Although the controversy over a unisensory versus a bisensory approach to training hearing-impaired children has not yet been satisfactorily resolved (Gaeth, 1967; Sanders, 1971), we must proceed in training hearing-impaired children with the realization that only on rare occasions will these children be placed in communicative situations in which they must rely exclusively on one sensory channel. In favorable listening environments where extraneous noise is limited, the hearing-impaired child will be able to rely primarily on auditory cues, using visual clues to supplement understanding of the message. However, in unfavorable settings (i.e., classrooms where ambient noise levels are high and less than optimum viewing conditions exist) the child must take advantage of cues which he can obtain through vision as well as audition. Since all hearing-impaired children will ultimately find themselves in surroundings which are less than ideal for the assimilation of strictly auditory or visual information, the training program should emphasize the integration of both audition and vision to achieve understanding of the message being conveyed.

AUDITORY TRAINING PROGRAMS

Systematic attempts to improve the auditory skills of hearing-impaired children date back to the work of the French physicist-educator, Jean Itard, in 1802. Since it is beyond the scope of this discussion to present all of the auditory training programs which have been developed since that time, emphasis will be given to a review of the classic auditory training outline by Carhart (1947) which forms the basis for many of the auditory training procedures currently in use today.

Carhart viewed auditory training for the young hearing-impaired child as an aid in (1) developing command of language, (2) instructing the child to speak and (3) encouraging better adjustment to the hearing world. His auditory training outline for children consisted of four major stages of development: (1) sound awareness, (2) gross discriminations, (3) broad discriminations among simple speech patterns and (4) fine discriminations of speech. In the first stage of training, the child's attention is focused on loud sounds which he encounters in everyday play situations. The second stage involves training the child to differentiate auditory events produced by noisemakers (i.e., bells, drums, cymbals, horns and whistles). Special attention is given to developing the child's ability to perceive differences in the frequency, intensity and sound composition of the stimuli used. Once the child has demonstrated skill in recognizing the presence of sound and perceiving gross differences between environmental stimuli, he is then trained to distinguish differences between vowel sounds with grossly dissimilar phonetic elements and between short phrases which are closely related to his everyday experiences. The fourth and final stage of Carhart's auditory training program focuses on repeated drills which train the child to recognize subtle differences between similar vowel and consonant sounds as well as integrating his expanding vocabulary to permit him quick and accurate understanding of connected speech.

The progression of teaching sound awareness, followed by gross discrimination of noisemakers and environmental sounds and then gross and fine speech discrimination is reflected in numerous other auditory training programs (Lowell and Stoner, 1960; Whitehurst, 1966; Griffiths, 1967; Boothroyd, 1971; Sanders, 1971). Procedures which are designed for the very young hearing-impaired child frequently employ noisemakers and recorded environmental sounds as means of training the auditory channel. The heavy emphasis placed upon nonspeech signals as training material is perhaps due, in large part, to the ease with which children respond to noisemakers that they can both see and manipulate to produce sound. Some serious questions concerning the use of this type of training material have been raised, however, which will be discussed later.

In contrast to the traditional auditory training procedures which are popular with many clinicians, some novel approaches to this component of an aural habilitation program have been developed. One of the approaches currently receiving attention from professionals interested in the habilitation of young hearing-impaired children is the verbotonal method (Guberina, 1964, 1967; Fellendorf, 1969; Asp, 1973). Originally developed in Yugoslavia by Petar Guberina as part of a system for teaching foreign languages to normal hearing college students, this method has been gaining popularity in the United States for use with both hearing-impaired children and adults.

The verbotonal method differs from traditional approaches to auditory training in that only speech, in the context of meaningful language experiences, is used as both the stimulus and the response. Attention is given to making modifications in the segmental (vowels and consonants) and suprasegmental (intonation, rhythm, pitch, intensity, etc.) features of the individual's speech. Initially, sophisticated electroacoustic equipment and extensive audiometric tests consisting of filtered and nonfiltered nonsense syllables are utilized to identify the individual's most sensitive area of hearing. Once the optimal field of hearing has been identified, multifiltered auditory training units are employed which are capable of producing the frequency response which is most appropriate for speech perception by that individual. In training young hearing-impaired children, the perception of speech by the child is facilitated through modifications which the clinician makes in one or several of the following perceptual parameters: (1) frequency, (2) intensity, (3) duration, (4) intonation, (5) rhythm, (6) tension of the articulators or (7) pause. Therapy activities center around the use of carefully selected speech materials which follow an orderly phonetic progression from low to high tonality. Intriguing body movements which correspond to the tension of the articulators in producing various sounds and rhythmical stimulations are also used for developing normal intonation and rhythm patterns in the child's speech. The likelihood that the child will develop intelligible speech and achieve the ultimate goal of the verbotonal method, that is, integration with hearing peers in the regular public school classroom, is enhanced when the normal production of these two suprasegmental features has been established.

Another approach to auditory training which does not adhere to traditional procedures is the auditory/language patterning program developed by Kretschmer (1974). The emphasis in this method is clearly on utilization of the auditory modality for language learning. Unlike Guberina's method where the concern focuses primarily on an analysis of the segmental and suprasegmental aspects of the hearing-impaired child's speech, Kretschmer's approach attempts to develop the child's knowledge and use of linguistic rules through auditory expansion and language rehearsal techniques so that he will eventually be able to put utterances together to form cohesive sentences. The linguistic input provided to the child in this training program is structured in such a manner so as to approximate the normal patterns of language growth found in children with normal hearing. The inclusion of nonlinguistic tasks, such as the recognition of environmental sounds, occurs only when such sounds relate to the specific therapy experiences used to develop a particular linguistic principle or model.

Clinical and nonclinical research data supporting the effectiveness of these nontraditional auditory training programs are sparse. The lack of information which offers comparisons between auditory training approaches or identifies the efficacy of one method over another for developing communication skills in hearing-impaired children may be the result of the difficulties researchers encounter in controlling a number of variables. For example, differences exist regarding the clinical skills and philosophical biases of the therapist, and the extent to which the parents of hearing impaired children implement therapy techniques outside of the therapy setting.

Despite these limitations, some studies have been completed which provide support for enrolling hearing-impaired children in either of these two programs. In a study by Craig, Craig and DiJohnson (1972), comparisons were made between the verbotonal method and traditional procedures used at the Western Pennsylvania School for the Deaf. The results of this investigation suggested that a group of children trained using the verbotonal method improved more in their ability to accurately produce speech than did the children trained using the more traditional procedures. A trend toward better speech quality was also noted for this group. A case study of a 12-year-old child with a congenital, profound, bilateral sensory-neural hearing loss conducted by Eisenberg and Santore (1976) indicated that verbotonal habilitation techniques employed for 2¹/₂ years resulted in improved speech perception, discrimination ability for phonetically balanced words and overall speech intelligibility. Kretschmer (1974) cites two studies which investigated the linguistic output of three children with varying degrees of hearing impairment who were trained using his auditory/language patterning procedures. The results of these studies suggest that this approach "can be an effective means to initiating linguistic acquisition in severely hearing-impaired children; particularly, in those children where initiation of educational programming has begun comparatively late" (p. 240).

As was mentioned earlier, questions have been raised by professionals concerning the use of nonlinguistic auditory signals, such as noise-makers and recorded environmental sounds, in auditory training programs for young hearing-impaired children. Asp (1973) contends that training a child to differentiate noisemakers is a gross form of discrimination where the child relies upon on-off clues and the duration of the signals. This type of discrimination task, he suggests, does not prepare the child for the linguistic discriminations he will need in perceiving speech. Ling (1974) also feels that progressing from gross to fine discrimination through the use of nonspeech stimuli followed by speech signals is inappropriate. Her reasoning is based upon research she reviews which indicates that the perception and recall of verbal and nonverbal materials involve different processes. Ling concludes that auditory training procedures developed to promote the acquisition of normal speech and language skills should be comprised of speech material which assists the child in learning to process long linguistic sequences.

The use of noisemakers is often justified as a means for teaching the young child to discriminate pitch differences. The assumption made by many clinicians is that certain noisemakers, a drum for example, constitute low frequency sounds while other noisemakers (i.e., a bell) are composed primarily of high frequency information. An investigation of the frequency components of 25 noisemakers by Bove and Flugrath (1973), however, revealed that 20 of them were unacceptable for the informal assessment of auditory sensitivity in infants due to the presence of multiple frequency components or spectral bands which were too broad to provide information concerning a baby's auditory sensitivity. Hodgson (1972) showed that a toy drum and a set of bells are broad-spectrum sounds with relatively little difference in their spectral composition.

The value of using nonlinguistic stimuli in auditory training procedures for young hearing-impaired children appears limited. While this is an enjoyable activity for the young child, gross environmental sound discrimination evidently does little to foster the growth of adequate communication skills. In general, gross discrimination tasks using environmental sounds should constitute only a minor portion of a child's auditory training program. The use of these exercises should be limited to activities which the parents can initiate in the home during the early months of their child's aural habilitation program. By doing so, it would be possible to achieve one of the two goals outlined in this chapter (i.e., training the child to perceive those environmental sounds which may necessitate changes in his behavior) and it would allow the parents to experience initial success with activities the clinician has encouraged them to employ.

Since it appears that the emphasis in auditory training should be placed on utilizing linguistic materials, a careful examination of the linguistic structures being presented to the child is required. Many approaches encourage the clinician and parents to "bathe the child in sound" through constant random verbalizations of activities going on around him. Achieving the goal of developing adequate communication skills through mastery of the linguistic rules of our language may be easiest if the parents and clinician adopt a strategy of language stimulation which approximates the pattern of language growth found in normal hearing children. As Kretschmer (1974) suggests, the sentence patterns developed by Blackwell (1971) and Streng (1972) may be useful in this regard. The Developmental Sentence Scoring Chart devised by Lee, Koenigsknecht and Mulhern, (1975) might also provide a useful guide to the clinician in determining the most appropriate linguistic structures to present to the young child auditorily.

In addition to a careful examination of the linguistic structures used in the therapy setting, it would appear important for the clinician to pay close attention to the phonetic makeup of the speech being used. For example, in the verbotonal method (Asp, 1973), the therapist makes the assumption that the hearing-impaired child is able to perceive low pitched sounds before high pitched sounds. Careful attention is given to teaching sounds according to a "phonetic progression" from low tonality (/bu/, /mu/, /pa/) to high tonality (/si/, /ʃi/). Since all phonemes can be arranged on a continuum which extends from low to high tonality, the clinician is provided with a guideline for introducing phonemes and words into the therapy setting in a particular order. Predominantly low tonality words, such as "blow," "pour," "mama" and "bottle," would be introduced before predominantly high tonality words, such as "see," "high" and "she."

AUDITORY TRAINING MATERIALS

Professionals interested in the habilitation of hearing-impaired individuals have devised a variety of auditory training materials. While it is not possible to list all of the resources which the audiologist has available to him, it is perhaps worthwhile to note some of the printed materials which this clinician has found useful in working with young hearing-impaired children. Since the mark of an effective clinician is one who is willing to improvise therapy techniques and continually search for more effective procedures for attaining therapy objectives, this brief review of auditory training materials is intended only to introduce the reader to some suggested techniques for improving a young child's listening skills.

Play It by Ear (Lowell and Stoner, 1960) is a collection of 36 auditory training games which are especially suitable for parents and clinicians to use with preschool hearing-impaired children. The manual is neatly divided into five sections emphasizing recognition of environmental sounds, music and speech sounds, as well as activities for direction and distance. The activities delineated in the section on speech sounds concentrate on developing the young child's skills at discriminating the segmental and suprasegmental aspects of speech. Whitehurst (1955, 1966) has developed a variety of auditory training materials which have become popular with clinicians. Her manual, *Auditory Training for Children,* consists of a series of carefully graded lessons which are appropriate for both parents and clinicians to use with the preschool or young school-age hearing-impaired child. For teenagers and hearing-impaired adults, Whitehurst has designed the *Auditory Training Manual* which includes a series of 40 lessons focusing on individual speech sounds. Another set of materials developed for hearing-impaired children over 10 years of age is the *Clinician's Handbook of Auditory Training* (Kelly, 1973). This workbook of graded exercises is designed to improve the child's listening skills, his discrimination of selected speech sounds and his auditory memory span. Sets of answer sheets accompany the handbook and permit the child to write his responses.

VISUAL TRAINING PROGRAMS

Visual communication training programs for hearing-impaired children have not received the attention from clinicians which auditory training programs have been given. Several factors can be identified which may explain why there has been limited emphasis placed upon procedures to develop the child's skills for visually processing information.

Language, as Jeffers and Barley (1971) state, "is an auditory phenomenon; one designed for hearing, not vision." Attempting to develop a child's communication skills through visual training is a difficult task due to the high percentage of movements of the tongue and lower jaw which are either obscure, invisible or identical movements made to produce another sound. The rapidity with which speech movements occur and individual differences in articulation patterns from speaker to speaker are additional factors which contribute to making speechreading an inferior means of acquiring information. The advances made in recent years in hearing aid technology, particularly in the design of ear-level instruments suitable for young children with severe hearing losses, have also contributed to a greater emphasis being placed on training the auditory modality rather than the visual modality as the vehicle for developing language skills.

The acoupedic approach (Pollack, 1970) is one example of a strictly aural-oral method in which the young hearing-impaired child is taught speech and language skills through the use of auditory cues alone. No formal instruction in lipreading is included in this program and the use of any form of manual communication, fingerspelling or natural gesturing is discouraged. Pollack believes that the child with a significant hearing loss can attain his full potential educationally, intellectually, socially and vocationally only if his hearing loss is identified at an early age, he is fitted with binaural amplification soon thereafter and he is rigorously trained to utilize his residual hearing, however limited it may be, for listening and developing speech and language skills.

Despite inherent limitations, training in visual communication would appear to be important, indeed necessary, for hearing-impaired children. One of the major goals of educational programs for hearing-impaired children today, particularly of those programs such as the acoupedic method where children learn through a unisensory (i.e., oral) approach, is the integration of these children into the regular public school classroom. The acoustical environment of the typical classroom, however, is often detrimental to learning through the use of auditory cues alone (see Chapter 38). If hearing-impaired children are to compete in an integrated educational setting, care must be taken to provide training programs which permit them to effectively utilize visual cues to supplement auditory information.

The traditional methods of lipreading instruction are generally classified as being either analytical or synthetic. Analytical approaches, such as the Meuller-Walle method (Bruhn, 1960) and the Jena method (Bunger, 1944) emphasize the rapid recognition of individual phonemes and syllables. In contrast synthetic approaches, perhaps best exemplified by the Nitchie (1912, 1930) method, stress recognition of complete thoughts and sentences rather than the identification of individual speech movements. For a more detailed discussion of lipreading methodologies, the reader is referred to Jeffers and Barley (1971) where a concise summary of the principles and instructional materials of each of these approaches is provided.

Few visual training programs for hearing-impaired children today adhere exclusively to techniques described in the traditional approaches to lipreading. Most often an eclectic approach, which includes principles and practice material from several different methods, is emphasized. The Kinzie (1931, 1936) method for hearing-impaired children and adults is one example of an eclectic approach which incorporates both synthetic and analytical principles. In their graded lessons for preschool and school-age children, the Kinzie sisters introduce speechreading materials consisting of short conversations, rhymes, sentence drills and story exercises to train the child's ability to synthesize visual information. For the older student, lessons are designed to train him to speechread individual speech movements, as well as single word and sentence drills and supplementary material consisting of stories and riddles.

Since our purpose in training visual communication is to provide the hearing-impaired child with cues which he can use to supplement auditory information, particularly when he is placed in an unfavorable listening environment such as the regular classroom, exercises in visual training for young hearing-impaired children should, whenever possible, be incorporated with auditory training exercises and language learning experiences. For example, preparing for lunchtime is a popular therapy activity for pre-schoolers. After a core vocabulary, such as *chair, table, cup, cookie, plate* and *spoon,* has been introduced and the child is able to identify each object, the clinician can give a series of instructions (i.e., *push your chair, pour the milk* or *eat the cookie*) first with auditory cues, then with visual cues alone and finally with both visual and auditory cues. While the child carries out each command, the clinician can then provide the appropriate linguistic input to the child by making statements of ongoing activity, such as, *Bobby is pushing the chair,* or *Susan is eating the cookie.*

For the older hearing-impaired child, formal speechreading lessons, such as those described by Jeffers and Barley (1971) or the integrated auditory training and lipreading exercises suggested by Whitehurst (1964) would be appropriate. However, the most beneficial training session would be one which incorporates new vocabulary from academic subjects, such as social studies, reading, geography and the natural sciences. Emphasis could be placed on improving the child's recognition of each new word first with auditory cues alone, then with visual cues alone and finally with both auditory and visual cues. Varying the distance and the angle of the child from the clinician and introducing distracting visual and auditory stimuli are additional modifications which can be made in the therapy setting to make the task more difficult for the child while preparing him for the less than optimal viewing and listening conditions he is likely to encounter in the classroom.

SUMMARY

The reader should be cautioned against concluding from this discussion that auditory and visual training constitutes the entire spectrum of an aural habilitation program for young hearing-impaired children. An aural habilitation program, by necessity, must encompass all aspects of a child's growth and development. Clinicians who provide habilitative services to these young children must be skilled not only in structuring effective auditory training and speechreading programs, but also in providing meaningful language learning experiences and effective parent counseling. The key to a successful habilitation program lies with the clinician who is willing to design, implement and modify procedures which meet the diverse needs of hearing-impaired children.

REFERENCES

Asp, C., The Verbo-Tonal Method as an Alternative to Present Auditory Training Techniques. In Wingo, J., and Holloway, G. (Eds.), *An Appraisal of Speech Pathology and Audiology: A Symposium*. Springfield, Ill.: Charles C Thomas, 1973.

Blackwell, P., *The Language Curriculum: Rhode Island School for the Deaf*. Providence: Rhode Island School for the Deaf, 1971.

Boothroyd, A., *Auditory Training*. Northampton, Mass.: Clarke School for the Deaf, 1971.

Bove, C., and Flugrath, J., Frequency components of noisemakers for use in pediatric audiological evaluation. *Volta Rev.*, 75, 551–556, 1973.

Bronfenbrenner, U., Is Early Intervention Effective? In Friedlander (Ed.) *Exceptional Infant*, Vol. 3, New York: Brunner-Mazel, 1975.

Bruhn, M., *The Mueller-Waller Method of Lipreading for the Hard of Hearing*. Washington, D. C.: Volta Bureau, 1960.

Bunger, A., *Speech Reading: Jena Method*. Danville, Ill.: The Interstate Press, 1944.

Carhart, R., Auditory Training. In Davis, H. (Ed.), *Hearing and Deafness: A Guide for the Layman*. New York: Holt, Rinehart & Winston, 1947.

Craig, W., Craig, H., and DiJohnson, A., Preschool verbotonal instruction for deaf children. *Volta Rev.*, 74, 236–246, 1972.

Eisenberg, D., and Santore, F., The verbotonal method of aural rehabilitation; a case study. *Volta Rev.*, 78, 16–22, 1976.

Fellendorf, G., The verbotonal method; questions and answers. *Volta Rev.*, 71, 213–224, 1969.

Gaeth, J., Learning with Visual and Audiovisual Presentations. In McConnell, F., and Ward, P.

(Eds.), *Deafness in Childhood*. Nashville, Tenn.: Vanderbilt University Press, 1967.

Griffiths, C., Auditory Training in the First Year of Life. In *Proceedings of the International Conference on Oral Education of the Deaf*, p. 758. Washington, D. C.: Volta Bureau, 1967.

Guberina, P., *Studies in the Verbo-Tonal System*. Columbus: The Ohio State University, 1964.

Guberina, P., The Use of Phonetic Rhythms in the Verbo-Tonal System. In *Proceedings of the International Conference on Oral Education of the Deaf*, pp. 730–732. Washington, D. C.: Volta Bureau, 1967.

Hodgson, W., Testing Infants and Young Children. In Katz, J. (Ed.), *Handbook of Clinical Audiology*. Baltimore: Williams & Wilkins, 1972.

Jeffers, J., and Barley, M., *Speechreading (Lipreading)*. Springfield, Ill.: Charles C Thomas, 1971.

John Tracy Clinic Correspondence Course for Parents of Preschool Deaf Children. Los Angeles: John Tracy Clinic, 1968.

Kelly, J. C.: *Clinician's Handbook of Auditory Training*. Washington, D. C.: A. G. Bell Association for the Deaf, Inc., 1973.

Kinzie, C., *Lip Reading for the Deafened Adult*. Chicago: The John Winston Co., 1931.

Kinzie, C., and Kinzie, R., *Lip Reading for Children (Grade I, II, III)*. Seattle: (no publisher), 1936.

Kretschmer, R., Auditory Training Procedures with Hearing-Impaired Preschool Children. In Donnelly, E. (Ed.), *Interpreting Hearing Aid Technology*. Springfield, Ill.: Charles C Thomas, 1974.

Lee, L., Koenigsknecht, R., and Mulhern, S., *Interactive Language Development Teaching*. Evanston, Ill.: Northwestern University Press, 1975.

Lenneberg, E., *Biological Foundations of Language*. New York: John Wiley & Sons, 1967a.

Lenneberg, E., Prerequisites for language acquisition. In *Proceedings of the International Conference on Oral Education of the Deaf*, pp. 1302–1362. Washington, D. C.: Volta Bureau, 1967b.

Ling, A. H., Sequential Processing in Hearing-Impaired Children. In Griffiths, C. (Ed.), *Proceedings of the International Conference on Auditory Techniques*. Springfield Ill.: Charles C Thomas, 1974.

Lowell, E., and Stoner, M., *Play It by Ear*. Los Angeles: John Tracy Clinic, 1960.

McConnell, F. (Ed.), *Proceedings of the Conference on Current Practices in the Management of Deaf Infants (0–3 Years)*. Nashville, Tenn.: Vanderbilt University Press, 1968.

Nitchie, E. B., *Lipreading: Principles and Practice*. New York: Frederick A. Stokes Co., 1912.

Nitchie, E. H., *New Lessons in Lip Reading*. Philadelphia: J. B. Lippincott Co., 1930.

Northcott, W. (Ed.), *Curriculum Guide: Hearing Impaired Children—Birth to Three Years—and Their Parents*. Washington, D. C.: A. G. Bell Association for the Deaf, Inc., 1972.

Pollack, D., *Educational Audiology for the Limited Hearing Infant*. Springfield, Ill.: Charles C Thomas, 1970.

Rollins, J., "I heard that!" auditory training at home. *Volta Rev.*, 74, 426–431, 1972.

Sanders, D., *Aural Rehabilitation*. Englewood Cliffs, N. J.: Prentice-Hall, 1971.

Streng, A., *Syntax, Speech and Hearing: Applied Linguistics for Teachers of Children with Language and Hearing Disabilities*. New York: Grune & Stratton, 1972.

Tervoort, B., Development of language and the "critical period," in the young deaf child; identification and management. *Acta Otolaryngol.*, Suppl. 206, 247–254, 1964.

Whitehurst, M., *Auditory Training Manual*. North Merrick, N. Y.: Hearing Rehabilitation, 1955.

Whitehurst, M., *Integrated Lessons in Lipreading and Auditory Training*. North Merrick, N. Y.: Hearing Rehabilitation, 1964.

Whitehurst, M., *Auditory Training for Children*. North Merrick, N. Y.: Hearing Rehabilitation, 1966.

chapter 48

EDUCATIONAL AUDIOLOGY

Verna V. Yater, Ph.D.

The public schools have been identified as the agents responsible for coordinating programs for hearing-impaired children. The classroom teacher and a team of specialists are needed to meet the various and varying needs of children with hearing losses. Trained personnel are needed to identify hearing loss in children, provide appropriate amplification and to serve on multidisciplinary teams charged with educational decision-making for the student.

Two specialists have emerged to initiate, coordinate and carry out the support services for public school children with hearing losses. These specialists are the educational audiologist and the hearing clinician. The two specialists also may be considered as part of a single specialty.

The term educational audiologist is frequently used and variously defined. One common aspect of the definitions is that this specialist is rooted in the profession of audiology. An audiologist working in a school serves as (1) a diagnostician of the hearing loss, (2) evaluator of amplification needs and (3) as a counselor for children and their families. In addition, he might also be charged with responsibility for (1) conducting a hearing conservation program, (2) consultation and monitoring of amplification needs or (3) consultation about the acoustical treatment of classrooms where hearing-impaired children are enrolled.

Because of the newness of educational audiology, its precise role and scope are not yet completely clear.

It is interesting to note that many states still name otologists as the designated professional to determine a child's eligibility for services, or to establish evidence of a hearing loss. Although the general profession of audiology is well established, in certain settings, the audiologist is not the person routinely deemed responsible by many state guidelines and regulations for making evaluations prior to placement of a child with a hearing loss.

In a recent survey of 130 directors of graduate programs in audiology, only 12% of the training programs reported that they were devising an option for school/educational audiology in their advanced degree programs (Carmean, 1976). Ten schools projected the date of program implementation to be within a year. The remaining directors who indicated current development of a school audiology program gave no date of program implementation.

In general, the program directors considered the basic coursework of a "clinical" audiologist to be necessary for the "school" audiologist. They pointed to a need for demonstrating competence in standard audiometric techniques, supervised practicum in diagnostic audiometry, aural rehabilitation, hearing aid evaluation procedures, counseling techniques, participation in planned observations of therapy as well as knowledge of anatomy and physiology of hearing and pathologies of the ear.

Other key areas deemed necessary for the school or educational audiologist by program directors, included knowledge of the physics of sound, competence in administering special site of lesion measurements, student teaching in speech and hearing therapy and demonstrated competence in electroacoustic measurement of audiometers.

Program directors frequently questioned the necessity of differentiating between "school" and "clinical" audiologists. The opinion was expressed that any audiologist should be a "complete" audiologist, capable of performing in the professional setting of his or her choice. While there existed an expressed need for educational audiologists, the directors felt that such specialists should be trained first as audiologists, and then in the educational aspects.

A second specialist, the hearing clinician, is needed to effect educational programming for children with a hearing loss. A hearing clinician functions as a consultant to regular school teachers and administrators, as well as acting as coordinator of ancillary services for students with hearing losses. He also provides direct individualized therapy services and management of student programs.

Direct services provided by hearing clinicians include programming to foster all aspects of speech and language development with major emphasis on syntax, morphology and semantics. They also include vocabulary development with major emphasis on "core" or "social" vocabulary. Thinking skills, including study skills, comprehension, creative and critical thinking in written and oral form, and coping skills, that is, the development of the student's ability to solve problems independently, are other aspects of direct service. Auditory training and speechreading may become part of the direct therapy services for young children or for a student who is a new hearing aid user.

Recognizing the need for various types of professionals is a first step in meeting the needs of children with a hearing loss. Neither state legislation nor certification nor personnel preparation as they now exist aid in providing optimal programming for children with a hearing loss. A movement for changes in both of these areas has already begun; further significant changes and improvements are needed.

DEVELOPMENT OF EDUCATIONAL AUDIOLOGY

Alpiner (1974) traced the historical development of educational audiology. He indicated that a major reason for the increased interest in educational audiology is the concern of audiologists with the placement and management of hearing-impaired children. Alpiner states that there has been dissatisfaction with the improper placement of children in traditional programs for the deaf. There was also concern for the youngsters who were being taught in regular classrooms and not receiving appropriate remediation. He was distressed because some children were provided with no services because of their geographical location. Thus, the primary push for educational audiology was the need for improved and expanded programming for hearing-impaired children.

O'Neill (1974) traces the need for audiologic services in the schools especially as it applies to hard of hearing children. He states that the school/educational audiologist is the logical professional to undertake services to children with a hearing loss in public schools. He suggests a core curriculum to help prepare such a professional.

There can be little doubt that the concept and practice of integration or mainstreaming are having an impact on the upsurge of interest in and development of educational audiology. In this chapter *mainstreaming* and *integration* are used synonymously. These terms refer to the process and product of getting hard of hearing and normal hearing children to interact. Usually, the strategy of mainstreaming is thought of as educational programming in which hearing-impaired children attend classes with normal hearing children on either a part- or full-time basis. Mainstreaming involves those children with a hearing loss who began their education in classes for the hearing impaired as well as those who started in a regular public school setting.

Neither the idea nor the practice of mainstreaming children into regular educational programs is new; however, national, state and local trends are providing an increased impetus for its implementation. The demand for increased services to hard of hearing children has been generated during the last several years. The Education for All Handicapped Children Act, passed by Congress in November 1975, demonstrated intensive federal concern with the issue of mainstreaming (Public Law 94-142, 1975). Most states have mandated some form of mainstreaming of students with exceptional needs into regular classrooms. These federal regulations are scheduled to be fully implemented by 1980.

Recent court decisions have focused attention on provisions for the least restrictive educational placement (Abeson and Bolick, 1974). One of the mandates ordered by Public Law 94-142, is to conduct an evaluation of the effectiveness of educating handicapped children in the least restrictive environment. It also ordered an evaluation of the effectiveness of procedures to prevent erroneous classification of children. Both of these will have relevance to programming and personnel needs for children with a hearing loss.

There is a definite need for professionals to serve hearing-impaired children in the schools, particularly the hard of hearing child. That need is evident from the number of children receiving services and those unserved.

SERVICE NEEDS

The need for increased services to children with a hearing loss is critical. The Bureau of Education for the Handicapped, U.S. Office of Education, cites an incidence rate of 3 in 4,000 children of school age, 5 to 19 years, who are deaf, 91 dB (ANSI-1969) hearing loss or greater in the better ear, and 1 in 200 persons of school age who are hard of hearing (Northcott, 1973). Data from Weintraub, Abeson and Braddock (1971) indicate that there are an estimated 261,000 hard of hearing children and 45,680 deaf children in the United States. Approximately 17% or 44,430 of these hard of hearing children are currently receiving services. Approximately 20,770 deaf children or 45% are receiving educational services. Clearly the need exists for expanding services for children with a hearing loss in the schools. Berg and Fletcher (1970) cite the critical need for services for hard of hearing children in the public schools and suggest many avenues for helping to meet this need.

It is not surprising that deaf children are faring better with regard to the numbers who are already served since the problem of identification would appear to be minimal. However, even service for 45% of the audiometrically deaf students is a startling figure when one considers that deafness is readily identifiable and is so critical as to not be ignored.

Until recently, many children with a hearing loss, even those who were categorized as hard of hearing, were educated in state schools for the deaf. A report released by the Office of Demographic Studies in Washington, D.C., in 1973 (Gentile, 1973), indicates that only 11% of 41,109 hearing-impaired students were integrated with hearing students. That percentage is startling. Even more startling is the fact that 49% of those 41,109 students were classified as hard of hearing on unaided audiograms. That is, they had hearing losses of up to 85 dB (ANSI-1969) in the better ear. Although almost 50% of the 41,000 students were classified as hard of hearing in audiometric terms, only 11% were integrated with hearing students. Forty-six percent of the hard of hearing children were located in residential schools for the deaf, 7% were in day schools for the deaf and 31% were in self-contained classes for the hearing impaired.

During the period of time covered by the survey conducted by the Office of Demographic Studies, it was evident that vast numbers of children with hearing losses in this country were still being educated in self-contained classes for hearing-impaired students. One must question whether the important needs of the child with a hearing loss are being met if he is not integrated into a regular public school classroom.

Responses to a questionnaire distributed by the staff of Project NEED (Bitter and Johnston, 1973; Bitter, Johnston, and Sorensen, 1973; Bitter and Mears, 1973) to administrators in schools for the deaf or classes for the hearing impaired, asking respondees to describe the philosophy of their programs toward integration of hearing-impaired children into regular classrooms, indicated the following responses. Integration was reported as their main goal by 45% of the respondents. Conditional integration accounted for another 34% of the responses. For example, some respondents did not believe in full-time integration immediately but preferred gradual integration over a period of time, beginning with social integration, then non-academic and finally academic integration. Thirteen percent of the administrators were not clear regarding their integrative goals and philosophies. Another 8% of the respondents were not committed to integration. So although 80% of the administrators in schools or classes for children with hearing losses were in favor of mainstreaming, only 11% of the hearing-impaired students in this country are actually integrated with hearing students.

When asked by the Project NEED staff what could be done to facilitate the integration of children with hearing losses who are not currently integrated, 67% of the responses indicacted personnel considerations. More than 23% of the respondees indicated that expanding knowledge regarding integration was of crucial importance. Twenty-one percent of the respondees indicated the need for improving programs, facilities, budget and increasing personnel. More than 11% indicated the need for improving communication, liaison, counseling and communication of goals. Administrative changes accounted for another 11% of the needs. Improving child skills which accounted for 28% of the responses also indirectly indicated a personnel need.

The results of the Project NEED questionnaire point to the need for administrators in schools and classes for the hearing impaired to change their atitudes toward integration of hearing-impaired children with their normal hearing peers.

LEGISLATIVE GUIDELINES AND CERTIFICATION

A look at state legislation, guidelines and certification requirements for personnel working with hearing-impaired children indicates some needed change. There are few specific requirements for audiologists working in school settings and virtually none for hearing clinicians, the two categories of personnel specifically needed under the mandate of least restrictive placement of hearing-impaired children. Very few states have specific requirements that an audiologist be certified by The American Speech and Hearing Association or that he be a licensed audiologist (Healey and Jones, 1973).

This problem of certification standards does not appear to have been appreciably altered since Roche and Neal (1972) indicated that some of the blame for lack of services for hard of hearing children rests on state certification agencies. According to these authors, if state educational agencies refuse or neglect to offer certification in all areas of specialty for hearing-impaired children, the unmet responsibilities are relegated to other specialists. Unfortunately these other specialists often do not have the training, experience nor time to provide the needed services.

In the matter of state certification, hearing clinicians have as few or fewer provisions than audiologists. State legislation rarely provides specifically for personnel certification or reimbursement for hearing clinicians serving students in a regular public school. In the few instances where legislative provisions are made, it is usually indicated that a hearing clinician is to be certified in the area of education of the deaf. It can be clearly demonstrated that the competencies of the hearing clinician/mainstreaming specialist are not the same as those of the classroom teacher of the hearing impaired. When provisions for certification of hearing clinicians are made at all they are usually slated to provide services to students with mild or moderate hearing losses and most often for children with minimal impairments. This severely limits potential services to children with more severe hearing impairments who have been shown to be capable of functioning in regular public schools (Yater, 1977).

Flexible certification standards with provision for periodic review and update should be provided for both the audiologist and hearing clinician. Provision should include the Master's level, ASHA certification in audiology or state licensure as the entry level certification standard for audiologists. ASHA certification standards for hearing clinicians need to be established. A committee representative of training programs, managers of programs for mainstreaming of children and of consumers including both parents and students receiving services needs to develop such certification standards.

The preparation of educational audiologists and hearing clinicians has such a vital influence on educational practices for hearing-impaired children that it cannot be overestimated. Personnel preparation must be strengthened.

PERSONNEL PREPARATION

There is a critical need for intensive training efforts to prepare personnel to work with hearing-impaired children. Training efforts are needed for both educational audiologists and hearing clinicians. As mentioned previously, about 80% of all hard of hearing children including 55% of children classified as audiometrically deaf are not yet receiving full educational services.

Training for audiologists is well established and can be partially met within the framework of traditional univeristy training settings. Modifications or additions to the training of clinical/traditional audiologists to act as school/educational audiologists might include internship experiences in public school settings for both assessment and habilitation approaches. The competencies emphasized by universities training educational audiologists are described below.

Training: Educational Audiologists-Hearing Clinicians

Training options for educational audiologists and hearing clinicians are limited. A look at some of the curriculum features of several universities now offering degrees or subspecialist training in educational audiology reveals a heavy emphasis on preparation in traditional audiology. There is need for expansion of course work specifically geared to educational audiology. California State University, Los Angeles, established a subcurriculum for audiology students interested in providing services in the public schools. The program was designed so that the student would also meet the academic requirements for the American Speech and Hearing Association's Certificate of Clinical Competence in Audiology (Jeffers et al., 1973).

The curriculum content of the educational audiology specialization at Utah State University is offered within the context of the curriculum of the College of Education, in particular the Department of Communication Disorders (Berg, 1974). It encompasses competencies from audiology, clinical processes, counseling, education of the hearing impaired, educational technology, general professional education, psychology, precision teaching and speech pathology.

The Utah State undergraduate program requires foundations for the educational audiology specialization from early childhood, general psychology, experimental psychology, physics, human physiology, communicative disorders and linguistics. The graduate program in educational audiology functions either as an extension of the undergraduate specialization or as an entity in itself. The Utah State program shows indications of being multifaceted, drawing from various disciplines, and does not appear to be restricted to clinical audiology per se.

Training options for hearing clinicians are very limited. Universities have not provided either the complete theoretical framework nor the internship options needed to train them. The role of a hearing clinician is a multifaceted one. Training should minimally encompass skills from language, speech, audiology, linguistics, human behavior, child and adolescent development, communications and public relations.

Hearing clinicians should have as part of their training a basic background in audiology. The training time and approach for areas in audiology should, however, be modified to the actual needs of the professionals being trained and less intensive training in some areas of audiology might be indicated.

Hearing clinicians need a background in linguistics which should include at least the basic concepts and methods involved in description of natural languages, syntax, descriptive and explanatory phonology, and semantics. It should also include the development of competencies and techniques in eliciting, collecting, and analyzing data.

In addition to traditional core courses in research and theory regarding language acquisition in children, it is important that a hearing clinician receive training and background in language analysis, programming and patterning at the elementary and secondary levels. Practice in those areas with hearing-impaired individuals from preschool through high school ages is essential.

Speech training needs to include a study of current theories and practices in articulation, voice and prosodic features. Skill practice during both the training and internship periods with children with all types of hearing losses is essential.

An extremely important facet of training for both the hearing clinician and the educational audiologist is the study of human behavior. This should include a study of skills related to pinpointing and shaping the behavior of others. There is a need to understand and practice direct interactional skills of communicating openly and nondefensively; coping with negative situations including defensive behaviors, resistance or refusal to listen, and learning to handle one's own feelings of frustration, hostility and inadequacy. Skill in identifying the impact of interactions and their effect on others, needs to be developed.

Part of the hearing clinician's job is to effectively communicate the child's needs to all concerned. He must integrate the efforts of the school, outside agencies and the parents on behalf of the child.

A knowledge of child and adolescent development is important in order to develop perspective in assessment, interaction, and skill building with the child with a hearing loss. Hearing clinicians need to be skilled in areas of auditory training and speechreading. The content of these areas should be mastered in considerably less time than is usually allotted to a quarter or semester of work. Emphasis should be placed on skill acquisition and application during training.

A practicum for a hearing clinician should include at least 500 hours of direct contact spread over at least a semester of service in a public school setting under the supervision of personnel experienced in mainstreaming. Direct experience must be provided in student assessment, skill profiling, and therapy in the areas of language, speech, vocabulary, auditory training, speechreading, thinking skills and coping skills. The hearing clinician needs experience in consulting with public school personnel and parents. He needs also sharpening of his observational skills, with which to perceive more fully the room environment, child/teacher interaction, peer interaction and behavior. Training should also include an introduction to community resources and to vocational guidance.

An intensive effort is needed to train new professionals as well as to retrain practicing professionals to assume new roles and responsibilities for mainstreaming. As the mandate for least restrictive placement of children is increasingly implemented, roles of some professionals will change. For example, teachers of the hearing impaired may assume increasing responsibilities as consultants to regular educators and other aspects of the role of the hearing clinician. Perhaps the training for hearing clinicians can be best met by nontraditional approaches.

Training Options

Some options for training and retraining educational audiologists and hearing clinicians and other professionals exist. Some of these options have already been described and others are being developed.

Consortiums

One of the best hopes for attaining the quality and type of educational preparedness necessary would be the creation of a model consortium of multiple university training programs and special education units of school programs providing consultation and direct services in the regular public schools. Cooperation between university training programs and school mainstreaming programs is needed to effect good training and education in both theoretical and practical aspects of educational programming for children with a hearing loss. Most individual universities in any one state will not have a pool of mainstreamed students from which to provide enough practicum or internship experience for graduate students to assure adequate practical skill development.

In a consortium situation, university staff members in various departments would ideally provide core courses in the designated need areas. Selected educational settings, would provide functional models of mainstreaming for purposes of practical training. A coordinator with joint responsibilities to the universities and the educational settings would administrate the program. This type of educational laboratory would bring together the theoretical and practical preparation for the student and provide feedback for needed modifications in the overall program.

The development of a model consortium requires the cooperation of many professionals in various settings to determine the training needs. The skills now being used by educational audiologists and hearing clinicians in the field are the logical starting bases for the development of core skill modules for training.

Personnel in training programs and in model school programs should provide important information for the consortium. Input from national organizations such as The American Speech and Hearing Association, the A. G. Bell Association for the Deaf, and the Council for Exceptional Children would be useful. Appraisal and evaluation of effectiveness of training and ongoing assessment of goals and objectives of the consortium should be part of the responsibility of selected university personnel, educational audiologists, hearing clinicians and trainees.

In-service Training

Few efforts have been directed at providing in-service training in the specific skills needed to work in mainstreaming settings, except as it exists in large programs for new staff members. Retraining professionals who are already knowledgeable and experienced in related areas (such as speech/language, education of the deaf, or traditional audiology) would help to solve personnel needs for educational audiologists and hearing clinicians.

The staff of Project NEED (Normal Educational Environment for the Hearing Impaired) (Bitter and Johnston, 1974) offered the following recommendations: "In-service training in integration procedures needs to be made available to special education teachers, speech and hearing clinicians, itinerant teachers, and educational audiologists to prepare them to more effectively perform in their new roles." They also suggested that workshops and organizational techniques in integrated programs should be made available. It was indicated that these workshops should deal with planning, scheduling, roles and responsibilities and communication skills. The Project NEED staff found lack of personnel to be one of the critical deficits in integration planning.

Program Evaluation

An organized system of program management and evaluation consultation is another manner of upgrading service to hearing impaired children. Experienced educational audiologists, hearing clinicians or program managers, wherever they exist, could use their knowledge and skills to help build programs which are just beginning or expanding. This would seem to be particularly important for those as yet unserved youngsters and for the vast numbers of hard of hearing children. Program development and management appear to be largely untapped resources. There is little reason why all new or developing programs need to grope in the darkness when resources already exist.

The program should include at least identification and assessment of children, referral, placement, reevaluation, dismissal and follow-up procedures, as well as direct and indirect services, in-service components, program evaluation and research. Consideration might be given to ways of utilizing already existing support personnel, helping to establish means and methods of doing in-service training with regular public school administrators, teachers and other school personnel.

In-service approaches and program management and consultation are both feasible methods for retraining or training of professionals to work with students with a hearing loss in least restrictive environments and to help upgrade programs. Both approaches need to be utilized immediately.

Mediated Training

Far too little use is currently being made of available human resources for manpower training from one region to another. One way to utilize such human resources is by increasing the use of mediated instruction including regular or videotaped television programs with input from school-service or university programs in varied geographical locations.

The use of videotapes for instructional purposes is limitless. Videotape has the advantage of repeated use and relative ease of reproduction. Using videotape, it is possible to film many types of skills needed by educational audiologists and hearing clinicians which may be viewed as often as necessary to learn a specific skill. For example, assessment procedures in audiology, language, speech or other communication areas might be filmed for skill acquisition practice. Demonstration therapy sessions and new methods could be taped for repeated training use. Classroom scenes could also be prepared for training purposes. For example, a child could be filmed utilizing various kinds of equipment or amplification systems in a regular public school. Or, one could show the ways of handling the problems of a child in an open classroom. Interviews with students who have been mainstreamed could be presented to help overcome a lack of experience base for professionals, which often takes years to accumulate. Students could state the attitudes, feelings, concerns, problems and solutions to mainstreaming that they have already faced. Professionals and others could glean factors significant to students from such tapes.

Videotaped comments of principals, teachers, counselors and other professionals prior to their first experience in working with a child with a hearing loss and after a selected number of months would provide comparison and hopefully insights for beginning educational audiologists and clinicians.

Educational audiologists and hearing clinicians doing different types of tasks, particularly those which would aid in pinpointing educational implications of a hearing loss, could be shown to prospective teachers and principals about to receive hearing impaired students in their schools or classes. Taped selected staffings, with counselors, teachers, principals, social workers, classroom demonstrations, and meetings with note-takers would also become useful training tools. Videotaped decision-making steps in selecting and placing students is another useful topic.

The major constraint in the use of mediated instruction is the time and cost consumed in production. Even large or cooperative school districts may not have personnel specifically assigned to such responsibilities. Universities often do not have the presence of experienced field staffs or children.

One solution to this problem would be a large scale funded project undertaken solely for the purpose of developing videotapes or other media projects in various mainstreaming programs and at universities or training centers. Such tapes could then be put into a bank or pool to be borrowed for a rental fee by personnel having need of such materials.

REFERENCES

Abeson, A., and Bolick, A., A Continuing Summary of Pending and Completed Litigation Regarding the Education of Handicapped Children. Reston, Council for Exceptional Children, 1974.

Alpiner, J., Educational audiology. *J. Rehabil. Audiol.*, 7, 50–54, 1974.

Berg, F., Educational audiology at Utah State University. *J. Rehabil. Audiol.*, 7, 40–49, 1974.

Berg, F., and Fletcher, S. (Eds.), *The Hard of Hearing Child*. New York: Grune & Stratton, 1970.

Bitter, G. B., and Johnston, K. A., A Review of Literature: Integration of Exceptional Children into Regular School Classes. Salt Lake City, Project NEED, 1973.

Bitter, G. B., and Johnston, K. A., Final Report Project NEED Facilitating the Integration of Hearing Impaired Children into Regular Public School Classes. Salt Lake City, University of Utah, 1974.

Bitter, G., Johnston, K., and Sorensen, R., Integration of the Hearing Impaired: Educational Issues. University of Utah, Project NEED, 1973.

Bitter, G., and Mears, E., Facilitating the integration of hearing impaired children into regular public school classes. *Volta Rev.*, 75, 13–22, 1973.

Carmean, D. M., Personal correspondence. Training procedures and certification requirements of school audiologists, a survey of training program directors, 1976.

Cozad, R. (Ed.), *The Speech Clinician and the Hearing Impaired Child*. Springfield, Ill.: Charles C Thomas, 1974.

Digest of State Laws and Regulations for School Language, Speech and Hearing Programs. Washington, D.C.: American Speech and Hearing Association, 1973.

Gentile, A., *Annual Survey of Hearing Impaired Children and Youth*. Washington, D.C.: Office of Demographic Studies, 1973.

Healey, W.. C., and Jones, S. A., *Project Upgrade: Model Regulations for School Language, Speech and Hearing Programs and Services*. Washington, D.C.: The American Speech and Hearing Association, 1973.

Jeffers, J., Trammell, J., Costilow, C., and Wall, H. V., The Development of a Prototype, Competency-Based Curriculum to Train Audiolo-

gists for Service in the Public Schools. California State University, Los Angeles, 1973.

Johnson, M., and Forbes, E., Bridging the Gap' Between Education and Audiology. Paper presented at the American Speech and Hearing Association Annual convention, Las Vegas, November, 1974.

Johnston, K. A., Perspectives on integration of children with limited hearing; consideration of current needs. *Lang. Speech Hear. Serv. Schools*, 5, 79–84, 1974.

Jones, S. A., and Healey, W. C., *Essentials of Program Planning, Development, Management, Evaluation: A Manual for School Speech, Hearing and Language Programs*. Washington, D.C.: American Speech and Hearing Association, 1973.

Martin, E. W., The right to education; issues facing the speech and hearing profession. *ASHA*, 17, 384–387, 1975.

Northcott, W. H., The integration of young deaf children into ordinary educational programs. *Except. Child.*, 35, 29–32, 1971.

Northcott, W. H., Tutoring a hearing impaired student in the elementary grades. *Volta Rev.*, 74, 432–435, 1972.

Northcott, W. H. (Ed.), *The Hearing Impaired Child in a Regular Classroom: Pre-school, Elementary and Secondary Years*. Washington, D.C.: Alexander Graham Bell Association for the Deaf, 1973.

Northcott, W. H., Normalization of the preschool child with hearing impairment. Symposium on sensori-neural hearing loss in children; early detection and intervention. *Otolaryngol. Clin. North Am.*, 8, 1, 1975.

O'Neill, J., The school-educational audiologist. *J. Rehabil. Audiol.*, 7, 31–39, 1974.

Pollack, D., *Educational Audiology for the Limited Hearing Infant*. Springfield, Ill.: Charles C Thomas, 1970.

Ptacek, P., A survey of the functions, uses, and training of specialized personnel in speech and hearing. *ASHA*, 15, 640–645, 1973.

Public Law 94-142. Education for All Handicapped Children Act of 1975, Washington, D.C., 1975.

Roche, A. R., and Neal, W. R., Jr., State certification policies and services for the hearing impaired. *Volta Rev.*, 74, 150–160, 1972.

Sanders, D., A case management approach to aural rehabilitation. *Hear. Speech News*, 39, 4–7, 1971.

Sanders, D. A., *Aural Rehabilitation*. Englewood Cliffs, N.J.: Prentice-Hall, 1971.

Watson, T. J., *The Education of Hearing Handicapped Children*. London: University of London Press, 1967.

Weintraub, F. J., Abeson, A. R., and Braddock, D. C., *State Law and Education of Handicapped Children: Issues and Recommendations*. Arlington, Va.: Council for Exceptional Children, 1971.

Yater, V., *Mainstreaming of Children with a Hearing Loss: Practical Guidelines and Implications*, Springfield, Ill.: Charles C Thomas, 1977.

Zink, G. D., Rehabilitative and educational audiology programming. *Lang. Speech Hear. Serv. Schools*, 4, 23–26, 1973.

chapter 49

ASSISTING THE ELDERLY CLIENT

Raymond H. Hull, Ph.D.

The boundaries of age as they relate to the term "aged" are ever changing due to the marvelous advances of medicine and related health maintenance. It is now becoming commonplace for individuals to live to ages that were thought impossible even 30 to 40 years ago. Although the boundaries of life expectancy continue to expand, the effects of the aging process on the sensory capabilities of man have not been altered appreciably. As persons in our society are enabled to live to a greater age, we must now look toward the maintenance and enhancement of those capabilities during their additional years.

One of the most devastating sensory deficits which accompanies the aging process is the deterioration of auditory function, or presbycusis. The inability to communicate in an efficient manner is the greatest problem elderly people have in attempting to cope with the world around them.

As stated in Chapter 35 of this text, presbycusis is a neurologic reality which is associated with other physical changes seen in the aged person. Each person's timetable for aging is different in its physical, social, and economic effects. The elderly individual who is devastated because he cannot understand what people are saying and is embarrassed by the confusions with which he must cope, may feel even greater despair when he finds that others his equal in years are experiencing little difficulty in interpreting auditory-verbal messages. He may feel confused and frustrated when he misunderstood the directions to the Senior Citizens Club outing and finds himself alone, far from the place he was supposed to be. Understandably, he may feel angry and dejected because he does not know where he went astray or was led astray. He is angry not only at himself for apparently not understanding the directions but also at his whole current life situation. He wonders what is happening to him that these situations are occurring with some regularity. He knows that he can hear people talk, but he is having difficulty "making sense out of it." It is not difficult for an otherwise alert elderly person to reason that the confusions are a result of growing older, but of greater concern are the thoughts that maybe he is losing his mind, or that senility is becoming a reality.

Since we all know others who have hearing difficulties, one could conclude that it may be an auditory problem. Many older persons wear hearing aids, but this often represents to elderly people the final sign that a person has grown "old." They also know many who have worn hearing aids but have found little help from them.

How does the audiologist help this person? The devastation of presbycusis is, in many cases, the last straw signaling the finality of aging for the elderly individual. The elderly client is, likewise, one of the most difficult with which to deal. The general frustrations involved in growing old, the lack of financial independence, the steady decline of physical capabilities, the resignation to confinement, and the final withdrawal from the communicating world make this client one of the audiologist's greatest challenges. The rehabilitative audiologist must accept that challenge if he/she is going to work with the elderly client in an effective manner toward rehabilitation. Many elderly clients with presbycusis can be rehabilitated. The audiologist must accept this challenge before initiating work with any hearing-impaired aged person.

The basic philosophy presented here is not new to our field. We have recognized for some time that any rehabilitative effort dealing with an elderly hearing-impaired client must be as unique and comprehensive as the hearing impairment itself (Alpiner, 1968; Barr, 1970; Pang and Fujikawa, 1969; Parker, 1969; Willeford, 1971). Therefore, the concepts presented in this chapter are neither complete nor final for all clients. The audiologist working with the geriatric client must be as innovative as he or she is competent. Each elderly person is, indeed, different, with differing physiologic and psychological problems accompanying the auditory deficit. The information presented here should be read with that fact in mind and modifications made for individual clients.

BEGINNINGS OF REHABILITATION

Hearing Aid Evaluation

Many elderly people have rejected the idea of wearing a hearing aid long before arriving at the audiology clinic. They may have come because their children have requested that they at least try an aid or because their spouses have reached the limits of their tolerance with communication breakdown and demanded an evaluation to determine if a hearing aid would help. We can assume that the elderly person who has consented to come for the hearing aid evaluation hopes that a hearing aid will allow him more efficient communication with others.

Many come with the hope that some problem will be discovered that can be helped medically.

Before arriving at the audiology clinic, the only knowledge many elderly persons have about hearing aids and diagnostic evaluations has come from a hearing aid dealer. The elderly client must understand that he is now dealing with the professional person who is trained in the assessment of hearing and the rehabilitation of those with hearing impairment. It is occasionally difficult to convince the aged person that your sole purpose is not to sell hearing aids.

Attempts at an effective hearing aid evaluation with an elderly hearing-impaired client can be extremely challenging and occasionally frustrating. The audiologist must remember that he is dealing with an individual who has probably heard normally in the past, led a relatively normal social life, may have been the supporter of the family, and had many friends. Now the elderly person may be retired; living on a fixed, smaller income; have few good friends who are now living; is having considerable difficulty communicating with his family because of decreased auditory function; and is frustrated and embittered at the whole process and devastation of becoming older. His feelings of desperation may be somewhat concealed but still evident. Again, the audiologist, probably a much younger person than the client, must gain the respect of the elderly person. If the audiologist is interpreted by the elderly client as "flippant, arrogant, or intolerant of his elders," much success in rehabilitative efforts may be lost. The elderly client's frustration in being unable to communicate, along with his many physical discomforts, may cause him to appear irritated or intolerant of the evaluative session. The elderly client may deny his apparent auditory difficulties and need for amplification by removing the blame from himself and placing it on the "younger generation" who do not speak clearly. "People seem to mumble nowadays," is a common statement by the elderly client.

The procedures utilized during the hearing aid evaluation will vary with the individual client. It is important to consider the elderly client's tolerance for the evaluation procedures. The procedures may need modification to compensate for the patient's physical limitations, potential fatigue, or emotional intolerance of the testing situation. The following procedures have been found generally tolerable and beneficial:

1. Initial test battery.
   a. Pure-tone air and bone conduction thresholds.
   b. Speech reception thresholds under phones.
   c. Assessment of auditory discrimination under phones for phonetically balanced words and sentences (CID Everyday Speech).
2. Extensive discussion regarding the preliminary results of the tests relative to the handicap of hearing impairment.
3. Referral to an appropriate physician with a commitment that referral of the client back to you, the audiologist, is expected for aural rehabilitative efforts.
4. Hearing aid evaluation:
   a. Discussion of the advantages and disadvantages of hearing aids and the fact that you would like to try different types of hearing aids to see if you *and* the client feel that amplification would be of benefit.
   b. Obtain a free field speech reception threshold.
   c. Free field auditory discrimination testing with phonetically balanced words and sentences (CID Everyday Speech).
   d. Free field speech reception thresholds with one or two representative post-auricle and one or two body-type aids. These should be carefully selected by the audiologist with reference to the degree and extent of the client's hearing loss.
   e. Retest of free field auditory discrimination (see item c) with the various hearing aids.
   f. If the preliminary results appear to indicate that amplification would benefit the person, the audiologist should instruct the client regarding the function of the hearing aids, how to change batteries, and other such intricacies. A family member should be present in case of communication or memory difficulties. The client is then sent home with one selected post-auricle and one body-type hearing aid utilized during the evaluation to compare and try them for at least one week to further determine their representative effectiveness in everyday life. Specific instructions regarding adjustments required for the use of the hearing aid and specific environments for trial should be made. A few suggested environments for trial of the hearing aids may include: (1) while watching television, (2) at church, (3) at any social gathering where the elderly person would feel comfortable wearing an aid and (4) while at a restaurant.

The client should be instructed to wear the hearing aid only if he/she desires to wear it. Emphasize that it is not mandatory to wear one in all environments suggested, but stress the desirability of trying them in as many situations as possible. Set an appointment for the client to return in one week. During the return visit, the client will be ready for extensive discussion regarding the benefits of amplification as it applies to him and not the generalities that were discussed during the initial evaluation the week prior.

In discussing the utilization of hearing aids with the elderly client and in selecting trial aids for consideration or purchase, the following should be considered:

1. *The Auditory Capabilities of the Client.* More and more we are finding that many elderly persons cannot utilize amplification well enough to warrant their being fitted with a hearing aid. Even though the pure tone configuration may indicate good prognosis for the use of amplification, auditory discrimination problems along with apparent central auditory processing dysfunction may contraindicate its use. The frustration of being able to hear speech more loudly, but still experiencing an inability to understand what is being said may make communication even more difficult than being without a hearing aid. The amplification of environmental noise and an elderly client's inability to separate noise from a primary signal may also cause increased anxiety and frustration.

Some elderly persons have purchased numbers of hearing aids from various dealers in the hope that one of them will successfully allow for more efficient communication. After spending large sums of money, the client may find that none of the aids provide sufficient benefit, and none of them are worn. "The dresser drawer syndrome" (Alpiner, 1974) is testimony to the caution that should surround the hearing aid evaluation of the elderly person. The audiologist must look carefully at the auditory capabilities of the aged client—not so much at the fact that hearing loss is present, but at whether a hearing aid will allow for more efficient auditory function. For some younger clients, a hearing aid may be viewed as providing benefits that are at least better than nothing at all. For many elderly clients, however, the frustrations resulting from an inappropriate hearing aid can be interpreted as worse than nothing at all.

2. *The Physical Capabilities of the Client.* The client's manual dexterity is an important consideration in selecting the type and size of the hearing aid. The elderly individual, fitted with a small post-auricle hearing aid, whose less than nimble fingers cannot manipulate the gain control, let alone a small telephone switch, will experience great frustration in attempting to wear the aid and in many instances will cease wearing it altogether. Many elderly persons have difficulty placing the small battery in the battery compartment. If the individual is unlucky enough to drop the battery, visual and other difficulties might interfere with its retrieval.

Body-type hearing aids generally allow for easier manipulation of the controls and require a larger battery size. Convincing the elderly client to accept the larger body-type aid is, however, another matter. It is often difficult for the elderly client to accept the need for amplification and the wearing of a hearing aid. The thought of using a large hearing aid is even more difficult to accept. It is important to compare the smaller post-auricle aid with the larger body-type aids during both the clinical and home trials. Once the elderly client determines that the ease of manipulation of the controls of the body-type aid, along with its acoustical characteristics, outweigh its disadvantages of size and wearability, counseling toward its use is facilitated. This is not to say that all elderly persons should be counseled toward the use of body-type hearing aids. Body aids are generally more beneficial for those with limited manual dexterity or visual problems or those who require the additional acoustic gain. Many active elderly persons can utilize smaller aids (post-auricle or all-in-the-ear). If one does appear to benefit the client, then of course it should be considered. Some recently developed body-type aids with rechargeable batteries are excellent for use by the less dexterous elderly person not only as a hearing aid for everyday use but also as an auditory trainer during rehabilitative therapy.

Hearing Aid Follow-Up

It is imperative that the hearing-impaired elderly person be involved in a vital aural rehabilitation program throughout the hearing aid evaluation and after the formal evaluation period is completed. If a hearing aid is, indeed, recommended, the client should be encouraged to wear it during speechreading sessions. Whether the client is wearing a trial aid or the aid he purchased, counseling about its use, discussions regarding the benefits and limitations of hearing aids, and suggestions for communicating in the everyday world should continue. This type of follow-up will greatly enhance the client's success in adapting to the use of amplification.

If it is found that the client cannot effectively utilize a hearing aid, the speechreading/auditory training alternatives should be employed without the use of amplification.

When effective hearing aid evaluation procedures are incorporated as a part of a total aural rehabilitation program for the elderly residing in a retirement home, it has virtually eliminated the exploitation of these patients by people who are simply interested in selling hearing aids (Hull and Traynor, 1975). The residents are therefore protected from high pressure sales practices and inappropriate fittings.

REHABILITATION PROCESS
Counseling the Elderly Client

Whether the client can benefit from amplification, his emotional acceptance of his auditory impairment and his desire for more efficient auditory function must be of primary concern to the audiologist. If the client does not appear to be able to cope emotionally with his auditory dysfunction or does not appear to desire exploration of possibilities for rehabilitation, then it is the responsibility of the audiologist to intervene as a counselor. The audiologist can show empathy as the elderly client describes his inability to understand what others are saying at church, at social gatherings, at Thanksgiving dinner, or while shopping, and the devastation he feels. The elderly client does not want sympathy from the counseling audiologist. The young audiologist who says, "I know just how you feel," when the elderly client describes his frustrations can expect to hear the client justifiably reply, "You do not know how I feel. You are not my age and are not experiencing my difficulties in communication." However, the audiologist must be able to relate to what the elderly person is saying through his knowledge of presbycusis and experiences in working with other elderly persons. The aged client may be envious of the young audiologist and might wonder how an individual so much his junior could possess the knowledge and understanding of his particular problem. The skilled rehabilitative audiologist should be able to overcome the barriers of age and deal with the specific auditory and related problems of the aged client through proper rapport. The client must be made to realize that the audiologist is there to listen and to discuss the problems which surround that particular client's auditory difficulties. The audiologist's purpose should be to help the client learn to function more efficiently with his auditory difficulties through effective counseling and through specific speechreading/auditory training.

Motivation toward participation in aural rehabilitation programs will occur only when the elderly client knows that the audiologist understands his auditory problems, concerns, and frustrations. Most importantly, the aged client must know that the audiologist feels that he can indeed be helped to communicate more efficiently. Motivation for some clients is more difficult to develop and maintain, especially when it concerns participation in aural rehabilitation efforts which can be difficult and sometimes only slightly rewarding from session to session.

Group Involvement

Group counseling can be most effective. The empathy and comradery which often develops within groups of hearing-impaired elderly clients can be very rewarding. Many realize for the first time that others have experienced similar frustrations and problems in communication. Effective counseling can result from such group catharsis. Until the elderly client realizes that his auditorily based problems are not unique to himself alone but are common also to others who are viable individuals, then effective aural rehabilitation can be difficult to initiate and maintain. These group techniques can work well both in a retirement center environment and in the community for more independent elderly persons.

Peer Involvement

Peer group pressure can be an effective technique for motivating the elderly client to attempt aural rehabilitation. Other elderly clients who have experienced success through aural rehabilitation programs can provide great encouragement to aged hearing-impaired clients who may be reluctant to participate. For those who express a seeming lack of desire to participate in aural rehabilitation because age or the feeling that these efforts should be concentrated on the younger person, peer group pressure from persons who would like to communicate with (talk to and be understood by) the potential client, can work effectively.

Family Involvement

It should be required that the elderly client's family be involved in counseling regarding his auditory difficulties, but this is frequently not possible. The elderly person who is placed in a retirement home because his son and daughter-in-law, for example, do not have the time to provide a meaningful home environment for him oftentimes indicates that they do not "have the time" to visit him or participate in such counseling activities. It is interesting, however, that lack of ability to communicate is often given as a reason for putting an aged family member in the retirement home. Yet, some families will not take the trouble to understand this communication problem. They report resulting anger on the part of their elderly family member and, in turn, anger and frustration on their part. They report that "Grandpa is getting confused." The term "confused" all too often takes on the connotation of "senility." He is placed in the retirement home so that he can be "looked after more carefully" or will be "more comfortable." The elderly person is then more devastated, being taken from his home and family and placed in a strange environment which he feels is terminal placement for him. No matter how nice the retirement home is, how good the meals, how stimulating the activities, it is not "home" to him and it never will be. The resulting depression that occurs can sometimes be fatal. If there is little or no involvement with the family from that time forth, the stay in the retirement home can be unbearable.

Effective aural rehabilitation, then, not only involves the hearing-impaired elderly client but also his family, i.e., a son or daughter who lives in the vicinity, the spouse, and of critical importance, the grandchildren. It is important that family counseling be conducted prior to the elderly person's placement in the retirement home since there is a possibility that such placement may be contraindicated. If, on the other hand, the elderly hearing-impaired client is first seen and evaluated after placement in the retirement home, then the family should be contacted as one of the initial steps in that client's aural rehabilitation program.

The following are suggested topics for discussion during the rehabilitative audiologist's meeting with family members:

1. What is presbycusis?
   a. How does it affect the elderly person's ability to communicate?
   b. The resulting frustrations on the part of the elderly person and those with whom he/she attempts to communicate.
2. Hearing aids.
   a. Why some elderly cannot utilize amplification on a day-to-day basis even though they appear to be hearing impaired.
   b. The benefits of amplification as part of a total aural rehabilitation program.
   c. How the hearing aid works.
3. How to more efficiently communicate with their hearing impaired family member.
   a. Speak at a slightly greater than normal intensity.
   b. Speak at a normal rate but not too rapidly.
   c. Do not speak to the elderly client at a greater distance than 6 feet but no less than 3 feet.
   d. Concentrate light on the speaker's face for greater visibility of lip movements, facial expression, and gestures.
   e. Do not speak to the elderly person unless you are visible to him, i.e., not from another room while he is reading the newspaper or watching television.
   f. Do not force the elderly person to listen to you when there is a great deal of environmental noise. That type of environment can be difficult for a younger normally hearing person, let alone an elderly individual with presbycusis.

If an elderly person's ability to communicate with his family can be enhanced, then a giant step toward other successes in aural rehabilitative efforts can be made.

SPEECHREADING/AUDITORY TRAINING

The approach to speechreading instruction recommended for use with the elderly client is by no means a traditional one. No matter how motivated the elderly client is toward learning to make more efficient use of residual hearing through speechreading instruction, that motivation will quickly fade if traditional analytic approaches of phoneme and word recognition are utilized to any extent. Analytical instruction regarding phoneme recognition in isolation and in the context of syllables and words is extremely difficult for young hearing-impaired clients, and even then those types of speechreading approaches must be questioned as to their real effectiveness. Assuming that the elderly clients involved in speechreading instruction possess normal or near normal language function, more meaningful approaches for the enhancement of their ability to receive and interpret verbal/auditory messages can be utilized.

The use of residual hearing should be stressed. If the elderly client can make use of a hearing aid, then it should be worn during speechreading sessions. If a hearing aid is not utilized by individual clients on a routine basis because they have not been able to make good use of amplification, for whatever reason, then a hearing aid is not advised during speechreading instruction, although voice should be used by the clinician. Therefore, all clients are forced to use their residual hearing. If an individual client appears to have the auditory capacity to wear a hearing aid but for some reason is having difficulty adjusting to its use, then speechreading sessions provide a good atmosphere for controlled trial of various amplification devices. Rechargeable body-type hearing aids with a flat frequency response have been found effective for use as wearable auditory trainers during speechreading instruction.

Effective speechreading lessons include (1) instruction regarding visually confusing phonemes; (2) the predictability of the English language in conversational speech; (3) the selection of important visual/auditory word clues from conversation that facilitate correct interpretation of meaning; and (4) instruction in facilitating environmental factors which allow for greater use of residual hearing and visual clues (Hull, 1969). These methods are also easily adapted for use in auditory training to provide an interesting and effective approach for this age group. Individuals with visual problems who are also hearing impaired are not excluded from the speechreading sessions. For these persons, the sessions become useful as auditory training therapy.

Extension of the more formalized speechreading/auditory training classes may include assignments that involve, at a beginning level:

1. Speaking to at least one other resident (person) at some time during each day (e.g., for 2 min) before the next speechreading class. They are instructed to record any difficulties in carrying on the conversations so the problems can be discussed at the next speechreading/auditory training class.
2. Residents are given assignments for practice regarding what they learned in speechreading class during special activities of the retirement center, at church, or at the Senior Citizens' Club.

In any aural rehabilitation program within a retirement center, carryover from the speechreading/auditory training class can be conducted by the activity director in the form of checker games, cards, or other activities. It is important that the audiologist and activity director work closely during these extensions of the aural rehabilitation program.

It is not recommended that speechreading sessions last longer than 45 to 60 min because of fatigue within this age group. Short "breaks" from intensive work are taken as needed during the sessions. The classes should meet at least once or twice a week, and should be limited to 8 to 10 members per class. It is recommended that as clients progress in their communication skills, advanced classes should be developed and new, less skilled clients be placed in beginning classes. Periodically it is good for a skilled member of an advanced class to visit a beginning class to demonstrate his skills. This tactic instills hope on the part of the beginning client and the desire to achieve similar skills in communication

At times, speechreading/auditory training classes can be used for purposes of socialization to promote a better atmosphere conducive to communication among residents within the retirement center. These socialization efforts are, however, necessarily structured as extensions of prior speechreading classes. The socializa-

tion aspects have also been found to be successful for use in conjunction with aural rehabilitation programs for the elderly within senior citizens' centers and other community programs. Other successful extensions of speechreading/auditory training classes include captioned films for the deaf which can be shown on a routine basis for all hearing-impaired elderly.

SPECIFIC SUGGESTIONS FOR INITIATION OF AURAL REHABILITATION PROGRAMS FOR THE ELDERLY CLIENT

Administration

Aural rehabilitation programs in the retirement center should be coordinated by the audiologist but should also involve persons who hold the following administrative positions: (1) the administrator of the retirement center, (2) the head of nursing, (3) the activity director, (4) the social worker and (5) the nurses' aides.

Administrative coordination is necessarily maintained by periodic meetings of the audiologist and the representatives of the retirement center listed above. These meetings, at least twice per year, should have as their purpose discussion of the maintenance and improvement of the program. The audiologist should, however, be in continual contact with the retirement center personnel regarding the program and progress of individual clients.

Funding

Funding of the aural rehabilitation program should come from the retirement center. Financial commitment on the center's part will provide for a more vital interest in its success. With appropriate medical prescriptions for diagnostic services, federal health insurance such as Medicare will provide payment for complete audiologic evaluations when conducted by an audiologist who is certified by the American Speech and Hearing Association and who has also applied for and received a provider number for administration of such services. Certain provisions may be forthcoming through federal health insurance which will make for greater ease in receiving payment for services by audiologists.

Payment for services by a retirement center can either be made on a per client basis or on a fee-for-services contract (a blanket fee for all services provided). The fee-for-services contract is generally more satisfactory, the amount being negotiable between the audiologist and the administration of the center on the basis of the number of clients seen or the types of services provided. If programs are being conducted at several centers, then a prorated fee can be established among them corresponding to the amount of time spent in individual centers and the number of clients who are participating.

Evaluation of Auditory Function

Once the administration of the center has given its approval for the initiation of the aural rehabilitation program, the first step is achieving as complete an audiometric evaluation as possible on residents whose health or mental state allow for such an evaluation. The procedures for complete evaluations are noted in Chapter 35. It is recommended that all residents who can be evaluated be initially screened for auditory problems. This evaluation should be conducted in as quiet an environment as possible, as this first evaluation will determine the need for further testing including hearing aid evaluation. The procedures for the initial evaluation consist of: (1) pure tone air-conduction threshold under phones, (2) impedance measurements (tympanometry and acoustic reflex) for the determination of the site of lesion and (3) screening for auditory discrimination difficulties by the use of monosyllabic words (25-word list) and 10 sentences (CID Everyday Speech).

After all current residents have been evaluated, new residents should be evaluated within 2 weeks after admittance to the retirement center. In this way, if hearing impairment is discovered, participation in the aural rehabilitation program can be initiated early. Early intervention not only encourages greater participation in the aural rehabilitation program but also tends to prevent the severe depression that affects many elderly when they are taken from their homes and placed in the retirement center.

Records of Progress

Complete records must be kept on each client. Results of audiometric evaluations should be kept not only in the client's master file but also in individual files kept by the audiologist. Communicative and social progress should be recorded for each client who participates in the aural rehabilitation program. One method which has been found to be successful is the use of individual client's social progress reports that are written jointly by the head nurse, the activity director, the social worker, and the audiologist. These contain reports of communicative progress made by the client and include, for example, an accounting of approximate number of times the client spoke with others, actively participated in social activities, went out to eat with family members, attended to his personal appearance, or increased his physical activity. Increased ability to communicate will generally reflect

upon many aspects of the elderly person's life. As the elderly person realizes that he can communicate more efficiently with others, he will often become more ambulatory, show a greater desire for improved personal appearance, and be more willing to venture into the world outside of the retirement center. These aspects are necessary to consider for a complete socio/communicative profile and should be jointly maintained by those who are in contact with the clients on a day-to-day basis.

IN-SERVICE TRAINING

An aware administrative and nursing staff are necessary to maintain an effective and workable aural rehabilitation program for the elderly in the retirement center. They must have knowledge of: (1) the devastation of hearing impairment on the aged person and (2) approaches for support of the aural rehabilitation program. One very effective way of assuring that the retirement center staff is aware of these problems and that a good working relationship is established is through inservice training. It has been found, however, that in-service training is beneficial not only for the retirement center staff but also the client.

Retirement Center Staff

As retirement centers traditionally have a rapid turnover in personnel, routine inservice training sessions should be conducted at least once or twice each month. The length of in-service sessions will vary with the topic of discussion, but at least 1 hour should be allotted. To be maximally effective, the in-service training should involve the nurses, nurses' aides (since they are more directly involved with the residents on a day-to-day basis), the activity director, social worker, and the director of the retirement center. It is not necessary for the retirement center director to be involved in all in-service sessions except when individual clients are being discussed.

Topics that are considered important for in-service training are as follows:

1. How the ear functions;
2. What is presbycusis;
3. The impact of presbycusis;
4. Hearing aids, their structure, care, advantages, and limitations with this population;
5. How to troubleshoot for simple hearing aid malfunction;
6. What is speechreading;
7. How to best communicate with the hearing-impaired elderly person; and
8. Staff discussions of individual hearing impaired residents and their progress in the aural rehabilitation program.

In essence, the in-service training provides the staff with insight into presbycusis, its complications, and information about the progress of residents participating in the aural rehabilitation program. It is essential for all new staff and previously employed staff members who have questions regarding residents to attend in-service training.

The Client

A type of "in-service" or continuing education effort that has been found extremely valuable as a part of an effective aural rehabilitation program are programs presented for the residents of the retirement center or for elderly persons in local senior citizens' clubs. The elderly person is personally interested in the process of aging and its effects on him physiologically and socially. Even though elderly persons often will not tolerate a long movie, lecture, or meeting, they will attend those meetings on the process of aging with eager anticipation. The content of this type of meeting is much the same as in-service with retirement center personnel, with modifications that allow for personal involvement and interaction between participants. Even though those elderly in attendance may be allowed to relate personal experiences regarding their own auditory difficulties, the purpose of such programs should not take on the image of group counseling. The purpose of such meetings may be the presentation of information about (1) the structure and function of the ear, (2) the impact of presbycusis on communication function, (3) hearing aids, their uses, and misuses, (4) why some elderly persons cannot use hearing aids, (5) hearing aid maintenance and trouble shooting, (6) how participation in aural rehabilitation programs will benefit them and (7) tips on how to more efficiently communicate with family and friends.

The elderly person is thus presented information that will allow for a better understanding of presbycusis, the aging process as related to hearing, how it affects him personally, and is encouraged to participate in the aural rehabilitation program. The basis for these meetings is the realization that one cannot limit the presentation of information about presbycusis strictly to those working with the elderly. It must also be taken to elderly persons who are forced to live with the effects of presbycusis so they, too, will have a better understanding of what is happening to them. These meetings also encourage greater participation by the elderly in aural rehabilitation programs.

PROGRAMS FOR THE WELL ELDERLY CLIENT IN THE COMMUITY

If all retirement centers within a given community work together to maintain an effective aural rehabilitation program for their elderly residents, then its viability increases manyfold. A unique program for the elderly has been established by the University of Northern Colorado, Area of Audiology, called "A Community-Wide Program in Geriatric Aural Rehabilitation" (Hull and Traynor, 1975). This program does not stop with the retirement center. Extension into the rest of the community is necessary if a complete aural rehabilitation program for the elderly is to exist.

A most efficient method for contacting elderly hearing-impaired persons in the community is through public interest talks by audiologists. Presentations can be made at the local community senior citizens' center and the Public Health Service Well Elderly Clinics (diagnostic health clinics) regarding hearing impairment and the effects of aging on the auditory mechanism. If interest is generated on the part of elderly persons, then auditory screening programs can be established to determine which persons will require complete diagnostic evaluations, hearing aid evaluations, and entrance into the aural rehabilitation program. The news media generally devote public service space for announcements concerning clinics for hearing evaluations for elderly persons. These screening clinics can be held, for example, at such familiar places as the local senior citizens' center. If a mobile unit with sound treated facilities is available, the testing sites can be established at several familiar sites for greater convenience for the elderly person.

The management principles which guide the aural rehabilitation program for the well elderly in the community should be similar to those discussed earlier in this chapter and include: (1) counseling techniques, (2) considerations regarding hearing aids, (3) inservice and (4) speechreading techniques. Modifications may necessarily be required when considering the social vitality and mobility of the well elderly client in the community.

Payment for diagnostic services may come from the client himself or, with a physician's prescription from the client's Federal health insurance. Payment for aural rehabilitative services is now being considered for coverage through Medicare. Until it is designated as a covered benefit, however, payment must be made by the client or agency sponsoring the client such as social services (welfare) or public health.

AFTER REHABILITATION?

Through aural rehabilitative efforts, we are attempting to improve the communicative capabilities of the hearing impaired elderly so that they may be able to function at a higher level socially and, perhaps, economically. We are, idealistically, looking toward individuals leaving the retirement center to once again reside in the community, to change the image of the retirement center to short-term care for some clients as opposed to long-term care (or terminal care) facilities. Realistically, not all clients will achieve the level of communicative competence that is required for independent living. Some may reach a level of skill that will allow for greater ease of auditory/verbal communication between client and family or friends. A few may leave the retirement center as independently functioning persons. The audiologist must realize, however, that many clients may achieve little success through his rehabilitative efforts. Some will achieve no increase in communicative function. The audiologist must also be able to face the death of clients. It behooves the audiologist not to concentrate upon the inevitability of death, but to look upon the rehabilitation as added life to the latter years of the aged client.

For those clients where success in increasing communicative function is achieved, what will the consequences be? For those who have the capability to work, what jobs are available? Vocational rehabilitation services offices have no authority to place individuals who are over age 65 on jobs, even if younger persons are not available. There are few, if any, small business loans available for persons over age 65 for even the smallest business ventures.

What social opportunities are available for elderly persons who have, perhaps, withdrawn from society in the past because of an inability to communicate with others? Perhaps persons who can function socially will institute the reawakening of old acquaintances and, for example, rejoin or reactivate membership in social organizations.

We must activate an interest toward opening avenues of participation for the elderly into our society occupationally, educationally, and socially. If aural rehabilitative efforts are effective and some elderly who were once tucked neatly away into a noncommunicating, nonfunctioning role begin to emerge again into society, opportunities for employment and social interaction must be offered them if they so desire. We must look beyond the fact that a much longer life has been given to the elderly. We have for too long looked at that gift of extended life as our ultimate goal for the aged person. If we are, indeed, adding more life to those additional years, we must also look toward allowing the elderly to function as productive citizens, to thus make use of the skills we are teaching them through our rehabilitative efforts. As work is expanded by audiologists toward aural rehabilitation for the approximately 17 million individuals over age 65 who possess some degree of hearing impairment, we must also look toward finding a place for them in our society. They were once functioning citizens and some will once again be seeking their place in the community.

REFERENCES

Alpiner, J., Audiologic problems of the aged. *Geriatrics,* 18, 19–26, 1968.

Alpiner, J., The feasibility of rehabilitating the hearing impaired elderly client. Paper presented at a Workshop on Hearing and Related Communication Disorders Among the Aged, Division of Long-Term Care, P.H.S., D.H.E.W., Denver, Colorado, 1974.

Barr, D., Aural rehabilitation and the geriatric patient. *Geriatrics,* 25, 111–113, 1970.

Hull, R., A linguistic approach to the teaching of speechreading: theoretical and practical application. Paper presented at the Annual Convention of the American Speech and Hearing Association, Chicago, 1969.

Hull, R., and Traynor, R., A community-wide program in geriatric aural rehabilitation. *ASHA,* 17, 33–34, 47–48, 1975.

Pang, L., and Fujikawa, S., Hearing impairment in the aged; incidence and management. *Hawaii Med. J.,* 29, 109–113, 1969.

Parker, W., Hearing and age. *Geriatrics,* 24, 151–157, 1969.

Willeford, J., The Geriatric Patient. In Rose, D. (Ed.), *Audiological Assessment,* Ch. 9, pp. 281–319. Englewood Cliffs, N.J.: Prentice-Hall, 1971.

AUTHOR INDEX

605

SUBJECT INDEX*

* In addition to the regular listings, all auditory tests can be found under the heading *Audiometric tests* and the diseases and disorders under *Disorders*.